CANCER 5

A COMPREHENSIVE TREATISE

CHEMOTHERAPY

CANCER 5

A COMPREHENSIVE TREATISE

CHEMOTHERAPY

FREDERICK F. BECKER, EDITOR

University of Texas System Cancer Center
M.D. Anderson Hospital and Tumor Institute
Houston, Texas

PLENUM PRESS • NEW YORK AND LONDON

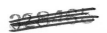

Library of Congress Cataloging in Publication Data

Main entry under title:

Chemotherapy.

  (Cancer; v. 5)
  Includes bibliographies and index.
  1. Cancer—Chemotherapy. 2. Antineoplastic agents. I. Becker, Frederick F. [DNLM:
1. Neoplasms. QZ200 C2143]
RC261.C263 vol. 5 [RC271.C5] 616.9'94'008s
ISBN 0-306-35205-2   [616.9'94'061]   77-1142

© 1977 Plenum Press, New York
A Division of Plenum Publishing Corporation
227 West 17th Street, New York, N.Y. 10011

Printed in the United States of America

Contributors

TO VOLUME 5

MARTIN A. APPLE, University of California Medical School, San Francisco, California

TERRY A. BEERMAN, Department of Pharmacology, Harvard Medical School, Boston, Massachusetts. Present address: Grace Cancer Drug Center, Roswell Park Memorial Institute, Buffalo, New York

ED CADMAN, Department of Medicine, Yale University School of Medicine, New Haven, Connecticut

ROBERT L. CAPIZZI, Yale University School of Medicine, New Haven, Connecticut

BRUCE A. CHABNER, Division of Cancer Treatment, National Cancer Institute, National Institutes of Health, Bethesda, Maryland

KELLY H. CLIFTON, Radiobiology Laboratories, Departments of Human Oncology and Radiology, University of Wisconsin Medical School, Madison, Wisconsin

WILLIAM A. CREASY, Departments of Internal Medicine and Pharmacology, Yale University School of Medicine, New Haven, Connecticut. Present address: Children's Hospital of Philadelphia and Department of Pharmacology, University of Pennsylvania School of Medicine, Philadelphia, Pennsylvania

IRVING H. GOLDBERG, Department of Pharmacology, Harvard Medical School, Boston, Massachusetts.

WILLIAM H. GREENE, Department of Internal Medicine, Yale University School of Medicine, New Haven, Connecticut

ION GRESSER, Institut de Recherches Scientifiques sur le Cancer, Villejuif, France

ROBERT E. HANDSCHUMACHER, Department of Pharmacology, Yale University School of Medicine, New Haven, Connecticut

DAVID G. JOHNS, Division of Cancer Treatment, National Cancer Institute, National Institutes of Health, Bethesda, Maryland

L. WAYNE KEISER, Yale University School of Medicine, New Haven, Connecticut

GERARD T. KENNEALEY, Section of Medical Oncology, Departments of Medicine and Pharmacology, Yale University School of Medicine, New Haven, Connecticut

Willi Kreis, Memorial Sloan–Kettering Cancer Center, New York, New York

G. A. LePage, McEachern Laboratory, University of Alberta, Edmonton, Canada

Craig A. Lindquist, Section of Medical Oncology, Yale University School of Medicine, New Haven, Connecticut

David B. Ludlum, Department of Pharmacology and Experimental Therapeutics, Albany Medical College, Albany, New York

W. Bruce Lundberg, Section of Medical Oncology, Yale University School of Medicine, New Haven, Connecticut

Frank Maley, Division of Laboratories and Research, New York State Department of Health, Albany, New York

John C. Marsh, Department of Internal Medicine, Yale University School of Medicine, New Haven, Connecticut

Malcolm S. Mitchell, Section of Medical Oncology, Departments of Medicine and Pharmacology, Yale University School of Medicine, New Haven, Connecticut

R. J. Papac, Yale University School of Medicine, New Haven, Connecticut, and West Haven Veterans Administration Hospital, West Haven, Connecticut

Raymond Poon, Department of Pharmacology, Harvard Medical School, Boston, Massachusetts. Present address: Division of Hematology, University of California, San Francisco General Hospital, San Francisco, California

Gerald L. Schertz, Department of Internal Medicine, Yale University School of Medicine, New Haven, Connecticut

Michael T. Shaw, Section of Medical Oncology, Yale University School of Medicine, New Haven, Connecticut

Roland T. Skeel, Section of Medical Oncology, Yale University School of Medicine, New Haven, Connecticut. Present Address: Section of Medical Oncology, Department of Medicine, Medical College of Ohio at Toledo, Toledo, Ohio

Robert D. Stebbins, Section of Medical Oncology, Yale University School of Medicine, New Haven, Connecticut

Jack R. Uren, Sidney Farber Cancer Institute, Harvard University, Boston, Massachusetts

Preface

The promise of chemotherapeutic control in the field of oncology seemed, in the beginning, no less bright than it had proven in the field of bacterial disease, and, therefore, its failures were felt all the more. Despite the serendipitous discoveries and inspired insights which tantalized us with striking remissions, or the rare tumors which proved to be fully susceptible to a given agent, in the main, there has been either total failure or a painfully slow acquisition of an armamentarium against a limited number of malignancies. To expect more, however, was the result of ignorance of the malignant cell, for, as has been described in the previous volumes of this series, the exploitable differences between malignant and normal cells are few or undiscovered. "Differences" is the "numerator" in this formula, but "exploitable" is the operational term, for, although a great number of differences between normal and malignant cells have been described, rarely are these differences observed in a vital metabolic pathway or a crucial macromolecular structure. Essentially, the basic metabolic pathways and nutritional requirements for normal and malignant cells are the same, resulting in the fact that no chemotherapeutic agent can successfully inhibit a function in the majority of malignant cells without adversely affecting a similar function in the normal cell.

It was, therefore, naive to expect a "magic bullet" which would select the malignant cell and destroy it. Our ignorance was compounded by a lack of understanding of the diversity of the cells within a tumor, some dormant, some performing the differentiated functions of their progenitors, and others acting as the stem cell pool. We were unaware of the enormous and multifaceted capacities of these cells to elude the effects of various agents or to rapidly acquire resistance.

This, then, is the challenge of tumor chemotherapy with its vast, but as yet unrealized, potential for the systemic destruction of malignancy. We must escape the need for the "fix" of serendipity and go beyond the slow acquisition via clinical testing. The future potential for chemotherapy must come in large part from a greater understanding of the subtle and intricate nature of the malignant cell. We must identify its unique characteristics, and target these for our attack. To achieve this objective, it is incumbent upon the investigator to turn to the basic sciences.

It is the purpose of this volume to examine the current state of chemotherapy from its basic science viewpoint. We have sought to emphasize the interactions of chemotherapeutic agents within the normal and malignant cell at the metabolic and molecular level and to analyze the response of the cells. The contributors repeatedly allude to strategies both for seeking new agents and for using those already available. They present means by which we may direct these agents to "home in" on the malignant cell alone, to penetrate that cell more effectively, to enhance specific metabolic activating pathways or to diminish those pathways which inhibit drug action. They delineate logical procedures to be used in predicting effective combinations of agents or ways in which to manipulate the structure of these substances to improve their effectiveness. Others suggest utilizing these same agents as probes for the very differences which might indicate the unique nature of the malignant cells. Where indicated, we have also included those clinical features which have broad implications for the area.

It is my belief that in this approach lies the promise of such therapy, that by understanding the cell's manipulation of the chemical agents introduced, we will be able to control their treatment, and, by understanding the nature of the neoplastic cell, we will ultimately be able to manipulate and eradicate the malignant cell itself.

Frederick F. Becker

Houston

Contents

General Principles of Chemotherapy

Factors That Influence the Therapeutic Response   1

GERARD T. KENNEALEY AND MALCOLM S. MITCHELL

Applications of Cell Kinetic Techniques to Human Malignancies   2

GERALD L. SCHERTZ AND JOHN C. MARSH

Toxicity of Chemotherapeutic Agents   3

ED CADMAN

Clinical Aspects of Resistance to Antineoplastic Agents   4

ROLAND T. SKEEL AND CRAIG A. LINDQUIST

Adjunctive Chemotherapy   5

MICHAEL T. SHAW AND ROBERT D. STEBBINS

Principles of Combination Chemotherapy   6

L. WAYNE KEISER AND ROBERT L. CAPIZZI

Intraarterial Chemotherapy   7

W. BRUCE LUNDBERG

Treatment of Malignant Disease in Closed Spaces   8

R. J. Papac

Supportive Care in the Cancer Patient   9

William H. Greene

Chemotherapeutic Agents

Alkylating Agents and the Nitrosoureas 10

David B. Ludlum

Purine Antagonists 11

G. A. LePage

Pyrimidine Antagonists   12

FRANK MALEY

Folate Antagonists   13

BRUCE A. CHABNER AND DAVID G. JOHNS

Plant Alkaloids   14

William A. Creasey

Antibiotics: Nucleic Acids As Targets in Chemotherapy   15

IRVING H. GOLDBERG, TERRY A. BEERMAN, AND RAYMOND POON

Enzyme Therapy   16

JACK R. UREN AND ROBERT E. HANDSCHUMACHER

Hydrazines and Triazenes   17

WILLI KREIS

Antitumor Effects of Interferon   18

ION GRESSER

The Physiology of Endocrine Therapy   19

KELLY H. CLIFTON

New Anticancer Drug Design: Past and Future Strategies

20

MARTIN A. APPLE

General Principles of Chemotherapy

Factors That Influence the Therapeutic Response

Gerard T. Kennealey and Malcolm S. Mitchell

1. Introduction

The use of drugs in the treatment of malignancies is of much more recent origin than the use of surgery or radiation therapy. The first recorded clinical trial of a chemotherapeutic agent took place in 1942, when nitrogen mustard was given to a patient with advanced lymphosarcoma (Goodman *et al.*, 1946). A dramatic but unfortunately brief tumor response was achieved in this patient. Later in that same decade, Sidney Farber observed what he termed an "acceleration phenomenon" in a retrospective analysis of children with acute leukemia treated with folate conjugates. This experience led him to a trial of folate antagonists, and in 1948, he reported dramatic responses in 10 of 16 children treated with the folate antagonist aminopterin (Farbet *et al.*, 1948).

Since these initial studies, the field of chemotherapy has grown tremendously, so that at the present time, a wide spectrum of human malignancies can be affected by the administration of antineoplastic drugs. Unfortunately, the response of diverse human malignancies to chemotherapy is neither uniform nor predictable. In some diseases such as choriocarcinoma and Hodgkin's disease, the response to chemotherapy is dramatic and often complete. In other diseases, such as carcinoma of the lung and kidney, fewer than 10% of patients respond, and the response is often partial and brief. This striking variability is seen even among patients with ostensibly identical tumors. When patients with similar histology,

Gerard T. Kennealey and Malcolm S. Mitchell • Section of Medical Oncology, Departments of Medicine and Pharmacology, Yale University School of Medicine, New Haven, Connecticut.

degree of tumor burden, and functional status are treated with the same drug regimen, a wide range in the degree of response is often noted.

Possible reasons underlying such a variation in the response of patients and tumors to chemotherapy are the subject of this introductory chapter. Factors relating to the tumor itself and factors relating to the response of the host to malignancy will be discussed, as well as general principles of and problems associated with treatment of the cancer patient with chemotherapy.

2. Tumor Factors

Small tumors are generally more responsive than large, bulky tumors of the same histological type, because more cells are in active nucleic acid or protein synthesis in small tumors. Also, since chemotherapy kills a *percentage* of tumor cells, rather than a large fixed *number* of cells, the chances of eradicating a tumor are better with a smaller tumor cell burden. While small tumors are not necessarily early tumors, but may simply be slow-growing, the host bearing a small tumor is usually in better physical condition, and therefore can tolerate the toxicity of chemotherapy more easily than a debilitated patient with extensive widespread metastases. For all these related reasons, treatment of tumors before they have become massive is advocated. Frequently, this means that therapy is indicated even for asymptomatic or only mildly symptomatic patients whose laboratory and radiological data show clear evidence of involvement with surgically or radiotherapeutically untreatable tumor. This is a matter of clinical judgment, since in the short run, chemotherapy often creates toxicity such as nausea, alopecia, and leukopenia, which must be balanced against possible long-term amelioration of symptoms that will undoubtedly arise due to the tumor. In the adjunctive therapy of postoperative patients with microscopic metastases, this is an especially important ethical decision, which is currently often resolved in favor of treatment. In any event, regardless of whether one treats before gross metastases are found or when disease is demonstrable, treatment of a severely debilitated patient as a heroic do-or-die attempt is usually futile, often highly dangerous, and should be avoided.

2.1. "Specific" Responsiveness to Drugs

Some tumors have a specific responsiveness to certain chemotherapeutic agents. Examples include the sensitivity of many acute lymphocytic leukemias to L-asparaginase, which deprives the leukemia cells of an essential nutrient, asparagine (Capizzi *et al.*, 1970). Unfortunately, many normal lymphocytes and pancreatic and liver cells are also affected by L-asparaginase. The strategy of designing more specific tumoricidal agents is a highly rational one, however difficult it is to accomplish. For reasons yet unknown to us, several tumors are sensitive to agents that are much less useful in most other disorders. *o,p'*-DDD has a highly limited range of action, affecting only adrenal cortical tumors, and mithramycin affects embryonal testicular tumors almost exclusively. Obversely, there are probably no tumors with intrinsic resistance to all therapeutic agents, but simply tumors for which the effective agent has not yet been found. Transitional cell carcinoma of the renal pelvis or bladder now responds to adriamycin (McGuire *et al.*, 1973), whereas other agents had hitherto been unsuccessful. Similarly, melanoma is influenced by dacarbazine (DTIC), the nitrosoureas, or hydroxyurea, and osteosarcoma responds to adriamycin or high-dose infusions of methotrexate (Jaffe *et al.*, 1974). The use of massive doses of drugs such as methotrexate or cyclophosphamide has also shown that tumors thought to have intrinsic resistance to these agents can often be treated successfully. Even when true drug resistance is manifest, after a period of treatment with an agent, very high doses of that agent may still be useful, as suggested by recent experience with cyclophosphamide in neuroblastoma (National Cancer Institute, unpublished data).

2.2. Location

The location of a tumor is of some importance in determining its responsiveness, particularly if it is in a "privileged" site. Relatively avascular regions may be protected from immunological rejection by the host, and from attack by agents that require transport by the blood to the tumor. Among such sites are the necrotic, relatively avascular center of a large tumor mass and such unusual sites of experimental tumors as a hamster cheekpouch or the anterior chamber of the eye. The "blood–brain barrier," which should more appropriately be designated the "blood–CSF barrier" or "blood–brain substance barrier" as the situation requires, is another instance in which location may hamper therapy. Agents that are lipid-soluble, such as the nitrosoureas, pass more freely into the brain substance through the Virchow-Robin spaces and are effective in treating tumors in or of the brain. On the other hand, adequate CSF levels of drugs can be achieved by many agents if the meninges are inflamed or if very high doses are used systematically to force the agent across. Methotrexate or cytarabine need not necessarily be given intrathecally to treat meningeal leukemia if high doses are used and cytocidal concentrations of the drugs are attained in the CSF, as measured by direct assay (Levitt *et al.*, 1971).

2.3. Conclusions

The nature of the tumor, i.e., its size, histological and biochemical characteristics, and location, determine its degree of responsiveness to chemotherapy. It is encouraging that many "drug-resistant" tumors may be treatable by altering the logistics of chemotherapy, suggesting that newer drugs and regimens can be devised for even the most devastating cancers currently unaffected by any agent.

6

GERARD T.
KENNEALEY
AND
MALCOLM S.
MITCHELL

3. Host Factors

The response of a patient to chemotherapy is determined by many factors. The characteristics of the tumor that affect the response to chemotherapy have been mentioned. In this section, the characteristics of the tumor-bearing host will be discussed.

3.1. Prior Therapy

One important point that must be considered in planning a program of chemotherapy is that most patients have had other antitumor therapy before presenting for drug treatment. The long-term effects of prior surgery, radiation therapy, or chemotherapy can profoundly influence the ability of a tumor-bearing host to tolerate and respond to various chemotherapeutic regimens.

3.1.1. Prior Surgery

Except for those who unfortunately first seek medical attention with advanced, inoperable disease, most patients with solid tumors have had some form of surgical treatment in an effort to control their disease prior to the consideration of chemotherapy. The interval between surgery and chemotherapy may vary widely from patient to patient, even with the same tumor. In carcinoma of the breast (Fisher *et al.*, 1975; Bonadonna *et al.*, 1976), and in pilot studies now with colon carcinoma and other tumors, chemotherapy has been instituted adjunctively in the immediate postoperative period, to eradicate presumed micrometastases in persons who are free of grossly detectable disease.

Since the first surgical adjuvant studies of carcinoma of the breast initiated in the late 1950s (Fisher *et al.*, 1968), there has been concern about the possible deleterious effects of chemotherapy in the immediate postoperative period. Most published animal studies (Farhat *et al.*, 1958; Conn *et al.*, 1957; Rath and Enquist, 1959) have indicated that perioperative administration of chemotherapy does not affect wound strength, although this opinion is not unanimous (Desprez and Kiehn, 1960). When this question was studied in man, Fisher *et al.* (1968) demonstrated no difference in the rate of local complications, including wound-healing and infection, between large groups of patients treated with surgery alone or surgery and thioTEPA in a surgical adjuvant study of carcinoma of the breast.

Another problem in the surgical patient, in theory at least, is the presence of depressed immunity in the immediate postoperative period. It has been known for many years that surgical stress decreases the resistance of experimental animals to exogenous inoculated tumor cells (Slawikowski, 1960). In humans, in whom such experiments are not possible, it has been shown that cell-mediated immunity, which is the most important antitumor immunity, may be impaired in the immediate postoperative period (Riddle and Berenbaum, 1967), when assessed by the response of lymphocytes to phytohemagglutinin. This temporary impairment has been postulated to lead to the aggressive tumor behavior that is occasionally seen postoperatively (Buinauskas *et al.*, 1958). This problem is usually not one of practical significance, since the effect of surgery on the immune system is short-lived, and indeed is probably much less than the effect of many antineoplastic agents on the immune system.

A more important problem that faces the chemotherapist in the postoperative patient is the physical and emotional debility that may be the unavoidable aftermath of aggressive ablative cancer surgery. The patient with head and neck cancer or the patient who has undergone a major gastrointestinal resection may have severe nutritional problems that will interfere with his subsequent management. Likewise, the postmastectomy patient or the patient with a colostomy may have such severe emotional difficulties as to make further therapy impossible. These problems will be discussed more fully below.

3.1.2. Radiation Therapy

Many cancer patients are seen by the chemotherapist following attempts at palliation or cure with radiotherapy. The damage to normal tissue that occurs in these patients following radiation therapy can seriously affect the patient's ability to tolerate chemotherapy.

From the point of view of a chemotherapist, the most important effect of radiation therapy is on the hematopoietic tissue of the normal bone marrow. In patients undergoing conventional supervoltage radiation, definite changes can be seen in the marrow as early as 3 days after starting therapy (Lehar *et al.*, 1966). At the end of 1 week, there is a predictable neutropenia, followed by thrombocytopenia in 2–3 weeks and a fall in the hematocrit by 2–3 months (Rubin, 1974). Unfortunately, the effect of radiation therapy on normal marrow is not always reversible, especially when the higher "curative" doses are used. Sykes *et al.* (1964a) have shown that 3000 rads administered to the sternal marrow will prevent repopulation by normal marrow elements. This dose does not, however, prevent tumor invasion of the irradiated marrow (Sykes *et al.*, 1964b). This is an important clinical problem in many patients who are referred for chemotherapy. For example, patients who have undergone high-dose radiation therapy to the pelvis, which contains about 40% of the active marrow in an adult (Ellis, 1961), usually cannot tolerate standard doses of cytotoxic agents. This problem is recognized in many chemotherapy protocols, in which reductions in the dose of cytotoxic drugs are made for patients who have had extensive prior radiation therapy. This problem assumes more serious proportions in the case of Hodgkin's disease, in which advanced disease may in some cases be cured with aggressive multidrug chemotherapeutic regimens such as MOPP (nitrogen mustard, oncovin, prednisone, and procarbazine) (DeVita *et al.*, 1970). Many patients with advanced Hodgkin's disease have been previously treated with total nodal irradiation, which encompasses the thoracic and lumbar vertebrae and part of the pelvis. These patients tolerate conventional doses of chemotherapy very poorly, and often require attenuated doses and protracted courses of therapy (Prosnitz *et al.*, 1976).

8

GERARD T.
KENNEALEY
AND
MALCOLM S.
MITCHELL

Radiation therapy may also have serious deleterious effects on other normal tissues. The acute effects of radiation therapy to normal tissues, i.e., the nausea and vomiting from radiation to the GI tract, are distressing but self-limited, and can be ameliorated by decreasing the dose per treatment or increasing the interval between treatments without altering the effectiveness of therapy. What is of more concern, however, as more and more people are surviving longer after radiation therapy, is the long-term effects of radiation therapy on normal tissue. This organ dysfunction is due in part to progressive vascular damage and interstitial fibrosis, and to a lesser degree to the normal effects of aging. In addition, the radiated organ may function adequately under normal conditions, only to deteriorate rapidly when subjected to further stress such as impairment of blood supply, inadequate nutrition, or aggressive cytotoxic chemotherapy. An example of the latter effect that has recently been noted (Samuels *et al.*, 1976; Iacovino *et al.*, 1976) is of patients who received bleomycin following mediastinal radiation. The pulmonary fibrosis that occasionally occurs with high doses of bleomycin was seen at much lower doses in these patients.

Table 1 lists some of the more common sequelae of radiation therapy that are encountered more than 6 months after completion of treatment. In recent years, the introduction of megavoltage units and a better understanding of dosimetry and the effects of radiation on normal tissue have led to a decrease in frequency of these complications. Despite these advances, however, problems such as these do occur, and can seriously affect the overall management of the patient with advanced cancer.

Radiation therapy—like surgery—is considered to be local treatment, and as noted above, most of the effects and complications of this therapeutic modality are confined to the radiated field. Recently, the attention of many investigators has been focused on the systemic effect of radiation on the immunocompetence of the patient. In 1965, Millard (1965) noted that lymphocytes from patients tested after pelvic radiation did not respond as well to mitogenic stimulation as they had

TABLE 1
Long-Term Effects of Radiation

Organ	Clinical problem
Salivary glands	Xerostomia
Esophagus	Ulcer, stricture
Stomach	Achlorhydria, "peptic ulcer," pyloric stenosis
Small intestine	Ulcer, perforation, stricture, malabsorption
Large intestine	Ulcer, perforation, stricture, fistula formation
Liver	Chronic symptoms uncommon
Kidney	Radiation nephritis, similar to other nephridites clinically
Bladder	Ulcers, contracture, dysuria, frequency
Lung	Pneumonitis, fibrosis
Heart	Pericarditis, rarely pancarditis
Bone	Arrested growth (in children)
CNS	Cerebral atrophy
Spinal cord	Transverse myelitis

prior to radiation. More recent studies (Stjernsward *et al.*, 1972; Braeman, 1973; Stratton *et al.*, 1975) have confirmed that radiation therapy can cause profound and long-lasting lymphopenia, and that this lymphopenia occurs primarily in the subpopulation of T lymphocytes—those derived from the thymus, which are thought to be responsible for cell-mediated immunity. In addition, the remaining lymphocytes have a decreased responsiveness to mitogenic stimuli (Thomas *et al.*, 1970; Cosimi *et al.*, 1973).

These *in vitro* studies, of course, do not prove that radiation is harmful, but they do suggest that the immunosuppression caused by local radiation therapy may have long-term, perhaps deleterious, effects on the body outside the field of treatment.

3.1.3. Prior Chemotherapy

Patients who have relapsed or failed to respond to a program of chemotherapy comprise one of the most difficult problems in oncology. These patients have often had major surgery or extensive radiation, or both, and their normal tissue may, as noted above, be severely compromised. Most patients are treated initially with the best available single agent or drug combination for their particular tumor. The failure of this first round of chemotherapy often forces the patient's physician to turn to "second-line" drug regimens. These regimens are usually less effective both in the percentage of patients who are helped and in the duration of response, and may be more toxic to the already debilitated patient. This is especially true if the patient has been entered in a Phase I or II drug study, in which proportionately less is known about toxicity than would be the case with conventional therapy. An example of this problem is observed in patients with advanced carcinoma of the breast who are treated with the "Cooper" (1969) regimen (cyclophosphamide, methotrexate, 5-fluorouracil, vincristine, and prednisone). Unfortunately, when patients fail to respond to or relapse after treatment with this highly effective drug regimen, they have been exposed to nearly every effective drug for their disease except adriamycin. For this reason, many investigators and cooperative groups are studying this regimen and other drug regimens to determine the minimal number of agents in the combination capable of achieving optimal results. In breast cancer, the deletion of prednisone (Canellos *et al.*, 1974) or prednisone and vincristine (Otis and Armentrout, 1975) from the "Cooper" regimen does not appear to affect the response rate. The principles of treatment with combination chemotherapy are discussed in greater detail in Chapter 6.

3.2. General Health

As has been mentioned above, the general health of a patient with malignancy plays an important role in determining his response to therapy. The chronological age of the patient must always be considered in planning the therapeutic approach. Elderly patients with a limited life span may not be suitable candidates

TABLE 2
Eastern Cooperative Oncology Group Performance Status

Grade	Status
0	Fully active, able to carry on all predisease performance without restriction. (Karnofsky 90–100)
1	Restricted in physically strenuous activity, but ambulatory and able to carry out work of a light or sedentary nature, e.g., light housework, office work. (Karnofsky 70–80)
2	Ambulatory and capable of all self-care, but unable to carry out any work activities. Up and about more than 50% of waking hours. (Karnofsky 50–60)
3	Capable of only limited self-care, confined to bed or chair more than 50% of waking hours. (Karnofsky 30–40)
4	Completely disabled. Cannot carry on any self-care. Totally confined to bed or chair. (Karnofsky 10–20)

for aggressive attempts at curative surgery. Similarly, the effects of aging on normal tissues may interfere with delivery of optimal doses of radiation therapy, and the decrease in bone marrow reserve that occurs with aging may require downward adjustment of the dose of chemotherapeutic agents, with a consequent decrease in therapeutic effect. While age may be an important consideration in determining a course of treatment, it must not be considered as a rigid contraindication to therapy. Every oncologist can recall elderly patients who have responded dramatically to chemotherapy. Indeed, Grann *et al.* (1974) have shown that in acute myelomonocytic leukemia, in which treatment to marrow aplasia is routine, responses occur in a significant percentage of elderly patients. What is more important than a patient's age is his functional status. A patient with cancer may be debilitated from the effects of the tumor or from its therapy. He may also be incapacitated from unrelated illnesses, such as diabetes, cardiovascular disease, pulmonary insufficiency, or a collagen vascular disease. Two commonly used

TABLE 3
Karnofsky Scale

Grade	Scale	Status
1	100%	Normal; no complaints, no evidence of disease.
2	90%	Able to carry on normal activity; minor signs or symptoms of disease.
3	80%	Normal activity with effort; some signs or symptoms of disease.
4	70%	Cares for self. Unable to carry on normal activity or to do active work.
5	60%	Requires occasional assistance, but is able to care for most of his needs.
6	50%	Requires considerable assistance and frequent medical care.
7	40%	Disabled; requires special care and assistance.
8	30%	Severely disabled; hospitalization is indicated, although death is not imminent.
9	20%	Hospitalization necessary; very sick, active supportive treatment necessary.
10	10%	Moribund; fatal processes progressing rapidly.

guidelines, the Eastern Cooperative Oncology Group (ECOG) Performance Status and the Karnofsky Scale (Tables 2 and 3), are very helpful in assessing the patient's functional impairment from his tumor or other disease processes. The correlation between functional status and response to therapy is a sound one, and the functional status of each patient should be critically assessed before embarking on any form of antineoplastic treatment.

3.2.1. Nutritional Factors

Anorexia, weight loss, and malnutrition are often the hallmarks of the patient with malignancy. This constellation may occur with advancing disease, or as a presenting manifestation of the tumor. It may be far out of proportion to the stage of the tumor. This "wasting away" is very distressing psychologically to the patient and his family, and is many times the most distressing complication of this disease. Often, the degree of wasting or loss of body tissues will exceed the actual weight loss, since patients with advancing malignancy may have significant intracellular and extracellular fluid retention in the absence of clinical edema (Waterhouse, 1963).

The cause of the cachexia of malignancy is not a single one, and may differ from patient to patient. In many cases, the reason for cachexia is obvious, especially in patients with GI tract involvement. The patient with head and neck cancer who has had a glossectomy or other mutilating surgery, the patient who has had radiation therapy that has destroyed his salivary glands and taste buds, the patient with a constricting lesion in the esophagus, the patient with lymphomatous involvement of the small intestine with resulting malabsorption—these patients present no problem in diagnosis. On the other hand, the patient with Hodgkin's disease or lung cancer has no obvious cause for the profound anorexia and weight loss that are often seen at presentation. The anorexia seen in these patients may be due in part to an aversion for the taste and smell of food that develops with malignant disease. DeWys and Walters (1975) have demonstrated that cancer patients have an aversion to the taste of meat protein and amino acids. Other workers have investigated the metabolic abnormalities that develop with advancing malignancy. In a recent review of this subject, Schein *et al.* (1975) concluded that the cachexia of malignancy resembles a state of insulin resistance, with glucose intolerance, increased gluconeogenesis, and an increase in amino acid degradation.

The treatment of nutritional problems in cancer patients is a difficult task, and one that has largely been neglected in the medical literature in comparison with other forms of supportive care such as blood product transfusions, antibiotic use, and infection prophylaxis. In some patients, the solution is easy. Upper GI tract obstruction may be relieved or bypassed to ensure delivery of adequate food and fluid to the stomach and small intestine. In patients who have an aversion to certain smells and tastes, an awareness of this aversion on the part of the patient and his family and the assistance of an experienced dietician can do much to alleviate the problem.

In patients in whom the etiology is not obvious, the task is more difficult. The cooperation of the patient, his physician, his family, a dietician, and at times a psychiatrist, is needed to encourage the maintenance of caloric intake. At times, this maintenance is still not possible, and in certain cases in which the patient's overall prognosis is otherwise good, intravenous hyperalimentation may be used as a temporary measure to improve nutrition. Copeland and Dudrick (1975) recently reviewed their experience with this mode of therapy, and found it to be useful in maintaining the patient's nutritional status during periods of intensive chemotherapy, radiation, and major GI surgery. This form of therapy, however, is not without risk. Common problems include catheter sepsis (Curry and Quie, 1971), often due to *Candida albicans*, and electrolyte abnormalities. Intravenous hyperalimentation is not a panacea for all patients, and should be used only in patients in whom there is reason to believe that the treatment of the underlying disease will be successful. In addition, parenteral hyperalimentation should be used only by physicians with experience in its use. As with all therapeutic endeavors, the complication rate associated with hyperalimentation is inversely proportional to the skill and experience of the user.

3.2.2. Immunologic Factors

The immunologic system plays an important but as yet incompletely understood role in arresting malignant disease. The immunologic defenses are threefold, consisting of antibody production, cell-mediated immunity, and interferon production. While the interactions among the different immune functions are quite complex, it appears that the cell-mediated or thymus-derived immune system plays the major role in preventing neoplastic disease. For a more complete discussion of tumor immunology, the reader is referred to a recent review by Mitchell (1976).

Evidence for a role of the immune system as a guardian against neoplastic disease is seen in the so-called "immunodeficiency diseases." In the Wiskott-Aldrich syndrome and in ataxia-telangiectasia, both of which are thymus-deficiency diseases, the incidence of malignancy is as high as 10%. Similarly, in patients who have received immunosuppressive agents following an organ transplant, there is a 5–6% incidence of *de novo* malignancy (Penn *et al.*, 1971), and there is a 4% incidence of new and apparently unrelated tumors in recipients who have been treated for preexisting cancers (Penn, 1976). There is also other circumstantial evidence that cancer results in part from a breakdown of the immunologic surveillance system. In mice, both delayed hypersensitivity reactions (reviewed by Makinodan *et al.*, 1971) and thymus-independent immune function (Gerbase-DeLima *et al.*, 1974) have been shown to decrease with age. Decreased responsiveness to dinitrochlorobenzene (DNCB) has also been demonstrated in a healthy population of elderly individuals (Waldorf *et al.*, 1968). Recently, Segre and Segre (1976) showed that "suppressor" T cells that interact with bone marrow–derived (B) cells to reduce antibody synthesis are *increased* in number in elderly mice. Since cancer by and large is a disease of the aged, these findings suggest that a decrease in immunologic activity may be partly responsible for this increased incidence of malignancy in the elderly.

Other workers (Catalona and Chretien, 1973) investigated the immune function in cancer patients and found that the ability to react to a new antigen (DNCB) was decreased in comparison with that of controls. These workers (Chretien *et al.*, 1973) were able to correlate the immune status of cancer patients assessed preoperatively with their prognosis. They found that the patients who had no evidence of disease at 3 years initially had a normal response of their lymphocytes to phytohemagglutinin.

These investigations have stimulated numerous clinical investigators to treat cancer patients by altering their immune status. Except for the use of BCG in melanoma (Eilber *et al.*, 1976) and in acute myeloblastic leukemia (Powles, 1976), most of the results to date have been disappointing. All these studies point to the next area of research endeavor—the field of cancer prevention. It is to be hoped that in the not too distant future, immunologists will be able to delineate and then correct the defect in the immune system that allows cancer to flourish.

3.2.3. *Psychosocial Factors*

The diagnosis of cancer presents many problems to the physician that are not seen in other chronic diseases. The mystique that still surrounds the diagnosis, the fear of pain and suffering, loss of sexual attractiveness, or impairment of bodily functions may aggravate an already difficult treatment program. The first problem that a physician faces is what to tell the patient who now carries the diagnosis of malignancy. Previously, this was a much-debated issue in the medical community. In 1953, Fitts and Ravdin (1953) surveyed 442 physicians in Philadelphia, and noted that two-thirds of them usually did not tell patients their diagnosis. In 1961, Oken (1961) polled 193 surgeons, internists, and general practitioners in the Chicago area, most of whom had academic affiliations, and found that 88% preferred not to inform cancer patients of their diagnosis. In the last decade, however, attitudes in the medical profession have changed dramatically. This change is in part due to the influence of Kubler-Ross (1969), who demonstrated that terminally ill patients need to talk about their diagnosis. It is also due to the increasing sophistication of the lay public concerning cancer and the possibilities of its cure, and to the increased requirement of informed consent for treatment of all medical problems. In a consultative oncology practice, we now very rarely see patients who are not fully informed of their diagnosis. Telling a patient his diagnosis with tact and in the least threatening manner means, however, that compassion is not lost, and helps to promote frank discussion of problems as they arise. Clearly, the physician must exercise judgment here in precisely what is said and how it is put. It is also important for the patient to realize that most cancers do not cause severe pain for prolonged periods. The patient must also be told that if severe pain should become a part of his illness, he will receive sufficient medication

14

GERARD T.
KENNEALEY
AND
MALCOLM S.
MITCHELL

to alleviate his suffering. In dealing with patients with advanced disease, hope and optimism should always be maintained, even though both the patient and his physician are tacitly aware of the ultimate outcome.

The treatment modalities used in the cancer patient may also lead to severe psychological problems. The first step for many cancer patients is surgery. The surgeon, while respected for his ability to potentially cure a patient, is also feared because he may interfere with the patient's integrity as a person. Different surgical procedures pose different psychological problems in the cancer patient. Surgery on the face and neck—often radical and deforming—in an attempt to cure leaves scars or deformities that are obvious to all as the hallmark of a cancer patient. The interference with speech or eating can compound the problem of the patient's self-image. In addition, many patients with head and neck cancer have a history of alcoholism and accompanying personality disorder that makes a postoperative adjustment very difficult even when the surgical procedure is successful. In these patients, the intensive efforts of the physician, nursing staff, social service, and often a psychiatrist need to be enlisted to ensure a successful adjustment to the mutilating surgery. It may also be helpful to have the patient seen by another patient who has made a successful adjustment to his disability.

Intensive perioperative counseling is also necessary for the mastectomy patient, who fears the loss of her sexual attractiveness and self-esteem as a woman following the removal of a breast. Exercises can usually be started in the immediate postoperative period to preserve function and decrease swelling in the adjacent extremity, and excellent prostheses that closely simulate normal breast tissue are now available. The widespread publicity surrounding the surgery on Mrs. Ford and Mrs. Rockefeller has helped many women both by encouraging earlier detection of this potentially curable disease and by removing some of the stigmata surrounding a mastectomy.

Another result of surgery that is difficult to accept is externalization of the GI tract, the "ostomies." The need for constant attention and the fear of leakage or odor are very distressing for most patients. Again, the compassion and attention of an ostomy nurse, and joining an ostomy club, are very helpful to patients with problems, psychological or physical.

The removal of the uterus or the ovaries in a woman, or a transurethral resection of the prostate or orchiectomy in a man, can lead to many psychological problems. While all these procedures result in sterility, they should not interfere with sexual function. A compassionate and factual discussion with the patient and his or her spouse preoperatively can do much to allay the patient's fears concerning sexual function.

When a patient must receive chemotherapy for his malignancy, an entirely different set of problems must be dealt with by the physician. Many patients know of someone who received chemotherapy—usually shortly before death—and they will be very depressed at the prospect of debilitating treatments for what they feel is a hopeless cause. Again, an attitude of realistic optimism is in order—discussing the possibilities with the patient and a responsible family member, with a truthful assessment of the risk and potential benefits of each form of therapy, is mandatory. The immediate side effects of chemotherapy can be as devastating to some patients as the disease itself, or as radical surgery. It is the duty of the medical oncologists to explain the side effects in as much detail as is necessary without unduly frightening the patient. Hair loss occurs with most chemotherapeutic agents, and patients should be informed of this loss and the need for a wig openly discussed. The nausea and vomiting that occur acutely with many agents can usually be alleviated by antiemetics (Moertel *et al.*, 1963). Patients should have a generous supply of antiemetics in both oral and suppository form to help ameliorate this acute toxicity.

Eventually, the patient's disease advances to the point at which no further treatment other than symptomatic therapy is contemplated. This is the most difficult time for the patient, his family, and his physician (White, 1969). If the patient is in the denial phase of his illness, the grim reality of his prognosis should not be inflicted upon him. However, the wasting of time and money looking for "cures" should be gently discouraged. At all times a responsible family member must be aware of the prognosis. Conversely, many times the patient is aware of his impending death, while the family persists in denial. It is the duty of the physician to assist the family in accepting the terminal phase of the illness, and thus provide better emotional support for the patient. During the terminal phase of the patient's illness, the physician who has been trained to battle disease may be tempted to withdraw, since the battle has been lost. This withdrawal can be very devastating to the terminal patient, and should never occur. The physician can do much simply by his continuing presence to alleviate the anxiety of the patient and his family as the time of death approaches.

3.2.4. Financial Factors

One of the most pressing concerns of the cancer patient is the fear that he will become a financial burden to his family. Unfortunately, these fears are often well founded. The cost of medical care in this country is high, and is continuing to increase faster than the rate of inflation. The cost of treatment of cancer is no exception. The patient receiving chemotherapy as an outpatient faces the prospect of frequent doctor visits, regular blood tests and nuclear medicine scans, and expensive medications. The patient who receives aggressive inpatient treatment may also face overwhelming costs for a prolonged hospitalization. A case in point is that of a 20-year-old man who recently received aggressive chemotherapy for acute nonlymphocytic leukemia at our institution. He required intensive hematological support and antibiotic treatment during the resulting marrow aplasia before achieving remission. His bill for the 7 weeks of hospitalization was $18,000. Fortunately, the majority of patients now have some form of medical insurance that covers the cost of inpatient hospitalization. Most insurance plans, however, do not provide coverage for medications and routine office visits, and this can be a source of great worry to the patient and his family.

The concern about the financial burden of cancer can lead to delay in diagnosis, refusal to accept treatment, or such severe emotional stress that successful treatment may be impaired. It is imperative that the physician who undertakes a plan of cancer treatment inquire carefully into the financial resources of every patient so as to anticipate any financial problems. The assistance of a competent social worker is mandatory in problem cases. The social worker should be aware of community resources that can be helpful, and is in a position to ascertain certain insurance benefits that the patient often is not aware of. She can also assist in application for veterans' benefits and union benefits (which are sometimes available), and can help in the application for various government programs, such as Title XIX, which can assist many lower-middle-income families. The social worker can also be helpful in arranging for medical assistance for the terminal patient at home, which is covered by many insurance plans. This kind of assistance often has the added benefit of decreasing the amount of time spent in a hospital, and thus decreases the total cost of medical care.

3.3. Support Facilities

Another factor that may influence the response to chemotherapy in advanced malignancy is the availability of adequate facilities to provide support for the patient during episodes of acute drug-induced illness. These problems usually occur during periods of bone marrow suppression, either planned, as in acute leukemia, or unplanned, as an unexpected toxicity of any one of numerous chemotherapeutic agents. To treat patients with chemotherapy for neoplastic disease, we feel that a number of support capabilities are required:

1. Platelet transfusion availability—necessary for episodes of drug-induced thrombocytopenia.
2. A competent bacteriology and fungal laboratory—vital for the acute diagnosis and treatment of severe infections that may occur during periods of drug-induced leukopenia, or as a result of obstruction by the malignant process.
3. Nearby radiation therapy—for treatment of brain or spinal cord metastases that may be needed on an urgent basis, for primary treatment of the tumor, or for palliation of painful bony metastases.
4. The availability of granulocyte transfusions—which appear to enhance survival in the infected granulocytopenic patient (see Chapter 9, Section 3.5.2), and may soon become a standard supportive measure, as have platelet transfusions in the last decade.

Because cancer chemotherapy at times requires intensive supportive care, it has recently been suggested that cancer can be treated competently only at a medical center. Robinson (1976), in a widely read popular magazine, has stated that "the average cancer patient is likely to be misdiagnosed by his local doctor and maltreated at his local hospital." While treatment at a medical center may be appropriate, or even necessary, in some cases, we believe that in a majority of cases, the difficulty and expense of travel do not justify a transfer of care to a cancer center. The number of well-trained oncologists in private practice has increased considerably in recent years, and will continue to increase in the near future. In addition, the support facilities enumerated above are available in many well-staffed community hospitals. There are exceptions, however. In patients who have failed conventional chemotherapy and whose functional status as defined above is adequate, experimental therapy at a well-equipped comprehensive cancer center is justified. The therapy may be helpful to the patient, and is also necessary to better understand the toxicity and spectrum of action of newer drugs or different dosage schedules. Patients who have very rare diseases may also be best evaluated and treated at centers where there is expertise in their particular illness.

There is one disease for which treatment at a comprehensive cancer center is strongly urged, and that is adult nonlymphocytic leukemia. This rare disease usually strikes in the prime of life, and if untreated, is usually fatal within 6 months. Current therapy is experimental, in that new drugs and drug combinations are constantly being tested. The therapy is aggressive, leading to bone marrow aplasia, with a prolonged risk of bleeding and sepsis. In addition, when complications occur, the expertise of specialists in multiple disciplines and highly skilled nursing care are necessary for a successful outcome. While these are often available in well-staffed community hospitals, it is axiomatic in medicine that seldom-encountered diseases or complications are usually poorly treated. For these reasons, we agree with Mosher *et al.* (1974) that this illness is best treated at a well-equipped cancer center.

4. Therapeutic Goals

As has been noted in the preceding sections, a number of tumor and host factors affect the therapeutic response of a host to a malignancy. These factors influence the chemotherapist in his approach to a particular patient with a particular tumor. Table 4 lists various tumors and their responsiveness to chemotherapy. In Category I are tumors in which chemotherapy can either effect a "cure" or a substantial increment in disease-free survival. In treating patients with one of these diseases, aggressive therapy with toxic medications and intensive supportive measures is indicated. Substantial morbidity and even mortality may be acceptable if the therapy can lead to cure or disease-free survival in many patients. The best example of this is acute lymphocytic leukemia in children in which even severe hematological toxicity is an acceptable risk (although not usually required) in the attainment of the goal of remission.

Category II encompasses a diverse group of malignancies with varying responses to therapy. In chronic myelocytic leukemia, chemotherapy may produce marked symptomatic improvement, but does not appear to influence survival. In small-cell anaplastic ("oat-cell") lung carcinoma, the response to chemotherapy alone, or more recently in combination with radiation therapy to

TABLE 4
Chemotherapeutic Potential in Malignant Disease

I. Tumors frequently curable by chemotherapy
   Choriocarcinoma
   Burkitt's lymphoma
   Advanced Hodgkin's disease
   Acute lymphocytic leukemia of children
   Testicular tumors
   Wilms's tumor
   Ewing's sarcoma
   Embryonal rhabdomyosarcoma
   Diffuse histiocytic lymphoma
II. Tumors in which remissions or increased survival are often achieved
   Acute nonlymphocytic leukemia
   Chronic myelocytic leukemia
   Chronic lymphocytic leukemia
   Multiple myeloma
   Non-Hodgkin's lymphoma
   "Head and neck" cancer
   Adenocarcinoma of the ovary
   Small-cell anaplastic lung cancer
   Soft-tissue sarcoma
   Neuroblastoma
   Adenocarcinoma of the colon and rectum
   Breast cancer
   Malignant melanoma
   Islet cell carcinoma
   Osteogenic sarcoma
III. Tumors with infrequent responses and no increase in survival
   Brain tumors
   GI adenocarcinoma (excluding colon–rectum)
   Bronchogenic carcinoma
   Cervical and uterine carcinoma
   Carcinoma of the kidney
   Carcinoma of the bladder
   Carcinoma of the prostate
   "Blast crisis" of chronic myelogenous leukemia
   Endocrine tumors
     adrenal
     thyroid
     carcinoid

the primary site (Hornback *et al.*, 1976), may be dramatic, but is often of short duration. In the non-Hodgkin's lymphomas, the effectiveness of therapy is more difficult to evaluate, since many patients have prolonged survival with minimal treatment, while others succumb quickly to their disease despite aggressive therapeutic maneuvers. Carcinoma of the breast, the most common tumor in women, is often responsive to chemotherapy. While there are no cures from chemotherapy in advanced breast carcinoma, the response to therapy, especially in soft-tissue disease, may be quite dramatic. Treatment of these diseases closely resembles the treatment of a chronic nonmalignant disease. While the life span is not always increased, the quality of life is often improved to the satisfaction of both the patient and his physician.

Category III comprises tumors in which chemotherapy is at present least useful. Responses to chemotherapy in these diseases are infrequent and usually of limited duration. It is here that Phase I (toxicity–dose) and Phase II (efficacy) drug trials are appropriate. In the treatment of these diseases, the physician must balance two goals: (1) to do no harm, by not shortening the patient's useful life span or increasing his discomfort; (2) to gain knowledge about new therapies that may be of ultimate benefit to many other patients. While these goals may occasionally come into conflict, usually they do not. A careful assessment of the patient's tumor burden, functional status, and, most important, his wishes and those of his family, will guide the physician in making a correct decision on the modality of therapy he offers to the patient.

These categories are not static. In adenocarcinoma of the colon and rectum, for example, Baker *et al.* (1975) recently demonstrated that the addition of a nitroso-urea (methyl CCNU) to the standard therapy with 5-fluorouracil has resulted in an increased response rate in advanced disease. Li and Ross (1976) showed a marked improvement in disease-free survival with adjunctive 5-fluorouracil after surgery for this type of tumor. More important, the introduction of a new agent through Phase I and II trials may rapidly change the outlook in tumors not only in the worst response category, but also in those that respond moderately to other agents, which may respond much better to the new drug. Such was the case for adriamycin in breast cancer.

5. New Problems

As more and more patients with cancer show longer survival following treatment with chemotherapeutic agents, we must become increasingly aware of the long-term effects of these medications.

5.1. Immunosuppressive and Carcinogenic Effects

The immunosuppressive effects of cytotoxic agents have been known for over half a century, since Hektoen and Corper (1921) demonstrated that mustard gas impairs the ability of rabbits to form antibodies to sheep erythrocytes. Most of the drugs used in the chemotherapy of malignancy have been shown to affect the immunologic system. The mechanisms of action are different for the different classes of drugs, but the end result is the same—interference with the proliferative capacity of the cells involved in the immune response. For a comprehensive treatment of the immunosuppressive potential of the various chemotherapeutic agents, the reader is referred to a recent monograph by Sartorelli and Johns (1974). The immunosuppressive capacity of chemotherapeutic agents is of great concern to the oncologist, since, as has been noted above, there is a markedly increased incidence of malignancies in patients who have received immunosuppressive therapy for nonmalignant conditions, i.e., transplant recipients. At present, many patients with nonmalignant conditions such as arthritis and occasionally those with psoriasis are being treated with immunosuppressive agents. These diseases may not significantly affect longevity, and the probable increased risk of malignancy due to immunosuppressive therapy in these patients is of great concern (Steinberg *et al.*, 1972). It should be emphasized, however, that intermittent therapy permits recovery of immunologic capacity. Also, several of the newer agents (bleomycin, DTIC, dimethylmyleran) are much less immunosuppressive than other agents.

In addition to the immunosuppressive potential, which may lead to an increased risk of malignancy, several of the anticancer drugs may be directly oncogenic. In animals, all the drugs that act by alkylation or by binding to DNA (the "alkylating" agents and antitumor antibiotics) have been shown to be carcinogenic. In addition, the antimetabolites such as methotrexate may act as "cocarcinogens" in animal systems by enhancing the carcinogenic effect of certain chemicals (reviewed by Harris, 1976). The use of one anticancer drug, chlornaphazine, was discontinued when high doses were shown to cause bladder cancer (Thiede and Christensen, 1969). Cycloposphamide, an alkylating agent used extensively for both malignant and nonmalignant conditions, has also been associated with malignancies of the bladder (Worth, 1971; Wall and Clausen, 1975). In addition, a number of other case reports of new cancers arising in patients treated with chemotherapy have recently appeared in the literature (reviewed by Harris, 1975; Penn, 1976). This potential carcinogenicity is of great concern now that the use of adjuvant chemotherapy is increasing. In breast cancer, women with four or more positive axillary nodes are being treated with either L-phenylalanine mustard (Fisher *et al.*, 1975) or a regimen containing cyclophosphamide (Bonadonna *et al.*, 1976)—both alkylating agents with known carcinogenic potential. In these patients, who have a 30% 5-year survival with surgery alone, careful long-term follow-up will be necessary to determine the risks and benefits of adjuvant chemotherapy (Costanza, 1975).

5.2. Specific Drug Effects

In addition to the immunosuppressive and carcinogenic potential of antineoplastic agents as a group, many of the individual drugs have been noted to have effects on normal tissues that may cause serious functional impairment in long-term survivors of chemotherapy. Since the antineoplastic agents will each be a subject of a more detailed analysis, only a brief description of the more important long-term problems will be presented here.

5.2.1. Alkylating Agents

These agents as a whole have been associated with oligospermia and azoospermia in many reports. These effects have been seen primarily with cytoxan and chlorambucil, which are the most commonly used oral agents. They were originally thought to be irreversible, but recent studies have demonstrated a return of spermatogenesis several years after discontinuation of therapy with cyclophosphamide (Sherins and DeVita, 1973) and chlorambucil (Cheviakoff *et al.*, 1973). Ovarian function is also affected by alkylating agents, amenorrhea being a common complication of therapy (Warne *et al.*, 1973). This complication may also be reversible, at least in some patients (Kumar *et al.*, 1972).

In addition to its effect on the reproductive system, cyclophosphamide has a deleterious effect on the urinary tract. Besides the hemorrhagic cystitis that may occur acutely, and the occurrence—rare, it is to be hoped—of bladder cancer noted above, chronic bladder fibrosis and vesicoureteral reflux may occur (Johnson and Meadows, 1971). This condition is usually seen following large doses, and fortunately is asymptomatic in many cases.

Busulfan, an alkylating agent used in chronic myelocytic leukemia, in addition to the expected effect on the marrow, may cause hyperpigmentation of the skin and an Addisonian-like syndrome. Its most serious long-term toxicity is to the lungs, where cough, fever, and dyspnea may herald the onset of irreversible pulmonary fibrosis. This condition may be fatal if not diagnosed and treated promptly (Podoll and Winkler, 1974).

5.2.2. Antitumor Antibiotics

The anthracycline antibiotics, daunorubicin and adriamycin, share with most anticancer agents acute GI toxicity, and may cause alopecia and bone marrow depression. The most significant long-term side effect of these agents is cardiotoxicity, manifested in its most severe form as fatal congestive heart failure. This congestive cardiomyopathy is characterized histologically by a decrease in the number of cardiac muscle cells and focal degeneration of the remaining myocardial cells (LeFrak *et al.*, 1973). This anthracycline cardiac toxicity is dose-related, and is usually not seen with a cumulative dose of less than 500–600 mg daunorubicin/M^2 and 500 mg adriamycin/M^2. In patients who have received mediastinal radiation, the incidence of cardiac toxicity is increased (Gilladoga *et al.*, 1976) and may occur at lower doses.

Bleomycin, another antitumor antibiotic, has clinically significant effects on the lungs. This pulmonary toxicity is manifest by fine rales on ausculation, dyspnea, tachypnea, and a nonproductive cough (Blum *et al.*, 1973). Radiographically, a diffuse interstitial pattern is seen; histologically, there are hyaline membranes, atypical proliferation of alveolar cells, and interstitial fibrosis, quite similar to the findings seen with busulfan. Clinically, this disease often has a fatal outcome if not recognized early. It is often difficult, however, to distinguish bleomycin lung toxicity from opportunistic infection or progression of the primary disease. Like that of the anthracyclines, the long-term pulmonary toxicity of bleomycin is dose-related, and is uncommon with a total dose of less than 400 units in the adult. A further similarity to the cardiotoxicity of the anthracyclines is the occurrence of pulmonary toxicity at lower doses in patients who have had prior radiotherapy (Samuels *et al.*, 1976).

5.2.3. Antimetabolites

Methotrexate, a folic acid antagonist, has been used for many years as a maintenance agent in acute lymphoblastic leukemia and for the treatment of nonmalignant diseases such as psoriasis. Because of continued therapy with methotrexate over a period of years in these and other diseases, the late effects of therapy on normal tissue have become a significant problem for the physician. The hepatic toxicity of methotrexate was first reported by O'Rourke *et al.*, (1964) in a patient with psoriasis. Long-term use of methotrexate has been associated with the development of hepatic fibrosis, and with cirrhosis leading to hepatic insufficiency (Dahl *et al.*, 1971). It has also been noted that hepatic fibrosis can be found by biopsy even in the absence of hepatomegaly or liver function abnormalities (Nesbit *et al.*, 1976). Fibrosis is the most common and most serious complication of methotrexate therapy, and it has been suggested that liver biopsies be done at frequent intervals to monitor the effect of this drug on hepatic function.

In addition to its effect on liver function, methotrexate has been shown to cause an acute pulmonic process, similar to that seen with bleomycin and busulfan, with diffuse interstitial infiltrates on the chest X ray (Evarts *et al.*, 1973). This is usually an acute self-limited process that responds to cessation of therapy, although Nesbit *et al.* (1976) reported a patient in whom an open lung biopsy one year after the acute illness showed marked interstitial fibrosis. Methotrexate may also have pronounced effects on the CNS when administered intrathecally in the prophylaxis or treatment of meningeal neoplasia, particularly leukemia or lymphoma. Studies of long-term survivors of childhood leukemia treated with intrathecal methotrexate have shown neurological sequelae varying from mild impairment to severe dementia and death (Meadows and Evans, 1976). These complications appear to be worse in patients who receive concomitant whole-brain radiation (Price and Jamieson, 1975). Less well known than these complications is the effect of methotrexate on the osseous system. Ragab *et al.* (1970) and O'Regan *et al.* (1973) reported bone pain and fractures in growing children receiving methotrexate therapy. The symptoms and X-ray changes (osteoporosis) regressed following discontinuation of methotrexate. The mechanism of this effect is unknown at present, although Nevinny *et al.* (1965) reported an increase in urinary and fecal calcium in some patients on methotrexate.

The purine analogues of 6-mercaptopurine and its derivative, azathioprine, have been associated with hepatotoxicity, which usually occurs within several months after initiation of therapy (Einhorn and Davidsohn, 1964). In most cases, the liver function abnormalities return to normal after cessation of therapy, although deaths have occurred (Clark *et al.*, 1960; Zarday *et al.*, 1972) with both drugs. The remaining commonly used antimetabolities, 5-fluorouracil and cytosine arabinoside, have no major long-term side effects.

5.2.4. Other Agents

The vinca alkaloids, especially vincristine, cause a peripheral neuropathy characterized by the loss of deep tendon reflexes, paresthesias, and distal musculature weakness. Ileus and cranial nerve abnormalities may also occur rarely (Sandler *et al.*, 1969). These side effects are self-limited and usually respond to cessation of therapy, although residua are sometimes seen.

The adrenal steroids, estrogens, progestins, and androgens are used frequently for treatment of breast cancer and other malignancies. Their side effects are well known, and will not be discussed here.

5.3. Summary

The treatment of neoplastic disease with chemotherapy is accompanied by substantial immediate and long-term morbidity to the patient. In each individual patient, the "risk–benefit ratio" needs to be carefully assessed to determine the best choice of drug and duration of therapy to attain the goal of therapy without undue hazard to the patient.

6. Conclusion

The progress that has been made in the 35 years since Goodman and Gilman's first use of nitrogen mustard in 1942 has been remarkable. Some diseases are curable and some are eminently treatable by chemotherapy. An entire medical specialty has evolved around the use of cytotoxic medication for cancer patients, and the American Board of Internal Medicine has conducted subspeciality board exams in Medical Oncology since 1972.

Unfortunately, much still remains to be accomplished. The currently used drug regimens for many malignancies are toxic to normal host tissues, and if improperly used can be lethal. Selective toxicity to tumor cells is still an elusive goal. Many diseases such as lung cancer are quite resistant to currently available chemotherapeutic agents. The reason for resistance of many tumors to chemotherapy is largerly unclear and is a major area of research by many investigators, and the complex interrelationship between the immune system of the patient and his malignancy is still another focus for intensive research. Yet, it is these intriguing complexities of the tumor–host–drug interrelationship, some of the details of which have been discovered, that have created so much interest among so many preclinical and clinical scientists. This scientific activity will, we trust, lead to significant therapeutic gains at an accelerated pace in the future.

7. References

BAKER, L. H., MATTER, R. TALLEY, R. AND VAITKEVICIUS, V., 1975, 5-FU vs. 5-FU and MeCCNU in gastrointestinal cancer, *Proc. Amer. Soc. Clin. Oncol.* **16**:229.
BLUM, R. H., CARTER, S. K., AND AGRE, K., 1973, A clinical review of bleomycin—a new antineoplastic agent, *Cancer* **31**:903.

BONADONNA, G., BRUSAMOLINO, E., VALAGUSSA, P., ROSSI, A., BRUGNATELLI, L., BRAMBILLA, C., DELENA, M., TANCINI, G., BAJETTA, E., MUSUMECI, R., AND VERONESI, N., 1976, Combination chemotherapy as an adjuvant treatment in operable breast cancer, *N. Engl. J. Med.* **294**:405.

BRAEMAN, J., 1973, Lymphocyte response after radiotherapy, *Lancet* **2**:683.

BUINAUSKAS, P., MCDONALD, G. O., AND COLE, W. H., 1958, Role of operative stress in the resistance of the experimental animal to inoculated cancer cells (and discussion of paper), *Ann. Surg.* **148**:642.

CANELLOS, G. P., DEVITA, V. T., GOLD, G. L., CHABNER, B. A., SCHEIN, P. S., AND YOUNG, R. C., 1974, Cyclical combination chemotherapy for advanced breast carcinoma, *Br. Med. J.* **1**:218.

CAPIZZI, R. L., BERTINO, J. R., AND HANDSCHUMACHER, R. E., 1970, L-Asparaginase, *Annu. Rev. Med.* **21**:433.

CATALONA, W. J., AND CHRETIEN, P. B., 1973, Abnormalities of quantitative dinitrochlorobenzene sensitization in cancer patients: Correlation with tumor stage and histology, *Cancer*, **31**:353.

CHEVIAKOFF, S., CALAMERA, J. C., MORGENFELD, M., AND MANCINI, R. E., 1973, Recovery of spermatogenesis in patients with lymphoma after treatment with chlorambucil, *J. Reprod. Fertil.* **33**:155.

CHRETIEN, P. B., CROWDER, W. L., GERTNER, H. R., SAMPLE, W. F., AND CATALONA, W. J. 1973, Correlation of preoperative lymphocyte reactivity with the clinical course of cancer patients, *Surg. Gynecol. Obstet.* **136**:380.

CLARK, P. A., HSIA, Y. E., AND HUNTSMAN, R. G., 1960, Toxic complications of treatment with 6-mercaptopurine, *Br. Med. J.* **1**:393.

CONN, J. H., LEB, S. M., AND HARDY, J. D., 1957, Effect of nitrogen mustard and thioTEPA on wound healing, *Surg. Forum* **8**:80.

COOPER, R., 1969, Combination chemotherapy in hormone resistant breast cancer, *Proc. Amer. Assoc. Cancer Res.* **10**:15.

COPELAND, E. M., III, AND DUDRICK, S. J., 1975, Cancer: Nutritional concepts, *Semin. Oncol.* **2**:329.

COSIMI, A. B., BRUNSTETTER, F. H., KEMMERER, W. T., AND MILLER, B. N., 1973, Cellular immune competence of breast cancer patients receiving radiotherapy, *Arch. Surg.* **107**:531.

COSTANZA, M., 1975, The problem of breast cancer prophylaxis, *N. Engl. J. Med.* **293**:1095.

CURRY, C. R., AND QUIE, P. G., 1971, Fungal septicemia in patients receiving parenteral hyperalimentation, *N. Engl. J. Med.* **285**:1221.

DAHL, M. G. C., GREGORY, M. M., AND SCHEUER, P. J., 1971, Liver damage due to methotrexate in patients with psoriasis, *Br. Med. J.* **1**:625.

DESPREZ, J. D., AND KIEHN, C. L., 1960, The effects of cytoxan (cyclophosphamide) on wound healing, *Plast. Reconstr. Surg.* **26**:301.

DEVITA, V. T., SERPICK, A. A., AND CARBONE, P. O., 1970, Combination chemotherapy in the treatment of advanced Hodgkin's disease, *Ann. Intern. Med.* **73**:881.

DEWYS, W. D., AND WALTERS, K., 1975, Abnormalities of taste sensation in cancer patients, *Cancer* **36**:1888.

EILBER, F. R., MORTON, D. L., AND HOLMES, E. C., 1976, Adjuvant immunotherapy with BCG in treatment of regional lymph node metastases from malignant melanoma, *N. Engl. J. Med.* **294**:237.

EINHORN, M., AND DAVIDSOHN, I., 1964, Hepatotoxicity of mercaptopurine, *J. Amer. Med. Assoc.* **188**:802.

ELLIS, R. E., 1961, The distributions of active bone marrow in the adult, *Phys. Med. Biol.* **5**:255.

EVARTS, C. S., WESTCOTT, J. L., AND BRAGG, D. C., 1973, Methotrexate therapy and pulmonary disease, *Radiology* **107**:539.

FARBER, S., DIAMOND, L. K., MERCER, R. D., SYLVESTER, R. J., JR., AND WOLFF, J. A., 1948, Temporary remissions in acute leukemia in children produced by folic acid antagonist, 4-aminopteroyl-glutamic acid (Aminopterin), *N. Engl. J. Med.* **238**:787.

FARHAT, S. M., AMER, N. S., WEEKS, B. S., AND MUSSELMAN, M. M., 1958, Effect of mechlorethamine hydrochloride (nitrogen mustard) on healing of abdominal wounds, *Arch. Surg.* **76**:749.

FISHER, B., RAVDIN, R. G., AUSMAN, R. K., SLACK, N. H., MOORE, G. E., AND NOER, R. J., 1968, Surgical adjuvant chemotherapy in cancer of the breast: Results of a decade of cooperative investigation, *Ann. Surg.* **168**:337.

FISHER, B., CARBONE, P., ECONOMOU, S. G., FRELICK, R., GLASS, A., LERNER, H., REDMOND, ZELEN, M., BAND, P., KATRYCH, D. L., WOLMARK, N., FISHER, E., et al., 1975, l-Phenalyalanine mustard (l-PAM) in the management of primary breast cancer, *N. Engl. J. Med.* **292**:117.

FITTS, W. T., JR., AND RAVDIN, I. S., 1953, What Philadelphia physicians tell their patients with cancer, *J. Amer. Med. Assoc.* **153**:901.

GERBASE-DELIMA, M., WILKINSON, J., SMITH, G. S., AND WALFORD, R. L., 1974, Age-related decline in thymic-independent immune function in a long-lived mouse strain, *J. Gerontol.* **29**:261.

GILLADOGA, A. C., MANUEL, C., TAN, C. T. C., WOLLNER, N., STERNBERG, S., AND MURPHY, M. L., 1976, The cardiotoxicity of adriamycin and daunomycin in children, *Cancer* **37**:1070.

GOODMAN, L. S., WINTROBE, M. M., DAMESHEK, W., GOODMAN, M. J., GILMAN, A., AND McLENNAN, M. T., 1946, Nitrogen mustard therapy, *J. Amer. Med. Assoc.* **132**:126.

GRANN, V., ERICHSON, R., FLANNERY, J., FINCH, S., AND CLARKSON, B., 1974, The therapy of acute granulocytic leukemia in patients more than fifty years old, *Ann. Intern. Med.* **80**:15.

HARRIS, C. C., 1975, Immunosuppressive anticancer drugs in man: Their oncogenic potential, *Radiology* **114**:163.

HARRIS, C. C., 1976, The carcinogenicity of anticancer drugs: A hazard in man, *Cancer* **37**:1014.

HEKTOEN, L., AND CORPER, H. J., 1921, Effect of mustard gas (dichlorethyl-sulphid) on antibody formation, *J. Infect. Dis.* **28**:279.

HORNBACK, N. B., EINHORN, L., SHIDNIA, H., JOE, B. T., KRAUSE, M., AND FURNAS, B., 1976, Oat cell carcinoma of the lung, early treatment results of combination radiation therapy and chemotherapy, *Cancer* **37**:2658.

IACOVINO, J. R., LEITNER, J., ABBAS, A. K., LOKICH, J. J., AND SNIDER, G. L., 1976, Fatal pulmonary reaction from low doses of bleomycin; an idiosyncratic tissue response, *J. Amer. Med. Assoc.* **235**:1253.

JAFFE, N., FREI, E., III, TRAGGIS, D., AND BISHOP, Y., 1974, Adjuvant methotrexate and citrovorum-factor treatment of osteogenic sarcoma, *N. Engl. J. Med.* **291**:994.

JOHNSON, W. W., AND MEADOWS, D. C., 1971, Urinary-bladder fibrosis and teleangiectasia associated with long-term cyclophosphamide therapy, *N. Engl. J. Med.* **284**:290.

KUBLER-ROSS, E., 1969, *On Death and Dying*, Macmillan, New York.

KUMAR, R., BIGGART, J. D., McEVOY, J., AND McGEOWN, M. G., 1972, Cyclophosphamide and reproductive function, *Lancet* **1**:1212.

LeFRAK, E. A., PITHA, J., ROSENHEIM, S., AND GOTTLIEB, J. A., 1973, A clinico-pathological analysis of adriamycin cardiotoxicity, *Cancer* **32**:302.

LEHAR, T. J., KIELY, J. M., PEASE, G. L., AND SCANLON, P. W., 1966, Effect of local irradiation on human bone marrow, *Amer. J. Roentgenol.* **99**:183.

LEVITT, M., NIXON, P. F., PINCUS, J. H., AND BERTINO, J. R., 1971, Transport characteristics of folates in cerebrospinal fluid; a study utilizing doubly labeled 5-methyltetrahydrofolate and 5-formyltetrahydrofolate, *J. Clin. Invest.* **50**:1301.

LI, M. C., AND ROSS, S. T., 1976, Chemoprophylaxis for patients with colorectal cancer, *J. Amer. Med. Assoc.* **235**:2825.

MAKINODAN, T., PERKINS, E. H., AND CHEN, M. G., 1971, Immunologic activity of the aged, *Adv. Gerontol. Res.* **3**:171.

McGUIRE, E. J., LYTTON, B., AND MITCHELL, M. S., 1973, Treatment of metastatic transitional cell carcinoma with adriamycin: A case report, *J. Urol.* **110**:384.

MEADOWS, A. T., AND EVANS, A. E., 1976, Effects of chemotherapy on the central nervous system, *Cancer* **37**:1079.

MILLARD, R. E., 1965, Effect of previous irradiation on the transformation of blood lymphocytes, *J. Clin. Pathol. (London)* **18**:783.

MITCHELL, M. S., 1976, An introduction to tumor immunology and immunotherapy, *Gynecol. Oncol.* **4**:1.

MOERTEL, C. G., REITEMEIER, R. J., AND GAGE, R. P., 1963, A controlled evaluation of antiemetic drugs, *J. Amer. Med. Assoc.* **186**:116.

MOSHER, M. B., TAUB, R. J., AND AVEDON, M., 1974, The private practice of medical oncology: An analysis, *Cancer Chemother. Rep.* **58**(1):759.

NESBIT, M., KRIVIT, W., HEYN, R., AND SHARP, W., 1976, Acute and chronic effects of methotrexate on hepatic, pulmonary, and skeletal systems, *Cancer*, **37**:1048.

NEVINNY, H. B., KRANT, M. J., AND MOORE, E. W., 1965, Metabolic studies of the effects of methotrexate, *Metabolism* **14**:135.

OKEN, D., 1961, What to tell cancer patients, *J. Amer. Med. Assoc.* **175**:1120.

O'REGAN, S., MELHORN, D. K., AND NEWMAN, A. J., 1973, Methotrexate-induced bone pain in childhood leukemia, *Amer. J. Dis. Child.* **126**:489.

O'ROURKE, R. A., AND ECKERT, G. E., 1964, Methotrexate-induced hepatic injury in an adult, *Arch. Intern. Med.* **113**:191.

OTIS, P. T., AND ARMENTROUT, S. A., 1975, Combination chemotherapy in metastatic carcinoma of the breast, *Cancer* **36**:311.

PENN, I., 1976, Second malignant neoplasms associated with immunosuppressive medications, *Cancer* **37**:1024.

PENN, I., HALGREMSON, G. C., AND STARZL, T. E., 1971, *De novo* malignant tumors in organ transplant recipients, *Transplant. Proc.* **3**:773.

PODOLL, L. N., AND WINKLER, S. S., 1974, Busulfan lung, *Amer. J. Roentgenol. Radium Ther. Nucl. Med.* **120**:151.

POWLES, R. L., 1976, Immunotherapy in the management of acute leukemia, *Br. J. Haematol.* **32**:145.

PRICE, R. A., AND JAMIESON, P. A., 1975. The central nervous system in childhood leukemia: II. Subacute leukoencephalopathy, *Cancer* **35**:306.

PROSNITZ, L. R., FARBER, L. R., FISCHER, J. J., BERTINO, J. R., AND FISCHER, D. B., 1976, Long-term remissions with combined modality therapy for advanced Hodgkin's disease, *Cancer* **37**:2826.

RAGAB, A. H., FRECH, R. S., AND VIETTI, T. J., 1970, Osteoporotic fractures secondary to methotrexate therapy of acute leukemia in remission, *Cancer* **25**:580.

RATH, H., AND ENQUIST, I. F., 1959, The effect of thioTEPA on wound healing, *Arch. Surg.* **79**:812.

RIDDLE, P. R., AND BERENBAUM, M. C., 1967, Postoperative depression of the lymphocyte response to phytohemagglutinin, *Lancet* **1**:746.

ROBINSON, D., 1976, Does your doctor know how to treat cancer? in: *Parade Magazine*, March 28, 1976, New York, p. 8.

RUBIN, P., 1974, The radiographic expression of radiotherapeutic injury: An overview, *Semin. Roentgenol.* **9**:5.

SAMUELS, M. L., JOHNSON, D. E., HOLOYE, P. Y., AND LANZOTTI, V. J., 1976, Large-dose bleomycin therapy and pulmonary toxicity: A possible role of prior radiotherapy, *J. Amer. Med. Assoc.* **235**:1117.

SANDLER, S. G., TOBIN, W., AND HENDERSON, E. S., 1969, Vincristine-induced neuropathy. Clinical study of fifty leukemic patients, *Neurology* **19**:367.

SARTORELLI, A. C., AND JOHNS, D. G. (eds.), 1974, *Antineoplastic and Immunosuppressive Agents*, Springer-Verlag, Berlin–Heidelberg–New York.

SCHEIN, P. S., MACDONALD, J. S., WATERS, C., AND HAIDAK, D., 1975, Nutritional complications of cancer and its treatment, *Semin. Oncol.* **2**:335.

SEGRE, D., AND SEGRE, S., 1976, Humoral immunity in aged mice. II. Increased suppressor T-cell activity in immunologically deficient old mice, *J. Immunol.* **116**:735.

SHERINS, R. J., AND DEVITA, V. T., JR., 1973, Effect of drug treatment for lymphoma on male reproductive capacity: Studies of men in remission after therapy, *Ann. Intern. Med.* **79**:216.

SLAWIKOWSKI, G. J. M., 1960, Tumor development in adrenalectomized rats given inoculations of aged tumor cells after surgical stress, *Cancer Res.* **20**:316.

STEINBERG, A. D. (moderator), 1972, Cytotoxic drugs in treatment of non-malignant diseases, *Ann. Intern. Med.* **76**:619.

STJERNSWARD, J., JONDAL, M., VANKY, F., WIGZELL, H., AND SEALY, R., 1972, Lymphopenia and change in distribution of human B and T lymphocytes in peripheral blood induced by irradiation for mammary carcinoma, *Lancet* **1**:1352.

STRATTON, J. A., BYFIELD, P. E., BYFIELD, J. E., SMALL, R. C., BENFIELD, J., AND PILCH, Y., 1975, A comparison of the acute effects of radiation therapy including or excluding the thymus on the lymphocyte subpopulations of cancer patients, *J. Clin. Invest.* **56**:88.

SYKES, M. P., SAVEL, H., CHU, F. C. H., BONADONNA, G., FARROW, J., AND MATHIS, H., 1964*a*, Long-term effects of therapeutic irradiation upon bone marrow, *Cancer* **17**:1144.

SYKES, M. P., CHU, F. C. H., SAVEL, H., BONADONNA, G., AND MATHIS, H., 1964*b*, The effects of varying dosages of irradiation upon sternal marrow regeneration, *Radiology* **83**:1084.

THIEDE, T., AND CHRISTENSEN, B. C., 1969, Bladder tumors induced by chlornaphazine, *Acta Med. Scand.* **185**:133.

THOMAS, J. W., COY, P., LEWIS, H. S., AND YUEN, A., 1970, Effect of therapeutic irradiation on lymphocyte transformation in lung cancer, *Cancer* **27**:1046.

WALDORF, D. S., WILLKENS, R. F., AND DECKER, J. L., 1968, Impaired delayed hypersensitivity in an aging population, *J. Amer. Med. Assoc.* **203**:831.

WALL, R. L., AND CLAUSEN, K. P., 1975, Carcinoma of the urinary bladder in patients receiving cyclophosphamide, *N. Engl. J. Med.* **293**:271.

WARNE, G. L., FAIREY, K. F., HOBBS, J. B., AND MARTIN, F. I. R., 1973, Cyclophosphamide-induced ovarian failure, *N. Engl. J. Med.* **289**:1159.

WATERHOUSE, C., 1963, Nutritional disorders in neoplastic disease, *J. Chron. Dis.* **16**:637.

WHITE, L. P. (ed.), 1969, Care of patients with fatal illness, *Ann. N. Y. Acad. Sci.* **164**:635.

WORTH, P. H., 1971, Cyclophosphamide and the bladder, *Br. Med. J.* **3**:182.

ZARDAY, Z., VEITH, J. F., GLIEDMAN, M. L., AND SOBERMAN, R., 1972, Irreversible liver damage after azathioprine, *J. Amer. Med. Assoc.* **222**:690.

2

Applications of Cell Kinetic Techniques to Human Malignancies

GERALD L. SCHERTZ AND JOHN C. MARSH

1. Introduction*

It is the purpose of this chapter to summarize methods that are currently and potentially available to measure the kinetics of cancer cells and to review data that are available for specific human neoplasms. The chapter includes information that influences the planning of treatment as well as information that reflects the response to therapy. A variety of techniques, both *in vitro* and *in vivo*, that have been developed in animal tumor systems are now being applied to human neoplasms. Lightdale and Lipkin (1975) reviewed some of these methods in Volume 3 of this series. Although much information on the kinetics of animal tumor systems is available, the extrapolation of such data is often speculative and

---

* Abbreviations of Terms Used. Phases of cell cycle: C is the cell cycle; T_c is the cell cycle time (or intermitotic time); G_1 is the pre-DNA synthesis phase; T_{G_1} is the time spent in pre-DNA synthesis phase; S is the DNA synthesis phase; T_s is the DNA synthesis time; G_2 is the post-DNA synthesis phase; T_{G_2} is the time spent in post-DNA synthesis phase; M is the mitosis; T_M is the mitotic time; and G_0 is the phase of proliferative rest. Other terms used are as follows: MI is the mitotic index; LI is the labeling index; GF is the growth fraction, ϕ is the cell loss factor; [^{3}H]TdR is tritium-labeled thymidine; [^{14}C]TdR is carbon-14-labeled thymidine; PLM is the percentage labeled mitosis (curve); DT is the observed tumor doubling time; DT_p is the potential tumor doubling time; N_s is the number of cells in S phase; P is the proliferating cell compartment; and Q is the quiescent cell compartment.

GERALD L. SCHERTZ AND JOHN C. MARSH ● Department of Internal Medicine, Yale University School of Medicine, New Haven, Connecticut.

misleading. Accordingly, we will restrict our discussion to specific information derived from human tumors or methods that are potentially available.

2. Currently Available Kinetic Techniques

2.1. Measurements of Tumor Size

Tumors that are visible or palpable on the body surface may be measured directly, although such measurement is usually possible only in two dimensions, rather than three. It is more common to measure lesions that are apparent on a chest film. An estimate of the volume of a spherical lesion is $V = \frac{4}{3}\pi r^3 = 4.2\,(d/2)^3$, where V is the volume, r is the radius, and d is the diameter. A 50% increase in the product of two diameters of a lesion is equal to an 84% increase in the volume.

If two measurements are made of the same lesion at separate times, the doubling time $DT = \log\frac{2}{3}\log(d_t/d_0)$, where d_0 is the original diameter, d_t is the second measurement, and t is the interval between measurements.

Doubling times for a wide variety of human tumors range from 66 hr to 745 days when measured in this way. They are distributed over a log normal distribution. Metastases from testicular tumors and lymphomas have shorter DTs than squamous cell carcinomas and adenocarcinomas on the average, but there is a wide overlap (Charbit *et al.*, 1971). Small-cell lung carcinomas have shorter DTs than large-cell undifferentiated ones, which in turn have shorter DTs than epidermoid and adenocarcinomas (M. J. Straus, 1974). Where directly compared, metastatic tumors usually have shorter DTs than their primary tumor of origin.

The DT is not constant for most tumors, but tends to increase with tumor size.

The DT has been correlated with duration of symptoms prior to diagnosis, and also with survival (Breur, 1966a). Tumors with short DTs also tend to be more sensitive to irradiation (Breur, 1966b). Of the various bronchogenic carcinomas, the small-cell undifferentiated variety, with the shortest DT (and highest labeling index [LI]) is clinically the most aggressive, most likely to be metastatic at the time of diagnosis, and most likely to respond to chemotherapy.

Lesions with either very short (<7 days) or very long (>500 days) DTs are benign, usually inflammations or benign tumors (M. J. Straus, 1974).

Similar DT measurements are potentially available on radionuclide scans, and have been reported for colonic tumors using serial barium enemas (Welin *et al.*, 1963).

2.2. Measurements of Tumor Size from Biological Markers

The growth or regression of a tumor may in some instances be measured by the changes in the amount of a biological marker associated with it. Some of these are not specific for a particular tumor, and thus their presence or absence may not be helpful diagnostically, but changes in the concentration or excretion of a marker may be very useful in following the course of the disease and response to therapy. Radioimmunoassay techniques have increased the sensitivity of some determinations of such markers by several orders of magnitude.

2.2.1. Human Chorionic Gonadotropin

Human chorionic gonadotropin (HCG) is secreted in large amounts by choriocarcinomas of the uterus in women, and by certain testicular tumors (generally those with choriocarcinoma elements) in men. Since the former are eminently curable with chemotherapy, the secretion of HCG is an important measurement of tumor response: it may fall to normal levels with therapy and remain there in patients who are cured. The response is less dramatic in patients who have an incomplete response, even though no tumor may be detectable by other means. A rise in the titer of the hormone may signal early relapse before detectable disease is evident. It is estimated that the hormone determination can detect 10^6–10^7 cells, while the smallest mass of tumor likely to be detected by radiologic or other means is 10^9 cells (Freedman, 1976). There may be a transient rise in HCG following successful lysis of tumor cells by therapy. While testicular tumors are less curable than uterine choriocarcinomas, HCG determinations are also of value in following the response to chemotherapy in the male tumors.

2.2.2. Carcinoembryonic Antigen

The glycoprotein carcinoembryonic antigen (CEA) is found in relatively large amounts on the surface of fetal foregut, liver, and pancreas, and in various endodermal cancers, particularly those of the GI tract. The serum concentration may be increased in cancers of the colon, stomach, pancreas, liver, lung, breast, bladder, prostate, endometrium, and ovary, as well as in neuroblastoma and osteosarcoma. Elevation is also found in the serum of some patients with ulcerative colitis, colorectal polyps, regional enteritis, emphysema, and alcoholic liver disease, and in chronic smokers and in pregnancy. The degree of elevation in tumors tends to be proportional to the extent of disease, and its value lies not so much in diagnosis as in monitoring the success of and relapse from treatment. Elevations in patients with colon carcinoma may fall to normal following successful resection and remain within the normal range in patients whose tumors are controlled, while the CEA may either not fall to normal or return rapidly to elevated values after an initial fall when the resection is less complete. Elevation may precede overt disease by several months, and provides an important indication for further therapy (Laurence and Neville, 1976).

2.2.3. α-1-Fetoprotein

The glycoprotein α-1-fetoprotein (AFP), like CEA, is a normal fetal protein, produced in the liver. As the sensitivity of assays has improved, it has become evident that about 80–95% of patients with hepatoma have elevated AFP serum concentrations. It is also found in increased amounts in the serum of most patients with testicular malignancies, and in significant but fewer patients with cancers of the colon, stomach, pancreas, and lung (Freedman, 1976). About one-third of patients with acute viral hepatitis may also have elevated values. Interestingly, most patients with GI cancers produce CEA or AFP, but not both. Serial changes in the concentration of this protein can also indicate the response to therapy.

2.2.4. Acid Phosphatase

Determination of the serum level of acid phosphatase can be helpful both in the diagnosis and following the response to treatment of advanced prostatic carcinoma. It is not elevated, however, in most patients with localized disease or in patients with very undifferentiated tumors. Although a fall in enzyme level may not occur in resistant patients, the level may sometimes fall following hormonal therapy or orchiectomy without a concomitant reduction in tumor mass (Laurence and Neville, 1976). Little correlation may be seen between serum acid phosphatase changes and tumor response to chemotherapy (Merrin *et al.*, 1976). Thus, the relationship of disease activity and enzyme levels is tenuous.

2.2.5. Regan Isoenzyme

This is an isoenzyme of alkaline phosphatase of placental origin. About 12% of patients with various types of cancer, generally in advanced stages, have this enzyme in their serum (Nathanson and Fishman, 1971). Less experience is currently available with it than with HCG, CEA, or AFP, and it is not known how useful it will be in following the response to therapy.

2.2.6. Hormones

Various hormones may be produced by human tumors and serve as biological markers of their activity. They include insulin, gastrin, parathormone, calcitonin, prolactin, ACTH, growth hormone, and gonadotropin. Although they are often associated with tumors of organs that normally secrete them, ectopic hormone production is also common, particularly in lung cancer (Laurence and Neville, 1976). Serial determinations of hormone production are potentially useful in following body tumor burden, but sufficient data in large numbers of patients are lacking.

2.3. Mitotic Index

The microscopic observation of an increased number of mitotic cells within some human tumor specimens was recognized early in the evolution of surgical pathology as one of many manifestations of malignancy. The frequency of mitoses appeared for some tumors to correlate roughly with the rate of tumor growth, a high proportion of mitoses being associated with a poor prognosis. Investigators of cell kinetics have attempted to quantitate mitotic activity, defining the mitotic index (MI) as the number of mitoses per 100 cells. Analysis demonstrates considerable variation among tumors of the same histological type and grade.

Explanations for this variation include: (1) possible variations in the duration of mitosis among actively proliferating cells; (2) sampling bias resulting from regional variation in growth rate and mitotic rate within tumors; (3) error induced by difficulty in distinguishing malignant cells from their supporting stromal tissues; and (4) the possible arrest of genetically damaged cells in mitosis, the MI thereby reflecting an accumulation of senescent cells, rather than cell proliferation.

Although MI determinations from routine biopsy specimens have found little utility, useful correlations exist for some specific tumors. In transitional-cell carcinoma of the bladder, the frequency of mitoses correlates with the histological grading. Well-differentiated tumors often have a MI less than 0.1, whereas more anaplastic tumors may have a MI 10–20 times higher (Fulker *et al.*, 1971). The quantitation of mitoses has had greater value as a kinetic probe when measured after administration of drugs known to arrest cells in mitosis (stathmokinetic techniques) or after the administration of radioactively labeled DNA precursors (percentage labeled mitosis technique).

2.4. Stathmokinetic Methods

Agents that are capable of causing metaphase arrest *in vivo* (such as colcemid, colchicine, and vincristine) can be used to quantitate the rate of cell entry into mitosis. Serial biopsies are obtained after exposure to the blocking agent. Mitotic time (T_M) and the rate of cell entry into metaphase can be calculated from a plot of MI (metaphase) against time (Lala, 1971). A knowledge of the initial MI and T_M permits calculation of cell birth rate and potential tumor doubling time, DT_p, by the following relationships:

$$\text{cell birth rate} = \text{MI}/T_M \tag{1}$$

$$\text{potential tumor doubling time} = \log_e 2 \, \frac{T_M}{\text{MI}} \tag{2}$$

Combinations of tritium-labeled thymidine ([³H]TdR) labeling with mitotic arrest can be applied to estimate other cell-cycle components (Lala, 1971). Several practical difficulties in the use of mitotic arresting agents, such as their ability to kill cells, make interpretation of data difficult (Tannock, 1965). Nonetheless, stathmokinetic techniques have been successfully applied in both rapidly proliferating (Iverson *et al.*, 1974) and slowly proliferating (Camplejohn *et al.*, 1973) human tumors, and conclusions correspond reasonably well with data obtained by [³H]TdR labeling techniques.

2.5. Labeling Index

The LI attempts to quantitate the percentage of cells in DNA synthesis at a given time. The percentage of total cells containing label is determined by autoradiography after a brief exposure to [³H]TdR either *in vivo* or *in vitro*. Three general methods have been applied to determine the LI in human tumors: (1) systemic venous or regional arterial infusion of [³H]TdR and subsequent preparation of autoradiographs from biopsied material; (2) local injection of [³H]TdR into a tumor mass, followed by needle aspiration or biopsy (Young and DeVita, 1970; Muggia *et al.*, 1974); (3) *in vitro* [³H]TdR incorporation by fresh tissue removed from the host. Recent refinements of *in vitro* techniques include use of high-specific-activity label, allowing brief incubation, single-cell suspensions from solid tumors, and Ficoll-Hypaque gradients to remove debris and nonviable cells (Livingston *et al.*, 1974; Braunschweiger *et al.*, 1976). Autoradiographs can be adequately exposed and interpreted within 24 hr of biopsy, potentially allowing therapeutic decisions based on cell kinetic data (Durie and Salmon, 1976; Schiffer *et al.*, 1976a).

The LI has recently been widely applied in the study of human malignancies as a rough index of proliferative activity. It is important to recognize that the LI is not simply a direct measurement of proliferation, but is related as well to the ratio of DNA synthesis time to cell cycle time (or intermitotic time) (T_s/T_c). Theoretically, cycling cells with a long DNA synthesis phase may have a higher LI than cells with a short DNA synthesis phase, although their rates of proliferation may be equivalent. The LI has the obvious advantage of requiring a single tissue sample. Serial LIs have been applied to human tumors to predict prognosis and response to chemotherapy (Livingston *et al.*, 1974; Greenberg and Holland, 1976; Hayes *et al.*, 1976; Thirlwell and Mansell, 1976; Sulkes *et al.*, 1976), and to detect recruitment and partial synchronization of cells (Barranco *et al.*, 1973; Klein and Lennartz, 1974; Costanzi, 1976). *In vitro* LI measurements, although generally preferable clinically to *in vivo* studies, assume that cells in the S phase continue DNA synthesis at the same rate *in vitro* as *in vivo*, and that the conditions of processing and incubation do not perturb the progression of cells through the S phase. Although rapid *in vitro* techniques often correspond well with published *in vivo* human data, simultaneous *in vitro–in vivo* studies of human tumors are not generally available. For some human solid tumors, the LI is higher at the tumor periphery than in the center of the tumor mass, emphasizing the importance of careful sampling in comparing patient groups (Shirakawa *et al.*, 1970). The LI is partially dependent on the technique of measurement, and data accrued by differing techniques cannot easily be compared.

The LI has now been measured in several hundred human neoplasms, leading to the following conclusions:

1. The LI is usually high in tumors with rapid rates of growth.
2. LIs vary considerably, even among tumors of the same type.
3. When considering all kinds of malignancy, those types with a higher mean LI tend to have a greater response rate to chemotherapy.
4. Within a particular tumor category, patient groups that respond to chemotherapy tend to have higher pretreatment LIs than nonresponders.

2.6. Percentage Labeled Mitosis

The technique of percentage labeled mitosis (PLM) is the definitive procedure for measuring the durations of phases of the cell cycle. Cells undergoing DNA synthesis *in vivo* are "flash"-labeled with [³H]TdR, and their progression through the mitotic phase is observed by the appearance of labeled mitotic figures on autoradiography. In essence, mitosis is used as a window to see a cohort of cells traverse the cell cycle. The durations of all phases of the cell cycle can be determined, at least theoretically, by the PLM technique (Fig. 1, top).

Unfortunately, the technique is impractical for most human tumor studies. It requires administration of [³H]TdR *in vivo* and cannot be done *in vitro*. A large number of serial tissue samples is required to define the curve. The technique is time-consuming due to the detailed microscopy required and to the low degree of labeling, which necessitates prolonged incubation of autoradiographs. Computer analysis is usually required to interpret results; such analysis usually assumes a log normal distribution of cells in pre-DNA-synthesis (G_1), S, and post-DNA-synthesis (G_2) phases (Barrett, 1966). Automated computer analysis produces a curve with a best fit to the data, and simultaneously generates mean values and standard errors of G_1, S, and G_2, and computes a mean T_c and a frequency distribution of intermitotic times (Steel and Hanes, 1971). Although these computer models are

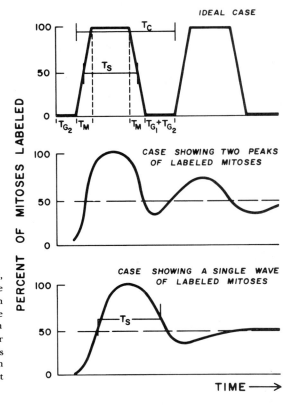

FIGURE 1. An idealized PLM curve (top), from which cell cycle parameters can be estimated. Significant damping is shown in the two bottom curves, which are more representative of data obtained from human tumors. (T_c) cell cycle time (or intermitotic time); (T_s) DNA synthesis time; (T_M) mitotic time; (T_{G_1}) time spent in pre-DNA synthesis phase; (T_{G_2}) time spent in post-DNA synthesis phase.

powerful tools, they make certain assumptions that may be erroneous for the tumor cell populations under study.

Most published human PLM curves have demonstrated marked "damping" of the curve with time (Fig. 1, middle). Data may define the first peak of labeled mitoses well, but information localizing the second peak may be less precise. The second peak is often absent, allowing definition of T_s but not of other phases or T_c (Fig. 1, bottom). This damping implies a very broad distribution of intermitotic times (Steel, 1972). In such cases, use of the terms *cell cycle* and *cell cycle time* may be inappropriate because they imply greater uniformity of cell behavior than the data warrant. The broad distribution of intermitotic times may be caused by reversibly damaged or dying cells, cell differentiation within the tumor, or selective cell loss from the tumor. Some cells capable of proliferating may temporarily reside out of cycle [in the phase of proliferative rest (G_0)] or have a prolonged residence in a specific phase, either mechanism contributing to the "damping."

Several investigators have obtained credible data in human malignancies by the technique of PLM. PLM data have been interpreted, however, in only a small and unrepresentative sampling of human tumors. Several studies in human tumors are technically inadequate for complete analysis (Steel, 1972). In an analysis of 30 studies in a variety of human solid tumors, intermitotic times varied widely, with a modal value of 48 hr, 90% between 15 and 120 hr. The duration of S was much more constant, with a modal value of 16 hr (Tubiana and Malaise, 1975). Although there are, understandably, few comparisons of PLM data before and after treatment of human tumors, a recent study demonstrated a faster rate of growth and a shortening of the intermitotic time by the PLM method in recurrent epidermoid carcinoma after therapy (Bresciani *et al.*, 1974).

Technical advances may make PLM studies more feasible in the future. The pharmacology, toxicology, and radiation dosimetry effects of [³H]TdR are now better understood, making the risk of drug administration ethically acceptable for tumor patients beyond the reproductive age (S. E. Straus and M. J. Straus, 1976). Localized intraarterial administration of high-specific-activity [³H]TdR into tumor feeder vessels can increase the intensity of labeling, allowing shorter incubation times. An automated television attachment to the microscope can now quantitate grain counts over cells automatically with acceptable accuracy.

2.7. Grain-Count-Halving

An alternative method of computing the intermitotic time (T_c) is the method of grain-count-halving. This technique may be useful in the absence of an adequate number of mitoses to compute PLM curves, since by this technique all labeled cells are counted at each time point. The T_c is assumed to be equal to the time required for halving of the highest mean grain count of labeled cells, since the number of grains over an individual cell is halved at mitosis. In cases in which simultaneous PLM data are available as well, the T_c calculated by both techniques shows comparable values (Clarkson *et al.*, 1965*a*). Although in theory this technique appears sound, there are several limitations to its application (Lala, 1971). Weakly labeled cells may cause false-negative assessment. Experiments of long duration may lead to reutilization of label in cells other than those initially labeled. Finally, the most significant limiting factor is the possible continuous transition of cells from a proliferative to a quiescent state.

2.8. Double-Labeling Techniques

Double-labeling of a cell population sequentially with [³H]TdR and carbon-14-labeled thymidine ([¹⁴C]TdR) can be used to measure the flux of cells into the DNA synthesis phase, and therefore to calculate T_s:

$$T_s = \frac{T_a(\% \,^{14}\text{C-labeled cells})}{\% \,^{3}\text{H-labeled cells}}$$

where T_a is the time between pulse labels. This technique relies on the different energy ranges of β emissions of ^{14}C and ^{3}H, ^{14}C producing grain tracks on autoradiographs in a plane well above those produced by ^{3}H. Scanning in different fields of focus allows independent enumeration of ^{14}C-labeled cells and cells labeled with ^{3}H alone. In animal experiments, this has generally been a combined *in vivo–in vitro* technique, the labeling being done with [³H]TdR *in vivo* and at short intervals later with [¹⁴C]TdR *in vitro* (Lala, 1971). Recently, the technique has been adapted to human tumor tissues entirely *in vitro*, cell suspensions being labeled initially with [³H]TdR, then with [¹⁴C]TdR (Schiffer and Braunschweiger, 1976). As with all *in vitro* labeling studies, it assumes well-preserved cell viability *in vitro* and no major alterations in cell cycle progression during the brief *in vitro* incubations. Ficoll-Hypaque gradient techniques may allow separation of viable cells from debris and dead cells (Braunschweiger *et al.*, 1976). The slow production of grains by ^{14}C and prolonged incubation times required for ^{14}C autoradiographs previously hampered their application. A system of gold activation of the photographic emulsion prior to development now allows assessment of double-labeling in 7 days (Braunschweiger *et al.*, 1976).

2.9. Growth Fraction

Any measurement of growth fraction (GF) assumes two compartments of a cell population: a dividing or proliferating (P) compartment, and a nonproliferating or quiescent (Q) compartment. Cells with very long intermitotic times are likely to be classified as nonproliferating. Clear separation of the two compartments is simplified if proliferating cells have a fairly uniform cell cycle. Despite obvious limitations of such a two-compartment model, the GF concept has been valuable, and is perhaps the single best parameter of the state of proliferation of a human tumor cell population (Malaise *et al.*, 1973).

Methods of estimating GF are not simple. In the past, most accepted methods have required *in vivo* [³H]TdR labeling. These methods include:

a. Repeated-Labeling Technique. A continuous or repeated pulse-labeling procedure with [³H]TdR to measure all cells passing through S in a time equal to the maximum duration of G_2 + mitosis $(M) + G_1$ should label all cycling cells. Such a GF is often measured as the LI at the end of a prolonged labeling period known to be longer than the average duration of the cell cycle from previous PLM data.

b. Labeled-Mitosis Technique. As waves of mitoses damp out because of variations in intermitotic times, the percentage of labeled mitoses reaches an equilibrium value that is equal to the ratio of cells in S (N_s) to cells in cycle (P), since mitosis is an attribute of the cycling population only (Lala, 1971). On the other hand, a simultaneous LI gives the ratio of cells in S (N_s) to all cells ($P + Q$). One can therefore compute GF by the following relationship:

$$\text{GF} = \frac{P}{P+Q} = \frac{(N_s)}{(P+Q)}\frac{(P)}{(N_s)} = \frac{\text{LI at equilibrium}}{\text{PLM at equilibrium}}$$

A simple correction can be made to compensate for growth of the population during the interval of observation (Lala, 1971).

c. Computation from Knowledge of Cell Cycle Stages. The ratio P/N_s can be computed in a cell population if measurements of T_c and T_s are available, for example, from the PLM technique or the double-labeling technique (Lala, 1971). For a steady-state population, the ratio of P/N_s is given directly by T_c/T_s. For a growing population, the age distribution of cells along the cycle must be known to calculate the fraction of cells in S. Since the age distribution of cells in the cycle is seldom available for human malignancies, this technique has not found application for studies in man.

d. PDP Assay. A fourth technique that can be applied *in vitro* estimates the GF by measuring the fraction of cells expressing nuclear-DNA-dependent DNA polymerase and nuclear priming-template activity (Nelson and Schiffer, 1973). Briefly, the method converts a standard biochemical assay for DNA polymerase to a slide assay utilizing unfixed cell smears or impressions. This is a slide autoradiographic procedure *in vitro* that correlates closely with simultaneous *in vivo* measurements in animals by alternate techniques mentioned above (Schiffer *et al.*, 1976*b*). The method is currently being applied to human tumor biopsy specimens (Schiffer and Braunschweiger, 1976).

2.10. Potential Doubling Time and Cell Loss Factor

Previously described kinetic measurements have focused on parameters of tumor cell growth, such as DT, MI, LI, GF, and phases of the cell cycle. In malignancies, particularly human malignancies, cell loss is a major factor accounting for the discrepancy between potential growth rate and observed growth rate. Basic methods compare a computed rate of production of new cells in the absence of cell loss (potential doubling time [DT_p] or birth rate) with observed tumor growth rate (observed doubling time [DT]) (Lala and Patt, 1966; Steel, 1967, 1968). The cell loss factor (ϕ) is defined by the ratio of cell loss to birth rate, and can be calculated by the following relationships:

$$\phi = \frac{\text{rate of cell loss}}{\text{rate of cell birth}} = 1 - \frac{DT_p}{DT}$$

$$DT_p = \log_e 2 \frac{T_M}{MI} = \lambda \frac{T_s}{LI}$$

in which λ represents a correction for the larger fraction of cells in earlier phases of the cell cycle in a growing cell population, and can be simply approximated by the value 0.75 in computations utilizing LI and T_s, such as data from double-labeling experiments (Steel, 1967). Measurements of cell loss for solid tumors generally require both volumetric DT and growth kinetic data obtained by stathmokinetic methods (MI and T_M) or labeling methods (LI and T_s). The DT for solid tumors is often approximated from the mean of values for volume DTs of similar tumors reported in the literature, rather than the volume DT of the individual tumor in question, which is frequently not available. Thus, the values of ϕ are only approximations or rough estimates, and must not be interpreted too rigidly.

In published data on human tumors, the rate of cell loss is generally greater than 50% ($\phi > 0.5$), often greater than 90%. Cell loss appears to be a factor of great importance in both rapidly proliferating and slowly proliferating tumor cell populations (Table 1). Measurement of cell loss neatly completes the balance sheet of tumor cell growth, but sheds little light on the mode of cell loss. Potential mechanisms such as overt necrosis, phagocytosis by macrophages, exfoliation, and spread to metastatic sites cannot be distinguished. The cell loss factor does not disclose where cell loss occurs in relation to the cell cycle. Cell loss may selectively occur from the nonproliferating or the proliferating cell compartment, or during a specific phase of the cell cycle. A combination of kinetic techniques can logically approach such problems (Lala, 1971), but detailed kinetic analysis of cell loss has not been pursued in depth for most human tumors.

TABLE 1

Tumor type	Volume DT	LI	GF	ϕ	Reference
Burkitt's lymphoma	66 hr	17%	0.90–1.0	0.69	Iverson *et al.* (1974)
Colonic adenocarcinoma	> 100 days	6%	0.35	> 0.8	Schiffer *et al.* (1976a)

2.11. DNA Distribution Techniques

GERALD L.
SCHERTZ
AND
JOHN C.
MARSH

Microspectrophotometric estimates of DNA in the nuclei of individual cells allow segregation of cells by DNA content (Kraemer *et al.*, 1973). Four compartments can be distinguished:

1. Cells with postmitotic DNA content ($2n$). This population is interpreted to represent either cells in G_1 or postmitotic, nonproliferating cells (G_0).
2. S-phase cells (greater than $2n$ and less than $4n$). These are assumed to be cells in DNA synthesis, although possibly cells arrested in the phase of DNA synthesis will be measured.
3. Cells with premitotic DNA content ($4n$). This population encompasses proliferating cells in G_2, cells arrested in G_2, and mitotic cells before separation.
4. Cells with greater than $4n$ DNA content. These are hyperdiploid cells.

Flow microfluorimetry (FMF) techniques permitting rapid automated analysis of approximately 10^5 monodispersed cells have widened the application of such techniques, particularly when combined with simultaneous cell size measurement and cellular protein content. DNA distribution curves, although rapid and easy to measure, are complicated by the presence of aneuploidy or polyploidy, and are difficult to apply to human solid tumors. A single DNA distribution curve can detect ploidy states, and roughly estimate the state of proliferation by measuring the relative size of the second compartment representing cells in DNA synthesis (Fig. 2). Serial samples can potentially measure the progresion of a perturbed cell

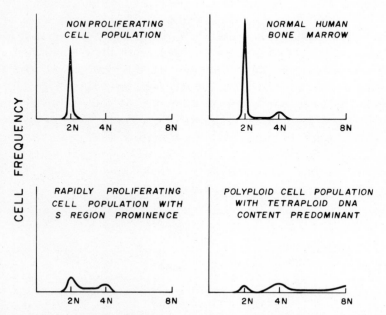

FIGURE 2. Idealized DNA distribution curves obtained by flow microfluorimetry for different populations.

population through the S phase, measure the duration of the S phase, and detect synchronization and recruitment phenomena. Simultaneous DNA distribution analysis of both tumor and vulnerable host tissues such as bone marrow may provide rationales for optimal scheduling of chemotherapy (Krishnan *et al.*, 1976).

2.12. Xenografts

There is currently considerable interest in the properties of human tumors transplanted into immune-deficient rodents. Several laboratories have achieved growth of xenografts with histology and growth rates stable on serial passage. Information on the response of xenograft tumors to treatment is now appearing (Smith, 1969; Berenbaum *et al.*, 1974; Cobb and Mitchley, 1974; Kopper and Steel, 1975). Interpretation of such data will depend on measurement of growth rate and cell population kinetics of such xenografts and comparisons with kinetic measurements from the original patients. Preliminary data suggest that xenograft tumors accelerate their growth, particularly by shortening the phase of DNA synthesis, in comparison with the original tumor, and may acquire some of the kinetic characteristics of the rodent host (Pickard *et al.*, 1975). This technique is potentially a guide to therapy for a specific patient whose tumor is grown in the xenograft systems (Kopper and Steel, 1975).

3. Kinetics of Specific Tumors

3.1. Acute Leukemia

More kinetic data are available for acute leukemia than for any other disease, reflecting the ease of repeated sampling and the diffuse nature of the disease, with similar LIs obtained at several bone marrow sites sampled simultaneously (Mauer and Fisher, 1966). Excellent reviews are available (Killman, 1968; Mauer, 1975).

3.1.1. Basic Kinetic Data

An early concept of the disease being one of rapid proliferation was shaken when low mitotic and stathmokinetic indices were described (Astaldi and Mauri, 1953), and discarded with many reports of low LI after *in vivo* or *in vitro* [^{3}H]TdR (Gavosto *et al.*, 1960; Mauer and Fisher, 1962; Clarkson *et al.*, 1965b; Saunders *et al.*, 1967; Killman, 1968). The *in vitro* method gives results similar to those obtained *in vivo*, at least when the time interval is 1 hr in children with acute lymphoblastic leukemia (ALL) (Saunders *et al.*, 1967). The LI of blasts in the bone marrow is nearly always greater than that of blasts in the blood in the same patient (Mauer and Fisher, 1962; Clarkson *et al.*, 1965b; Faadi *et al.*, 1967). Large cells have higher LI values than small ones, both in ALL (Mauer *et al.*, 1969) and in acute myeloblastic leukemia (AML) (Greenberg *et al.*, 1972), and it has been suggested that small cells represent the noncycling (G_0) cells, which are relatively resistant to chemotherapy. Certainly there is marked variation in LI values, cell cycle parameters derived from PLM curves, and estimated GF among different patients with the same disease and in the same patient at different times. Higher LI values have been reported in patients in early relapse (Saunders *et al.*, 1967; Faadi *et al.*, 1967), as compared with initial diagnosis.

Most PLM curves have been very rapidly damped, thus confirming the heterogeneity of cell cycle times. The derived cell cycle parameters (T_c, T_s) are longer than those for normal bone marrow cells (Clarkson *et al.*, 1967; Killmann *et al.*, 1963; Saunders *et al.*, 1967), although the values for large leukemic myeloblasts approach those for normal myeloblasts (Greenberg *et al.*, 1972). Pulse cytofluorimetry has indicated a smaller fraction of AML cells in the S, G_2, and M phases, as compared with normal marrow cells (Hillen *et al.*, 1975). Cell cycle measurements have also been made in one patient by Momparler (1974, 1976), by following the rate of fall of blood blasts following multiple doses of cytosine arabinoside. Although a majority of AML blasts are unlabeled with a brief exposure to [^{3}H]TdR, with continuous infusion, it is possible to label 88–93% after 8–10 days, and 92–99% after 3 weeks (Clarkson, 1969). These residual unlabeled cells must be of considerable importance in determining resistance to therapy and relapse of disease.

3.1.2. Effects of Antileukemic Agents on Cell Kinetics

A variety of agents have been studied, both alone and in combination, to ascertain their effect on the kinetics of leukemic cells and, it is hoped, to use this information to design more appropriate chemotherapeutic regimens (Lampkin *et al.*, 1972; Killmann, 1974).

a. Single Agents

Corticosteroids. These agents cause a fall in the LI in patients with ALL, an effect not observed in AML or normal marrow (Lampkin *et al.*, 1969*b*; Ernst and Killmann, 1970). The MI falls later, or is unchanged. Both proliferating and nonproliferating cells are killed. The effect on proliferating cells appears to be an inhibition of the progression of cells from G_1 into the S phase of the cycle.

L-Asparaginase. This agent also appears to be specific for lymphoblasts, killing both proliferating and nonproliferating cells, the former more rapidly (Saunders, 1972; Killmann, 1974). The data of Saunders (1972) suggests an inhibition of entrance of cells into the S phase, since LI is reduced more rapidly than MI, but other data have been cited to suggest that the main effect is during S, and that the G_1–S transition is not affected (Killmann, 1974).

Daunomycin. This drug can kill myeloblasts directly, but the most sensitive ones are in the S phase (Stryckmans *et al.*, 1973). Blocking in G_1 and G_2 has also been described. In contrast to prednisone and L-asparaginase, the MI falls earlier than the LI, suggesting a block in G_2 (Killmann, 1974).

Cyclophosphamide. This alkylating agent inhibits DNA synthesis, arrests cells in *M*, and inhibits the transition into *S* (Lampkin *et al.*, 1971).

Methotrexate. The LI of bone marrow myeloblasts rises while the MI falls, an effect amplified by repeated doses (Ernst and Killmann, 1971). This can be interpreted as inhibition of the progression of cells through the *S* phase, but not prevention of the entry from G_1 into *S*. The arrest of cells in *S* was related to the duration of *S*. In higher doses, the duration of the block is longer. The release of the block may result in a synchronized population of remaining cells (Lampkin *et al.*, 1971).

Cytosine Arabinoside. This drug is known primarily to inhibit DNA synthesis, although through a different mechanism than that of methotrexate. The immediate effect in both myeloblasts and lymphoblasts is to decrease the LI, MI, and grain count (Lampkin *et al.*, 1969*a, b,* 1976; Ernst *et al.*, 1973). Recovery of LI tends to occur before MI, suggesting synchronization, although the degree to which this develops is variable (Lampkin *et al.*, 1976). The recovery of proliferating cells in AML is more rapid than after methotrexate (Ernst *et al.*, 1973). The entry of cells into *S* from G_1 appears to be unaffected. Overshoots of LI in the recovery phase are less frequent in AML than in ALL. The effects on LI and MI are more profound with continuous infusion than with an intravenous bolus (Killmann, 1974).

An increased generation time in AML after the drug has been reported (Clarkson, 1969), using the grain-count-halving method, thought to be due either to selective killing of proliferating cells or to sublethal injury with slowing of the cell cycle of surviving proliferating cells.

The red cell precursors, but not the myeloid precursors, of normal bone marrow were reported to be synchronized by the drug (Lampkin *et al.*, 1971).

Vincristine. Significant arrest of cells in mitosis occurs with this drug, and their subsequent recovery (and synchronization) or death is dose-related (Mauer, 1975). After administration of the drug to patients with ALL, the MI reaches a maximum at 12–24 hr, while the LI falls at 24–48 hr (Lampkin *et al.*, 1969*b*). Resting cells may well be prevented from reentering the cell cycle (Lampkin *et al.*, 1972). Similar events occur in AML (Killmann, 1974).

b. Combination Therapy

Most therapeutic regimens for acute leukemia now involve multiple drugs. Kinetic data are available in man for several combinations. The use of cytosine arabinoside to synchronize and recruit populations has been studied, with the addition of other drugs or repeated infusions of cytosine arabinoside subsequently.

Cytosine Arabinoside and Vincristine. The addition of vincristine at a time when some recovery of MI occurs after cytosine arabinoside results in a sustained increase in MI, presumably due to synchronization and recruitment by the former drug (Lampkin *et al.*, 1971, 1972). The effect was less in AML than in ALL.

Cytosine Arabinoside and Methotrexate. Here, too, evidence of synchronization and recruitment was seen after cytosine arabinoside, but the clinical results were disappointing in both AML and ALL (Lampkin *et al.*, 1971, 1972). No correlation of kinetic data and response was found in another study utilizing these agents (Murphy *et al.*, 1976).

Cytosine Arabinoside Bolus Plus Infusions. Lampkin *et al.* (1976) reported the use of a priming dose of cytosine arabinoside followed by infusions of the same agent to produce a high number of remissions in AML in children and adults. Not all patients had documented synchronization by serial LI studies.

Cytosine Arabinoside, Methotrexate–Leucovorin, and Vincristine. A group of patients with AML were treated with cytosine arabinoside in several schedules. At 48 hr after the end of the drug, methotrexate with vincristine and leucovorin were given. Response occurred most frequently in those patients who had an increase in LI at 48 hr, evidence of presumed synchronization and recruitment (Vogler *et al.*, 1974; Kremer *et al.*, 1976).

3.1.3. Other Attempts to Synchronize or Recruit Leukemic Cells

Extracorporeal irradiation of the blood in AML has resulted in increased LI values of bone marrow blasts (Chan *et al.*, 1969; Ernst *et al.*, 1971; Chan and Hayhoe, 1971). Leukophoresis with exchange transfusion or a cell separator has had variable effects on the LI (Lampkin *et al.*, 1971; Reich *et al.*, 1971; Hoelzer *et al.*, 1974).

3.1.4. Do Cell Kinetic Studies Predict Response in Acute Leukemia?

Pretreatment studies have been used to attempt a correlation with response. The LI has been used most often, and the data are conflicting. The initial bone marrow LI has been reported to correlate with the achievement of remission in both kinds of adult leukemia (Hart *et al.*, 1973, 1974, 1975) and in AML (Vogler *et al.*, 1974; Zittoun *et al.*, 1975). The correlation was better in patients with adult AML than in those with ALL (Hart *et al.*, 1974). No relationship between initial LI and response was found in AML by Burke and Owens (1971), Crowther *et al.* (1975), Kremer *et al.* (1976), and Arlin *et al.* (1976). A similar lack of correlation was found in studies of both kinds of acute leukemia (Faadi *et al.*, 1967; Cheung *et al.*, 1972; Faille *et al.*, 1973), and in ALL (Saunders *et al.*, 1967). Gavosto and Maresa (1975) reported that a high LI was associated with a shorter survival in ALL, but not in AML. Some of the patients reported by Vogler *et al.* (1974) to show a correlation between LI and response were included in the larger study of Kremer *et al.* (1976), which did not show this relationship.

The combination of high LI for [³H]TdR and [³H]cytosine arabinoside in leukemic myeloblasts was found to correlate with subsequent remission by Burke and Owens (1971), while either label alone did not.

The presence of a large number of cells (more than 15%) in S, G₂, and M, as determined by pulse cytophotometry, was found to be associated with a very high likelihood of remission in patients with AML (Hillen *et al.*, 1975).

The duration of remission has been reported to correlate inversely with LI, both in adult AML and ALL (Hart *et al.*, 1975) and in AML (Crowther *et al.*, 1975).

Serial changes in LI following therapy have also been studied as a measurement of possible recruitment or synchronization. The LI 48 hr after cytosine arabinoside has been reported to be significantly increased in responding AML patients compared with pretreatment values, but not in nonresponders (Kremer *et al.*, 1976). Responding patients with both AML and ALL were reported to have increased LI values of nonerythroid cells in the marrow, compared with nonresponders, 3 weeks after the initiation of therapy (Cheung *et al.*, 1972).

The value of cytokinetic studies in predicting prognosis or dictating the timing of therapy is not yet firmly established. The variability of the data regarding initial LI makes such prediction unreliable, although this may be related in part to the different treatments used. Clearly, more studies using newer techniques, such as flow microfluorimetry, and changes following therapy will be done, and may improve the ability to predict the therapeutic outcome.

3.2. Chronic Myelocytic Leukemia

The LI of chronic myelocytic leukemia (CML) blood leukocytes is high compared with the LI of those in normal blood, since CML blood leukocytes consist of many granulocyte precursors capable of DNA synthesis (Bond *et al.*, 1959). The LI of CML myeloblasts is lower in the blood than in the bone marrow (Ogawa *et al.*, 1970; Baccarani and Killmann, 1972), similar to the situation in acute leukemia, although the absolute values for LI of blood myeloblasts are higher in CML than in AML (Killmann, 1965; Schmid *et al.*, 1967). While the LIs of bone marrow promyelocytes and myelocytes in CML are similar to those of normal precursors, the LI and MI of myeloblasts in this disease, even at the time of diagnosis, are lower (Ogawa *et al.*, 1970; Baccarani and Killmann, 1972). Gavosto *et al.* (1964) reported that the LI falls in CML as the percentage of blasts in the marrow increases. It has been suggested that a subpopulation of abnormal myeloblasts is already established in the marrow at the time of diagnosis. The T_M and T_s derived from stathmokinetic data suggested that T_M was longer and T_s shorter than those of normal cells (Baccarani and Killmann, 1972). An inverse relationship between the LI of marrow blasts and blood total leukocyte count has been reported (Stryckmans *et al.*, 1975).

There are as yet no data that relate kinetic values in this disease or in its acute terminal phase to response to treatment or survival.

GERALD L.
SCHERTZ
AND
JOHN C.
MARSH

3.3. Chronic Lymphocytic Leukemia

Early studies of the blood in chronic lymphocytic leukemia (CLL) revealed an increased total LI of the blood, due to labeling of large mononuclear cells of the kind that are found in smaller numbers in normal blood. Small lymphocytes in both blood and bone marrow are not labeled (Bond *et al.*, 1959). The overall LI of CLL lymph nodes was 0.3–1.5%, but that of the large blast cells was 19–46%, similar to values found in normal lymph nodes (Cooper *et al.*, 1968). The 24-hr uptake of [^{3}H]TdR by CLL blood leukocytes has been reported to correlate with the need for treatment and survival (Lopez-Sandoval *et al.*, 1974).

3.4. Multiple Myeloma

3.4.1. Total-Body Tumor Cell Number

Before discussing the kinetics of myeloma, it is worth describing a technique used to obtain an estimate of total tumor mass. It is possible to estimate the total number of myeloma cells in those cases (the vast majority) that are associated with the production of a specific immunoglobulin, or fraction thereof. This estimate is made by measuring the production rate of the protein *in vivo* using labeled immunoglobulin, or calculating it from the plasma volume, the serum concentration of the protein, and the fractional catabolic rate. The rate of synthesis of this "M" protein *in vitro* is measured by the identification of new protein formed from a known number of myeloma cells in aspirated bone marrow. The total-body number of myeloma cells is then calculated from the ratio of the *in vivo* synthetic rate to the *in vitro* rate expressed per cell (Salmon and Durie, 1975).

3.4.2. Cellular Kinetics

The LI at diagnosis of myeloma, both *in vivo* and *in vitro*, is low, usually ranging from less than 1 to 7% (Killmann *et al.*, 1962; Drewinko *et al.*, 1974; Salmon, 1975). Patients with low tumor mass at diagnosis have tended to have higher values (Drewinko *et al.*, 1974), and in a serial study, a halving of the LI was reported in association with doubling of the tumor cell number (Salmon, 1975). The LI of normal bone marrow plasma cells is usually zero, or at most 2% (Drewinko *et al.*, 1974).

Values for T_c derived from *in vivo* data and serial grain counts were 2–6 days (Killmann *et al.*, 1962), with a DT at the time of diagnosis estimated to be 4–6 months (Salmon and Smith, 1970). Data have been presented to support the concept that myeloma cells follow Gompertzian kinetics, in which the growth rate is steadily decreasing (Sullivan and Salmon, 1972), rather than exponential growth, which has been suggested from serial studies of the serum "M" protein concentration (Hobbs, 1975). According to the Gompertzian concept, back-calculations have suggested an initial doubling time of 1–3 days with a preclinical growth period of about 5 years (Salmon and Durie, 1975).

Effective therapy with non-cell-cycle-specific therapy (alkylating agents) has been accompanied by a reduction in tumor cell number, as well as some very impressive increases in LI (Salmon and Smith, 1972; Drewinko et al., 1974; Alberts and Golde, 1974; Salmon, 1975). In one study, nonresponders showed no increase in LI as a group (Drewinko et al., 1974), but other workers reported variable increases in LI without significant tumor cell reduction, and related it to true prereplicative DNA synthesis, rather than DNA repair (Alberts and Golde, 1974; Salmon, 1975). This increase in LI and presumably the GF has given rise to hopes that cycle-specific agents, such as vincristine, cytosine arabinoside, and hydroxyurea, would find clinical utility following initial therapy with alkylating agents. These agents are just beginning to be used in this way (Salmon, 1975; Lee et al., 1974).

3.5. Lymphomas

The wide spectrum of clinical behavior and morphology of the lymphomas has complicated interpretation of their kinetic behavior. Regardless of interesting postulates, there is little information on LI and durations of phases of the cell cycle. Aneuploidy complicates interpretation of DNA content distribution data. Morphologically, lymphomas with a predominance of large cells, such as Burkitt's lymphoma, histiocytic lymphoma, and lymphocyte-depleted Hodgkin's disease, tend to be the most aggressive. Conversely, the small-cell lymphomas have a more favorable prognosis. Available kinetic data generally confirm that large-cell lymphomas are rapidly proliferating. Burkitt's lymphoma is an extreme example, with GF approaching 100% (Cooper et al., 1966; Iverson et al., 1974). Large-cell lymphomas frequently exhibit high LIs; DNA content distributions show a predominance of cells in the S region (Cooper et al., 1968; Peckham and Cooper, 1970). The volume DTs can be less than 10 days in recticulum-cell sarcoma (Peckham and Steel, 1972). Cell cycle parameters from PLM data in one case after in vivo [^{3}H]TdR were an estimated T_c of 53 hr, T_{G_1} of 32 hr, and T_s of 14 hr, with an estimated GF of less than 50%. In one study, lymphocyte-depleted Hodgkin's disease had the highest LI among the various Hodgkin's disease subtypes (Peckham and Cooper, 1973). Reed-Sternberg cells may be markers of rapid proliferation, arising through acytokinesis and endoreduplication (Peckham and Cooper, 1970; Shackney, 1976). These basic issues may be approached in the near future by application of physical cell-separation techniques and flow microfluorimetry (Shackney, 1976).

3.6. Breast Carcinoma

Kinetic data for breast carcinoma, particularly for primary breast lesions studied by in vitro techniques, have accumulated rapidly in the last 5 years. Volume DTs have been estimated at 85 days (Gershon-Cohen et al., 1963) and 105 days (Kusama et al., 1972) for primary lesions, and 40 days for local recurrences (Philippe and Legal, 1968). All studies of volume DTs show a wide distribution of values. In one study, DTs of primary lesions correlated directly with age of patients, duration of preoperative findings, and duration of survival following mastectomy (Kusama *et al.*, 1972). An intriguing alternative approach roughly estimates DTs from statistics on duration of survival from "curative" breast surgery to death secondary to recurrent disease, assuming that residual clonogenic cells multiply from 1 to 10^{12} during that interval. DT values in the range of 30–90 days result (Skipper, 1971).

Only a small number of metastatic breast lesions have been studied by the PLM method (Young and DeVita, 1970; Terz *et al.*, 1971). A method to determine LI from needle aspirates of breast lesions and their metastases was recently described (Nordenskjöld *et al.*, 1974). Several investigators are now performing *in vitro* LIs from primary breast lesions removed at surgery (Silvestrini *et al.*, 1974; Meyer and Bauer, 1975; Schiffer *et al.*, 1976a). Companion studies show comparable *in vitro* and *in vivo* results in mouse solid tumors. All studies have shown a wide distribution of LIs. Two groups have used double-labeling techniques allowing simultaneous determination of LI, duration of S phase, and DT_p (Silvestrini *et al.*, 1974; Schiffer *et al.*, 1976a). Although single measurements for individual patients are unlikely to aid in the management of primary breast carcinoma, serial labeling indices of recurrent lesions may in the future help guide chemotherapy (Sky-Peck, 1971; Sulkes *et al.*, 1976).

3.7. Colon Carcinoma

Previous kinetic studies of normal colonic mucosa of man and rodents have defined an orderly and relatively rapid process of cell division within crypts, migration of cells to colonic villi; and eventual cell loss into the intestinal lumen, resulting in a steady-state condition with a mucosal turnover rate of 4–8 days (Lipkin, 1973). Several studies show that cell proliferation is more rapid in normal mucosa than in colonic tumors (Hoffman and Post, 1967; Bottomly and Cooper, 1973; Camplejohn *et al.*, 1973), whereas one recent study that simultaneously compared tumors and adjacent healthy-appearing mucosa refutes this finding (Bleiberg and Galand, 1976). S-phase duration is significantly longer in carcinomas than in normal mucosa (Hoffman and Post, 1967; Bleiberg and Galand, 1976). Atypical spatial distributions of proliferating cells have been observed in several diseases associated with an increased incidence of colonic carcinoma: villous and adenomatous polyps (Cole and McKalen, 1961; Bleiberg and Galand, 1974), familial polyposis (Bleiberg *et al.*, 1972; Deschner and Lipkin, 1975), and ulcerative colitis (Bleiberg *et al.*, 1970). Disordered proliferation of colonic mucosal cells and prolongation of S-phase duration may be premalignant mucosal changes, but are by no means specific for malignancy, and demonstration of these abnormalities has not found clinical utility thus far (Lipkin *et al.*, 1970).

In contrast to the rapid proliferation of normal mucosa, colon carcinomas are quite slow-growing. Serial barium enema studies have demonstrated a mean volume DT of 620 days (Welin *et al.*, 1963). Pulmonary metastases from the colon and rectum appear to grow more rapidly, with a volume DT of 109 days reported (Spratt, 1965). A high cell loss factor is largely responsible for this slow growth (Camplejohn *et al.*, 1973). Normal mucosa is, of course, in a steady-state in which cell birth balances cell loss ($\phi = 1$). In tumors, this balance is lost, and a cell loss factor that is quite high but less than unity accounts for the slow but progressive enlargement of colonic malignancies. Indices of cell proliferation such as MI, LI, and GF have not been correlated thus far with Dukes staging or prognosis, but such clinical correlations are incomplete (Camplejohn *et al.*, 1973).

Xenografts of human colonic carcinomas transplanted into immune-deprived rodents appear to reproduce the histology and kinetic behavior of their parent tumor (Pickard *et al.*, 1975; Lamerton, 1976). Such explants may eventually permit the selective use of anticancer drugs known to be effective against xenografts derived from progeny of the parent human tumor.

3.8. Lung Carcinoma

The size of primary lung tumors can be easily measured, and reliable data are available to assess volume DT (Charbit *et al.*, 1971; Straus, 1974). Small-cell carcinoma has a short DT (33 days), in contrast to adenocarcinoma (187 days), epidermoid carcinoma (103 days), and undifferentiated carcinoma (100 days) (Straus, 1974). Short DTs have correlated with a brief clinical course and poor prognosis. Labeling studies have usually been performed on metastatic skin lesions or bone lesions, and have seldom produced adequate PLM curves. A technique involving local injection of [^{3}H]TdR followed by aspiration has generated a larger body of data on LIs, particularly for small-cell carcinoma (Muggia and DeVita, 1972; Muggia *et al.*, 1974). Small-cell carcinoma demonstrates a higher LI (in the range of 24%) than adenocarcinoma and epidermoid carcinoma (Muggia, 1973). Other cell types may occasionally have an initial LI comparable to small-cell carcinoma. Repeated thymidine pulse-labeling suggests a rank order or rate of labeling with small-cell most rapid and adenocarcinoma least rapid, probably a reflection of GF (Muggia *et al.*, 1974). Rapid *in vitro* assays of LIs of primary lung tumors correlate reasonably well with data accumulated for metastatic lesions (Schiffer *et al.*, 1976*a*). All histological types have had cell loss factors calculated to be greater than 90%.

Such kinetic studies have helped to distinguish small-cell carcinoma from other primary lung tumors as a rapidly proliferating tumor that responds to chemotherapy. Preliminary data suggest that among patients with small-cell carcinoma, those with the highest LIs are most likely to respond to therapy which is composed in part of cycle- or phase-specific agents (Muggia *et al.*, 1974). DTs and LIs are often obtainable for lung cancer patients, and may provide a better correlation with survival and response to therapy than does DT alone. The GF can be estimated from DT and LI if one has a rough estimate of duration of phases of the cell cycle (Malaise *et al.*, 1973). GF appears to be the single kinetic parameter that correlates best with growth rate. Selection of patients with "poor histology" but with evidence of high GF may segregate a portion of patients with adenocarcinoma, epidermoid carcinoma, or undifferentiated lung carcinoma who would benefit from aggressive therapy.

3.9. Head and Neck Cancer

Tumors of the head and neck region may be suitable for kinetic analysis by *in vivo* labeling techniques because of two characteristics of malignancies in this region of the body: (1) tumors are often easily accessible for repeated biopsy; and (2) the arterial supply of head and neck tumors is often accessible, allowing regional perfusion with [^{3}H]TdR, resulting in intensive labeling of dividing cells. A recent study utilized pulse-labeling with [^{3}H]TdR through a permanent indwelling catheter in the carotid artery followed by serial biopsies (Bresciani and Nervi, 1976). Data from 10 of 22 total attempted procedures were adequate for classic computer-processed PLM analysis. Mean intermitotic times (T_c) ranged from 52 to 88 hr, with an average of 68 hr. The mean duration of DNA synthesis (T_s) ranged from 18 to 34 hr, with an average of 25 hr. LIs *in vivo* ranged from 11% to 36%, with an average value of 17.4%. The cell loss factor based on an average observed tumor DT of 21 days ranged from 0.78 to 0.93. Although the distribution of intermitotic times was generally very broad, an occasional tumor demonstrated a very narrow distribution (Bresciani *et al.*, 1974). Interestingly, there was no obvious relationship between LI and other cell cycle parameters. Two tumors studied both before and after therapy demonstrated more rapid proliferation in recurrent tumors than the initial primary lesions. Microfluorimetric DNA content analysis of squashed biopsy specimens demonstrated that some tumors are diploid, whereas others are polyploid; more undifferentiated epidermoid tumors most likely demonstrate polyploidy.

Basic data such as the studies reported above have led to therapeutic trials utilizing bleomycin as a possible synchronizing agent, followed by appropriately timed cell-cycle-specific agents (Costanzi, 1976). Bleomycin in low dose reversibly inhibits cells at the $S-G_2$ boundary (Barranco *et al.*, 1973). Early data, although encouraging, are too preliminary to be conclusive.

3.10. Malignant Melanoma

Melanoma has been frequently investigated by classic kinetic techniques, largely because of accessibility of lesions for biopsy. It behaves clinically as a moderately rapidly proliferating tumor. Although serial measurements of primary lesions are not available, pulmonary metastases have a mean volume DT of 42 days (Nathanson *et al.*, 1967), shorter than most solid tumors metastasizing to lung and exceeded by small-cell carcinoma of the lung, metastatic embryonal tumor, and some lymphomas. Data from independent sources suggest kinetic homogeneity among tumors in different individuals. Three studies of cutaneous nodules by the PLM method demonstrate T_s averaging 24 hr and T_c averaging 3 days with minimal variation (Shirakawa *et al.*, 1970; Young and DeVita, 1970; Terz *et al.*, 1971). Simultaneous sampling of small nodules and the periphery of large nodules in the same host shows equivalent LI and MI. Values in the center of large nodules, however, are approximately one-third less than those at the periphery, presumably reflecting more intense proliferative activity in the well-vascularized area (Shirakawa *et al.*, 1970).

Several studies indicate that the LI predicts the response of disseminated melanoma to therapy (Hart *et al.*, 1972; Murphy *et al.*, 1975; Thirlwell and Mansell, 1976). High LI values prior to therapy correlate with a greater probability of response to therapy. Unequivocal responders have a lower LI after therapy. Rapid *in vitro* LI methods may allow tailoring of therapy to individual patients. Attempts to produce synchrony of melanoma cells *in vivo* may find clinical application (Barranco *et al.*, 1973). Bleomycin has been slowly infused into patients with melanoma, producing an accumulation of melanoma cells in S, as demonstrated by serial increases of *in vitro* LI during drug infusion. The definitive studies in human melanoma to demonstrate synchronous kinetic behavior after removal of bleomycin "blockade" are not yet available. Partial synchronization might well be exploited therapeutically by administration of the synchronizing agent, followed at an appropriate interval by phase-specific cytotoxic agents.

3.11. Miscellaneous Tumors

Cell kinetic data were obtained with the PLM method after *in vivo* [^{3}H]TdR in a patient with ovarian cancer and ascites before and after chemotherapy. The T_c, T_s, and T_{G_1} all decreased, while the LI increased. It was suggested that in association with reduction of ascitic cell number, recruitment had occurred (Sheehy *et al.*, 1974).

Cell cycle parameters from two cases of invasive carcinoma of the cervix were derived from PLM curves obtained from *in vivo* [^{3}H]TdR labeling and multiple biopsies. The majority of labeled cells were at the periphery of the tumor. Intermitotic times were low (14 and 15 hr), with remarkably low values for G_1 (1.1 and 1.5 hr), not unlike values cited for normal cervix (Bennington, 1969).

Cell cycle parameters have been reported for basal-cell carcinomas of the skin, obtained from intratumor (Weinstein and Frost, 1970) and intravenous (Frindel *et al.*, 1968) [^{3}H]TdR injection.

Bladder carcinomas have been studied by *in vitro* labeling of biopsy specimens (Levi *et al.*, 1969) and biopsy following administration of colcemid, to allow calculation of DT_p (Fulker *et al.*, 1971). LI did not correlate with tumor stage or histology, but the stathmokinetic technique did, with poorly differentiated lesions having short DT_p (2–6 days) compared with well-differentiated ones (22 days).

Neuroblastomas have been studied by the stathmokinetic technique, with a median DT_p value of 4.2 days (Ahern and Buck, 1971). Cell cycle times were derived from a PLM curve in one patient, with serial biopsy of a metastasis. The T_s

was 28 hr, and the estimated T_c was 35–40 hr (Wagner and Käser, 1970). Recent LI and MI studies of marrow tumor cells following therapy have been correlated with the response to therapy, in that an increase in these values heralded a good response (Hayes *et al.*, 1976).

4. Conclusions

The application of cell kinetic techniques to human tumors is still in its infancy. The relevance of cell kinetics to cancer treatment has been limited in the past by poor methodology, unwarranted assumptions, inappropriate application of animal data to human disease, marked heterogeneity of values for various tumors, and overlap with the kinetics of normal tissues (Hall, 1971; Van Putten, 1974). Clearly, this area of research should not assume priority over studies of the specific biochemical sensitivity of malignant cells to chemotherapeutic agents. At the same time, dismissing the role of cell kinetics in clinical-therapy planning as totally irrelevant is premature and erroneous. Information about human tumors thus far is largely descriptive, but several meaningful concepts have emerged. Clinical cancers often have long cell cycle times compared with normal, with a significant number of cells not in cycle, and with a large component of cell loss. As methods of tumor measurement become more sensitive, it is likely that more valuable data will become available. The correlation between the response to treatment and changes in such easily and (now) rapidly measured parameters as labeling indices that has been described for acute leukemia and neuroblastoma seems especially encouraging, and such changes may well be more important than pretreatment values. The striking increase in the LI after therapy in multiple myeloma suggests that increases in the GF occur with reduction of total tumor mass, and supports the hypothesis of Gompertzian kinetics. It is very likely that this information may produce improved utilization of cycle-active agents. Evidence for synchronization of cells in cycle and recruitment of resting tumor cells into cycle is beginning to be presented, and it should be possible in the future to take advantage of these developments therapeutically.

5. References

AHERN, W., AND BUCK, P., 1971, The potential cell population doubling time in neuroblastoma and nephroblastoma, *Br. J. Cancer* **25**:691.

ALBERTS, D. S., AND GOLDE, D. W., 1974, DNA synthesis in multiple myeloma cells following cell cycle–nonspecific chemotherapy, *Cancer Res.* **34**:2911.

ARLIN, Z., GEE, T., DOWLING, M., CAMPBELL, J., AND CLARKSON, B., 1976, Significance of pulse ³H-thymidine labeling index (LI) in adult acute myeloid leukemia (AML), *Proc. Amer. Assoc. Cancer Res. Amer. Soc. Clin. Oncol.* **17**:296.

ASTALDI, D., AND MAURI, C., 1953, Recherches sur l'activite proliferative de l'hemocytoblaste de la leucemie aigué, *Rev. Belge Pathol. Med. Exp.* **23**:69.

BACCARANI, M., AND KILLMANN, S. A., 1972, Cytokinetic studies in chronic myeloid leukaemia: Evidence for early presence of abnormal myeloblasts, *Scand. J. Haematol.* **9**:283.

BARRANCO, S. C., LUCE, J. K., ROMSDAHL, M. M., AND HUMPHREY, R. M., 1973, Bleomycin as a possible synchronizing agent for human tumor cells *in vivo*, *Cancer Res.* **33**:882.

BARRETT, J. C., 1966, A mathematical model of the mitotic cycle and its application to the interpretation of percentage labeled mitosis data, *J. Natl. Cancer Inst.* **37**:443.

BENNINGTON, J. L., 1969, Cellular kinetics of invasive squamous carcinoma of the human cervix, *Cancer Res.* **29**:1082.

BERENBAUM, M. C., SHEARD, C. E., REITTIC, AND BUNDICK, R. V., 1974, The growth of human tumours in immunosuppressed mice and their response to chemotherapy, *Br. J. Cancer* **30**:13.

BLEIBERG, H., AND GALAND, P., 1974, Autoradiographic measurement of the cellular proliferation in the digestive tract. Hypothesis concerning the malignant degeneration of atrophic mucosas, *Acta Gastro-Enterol. Belg.* **37**:475.

BLEIBERG, H., AND GALAND, P., 1976, *In vitro* autoradiographic determination of cell kinetic parameters in adenocarcinomas and adjacent healthy mucosa of the human colon and rectum, *Cancer Res.* **36**:325.

BLEIBERG, H., MAINGUET, P., GALAND, P., CHRETIEN, J., AND DUPONT-MAIRESSE, N., 1970, Cell renewal in the human rectum. *In vivo* autoradiographic study on active ulcerative colitis, *Gastroenterology* **58**:851.

BLEIBERG, H., MAINGUET, P., AND GALAND, P., 1972, Cell renewal in familial polyposis: Comparison between polyps and healthy mucosa, *Gastroenterology* **63**:240.

BOND, V. P., FLEIDNER, T. M., CRONKITE, E. P., RUBINI, J. R., BRECHER, G., AND SCHORK, P., 1959, Proliferative potentials of bone marrow and blood cells studied by *in vitro* uptake of tritiated thymidine, *Acta Haematol.* **21**:1.

BOTTOMLY, J. P., AND COOPER, E. H., 1973, Cell proliferation in colonic mucosa and carcinoma of the colon, *Proc. R. Soc. Med.* **66**:1183.

BRAUNSCHWEIGER, P. G., POULAKOS, L., AND SCHIFFER, L. M., 1976, *In vitro* labeling and gold activating autoradiography for determination of labeling index and DNA synthesis times of solid tumors, *Cancer Res.* **36**:1748.

BRESCIANI, F., AND NERVI, C., 1976, Cell population kinetics and growth of squamous cell carcinomas in man, in: *Growth Kinetics and Biochemical Regulation of Normal and Malignant Cells*, 29th Annual Symposium on Fundamental Cancer Research, Houston, Texas.

BRESCIANI, F., PAOLUZI, R., BENASSI, M., NERVI, C., CASALE, C., AND ZIPORO, E., 1974, Cell kinetics and growth of squamous cell carcinomas in man, *Cancer Res.* **34**:2405.

BREUR, K., 1966*a*, Growth rate and radiosensitivity of human tumors. I. Growth rate of human tumors, *Eur. J. Cancer* **2**:157.

BREUR, K., 1966*b*, Growth rate and radiosensitivity of human tumors. II. Radiosensitivity of human tumors, *Eur. J. Cancer* **2**:173.

BURKE, P. J., AND OWENS, A. H., 1971, Attempted recruitment of leukemic myeloblasts to proliferative activity by sequential drug treatment, *Cancer* **28**:830.

CAMPLEJOHN, R. S., BONE, G., AND AHERNE, W., 1973, Cell proliferation in rectal carcinoma and rectal mucosa—a stathmokinetic study, *Eur. J. Cancer* **9**:577.

CHAN, B. W. B., AND HAYHOE, F. G. J., 1971, Changes in proliferative activity of marrow leukemic cells during and after extracorporeal irradiation of blood, *Blood* **37**:657.

CHAN, B. W. B., HAYHOE, F. G. J., AND BULLIMORE, J. A., 1969, Effect of extracorporeal irradiation of the blood on bone marrow activity in acute leukaemia, *Nature (London)* **221**:972.

CHEUNG, W. H., RAI, K. R., AND SAWITSKY, A., 1972, Characteristics of cell proliferation in acute leukemia, *Cancer Res.* **32**:939.

CHARBIT, A., MALAISE, E. P., AND TUBIANA, M., 1971, Relation between the pathologic nature and the growth rate of human tumours, *Eur. J. Cancer* **7**:307.

CLARKSON, B. D., 1969, Review of recent studies of cellular proliferation in acute leukemia, in: *Human Tumor Cell Kinetics*, National Cancer Institute Monograph No. 30 (S. Perry, ed.), p. 81, Bethesda, Maryland.

CLARKSON, B. OTA, K., OHKITA, T., AND O'CONNOR, A., 1965*a*, Kinetics of proliferation of cancer cells in neoplastic effusions in man, *Cancer* **18**:1189.

CLARKSON, B., OHKITA, T., OTA, K., AND O'CONNOR, A., 1965*b*, Studies of cellular proliferation in acute leukemia, *J. Clin. Invest.* **44**:1035.

CLARKSON, B., OHKITA, T., OTA, K., AND FRIED, J., 1967, Studies of cellular proliferation in human leukemia. I. Estimation of growth rates of leukemia and normal hematopoietic cells in two adults with acute leukemia given single injections of tritiated thymidine, *J. Clin. Invest.* **46**:506.

COBB, L., AND MITCHLEY, B. C. U., 1974, Development of a method for assessing the antitumor activity of chemotherapeutic agents using human tumor xenografts, *Cancer Chemother. Rep.* **58:**645.

COLE, J. W., AND MCKALEN, A., 1961, Observations of cell renewal in human rectal mucosa *in vivo* with thymidine ³H, *Gastroenterology* **41:**122.

COOPER, E. H., FRANK, G. L., AND WRIGHT, D. H., 1966, Cell proliferation in Burkitt tumours, *Eur. J. Cancer* **2:**377.

COOPER, E. H., PECKHAM, M. J., MILLARD, R. E., HAMLIN, I. M. E., AND GERARD-MARCHANT, R., 1968, Cell proliferation in human malignant lymphomas. Analysis of labelling index and DNA content in cell populations obtained by biopsy, *Eur. J. Cancer* **4:**287.

COSTANZI, J., 1976, Bleomycin infusion as a potential synchronizing agent in carcinoma of the head and neck, *Amer. Assoc. Cancer Res. Amer. Soc. Clin. Oncol.* **17:**11.

CROWTHER, D., BEARD, M. E. J., BATEMAN, C. J. T., AND SEWELL, R. L., 1975, Factors influencing prognosis in adults with acute myelogenous leukemia, *Br. J. Cancer* **32:**456.

DESCHNER, E. E., AND LIPKIN, M., 1975, Proliferative patterns in colonic mucosa in familial polyposis, *Cancer* **35:**413.

DREWINKO, B., BROWN, B. W., HUMPHREY, R., AND ALEXANIAN, R., 1974, Effect of chemotherapy on the labelling index of myeloma cells, *Cancer* **34:**526.

DURIE, B. G. M., AND SALMON, S. E., 1976, High speed scintillation autoradiography, *Science* **190:** 1093.

ERNST, P., AND KILLMANN, S. A., 1970, Perturbation of generation cycle of human leukemic blast cells by cytostatic therapy *in vivo*: Effect of corticosteroids, *Blood* **36:**689.

ERNST, P., AND KILLMANN, S. A., 1971, Perturbation of generation cycle of human leukemic myeloblasts *in vivo* by methotrexate, *Blood* **38:**689.

ERNST, P., ANDERSEN, V., AND KILLMANN, S. A., 1971, Cell cycle effect of extracorporeal irradiation of the blood in acute myeloid leukaemia, *Scand. J. Haematol.* **8:**21.

ERNST, P., FAILLE, A., AND KILLMANN, S. A., 1973, Perturbation of cell cycle of human leukaemic myeloblasts *in vivo* by cytosine arabinoside, *Scand. J. Haematol.* **10:**209.

FAADI, M. D., COOPER, E. H., AND HARDISTY, R. M., 1967, DNA synthesis and DNA content of leucocytes in acute leukaemia, *Nature (London)* **216:**134.

FAILLE, A., NAJEAN, Y., AND BERNARD, J., 1973, Capacité de proliferation des cellules leucémiques de la moelle humanine, *Nouv. Presse Med.* **2:**889.

FREEDMAN, S. O., 1976, Antigens in tumors, in: *Scientific Foundations in Oncology* (T. Symington and R. L. Carter, eds.), p. 505, William Heinemann Medical Books, London.

FRINDEL, E., MALAISE, E., AND TUBIANA, M., 1968, Cell proliferation kinetics in five human solid tumors, *Cancer* **22:**611.

FULKER, M. J., COOPER, E. H., AND TANAKA, T., 1971, Proliferation and ultrastructure of papillary transitional cell carcinoma of the human bladder, *Cancer* **27:**71.

GAVOSTO, F., AND MARESA, P., 1975, Aspects of cell kinetics in acute leukemia with relationship to prognosis, *Adv. Biosci.* **14:**329.

GAVOSTO, F., MARAINI, G., AND PILERI, A., 1960, Proliferative capacity of acute leukemia cells, *Nature (London)* **187:**611.

GAVOSTO, F., PILERI, A., BACHI, C., AND PEGORARO, L., 1964, Proliferation and maturation defect in acute leukemia cells, *Nature (London)* **203:**92.

GERSHON-COHEN, J., BERGER, S. M., AND KLICKSTEIN, H. S., 1963, Roentgenography of breast cancer moderating concept of "biologic predeterminism," *Cancer* **16:**961.

GREENBERG, M. L., AND HOLLAND, J., 1976, Kinetic studies of vincristine (VCR) infusions in man, *Proc. Amer. Assoc. Cancer Res. Amer. Soc. Clin. Oncol.* **17:**189.

GREENBERG, M. L., CHANANA, A. D., CRONKITE, E. P., GIACOMELLI, G., RAI, K. R., SCHIFFER, L. M., STRYCKMANS, P. A., AND VINCENT, P. C., 1972, The generation time of human leukemic myeloblasts, *Lab. Invest.* **26:**245.

HALL, T. C., 1971, Limited role of cell kinetics in clinical cancer chemotherapy, in: *Prediction of Response in Cancer Therapy*, National Cancer Institute Momograph No. 34 (T. Hall, ed.), p. 15, Bethesda, Maryland.

HART, J. S., HO, D. H., GEORGE, S. L., SALEM, P., GOTTLIEB, J. A., AND FREI, E., III, 1972, Cytokinetic and molecular pharmacology studies of arabinosylcytosine in metastatic melanoma, *Cancer Res.* **32:**2711.

HART, J. S., GEORGE, S. L., AND FREI, E., III, 1973, Cytokinetic studies and clinical correlates in adult acute leukemia, *Proc. Amer. Assoc. Cancer Res.* **14:**54.

HART, J. S., FREIREICH, E. J., AND FREI, E., III, 1974, Prognostic significance of pretreatment (pre-rx) proliferative activity in adult acute leukemia (AAL), *Proc. Amer. Assoc. Cancer Res.* **15**:73.

HART, J. S., FREIREICH, E. J., McCREDIE, K. B., SPEER, J. F., AND COPELAND, M. M., 1975, Significance of marrow leukemic cell infiltrate (LCI) and labeling index (LI) in adult acute leukemia (AAL), *Proc. Amer. Assoc. Cancer Res.* **16**:200.

HAYES, A., GREEN, A., AND MAUER, A., 1976, Cell kinetic studies in children with neuroblastoma, *Proc. Amer. Assoc. Cancer Res. Amer. Soc. Clin. Oncol.* **17**:121.

HILLEN, H., WESSELS, J., AND HAANEN, C., 1975, Bone-marrow-proliferation patterns in acute myeloblastic leukaemia determined by pulse cytophotometry, *Lancet* **1**:609.

HOBBS, J. R., 1975, Monitoring myelomatosis, *Arch. Intern. Med.* **135**:125.

HOELZER, D., KURRLE, E., DIETRICH, M., MEYER-HAMME, K. D., AND FLIEDNER, T. M., 1974, The effect of continuous cell removal on blast cell kinetics in acute leukaemia, *Scand. J. Haematol.* **12**:311.

HOFFMAN, J., AND POST, J., 1967, *In vivo* studies of DNA synthesis in human normal and tumor cells, *Cancer Res.* **27**:898.

IVERSON, O. H., IVERSON, U., ZIEGLER, J. L., AND BLUMING, A. Z., 1974, Cell kinetics in Burkitt lymphoma, *Eur. J. Cancer* **10**:155.

KILLMANN, S.-A., 1965, Proliferative activity of blast cells in leukemia and myelofibrosis. Morphological differences between proliferating and non-proliferating blast cells, *Acta Med. Scand.* **178**:263.

KILLMANN, S.-A., 1968, Acute leukemia: The kinetics of leukemic blast cells in man—an analytic review, *Ser. Haematol.* **1**:38.

KILLMANN, S.-A., 1974, Effect of cytostatic drugs on the kinetics of leukemic blast cells in man, *Schweiz. Med. Wochenschr.* **104**:278.

KILLMANN, S.-A., CRONKITE, E. P., AND FLIEDNER, T. M., 1962, Cell proliferation in multiple myeloma studied with tritiated thymidine *in vivo*, *Lab. Invest.* **11**:845.

KILLMANN, S.-A., CRONKITE, E. P., ROBERTSON, J. S., FLIEDNER, T. M., AND BOND, V. P., 1963, Estimation of phases of the life cycle of leukemic cells from labeling in human beings *in vivo* with tritiated thymidine, *Lab. Invest.* **12**:671.

KLEIN, H. O., AND LENNARTZ, K. L., 1974, Chemotherapy after synchronization of tumor cells, *Semin. Hematol.* **11**:203.

KOPPER, L., AND STEEL, G. G., 1975, The therapeutic response of three human tumor lines maintained in immune-suppressed mice, *Cancer Res.* **35**:2704.

KRAEMER, P. M., DEAVOR, L. L., CRISSMAN, H. A., STEINKAMP, J. A., AND PETERSEN, D. F., 1973, On the nature of heteroploidy, *Cold Spring Harbor Symp. Quant. Biol.* **38**:133.

KREMER, W. B., VOGLER, W. R., AND CHAN, Y.-K., 1976, An attempt at synchronization of marrow cells in acute leukemia. Relationship to therapeutic response, *Cancer* **37**:390.

KRISHAN, A., TATTERSALL, M. H. N., AND PAIKA, K., 1976, Flow microfluorimetric patterns of human bone marrow and tumor cells in response to cancer chemotherapy, *Proc. Amer. Assoc. Cancer Res. Amer. Soc. Clin. Oncol.* **17**:272.

KUSAMA, S., SPRATT, J. S., JR., DRAEGER, W. L., WATSON, F. R., AND CUNNINGHAM, C., 1972, The gross rates of growth of human mammary carcinoma, *Cancer* **30**:594.

LALA, P. K., 1971, Studies in tumour cell population kinetics, *Methods Cancer Res.* **6**:4.

LALA, P. K., AND PATT, H. M., 1966, Cytokinetic analysis of tumor growth, *Proc. Natl. Acad. Sci. U.S.A.* **56**:1735.

LAMERTON, L. F., 1976, Growth kinetics of human solid tumors in immuno-suppressed mice, in: *Growth Kinetics and Biochemical Regulation of Normal and Malignant Cells*, 29th Annual Symposium on Fundamental Cancer Research, Houston, Texas.

LAMPKIN, B. C., NAGAO, T., AND MAUER, A. M., 1969a, Synchronization of the mitotic cycle in acute leukemia, *Nature (London)* **222**:1274.

LAMPKIN, B. C., NAGAO, T., AND MAUER, A. M., 1969b, Drug effect in acute leukemia, *J. Clin. Invest.* **48**:1124.

LAMPKIN, B. C., NAGAO, T., AND MAUER, A. M., 1971, Synchronization and recruitment in acute leukemia, *J. Clin. Invest.* **50**:2204.

LAMPKIN, B. C., McWILLIAMS, N. B., AND MAUER, A. M., 1972, Cell kinetics and chemotherapy in acute leukemia, *Semin. Hematol.* **9**:211.

LAMPKIN, B., McWILLIAMS, N. B., MAUER, A. M., FLESSA, H. C., HAKE, D. A., AND FISHER, V., 1976, Manipulation of the mitotic cycle in the treatment of acute myelogenous leukemia, *Br. J. Haematol.* **32**:29.

LAURENCE, D. J. R., AND NEVILLE, A. M., 1976, Biological markers, in: *Scientific Foundations in Oncology* (T. Symington and R. L. Carter, eds.), p. 594, William Heinemann Medical Books, London.

LEE, B. J., SAHAKIAN, G., CLARKSON, B. D., AND KRAKOFF, I. H., 1974, Combination chemotherapy of multiple myeloma with alkeran, cytoxan, vincristine, prednisone, and BCNU, *Cancer* **33**:533.

LEVI, P. E., COOPER, E. H., ANDERSON, C. K., AND WILLIAMS, R. E., 1969, Analyses of DNA content. Nuclear size and cell proliferation of tansitional cell carcinoma in man, *Cancer* **23**:1074.

LIGHTDALE, C., AND LIPKIN, M., 1975, Cell division and tumor growth, in: *Cancer, A Comprehensive Treatise*, Vol. 3, *Biology of Tumors: Cellular Biology and Growth* (F. F. Becker, ed.), p. 201, Plenum Press, New York.

LIPKIN, M., 1973, Proliferation and differentiation of gastrointestinal cells, *Physiol. Rev.* **53**:891.

LIPKIN, M., BELL, B., STALDER, C., AND TRONCALE, F., 1970, The development of abnormalities of growth in colonic epithelial cells of man, in: *Carcinoma of the Colon and Antecedent Epithelium* (W. Burdette ed.), Charles C. Thomas, Springfield, Illinois.

LIVINGSTON, R. B., AMBROSE, U., GEORGE, S., FREIREICH, E. J., AND HART, J., 1974, *In vitro* determination of thymidine-^{3}H labelling index in human solid tumors, *Cancer Res.* **34**:1376.

LOPEZ-SANDOVAL, R. MOAYERI, H., AND SOKAL, J. E., 1974, *In vitro* leukocyte uptake in chronic lymphocytic leukemia, *Cancer Res.* **34**:146.

MALAISE, E. P., CAVAUDRA, N., AND TUBIANA, M., 1973, The relationship between growth rate, labelling index and histological type of human solid tumours, *Eur. J. Cancer* **9**:305.

MAUER, A. M., 1975, Cell kinetics and practical consequences for therapy of acute leukemia, *N. Engl. J. Med.* **292**:389.

MAUER, A. M., AND FISHER, V., 1962, Comparison of the proliferative capacity of acute leukaemia cells in bone marrow and blood, *Nature (London)* **193**:1085.

MAUER, A. M., AND FISHER, V., 1966, Characteristics of cell proliferation in four patients with untreated acute leukemia, *Blood* **28**:428.

MAUER, A. M., SAUNDERS, E. F., AND LAMPKIN, B. C., 1969 Possible significance of nonproliferating leukemic cells, in: *Human Tumor Cell Kinetics, National Cancer Institute Monograph No. 30* (S. Perry ed.), p. 63, Bethesda, Maryland.

MERRIN, C., ETRA, W., WAJSMAN, Z., BAUMGARTNER, G., AND MURPHY, G., 1976, Chemotherapy and advanced carcinoma of the prostate with 5-fluorouracil, cyclophosphamide, and adriamycin, *J. Urol.* **115**:86.

MEYER, J. S., AND BAUER, W. C., 1975, *In vitro* determination of tritiated thymidine labeling index (LI), *Cancer* **36**:1374.

MOMPARLER, R. L., 1974, A model for the chemotherapy of acute leukemia with 1-β-D-arabinofuranosylcytosine, *Cancer Res.* **34**:1775.

MOMPARLER, R. L., 1976, Estimation of cell cycle parameters of clonogenic leukemic cells *in vivo* using chemotherapeutic agents, in: *Growth Kinetics and Biochemical Regulation of Normal and Malignant Cells*, 29th Annual Symposium on Fundamental Cancer Research, Houston, Texas.

MUGGIA, F. M., 1973, Correlation of histologic types with cell kinetic studies in lung cancer, *Cancer Chemother. Rep.* **4**:69.

MUGGIA, F. M., AND DEVITA, V. T., 1972, *In vivo* tumor cell kinetic studies on the use of local thymidine injection followed by fine-needle aspiration, *J. Lab. Clin. Med.* **80**:297.

MUGGIA, F. M., KROZOSKI, S. K., AND HANSEN, H. H., 1974, Cell kinetic studies in patients with small cell carcinoma of the lung, *Cancer* **34**:1683.

MURPHY, W. K., LIVINGSTON, R. B., RUIZ, V. G., GERCOVICH, F. G., GEORGE, S. L., HART, J. S., AND FREIREICH, E. J., 1975, Serial labelling index determination as a predictor of response in human solid tumors, *Cancer Res.* **35**:1438.

MURPHY, S., DAHL, G., RIVERA, G., MAUER, A., AND SIMONE, J., 1976, Cytokinetic observations on the effects of either simultaneous or sequential administration of cytosine arabinoside (ara-C) and methotrexate (MTX) in childhood lymphocytic leukemia in relapse, *Proc. Amer. Assoc. Cancer Res.* **17**:121.

NATHANSON, L., AND FISHMAN, W. H., 1971, New observations on the Regan isoenzyme of alkaline phosphotase in cancer patients, *Cancer* **27**:1388.

NATHANSON, L., HALL, T. C., VAWTER, G. F., AND FARBER, S., 1967, Melanoma as a medical problem, *Arch. Intern. Med.* **119**:479.

NELSON, J. S. R., AND SCHIFFER, L. M., 1973, Autoradiographic detection of DNA polymerase containing nuclei in Sarcoma 180 Ascites cells, *Cell Tissue Kinet.* **6**:45.

NORDENSKJÖLD, B., ZETTERBERG, A. L., AND LOWHAGER, T., 1974, Measurement of DNA synthesis by ³H-thymidine incorporation into needle aspirates from human tumors, *Acta Cytol.* (*Baltimore*) **18**:215.

OGAWA, M., FRIED, J., SAKAI, Y., STRIFE, A., AND CLARKSON, B., 1970, Studies of cellular proliferation in human leukemia. VI. The proliferative activity, generation time and emergence time of neutrophilic granulocytes in chronic granulocytic leukemia, *Cancer* **25**:1031.

PECKHAM, M. J., AND COOPER, E. H., 1970, The pattern of cell growth in reticulum cell sarcoma and lymphosarcoma, *Eur. J. Cancer* **6**:453.

PECKHAM, M. J., AND COOPER, E. H., 1973, Cell proliferation in Hodgkin's disease, in: *International Symposium on Hodgkin's Disease, National Cancer Institute Monograph No. 36* (J. O'Brien, ed.), p. 179, Bethesda, Maryland.

PECKHAM, M. F., AND STEEL, G. C., 1972, Cell kinetics in reticulum cell sarcoma, *Cancer* **29**:1724.

PHILIPPE, E., AND LEGAL, T., 1968, Growth of seventy-eight recurrent mammary carcinomas, *Cancer* **21**:461.

PICKARD, R. G., COBB, L. M., AND STEEL, G. G., 1975, The growth kinetics of xenografts of human colorectal tumours in immune-deprived mice, *Br. J. Cancer* **31**:36.

REICH, L., OHARA. K., STOERZINGER, P., AND CLARKSON, B., 1971, Effect of massive leukophoresis on proliferation in acute myeloblastic leukemia, *Proc. Amer. Assoc. Cancer Res.* **12**:25.

SALMON, S. E., 1975, Expansion of the growth fraction in multiple myeloma with alkylating agents, *Blood* **45**:119.

SALMON, S. E., AND DURIE, B. G. M., 1975, Cellular kinetics in multiple myeloma, *Arch. Intern. Med.* **135**:131.

SALMON, S. E., AND SMITH, B. A., 1970, Immunoglobin synthesis and total body tumor cell number in IgG multiple myeloma, *J. Clin. Invest.* **49**:1114.

SALMON, S. E., AND SMITH, B. A., 1972, Induction of tumor-susceptibility to cycle-active agents in IgG multiple myeloma, *Clin. Res.* **20**:570.

SAUNDERS, E. F., 1972, The effect of L-asparaginase on the nucleic acid metabolism and cell cycle of human leukemia cells, *Blood* **39**:575.

SAUNDERS, E. F., LAMPKIN, B. C., AND MAUER, A. M., 1967, Variation of proliferative activity in leukemic cell populations of patients with acute leukemia, *J. Clin. Invest.* **46**:1356.

SCHIFFER, L. M., AND BRAUNSCHWEIGER, P. G., 1976, Cytokinetics of human breast cancer: Primary in metastatic lesions, *Proc. Amer. Assoc. Cancer Res. Amer. Soc. Clin. Oncol.* **17**:238.

SCHIFFER, L. M., BRAUNSCHWEIGER, P. G., AND POULAKOS, L., 1976a, Studies on the cell kinetics of human solid tumors, in: *Growth Kinetics and Biochemical Regulation of Normal and Malignant Cells*, 29th Annual Symposium on Fundamental Cancer Research, Houston, Texas.

SCHIFFER, L. M., MARKOE, A. M., AND NELSON, J. S. R., 1976b, Estimation of tumor growth fraction in murine tumors by the primer-available DNA-dependent DNA polymerase assay, *Cancer Res.* **36**:2415.

SCHMID, J. R., OESCHLIN, R. J., FRICK, P. F., AND MOESCHLIN, S., 1967, Cell proliferation in leukemia during relapse and remission. II. DNA synthesis of leukemic cells in peripheral blood *in vitro*, *Acta Haematol.* **37**:16.

SHACKNEY, S. E., 1976, Interrelationship among the DNA content distribution, cell kinetics, and cell morphology, in: *Growth Kinetics and Biochemical Regulation of Normal and Malignant Cells*, 29th Annual Symposium on Fundamental Cancer Research, Houston, Texas.

SHEEHY, P. F., FRIED, J., WINN, R., AND CLARKSON, B. D., 1974, Cell cycle changes in ovarian cancer after arabinosylcytosine, *Cancer* **33**:28.

SHIRAKAWA, S., LUCE, J., TANNOCK, I., AND FREI, E., III, 1970, Cell proliferation in human melanoma, *J. Clin. Invest.* **49**:1188.

SILVESTRINI, R., SANFILIPPO, O., AND TEDESCO, G., 1974, Kinetics of human mammary carcinomas and the correlations with the cancer and the host characteristics, *Cancer* **34**:1252.

SKIPPER, H. E., 1971, Kinetics of mammary tumor cell growth and implications for therapy, *Cancer* **28**:1470.

SKY-PECK, H., 1971, Effects of chemotherapy on the incorporation of ³H-thymidine into DNA of human neoplastic tissue, in: *Prediction of Response in Cancer Therapy, National Cancer Institute Monograph No. 34* (T. Hall, ed.), p. 197, Bethesda, Maryland.

SMITH, G. M. R., 1969, The effect of cytotoxic agents on human tumours transplanted to the hamster cheek pouch, *Br. J. Cancer* **23**:78.

58

GERALD L.
SCHERTZ
AND
JOHN C.
MARSH

SPRATT, J. S., JR., 1965, The rates and patterns of growth of neoplasms of the large intestine and rectum, *Surg. Clin. N. Amer.* **45**:1103.

STEEL, G. G., 1967, Cell loss as a factor in the growth rate of human tumours, *Eur. J. Cancer* **3**:381.

STEEL, G. G., 1968, Cell loss from experimental tumors, *Cell Tissue Kinet.* **1**:193.

STEEL, G. G., 1972, The cell cycle in tumours: An examination of data gained by the technique of labelled mitoses, *Cell Tissue Kinet.* **5**:87.

STEEL, G. G., AND HANES, S., 1971, The technique of labelled mitoses: Analysis by automatic curve-fitting, *Cell Tissue Kinet.* **4**:93.

STRAUS, M. J., 1974, The growth characteristics of lung cancer and its application to treatment design, *Semin. Oncol.* **1**:167.

STRAUS, S. E., AND STRAUS, M. J., 1976, The pharmacokinetics and radiation hazard of tritiated thymidine in man, *Proc. Amer. Assoc. Cancer Res. Amer. Soc. Clin. Oncol.* **17**:8.

STRYCKMANS, P. A., MANASTER, J., LACHAPELLE, F., AND SOCQUET, M., 1973, Mode of action of chemotherapy *in vivo* on human acute leukemia. I. Daunomycin, *J. Clin. Invest.* **52**:126.

STRYCKMANS, P., DEBUSSCHER, L., PELTZER, T., AND SOCQUET, M., 1975, Variations of the proliferative activity of leukemia myeloblasts related to stage of the disease, *Blood Cells* **1**:217.

SULKES, A., LIVINGSTON, R., AND TAYLOR, G., 1976, Pre-treatment labeling index (LI%) in breast carcinoma patients as a predictor of response to combination chemotherapy (cc), *Proc. Amer. Assoc. Cancer Res. Amer. Soc. Clin. Oncol.* **17**:59.

SULLIVAN, P. W., AND SALMON, S. E., 1972, Kinetics of tumor growth and regression in IgG multiple myeloma, *J. Clin. Invest.* **51**:1697.

TANNOCK, I. F., 1965, A comparison of the relative efficiencies of various metaphase arrest agents, *Exp. Cell Res.* **47**:345.

TERZ, J. J., CURUTCHET, H. P., AND LAWRENCE, W. J., 1971, Analysis of the cell kinetics in five human solid tumors, *Cancer* **28**:1100.

THIRLWELL, M. P., AND MANSELL, P. W. A., 1976, A correlation of clinical response with *in vitro* pre-chemotherapy labeling indices % (PLI) in human solid tumors, *Proc. Amer. Assoc. Cancer Res. Amer. Soc. Clin. Oncol.* **17**:307.

TUBIANA, M., AND MALAISE, E., 1975, Growth rate and cell kinetics in human tumours: Some prognostic and therapeutic implications, in: *Scientific Foundations in Oncology* (T. Symington and R. L. Carter, eds.), p. 126, William Heinemann Medical Books, London.

VAN PUTTEN, L. M., 1974, Are cell kinetic data relevant for the design of tumor chemotherapy schedule?, *Cell Tissue Kinet.* **7**:493.

VOGLER, W. R., COOPER, L. E., AND GROTH, D. P., 1974, Correlation of cytosine arabinoside-induced increment in growth fraction of leukemic cells with clinical response, *Cancer* **33**:603.

WAGNER, H. P., AND KÄSER, H., 1970, Cell proliferation in neuroblastoma, *Eur. J. Cancer* **6**:369.

WEINSTEIN, G. D., AND FROST, P., 1970, Cell proliferation in human basal cell carcinoma, *Cancer Res.* **30**:724.

WELIN, S., YOUKER, J., AND SPRATT, J. S., 1963, The rates and patterns of growth of 375 tumours of the large intestine and rectum observed serially by double contrast enema studies (Malmö technique), *Amer. J. Roentgenol.* **90**:673.

YOUNG, R. C., AND DEVITA, V., 1970, Cell cycle characteristics of human solid tumors *in vivo*, *Cell Tissue Kinet.* **3**:285.

ZITTOUN, R., BOUCHARD, M., FACQUET-DANIS, J., PERCIE-DU-SERT, M., AND BOUSSER, J., 1975, Prediction of the response to chemotherapy in acute leukemia, *Cancer* **35**:507.

3

Toxicity of Chemotherapeutic Agents

ED CADMAN

1. Introduction

Effective chemotherapeutic agents are limited in their clinical use by the effects they produce on normal cells. The ratio of the doses at which therapeutic effect and toxicity occur is referred to as the *therapeutic index*. Ideally, one would like to have at his disposal drugs that have a higher therapeutic index, i.e., maximum therapeutic benefit with virtually no toxicity. But since this ideal situation has not been achieved, we must remain cognizant of the various toxicities of the chemotherapeutic drugs so that these agents can be used as effectively as possible. Each drug has unique antitumor properties and, as would be expected, unique toxicities. Some toxicity is acute, some delayed, but it is always present. This chapter is a review of these toxicities.

2. Gastrointestinal Toxicity

Nausea and vomiting are perhaps the most obvious manifestations of drug toxicity that a cancer patient experiences. Their effect can be so great that some patients refuse further treatments to avoid the emotional and physical pains associated with the recurrent sick feeling and emesis. Fortunately, not all drugs produce this untoward effect—but several do.

Alkylating agents generally produce nausea and vomiting of varying degrees. Generally, the less the dose administered, the less severe the effect. Some combination programs that utilize oral agents produce definitely less nausea and vomiting in comparison with equivalent doses given by intravenous bolus (Bagley *et al.*, 1972; Stutzman *et al.*, 1966; Solomon *et al.*, 1963).

ED CADMAN ● Department of Medicine, Yale University School of Medicine, New Haven, Connecticut.

Nitrogen mustard, which is administered only by vein, produces nausea and vomiting in nearly all patients (Wintrobe and Huguley, 1948; Dameshek *et al.*, 1949; Karnofsky, 1950). The symptoms generally occur 3–6 hr after drug administration and may persist for as long as 36 hr, but have generally subsided by 12–18 hr.

Cyclophosphamide, when administered in doses designed to produce marrow hypoplasia (60 or 120 mg/kg), results in 100% nausea and vomiting (Buckner *et al.*, 1972). However, when the dose is decreased to therapeutic levels (30–40 mg/kg), nausea and vomiting are not a major deterrent, although they occur in a majority of patients (Höst and Nissen-Meyer, 1960; Coggins *et al.*, 1959; Davis *et al.*, 1969). If an equivalent dose is administered orally, there is considerably less trouble with nausea and vomiting (Solomon *et al.*, 1963; Jacobs *et al.*, 1968). As little as 100 mg/kg orally may result in transient nausea and abdominal pain, but rarely vomiting (Fosdick *et al.*, 1968).

Chlorambucil, which is administered only orally, results in mild (Ezdinli and Stutzman, 1965; Masterson *et al.*, 1960) or no nausea and vomiting (Rundles *et al.*, 1959).

Busulfan and melphalan, both oral agents, have little appreciable GI toxicity (Louis *et al.*, 1956; Galton *et al.*, 1958; Haut *et al.*, 1961; Brook *et al.*, 1964; Frick *et al.*, 1968). Although 30% of women who received melphalan in the National Adjuvant Breast Study complained of nausea and vomiting, only 9 of 64 episodes of GI toxicity were considered "severe." It is of amusing interest that 11% of the placebo group had similar symptoms (Fisher *et al.*, 1975).

Methotrexate (MTX) administered once or twice weekly in conventional doses (30 mg/M^2) seldom results in nausea or vomiting, although on occasion stomatitis has occurred (Acute Leukemia Group B, 1969). When smaller doses of MTX (20 mg) are given daily for 5 or more days, nearly all patients develop stomatitis, but generally very little nausea or vomiting (Lamb *et al.*, 1964). Intravenous infusions of MTX (96 mg/M^2) over 48–72 hr produce marked oral ulcerations and mild nausea and vomiting, necessitating a shortening of the infusion time (Djerassi *et al.*, 1967). The stomatitis is not a major problem, however, when similar doses of MTX are administered weekly (Condit, 1960).

There is experimental evidence that corroborates the clinical observation of increased toxicity from prolonged MTX. Chabner and Young (1973) showed that prolonged serum MTX concentrations of greater than 10^{-8} M always resulted in depressed incorporation of [^{3}H]UdR in bone marrow and GI mucosal cells of mice. The dose of MTX is not as important as the duration of the infusion. Goldie *et al.* (1972) did not observe any toxicity if the MTX infusions were 30 hr or less. Toxicity became evident only following infusions of 36 hr or more, irrespective of total dose. Small doses given over 48 hr were much more toxic than larger doses given over considerably shorter periods. It is now well established that for leucovorin to be most effective, it must be given no later than 36–44 hr. These observations are related to the known rapid renal excretion of MTX. At moderate single doses the serum concentration of MTX will fall below the toxic level (10^{-8} M) before the critical duration of exposure is exceeded.

With the use of much higher doses of MTX, stomatitis can become the limiting toxicity, especially in patients who do not receive adequate leucovorin or have a delayed excretion of drug because of renal impairment. In addition, high-dose MTX may result in other GI side effects not observed with the lower doses. Vogler and Jacobs (1971) reported the frequent complaint of anorexia and mild nausea and vomiting following a rapid intravenous infusion of 100–300 mg MTX/M². The leucovorin rescue, which generally prevented the stomatitis, did not influence these new side effects. Similar GI side effects were reported by Pratt *et al.* (1974) following 100–500 mg MTX/kg. They also observed one episode of severe abdominal discomfort during an infusion of 500 mg/kg.

All the patients Rosen *et al.* (1974) treated with 100–750 mg MTX/kg experienced anorexia. Of 87 infusions, 81 resulted in oral mucositis in spite of leucovorin. This was usually evident by day 3 and maximal by day 5, which precedes, and can predict, the subsequent fall in white blood count. In 9 instances, the ulcerations resulted in a secondary oral cellulitis (Rosen *et al.*, 1974). Only 5 of 20 patients with osteogenic sarcoma treated with 1.5–7.5 g/M² by Jaffe *et al.* (1974) developed stomatitis. This difference in frequency of stomatitis may represent the higher doses of leucovorin used by Jaffe and co-workers—9–15 mg/M² i.m. every 6 hr × 12 vs. 9 mg every 6 hr × 12 p.o.

6-Mercaptopurine (6-MP), which is generally administered orally at a dose of 2.5 mg/kg per day, has very minimal GI toxicity (Newton, 1954; Farber, 1954). When the daily dose exceeds 3 mg/kg, anorexia, nausea, vomiting, and stomatitis increase in frequency (Hall *et al.*, 1954). The other clinically used purine analogue, 6-thioguanine, also has a very mild effect on the GI system.

5-Fluorouracil (5-FU), when administered intravenously at 15 mg/kg × 5 days followed by 7.5 mg/kg on alternate days in three large studies, resulted in the following GI toxicity: nausea, 78–90%; vomiting, 50–65%; stomatitis, 63–75%; and diarrhea, 34–85% (Kennedy and Theologides, 1961; Rochlin *et al.*, 1962; Moertel *et al.*, 1964). The GI toxicity is markedly reduced when the drug is given weekly. Only 2 of 67 and 5 of 56 patients who received weekly 15 mg/kg and 20 mg/kg, respectively, developed stomatitis or diarrhea. There was some anorexia and occasional vomiting (Horton *et al.*, 1970).

The major GI toxicity of cytosine arabinoside (Ara-C) is nausea and vomiting, the frequency of which appears to be dose-related, being 19% at 100 mg/M² daily to 40% at 3.5 mg/kg daily (a larger equivalent dose) (Ellison *et al.*, 1968; Davis *et al.*, 1974). Bodey *et al.* (1974), however, found very little GI toxicity in 57 patients who received 200 mg Ara-C/M² per day; 86% had no GI symptoms. When given subcutaneously, 5 mg/kg resulted in 16 of the 18 patients becoming nauseated or vomiting, although no local reaction occurred. The symptoms began 2–4 hr after drug injection, and subsided 3–5 hr later (Savel and Burns, 1969). The recent use of gram doses of Ara-C has surprisingly not resulted in a worsening of the GI symptomatology (personal observation). Mucositis and diarrhea are not observed following Ara-C.

Vinblastine (Vlb), when given in conventional doses of 0.1–0.2 mg/kg i.v. weekly, rarely produces nausea or vomiting (J. M. Hill and Loeb, 1961). A small number of patients will experience a paralytic ileus at this dose (Wright *et al.*, 1963). Nausea and vomiting do occur when the dose is escalated to 0.3 mg/kg or above (Frei *et al.*, 1961). Paralytic ileus, which in itself can be life-threatening, especially in leukopenic patients, occurs more frequently after much larger doses—0.3–0.6 mg/kg. Vomiting did not appear to occur more often at these higher doses (Frost *et al.*, 1962; Samuels and Howe, 1970; Samuels *et al.*, 1975*a, b*).

Vincristine (VCR), which has greater neurotoxicity than vinblastine, can also result in ileus. Constipation and abdominal cramps occurred in 15% and 12% of 103 patients who received from 1 to 7 mg VCR. Diarrhea and vomiting, however, occurred in only 2 patients (D. V. Desai *et al.*, 1970). These abdominal symptoms have been previously documented by Martin (1963) following the same weekly dose; 12 of 19 patients were affected. Other investigations have repeatedly documented the rather consistent occurrence of bowel ileus, constipation, and abdominal pain (Carey *et al.*, 1963; Haggard *et al.*, 1968).

Actinomycin D, when used in the standard dose of 450 mg/M^2 per day×5, results in nausea and vomiting in most patients. The onset is generally a few hours following the infusion, and the effects last for approximately 24 hr (Frei, 1974).

Following the rapid infusion of mithramycin (25–50 μg/kg per day), there is immediate anorexia and nausea, with or without emesis, that persists for several hours. The GI symptoms were noted in 42 (89%) of 47 patients (Kennedy, 1970*a*). Of 99 patients treated with a similar dose, but given over 24 hr, G. J. Hill, II *et al.* (1972) observed severe vomiting in 38 patients and nausea with emesis in 25 patients. Although there was a dramatic decrease in the subsequent coagulopathy and hepatic and renal abnormalities following the same dose when given every other day, the GI effects were the same (Kennedy, 1970*b*). Stomatitis and diarrhea have been reported in less than 10% of patients treated with mithramycin (Brown and Kennedy, 1965; Ream *et al.*, 1968).

The GI manifestations of bleomycin, 15–25 mg/M^2 weekly or twice a week, are anorexia, nausea, vomiting, and mucositis. The reported frequency varies somewhat, but ranges between 5 and 30%. It is often part of the generalized hyperpyrexia syndrome, and is rarely a cause of cessation of therapy (Blum *et al.*, 1973; Mosher *et al.*, 1972; Ohnuma *et al.*, 1972; Yagoda *et al.*, 1972). There is apparently no greater GI toxicity from 30 units of bleomycin given in 24-hr infusions for 5 continuous days (Samuels *et al.*, 1975*a, b*).

Most patients who receive daunomycin, 1 mg/kg per day×5, develop nausea and vomiting. Some patients have complained of abdominal pain and diarrhea (Bornstein *et al.*, 1969). GI toxicity appears to be less following lower doses, 25 mg/M^2 per day×3; 7 of 67 patients developed stomatitis only (Holton *et al.*, 1969).

Adriamycin, which differs from daunomycin by a hydroxyl group, results in nausea in most patients and vomiting in 50–60%. Erythema and ulceration of the buccal mucosa occur in approximately 75% of patients (Wang *et al.*, 1971; Tan *et al.*, 1973; Blum and Carter, 1974; Bonadonna *et al.*, 1975; Gottlieb *et al.*, 1973).

cis-Platinum, irrespective of dose or schedule, produces nausea in all patients and vomiting in most (Higsby *et al.*, 1973, 1974; Talley *et al.*, 1973; Ellerby *et al.*,

1974). These symptoms generally begin 2–5 hr after the injection, and rarely continue beyond 4 hr (Ellerby *et al.*, 1974).

The nitrosourea compounds all produce nausea and vomiting in most patients. CCNU, 100–130 mg/M^2 i.v. every 6 weeks, resulted in GI toxicity in all 141 patients to whom it was given (H. H. Hansen *et al.*, 1971; Klaassen and Rapp, 1974; Stolinsky *et al.*, 1975; Hoogstraten *et al.*, 1973). Methyl-CCNU, when given at doses above 170 mg/M^2 p.o., produced these same GI effects consistently (Young *et al.*, 1973). BCNU has identical GI toxicity (DeVita *et al.*, 1965; Young *et al.*, 1971; Godfrey and Rentschler, 1973). The nausea and vomiting generally commence a few hours after drug administration and last 4–6 hr.

Most patients who take procarbazine, 100–300 mg/day, experience nausea and vomiting (75–95%). It generally occurs during the first few days of therapy, and often lessens despite continued treatment (Mathé *et al.*, 1963; Brunner and Young, 1965; M. M. Hansen *et al.*, 1966; Stolinsky *et al.*, 1970; Martz *et al.*, 1963). If vomiting persists, dose reduction is generally effective in decreasing symptoms (Todd, 1965; Samuels *et al.*, 1967). Stomatitis is very rare, occurring in only 3 of 50 patients (Stolinsky *et al.*, 1970).

Although nausea and vomiting occur in approximately 25% of patients who take 25–50 mg hydroxyurea/kg per day (Thurman *et al.*, 1963), this effect is generally very mild (Fishbein *et al.*, 1964).

Between half and two-thirds of patients who receive L-asparaginase experience nausea and vomiting shortly after the infusion (Haskell *et al.*, 1969*a*, *b*; Pratt *et al.*, 1970; Oettgen *et al.*, 1970). These GI symptoms may also be part of a generalized hypersensitivity reaction that occurs after repeated doses (Oettgen *et al.*, 1970).

Nausea and vomiting occur in nearly all patients who receive daily imidazole carboxamide (DTIC) (Falkson *et al.*, 1972; Costanza *et al.*, 1972; Gerner and Moore, 1973; G. J. Hill, II, *et al.*, 1974). The symptoms begin shortly after the first infusion and tend to decrease in severity with each successive injection, disappearing by the 4th or 5th day (Frei *et al.*, 1972).

Streptozotocin, a chemotherapeutic agent that may be limited in clinical usefulness to the treatment of the islet cell carcinomas, produces nausea and vomiting in nearly all patients (87%). Symptoms usually appear 1–4 hr after drug infusion. Patient tolerance tends to improve with each succeeding dose of a 5-day treatment schedule (Schein *et al.*, 1974; Broder and Carter, 1973).

The common antiemetics do little to ameliorate chemotherapeutic-induced nausea and vomiting. Cannabis (marijuana) has recently been shown to provide complete protection against these untoward GI symptoms (Sallan *et al.*, 1975). This finding is most encouraging, and, if cultivated properly, would eliminate a most uncomfortable side effect of chemotherapy.

3. Cutaneous Reactions

Cutaneous reactions are of clinical interest, but seldom a cause of great concern, with the exception of the severe local tissue necrosis that may occur if certain drugs extravasate from the infusion site.

Nitrogen mustard (Wintrobe and Huguley, 1948), adriamycin (Tan *et al.*, 1973; Wang *et al.*, 1971), daunomycin (Holton *et al.*, 1969; Bornstein *et al.*, 1969), actinomycin D (Frei, 1974), vinblastine (Wright *et al.*, 1963), and vincristine (Selawry and Hananian, 1963) all result in severe local reaction if they infiltrate the local tissues. Occasionally, the area becomes very necrotic, resulting in a fibrotic contracture that limits joint motion. Even without extravasation, nitrogen mustard (Jacobs *et al.*, 1968; Mrazek and Wachowski, 1955; Jacobson *et al.*, 1946), vinblastine (J. M. Hill and Loeb, 1961; Warwick *et al.*, 1961), mithramycin (G. J. Hill, II, *et al.*, 1972), adriamycin (Etcubanas and Wilbur, 1974), DTIC (Falson *et al.*, 1972), and BCNU (DeVita *et al.*, 1965; Young *et al.*, 1971) can produce local pain in the veins into which they are infused, occasionally leading to a local thrombophlebitis.

Bleomycin can produce a morbiliform rash, urticaria, erythematous swelling, or pruritis within $\frac{1}{2}$–3 hr following intravenous or intramuscular administration. Hyperpigmentation and hyperkeratosis, especially of the palms and fingers, tend to develop as the treatments are continued, being present in 75% of patients who have received 400–500 mg total of the drug (Blum *et al.*, 1973; Mosher *et al.*, 1972; Yagoda *et al.*, 1972; Ohnuma *et al.*, 1972).

Hyperpigmentation of the skin, which is indistinguishable from the melanosis of Addison's disease, occurs in some patients who have been treated with busulfan for long periods (Galton, 1953; Petrakis *et al.*, 1954; Greig, 1956; Haut *et al.*, 1961; Kyle *et al.*, 1961; R. G. Desai, 1965). Skin biopsy has not demonstrated an increase in number of melanocytes, but the increased pigment was dopa-positive, and therefore probably melanin (Kyle *et al.*, 1961). Vivacqua *et al.* (1967) studied the pituitary–adrenal axis of the two patients who developed hyperpigmentation while on long-term busulfan. One patient had agnogenic myeloid metaplasia, the other polycythemia vera. There was evidence of adrenal insufficiency secondary to reduced pituitary reserve of ACTH. This is the opposite of what one would have thought if the hyperpigmentation was secondary to increased ACTH levels.

Hyperpigmentation has been described following cyclophosphamide (Thurman *et al.*, 1964), actinomycin (Frei, 1974; Epstein and Lutzner, 1969), 5-FU (Rochlin *et al.*, 1962; Kennedy and Theologides, 1961), and adriamycin (O'Bryan *et al.*, 1973; Rothberg *et al.*, 1974), but this effect is apparently not common. Occasionally, the hyperpigmentation following 5-FU may be of the epidermis overlying veins used for repeated infusions (Hrushesky, 1976).

Maculopapular dermatitis has also been noted following chlorambucil (Ezdinli and Stutzman, 1965; Koler and Forsgren, 1958), melphalan (Hoogstraten *et al.*, 1969), hydroxyurea (Thurman *et al.*, 1963), and CCNU (Stolinsky *et al.*, 1975), but it is very uncommon.

Actinomycin D has been associated with an erythematous rash and subsequent folliculitis in 9 of 11 patients (Epstein and Lutzner, 1969), which is the postulated mechanism of hair loss following this drug.

A maculopapular generalized skin reaction can follow the use of MTX, whether the drug is given orally in conventional doses (Lamb *et al.*, 1964; Berlin *et al.*, 1963; Brewer *et al.*, 1964) or in high intravenous doses that require leucovorin rescue (Jaffe *et al.*, 1974; Djerassi *et al.*, 1972; Pratt *et al.*, 1974). The frequency of the erythematous rash increases when the MTX is given by infusion over 48 hr, as compared with bolus administration (Djerassi *et al.*, 1967). Biopsy of the lesion demonstrated the pathology to be that of a vasculitis (Capizzi *et al.*, 1970). Occasionally, a very life-threatening bullous eruption has been reported. One patient with osteogenic sarcoma was receiving high doses of MTX with leucovorin rescue (Rosen *et al.*, 1974); the other was a psoriatic patient taking daily MTX (Lyell, 1967). A violaceous, blanching, painful erythematous reaction localized to areas of a recent but resolved solar burn did develop in a patient 24 hr after 100 mg MTX/kg i.v. Previous radiation areas were spared, and other toxicity was absent (Corder and Stone, 1976).

Approximately 10–20% of patients receiving 5-FU will develop during the later weeks of therapy a dry scaling form of dermatitis. This dermatitis may also affect the mucous membranes to a certain extent, often promoting the subsequent development of epistaxis (Kennedy and Theologides, 1961; Weiss *et al.*, 1961; Ansfield *et al.*, 1962; Ivy, 1962; Rochlin *et al.*, 1962; Moertel *et al.*, 1964; Greenwald, 1975).

Urticaria, a manifestation of the allergic reaction to L-asparaginase, occurs in approximately one-third of patients, generally after several doses have been administered (Tallal *et al.*, 1970; Oettgen *et al.*, 1970; Haskell *et al.*, 1969*a, b*; Killander *et al.*, 1976).

A facial flush is very common immediately following the infusion of mithramy- cin (Brown and Kennedy, 1965), and only rarely follows adriamycin (Benjamin *et al.*, 1974), BCNU (DeVita *et al.*, 1965; Young *et al.*, 1971), and DTIC (Falkson *et al.*, 1972). The mithramycin dermatologic reaction is quite unique, consisting of an initial pink flush of the face and neck, which then progresses to a deeper plethora, facial edema, and coarsening of facial features (Brown and Kennedy, 1965; Ream *et al.*, 1968; Kennedy, 1970*a, b*).

Procarbazine is associated very rarely with a skin eruption. Of 40 patients treated with 300 mg orally (Todd, 1965), 2 developed a punctate erythematous rash on the legs. Of the 44 patients Mathé *et al.* (1963) treated, 2 had symptoms of a pruritic dermatologic reaction. Of the 15 patients to whom Brunner gave procarbazine, in only 2 was a subsequent dermatitis noted (Brunner and Young, 1965). Dermatitis was present in 1 of 50 patients that Stolinsky reported. It was severe enough, however, to force discontinuation of therapy (Stolinsky *et al.*, 1970). Urticaria has been recorded twice (Martz *et al.*, 1963; Jones *et al.*, 1972). Jones also reported a second patient who developed arthralgia and a generalized erythematous maculopapular eruption, which recurred when the patient was later rechallenged with procarbazine. An acute reaction following the intravenous administration of procarbazine, which consisted in temperature elevation to 40°C and generalized rash, developed in 3 of 35 patients. This acute reaction did not recur when the drug was readministered orally (M. M. Hansen *et al.*, 1966), and has not been reported by others following oral use of this drug.

An interesting syndrome has occurred following the ingestion of alcohol by patients who are taking procarbazine. Mathé *et al.* (1963) first noted that 5 of their patients complained of a "flush syndrome" when they drank wine following the hydrazine injection; there was a transient but marked facial erythema. Todd

(1965) reported the same syndrome in 2 of his 40 patients who were receiving oral hydrazine. It is thought that procarbazine may prevent intermediate metabolism of alcohol in some patients, allowing the buildup of acetaldehyde, which, in fact, is the toxin responsible for this syndrome.

Icterus does occur with the chronic use of 6-MP (Farber, 1954). It is a consequence of the hepatic toxicity of this drug, which is discussed in Section 6.

On occasion, radiation treatments are not interrupted for the administration of chemotherapy. Certain patients treated either concurrently or sequentially may develop a severe local inflammatory response of the skin exposed to radiation. The first drug with which this response was observed was actinomycin D (D'Angio, 1962, 1969). Recently, this same phenomenon has been seen with adriamycin when it is given in conjunction with radiotherapy (Cassady et al., 1975). A strange acute erythema and hyperpigmentation reaction may appear at cutaneous sites that had prior exposure to irradiation. This phenomenon is often referred to as a *recall reaction*. Actinomycin is again the main offender (Liebner, 1962; Donaldson et al., 1974; D'Angio, 1969; Tefft et al., 1976); however, it has also occurred following adriamycin (Cassady et al., 1975; Donaldson et al., 1974; Etcubanas and Wilbur, 1974; Wang et al., 1971) and 5-FU (Kennedy and Theologides, 1961).

Cyclophosphamide generally has no skin toxicity; however, Santos et al. (1972) did describe 6 of 12 patients who developed a patchy morbiliform erythematous nonpruritic rash 1–4 days following 60 mg/kg per day×4 in preparation for marrow transplants. Urticaria has also been described following cyclophosphamide (Lakin and Cahili, 1976).

4. Fever

Fever that is associated with leukopenia and infection is often an early manifestation of drug toxicity. Fever may also be part of generalized acute drug reaction and unrelated to leukopenia.

Rosen (Rosen et al., 1974) noted that his patients who received MTX, 100–750 mg/kg i.v. over 4 hr, had a 0.5–1.0°C temperature elevation that occurred on days 1–3 after every infusion. When the dose was much lower but infused over the same time (100–300 mg/M^2), only 1 of 113 patients developed a fever (Vogler and Jacobs, 1971). Djerassi made no mention of fever following the 6-hr infusion of from 1 to 24 g MTX (Djerassi et al., 1972). Pratt did not report fever after a similar infusion of 50–500 mg/kg (Pratt et al., 1974), nor did Jaffe after 1.5–7.5 g MTX (Jaffe et al., 1974). The most likely explanation for no reported temperature elevations following MTX in these studies is that since elevation is so mild and asymptomatic, many observers did not obtain temperatures following the MTX infusion as Rosen did.

Hyperpyrexia of a mild degree did comprise part of the symptom complex of patients who developed MTX pulmonary toxicity. This hyperpyrexia, however, generally occurred after rather prolonged MTX use (Everts et al., 1973). Temperature elevation is not, however, part of the insidious onset of MTX hepatitis or cirrhosis (Hersh *et al.*, 1966; Weinstein *et al.*, 1973), nor is fever present with the syndrome of mercaptopurine hepatotoxicity (Shorey *et al.*, 1968).

The only alkylating agent that is documented to cause a febrile reaction is nitrogen mustard. Dameshek reported in his superb evaluation of the effects of nitrogen mustard in 1949 that 6.8% of the 50 patients had fever and 12% chills (Dameshek *et al.*, 1949). Large intravenous boluses of cytoxan, 60–120 mg/kg, were not associated with hyperpyrexia (Buckner *et al.*, 1974*a*, *b*).

Without equivocation, the hyperpyrexia following bleomycin is the highest (103–105°F), and is often associated with violent chills. The fever generally develops between 4 and 10 hr following either intramuscular or intravenous administration of the drug, and can persist for up to 48 hr. It occurs in up to 60% of patients who receive bleomycin. Fortunately, it tends to lessen in severity with successive doses (Mosher *et al.*, 1972; Yagoda *et al.*, 1972; Ohnuma *et al.*, 1972; Samuels *et al.*, 1975*a*, *b*). Although it generally does not represent any known long-term toxicity, the 4 patients who have succumbed to an acute fulminate reaction all had profound hyperpyrexia. In addition, they had accompanying hypotension and irreversible cardiorespiratory collapse. All these 4 patients had lymphoma, and had received a dose of 25 mg/M² or greater (Blum *et al.*, 1973).

Mithramycin, when administered daily, 25 μg/kg per day $\times$ 5, produces a mild febrile reaction in 75–89% of patients, with the temperature rising to 99.5–101°F, with an occasional rise to 102–103°F (Brown and Kennedy, 1965; Kennedy, 1970*b*). Because the daily dose schedule proved too toxic, an every-other-day dose schedule is now used. When mithramycin is administered in this fashion, the febrile reaction has decreased to a frequency of 13% or less (Kennedy, 1970*b*; G. J. Hill, II *et al.*, 1972).

A rare fever and chill reaction has been reported following adriamycin and daunomycin. The reaction is unassociated with any catastrophic event (Bonadonna *et al.*, 1969, 1970; Benjamin *et al.*, 1974; Evans *et al.*, 1974). Following intravenous procarbazine, a temperature elevation to 40°C associated with a generalized delicate rash was reported to have occurred in 3 patients after the 5th, 5th, and 6th dose, respectively (M. M. Hansen *et al.*, 1966). Jones reported that 1 patient who developed eosinophilia, pulmonary infiltrates, and a rash also had the sudden onset of a fever and rigor (Jones *et al.*, 1972).

Although a febrile reaction of 1°C or more has been associated with L-asparaginase therapy in 40–66% of patients, seldom is it as severe as that seen following bleomycin (Haskell *et al.*, 1969*a*, *b*; Oettgen *et al.*, 1970; Pratt *et al.*, 1970).

DTIC has also been reported to result in mild fever (Falkson *et al.*, 1972; Gottlieb and Serpick, 1971).

5. Alopecia

Alopecia is a bothersome side effect of some chemotherapeutic agents only in the sense that it tends to be a constant reminder to the patient and his family and friends that he has cancer. The emotional consequences can be very great in some patients; however, most accept this side effect as inconsequential compared with the other adverse effects the drug may also produce, mainly nausea, vomiting, loss of sensation, muscular weakness, cardiac damage, and the ever-lurking threat of leukopenia and thrombocytopenia, which can allow devastating infection or hemorrhage to occur.

Cyclophosphamide is the only alkylating agent that results in significant hair loss. With the use of high intravenous doses, 60–120 mg/kg, all patients experience loss of all scalp hair (Buckner *et al.*, 1974*a*, *b*). When the dose is reduced to 100–300 mg/day i.v., only approximately 20% of patients experience this untoward effect (Wall and Conrad, 1961). The chronic daily administration of 100 mg orally results only in thinning of the hair, not total loss (Fosdick *et al.*, 1968). In one study that compared vinblastine, 0.15 mg/kg per week i.v., with cyclophosphamide, 2 mg/kg per day, for the treatment of lymphoma, alopecia developed in 5 of 50 patients following vinblastine, and in 4 of 46 patients receiving cyclophosphamide (Stutzman *et al.*, 1966). The hair loss is never permanent, and in fact the hair generally regrows despite continued therapy.

Nitrogen mustard (Wintrobe and Huguley, 1948; Dameshek *et al.*, 1949), melphalan (Frick *et al.*, 1968; Fisher *et al.*, 1975), busulfan (Haut *et al.*, 1961; Louis *et al.*, 1956), and chlorambucil (Masterson *et al.*, 1960) do not result in alopecia.

Alopecia following the chronic use of MTX does occur. It is generally patchy or a diffuse thinning, often not noticed by the casual observer (Lamb *et al.*, 1964). Since the hair bulb has a cell turnover rate of close to 24 hr (Van Scott *et al.*, 1963), MTX can temporarily inhibit cellular activity (Van Scott *et al.*, 1957). As a consequence, a constriction in the hair shaft results as a documentation of the MTX inhibition. This constriction renders the shaft weak, and as the hair resumes growth, it may break, leaving the patient with patchy hair loss or thinning. Hair loss was not mentioned in four recent reports using high-dose MTX and leucovorin rescue (Djerassi *et al.*, 1967, 1972; Vogler and Jacobs, 1971; Rosen *et al.*, 1974).

5-FU produces varying degrees of alopecia in 5–57% of patients who begin the 5-day regimen of 15 mg/kg i.v. (Ansfield *et al.*, 1962; Moertel *et al.*, 1964; Weiss *et al.*, 1961; Kennedy and Theologides, 1961). It invariably occurs at the onset of therapy, is seldom total, and regrows despite persistent 5-FU (Kennedy and Theologides, 1961; Rochlin *et al.*, 1962).

The vinca alkaloids may cause transient loss of hair, which also regrows during continued therapy. With the use of standard doses of vinblastine (0.1–0.15 mg/kg every 1–3 days), 2 of 120 (Warwick *et al.*, 1961), 3 of 65 (J. M. Hill and Leob, 1961), 14 of 265 (Wright *et al.*, 1963), 5 of 33 (Frost *et al.*, 1962), and 2 of 112 patients (Frei *et al.*, 1961) developed alopecia. Samuels noted significant hair loss in 15 of 32 patients who received 0.35–0.40 mg/kg every 3 weeks i.v. (Samuels and Howe, 1970).

Patients treated with vincristine develop alopecia slightly more often than do patients who receive vinblastine: 9 of 19 (Martin and Compston, 1963), 12 of 26 (Carey *et al.*, 1963), 17 of 62 (Shaw and Bruner, 1964), 21 of 94 (Haggard *et al.*, 1968), and 12 of 103 (D. V. Desai *et al.*, 1970).

As a consequence of the folliculitis that some persons develop following actinomycin D, mild hair loss may result (Epstein and Lutzner, 1969; Frei, 1974).

Hair loss follows chronic use of bleomycin. Initially, it is usually very slight, but as repeated courses of treatment continue, nearly complete alopecia is seen (Ohnuma *et al.*, 1972; Yagoda *et al.*, 1972). Often, the higher the dose used, the sooner and more complete is the alopecia (Samuels *et al.*, 1975a). It is not unusual for new but darker hair to reappear 2–3 months later (Yagoda *et al.*, 1972).

Of the anthracycline antibiotic tumor agents, adriamycin results in alopecia in more than 80% of patients treated (Tan *et al.*, 1973; Wang *et al.*, 1971; Bonadonna *et al.*, 1970, 1975), which is considerably greater than the incidence observed following daunomycin. Although alopecia has been reported following daunomycin (Bornstein *et al.*, 1969), some observers have not noticed the hair loss (Holton *et al.*, 1969).

BCNU has also been associated with alopecia (Young *et al.*, 1971). None of the other agents covered in this review is associated with alopecia.

6. Hepatic Toxicity

Hepatic toxicity from chemotherapeutic agents ranges from only transient enzyme elevations, as seen with cytosine arabinoside (Bodey *et al.*, 1974), DTIC (Nathanson *et al.*, 1971; Gottlieb and Serpick, 1971), hydroxyurea (Thurman *et al.*, 1963), and the nitrosoureas (Hoogstraten *et al.*, 1973; Young *et al.*, 1971, 1973), to the permanent cirrhotic changes that follow prolonged MTX use (Podurgiel *et al.*, 1973) and necrosis subsequent to 6-MP (Clark *et al.*, 1960).

Hepatic necrosis was documented as early as 1954 following 6-MP in mice and rats (Philips *et al.*, 1957). During that same year, Farber reported 6 patients who became icteric while taking 6-MP. In each instance, it subsided when the drug was withheld (Farber, 1954). Philips *et al.* (1957) also noted that dogs given 6-MP did not develop much liver necrosis, but instead the bile canaliculi were engorged, suggestive of cholestasis. In 1959, McIlvanie and MacCarthy (1959) reported 4 patients with leukemia who became jaundiced after receiving dosages of 6-MP that were greater than the recommended dose of 2.5 mg/kg. The jaundice promptly cleared with discontinuance of 6-MP. Histological examination of two liver specimens demonstrated pronounced bile stasis without focal necrosis, reminiscent of biliary stasis secondary to chlorpromazine (McIlvanie and MacCarthy, 1959). Others have subsequently reported the association of chronic 6-MP use in leukemic patients with jaundice and liver histology showing bile stasis and occasional hepatic necrosis (Clark *et al.*, 1960; Einhorn and Davidsohn, 1964). This toxic effect is not limited to patients with leukemia; it has also been observed in patients with chronic active hepatitis (Krawitt *et al.*, 1967), membranous glomerulonephritis, and systematic lupus erythematosus (Shorey *et al.*, 1968).

The serum glutamicoxolate transminase (SGOT) and alkaline phosphatase are generally only minimally elevated. Although total bilirubin as high as 26.8 mg/100 ml has been reported, the values are generally between 3 and 7 mg/100 ml (Einhorn and Davidsohn, 1964; Shorey *et al.*, 1968).

Azathioprine, the active metabolite of which is 6-MP, has been associated with reversible elevations of SGOT and alkaline phosphatase in patients with "autoimmune" diseases (Cordley et al., 1966) and renal transplants (Starzl et al., 1971; Zarday et al., 1972).

Shortly after the clinical use of MTX in childhood leukemia, there was a suggestion that this drug may lead to hepatic fibrosis (Colsky et al., 1955). A review of 333 cases of leukemia by R. V. P. Hutter and co-authors in 1960 noted that hepatic fibrosis was present in nearly 80% of patients who had received antifolates, steroids, and antipurines, as compared with its presence in only 30% of patients who had not received these drugs (R. V. P. Hutter et al., 1960). Since 6-MP had not been shown to lead to hepatic fibrosis, the finding was due either to antifolates or to the combination with 6-MP.

It is well established that the prolonged use of MTX in patients with psoriasis can lead to a range of hepatotoxicity culminating in cirrhosis in a small but significant number of patients (Coe and Bull, 1968; Epstein and Croft, 1969; Muller et al., 1969; Almeyda et al., 1971; Millward-Sadler and Ryan, 1974; Reese et al., 1974). Dahl et al. (1971) reported that of 37 patients with psoriasis who received continuous low-dose MTX, 19% developed cirrhosis, 27% hepatic fibrosis, and 46% minor abnormalities, which consisted of fatty change, polymorphonuclear cell infiltration, and extensive hepatic nuclei vacuolation. Only 3 patients (8%) had normal hepatic histology. The progression to cirrhosis appears to be related not only to the total dose administered, but also to whether MTX is given intermittently or chronically. Dahl et al. (1972) found that the prevalence of cirrhosis and fibrosis was significantly higher in those patients who received frequent small doses of MTX than in those who had the same total dose, but given intermittently. A similar observation was reported from the Mayo Clinic in 1973 (Podurgiel et al., 1973).

In the group of 22 patients treated by Dahl et al. (1972) with frequent small doses of MTX (2.5 mg p.o. daily 2–5 days/week), the mean duration of treatment in patients with nonspecific histology was 11.6 ± 2.4 months; in those with hepatic fibrosis, it was 33.3 ± 7.1 months; in those with cirrhosis, it was 48.3 ± 6.7 months. Each successive group was significantly different from the next worse histologic group: $P < 0.05$ and < 0.001, respectively. There was no cirrhosis encountered in the 14 patients who received intermittent large doses (10–25 mg p.o. or i.m. every 1–4 weeks). Two did have hepatic fibrosis, however. Although the hepatic enzymes are of little value in predicting the amount of liver damage (Podurgiel et al., 1973; Roenigk et al., 1971), the clinical observation that all patients who had hepatic fibrosis or cirrhosis also had hepatomegaly was noted by Dahl et al. (1972).

The international cooperative study that examined a study population of 550 psoriatic patients receiving MTX corroborated the earlier association of hepatic fibrosis and daily MTX. Of the 247 patients whose liver biopsies revealed fibrosis or cirrhosis, 88 had no history or laboratory abnormalities to suggest any hepatic injury. Another 69 patients had only one abnormality, and the results suggested that the BSP retention test was perhaps the most sensitive indication (Weinstein et al., 1973).

Elevations of hepatic enzymes are quite common following the initial onset of therapy with MTX. In 1965, Hersh *et al.* (1965) evaluated 10 patients receiving 10–22 mg/M^2 per day × 5 and 12 patients receiving 25 mg/M^2 per 4 days × 6 weeks. With each successive course of MTX, the mean serum glutamicpyruvictransaminase (SGPT), SGOT, and lactic dehydrogenase (LDH) rose abnormally higher. The values in those patients who were treated daily were greater than in those who received their therapy intermittently. All abnormalities resolved completely within 1 month after cessation of therapy. Of 10 patients who had liver biopsies performed during the period of elevated hepatic enzymes, 6 had a partial inflammation, 3 had fatty degeneration, and 1 was normal. There was no necrosis. No patient in the study had any signs or symptoms to suggest hepatic toxicity (Hersh *et al.*, 1965). These clinical and pathological findings of MTX hepatotoxicity are in distinct contrast to those secondary to 6-MP, which is in large part a cholestatic process resulting in elevations of bilirubin. Bilirubin is seldom elevated in MTX hepatotoxicity, although it does occur (Jaffe *et al.*, 1974; Rosen *et al.*, 1974).

Toxic hepatitis with jaundice was reported, however, in 2 of 10 patients who were treated with 3-day infusions of MTX, 96 mg/M^2. When 180 mg/M^2 was given over 4 hr on 2 consecutive days, there was an elevation of SGOT in 2 of 4 patients that did not return to normal for 2 weeks (Djerassi *et al.*, 1967). Only 1 of 156 patients treated with MTX, 100–300 mg/M^2 p.o. in divided doses over 24 hr, followed by leucovorin rescue, had an SGOT elevation (Vogler and Jacobs, 1971). However, with the use of much larger doses of MTX, 100–750 mg/kg i.v., it is the rule to have an elevated SGOT that returns to normal in all patients by day 14 (Rosen *et al.*, 1974; Pratt *et al.*, 1974). Rosen *et al.* (1974) also noted that on 11 occasions, when the SGOT exceeded 200 U following the MTX, there was also an elevation of bilirubin, 1.6–6.4 mg/100 ml, which returned to normal values along with the SGOT. The duration of the MTX infusion appeared to correlate more with the degree of SGOT elevation than did the total dose given. This may represent the greater hepatic damage following prolonged serum concentrations of MTX analogous to the bone marrow and GI toxicity that increases with prolonged serum concentrations of this drug.

Mithramycin is undoubtedly the most acutely hepatotoxic chemotherapeutic agent currently in use. Patients who are treated with 25–50 μg/kg per day × 5 all experience elevations of hepatic enzymes. Only approximately 50% of the patients have a modest elevation of alkaline phosphatase, but 100% have increases in SGOT, SGPT, and LDH, often into the thousands. The greatest increase in LDH has been 63,000 International Units/liter. Bilirubin elevation does not occur.

The abnormalities begin with the first 24 hr, reaching a peak often by 48 hr, and then return to normal levels by 4–21 days. The hepatic histology during this time is that of acute liver necrosis. There is vacuolization of liver cells and fatty metamorphosis. Normal liver cells can be found, but are unusual (Brown and Kennedy, 1965; Kennedy, 1970*b*; Ream *et al.*, 1968). Probably also as a result of the acute liver necrosis, clotting factors II, V, VII, and X are depressed (Monto *et al.*, 1969), as well as the prothrombin time being elevated. This effect plus the marked thrombocytopenia are major factors leading to the unique coagulopathy that occurs following mithramycin therapy. When the dose is given every other day for 3 doses, there is a marked reduction in hepatic toxicity and complete disappearance of the hemorrhagic diathesis. The LDH continues to become elevated, but generally not above 2000 International Units/liter, which is the recommended elevation not to be exceeded.

A mild elevation of all liver enzymes and bilirubin occurs in approximately 50% of patients who receive L-asparaginase, irrespective of dose, and whether it is given daily or weekly. In addition, there is generally a decrease in clotting factors II, V, VII, IX, and X; hypoalbumina; and hypocholesterolemia, presumably from lack of hepatic production. None of the abnormalities is permanent (Oettgen *et al.*, 1970; Haskell *et al.*, 1969a, b; Pratt *et al.*, 1970).

Two patients had liver biopsies during their therapy. One showed the effects of a toxic hepatitis with some fatty changes; the other consisted of fatty degeneration (Haskell *et al.*, 1969a, b). Two other patients who died during therapy had a similar histological pattern (Pratt *et al.*, 1970). In one other patient, a subsequent biopsy following cessation of therapy did show improvement (Haskell *et al.*, 1969a, b). In two studies, however, fatty metamorphosis was still present in 40 of 55 (Oettgen *et al.*, 1970) and 27 of 31 patients (Pratt and Johnson, 1971), many of whom had not had L-asparaginase for months.

Alkylating agents do not characteristically have hepatic toxicity as a side effect. However, one patient who was receiving chlorambucil, 14 mg/day, did develop an allergic drug reaction that consisted of a rash, enlarged nodes, jaundice, and a tender liver, all of which subsided with discontinuance of therapy. The signs and symptoms abruptly returned when rechallenged with the drug at a later date (Koler and Forsgren, 1958). One autopsy study of 6 patients who were taking chlorambucil did show hepatic findings consistent with a toxic hepatitis (Amromin *et al.*, 1962). But patients who come to autopsy undoubtedly have many other possible causes for hepatitis. Hepatitis is not a common problem of the many patients with chronic lymphocytic leukemia who are taking chlorambucil.

One patient receiving cyclophosphamide had a transient rise in hepatic enzymes that abated with discontinuance of the drug (Fernbach *et al.*, 1962).

Streptozotocin will cause elevations of liver enzymes 1 or 2 days following the completion of a 5-day treatment. There are no symptoms, and prompt return to normal always occurs. Liver histology has failed to show any abnormalities (Schein *et al.*, 1974).

7. Pulmonary Toxicity

Pulmonary toxicity is not a common side effect of most chemotherapeutic agents; however, three of these drugs can produce devastating damage to the lungs.

Bleomycin does cause significant radiographic and physiological changes in approximately 10% of patients who receive this drug (Blum *et al.*, 1973). Anatomical changes were found by Luna *et al.* (1972) to be present in 12 of 35 (30%)

patients who had received bleomycin. These changes were consistent with those found due to many other agents that afflict the pulmonary parenchyma: fibrinous exudate, hyaline membranes, and interstitial and intraalveolar fibrosis. Similar findings have been seen by others (Bedrossian et al., 1973; Yagoda et al., 1972).

Radiographic findings routinely show a diffuse, occasionally miliary, but generally interstitial infiltrate located predominantly basally (Yagoda et al., 1972; Blum et al., 1973; Pascual et al., 1973). Pulmonary function is often abnormal, with the forced vital capacity and diffusing capacity being decreased (Mosher et al., 1972; Pascaul et al., 1973). In a few patients, these physiological abnormalities did not progress with subsequent doses, and, in fact, returned to normal in 2 of 11 patients (Mosher et al., 1972). The pulmonary function abnormalities tend to occur before radiographic evidence of lung damage has taken place. Of the 14 patients followed by Mosher and co-workers with serial pulmonary function tests, 11 developed significant abnormalities that were not associated with total dose. Permanent parenchymal damage can result, however. The risk of developing this complication is about 3–5% with cumulative doses below 450 mg. There is a definite increase in frequency that approaches 20% at totals exceeding this dosage (Blum et al., 1973).

Death from the pulmonary damage has been reported in at least 12 patients (Blum et al., 1973; Samuels et al., 1976). It is therefore recommended that a total cumulative dose of 450–500 mg not be exceeded.

There are no consistently effective ways of treating the pulmonary damage once it is present. Anecdotal reports of the beneficial use of corticosteroids in some patients with pulmonary toxicity from bleomycin have appeared (Yagoda et al., 1972; Ohnuma et al., 1972). Steroids may be helpful if started at the first evidence of pulmonary toxicity in conjunction with discontinuing the bleomycin.

Since the first description of interstitial pulmonary fibrosis following busulfan therapy by Oliner et al. (1961), there have been 19 other cases reported (Leake et al., 1963; Koss et al., 1965; Harrold, 1966; Smalley and Wall, 1966; Heard and Cooke, 1968; Min and Gyorkey, 1968; Littler et al., 1969; Feingold and Koss, 1969; Burns et al., 1970; Castleman and McNeely, 1971; Kirshner and Esterly, 1971; Podoll and Winkler, 1974). Of these 19 patients, 16 had respiratory insufficiency. The symptomatology in almost all patients consisted of dyspnea, cough, and fever. On examination, there was generally skin hyperpigmentation and pulmonary rales. Chest X-rays demonstrated bilateral infiltrates suggestive of an interstitial process, although they were not necessarily diffuse. Biopsy or autopsy showed an interstitial fibrotic process, occasionally a vasculitis, and rarely small areas of calcification.

The duration of therapy ranged from 13 to 123 months, with a mean of 50 months. Death was often due to respiratory failure; survival from onset of symptoms ranged from a few days to 24 months, with a mean of 4.6 months. Corticosteroid therapy did not appear to be beneficial.

Methotrexate pulmonary toxicity was suddenly brought into focus in 1969 when Acute Leukemia Group B (1969) reported that 38 of their 93 children who were receiving maintenance MTX developed a pneumonitis, of which 3 died.

Since then, there have been 25 cases reported (Clarysse *et al.*, 1969; I. R. Schwartz and Kajani, 1969; J. H. Robertson, 1970; G. C. Goldman and Moschella, 1971; Filip *et al.*, 1971; Pasquinucci *et al.*, 1971; Whitcomb *et al.*, 1972; Everts *et al.*, 1973). Although most patients had acute lymphocytic leukemia, 1 had oat-cell carcinoma of the lung (Whitcomb *et al.*, 1972), 1 pemphigus vulgaris, 1 mycosis fungoides (G. C. Goldman and Moschella, 1971), and 1 psoriasis (Filip *et al.*, 1971).

The syndrome was of an acute onset, often within days to a few months from the onset of MTX therapy. There was marked dyspnea, nonproductive cough, low-grade temperature, and cyanosis. Dry rales were always present on chest auscultation. Eosinophilia was present in nearly 75% of patients. Radiographic examination generally demonstrated a confluent interstitial pattern with rare nodular densities up to 0.4 mm (Everts *et al.*, 1973).

Although there have been dramatic improvements in symptoms and arterial oxygenation within hours following corticosteroids (Whitcomb *et al.*, 1972; I. R. Schwartz and Kajani, 1969; G. C. Goldman and Moschella, 1971), even without any specific therapy, the symptoms and radiographic changes generally resolve within 1 week. Unlike the pulmonary toxicity from melphalan and bleomycin, patients seldom succumb from their pulmonary insult.

Biopsy specimens show filling of alveolar spaces filled with large mononuclear cells, arteriolar cuffing with polymorphonuclear cells, and small cellular nodular aggregates. Occasionally, there has been a mild interstitial fibrosis, certainly nothing like that observed following melphalan (Everts *et al.*, 1973).

Occasional patients receiving MTX have developed a transient painful pleuritis or peritonitis or both. These symptoms are generally unassociated with other signs of MTX toxicity (Berlin *et al.*, 1963), and resolve spontaneously over a few days.

Cyclophosphamide has been associated with a diffusely infiltrative chest radiograph in 5 patients (Castleman *et al.*, 1972; Hunt, 1972; Rodin et al., 1970; Karnofsky, 1967; Andre *et al.*, 1967). The diagnoses were: reticulum sarcoma, Hodgkin's disease, mycosis fungoides, lymphosarcoma. Each had also received vincristine and prednisone. The onset of symptoms was acute, with death following shortly. Pulmonary histology demonstrated interstitial infiltrates of polymorphonuclear cells without fibrosis.

Procarbazine has been associated in one patient with persistent fever, nonproductive cough, and dyspnea. The chest radiograph demonstrated a right pleural effusion and bilateral basal interstitial infiltrates. The signs and symptoms abated abruptly with stoppage of the drug. A rechallenge with procarbazine 1 month later resulted in an abrupt return of the initial syndrome (Jones *et al.*, 1972).

Intrapleural administration of nitrogen mustard is often used for local control of malignant pleural effusions. Local pain and subsequent leukopenia from systemic drug absorption are well-recognized hazards of this therapy. In one woman with metastatic breast cancer, the instillation of nitrogen mustard into the left pleural space resulted in unilateral pulmonary diffuse interstitial infiltrate. The fever and pulmonary reaction subsided over 4 days (Goodman and Shanser, 1976).

Shortly after daunomycin began clinical trials, there was evidence of cardiac toxicity. Tan *et al.* (1967) reported that of 19 children who had received a total dose that exceeded 25 mg/kg, 7 of 14 who died developed cardiopulmonary symptoms. These symptoms were characterized by tachycardia, occasional arrhythmia, and congestive heart failure. Bonadonna and Monfardini (1969), however, noted a different syndrome in adults. Of 16 adults who had received this drug, 5 developed acute cardiac insufficiency characterized by hypotension and not congestive heart failure. Of these patients, 4 died within 24 hr of the onset of symptoms. No patient responded to the use of digitalis. Their total dose of daunomycin ranged from 2.2 to 8.0 mg/kg. Others have also observed this difference in cardiac toxicity between adults and children (Malpas and Scott, 1968, 1969; Marmont *et al.*, 1969; Bonadonna and Monfardini, 1969; Mathé *et al.*, 1967).

Acute Leukemia Group B (1969) documented daunomycin cardiac toxicity in 17 of 187 (9.9%) children with acute lymphocytic leukemia who had received the drug as part of a maintenance therapy program. A simultaneous randomized group of children who did not get daunomycin did not have a single case of cardiac decompensation. The total dose received ranged from 360 to 1260 mg/M^2, with a mean of 780 mg/M^2. The interval from the first injection of daunomycin to the onset of cardiac failure ranged from 105 to 1348 days, with a median of 518 days. The interval from the last injection to onset of cardiac failure was 11–280 days, with a median of 79 days. Of patients who developed cardiac toxicity, 70% did so within 100 days of their last dose. The heart failure developed suddenly in all 17 patients, each of whom had ECG abnormalities. Systolic time intervals were abnormally prolonged in the 3 children in whom it was measured. Only 2 patients recovered normal functional status, 6 died of inexorable congestive heart failure, 3 improved with appropriate therapy, while 6 showed no improvement despite the use of diuretics and digitalis preparations. Microscopic cardiac examination showed there to be severe cellular degeneration, many "ghost" cells, and interstitial edema (Halazun *et al.*, 1974). Similar myocardial degeneration in association with fibrosis had been observed previously following this drug (Ripault and Jacquillat, 1967).

Adriamycin, hydroxydaunorubicin, in addition to producing predictable leukopenia, alopecia, nausea, vomiting, and mucositis, can result in the insidious onset of irreversible congestive failure (Benjamin, 1975). The overall frequency of cardiac toxicity following this drug is 1.8%, but only 0.3% of patients who received doses of 500 mg/M^2 or less. The frequency increases dramatically with dose escalation: 11% with doses between 501 and 600 mg/M^2, and to 31% when the dose exceeds 600 mg/M^2. A review of the reported cases to 1975 found that 61% of patients who had received more than 550 mg adriamycin/M^2 developed a cardiomyopathy (Minow *et al.*, 1975). Therapy is that used for other cardiomyopathies—bed rest, diuretics, and inotropic agents, none of which may be effective in reversing the gradual progression to death. There is reason, however, to be optimistic that some will benefit (Cortes *et al.*, 1975).

The ECG tracing of patients with the adriamycin failure syndrome characteristically shows low voltage, as would be expected in cardiomyopathies attributable to other causes (Minow *et al.*, 1975; Lefrak *et al.*, 1975; Gilladoga *et al.*, 1975). In addition, there are often arrhythmias, T-wave flattening, and prolonged QT intervals during the infusion of adriamycin. These transient ECG abnormalities have not been shown to predict subsequent development of the cardiomyopathy (Gilladoga *et al.*, 1975; Bonadonna *et al.*, 1969; Middleman *et al.*, 1971; Cortes *et al.*, 1975). The systolic time interval (STI), which is a quick method for determining the efficiency of the heart in performing its blood-pumping function, has been used to detect early cardiotoxicity (Rinehart *et al.*, 1974). The STI is a measure of the ratio of the preejection period (PEP) to the time of left ventricular ejection (LVET) (Weissler *et al.*, 1968, 1969). Patients who have congestive heart failure (CHF) or a cardiomyopathy have a prolonged PEP and a shortened LVET; as a consequence, the STI (PEP/LVET) is prolonged. Rinehart *et al.* (1974) found a prolongation of the STI in 48 of 54 patients who were receiving adriamycin. This prolongation often occurred shortly after each dose, returning to normal prior to the next infusion. The STI is probably too sensitive a test to use routinely to follow the cardiac effects of adriamycin. It may also lack predictability of the eventual long-term cardiac effects, as demonstrated by the occasional patient who develops a sudden onset of CHF without previously having had a prolonged STI (Minow *et al.*, 1975).

Light microscopy shows there to be a paucity of normal myocardial fibers in the hearts of patients who had congestive cardiomyopathy. There is abundant new cellular degeneration and interstitial edema present in the hearts of patients who expired during the acute episode. An inflammatory reaction is conspicuously absent (Lefrak *et al.*, 1973).

Prior mediastinal irradiation and the concomitant use of cyclophosphamide apparently render the myocardium more susceptible to adriamycin. The cardiomyopathy unquestionably develops at lower cumulative doses in these circumstances. The lower threshold level appears to be 450 mg/M^2 if there has been prior mediastinal irradiation or if there is concurrent cyclophosphamide therapy (Minow *et al.*, 1975; Gilladoga *et al.*, 1976). It is recommended that adriamycin not exceed 550 mg/M^2 total cumulative dose when given alone, or 450 mg/M^2 if cyclophosphamide is also being used to treat the patient or if there has been prior mediastinal or cardiac irradiation.

High doses of cyclophosphamide can produce ECG changes and acute myocardial necrosis.

Doses of 120 mg/M^2 consistently produce nonspecific T-wave changes and voltage diminution during the first few weeks following the infusion in approximately a third of patients. Serum creatinine phosphokinase values are also generally elevated in these patients (Buckner *et al.*, 1972; Mullins *et al.*, 1975). Physical examination of the cardiovascular system of these patients does not suggest imminent failure. With lower doses (60 mg/kg), Buckner *et al.* (1972)

found no ECG changes in the 7 patients given this dose. However, when the dose of cyclophosphamide was increased to 240 mg/M^2 given over 4 days, both Buckner *et al.* (1972) and Santos *et al.* (1972, 1973) observed the evolution of heart failure and death over 1 to 2 weeks. Buckner and co-workers' patient had hemorrhagic necrosis of the myocardium. Some of the bone marrow transplant patients treated at the National Cancer Institute (Buja *et al.*, 1976) also had a myocardial hemorrhagic necrotic process at the time of death. Occasionally, this process was quite extensive and thought to be cyclophosphamide-related. Of 22 patients, 2 died within days after transplantation, and were felt to have succumbed to the cardiac effects of the cyclophosphamide. The identical pathological finding of hemorrhagic myocardial necrosis has been seen following large doses of cyclophosphamide in dogs (O'Connell and Berenbaum, 1974) and rhesus monkeys (Storb *et al.*, 1970).

There is no doubt that the large doses of cyclophosphamide that are used in preparation for bone marrow transplants are very cardiotoxic. The lower therapeutic doses are apparently free of any known deleterious effect on the heart.

Routine ECG examinations in patients who were receiving 100–750 mg MTX/kg demonstrated transient nonspecific changes similar to those seen following adriamycin. Those patients who subsequently received adriamycin at a later time had a frequency of ECG abnormalities 3 times the frequency of that seen in patients receiving adriamycin without prior administration of high doses of MTX (Rosen *et al.*, 1974).

Of 43 patients who received hydroxyurea (60 mg/kg per day), 2 developed nonspecific ECG changes. No permanent cardiac sequelae developed (Thurman *et al.*, 1963).

9. Renal Toxicity

Cyclophosphamide is the only alkylating agent that has resulted in renal toxicity. With conventional therapeutic doses, 1–2 g/M^2 i.v. weekly or orally in divided doses, or chronic lower doses daily, there is occasionally the development of a hemorrhagic cystitis. In most large series of patients treated with cyclophosphamide, the incidence of hemorrhagic cystitis is 10% or less (Höst *et al.*, 1961; Davis *et al.*, 1969; Fosdick *et al.*, 1968; Coggins *et al.*, 1960; Fernbach *et al.*, 1962; Bagley *et al.*, 1972; Lawrence *et al.*, 1975). The time of onset of the cystitis can be from less than 1 month (Davis *et al.*, 1969) to more than 29 months (Liedberg *et al.*, 1970) from the initiation of therapy. Dysuria and frequency are the initial symptoms, followed by hematuria, which is generally mild. There is never evidence of renal parenchymal function abnormality or infection. The disappearance of all symptoms and hematuria generally requires 4–6 weeks (Davis *et al.*, 1969; Fernbach *et al.*, 1962). There are generally recurrent symptoms with resumption of the drug.

With the use of intravenous cyclophosphamide, the onset of symptoms is generally prompt, occurring within 24–48 hr (Coggins *et al.*, 1960; Buckner *et al.*, 1974*a, b*), and often subsiding within 2 weeks (Buckner *et al.*, 1972). Larger doses of cyclophosphamide (60–120 mg/kg) result in a higher fraction of patients who develop this syndrome: 27 of 43 (Buckner *et al.*, 1972), 5 of 30 (Buckner *et al.*, 1974*a, b*), 4 of 12 (Santos *et al.*, 1972), and 5 of 20 (Mullins *et al.*, 1975). This occurred despite administration of 6–8 liters of a saline infusion the first 24 hr following the injection of cyclophosphamide.

Although most patients who experience this uncomfortable complication recover without any symptomatic sequelae, deaths from massive unstoppable hemorrhage have occurred (Liedberg *et al.*, 1970; A. M. Hutter *et al.*, 1969; Berkson *et al.*, 1973; Lawrence *et al.*, 1975). Occasionally, 50 and 60 units of blood have been required over a period of weeks to maintain an acceptable hematocrit (Riggenbach *et al.*, 1968; Reynolds *et al.*, 1969).

An intravenous pyelogram (IVP) often shows the bladder contracted, with irregular densities that represent blood clots (Pearlman, 1966; Reynolds *et al.*, 1969). Occasionally, a ureter may be occluded at the ureterovesicle junction (Pearlman, 1966). Blood clots, multiple mucosal ulcerations, and bleeding are often visualized by cystoscopic exam (Anderson *et al.*, 1967; Berkson *et al.*, 1973; Perlman, 1966).

In instances in which hemorrhage persists, urinary diversion has been necessary to prevent continued urine contact with the bladder mucosa. The means of achieving this diversion has been bilateral ureteral catheter placement (Riggenbach *et al.*, 1968; Reynolds *et al.*, 1969) or surgical diversion (Anderson *et al.*, 1967; Berkson *et al.*, 1973; Marsh *et al.*, 1971). Biopsy or autopsy specimens invariably show inflammation, diffuse capillary proliferation, fibrosis, denuded mucosa, and ulcerations that often extend through the bladder wall (A. M. Hutter *et al.*, 1969; Reynolds *et al.*, 1969; Berkson *et al.*, 1973; George, 1963). An autopsy study of 40 bladders from patients who had received cyclophosphamide found that 10 were fibrotic; of these, 3 also exhibited mucosal telangiectasia. Of these patients, 5 had been asymptomatic. Of major interest was that all 10 patients had been given intravenous drug, with the total dose exceeding 6 g/M^2 (W. W. Johnson and Meadows, 1971).

There has been documentation of the excretion of bizarre transitional epithelial cells following cyclophosphamide (Aptekar *et al.*, 1972). It was not surprising, therefore, that 7 patients who had been receiving cyclophosphamide for long periods developed bladder cancer (Worth, 1971; Wall and Clausen, 1975; Richtsmeier, 1975). The hemorrhagic cystitis and bladder cancer following cyclophosphamide may be related to the excretion and accumulation of active cyclophosphamide metabolites in the urine. Approximately 60% of the active form of cyclophosphamide is excreted in 1 or 2 days (Bagley *et al.*, 1973; Milner and Sullivan, 1967; Mouridsen *et al.*, 1976). This being the case makes it very logical therapy to administer large quantities of fluid following cyclophosphamide, especially after an intravenous bolus of the drug, the purpose being to dilute and decrease the exposure of the bladder epithelium to a potentially toxic agent.

Cyclophosphamide has also been shown to cause temporary water retention, especially following large intravenous doses of 60–120 mg/kg (Buckner et al., 1972; Mullins et al., 1975; Santos et al., 1972). This physiological effect of water retention was studied by DeFronzo et al. (1973, 1974). They observed a decrease in serum osmolarity of 41 mosmole/liter and a rise in urine osmolarity up to 798 mosmole/liter. These effects occurred 4–12 hr after the infusion of cyclophosphamide. Whether this was a direct effect on the kidney or a result of an alteration of antidiuretic hormone was not resolved.

Methotrexate (0.5–3.0 mg/kg i.v. every 2 weeks) has been found to have a direct toxic effect on the kidney. There was a transient increase in BUN and a decrease in inulin clearance on PAH secretion, indicating an adverse effect on glomerular filtration and renal tubular secretion. The kidneys of 3 patients who expired from the other effects of methotrexate toxicity had extensive tubular necrosis (Condit et al., 1969). Similar pathologic and kidney changes have been observed in dogs following MTX in high doses (Patel et al., 1969). Recent additional information has shown that after gram doses of MTX, there is, in fact, precipitated MTX in the tubular lumens in those patients who experienced renal impairment following the infusion of MTX (Frei et al., 1975). Pathologically, there was tubular dilation, a situation that is analogous, at least in part, to uric acid nephropathy.

Mithramycin has produced a transient elevation of BUN, proteinuria, and a decreased specific gravity in some patients. Oliguria or anuria does not occur (Brown and Kennedy, 1965). Kennedy reported in 1970 (Kennedy, 1970a, b) that following the same dose they had used earlier (25–50 μg/kg per day × 5), 40% of patients had a BUN elevation greater than 25 mg/100 ml. Six patients died of renal failure. In the others who developed azotemia, the creatinine clearance remained abnormal for weeks or months. There was microscopic evidence of tubular atrophy. With the subsequent use of 50 μg/kg every other day for only 3 days, only 21% of 23 patients developed a transient BUN elevation, which never exceeded 45 mg/100 ml. There were no deaths (Kennedy, 1970a, b). Other observers have documented the marked decrease in renal toxicity with the use of lower doses of mithramycin (G. J. Hill, II, et al., 1972; Ream et al., 1968).

Azotemia (BUN >20 mg/100 ml) occurs in approximately 40–50% of patients who receive L-asparaginase, irrespective of dose schedule (Pratt et al., 1970; Haskell et al., 1969a, b; Wilson et al., 1975). Occasionally, there has been oliguria and marked azotemia, which contributed to the patient's death (Haskell et al., 1969a, b). This occurrence is distinctly unusual, since the BUN generally returns to normal levels by the 2nd or 3rd week despite continued therapy (Oettgen et al., 1970).

cis-Platinum has also been noted to result in azotemia. The azotemia is to a certain extent dose-related, being 100% at doses greater than 17.5 mg/M² per day × 5, but 50% at doses less than 12 mg/M² per day × 5. The abnormality generally begins within 1–2 weeks, reaching a peak level at 3 weeks. The abnormality may be quite prolonged (Talley et al., 1973). Higby et al. (1973) noted that with the first course of cis-platinum (20 mg/M² per day × 5), renal impairment developed in 3 of 9 patients. In 9 patients who had a second course of therapy, however, 7 developed renal toxicity, which was irreversible in 1. Renal tubular necrosis was present histologically in the 2 patients who died during the study, neither from the renal toxicity. Because of the possibility that a component of the effects on the renal tubules may be from the drug in the tubular fluid, it is recommended that diuresis be instituted during *cis*-platinum therapy.

Streptozotocin is a tubule toxin; this adverse effect is most commonly the factor limiting its further use. In the majority of patients, there is a mild, asymptomatic reversible lesion. The earliest manifestation is proteinuria (28%) and decreased glomerular filtration (27%). Other changes are hypophosphatemia, elevated BUN, renal glucosuria, and renal tubular acidosis. Occasionally, the tubular damage may be of such severity that the proteinuria reaches 10 g/day. Some patients have succumbed from the renal failure. In these cases, the renal histology has been that of cellular degeneration and tubular necrosis (Schein *et al.*, 1974; Broder and Carter, 1973).

10. Coagulopathy

Mithramycin, a useful drug for the treatment of testicular cancers, has been associated with a life-threatening coagulopathy. Of 58 patients who received 25–50 μg/kg per day until toxicity ensued, 13 died as a result of drug-induced hemorrhage (Kennedy, 1970*a*). Thrombocytopenia, which was less than 50,000/mm³ in only 6 of these patients, was a contributory but not the major factor in the diffuse hemorrhaging. Three previous patients with testicular cancer treated in 1965 with the same dose regimen died of gastric hemorrhage (Kennedy *et al.*, 1965). Similar treatment programs that used daily mithramycin had evidence of a hemorrhagic diathesis, which resulted in death in approximately 30% of the patients (G. J. Hill, II *et al.*, 1972; Ream *et al.*, 1968). This marked frequency of deaths following daily mithramycin resulted in the development of an alternate-day program 50 μg/kg every other day × 3. Kennedy (1970*a*) found the frequency of hemorrhage reduced from 43% to no cases while maintaining the same therapeutic effectiveness with the alternate-day schedule. Monto *et al.* (1969) demonstrated not only that the coagulopathy and hemorrhage were related to dose (2 of 3 patients at 50 μg/kg per day vs. 2 of 36 patients at 37.5 μg/kg per day), but also that the frequency of hemorrhage increased with successive courses of therapy.

The exact nature of this hemorrhagic diathesis following mithramycin therapy is not fully understood. Depression of clotting factors II, V, VII, and X occurs regularly, in addition to moderate thrombocytopenia (50–100,000/mm³). Perhaps the major initiator of the bleeding is the vascular damage that has been observed in most of the small vessels after mithramycin infusions (Monto *et al.*, 1969). There is no evidence that disseminated intravascular coagulation is occurring. The treatment is that of platelet and red cell support. Vitamin K₁ (phytonadione) has been of little or no value, probably because while factors II, VII, and X are vitamin K–dependent, factor V and others are not.

Temporary cessation of mithramycin therapy because of hemorrhagic toxicity
can be guided by (1) marked facial flush and edema (which are associated with the
subsequent development of coagulopathy); (2) persistent epistaxis, which often
precedes major bleeding elsewhere; (3) platelet count less than 50,000/mm^3;
and (4) prolonged prothrombin time (Monto *et al.*, 1969; Kennedy, 1970*a, b*).

Most patients (75%) who are receiving L-asparaginase develop abnormal clotting parameters. Seldom is there bleeding of any major clinical significance
(Haskell *et al.*, 1969*a, b*; Gralnick and Henderson, 1971). Close analysis by Gralnick and Henderson (1971) of 13 patients treated with L-asparaginase found there
to be abnormalities of blood coagulation and fibrinolysis in each patient. The
serum levels of fibrinogen, clotting factors V, VII, VIII, IX, and plasminogen
were all decreased. Fibrinogen degradation products were present in the serum.
The physiological disturbance appeared to be that of limited disseminated
intravascular coagulation, possibly in concert with impaired coagulation factor
synthesis. The hemorrhagic problems following L-asparaginase are relatively
minor compared with the catastrophic hemorrhages that have been observed
following mithramycin.

11. Nervous System Toxicity

The neurotoxic effects of vincristine and vinblastine have been well recognized
since these drugs were introduced for the treatment of neoplastic disease in 1962
(Armstrong *et al.*, 1962). The clinical features of the neurotoxicity produced by
vincristine have been described in exquisite detail by Sandler *et al.* (1969) and
Casey *et al.* (1973).

The manner in which the effect of vincristine on the nervous system manifests
itself does appear to be rather predictable. The first changes are often loss of ankle
jerks and depression of other tendon reflexes. Areflexia occurs in about 50% of
patients who receive weekly vincristine, but it is not always a precursor of motor
weakness or near-paralysis (Casey *et al.*, 1973). This is then followed by distal
extremity parasthesias, which are generally a forewarning of the muscular weakness that often follows. The parasthesias and loss of superficial sensation are
almost exclusively limited to the very distal portion of limbs, seldom extending
proximally beyond the wrists or ankles. Rarely, muscle pains have occurred
(Martin and Compston, 1963; Casey *et al.*, 1973; Johnston and Novales, 1961).

Motor weakness, which can be extremely disabling, requires dose reduction
whenever it is observed. The initial symptom is usually clumsiness of the hands.
Examination invariably points out the impressive weakness, first, of extensor
muscles of the fingers, and a short time later, those of the wrist (Casey *et al.*, 1973).
Generally, the extensor muscles of the feet are similarly involved at the same time,
which can be detected clinically by the loud, slapping gait. Although these muscle
groups can have profound loss of strength, other major muscle groups are
generally spared. Occasionally, however, the proximal muscles may become weak,

leading to difficulty in climbing stairs and walking (D. V. Desai *et al.*, 1970; Casey *et al.*, 1973), but they are never as weak as the more distal muscle groups (Casey *et al.*, 1973). Weakness of this severity often progresses rapidly. Cessation of therapy will lead to gradual improvement, but complete symptomatic resolution may require up to 4 months (Martin and Compston, 1963; Sandler *et al.*, 1969). Slight muscle weakness detectable by meticulous physical exam and persistent absence of ankle reflexes may exist for much longer periods (Casey *et al.*, 1973). These neurotoxic effects of vincristine are definitely dose-related (D. V. Desai *et al.*, 1970; Sandler *et al.*, 1969; Casey *et al.*, 1973).

Cranial nerve paresis of III, VI, and VII has been documented to occur following vincristine therapy in children (Albert *et al.*, 1967; Sandler *et al.*, 1969; Selawry and Hananian, 1963). Albert *et al.* (1967) noted this adverse effect in 20 of 40 children, while D. V. Desai *et al.* (1970) were unable to detect any cranial nerve paresis in 103 adults. The most common ocular abnormalities secondary to vincristine reported by Albert and co-workers were ptosis, III nerve (14 patients); lateral rectus paresis, VI nerve (13 patients); facial palsy, VII nerve (6 patients); and corneal hypesthesia, V nerve (2 patients). Others have also noted these cranial nerves to be most frequently affected from vincristine (Sandler *et al.*, 1969; Selawry and Hananian, 1963). These changes will subside after discontinuance of vincristine.

Other neurological side effects reported following vincristine include arthralgias, myalgias and jaw pain, ileus, and urinary retention, especially in older males (Carey *et al.*, 1963; Martin and Compston, 1963; Sandler *et al.*, 1969). The jaw pain, which can be severe, usually occurs after the first or second injection (Haggard *et al.*, 1968), and is apparently not dose-related.

Seizures associated with vincristine use and in the absence of hyponatremia have been reported (Hreshchyshyn, 1963; F. L. Johnson *et al.*, 1973). Confusion (Karon *et al.*, 1962) and hallucinations (Mittelman *et al.*, 1963) have been thought rarely to be secondary to vincristine.

Vinblastine can also produce similar effects on the nervous system, but generally in considerably fewer patients than does vincristine—10% vs. 100% (Wright *et al.*, 1963; Frost *et al.*, 1962). Confusion and lethargy following the infusion appear in approximately 1–10% of patients (Warwick *et al.*, 1961; Wright *et al.*, 1963; Frei, 1961; J. M. Hill and Loeb, 1961). Depression has also been noted (Johnston and Novales, 1961).

Seizures are rarely encountered following vinblastine (Warwick *et al.*, 1961; Frei *et al.*, 1961). With the larger doses that are currently used for the treatment of nonseminomatous testicular carcinoma, myalgias have been frequently observed, as well as occasional jaw pains. Cranial nerve paresis is distinctly absent (Samuels and Howe, 1970; Samuels *et al.*, 1975*a, b*).

The syndrome of inappropriate antidiuretic hormone secretion (SIADH) was first clinically recognized in 1957 by W. B. Schwartz *et al.* (1957). Since then, it has been associated with various disease entities, among which are neoplastic tumors (Vorherr, 1974), pneumonia (Rosenow *et al.*, 1972), acute CNS trauma (Joynt *et al.*, 1965; Richards *et al.*, 1971), and recently the use of vincristine. There have been 9 reported cases of clinical SIADH (Table 1). In each case, the complication occurred shortly after the onset of therapy with vincristine, but not necessarily following the first dose. The patients were symptomatic within the week after the drug administration. There was also a profound effect on the peripheral nervous system, such as absent reflexes and ileus, which are characteristically not seen quite so soon after the initial use of vincristine. Lethargy was present in all patients, seizures in most. There were no deaths, and the electrolyte and water abnormalities were generally corrected within 1–2 weeks.

G. L. Robertson *et al.* (1973) measured serum vasopression and found it elevated in their patients. Of interest were normal levels in patients receiving vincristine who did not have neuropathy. Stuart *et al.* (1975) documented an elevation of urine ADH excretion in their patient that decreased progressively with each successive weekly dose of vincristine. By the 8th dose, there was no longer an appreciable rise.

Vincristine probably acts in certain susceptible individuals to cause the release of inappropriately large quantities of ADH, which results in the retention of water by the kidney, hyponatremia, and ultimately the signs and symptoms characteristic of this syndrome.

Cerebellar ataxia has been intermittently observed in patients receiving 5-FU. Of 56 patients who were given 20 mg/kg weekly, 4 developed a mild reversible cerebellar ataxia, while there were no symptoms observed in the 121 who got 7.5–15 mg/kg (Horton *et al.*, 1970). Moertel *et al.* (1964) had previously noted the frequent occurrence of a cerebellar ataxia in the absence of other neurological abnormalities in those patients whose 5-FU therapy had fortuitously become long-term. This neurotoxicity of 5-FU appears to be potentiated if hydroxyurea is given simultaneously (Lokich *et al.*, 1975).

Mithramycin was reported to produce a bizzare behavioral change in patients that began shortly after the infusion had been completed. It generally consisted of headache, irritability, akathisia, agitation, and lethargy (Kennedy, 1970*a*, *b*). This same reaction had been noted previously (Ream *et al.*, 1968). When Kennedy changed the dose schedule of mithramycin from 50 μg/kg per day to 50 μg/kg every other day, the frequency of these annoying reactions decreased from 76% to 47% (Kennedy, 1970*a*). G. J. Hill, II *et al.* (1972) observed only 6 of 99 patients with a similar syndrome when the patients were given 30 μg/kg per day of the drug. It would appear that the CNS toxicity of mithramycin is time- or dose-related, or both.

Bleomycin is not considered to have any major nervous system toxicity; however, generalized headache beginning 2–8 hr following each dose and lasting 8–24 hr does occur in approximately 10% of patients (Yagoda *et al.*, 1972).

Adriamycin has produced drowsiness rarely (Benjamin, 1975).

Tinnitus occurs following *cis*-platinum in a minority of patients, and is also associated with a high-frequency hearing loss (Higby *et al.*, 1973, 1974; Talley *et al.*, 1973). With careful monitoring of hearing with routine audiograms, approximately 50% of patients will experience a deficit in the high-frequency range (Ellerby *et al.*, 1974).

TABLE 1

Summary of Patients Reported to Have SIADH Following Vincristine

Patient			Diagnosis[a]	ADH measured?	VCR dose	Days after last VCR to SIADH	Days for correction of SIADH	Other CNS effects[b]	Lowest Na$^+$	Reference
No.	Age	Sex								
1	11	M	Rhabdomyosarcoma	No	0.5 mg/wk then 0.07 mg/kg · wk × 8	~3	4	Coma Abs. DTR Paralysis Seizure Ptosis	120	Fine *et al.* (1966)
2	7	M	ALL	No	2 mg/M² on days 1 & 9	2	7	Seizure Coma	120	Slater *et al.* (1969)
3	34	M	ALL	No	(2 mg/M² 3 mo before) 2 mg/M² · wk × 2	~3	3	Abs. DTR Paresthesia Lethargy Ileus	125	Meriwether (1971)
4	52	F	RCS	No	2.25 mg × 2	7	3	Disorientation Dysarthria Abs. DTR	98	Oldham and Pomeroy (1972)

5	3.5	F	Wilm's tumor	Yes↑ (bioassay) 4.1 μU/ml[c]	0.5 mg/kg × 1	5	13	Anorexia Lethargy ↓DTR	118	Suskind et al. (1972)
6	54	M	AML	No	4 mg	3	7	Ileus Confusion Neuropathy	106	Cutting (1971)
7	2.5	M	Leukemia (type?)	No	0.1 mg/kg · wk, 2 doses	3	6	Ileus Abs. DTR Lethargy	112	Nicholson and Feldman (1972)
8	50	M	Lymphosarcoma cell leukemia	Yes↑ 5.8–8.8 μU/ml[c]	2 mg/wk	7	14	↓DTR Ileus Confusion	113	G. L. Robertson et al. (1973)
9	4	F	ALL	Yes↑ 284 mU/TV (urine)	2 mg/M² · wk × 2	7 after 1st VCR	9	Seizure Ileus	118	Stuart et al. (1975)

[a] (ALL) acute lymphocytic leukemia; (AML) acute myelogenous leukemia; (RCS) reticulum-cell sarcoma.
[b] (Abs. DTR) absent deep tendon reflex.
[c] Normal values 0.4 ± 0.6 μU/ml.

Methyl-CCNU can rarely produce a metabolic encephalopathy with EEG changes consistent with that diagnosis. The patients were confused and disoriented and often had delusions that began within 1 day after drug ingestion and lasted 2–14 days (Tranum *et al.*, 1975). This effect has not been observed with the other nitrosourea compounds.

Procarbazine has been reported to cause CNS depression manifested as mild drowsiness (Brunner and Young, 1965) or lethargy (Stolinsky *et al.*, 1970). Occasionally, profound stupor with diffusely abnormal EEGs and normal CSF analysis has also been seen (Brunner and Young, 1965). Euphoria has also been observed on occasion (Todd, 1965). Other nervous system problems related to procarbazine use have been paresthesias, ataxia, and myalgias (Brunner and Young, 1965; Samuels *et al.*, 1967; Stolinsky *et al.*, 1970).

L-Asparaginase predictably has CNS toxicity, which generally consists of lethargy and confusion. Acute psychosis (Wilson *et al.*, 1975) and disorientation (Haskell *et al.*, 1969*a, b*) have occurred. A syndrome indistinguishable from alcoholic delirium tremens has also been reported (Haskell *et al.*, 1969*a, b*). EEGs, when obtained, have been diffusely abnormal, similar to those seen following procarbazine (Haskell *et al.*, 1969*a, b*; Wilson *et al.*, 1975). Although Haskell *et al.* (1969*a, b*) noted the nervous system aberrations only in children, Oettgen *et al.* (1970) observed the changes in 48 of 147 trials with children, and 71 of 156 trials with adults. L-Asparaginase apparently affects 30–40% of patients receiving the drug, adults perhaps more frequently than children.

DTIC has caused a mild confusion in some patients (Gottlieb and Serpick, 1971). The confusion is certainly not of the same magnitude as that seen with some of the other agents.

Although Brewer *et al.* (1964) noted myalgias and mental depression in 12 and 9 patients, respectively, from a total of 28 who received MTX, Vogler and Jacobs (1971) did not mention any nervous system abnormalities after 100–300 mg MTX/M^2. Pratt *et al.* (1974) specifically stated that no nervous system toxicity occurred in children after 50–500 mg MTX/kg.

The use of intrathecal MTX to combat meningeal leukemia or meningeal carcinomatosis is standard therapy (C. B. Hyman *et al.*, 1965; Sullivan *et al.*, 1969). It is not uncommon (60%) for patients to develop a sterile arachnoiditis and mild pleocytosis with clinical meningismus, headache, and an occasional low fever (Geiser *et al.*, 1975). Severe reactions, however, presumably from the MTX, have occurred.

Quadraplegia has occurred in 2 patients. One reaction was immediate (Bleyer *et al.*, 1973); the other occurred 24 hr after the intrathecal MTX administration (Baum *et al.*, 1971). Paraplegia occurred in 8 patients, developing immediately in 3 (Bagshawe *et al.*, 1969; Back, 1969; Saiki *et al.*, 1972), and 6–48 hr following the instillation of the drug in the remaining 5 patients (Pasquinucci *et al.*, 1970; Sullivan *et al.*, 1969; Baum *et al.*, 1971; Luddy and Gilman, 1973; Gagliano and Costanzi, 1976). One patient had an immediate but transient weakness and anesthesia of the right leg following MTX. It reoccurred following intrathecal cytosine arabinoside (Bagshawe *et al.*, 1969); other than this reversible reaction,

the others were permanent. All patients had leukemia; 3 were receiving prophylactic therapy (Baum *et al.*, 1971; Luddy and Gilman, 1973). The doses of
MTX ranged from 5 to 40 mg.

Bleyer *et al.* (1973) eloquently described 5 patients with various neurotoxic
symptoms following intrathecal MTX. In each toxic patient, the concentration of
MTX in the CSF was elevated for prolonged periods as compared with nontoxic
controls ($>10^{-8}$ mole for >5 days).

A necrotizing encephalopathy following the intraventricular administration of
MTX has been reported in 3 patients (Shapiro *et al.*, 1973). Autopsy evaluation
demonstrated fibrinoid degeneration, coagulation necrosis, and a reactive
astrocytosis of the periventricular white matter. The cause was postulated to be
from high local concentrations of the drug that diffused through the ventricular
walls.

The chronic systemic use of MTX may also have deleterious effects on the CNS.
Long-term follow-up of 23 children who received MTX for at least 2 years and
were alive for 5 or more years following the onset of therapy revealed that 14 of
these children had neurological abnormalities (Meadows and Evans, 1976). Of
these 14, the 4 patients who had severe impairment—seizures, paraplegia, and
dementia—had received other drugs in addition to MTX. Three had also been
treated with cranial irradiation. Brain biopsies of 3 of these children revealed
gliosis. A total of 10 children had either mild EEG changes or mild neurological
deficits; 3 had received cranial irradiation, 1 had received intrathecal MTX, and 2
had been treated with both. Of the 9 normal children, none had been treated with
irradiation, and only 2 were given intrathecal MTX; one child was given only 6
injections; the other was treated intermittently for 2 years.

Price and Jamieson (1975) reviewed the brains of 231 children from St. Jude's
Children's Hospital, spanning the years 1962–1974. Of this total,13 were found to
have specific degenerative changes in the white matter. The common clinical
features of these 13 children were greater than 2000 rads of cranial irradiation,
and systematic MTX given shortly following the radiation treatments. A similar
report also confirmed the association of radiation followed by MTX with necrotizing leukoencephalopathy (Rubenstein *et al.*, 1975).

In addition to these irreversible long-term neural tissue changes, there are also
acutely toxic reactions involving the nervous system that are generally reversible.
Intrathecal use of MTX may result in an acute toxic syndrome characterized by
nausea, vomiting, headache, and fever. These symptoms often persist for 5 days
(Geiser *et al.*, 1975; Duttera *et al.*, 1973). The CSF generally has increased numbers
of lymphocytes, but normal glucose and protein. Geiser and co-workers noted the
frequency of this toxic syndrome to drop from 61% to 20% if the MTX were
dissolved in Elliot's B Solution; however, Duttera and co-workers did not make the
same observation.

There is little doubt that intrathecal MTX is a toxic agent, not only acutely, but
possibly chronically as well. With high doses of systematic MTX followed by
leucovorin, MTX will enter the CSF in quantities sufficient to provide prophylaxis
against leukemia (Wang *et al.*, 1976). This treatment approach may obviate the

acute toxic syndrome, especially if the reaction is secondary to the diluent in which the MTX is dissolved for intrathecal administration. However, if the delayed mental impairments and leukoencelphalopathy are a manifestation of a radiation–MTX schedule, then this latter problem may not be improved on.

CNS toxicity from alkylating agents is generally not a recognized clinical problem. Coma and hyperpyrexia did occur twice in a single patient following intravenous nitrogen mustard. The patient recovered completely on each occasion (Bethlenfalvay and Bergin, 1972). Headaches are not uncommon, however (Dameshek *et al.*, 1949).

12. Effects on Serum Electrolytes

Cyclophosphamide in doses of 60 mg/kg and more uniformly causes fluid retention, which in some patients requires diuretics and inotropic agents to lessen symptoms of fluid overload (Buckner *et al.*, 1972; Mullins *et al.*, 1975). The exact cause is unknown, but the physiological derangements are compatible with the SIADH (DeFronzo *et al.*, 1973). In only 1 of 3 patients was the serum vasopressin concentration appropriately elevated to explain the clinical observations (DeFronzo *et al.*, 1974).

Mithramycin may cause hypocalcemia, which on occasion is associated with tetany (Brown and Kennedy, 1965). The drug is, in fact, also used clinically to lower calcium acutely when saline diuresis and prednisone are not effective or appropriate.

Hyperkalemia does occur following effective chemotherapy in certain rapidly proliferating neoplasms (Table 2). This hyperkalemia is not a direct toxic effect of the drug used, but rather is a consequence of rapid cellular lysis. The hyperkalemia invariably occurs in the presence of renal compromise. The pathophysiology is such that the cells release large quantities of potassium as they undergo dissolution secondary to chemotherapy. But in the presence of mild renal

TABLE 2
Hyperkalemia Following Cellular Lysis

	Patient			Potassium		BUN		
No.	Diagnosis[a]	Age	Sex	Before	After	Before	After	Reference
1	Burkitt	30	M	4.5	8.5	20	93	Arseneau *et al.* (1973)
2	Burkitt	8	F	4.0	8.9	8	80	Arseneau *et al.* (1973)
3	Burkitt	6	M	4.6	7.8	21	177	Arseneau *et al.* (1973)
4	Burkitt	27	F	3.8	6.0	35	60	Arseneau *et al.* (1973)
5	ALL	17	M	4.4	9.8	90	203	Fennelly *et al.* (1974)
6	ALL	50	F	—	7.0	15	119	Gold and Fritz (1957)
7	ALL	8	M	—	7.5	—	212	Gold and Fritz (1957)
8	PDL	76	M	5.8	6.8	63	120	Muggia (1973)

[a](ALL) acute lymphocytic leukemia; (PDL) poorly differentiated lymphoma.

TABLE 3

Hyperphosphatemia and Hypocalcemia Following Cellular Lysis

No.	Diagnosis[a]	Age	Sex	Calcium Before	Calcium After	Phosphorus Before	Phosphorus After	BUN Before	BUN After	Reference
1	Burkitt	6	M	9.8	2.4	5	28	21	177	Brereton et al. (1975)
2	Burkitt	4	M	9.4	5.2	2.1	16	2	—	Brereton et al. (1975)
3	Burkitt	27	M	10.0	6.3	3	19.6	22	100	Cadman et al. (1977b)
4	ALL	16	M	9.3	7.0	6.7	10.2	18	26	Zuzman et al. (1973)
5	ALL	6	M	10.4	5.1	3.2	15.5	25	74	Zuzman et al. (1973)
6	ALL	—	—	—	6.8	—	6.4	—	37	Jaffe et al. (1972)
7	ALL	—	—	—	4.8	—	12	—	63	Jaffe et al. (1972)
8	ALL	—	—	—	4.3	—	21.2	—	94	Jaffe et al. (1972)
9	ALL	—	—	—	5.0	—	16.5	—	74	Jaffe et al. (1972)
10	ALL	50	F	—	8.1	—	21.9	17	114	Gold and Fritz (1957)
11	ALL	8	M	—	4.6	—	24.2	—	212	Gold and Fritz (1957)
12	ALL	3	M	—	3.8	—	17.4	—	—	Armata and Depowska (1974)
13	ALL	19	M	10	5.4	1.5	10.2	18	45	Clarkson et al. (1973)
14	PDL	74	M	9.3	7.9	2.6	11.6	39	75	Muggia et al. (1974)

[a](ALL) acute lymphocytic leukemia; (PDL) poorly differentiated lymphoma.

compromise, a major homeostatic mechanism is malfunctioning; i.e., the potassium cannot be excreted in adequate quantities. The problem is rare but potentially serious, since several patients have died suddenly of cardiac arrest. Anticipation of the problem is the major step in treatment. The use of potassium exchange ions, alkalization, glucose, and insulin—and, in refractory situations, dialysis—may be of benefit if the potassium begins to reach dangerously high concentrations.

Hyperphosphatemia and hypocalcemia, which are presumably a consequence of the elevated phosphorus, have also been observed following the rapid lysis of large numbers of neoplastic cells (Table 3). The sequence of events is postulated to be an outpouring of intracellular phosphates, which then cause precipitation and subsequent lowering of the serum calcium. Again, a major factor in patients who develop this complication is impaired renal function, and therefore less phosphate excretion than would normally have occurred. In fact, studies of phosphate metabolism in children with lymphoblastic leukemia and normal renal function have shown that following chemotherapy, there is a transient but significant rise of the serum phosphorus. The urinary excretion, which is a major mechanism of lowering the elevated phosphorus, is expectedly increased (Zuzman *et al.*, 1973).

13. Sterility

Amenorrhea occurs frequently following the aklylating agents myleran (Greig, 1956; Louis *et al.*, 1956; Galton *et al.*, 1958), chlorambucil (Ezdinli and Stutzman, 1965), and cyclophosphamide (Warne *et al.*, 1973; Uldall *et al.*, 1972; J. J. Miller, III *et al.*, 1971; Fosdick *et al.*, 1968). This effect has also been observed following procarbazine (Brunner and Young, 1965) and vinblastine (Sobrinho *et al.*, 1971).

Daily cyclophosphamide produces amenorrhea generally within 7 months of onset of therapy. Even after 12 months without any drug, only 1 of 9 patients had resumption of menses (Uldall *et al.*, 1972). Others have confirmed the frequency, time of onset, and general persistence of ovarian failure (Warne *et al.*, 1973). The ovarian histology of such women consistently showed destruction (Morgenfeld *et al.*, 1972; J. J. Miller, III *et al.*, 1971). Hormonal changes have confirmed that the amenorrhea was primary, not pituitary in origin (Warne *et al.*, 1973). Pregnancy has occurred while patients have been taking daily cyclophosphamide, but it is distinctly unusual. Warne *et al.* (1973) described 3 such women, 2 of whom had taken the drug continuously for 26 and 28 months.

Chlorambucil has been shown to cause testicular germinal epithelium to atrophy. The endocrine-secreting component of the testis, Sertoli cells, escapes unscathed. Recovery of azoospermia may not occur (Richter *et al.*, 1970), although there are exceptions. Azoospermia occurred in all 31 patients studied by Fairley *et al.* (1972) who had been receiving cyclophosphamide for 6 months or longer. Testicular biopsy in 5 during this period demonstrated only Sertoli cells. Of 10

TABLE 4

Effect of Chemotherapeutic Agents on Sterility in Humans

Drug	Effect[a] Oligospermia/ azoospermia	Amenorrhea
Chlorambucil	+	+
Cyclophosphamide	+	+
Busulfan	−	+
Vinblastine	−	+(3 cases)
Procarbazine	−	+(1 case)

[a](+) present; (−) no information.

men reexamined from 3 to 19 months following discontinuation of therapy, 2 had mature spermatozoa, although in reduced numbers. Others have also documented that 100% of males who receive cyclophosphamide for approximately 6 months become sterile (Qureshi *et al.*, 1972; D. G. Miller, 1971) (Table 4).

An important observation made by Arneil (1972) was that 27 prepubertal children, boys and girls, did not show histological evidence of gonadal toxicity from cyclophosphamide. Recently, Siris *et al.* (1976) unequivocally demonstrated return of normal hypothalamic pituitary–ovarian function in 16 of 17 girls who received aggressive prepubertal chemotherapy, which included cyclophosphamide, for acute leukemia. Of the 11 girls who were treated during the pubertal age, 7 had spontaneous menarche, while 5 of 7 postmenarchal-treated girls had normal menses return. Several have become pregnant.

The current widespread use of cyclophosphamide in combination treatment for lymphoma and the lengthy survivals that are not expected brings concerns regarding the capability of fertility at a later date. Libido and potency are unaffected by therapy, although azoospermia is the rule. Of 16 men studied by Sherins and DeVita (1973), 2 had minimal and 4 complete spermatogenesis following a 2–7 year remission. Their information suggests that spermatogenesis may return 2 years following completion of therapy.

14. Immunosuppression

The antineoplastic agents that have been documented to depress the immune system in humans are presented in Table 5. Cyclophosphamide is considered to have the greatest immunosuppressive potential. Azathioprine, which is used as an immunosuppressive agent in organ transplants and autoimmune diseases, is not included in Table 5.

TABLE 5

Antineoplastic Agents That Cause Immunosuppression in Humans

Agent	Degree[a]	References
Alkylating agents		
Nitrogen mustard	+ +	Santos (1967)
Chlorambucil	+	Braeman (1972)
Cyclophosphamide	+ + +	Santos *et al.* (1964), Hersh and Oppenheim (1967)
Melphalan	+	Santos (1967)
Busulfan	NI	
Antimetabolites		
Methotrexate	+	Santos *et al.* (1964), Hersh *et al.* (1965), Mitchell *et al.* (1969)
Mercaptopurine	+ +	Santos *et al.* (1964), Hersh *et al.* (1965), Levin *et al.* (1964)
Thioguanine	NI	
Fluorouracil	+	Mitchell and DeConti (1970), Santos *et al.* (1964)
Cytosine arabinoside	+	Mitchell *et al.* (1969)
Plant alkaloids		
Vinblastine	+[b]	Aisenberg and Wilkes (1964)
Vincristine	+[b]	
Antibiotics		
Actinomycin D	+	Al-Sarraf *et al.* (1970), Hirschhorn *et al.* (1963)
Mithramycin	0	Santos (1967)
Bleomycin	0	Lehane *et al.* (1975)
Daunomycin	+	Whang-Peng *et al.* (1969)
Adriamycin	NI	
Metals		
Platinum	NI	
Miscellaneous		
CCNU	NI	
BCNU	+	Santos (1967)
Methyl CCNU	NI	
Procarbazine	NI	
Hydroxyurea	NI	
L-Asparaginase	+	Ohno and Hersh (1970)
DTIC	+	Bruckner *et al.* (1974)

[a] (+, + +, + + +) present; (0) absent; (NI) no information.
[b] Studied in mice.

15. Bone Marrow Toxicity

Most drugs are limited in their doses and schedule by the effects produced on marrow production of hematopoietic cells. Bleomycin (Yagoda *et al.*, 1972) and vincristine (Carey *et al.*, 1963) are free of any significant bone marrow depression.

Even the larger doses of bleomycin infused in combination with other agents for treating testicular tumors do not seem to potentiate bone marrow toxicity (Samuels *et al.*, 1975*a*, *b*). Vinblastine, unlike vincristine, does produce bone marrow depression (Warwick *et al.*, 1961; Costa *et al.*, 1963), but the depression is severe only when the drug is given in large doses (Samuels and Howe, 1970).

cis-Platinum (Talley *et al.*, 1973; Higby *et al.*, 1973), L-asparaginase (Haskell *et al.*, 1969*a*, *b*), and streptozotocin (Schein *et al.*, 1974; Broder and Carter, 1973) have minimal to mild effects on the bone marrow. The platinum toxicity may be cumulative, however.

Generally, the effects of the chemotherapeutic drugs are noted in all the cellular elements of the bone marrow. In moderate doses, however, which are often used therapeutically, cyclophosphamide distinctly depresses platelets less than the white blood cells (Bergsagel *et al.*, 1968; Wall and Conrad, 1961; Pegg, 1963).

The nadir blood count following bolus doses of chemotherapeutic agents is generally between 7 and 14 days, with recovery by day 21 or 28. The nitrosourea compounds, however, are unique in that the nadir counts may occur between 2 and 4 weeks, with return to normal occasionally requiring 6 weeks. The platelet nadir is often sooner and lower than the white count depression would suggest. The other major effect to be cognizant of when using the nitrosourea drugs is the cumulative bone marrow toxicity. The pancytopenia may become more profound and last longer with successive treatments, requiring reduction of dose (Young *et al.*, 1971, 1973; Hoogstraten *et al.*, 1973; DeVita *et al.*, 1965; Tranum *et al.*, 1975).

Megaloblastic changes of bone marrow cells have been noted to be present following MTX (Speck *et al.*, 1967), hydroxyurea (Thurman *et al.*, 1963; Fishbein *et al.*, 1964), Ara-C (Bell *et al.*, 1966), and 6-MP (Gaffney and Cooper, 1954). Bonadonna *et al.* (1970) reported a mild degree of megaloblastosis in a few patients given adriamycin.

16. Miscellaneous Toxic Effects

A syndrome resembling adrenocortical insufficiency occurs after prolonged busulfan use in a minority of patients (Kyle *et al.*, 1961; Harrold, 1966; Ward *et al.*, 1965). Pituitary insufficiency secondary to diminished pituitary ACTH release was found in two patients. The physiological abnormalities and clinical features of weight loss, anorexia, fatigue, and hyperpigmentation corrected after the drug was discontinued (Vivacqua *et al.*, 1967).

Combinations of various drugs with or without radiation may have untoward effects that neither alone possesses.

Allopurinol, which inhibits xanthinoxidase, when given with 6-MP or azathioprine, will decrease the metabolism of the active forms of these drugs, which require this enzyme for degradation. As a consequence, severe bone marrow toxicity may occur (Elion *et al.*, 1963; Rundles, 1966).

The deleterious effects of adriamycin plus cyclophosphamide and adriamycin plus cardiac irradiation were mentioned in Section 8. The concomitant use of

TABLE 6
Acute Toxicity of Chemotherapeutic Agents

Agent	GI	Skin	Fever	Alopecia	Bone marrow	Liver	Lung
Alkylating agents							
Nitrogen mustard	+ + + +	Local necrosis, vein pain	+	0	+	0	Unilateral infiltrate in 1 pt.
Chlorambucil	+	Dermatitis	0	0	±	±	
Cyclophosphamide	+ +	↑Pig. ±	0	+ + + +	+ Fewer plts.	Tran. ↑Enz. 1 pt.	Infiltrate in 5 pts.
Melphalan	+	Dermatitis	0	0	+	0	
Busulfan	0	↑Pig. ±	0	0	+	0	Infiltrate Fibrosis, nonreversible
Antimetabolites							
Methotrexate HD	s[a]+ +	Dermatitis	+	±	+	↑SGOT	Infiltrate, reversible
LD	s +	Vasculitis	0		Megaloblast	Fib/cir	
Mercaptopurine	±	Icterus	0	0	+ Megaloblast	Cholostalic ↑Bili	
Thioguanine	±	0	0	0	+	0	
Fluorouracil Daily	+ +	Dermatitis	0	+	+	0	
Weekly	±	↑ Pig. ±					
Cytosine arabinoside	+	0	0	0	+ Megaloblast	↑SGOT ±	
Plant alkaloids							
Vinblastine	±	Local nec.	0	+	0	0	
Vincristine	±	Local nec.	0	+ +	0	0	
Antibiotics							
Actinomycin D	+ + +	Folliculitis	0	±	+		
Mithramycin	s + +	Flush	+ + 101–103	0	+	↑LDH, SGOT Acute nec.	
Bleomycin	s +	Dermatitis Urticaria ↑ Pig.	+ + + + 103–105	+ +	0		Fibrosis, nonreversible
Daunomycin	s +	Local nec.		+	+		
Adriamycin	s + +	Local nec. ↑ Pig. ±	+	+ + + +	+		
Metals							
Platinum	+ + +	0	0	0	±		
Miscellaneous							
CCNU	+ +	0	0	0	+ Prolonged	Tran. ↑Enz.	
BCNU	+ +	0	0	0	+ Prolonged	Tran. ↑Enz.	
Methyl CCNU	+ +	0	0	0	+ Prolonged	Tran. ↑Enz.	
Procarbazine	s + +	Dermatitis Urticaria	±	0	+		Infiltrates in 1 pt.
Hydroxyurea	+	Dermatitis	0	0	+ Megaloblasts	Hepat. ?	
ʟ-Asparaginase	+ +	Urticaria	+ +	0	±	Mild ↑ enz. Fat	
Imidazole carboxamide	+ + + +	Local pain	+	0	+	Tran. ↑Enz.	
Streptozotocin	+ + +	0	0	0	±	Tran. ↑Enz.	

[a]s, stomatitis.

TABLE 6—*continued*

Agent	Heart	Kidney	Coagu-lopathy	Electro-lytes	CNS	Misc.
Alkylating agents						
Nitrogen mustard					± Headache	
Chlorambucil						
Cyclophosphamide	240 mg/kg acute necrosis	Cystitis, fibrosis, bladder tumor		Hyponatremia with large doses	SIADH	
Melphalan						
Busulfan						
Antimetabolites						
Methotrexate HD		↑BUN				Pleuritis
LD		Tube nec. Sludge				Peritonitis
Mercaptopurine						
Thioguanine						
Fluorouracil Daily					Ataxia	
Weekly						
Cytosine arabinoside						
Plant alkaloids						
Vinblastine					↓Reflexes Ileus	Myalgias
Vincristine				Hyponatremia	Same Seizures SIADH	Jaw pain
Antibiotics						
Actinomycin D						
Mithramycin		↑BUN	↓Fib ↓II, VII V, X	↓Ca^{2+}	Dizziness Lethargy Headache	Acute react.
Bleomycin						Acute react.
Daunomycin	Child—CHF Adult—acute					
Adriamycin	CHF—61% if >550 mg/M^2				Drowsiness	
Metals						
Platinum	CHF+ECG 1 pt.	Prolonged ↑BUN Tub. nec.			Tinnitus	
Miscellaneous						
CCNU						
BCNU						
Methyl CCNU						
Procarbazine					Lethargy Neuritis	
Hydroxyurea						
L-Asparaginase		↑BUN, reversible	↓Fib ↓V, VII VIII, IX		Lethargy $\frac{1}{3}$	Pancreatitis Acute react.
Imidazole carboxamide						
Streptozotocin		↑BUN Fanconi syn.				

actinomycin D during radiation therapy can result in an enhanced dermal erythema at the radiation port (D'Angio, 1962, 1969; D'Angio *et al.*, 1959). Similar effects at prior irradiation skinports have occurred following adriamycin (Cassady *et al.*, 1975; Donaldson *et al.*, 1974; Etcubanas and Wilbur, 1974; Wang *et al.*, 1971) and 5-FU (Kennedy and Theologides, 1961).

The flush syndrome that occurs with alcohol and procarbazine was also mentioned (see Section 3).

Recently, aseptic necrosis of the femoral head has been observed in lymphoma patients who have received CVPP (cyclophosphamide, vincristine, procarbazine, and prednisone)—4 patients (Sweet *et al.*, 1976), and MOPP (same drug combination, except with nitrogen mustard substituted for cyclophosphamide)—4 patients (Ihde and DeVita, 1975).

The long-term use of MTX has resulted in osteoporosis, hairline fractures, and bone pain in some children. The problem resolves after MTX is discontinued (Ragab *et al.*, 1970; O'Regan *et al.*, 1973; Nesbit *et al.*, 1976).

There is reason to suspect that the combination of 5-FU and hydroxyurea may be neurotoxic. Lokich *et al.* (1975) found that 21% (4 of 19) of patients given this combination developed acute cerebellar ataxia. The hydroxyurea may be potentiating the 5-FU neurotoxicity by a variety of possible mechanisms.

A non-Coombs hemolytic anemia has been seen following cyclophosphamide (Yonet *et al.*, 1967). Samuels *et al.* (1975*b*) noted that following the large doses of vinblastine and bleomycin, a falling hemoglobin and a rising bilirubin developed in 30% of patients. In at least 1 patient, it was clear there was hemolysis.

Eosinophilia has been observed rarely following the use of mithramycin (G. J. Hill, II *et al.*, 1972), DTIC (Gottlieb and Serpick, 1971), streptozotocin (Schein *et al.*, 1974), 6-MP (G. A. Hyman *et al.*, 1954), and procarbazine (Martz *et al.*, 1963; Jones *et al.*, 1972).

The hypersensitivity reactions that occur in 15–28% of patients treated with L-asparaginase are associated with the appearance of L-asparaginase antibodies. The syndrome consists of the rapid onset of urticaria, chills, fever, flushing, fall in blood pressure, and dyspnea. Epinephrine ameliorates the symptoms (Killander *et al.*, 1976).

17. Second Malignancies

There is great concern that the effective cytotoxic therapy that allows long clinical remissions of some cancers may induce another. There is little doubt that acute nonlymphocytic leukemia following the therapy of Hodgkin's disease is occurring at an alarming frequency—109 cases reported by 1976 (Cadman *et al.*, 1977*a*). Similar observations have been noted with multiple myeloma (Kyle *et al.*, 1975; Rosner and Grünwald, 1974; Karchmer *et al.*, 1974). In addition, the use of alkylating agents has also been associated with the development of acute nonlymphocytic leukemia in chronic lymphocytic leukemia (Catovsky and Galton, 1971; Cardamone *et al.*, 1974; Castro *et al.*, 1973), primary amyloidosis (Kyle *et al.*, 1974), lung cancer (Garfield, 1970), cold agglutinin syndrome (Stavem and Harboe, 1971), macroglobulinemia (Petersen, 1973), Wegener's granulomatosis (Westberg and Swolin, 1976), breast cancer (Carey *et al.*, 1967; Perlman and Walker, 1973; Davis *et al.*, 1973), and ovarian cancer (Kaslow *et al.*, 1972; Allen, 1970; Smit and Muler, 1970; Greenspan and Tung, 1974).

Second malignancies (generally histiocytic lymphoma) are common in renal transplant patients who are immunosuppressed and receiving azathioprine (McKhann, 1969).

This complication is unfortunate. But when one contrasts the potential benefits to many patients, especially those who remain free of cancer following the use of cytotoxic drugs, with the few second malignancies that may develop, it becomes clear that this is a risk worth taking. The second malignancy is apparently the ultimate price required for success. Because the second malignancy is a real threat following long-term chemotherapy, especially the alkylating drugs, one must seriously question their prolonged use in nonmalignant diseases that have a projected long survival.

The various toxicities of the chemotherapeutic agents have been presented in hopes that better use and a clearer understanding of their limitations can be appreciated. A summary is presented in Table 6.

The steroids and hormones were not included in this chapter, nor were the teratogenic or mutagenic effects of chemotherapeutic drugs.

18. References

ACUTE LEUKEMIA GROUP B, Acute lymphocytic leukemia in children, *J. Amer. Med. Assoc.* **207**: 923.

AISENBERG, A. C., AND WILKES, B., 1964, Studies on the suppression of immune responses by the periwinkle alkaloids vincristine and vinblastine, *J. Clin. Invest.* **43**:2394.

ALBERT, D. M., WONG, V. G., AND HENDERSON, E. S., 1967, Ocular complications of vincristine therapy, *Arch. Ophthalmol.* **78**:709.

ALLEN, W. S. A., 1970, Acute myeloid leukemia after treatment with cytostatic agents, *Lancet* **2**:775.

ALMEYDA, J., BARNARDO, D., AND BAKER, H., 1971, Drug reactions XV: Methotrexate, psoriasis and the liver, *Br. J. Dermatol.* **85**:302.

AL-SARRAF, M., WONG, P., SARDESAL, S., AND VAITKEVICIUS, V. K., 1970, Clinical immunologic responsiveness in malignant disease, *Cancer* **26**:262.

AMROMIN, G. D., DELIMAN, R. M., AND SHANBROM, E., 1962, Liver damage after chemotherapy for leukemia and lymphoma, *Gastroenterology* **42**:401.

ANDERSON, E. E., COBB, O. E., AND GLENN, J. F., 1967, Cyclophosphamide hemorrhagic cystitis, *J. Urol.* **97**:857.

ANDRE, M. R., ROCHANT, H., DREYFUS, B., DUHAMEL, G., AND PECHERE, J.-Cl., 1967, Fibrose interstitielle diffuse du poumon au cours d'une maladie de Hadgkin traitée par des doses élevées d'endoxan, *Soc. Méd. Hôp. Paris* **118**:1133.

ANSFIELD, F. J., SCHROEDER, J. M., AND CURRERI, A. R., 1962, Five years clinical experience with 5-fluorouracil, *J. Amer. Med. Assoc.*, **181**:295.

APTEKAR, R. G., SALISBURY, K. W., STEINBERG, A. D., AND MYERS, G. H., JR., 1972, Cyclophosphamide-induced, nonhemorrhagic cystitis with abnormal bladder cells, *Arthritis Rheum.* **15**:530.

ARMATA, J., AND DEPOWSKA, T., 1974, Hyperphosphatemia and hypercalcemia in neoplastic disorders, *N. Engl. J. Med.* **290**:858.

ARMSTRONG, J. G., DYKE, R. W., AND FOUTS, P. J., 1962, Initial clinical experience with leucocristine, a new alkaloid from *Vinca rosea, Proc. Amer. Assoc. Cancer Res.* **3**:301.

ARNEIL, G. C., 1972, Cyclophosphamide and the prepubertal testis, *Lancet* **2**:1259.

ARSENEAU, J. C., BAGLEY, C. M., ANDERSON, T., AND CANELLOS, G. P., 1973, Hyperkalemia, a sequel to chemotherapy of Burkitt's lymphoma, *Lancet* **1**:10.

BACK, E. H., 1969, Death after intrathecal methotrexate, *Lancet* **2**:1005.

BAGLEY, C. M., JR., DEVITA, V. T., JR., BERARD, C. W., AND CANELLOS, G. P., 1972, Advanced lymphosarcoma: Intensive cyclical combination chemotherapy with cyclophosphamide, vincristine, and prednisone, *Ann. Intern. Med.* **76**:227.

BAGLEY, C. M., JR., BOSTICK, F. W., AND DEVITA, V. T., JR., 1973, Clinical pharmacology of cyclophosphamide, *Cancer Res.*, **33**:226.

BAGSHAWE, K. D., MAGRATH, I. T., AND GOLDING, P. R., 1969, Intrathecal methotrexate, *Lancet* **2**:1258.

BAUM, E. S., KOCH, H. F., CORBY, D. G., AND PLUNKET, D. C., 1971, Intrathecal methotrexate, *Lancet* **1**:649.

BEDROSSIAN, C. W. M., LUNA, M. A., MACKAY, B., AND LICHTIGER, B., 1973, Ultrastructure of pulmonary bleomycin toxicity, *Cancer* **32**:44.

BELL, W. R., WHANG, J. J., CARBONE, P. P., BRECHER, G., AND BLOCK, J. B., 1966, Cytogenic and morphologic abnormalities in human bone marrow cells during cytosine arabinoside therapy, *Blood* **27**:771.

BENJAMIN, R. S., 1975, A practical approach to adriamycin (NSC-123127) toxicology, *Cancer Chemother. Rep.* **6**:191.

BENJAMIN, R. S., WIERNIK, P. H., AND BACHUR, N. R., 1974, Adriamycin chemotherapy—efficacy, safety, and pharmacologic basis of an intermittent single high-dosage schedule, *Cancer* **33**:19.

BERGSAGEL, D. E., ROBERTSON, G. L., AND HASSELBACK, R., 1968, Effect of cyclophosphamide on advanced lung cancer and the hematological toxicity of large intermittent intravenous doses, *Can. Med. Assoc. J.* **98**:532.

BERKSON, B. M., LOME, L. G., AND SHAPIRO, I., 1973, Severe cystitis induced by cyclophosphamide: Role of surgical management, *J. Amer. Med. Assoc.* **225**:605.

BERLIN, N. I., RALL, D., MEAD, J. A. R., FREIREICH, E. J., VAN SCOTT, E., HERTZ, R., AND LIPSETT, M. B., 1963, Folic acid antagonists: Effects on the cell and the patient—combined clinical staff conference at the National Institutes of Health, *NIH Clin. Staff Conf., Ann. Int. Med.* **59**:931.

BETHLENFALVAY, N. C., AND BERGIN, J. J., 1972, Severe cerebral toxicity after intravenous nitrogen mustard therapy, *Cancer* **29**:366.

BLEYER, W. A., DRAKE, J. C., AND CHABNER, B. A., 1973, Neurotoxicity and elevated cerebrospinal-fluid methotrexate concentration in meningeal leukemia, *N. Engl. J. Med.* **289**:770.

BLUM, R. H., AND CARTER, S. K., 1974, Adriamycin: A new anticancer drug with significant clinical activity, *Ann. Intern. Med.* **80**:249.

BLUM, R. H., CARTER, S. K., AND AGRE, K., 1973, A clinical review of bleomycin—a new antineoplastic agent, *Cancer* **31**:903.

BODEY, G. P., COLTMAN, C. A., FREIREICH, E. J., BONNET, J. D., GEHAN, E. A., HAUT, A. B., HEWLETT, J. S., McCREDIT, K. B., SAIKI, J. H., AND WILSON, H. E., 1974, Chemotherapy of acute leukemia: Comparison of cytarabine alone and in combination with vincristine, prednisone, and cyclophosphamide, *Arch. Intern. Med.* **133**:260.

BONADONNA, G., AND MONFARDINI, S., 1969, Cardiac toxicity of daunorubicin, *Lancet* **1**:837.

BONADONNA, G., MONFARDINI, S., DELENA, M., AND FOSSATI-BELLANI, F., 1969, Clinical evaluation of adriamycin, a new antitumour antibiotic, *Br. Med. J.* **3**:503.

BONADONNA, G., MONFARDINI, S., DELENA, M., FOSSATI-BELLANI, F., AND BERETTA, G., 1970, Phase I and preliminary phase II evaluation of adriamycin (NSC-123127), *Cancer Res.* **30**:2572.

BONADONNA, G., BERETTA, G., TANCINI, G., BRAMBILLA, C., BAJETTA, E., DEPALO, G. M., DELENA, M., FOSSATI-BELLANI, F., GASPARINI, M., VALAGUSSA, P., AND VERONESI, U., 1975, Adriamycin (NSC-123127) studies at the Istituto Nazionale Tumori, Milan, *Cancer Chemother. Rep.* **6**:231.

BORNSTEIN, R. S., THEOLOGIDES, A., AND KENNEDY, B. J., 1969, Daunorubicin in acute myelogenous leukemia in adults, *J. Amer. Med. Assoc.* **207**:1301.

BRAEMAN, J., 1972, P. H. A. response and cytotoxic drugs, *Lancet* **2**:818.

BRERETON, H. D., ANDERSON, T., JOHNSON, R. E., AND SCHEIN, P. S., 1975, Hyperphosphatemia and hypocalcemia in Burkitt lymphoma, *Arch. Intern. Med.* **135**:307.

BREWER, J. I., GERBIE, A. B., DOLKART, R. E., SKOM, J. H., NAGLE, R. G., AND TOROK, E. E., 1964, Chemotherapy in trophoblastic diseases, *Amer. J. Obstet. Gynecol.* **90**:566.

BRODER, L. E., AND CARTER, S. K., 1973, Pancreatic islet cell carcinoma: Results of therapy with streptozotocin in 52 patients, *Ann. Intern. Med.* **78**:108.

BROOK, J., BATEMAN, J. R., AND STEINFELD, J. L., 1964, Evaluation of melphalan (NSC-8806) in treatment of multiple myeloma, *Cancer Chemother. Rep.* **36**:25.

BROWN, J. H., AND KENNEDY, B. J., 1965, Mithramycin in the treatment of disseminated testicular neoplasms, *N. Engl. J. Med.* **272**:111.

BRUCKNER, H. W., MOKYR, M. B., AND MITCHEKK, M. S., 1974, Effect of 5-(3,3-dimethyl-1-triazeno) imidazole-4-carboxamide on immunity in patients with malignant melanoma, *Cancer Res.* **34**:181.

BRUNNER, K. W., AND YOUNG, C. W., 1965, A methylhydrazine derivative in Hodgkin's disease and other malignant neoplasms, *Ann. Intern. Med.* **63**:69.

BUCKNER, C. D., RUDOLPH, R. H., FEFER, A., CLIFT, R. A., EPSTEIN, R. B., FUNK, D. D., NEIMAN, P. E., SLICHTER, S. J., STORB, R., AND THOMAS, E. D., 1972, High-dose cyclophosphamide therapy for malignant disease: Toxicity, tumor response, and the effects of stored autologous marrow, *Cancer* **29**:357.

BUCKNER, C. D., BRIGGS, R., CLIFT, R. A., FEFER, A., FUNK, D. D., GLUCKSBERG, H., NEIMAN, P. E., STORB, R., AND THOMAS, E. D., 1974a, Intermittent high-dose cyclophosphamide (NSC-26271) treatment of stage III ovarian carcinoma, *Cancer Chemother. Rep.* **58**:697.

BUCKNER, C. D., CLIFT, R. A., FEFER, A., FUNK, D. D., GLUCKSBERG, H., NEIMAN, P. E., PAULSEN, A., STORB, R., AND THOMAS, E. D., 1974b, High-dose cyclophosphamide (NSC-26271) for the treatment of metastatic testicular neoplasms, *Cancer Chemother. Rep.* **58**:709.

BUJA, L. M., FERRANS, V. J., AND GRAW, R. G., 1976, Cardiac pathologic findings in patients treated with bone marrow transplantation, *Hum. Pathol.* **7**:17.

BURNS, W. A., MCFARLAND, W., AND MATTHEWS, M. J., 1970, Busulfan-induced pulmonary disease: Report of a case and review of the literature, *Amer. Rev. Respir. Dis.* **101**:408.

CADMAN, E. C., CAPIZZI, R. L., AND BERTINO, J. R., 1977a, Acute non-lymphocytic leukemia: A delayed complication of Hodgkin's disease therapy, *Cancer* (in press).

CADMAN, E. C., LUNDBERG, W. B., AND BERTINO, J. R., 1977b, Hyperphosphatemia in a patient with Burkitt's lymphoma and Burkitt cell leukemia, *Amer. J. Med.* (in press).

CAPIZZI, R. L., DECONTI., R. C., MARSH, J. C., AND BERTINO, J. R., 1970, Methotrexate therapy of head and neck cancer: Improvement in therapeutic index by the use of leucovorin "rescue," *Cancer Res.* **30**:1782.

CARDAMONE, J. M., KIMMERLE, R. I., AND MARSHALL, E. Y., 1974, Development of acute erythroleukemia in B-cell immunoproliferative disorders after prolonged therapy with alkylating drugs, *Amer. J. Med.* **57**:836.

CAREY, R. W., HALL, T. C., AND FINKEL, H. E., 1963, A comparison of two dosage regimens for vincristine, *Cancer Chemother. Rep.* **27**:91.

CAREY, R. W., HOLLAND, J. F., AND SHEEHE, P. R., 1967, Association of cancer of the breast and acute myelocytic leukemia, *Cancer* **20**:1080.

CASEY, E. B., JELLIFE, A. M., LE QUESNE, P. M., AND MILLETT, Y. L., 1973 Vincristine neuropathy: Clinical and electrophysiological observations, *Brain* **96**:69.

CASSADY, J. R., RICHTER, M. P., PIRO, A. J., AND JAFFE, N., 1975, Radiation–adriamycin interactions: Preliminary clinical observations, *Cancer* **36**:946.

CASTLEMAN, B., AND MCNEELY, 1971, Case records of the Massachusetts General Hospital, *N. Engl. J. Med.* **285**:847.

CASTLEMAN, B., SCULLY, R. E., AND MCNEELY, B. U., 1972, Case records of the Massachusetts General Hospital, *N. Engl. J. Med.* **286**:1405.

CASTRO, G. A. M., CHURCH, A., AND PECHET, L., 1973, Leukemia after chemotherapy of Hodgkin's disease, *N. Engl. J. Med.* **289**:103.

CATOVSKY, D., AND GALTON, D. A. G., 1971, Myelomonocytic leukemia supervening on chronic lymphocytic leukemia, *Lancet* **1**:478.

CHABNER, B. A., AND YOUNG, R. C., 1973, Threshold methotrexate concentration for *in vivo* inhibition of DNA synthesis in normal and tumorous target tissues, *J. Clin. Invest.* **52**:1804.

CLARK, P. A., HSIA, Y. E., AND HUNTSMAN, R. G., 1960, Toxic complications of treatment with 6-mercaptopurine, *Br. Med. J.* **1**:393.

CLARKSON, D. R., BLONDIN, J., AND CRYER, P. E., 1973, Phosphate depletion and glucocorticoid-induced hyperphosphatemia in lymphoblastic leukemia, *Metabolism* **22**:611.

CLARYSSE, A. M., CATHEY, W. J., CARTWRIGHT, G. E., AND WINTROBE, M. M., 1969, Pulmonary disease complicating intermittent therapy with methotrexate, *J. Amer. Med. Assoc.* **209**:1861.

COE, R. O., AND BULL, F. E., 1968, Cirrhosis associated with methotrexate treatment of psoriasis, *J. Amer. Med. Assoc.* **206**:1515.

COGGINS, P. R., RAVDIN, R. G., AND EISMAN, S. H., 1959, Clinical pharmacology and preliminary evaluation of Cytoxan (cyclophosphamide), *Cancer Chemother. Rep.* **3**:9.

COGGINS, P. R., RAVDIN, R. G., AND EISMAN, S. H., 1960, Clinical evaluation of a new alkylating agent: Cytoxan (cyclophosphamide), *Cancer* **13**:1254.

COLSKY, J., GREENSPAN, E. M., AND WARREN, T. N., 1955, Hepatic fibrosis in children with acute leukemia after therapy with folic acid antagonists, *Arch. Pathol.* **59**:198.

CONDIT, P. T., 1960, Studies on the folic acid vitamins: II. The acute toxicity of amethopterin in man, *Cancer* **12**:222.

CONDIT, P. T., CHANES, R. E., AND JOEL, W., 1969, Renal toxicity of methotrexate, *Cancer* **23**:126.

CORDER, M. P., AND STONE, W. H., 1976, Failure of leucovorin rescue to prevent reactivation of a solar burn after high dose methotrexate, *Cancer* **37**:1660.

CORDLEY, C. C., LESSNER, H. E., AND LARSEN, W. E., 1966, Azathioprine therapy of "autoimmune" diseases, *Amer. J. Med.* **41**:404.

CORTES, E. P., LUTMAN, G., WANKA, J., WANG, J. J., PICKREN, J., WALLACE, J., AND HOLLAND, J. F., 1975, Adriamycin (NSC-123127) cardiotoxicity: A clinicopathologic correlation, *Cancer Chemother. Rep.* **6**:215.

COSTA, G., CARBONE, P. P., GOLD, G. L., OWENS, A. H., JR., MILLER, S. P., KRANT, M. J., AND BONO, V. H., JR., 1963, Clinical trial of vinblastine in multiple myeloma, *Cancer Chemother. Rep.* **27**:87.

COSTANZA, M. E., NATHANSON, L., LENHARD, R., WOLTER, J., COLSKY, J., OBERFIELD, R. A., AND SCHILLING, A., 1972, Therapy of malignant melanoma with an imidazole carboxamide and bis-chloroethyl nitrosourea, *Cancer* **30**:1457.

CUTTING, H. O., 1971, Inappropriate secretion of antidiuretic hormone secondary to vincristine therapy, *Amer. J. Med.* **51**:269.

DAHL, M. G. C., GREGORY, M. M., AND SCHEUER, P. J., 1971, Liver damage due to methotrexate in patients with psoriasis, *Br. Med. J.* **1**:625.

DAHL, M. G. C., GREGORY, M. M., AND SCHEUER, P. J., 1972, Methotrexate hepatotoxicity in psoriasis—comparison of different dose regimens, *Br. Med. J.* **1**:654.

DAMESHEK, W., WEISFUSE, L., AND STEIN, T., 1949, Nitrogen mustard therapy in Hodgkin's disease, *Blood* **4**:338.

D'ANGIO, G. J., 1962, Clinical and biologic studies of actinomycin D and roentgen irradiation, *Amer. J. Roentgenol.* **87**:106.

D'ANGIO, G. J., 1969, The use of combined actinomycin D and radiotherapy in children with Wilms' tumor, in: *Frontiers in Radiation Therapy and Oncology*, pp. 174–180, S. Karger, Basel and New York,

D'ANGIO, G. J., FARBER, S., AND MADDOCK, C. L., 1959, Potentiation of x-ray effects by actinomycin D, *Radiology* **73**:175.

DAVIS, H. L., JR., RAMIREZ, G., KORBITZ, B. C., AND ANSFIELD, F. J., 1969, Advanced lung cancer treated with cyclophosphamide, *Dis. Chest* **56**:494.

DAVIS, H. L., JR., PROUT, M. N., AND McKENNA, P. J., 1973, Acute leukemia complicating metastatic breast cancer, *Cancer* **31**:543.

DAVIS, H. L., JR., ROCHLIN, d. b., B., WEISS, A. J., WILSON, W. L., ANDREWS, N. C., MADDEN, R., AND SEDRANSK, N., 1974, Cytosine arabinoside (NSC-63878) toxicity and antitumor activity in human solid tumors, *Oncology* **29**:190.

DeFRONZO, R. A., BRAINE, H., COLVIN, M., AND DAVIS, P. J., 1973, Water intoxication in man after cyclophosphamide therapy: Time course and relation to drug activation, *Ann. Intern. Med.* **78**:861.

DeFRONZO, R. A., COLVIN, O. M., BRAINE, H., ROBERTSON, G. L., AND DAVIS, P. J., 1974, Cyclophosphamide and the kidney, *Cancer* **33**:483.

DESAI, D. V., EZDINLI, E. Z., AND STUTZMAN, L., 1970, Vincristine therapy of lymphomas and chronic lymphocytic leukemia, *Cancer* **26**:352.

DESAI, R. G., 1965, Pigmentation after busulfan therapy, *N. Engl. J. Med.* **272**:808.

DeVITA, V. T., CARBONE, P. P., OWENS, A. H., JR., GOLD, G. L., KRANT, M. J., AND EDMONSON, J., 1965, Clinical trials with 1,3-bis(2-chloroethyl)-1-nitrosourea, NSC-409962, *Cancer Res.* **25**:1876.

DJERASSI, I., FARBER, S., ABIR, E., AND NEIKIRK, W., 1967, Continuous infusion of methotrexate in children with acute leukemia, *Cancer* **20**:233.

DJERASSI, I., ROMINGER, C. J., KIM, J. S., TURCHI, J., SUVANSRI, U., AND HUGHES, D., 1972, Phase I study of high doses of methotrexate with citrovorum factor in patients with lung cancer, *Cancer* **30**:22.

DONALDSON, S. S., GLICK, J. M., AND WILBUR, J. R., 1974, Adriamycin activating a recall phenomenon after radiation therapy, *Ann. Intern. Med.* **81**:407.

DUTTERA, M. J., BLEYER, W. A., POMEROY, T. C., LEVENTHAL, C. M., AND LEVENTHAL, B. G., 1973, Irradiation, methotrexate toxicity, and the treatment of meningeal leukaemia, *Lancet* **2**:703.

EINHORN, M., AND DAVIDSOHN, I., 1964, Hepatotoxicity of mercaptopurine *J. Amer. Med. Assoc.* **188**:802.

ELION, G. B., CALLAHAN, S., NATHAN, H., BIEBER, S., RUNDLES, R. W., AND HITCHINGS, G. H., 1963, Potentiation by inhibition of drug degradation: 6-Substituted purines and xanthine oxidase, *Biochem. Pharmacol.* **12**:85.

ELLERBY, R. A., DAVIS, H. L., JR., ANSFIELD, F. J., AND RAMIREZ, G., 1974, Phase I clinical trial of combined therapy with 5-FU (NSC-19893) and *cis*-platinum (II) diaminedichloride (NSC-119875), *Cancer* **34**:1005.

ELLISON, R. R., HOLLAND, J. F., WEIL, M., JACQUILLAT, C., BOIRON, M., BERNARD, J., SAWITSKY, A., ROSNER, F., GUSSOFF, B., SILVER, R. T., KARANAS, A., CUTTNER, J., SPURR, C. L., HAYES, D. M., BLOM, J., LEONE, L. A., HAURANI, F., KYLE, R., HUTCHISON, J. L., FORCIER, R. J., AND MOON, J. H., 1968, Arabinosyl cytosine: A useful agent in the treatment of acute leukemia in adults, *Blood* **32**:507.

EPSTEIN, E. H., JR., AND CROFT, J. D., JR., 1969, Cirrhosis following methotrexate administration for psoriasis, *Arch. Dermatol.* **100**:531.

EPSTEIN, E. H., JR., AND LUTZNER, M. A., 1969, Folliculitis induced by actinomycin D, *N. Engl. J. Med.* **281**:1094.

ETCUBANAS, E., AND WILBUR, J. R., 1974, Uncommon side effects of adriamycin (NSC-123127), *Cancer Chemother. Rep.* **58**:757.

EVANS, A. E., BAEHNER, R. L., CHARD, R. L., JR., LEIKIN, S. L., PANG, E. M., AND PIERCE, M., 1974, Comparision of daunorubicin (NSC-83142) with adriamycin (NSC-123127) in the treatment of late-stage childhood solid tumors, *Cancer Chemother. Rep.* **58**:671.

EVERTS, C. S., WESTCOTT, J. L., AND BRAGG, D. G., 1973, Methotrexate therapy and pulmonary disease, *Radiology* **107**:539.

EZDINLI, E. Z., AND STUTZMAN, L., 1965, Chlorambucil therapy for lymphomas and chronic lymphocytic leukemia, *J. Amer. Med. Assoc.* **191**:100.

FAIRLEY, K. F., BARRIE, J. U., AND JOHNSON, W., 1972, Sterility and testicular atrophy related to cyclophosphamide therapy, *Lancet* **1**:568.

FALKSON, G., VAN DER MERWE, A. M., AND FALKSON, H. C., 1972, Clinical experience with 5-[3,3-bis(2-chloroethyl)-1-triazeno]imidazole-4-carboxamide (NSC-82196) in the treatment of metastatic malignant melanoma, *Cancer Chemother. Rep.* **56**:671.

FARBER, S., 1954, Summary of experience with 6-mercaptopurine, *Ann. N.Y. Acad. Sci.* **60**:412.

FEINGOLD, M. L., AND KOSS, L. G., 1969, Effects of long-term administration of busulfan, *Arch. Intern. Med.* **124**:66.

FENNELLY, J. J., SMYTH, H., AND MULDOWNEY, F. P., 1974, Extreme hyperkalemia due to rapid cell lysis of leukemia cells, *Lancet*, **1**:27.

FERNBACH, D. J., SUTOW, W. W., THURMAN, W. G., AND VIETTI, T. J., 1962, Clinical evaluation of cyclophosphamide: A new agent for the treatment of children with acute leukemia, *J. Amer. Med. Assoc.* **182**:140.

FILIP, D. J., LOGUE, G. L., HARLE, T. S., AND FARRAR, W. H., 1971, Pulmonary and hepatic complications of methotrexate therapy of psoriasis, *J. Amer. Med. Assoc.* **216**:881.

FINE, R. N., CLARKE, R. R., AND SHORE, N. A., 1966, Hyponatremia and vincristine therapy, *Amer. J. Dis. Child.* **112**:256.

FISHBEIN, W. N., CARBONE, P. P., FREIREICH, E. J., MISRA, D., AND FREI, E., III, 1964, Clinical trials of hydroxyurea in patients with cancer and leukemia, *Clin. Pharmacol. Ther.* **5**:574.

FISHER, B., CARBONE, P., ECONOMOU, S. G., FRELICK, R., GLASS, A., LERNER, H., REDMOND, C., ZELEN, M., BAND, P., KATRYCH, D. L., WOLMARK, N., AND FISHER, E. R., 1975, 1-Phenylalanine mustard (L-PAM) in the management of primary breast cancer: A report of early findings, *N. Engl. J. Med.* **292**:117.

FOSDICK, W. M., PARSONS, J. L., AND HILL, D. F., 1968, Long-term cyclophosphamide therapy in rheumatoid arthritis, *Arthritis Rheum.* **11**:151.

FREI, E., III, 1974, The clinical use of actinomycin, *Cancer Chemother. Rep.* **58**:49.

FREI, E., III, RRANZINO, A., SHNIDER, B. I., COSTA, G., COLSKY, J., BRINDLEY, C. O., HOSLEY, H., HOLLAND, J. F., GOLD, G. L., AND JONSSON, U., 1961, Clinical studies of vinblastine, *Cancer Chemother. Rep.* **12**:125.

FREI, E., III, LUCE, J. K., TALLEY, R. W., VAITKEVICIUS, V. K., AND WILSON, H. E., 1972, 5-(3,3-Dimethyl-1-triazeno)imidazole-4-carboxamide (NSC-45388) in the treatment of lymphoma, *Cancer Chemother. Rep.* **56**:667.

FREI, E., III, JAFFE, N., TATTERSALL, M. H. N., PITMAN, S., AND PARKER, L., 1975, New approaches to cancer chemotherapy with methotrexate, *N. Engl. J. Med.* **292**:846.

FRICK, H. C., II, TRETTER, P., TRETTER, W., AND HYMAN, G. A., 1968, Disseminated carcinoma of the ovary treated by L-phenylalanine mustard, *Cancer* **21**:508.

FROST, J. W., GOLDWEIN, M. I., AND BRYAN, J. A., 1962, Clinical experience with vincaleukoblastine in far-advanced Hodgkin's disease and various malignant states, *Ann. Inter. Med.* **56**:854.

GAFFNEY, P. C., AND COOPER. W. M., 1954, A clinical study of 6-mercaptopurine, *Ann. N.Y. Acad. Sci.* **60**:478.

GAGLIANO, R. G., AND COSTANZI, J. J., 1976, Paraplegia following intrathecal methotrexate, *Cancer* **37**:1663.

GALTON, D. A. G., 1953, Myleran in chronic myeloid leukaemia: Results of treatment, *Lancet* **1**:208.

GALTON, D. A. G., TILL, M., AND WILTSHAW, E., 1958, Busulfan (1,4-dimethanesulfonyloxybutane, myleran): Summary of clinical results, *Ann. N.Y. Acad. Sci.* **68**:967.

GARFIELD, D. H., 1970, Acute erythromegakaryocytic leukemia after treatment with cytostatic agents, *Lancet* **2**:1037.

GEISER, C. F., BISHOP, Y., JAFFE, N., FURMAN, L., TRAGGIS, D., AND FREI, E., III, 1975, Adverse effects of intrathecal methotrexate in children with acute leukemia in remission, *Blood* **45**:189.

GEORGE, P., 1963, Haemorrhagic cystitis and cyclophosphamide, *Lancet* **2**:942.

GERNER, R. E., AND MOORE, G. E., 1973, Study of 5-(3,3-dimethyl-1-triazeno)imidazole-4-carboxamide (NSC-45388) in patients with disseminated melanoma, *Cancer Chemother. Rep.* **57**:83.

GILLADOGA, A. C., MANUEL, C., TAN, C. C., WOLLNER, N., AND MURPHY, M. L., 1975, Cardiotoxicity of adriamycin (NSC-123127) in children, *Cancer Chemother. Rep.* **6**:209.

GILLADOGA, A. C., MANUEL, C., TAN, C. T. C., WOLLNER, N., STERNBERG, S. S., AND MURPHY, M. L., 1976, The cardiotoxicity of adriamycin and daunomycin in children, *Cancer* **37**:1070.

GODFREY, T. E., KING, A., AND RENTSCHLER, R., 1973, 1,3-bis(2-chloroethyl)-1-nitrosourea: Effects on advanced ovarian carcinoma, *Amer. J. Obstet. Gynecol.* **115**:576.

GOLD, G. L., AND FRITZ, R. D., 1957, Hyperuricemia associated with the treatment of acute leukemia, *Ann. Intern. Med.* **47**:428.

GOLDIE, J. H., PRICE, L. A., AND HARRAP, K. R., 1972, Methotrexate toxicity: Correlation with duration of administration, plasma levels, dose and excretion pattern, *Eur. J. Cancer* **8**:409.

GOLDMAN, G. C., AND MOSCHELLA, S. L., 1971, Severe pneumonitis occurring during methotrexate therapy, *Arch. Dermatol.* **103**:194.

GOLDMAN, R., BASSETT, S. H., AND DUNCAN, G. B., 1954, Phosphorus excretion in renal failure, *J. Clin. Invest.* **33**:1623.

GOODMAN, L. R., AND SHANSER, J. D., 1976, Unilateral pulmonary edema: An unusual complication of nitrogen mustard therapy, *Radiology* **120**:166.

GOTTLIEB, J. A., AND SERPICK, A. A., 1971, Clinical evaluation of 5-(3,3-dimethyl-1-triazeno)imidazole-4-carboxamide in malignant melanoma and other neoplasms: Comparison of twice-weekly and daily administration schedules, *Oncology* **25**:225.

GOTTLIEB, J. A., GUTTERMAN, J. U., McCREDIE, K. B., RODRIGUEZ, V., AND FREI, E., III, 1973, Chemotherapy of malignant lymphoma with adriamycin, *Cancer Res.* **33**:3024.

GRALMICK, H. R., AND HENDERSON, E., 1971, Hypofibrinogenemia and coagulation factor deficiencies with L-asparaginase treatment, *Cancer* **27**:1313.

GREENSPAN, E. M., AND TUNG, B. G., 1974, Acute myeloblastic leukemia after cure of ovarian cancer, *J. Amer. Med. Assoc.* **230**:418.

GREENWALD, E. S., 1975, Fluorouracil, *J. Amer. Med. Assoc.* **232**:1126.

GREIG, H. B. W., 1956, Myleran in the treatment of chronic myeloid leukaemia, *Acta Haematol.* **16**:171.

HAGGARD, M. E., FERNBACH, D. J., HOLCOMB, T. M., SUTOW, W. W., VIETTI, T. J., AND WINDMILLER, J., 1968, Vincristine in acute leukemia of childhood, *Cancer* **22**:438.

HALAZUN, J. F., WAGNER, H. R., GAETA, J. F., AND SINKS, L. F., 1974, Daunorubicin cardiac toxicity in children with acute lymphocytic leukemia, *Cancer* **33**:545.

HALL, B. E., RICHARDS, M. D., WILLETT, F. M., AND FEICHTMEIR, T. V., 1954, Clinical experience with 6-mercaptopurine in human neoplasia, *Ann. N.Y. Acad. Sci.* **60**:374.

HANSEN, H. H., SELAWRY, O. S., MUGGIA, F. M., AND WALKER, M. D., 1971, Clinical studies with 1-(2-chloroethyl)-3-cyclohexyl-1-nitrosourea (NSC-79037), *Cancer Res.* **31**:223.

HANSEN, M. M., HERTZ, H., AND VIDEBAEK, Aa., 1966, Use of a methyl hydrazine derivative (Natulan), especially in Hodgkin's disease, *Acta Med. Scand.* **180**:211.

HARROLD, B. P., 1966, Syndrome resembling Addison's disease following prolonged treatment with busulphan, *Br. Med. J.* **1**:463.

HASKELL, C. M., CANELLOS, G. P., LEVENTHAL, B. G., CARBONE, P. P., BLOCK, J. B., SERPICK, A. A., AND SELAWRY, O. S., 1969a, L-Asparaginase: Therapeutic and toxic effects in patients with neoplastic disease, N. Engl. J. Med. 281:1028.

HASKELL, C. M., CANELLOS, G. P., LEVENTHAL, B. G., CARBONE, P. P., SERPICK, A. A., AND HANSEN, H. H., 1969b, L-Asparaginase toxicity, Cancer Res. 29:974.

HAUT, A., ABBOTT, W. S., WINTROBE, M. M., AND CARTWRIGHT, G. E., 1961, Busulfan in the treatment of chronic myelocytic leukemia. The effect of long term intermittent therapy, Blood, 17:1.

HEARD, B. E., AND COOKE, R. A., 1968, Busulphan lung, Thorax 23:187.

HERSH, E. M., AND OPPENHEIM, J. J., 1967, Inhibition of in vitro lymphocyte transformation during chemotherapy in man, Cancer Res. 27:98.

HERSH, E. M., CARBONE, P. P., WONG, V. G., AND FREIREICH, E. J., 1965, Inhibition of the primary immune response in man by anti-metabolites, Cancer Res. 25:997.

HERSH, E. M., WONG, V. G., HENDERSON, E. S., AND FREIREICH, E. J., 1966, Hepatotoxic effects of methotrexate, Cancer 19:600.

HIGBY, D. J., WALLACE, H. J., JR., AND HOLLAND, J. F., 1973, cis-Diamminedichloroplatinum (NSC-119875): A phase I study, Cancer Chemother. Rep. 57:459.

HIGBY, D. J., WALLACE, H. J., JR., ALBERT, D., AND HOLLAND, J. F., 1974, Diamminodichloroplatinum in the chemotherapy of testicular tumors, J. Urol. 112:100.

HILL, G. J., II, SEDRANSK, N., ROCHLIN, D., BISEL, H., ANDREWS, N. C., FLETCHER, W., SCHROEDER, J. M., AND WILSON, W. L., 1972, Mithramycin (NSC-24559) therapy of testicular tumors, Cancer 30:900.

HILL, G. J., II, RUESS, R., BERRIS, R., PHILPOTT, G. W., AND PARKIN, P., 1974, Chemotherapy of malignant melanoma with dimethyl triazeno imidazole carboxamide (DTIC) and nitrosourea derivatives (BCNU, CCNU), Ann. Surg. 180:167.

HILL, J. M., AND LOEB, E., 1961, Treatment of leukemia, lymphoma, and other malignant neoplasms with vinblastine, Cancer Chemother. Rep. 15:41.

HIRSCHHORN, K., BACH, F., AND KOLODNY, R. L., 1963, Immune response and mitosis of human peripheral blood lymphocytes in vitro, Science 142:1185.

HOLTON, C. P., VIETTI, T. J., NORA, A. H., DONALDSON, M. H., STUCKEY, W. J., JR., WATKINS, W. L., AND LANE, D. M., 1969, Clinical study of daunomycin and prednisone for induction of remission in children with advanced leukemia, N. Engl. J. Med. 280:171.

HOOGSTRATEN, B., COSTA, J., CUTTNER, J., FORCIER, R. J., LEONE, L. A., HARLEY, J. B., AND GLIDEWELL, O. J., 1969, Intermittent melphalan therapy in multiple myeloma, J. Amer. Med. Assoc. 209:251.

HOOGSTRATEN, B., GOTTLIEB, J. A., GAOILI, E., TUCKER, W. G., TALLEY, R. W., AND HAUT, A., 1973, CCNU (1,[2-chloroethyl]-3-cyclohexyl-1-nitrosourea, NSC-79037) in the treatment of cancer, Cancer 32:38.

HORTON, J., OLSON, K. B., SULLIVAN, J., REILLY, C., SHNIDER, B., AND THE EASTERN COOPERATIVE ONCOLOGY GROUP, 1970, 5-Fluorouracil in cancer: An improved regimen, Ann. Intern, Med. 73:897.

HÖST, H., AND NISSEN-MEYER, R., 1960, A preliminary clinical study of cyclophosphamide, Cancer Chemother. Rep. 9:47.

HRESHCHYSHYN, M. M., 1963, Vincristine treatment of patients with carcinoma of the uterine cervix, Proc. Amer. Assoc. Cancer Res. 4:29.

HRUSHESKY, W. J., 1976, Serpentine supravenous fluorouracil hyperpigmentation, J. Amer. Med. Assoc. 236:138.

HUNT, K. K., JR., 1972, Post-cyclophosphamide pneumonitis, N. Engl. J. Med. 287:668.

HUTTER, A. M., JR., BAUMAN, A. W., AND FRANK, I. N., 1969, Cyclophosphamide and severe hemorrhagic cystitis, N.Y. J. Med. 69:305.

HUTTER, R. V. P., SHIPKEY, F. H., TAN, C. T. C., MURPHY, M. L., AND CHOWDHURY, M., 1960, Hepatic fibrosis in children with acute leukemia: A complication of therapy, Cancer 13:288.

HYMAN, C. B., BOGLE, J. M., BRUBAKER, C. A., WILLIAMS, K., AND HAMMOND, D., 1965, Central nervous system involvement by leukemia in children. II. Therapy with intrathecal methotrexate, Blood 23:13.

HYMAN, G. A., GELLHORN, A., AND WOLFF, J. A., 1954, The therapeutic effect of mercaptopurine in a variety of human neoplastic diseases, Ann. N.Y. Acad. Sci. 60:430.

IHDE, D. C., AND DEVITA, V. T., 1975, Osteonecrosis of the femoral head in patients with lymphoma treated with intermittent combination chemotherapy (including corticosteroids), Cancer 36:1585.

IVY, H. K., 1962, Treatment of breast cancer with 5-fluorouracil, *Ann. Intern. Med.* **57:**598.

JACOBS, E. M., PETERS, F. C., LUCE, J. K., ZIPPIN, C., AND WOOD, D. A., 1968, Mechlorethamine HCl and cyclophosphamide in the treatment of Hodgkin's disease and the lymphomas, *J. Amer. Med. Assoc.* **203:**104.

JACOBSON, L. O., SPURR, C. L., BARRON, E. S. G., SMITH, T., LUSHBAUGH, C., AND DICK, G. F., 1946, Nitrogen mustard therapy: Studies on the effect of methyl-bis(beta-chloroethyl) amine hydrochloride on neoplastic diseases and allied disorders, *J. Amer. Med. Assoc.* **132:**263.

JAFFE, N., KIM, B. S., AND VAWTER, G. F., 1972, Hypocalcemia—a complication of childhood leukemia, *Cancer* **29:**392.

JAFFE, N., FREI, E., III, TRAGGIS, D., AND BISHOP, Y., 1974, Adjuvant methotrexate and citrovorum-factor treatment of osteogenic sarcoma, *N. Engl. J. Med.* **29:**994.

JOHNSON, F. L., BERNSTEIN, I. D., HARTMANN, J. R., AND CHARD, R. L., 1973, Seizures associated with vincristine sulfate therapy, *J. Pediatr.* **82:**699.

JOHNSON, W. W., AND MEADOWS, D. C., 1971, Urinary bladder fibrosis and telangiectasia associated with long-term cyclophosphamide therapy, *N. Engl. J. Med.* **284:**290.

JOHNSTON, B., AND NOVALES, E. T., 1961, The use of Velban (vinblastine sulfate) in metastatic carcinoma of the breast, *Cancer Chemother. Rep.* **12:**109.

JONES, S. E., MOORE, M., BLANK, N., AND CASTELLINO, R. A., 1972, Hypersensitivity to procarbazine (Matulane) manifested by fever and pleuropulmonary reaction, *Cancer* **29:**498.

JORGENSEN, E. O., MALKASIAN, G. D., WEBB, M. J., AND HAHN, R. G., 1973, Pilot study evaluating 1,3-bis(2-chloroethyl)-1-nitrosourea in the treatment of advanced ovarian carcinoma, *Amer. J. Obstet. Gynecol.* **116:**769.

JOYNT, R. J., AFIFI, A., AND HARBISON, J., 1965, Hyponatremia in subarachnoid hemorrhage, *Arch. Neurol.* **13:**633.

KARCHMER, R. K., AMARE, M., AND LARSEN, W. E., 1974, Alkylating agents as leukemogens in multiple myeloma, *Cancer* **33:**1103.

KARNOFSKY, D. A., 1950, Nitrogen mustards in the treatment of neoplastic disease, *Adv. Intern. Med.* **4:**1.

KARNOFSKY, D. A., 1967, Late effects of immunosuppressive anticancer drugs, *Fed. Proc. Fed. Amer. Soc. Exp. Biol.* **26:**925.

KARON, M. R., FREIREICH, E. J., AND FREI, E., III, 1962, A preliminary report on vincristine sulfate—a new active agent for the treatment of acute leukemia, *Pediatrics* **30:**791.

KASLOW, R. A., WISCH, N., AND GLASS, J. L., 1972, Acute leukemia following cytotoxic chemotherapy, *J. Amer. Med. Assoc.* **219:**75.

KENNEDY, B. J., 1970*a*, Metabolic and toxic effects of mithramycin during tumor therapy, *Amer. J. Med.* **49:**494.

KENNEDY, B. J., 1970*b*, Mithramycin therapy in advanced testicular neoplasms, *Cancer* **26:**755.

KENNEDY, B. J., AND THEOLOGIDES, A., 1961, The role of 5-fluorouracil in malignant disease, *Ann. Intern. Med.* **55:**719.

KILLANDER, D., DOHLWITZ, A., ENGSTEDT, L., FRANZEN, S., GAHRTON, G., GULLBRING, B., HOLM, G., HOLMGREN, A., HÖGLUND, S., KILLANDER, A., LOCKNER, D., MELLSTEDT, H., MOE, P. J., PALMBLAD, J., REIZENSTEIN, P., SKÅRBERG, K.-O., SWEDBERG, B., UDÉN, A.-M., WADMAN, B., WIDE, L., AND ÅHSTRÖM, L., 1976, Hypersensitive reactions and antibody formation during L-asparaginase treatment of children and adults with acute leukemia, *Cancer* **37:**220.

KIRSCHNER, R. H., AND ESTERLY, J. R., 1971, Pulmonary lesions associated with busulfan therapy of chronic myelogenous leukemia, *Cancer* **27:**1074.

KLAASSEN, D. J., AND RAPP, E., 1974, Phase II study of CCNU (NSC-79037) in the treatment of advanced gastrointestinal cancer, *Cancer Chemother. Rep.* **58:**667.

KOLER, R. D., AND FORSGREN, A. L., 1958, Hepatotoxicity due to chlorambucil, *J. Amer. Med. Assoc.* **167:**316.

KOSS, L. G., MELAMED, M. R., AND MAYER, K., 1965, The effect of busulfan on human epithelia, *Amer. J. Clin. Pathol.* **44:**385.

KRAWITT, E. L., STEIN, J. H., KIRKENDALL, W. M., AND CLIFTON, J. A., 1967, Mercaptopurine hepatotoxicity in a patient with chronic active hepatitis, *Arch. Intern. Med.* **120:**729.

KYLE, R. A., SCHWARTZ, R. S., OLINER, H. L., AND DAMESHEK, W., 1961, A syndrome resembling adrenal cortical insufficiency associated with long-term busulfan (Myleran) therapy, *Blood* **18:**497.

KYLE, R. A., PIERRE, R. V., AND BAYRD, E. D., 1974, Primary amyloidosis and acute leukemia associated with melphalan therapy, *Blood* **44:**333.

KYLE, R. A., PIERRE, R. V., AND BAYRD, E. D., 1975, Multiple myeloma and acute leukemia associated with alkylating agents, *Arch. Intern. Med.* **135**:185.

LAKIN, J. D., AND CAHILI, R. A., 1976, Generalized urticaria to cyclophosphamide: Type I hypersensitivity to an immunosuppressive agent, *J. Allergy Clin. Immunol.* **58**:160.

LAMB, E. J., MORTON, D. G., AND BYRON, R. C., 1964, Methotrexate therapy of choriocarcinoma and allied tumors, *Amer. J. Obstet. Gynecol.* **90**:317.

LAWRENCE, H. J., SIMONE, J., AND AUR, R. J. A., 1975, Cyclophosphamide-induced hemorrhagic cystitis in children with leukemia, *Cancer* **36**:1572.

LEAKE, E., SMITH, W. G., AND WOODLIFF, H. J., 1963, Diffuse interstitial pulmonary fibrosis after busulphan therapy, *Lancet* **2**:432.

LEFRAK, E. A., PITHA, J., ROSENHEIM, S., AND GOTTLIEB, J. A., 1973, A clinicopathologic analysis of adriamycin cardiotoxicity, *Cancer* **32**:302.

LEFRAK, E. A., PITHA, J., ROSENHEIM, S., O'BRYAN, R. M., BURGESS, M. A., AND GOTTLIEB, J. A., 1975, Adriamycin (NSC-123127) cardiomyopathy, *Cancer Chemother. Rep.* **6**:203.

LEHANE, D. E., HURD, E., AND LANE, M., 1975, The effects of bleomycin on immunocompetence in man, *Cancer Res.* **35**:2724.

LEVIN, R. H., LANDY, M., AND FREI, E., III, 1964, The effect of 6-mercaptopurine on immune response in man, *N. Engl. J. Med.* **271**:16.

LIEBNER, E. J., 1962, Actinomycin D and radiation therapy, *Amer. J. Roentgenol.* **89**:94.

LIEDBERG, C.-F., RAUSING, A., AND LANGELAND, P., 1970, Cyclophosphamide hemorrhagic cystitis, *Scand. J. Urol. Nephrol.* **4**:183.

LITTLER, W. A., KAY, J. M., HASLETON, P. S., AND HEATH, D., 1969, Busulphan lung, *Thorax* **24**:639.

LOKICH, J. J., PITMAN, S. W., AND SKARIN, A. T., 1975, Combined 5-fluorouracil and hydroxyurea therapy for gastrointestinal cancer, *Oncology* **32**:34.

LOUIS, J., LIMARZI, L. R., AND BEST, W. R., 1956, Treatment of chronic graulocytic leukemia with Myleran, *Arch. Intern. Med.* **97**:299.

LUDDY, R. E., AND GILMAN, P. A., 1973, Paraplegia following intrathecal methotrexate, *J. Pediatr.* **83**:988.

LUNA, M. A., BEDROSSIAN, C. W. M., LICHTIGER, B., AND SALEM, P. A., 1972, Interstitial pneumonitis associated with bleomycin therapy, *Amer. J. Clin. Pathol.* **58**:501.

LYELL, A., 1967, Psoriasis and folid acid antagonists, *Br. J. Dermatol.* **79**:367.

MALPAS, J. S., AND SCOTT, R. B., 1968, Rubidomycin in acute leukaemia in adults, *Br. Med. J.* **3**:227.

MALPAS, J. S., AND SCOTT, R. B., 1969, Daunorubicin in acute myelocytic leukaemia, *Lancet* **1**:469.

MARMONT, A. M., DAMASIO, E., AND ROSSI, F., 1969, Cardiac toxicity of daunorubicin, *Lancet* **1**:837.

MARSH, F. P., VINCE, F. P., POLLOCK, D. J., AND BLANDY, J. P., 1971, Cyclophosphamide necrosis of bladder causing calcification, contracture and reflux; treated by colocystoplasty, *Br. J. Urol.* **43**:324.

MARTIN, J., AND COMPSTON, N., 1963, Vincristine sulphate in the treatment of lymphoma and leukaemia, *Lancet* **2**:1080.

MARTZ, B., D'ALESSANDRI, A., KEEL, H. J., AND BOLLAG, W., 1963, Preliminary clinical results with a new antitumor agent RO 4-6467 (NSC-77213), *Cancer Chemother. Rep.* **33**:5.

MASTERSON, J. G., CALAME, R. J., AND NELSON, J., 1960, A clinical study on the use of chlorambucil in the treatment of cancer of the ovary, *Amer. J. Obstet. Gynecol.* **79**:1002.

MATHÉ, G., SCHWEISGUTH, O., SCHNEIDER, M., AMIEL, J. L., BERUMEN, L., BRULE, G., CATTAN, A., AND SCHWARZENBERG, L., 1963, Methyl-hydrazine in treatment of Hodgkin's disease and various forms of haematosarcoma and leukaemia, *Lancet* **2**:1077.

MATHÉ, G., SCHWARZENBERG, L., SCNEIDER, M., SCHLUMBERGER, J. R., HAYAT, M., AMIEL, J. L., CATTAN, A., AND JASMIN, C., 1967, Acute lymphoblastic leukaemia treated with a combination of prednisone, vincristine, and rubidomycin, *Lancet* **2**:380.

MCILVANIE, S. K., AND MACCARTHY, J. D., 1959, Hepatitis in association with prolonged 6-mercaptopurine therapy, *Blood* **14**:80.

MCKHANN, C. F., 1969, Primary malignancy in patients undergoing immunosuppression for renal transplantation, *Transplantation* **8**:209.

MEADOWS, A. T., AND EVANS, A. E., 1976, Effects of chemotherapy on the central nervous system, *Cancer* **37**:1079.

MERIWETHER, W. D., 1971, Vincristine toxicity with hyponatremia and hypochloremia in an adult, *Oncology* **25**:234.

MIDDLEMAN, W., LUCE, J., AND FREI, E., III, 1971, Clinical trials with adriamycin, *Cancer* **28**:844.

MILLER, D. G., 1971, Alkylating agents and human spermatogenesis, *J. Amer. Med. Assoc.* **217**:1662.

MILLER, J. J., III, WILLIAMS, G. F., AND LEISSRING, J. C., 1971, Multiple late complications of therapy with cyclophosphamide, including ovarian destruction, *Amer. J. Med.* **50:**530.

MILLWARD-SADLER, G. H., AND RYAN, T. J., 1974, Methotrexate induced liver disease in psoriasis, *Br. J. Dermatol.* **90:**661.

MILNER, A. N., AND SULLIVAN, M. P., 1967, Urinary excretion of cyclophosphamide (NSC-26271) and its metabolites: Evidence for the existence of an "active" cyclic metabolite, *Cancer Chemother. Rep.* **51:**343.

MIN, K.-W., AND GYORKEY, F., 1968, Interstitial pulmonary fibrosis. Atypical epithelial changes and bronchiolar cell carcinoma following busulfan therapy, *Cancer* **22:**1027.

MINOW, R. A., BENJAMIN, R. S., AND GOTTLIEB, J. A., 1975, Adriamycin (NSC-123127) cardiomyopathy—an overview with determination of risk factors, *Cancer Chemother. Rep.* **6:**195.

MITCHELL, M. S., AND DeCONTI, R. C., 1970, Immunosuppression by 5-fluorouracil, *Cancer* **26:**884.

MITCHELL, M. S., WADE, M. E., DeCONTI, R. C., BERTINO, J. R., AND CALABRESI, P., 1969, Immunosuppressive effects of cytosine arabinoside and methotrexate in man, *Ann. Intern. Med.* **70:**535.

MITTELMAN, A., GRINBERG, R., AND DAO, T. L., 1963, Clinical experience with vincristine in women with breast cancer, *Proc. Amer. Assoc. Cancer Res.* **4:**44.

MOERTEL, C. G., REITEMEIER, R. J., AND HAHN, R. G., 1964, Fluorinated pyrimidine therapy of advanced gastrointestinal cancer, *Gastroenterology* **46:**371.

MONTO, R. W., TALLEY, R. W., CALDWELL, M. J., LEVIN, W. C., AND GUEST, M. M., 1969, Observations on the mechanism of hemorrhagic toxicity in mithramycin (NSC-24559) therapy, *Cancer Res.* **29:**697.

MORGENFELD, M. C., GOLDBERG, V., PARISIER, H., BUGNARD, S. C., AND BUR, G. E., 1972, Ovarian lesions due to cytostatic agents during the treatment of Hodgkin's disease, *Surg. Gynecol. Obstet.* **134:**826.

MOSHER, M. B., DeCONTI, R. C., AND BERTINO, J. R., 1972, Bleomycin therapy in advanced Hodgkin's disease and epidermoid cancers, *Cancer* **30:**56.

MOURIDSEN, H. T., FABER, O., AND SKOVSTED, L., 1976, The metabolism of cyclophosphamide: Dose dependency and the effect of long-term treatment with cyclophosphamide, *Cancer* **37:**665.

MRAZEK, R. G., JR., AND WACHOWSKI, T. J., 1955, Hematopoietic depression from nitrogen mustard and triethylene melamine, *J. Amer. Med. Assoc.* **159:**160.

MUGGIA, F. M., 1973, Hyperkalemia and chemotherapy, *Lancet* **1:**602.

MUGGIA, F. M., CHIA, G. A., AND MICKLEY, D. W., 1974, Hyperphosphatemia and hypercalcemia in neoplastic disorders, *N. Engl. J. Med.* **290:**858.

MULLER, S. A., FARROW, G. M., AND MARTALOCK, D. L., 1969, Cirrhosis caused by methotrexate in the treatment of psoriasis, *Arch. Dermatol.* **100:**523.

MULLINS, G. M., ANDERSON, P. N., AND SANTOS, G. W., 1975, High dose cyclophosphamide therapy in solid tumors: Therapeutic, toxic, and immunosuppressive effects, *Cancer* **36:**1950.

NATHANSON, L., WOLTER, J., HORTON, J., COLSKY, J., SHNIDER, B. I., AND SCHILLING, A., 1971, Characteristics of prognosis and response to an imidazole carboxamide in malignant melanoma, *Clin. Pharmacol. Ther.* **12:**955.

NESBIT, M., KRIVIT, W., HEYN, R., AND SHARP, H., 1976, Acute and chronic effects of methotrexate on hepatic, pulmonary, and skeletal systems, *Cancer* **37:**1048.

NEWTON, W. A., JR., 1954, Clinical experience using 6-mercaptopurine in childhood leukemia, *Ann. N.Y. Acad. Sci.* **60:**468.

NICHOLSON, R. G., AND FELDMAN, W., 1972, Hyponatremia in association with vincristine therapy, *Canad. Med. Assoc. J.* **106:**356.

O'BRYAN, R. M., LUCE, J. K., TALLEY, R. W., GOTTLIEB, J. A., BAKER, L. H., AND BONADONNA, G., 1973, Phase II evaluation of adriamycin in human neoplasia, *Cancer* **32:**1.

O'CONNELL, T. X., AND BERENBAUM, M. C., 1974, Cardiac and pulmonary effects of high doses of cyclophosphamide and isophosphamide, *Cancer Res.* **34:**1586.

OETTGEN, H. F., STEPHENSON, P. A., SCHWARTZ, M. K., LEEPER, R. D., TALLAL, L., TAN, C. C., CLARKSON, B. D., GOLBEY, R. B., KRAKOFF, I. H., KARNOFSKY, D. A., MURPHY, M. L., AND BURCHENAL, J. H., 1970, Toxicity of *E. coli* L-asparaginase in man, *Cancer* **25:**253.

OHNO, R., AND HERSH, E. M., 1970, Immunosuppressive effects of L-asparaginase, *Cancer Res.* **30:**1605.

OHNUMA, R., SELAWRY, O. S., HOLLAND, J. F., DeVITA, V. T., SHEDD, D. P., HANSEN, H. H., AND MUGGIA, F. M., 1972, Clinical study with bleomycin: Tolerance to twice weekly dosage, *Cancer* **30:**914.

OLDHAM, R. K., AND POMEROY, T. C., 1972, Vincristine-induced syndrome of inappropriate secretion of antidiuretic hormone, *South. Med. J.* **65**:1010.

OLINER, H., SCHWARTZ, R., RUBIO, F., AND DAMESHEK, W., 1961, Interstitial, pulmonary fibrosis following busulfan therapy, *Amer. J. Med.* **31**:134.

O'REGAN, S., MELHORN, D. K., AND NEWMAN, A. J., 1973, Methotrexate-induced bone pain in childhood leukemia, *Amer. J. Dis. Child.* **126**:489.

PASCUAL, R. S., MOSHER, M. B., RAJINDER, S. S., DECONTI, R. C., AND BOUHUYS, R. S., 1973, Effects of bleomycin on pulmonary function in man, *Amer. Rev, Respir. Dis.* **108**:211.

PASQUINUCCI, G., FARDINI, R., AND FEDI, F., 1970, Intrathecal methotrexate, *Lancet* **1**:309.

PASQUINUCCI, G., FERRARA, P., AND CASTELLARI, R., 1971, Daunorubicin treatment of methotrexate pneumonia, *J. Amer. Med. Assoc.* **216**:2017.

PATEL, D. D., MORGENTHALER, F. R., KHAZEI, A. M., GRIMALDI, R., AND WATKINS, E., JR., 1969, Methotrexate excretion patterns and renal toxicity, *Arch. Surg.* **98**:305.

PEARLMAN, C. K., 1966, Cystitis due to Cytoxan: Case report, *J. Urol.* **95:**713.

PEGG, D. E., 1963, The hematological side effects of cyclophosphamide and a discussion of autologous bone marrow grafting after cancer chemotherapy, *Cancer Chemother. Rep.* **27**:39.

PERLMAN, M., AND WALKER, R., 1973, Acute leukemia following cytotoxic chemotherapy, *J. Amer. Med. Assoc.* **224**:250.

PETERSEN, H. S., 1973, Erythroleukemia in a melphalan-treated patient with primary macroglobulinemia, *Scand. J. Haematol.* **10**:5.

PETRAKIS, N. L., BIERMAN, H. R., KELLY, K. H., WHITE, L. P., AND SHIMKIN, M. B., 1954, The effect of 1,4-dimethanesulfonyloxybutane (GT-41 or Myleran) upon leukemia, *Cancer* **7**:383.

PHILIPS, F. S., STERNBERG, S. S., HAMILTON, L., AND CLARKE, D. A., 1957, The toxic effects of 6-mercaptopurine and related compounds, *Ann. N.Y. Acad. Sci.* **60**:283.

PODOLL, L. N., AND WINKLER, S. S., 1974, Busulfan lung: Report of two cases and review of the literature, *Amer. J. Roentgenol.* **120**:151.

PODURGIEL, B. J., MCGILL, D. B., LUDWIG, J., TAYLOR, W. F., AND MULLER, S. A., 1973, Liver injury associated with methotrexate therapy for psoriasis, *Mayo Clin. Proc.* **48**:787.

PRATT, C. B., AND JOHNSON, W. W., 1971, Duration and severity of fatty metamorphosis of the liver following L-asparaginase therapy, *Cancer* **28**:361.

PRATT, C. B., SIMONE, J. V., ZEE, P., AUR, J. J. A., AND JOHNSON, W. W., 1970, Comparison of daily versus weekly L-asparaginase for the treatment of childhood acute leukemia, *J. Pediatr.* **77**:474.

PRATT, C. B., ROBERTS, D., SHANKS, E. C., AND WARMATH, E. L., 1974, Clinical trials and pharmacokinetics of intermittent high-dose methotrexate—"leucovorin rescue" for children with malignant tumors, *Cancer Res.* **34**:3326.

PRICE, R. A., AND JAMIESON, P. A., 1975, The central nervous system in childhood leukemia. II. Subacute leukoencephalopathy, *Cancer* **35**:306.

QURESHI, M. S. A., PENNINGTON, J. H., GOLDSMITH, H. J., AND COX, P. E., 1972, Cyclophosphamide therapy and sterility, *Lancet* **2**:1290.

RAGAB, A. H., FRECH, R. S., AND VIETTI, T. J., 1970, Osteoporotic fractures secondary to methotrexate therapy of acute leukemia in remission, *Cancer* **25**:580.

REAM, N. W., PERLIA, C. P., WOLTER, J., AND TAYLOR, S. G., III, 1968, Mithramycin in disseminated germinal testicular cancer, *J. Amer. Med. Assoc.* **204**:96.

REESE, L. T., GRISHAM, J. W., AACH, R. D., AND EISEN, A. Z., 1974, Effects of methotrexate on the liver in psoriasis, *J. Invest. Dermatol.* **62**:597.

REYNOLDS, R. D., SIMERVILLE, J. J., OHARA, D. D., HART, J. B., AND PARKINSON, J. E., 1969, Hemorrhagic cystitis due to cyclophosphamide, *J. Urol.* **101**:45.

RICHARDS, D. E., WHITE, R. J., AND YASHON, D., 1971, Inappropriate release of ADH in subdural hematoma, *J. Trauma* **11**:758.

RICHTER, P., CALAMERA, J. C., MORGENFELD, M. C., KIERSZENBAUM, A. L., LAVIERI, J. C., AND MANCINI, R. E., 1970, Effect of chloramucil on spermatogenesis in the human with malignant lymphoma, *Cancer* **25**:1026.

RICHTSMEIER, A. J., 1975, Urinary-bladder tumors after cyclophosphamide, *N. Engl. J. Med.* **293**:1045.

RIGGENBACH, R., BARRETT, O., JR., AND SHOWN, T., 1968, Hemorrhagic cystitis due to cyclophosphamide: Report of two cases, *South. Med. J.* **61**:139.

RINEHART, J. J., LEWIS, R. P., AND BALCERZAK, S. P., 1974, Adriamycin cardiotoxicity in man, *Ann. Intern. Med.* **81**:475.

RIPAULT, J., WEIL, M., AND JACQUILLAT, Cl., 1967, Étude nécropsique de quatre malades traités par la rubidomycine, *Pathol. Biol.* **15**:955.

ROBERTSON, G. L., BHOOPALAM, N., AND ZELKOWITZ, L. J., 1973, Vincristine neurotoxicity and abnormal secretion of antidiuretic hormone, *Arch. Intern. Med.* **132**:717.

ROBERTSON, J. H., 1970, Pneumonia and methotrexate, *Br. Med. J.* **2**:156.

ROCHLIN, D. B., SHINER, J., LANGDON, E., AND OTTOMAN, R., 1962, Use of 5-fluorouracil in disseminated solid neplasms, *Ann. Surg.* **156**:105.

RODIN, A. E., HAGGARD, M. E., AND TRAVIS, L. B., 1970, Lung changes and chemotherapeutic agents in childhood: Report of a case associated with cyclophosphamide therapy, *Amer. J. Dis. Child.* **120**:337.

ROENIGK, H. H., JR., BERGFELD, W. F., ST. JACQUES, R., OWENS, F. J., AND HAWK, W. A., 1971, Hepatotoxicity of methotrexate in the treatment of psoriasis, *Arch. Dermatol.* **103**:250.

ROSEN, G., SUWANSIRIKUL, S., KWON, C., TAN, C., WU, S. J., BEATTIE, E. J., JR., AND MURPHY, M. L., 1974, High-dose methotrexate with citrovorum factor rescue and adriamycin in childhood osteogenic sarcoma, *Cancer* **33**:1151.

ROSENOW, E. C., III, SEGAR, W. E., AND ZEHR, J. E., 1972, Inappropriate antidiuretic hormone secretion in pneumonia, *Mayo Clin. Proc.* **47**:169.

ROSNER, F., AND GRÜNWALD, H., 1974, Multiple myeloma terminating in acute leukemia: Report of 12 cases and review of literature, *Amer. J. Med.* **57**:927.

ROTHBERG, H., PLACE, C. H., AND SHTEIR, O., 1974, Adriamycin (NSC-123127) toxicity: Unusual melanotic reaction, *Cancer Chemother. Rep.* **58**:749.

RUBINSTEIN, L. J., HERMAN, M. M., LONG, T. F., AND WILBUR, J. R., 1975, Disseminated necrotizing leukoencephalopathy: A complication of treated central nervous system leukemia and lymphoma, *Cancer* **35**:291.

RUNDLES, R. W., 1966, Effects of allopurinol on 6-mercaptopurine therapy in neoplastic diseases, *Ann. Rheum. Dis.* **25**:655.

RUNDLES, R. W., GRIZZLE, J., BELL, W. N., CORLEY, C. C., FROMMEYER, W. B., GREENBERG, B. G., HUGULEY, C. M., JAMES, G. W., III, JONES, R., JR., LARSEN, W. E., LOEB, V., LEONE, L. A., PALMER, J. G., RISER, W. H., JR., AND WILSON, S. J., 1959, Comparison of chlorambucil and Myleran in chronic lymphocytic and granulocytic leukemia, *Amer. J. Med.* **27**:424.

SAIKI, J. H., THOMPSON, S., SMITH, F., AND ATKINSON, R., 1972, Paraplegia following intrathecal chemotherapy, *Cancer* **29**:370.

SALLAN, S. E., ZINBERG, N. E., AND FREI, E., III, 1975, Antiemetic effect of delta-9-tetrahydrocannabinol in patients receiving cancer chemotherapy, *N. Engl. J. Med.* **293**:795.

SAMUELS, M. L., AND HOWE, C. D., 1970, Vinblastine in the managment of testicular cancer, *Cancer* **25**:1009.

SAMUELS, M. L., LEARY, W. V., ALEXANIAN, R., HOWE, C. D., AND FREI, E., III, 1967, Clinical trials with *N*-isopropyl-α-(2-methylhydrazino)-*p*-toluamide hydrochloride in malignant lymphoma and other disseminated neoplasia, *Cancer* **20**:1187.

SAMUELS, M. L., HOLOYE, P. Y., AND JOHNSON, D. E., 1975a, Bleomycin combination chemotherapy in the management of testicular neoplasia, *Cancer* **36**:318.

SAMUELS, M. L., JOHNSON, D. E., AND HOLOYE, P. Y., 1975b, Continuous intravenous bleomycin (NSC-125066) therapy with vinblastine (NSC-49842) in stage III testicular neoplasia, *Cancer Chemother. Rep.* **59**:563.

SAMUELS, M. L., JOHNSON, D. E., HOLOYE, P. Y., AND LANZOTTI, V. J., 1976, Large-dose bleomycin therapy and pulmonary toxocity: A possible role of prior radiotherapy, *J. Amer. Med. Assoc.* **235**:1117.

SANDLER, S. G., TOBIN, W., AND HENDERSON, E. S., 1969, Vincristine-induced neuropathy: A clinical study of fifty leukemic patients, *Neurology* **19**:367.

SANTOS, G. W., 1967, Immunosuppressive drugs I, *Fed. Proc. Fed. Amer. Soc. Exp. Biol.* **26**:907.

SANTOS, G. W., OWENS, A. H., JR., AND SENSENBRENNER, L. L., 1964, Effects of selected cytotoxic agents on antibody production in man: A preliminary report, *Ann N.Y. Acad. Sci.* **114**:404.

SANTOS, G. W., SENSENBRENNER, L. L., BURKE, P. J., MULLINS, G. M., BIAS, W. B., TUTSCHKA, P. J., AND SLAVIN, R. E., 1972, The use of cyclophosphamide for clinical marrow transplantation, *Transplant. Proc.* **4**:559.

SANTOS, G. W., SENSENBRENNER, L. L., BURKE, P. J., COLVIN, M., A. H., JR., BIAS, W. B., AND SLAVIN, R. E., 1973, Marrow transplantation in man following cyclophosphamide, *Transplant. Proc.* **3**:400.

SAVEL, H., AND BURNS, S. L., 1969, Cytosine arabinoside (NSC-63878) given subcutaneously to patients with cancer, *Cancer Chemother. Rep.* **53**:153.

SCHEIN, P. S., O'CONNELL, M. J., BLOM, J., HUBBARD, S., MAGRATH, I. T., BERGEVIN, P., WIERNIK, P. H., ZIEGLER, J. L., AND DEVITA, V. T., 1974, Clinical antitumor activity and toxicity of streptozotocin (NSC-85998), *Cancer* **34**:993.

SCHWARTZ, I. R., AND KAJANI, M. K., 1969, Methotrexate therapy and pulmonary disease, *J. Amer. Med. Assoc.* **210**:1924.

SCHWARTZ, W. B., BENNETT, W., CURELOP, S. AND BARTTER, F. C., 1957, A syndrome of renal sodium loss and hyponatremia probably resulting from inappropriate secretion of antidiuretic hormone *Amer. J. Med.* **23**:529.

SELAWRY, O. S., AND HANANIAN, J., 1963, Vincristine treatment of cancer in children, *J. Amer. Med. Assoc.* **183**:741.

SHAPIRO, W. R., CHERMIK, N. L., AND POSNER, J. B., 1973, Necrotizing encephalopathy following intraventricular instillation of methotrexate, *Arch. Neurol.* **28**:96.

SHAW, R. K., AND BRUNER, J. A., 1964, Clinical evaluation of vincristine (NSC-67574), *Cancer Chemother. Rep.* **42**:45.

SHERINS, R. J., AND DEVITA, V. T., 1973, Effect of drug treatment for lymphoma on male reproductive capacity, *Ann. Intern. Med.* **79**:216.

SHOREY, J., SCHENKER, S., SUKI, W. N., AND COMBES, B., 1968, Hepatotoxicity of mercaptopurine, *Arch. Intern. Med.* **122**:54.

SIRIS, E. S., LEVENTHAL, B. G., AND VAITUKAITIS, J. L., 1976, Effects of childhood leukemia and chemotherapy on puberty and reproductive function in girls, *N. Engl. J. Med.* **294**:1143.

SLATER, L. M., WAINER, R. A., AND SERPICK, A. A., 1969, Vincristine neurotoxicity with hyponatremia, *Cancer* **23**:122.

SMALLEY, R. V., AND WALL, R. L., 1966, Two cases of busulfan toxicity, *Ann. Intern. Med.* **64**:154.

SMIT, C. G. S., AND MULER, L., 1970, Acute myeloid leukemia after treatment with cytostatic agents, *Lancet*, **2**:671.

SOBRINHO, L. G., LEVINE, R. A., AND DECONTI, R. C., 1971, Amenorrhea in patients with Hodgkin's disease treated with antineoplastic agents, *Amer. J. Obstet. Gynecol.* **109**:135.

SOLOMON, J., ALEXANDER, M. J., AND STEINFELD, J. L., 1963, Cyclophosphamide: A clinical study, *J. Amer. Med. Assoc.* **183**:165.

SPECK, B., KIELY, J. M., AND PEASE, G. L., 1967, Hematopoietic effects of a folate antagonist in man, *Cancer* **20**:225.

STARZL, T. E., PENN, I., SCHROTER, G., PUTNAM, C. W., HALGRIMSON, C. G., MARTINEAU, G., AMEMIYA, H., AND GROTH, C. G., 1971, Cyclophosphamide and human organ transplantation, *Lancet* **2**:70.

STAVEM, P., AND HARBOE, M., 1971, Acute erythroleukemia in a patient treated with melphalan for cold agglutinin syndrome, *Scand. J. Haematol.* **8**:375.

STOLINSKY, D. C., SOLOMON, J., PUGH, R. P., STEVENS, A. R., JACOBS, E. M., IRWIN, L. E., WOOD, D. A., STEINFELD, J. L., AND BATEMAN, J. R., 1970, Clinical experience with procarbazine in Hodgkin's disease, reticulum cell sarcoma, and lymphosarcoma, *Cancer* **26**:984.

STOLINSKY, D. C., BULL, F. E., PAJAK, T. F., AND BATEMAN, J. R., 1975, Trial of 1-(2-chloroethyl)-3-cyclohexyl-1-nitrosourea (CCNU; NSC-79037) in advanced bronchogenic carcinoma, *Oncology* **31**:288.

STORB, R., BUCKNER, C. D., DILLINGHAM, L. A., AND THOMAS, E. D., 1970, Cyclophosphamide regimens in rhesus monkeys with and without marrow infusion, *Cancer Res.* **30**:2195.

STUART, M. J., CUASO, C. MILLER, M., AND OSKI, F. A., 1975, Syndrome of recurrent increased secretion of antidiuretic hormone following multiple doses of vincristine, *Blood*, **45**:315.

STUTZMAN, L., EZDINLI, E. Z., AND STUTZMAN, M. A., 1966, Vinblastine sulfate vs. cyclophosphamide in the therapy for lymphoma, *J. Amer. Med. Assoc.* **195**:111.

SULLIVAN, M. P., VIETTI, T. J., FERNBACH, D. J., GRIFFITH, K. M., HADDY, T. B., AND WATKINS, W. L., 1969, Clinical investigations in the treatment of meningeal leukemia: Radiation therapy regimens vs. conventional intrathecal methotrexate, *Blood* **34**:301.

SUSKIND, R. M., BRUSILOW, S. W., AND ZEHR, J., 1972, Syndrome of inappropriate secretion of antidiuretic hormone produced by vincristine toxicity (with bioassay of ADH level), *J. Pediatr.* **81**:90.

SWEET, D. L., ROTH, D. G., DESSER, R. K., MILLER, J. B., AND ULTMAN, J. E., 1976, Avascular necrosis of the femoral head with combination therapy, *Ann. Intern. Med.* **85**:67.

TALLAL, L., TAN, C., OETTGEN, H., WOLLNER, N., MCCARTHY, M., HELSON, L., BURCHENAL, J., KARNOFSKY, D., AND MURPHY, M. L., 1970, *E. coli* L-asparaginase in the treatment of leukemia and solid tumors in 131 children, *Cancer* **25**:306.

TALLEY, R. W., O'BRYAN, R. M., GUTTERMAN, J. U., BROWNLEE, R. W., AND MCCREDIE, K. B., 1973, Clinical evaluation of toxic effects of *cis*-diamminedichloroplatinum (NSC-119875)—Phase I clinical study, *Cancer Chemother. Rep.* **57**:465.

TAN, C., TASAKA, H., YU, K.-P., MURPHY, M. L., AND KARNOFSKY, D. A., 1967, Daunomycin, an antitumor antibiotic in the treatment of neoplastic disease, *Cancer* **20**:333.

TAN, C., ETCUBANAS, E., WOLLNER, N., ROSEN, G., GILLADOGA, A., SHOWEL, J., MURPHY, M. L., AND KRAKOFF, I. H., 1973, Adriamycin—an antitumor antibiotic in the treatment of neoplastic diseases, *Cancer* **32**:9.

TEFT, M., LATTIN, P. B., JEREB, B., CHAM, W., GHAVIMI, F., ROSEN, G., EXELBY, P., MARCOVE, R., MURPHY, M. L., AND D'ANGIO, G. J., 1976, Acute and late effects on normal tissues following combined chemo- and radiotherapy for childhood rhabdomyosarcoma and Ewing's sarcoma, *Cancer* **37**:1201.

THURMAN, W. G., BLOEDOW, C., HOWE, C. D., LEVIN, W. C., DAVIS, P., LANE, M., SULLIVAN, M. P., AND GRIFFITH, K. M., 1963, A phase I study of hydroxyurea, *Cancer Chemother. Rep.* **29**:103.

THURMAN, W. G., FERNBACH, D. J., SULLIVAN, M. P., AND SOUTHWEST CANCER CHEMOTHERAPY STUDY GROUP, 1964, Cyclophosphamide therapy in childhood neuroblastoma, *N. Engl. J. Med.* **270**:1336.

TODD, I. D. H., 1965, Natulan in management of late Hodgkin's disease, other lymphoreticular neoplasms, and malignant melanoma, *Br. Med. J.* **1**:628.

TRANUM, B. L., HAUT, A., RIVKIN, S., WEBER, E., QUAGLIANA, J. M., SHAW, M., TUCKER, W. G., SMITH, F. E., SAMSON, M., AND GOTTLIEB, J., 1975, A phase II study of methyl CCNU in the treatment of solid tumors and lymphomas: A Southwest Oncology Group study, *Cancer* **35**:1148.

ULDALL, P. R., KERR, D. N. S., AND TACCHI, D., 1972, Sterility and cyclophosphamide, *Lancet* **1**:693.

VAN SCOTT, E. J., REINERTSON, R. P., AND STEINMULLER, R., 1957, The growing hair roots of the human scalp and morphologic changes therein following amethopterin therapy, *J. Invest. Dermatol.* **29**:197.

VAN SCOTT, E. J., EKEL, T. M., AND AUERBACH, R., 1963, Determinants of rate and kinetics of cell division in scalp hair, *J. Invest. Dermatol.* **41**:269.

VIVACQUA, R. J., HAURANI, F. I., AND ERSLEV, A. J., 1967, "Selective" pituitary insufficiency secondary to busulfan, *Ann. Intern. Med.* **67**:380.

VOGLER, W. R., AND JACOBS, J., 1971, Toxic and therapeutic effects of methotrexate–folinic acid (leucovorin) in advanced cancer and leukemia, *Cancer* **28**:894.

VORHERR, H., 1974, Para-endocrine tumor activity with emphasis on ectopic ADH secretion, *Oncology* **29**:382.

WALL, R. L., AND CLAUSEN, K. P., 1975, Carcinoma of the urinary bladder in patients receiving cyclophosphamide, *N. Engl. J. Med.* **293**:271.

WALL, R. L., AND CONRAD, F. G., 1961, Cyclophosphamide therapy, *Arch. Intern. Med.* **108**,178.

WANG, J. J., CORTES, E., SINKS, L. F., AND HOLLAND, J. F., 1971, Therapeutic effect and toxicity of adriamycin in patients with neoplastic disease, *Cancer* **28**:837.

WANG, J. J., FREEMAN, A. I., AND SINKS, L. F., 1976, Treatment of acute lymphocytic leukemia by high-dose intravenous methotrexate, *Cancer Res.* **36**:1441.

WARD, H. N., KONIKOV, N., AND REINHARD, E. H., 1965, Cytologic dysplasia occurring after busulfan (Myleran) therapy, *Ann. Intern. Med.* **63**:654.

WARNE, G. L., FAIRLEY, K. F., HOBBS, J. B., AND MARTIN, F. I. R., 1973, Cyclophosphamide-induced ovarian failure, *N. Engl. J. Med.* **289**:1159.

WARWICK, O. H., ALISON, R. E., AND DARTE, J. M. M., 1961, Clinical experience with vinblastine sulfate, *Can. Med. Assoc. J.* **85**:579.

WEINSTEIN, G., ROENIGK, H., MAIBACH, H., AND COSMIDES, J., 1973, Psoriasis–liver–methotrexate interactions, *Arch. Dermatol.* **108**:36.

WEISS, A. J., JACKSON, L. G., AND CARABASI, R., 1961, An evaluation of 5-fluorouracil in malignant disease, *Ann. Intern. Med.* **55**:731.

WEISSLER, A. M., HARRIS, W. S., AND SCHOENFELD, C. D., 1968, Systolic time intervals in heart failure in man, *Circulation* **37**:149.

WEISSLER, A. M., HARRIS, W. S., AND SCHOENFELD, C. D., 1969, Bedside technics for the evaluation of ventricular function in man, *Amer. J. Cardiol.* **23**:577.

WESTBERG, N. G., AND SWOLIN, B., 1976, Acute myeloid leukaemia appearing in two patients after prolonged continuous chlorambucil treatment for Wegener's granulomatosis, *Acta Med. Scand.* **199**:373.

WHANG-PENG, J., LEVENTHAL, B. G., ADAMSON, J. W., AND PERRY, S., 1969, The effect of daunomycin on human cells *in vivo* and *in vitro*, *Cancer* **23**:113.

WHITCOMB, M. E., SCHWARZ, M. I., AND TORMEY, D. C., 1972, Methotrexate pneumonitis: Case report and review of the literature, *Thorax* **27**:636.

WILSON, W. L., WEISS, A. J., AND RAMIREZ, G., 1975, Phase I study of L-asparaginase (NSC-109229), *Oncology* **32:**109.

WINTROBE, M. M., AND HUGULEY, C. M., JR., 1948, Nitrogen-mustard therapy for Hodgkin's disease, lymphosarcoma, the leukemias, and other disorders, *Cancer* **1:**357.

WORTH, P. H. L., 1971, Cyclophosphamide and the bladder, *Br. Med. J.* **3:**182.

WRIGHT, T. L., HURLEY, J., KORST, D. R., MONTO, R. W., ROHN, R. J., WILL, J. J., AND LOUIS, J., 1963, Vinblastine in neoplastic disease, *Cancer Res.* **23:**169.

YAGODA, A., MUKHERJI, B., YOUNG, C., ETCUBANAS, E., LAMONTE, C., SMITH, J. R., TAN, C. T. C., AND KRAKOFF, I. H., 1972, Bleomycin, an antitumor antibiotic, *Ann. Intern. Med.* **77:**861.

YONET, H. M., VIGLIANO, E. M., AND HOROWITZ, H. I., 1967, Acute hemolytic anemia associated with administration of alkylating agents: Report of two cases due to cyclophosphamide and review of the literature, *Amer. J. Med. Sci.* **254:**48.

YOUNG, R. C., DEVITA, V. T., SERPICK, A. A., AND CANELLOS, G. P., 1971, Treatment of advanced Hodgkin's disease with [1,3bis(2-chloroethyl)-1-nitrosourea] BCNU, *N. Engl. J. Med.* **285:**475.

YOUNG, R. C., WALKER, M. D., CANELLOS, G. P., SCHEIN, P. S., CHABNER, B. A., AND DEVITA, V. T., 1973, Initial clinical trials with methyl CCNU 1-(2-chloroethyl)-3-(4-methyl cyclohexyl)-1-nitrosourea (MeCCNU), *Cancer* **31:**1164.

ZARDAY, A., VEITH, F. J., GLIEDMAN, M. L., AND SOBERMAN, R., 1972, Irreversible liver damage after azathioprine, *J. Amer. Med. Assoc.* **222:**690.

ZUZMAN, J., BROWN, D. M., AND NESBIT, M. E., 1973, Hyperphosphatemia, hyperphosphaturia and hypocalcemia in acute lymphoblastic leukemia, *N. Engl. J. Med.* **289:**1335.

4

Clinical Aspects of Resistance to Antineoplastic Agents

ROLAND T. SKEEL AND CRAIG A. LINDQUIST

1. General Considerations

Were it not for the resistance of human tumors to antineoplastic agents, disseminated cancer would not be a clinical problem, and in fact surgery and radiotherapy would be passé. All too familiar to the layperson, physician, and biomedical scientist, however, is the fact that most disseminated cancers respond little, if at all, to systemic chemotherapy, and among those cancers that are initially responsive, the duration of clinical benefit is more often marked by months than years. Thus, those whose aim is to discover the means for successfully treating cancers have had to contend with drug resistance.

The study of drug resistance has covered a broad biological spectrum, from enzymes and membranes through the intact—save for cancer—patient. In this chapter, we will discuss general mechanisms of resistance, as well as resistance to a variety of clinically useful chemotherapeutic agents. Finally, we will discuss ways of overcoming and possibly exploiting drug resistance.

In the most fundamental sense, resistance and selectivity are opposite sides of the same coin. The problem of resistance is not simply to find a drug (chemical) that can kill cells. Irreversibly cytotoxic drugs are easily found. The problem,

ROLAND T. SKEEL AND CRAIG A. LINDQUIST ● Section of Medical Oncology, Yale University School of Medicine, New Haven, Connecticut. Dr. Skeel's present address is: Section of Medical Oncology, Department of Medicine, Medical College of Ohio at Toledo, Toledo, Ohio.

rather, is to find a drug that can selectively kill neoplastic cells while preserving intact—or at least in a reparable state—the essential host cells and their integrated function.

Among the useful chemotherapeutic agents, virtually none is without toxicity to one or more host tissues or systems when the drugs are given in therapeutic doses. All antineoplastic drugs, therefore, lack exclusive selectivity for the cancer tissue, and to a corresponding degree the cancer is resistant. Regardless whether the major host toxicity is on the bone marrow, the epithelial lining of the gut, the nervous system, or the heart, if the drug administration (dose, schedule, route) is limited by adverse host effect, and within that limitation the cancer does not respond, whether initially or with subsequent treatment, then a state of drug resistance exists.

One of the difficulties in studying resistance is that we know very little about what is fundamentally responsible for the increased sensitivity of human tumors to antineoplastic agents as compared with normal tissues, particularly those normal tissues that are rapidly dividing, such as the bone marrow and gut. Even in animal tumor systems, this increased sensitivity is in most circumstances poorly understood. For example, while we can demonstrate that there is a greater sensitivity to methotrexate of L1210 leukemia than of the gut mucosa, which in turn is more sensitive than the bone marrow (Chabner and Young, 1973) as measured by incorporation of tritium-labeled deoxyuridine into DNA, the greater sensitivity is not readily explained on the basis of known pharmacological, biochemical, or kinetic differences between these tissues. For actinomycin D, it has been demonstrated that there are persistent high concentrations localized in spleen, thymus, and Ridgeway osteogenic sarcoma in AKR mice, all of which are considered highly sensitive to the agent. Less persistent levels are found in salivary gland and small intestine, liver, and 7,12-dimethyl benz(α)anthracene-induced spindle-cell sarcoma, which are progressively moderately sensitive to insensitive to the drug (Schwartz et al., 1968). But again, the precise reasons have not been clarified, despite the demonstration of some quantitative differences in cell-surface glycoprotein between parent and actinomycin-D-induced resistant murine tumors (Kessel and Bosmann, 1970).

There are some circumstances in model systems in which marked quantitative differences between normal and neoplastic cells can be demonstrated, such as the enhanced transport and accumulation of the triazine antifol triazinate in Walker 256 carcinoma cells in comparison with the accumulation in normal rat tissues (Cashmore et al., 1975), but the reasons for the transport differences are not known. Such enhanced transport has not been observed in human leukemias or solid tumors tested thus far (Skeel et al., 1976).

The one clinically useful drug for which there is a fairly clear biochemical reason for the difference in sensitivity between cancer cells and normal marrow cells, at least in the mouse, is L-asparaginase (Prager and Bachynsky, 1968). It has been found that sensitive tumor cells lack significant asparagine synthetase activity following asparaginase treatment, while normal tissues (and resistant tumors) can derepress asparagine synthesis, and thus be protected from asparagine depletion.

This difference is also found between sensitive and resistant human leukemia cells (Haskell and Canellos, 1969; Haskell *et al.*, 1970).

115

CLINICAL
ASPECTS OF
RESISTANCE TO
ANTINEOPLASTIC
AGENTS

A second problem in studying resistance in humans is that of obtaining sufficient and repetitive sampling of tumors to document a biochemical mechanism of resistance and then proving the patient is resistant to an individual drug. The sampling problem has limited most studies of resistance in humans to leukemia, since response or lack of response can be easily quantitated, and repeated sampling of blood or bone marrow for isolation of leukemia cells is easily accomplished.

Obtaining adequate samples from patients with solid tumor is more difficult because: (1) frequent visceral or other internal location makes repetitive sampling impossible; (2) tumor composition and viability may be quite variable, due to admixtures of reactive and normal tissue with tumor cells, nonrepresentative anaplasia of the biopsy, and uncertain viability, which in turn depends on the blood supply and other factors. If tissue is available, biochemical studies, such as measurement of drug uptake and nucleoside incorporation, are more difficult to perform because of the problems encountered in obtaining uniform cell suspensions. This problem can be circumvented if the patient has a cellular pleural or peritoneal effusion, but this opportunity is more the exception than the rule.

Proving that a patient is resistant to a single drug is not as simple in human as in animal tumors. For one thing, most patients are now treated on programs that include multiple drugs, so that it is not possible to know whether a tumor was originally sensitive to a specified drug alone, and to what degree the development of clinical resistance is related to a change in responsiveness to that drug. Second, if one is able to use a single drug, criteria for sensitivity/resistance are not easily established. Moreover, while one can document cell kill in leukemia with some reliability, response to therapy in patients with solid tumors is more difficult to quantitate because of tumor location and inadequacy of methods to measure cell kill.

2. Basic Mechanisms of Resistance

Resistance to chemotherapeutic agents is customarily considered to be either natural (i.e., initial unresponsiveness) or acquired. Neither category is mutually exclusive, and resistance acquired after initial successful treatment may occur for the same reason as natural resistance.

2.1. Natural Drug Resistance

Natural resistance may be defined as a lack of tumor response to a given drug regimen despite significant host toxicity. One can postulate four major groups of reasons that tumor cells may be naturally resistant to a drug (Table 1): kinetic, biochemical, pharmacological, and nonselectivity.

TABLE 1
Basic Mechanisms of Resistance to Chemotherapy[a]

A. Kinetic reasons
    1. Because of cell kinetics (growth fraction, generation time, rate of cell loss), drug schedule may be wrong.
    2. Tumor may be in "plateau phase" of growth and refractory to cell-cycle-specific agents.

B. Biochemical reasons
    1. Tumor may be unable to "activate" drug, i.e., convert it to active form.
    2. Tumor may be able to "inactivate" drug.
    3. Tumor may be located in a site in which substrates (e.g., liver and asparaginase) that bypass drug block are available.

C. Pharmacological reasons
    1. Inadequate blood levels (poor absorption, increased excretion or catabolism, drug interactions).
    2. Poor transport into certain body tissues (e.g., CNS).
    3. Poor transport into tumor cells.

D. Nonselectivity reasons

[a] From Bertino and Skeel (1973).

2.1.1. Kinetic Reasons

Resistance based on cell population kinetics is consequent to the fact that as tumors increase in size, the fraction of viable cells undergoing active cell division decreases. This results in a decrease in the sensitivity to antimetabolites and other drugs that show cell-cycle specificity (Schabel, 1969). Such resistance has been termed "temporary" (Skipper, 1974) because it is presumably dependent on the number of cells in a given volume that can be altered by surgery, radiotherapy, or the addition of other drugs. The effect of such combination approaches will be discussed in Section 5.3. It is worth pointing out here, however, that despite our ability to reduce cell burden, sensitivity to cell-cycle-specific agents does not always return. For example, treatment of advanced L1210 leukemia with a single high dose of cyclophosphamide does not restore the sensitivity to treatment every 3 hr for 24 hr on every 4th day, which is able to cure many mice with early disease (Kline *et al.*, 1972). The proliferative state of the cell does play a major role in sensitivity to chemotherapeutic agents, however, and appears to be responsible, at least in part, for the presence or absence of natural resistance/sensitivity (Bruce *et al.*, 1966; Venditti, 1971; Bruce and Meeker, 1967; Goldin *et al.*, 1956). Biochemical changes that accompany the kinetic changes, other than the obvious ones that simply reflect a changed distribution of cells, may also play a role (Hryniuk *et al.*, 1969), and these changes deserve further investigation.

Studies in humans relating proliferative rate to response have been limited. In myeloma, more rapidly responding tumors have a poorer prognosis (Hobbs, 1969), suggesting that a tumor with a high proliferative fraction is more responsive, but—unless cured, as Burkitt's lymphoma may be—is likely to regrow rapidly and result in the patient's death. That this is so emphasizes the clinical paradox that a rapid response to chemotherapy is not necessarily a favorable sign, and may, in fact, forbode a rapid recurrence when resistance emerges. Later studies have shown a marked correlation between increasing myeloma cell mass (measured using the total-body and the cellular M-component synthetic rates) and worsening prognosis (Durie and Salmon, 1975). Studies in other human tumors have not been as elaborate, although knowledge of cell kinetics in leukemia has significant effect on the design of chemotherapeutic programs (Mauer, 1975; Lampkin *et al.*, 1972). Studies in nonhematologic malignancies have been more variable, and it has been difficult to establish correlations between the type of tumor response to therapy and the kinetics of the cell components (Terz *et al.*, 1971) that are of help in designing treatment programs. Thus, for nonhematologic malignancies, treatment plans have had to rely heavily on animal models combined with empirical clinical observations.

117

CLINICAL
ASPECTS OF
RESISTANCE TO
ANTINEOPLASTIC
AGENTS

2.1.2. Biochemical Reasons

Among the biochemical reasons that a tumor may not be sensitive to a drug are the following: (1) inability of the tumor to activate the drug, e.g., conversion of purine and pyrimidine analogues to nucleosides and nucleotides; (2) ability of the tumor or host to inactivate the drug, e.g., deamination of cytosine arabinoside; and (3) location of the tumor in a site in which substrates are available that bypass the drug block, such as is seen in the relative resistance of L5178Y cells in the liver (Fulkerson and Handschumacher, personal communication) to L-asparaginase therapy due to the homeostatic production of L-asparaginase by neighboring liver cells (Woods and Handschumacher, 1971). Specific biochemical reasons for drug resistance will be discussed in greater detail in Sections 3 and 4.

2.1.3. Pharmacological Reasons

Certain pharmacological considerations may also explain natural drug resistance. Blood levels may be inadequate because of poor absorption or increased excretion or catabolism. In a strict sense, this is not true resistance, since inadequate blood levels would not be associated with host toxicity, but to the degree that the insufficient levels are not appreciated by the clinician, the tumor will appear resistant to the drug administration. Such variability among patients has resulted in the provision in many treatment programs for escalation and deescalation of dose, depending on host toxicity, in order to achieve the maximum tolerated and, it is hoped, optimal dose for therapy.

Poor transport into the target cell or into certain host organs and tissues may also lead to tumor unresponsiveness. This problem has probably been studied most extensively in acute lymphocytic leukemia of childhood, during the course of which the development of meningeal leukemia formerly was a common mode of relapse, 40% of patients developing this complication prior to the institution of "CNS prophylaxis" (Evans and Craig, 1964). Because the brain and subarachnoid space exclude many chemotherapeutic agents (Rall *et al.*, 1962; Levitt *et al.*, 1971; Broder and Rall, 1972), they have been called "sanctuaries" for leukemic and other malignant cells. This phenomenon has been best studied in experimental solid tumors, in which it has been observed that while at the center of a tumor mass in the brain, there is essentially no barrier to the entry of compounds that are normally excluded from the brain, at the growing edge of the tumor, where there is an admixture of tumor and normal brain cells, the barrier is nearly intact. Thus, where there are the most proliferative cells and the greatest need, the least drug is found (Broder and Rall, 1972).

Resistance due to poor transport into the tumor cell *per se* will be considered under individual agents when appropriate. For a thorough discussion of basic mechanisms and the relationship between uptake of drugs and resistance, the review by Goldman (1973) is recommended.

2.1.4. Nonselectivity Reasons

Invoking nonselectivity as a reason for natural resistance is in a sense begging the question, since it is a way of saying that many tumors are unresponsive *de novo* to chemotherapeutic agents for unknown reasons. On the other hand, it also emphasizes a fundamental fact: that, excluding variable host organ sensitivity to some agents on the basis of different cell kinetics, very little of the basis for selectivity is known. Even for the most effective chemotherapeutic agents, the therapeutic margin is generally quite narrow, the maximum tolerated dose most often being limited by marrow or gut toxicity. Given the little that is known about the biochemical differences between normal and malignant cells, it is not surprising that more specific, target-directed agents have not been found.

2.2. Acquired Drug Resistance

Acquired drug resistance may be defined as a lack of response of a tumor to a given drug regimen to which it was previously responsive. Acquired drug resistance can most easily be viewed as the selection of a mutant tumor cell clone, resistant on the basis of one of the previously described basic mechanisms of resistance. Other mechanisms such as gene derepression and enzyme induction may also play a role.

In relating the mechanisms of drug resistance found in experimental models to resistance found in the human situation, it is important to note that the usual method of producing drug resistance in transplanted animal tumor is by serial passage through drug-treated mice. Thus, a high degree of resistance may be produced, the mechanism for which may or may not have relevance to the clinical situation. Studies of the type reported by Schrecker *et al.* (1971), in which resistance is produced in a single animal during continuous drug treatment, are more analogous to the human situation, and the mechanism thus found may therefore be more relevant.

As has been pointed out before, not all mechanisms of acquired drug resistance are related to the mechanism of action of the drug; changes in the cell membrane, inactivation of drug by host tissues, or changes in kinetics of the growth of the

119

CLINICAL
ASPECTS OF
RESISTANCE TO
ANTINEOPLASTIC
AGENTS

TABLE 2
Acquired Drug Resistance[a]

A. Related to the mechanism of action
 1. Increased activity of a target enzyme
 2. Altered affinity of a target enzyme (receptor) for the drug
 3. Decreased activation of the drug
 4. Increased activation of the drug
 5. Increased utilization of alternate metabolic pathway
 6. Rapid repair of drug-induced lesion

B. Not related to the mechanism of action
 1. Impaired cellular transport
 2. Increased inactivation of drug
 3. Change in kinetics of tumor growth

---

[a] From Bertino and Skeel (1973).

tumors may also lead to acquired drug resistance (Bertino and Skeel, 1973) (Table 2).

3. Drug Resistance in Human Leukemia

3.1. Thiopurines

Acquired resistance to 6-thiopurines in animal model systems has most frequently been associated with a loss or marked decrease in the activity of the anabolic enzyme hypoxanthine-guanine phosphoribosyl transferase (HGPRT), which is required to convert the 6-thiopurines into their active nucleotides, and there is a good correlation between the capacity of animal leukemias for conversion of 6-mercaptopurine (6-MP) into nondiffusible metabolites (nucleotides) and *in vivo* drug responsiveness (Kessel and Hall, 1969). Uptake of the 6-MP by all cell lines is a rapid process, yielding equimolar ratios in the medium and cell. Increased catabolism has also been observed to be associated with thioguanine resistance in the murine sarcoma 180 (Bieber and Sartorelli, 1964).

Studies in human acute leukemia (Davidson and Winter, 1964; Rosman and Williams, 1973; Rosman *et al.*, 1974) have shown that only occasional ($\sim 10\%$) resistant patients with acute nonlymphocytic leukemia (ANLL) have a marked decrease in HGPRT, while some others ($\sim 25\%$) have a relative deficiency as defined by an adenine phosphoribosyl transferase/HGPRT (A/H) ratio greater than 3 S.D.s from the average for untreated patients. This mechanism did not appear to account for resistance in any patients with acute lymphocytic leukemia (ALL). Mutant enzymes with altered affinity for 5-phosphoribosyl-1-pyrophosphate, particularly when 6-MP was used as substrate, have been seen in human leukemia (Rosman and Williams, 1973), but apparently are uncommon.

Increased catabolic activity has been found in several other patients. Particulate-bound alkaline phosphatase activity was significantly elevated in 2 of

11 resistant ANLL and 6 of 7 resistant ALL patients (Rasman *et al.*, 1974). Increased alkaline phosphatase activity tended to occur in resistant patients with normal A/H ratios. Either kind of change in resistant cells would be consistent with the observations of Kessel and Hall (1969), who reported that leukemia cells from patients who were resistant to 6-mercaptopurine achieved lower rates of conversion to nondiffusible products (nucleotides) of [8-^{14}C]6-mercaptopurine than did cells from sensitive patients. Permeability to 6-MP did not vary between sensitive and resistant human leukemia cells.

3.2. Cytosine Arabinoside

Cytosine arabinoside (Ara-C) is a synthetic nucleoside that in the past 10 years has become the single most important and most widely used agent in the treatment of adult ANLL. While it has been effective as a single agent and in combination for induction of remission of ANLL, its effectiveness for remission maintenance is limited, and some would argue that chemotherapy maintenance in this disease is without value (Embury *et al.*, 1974). In a sense, this view is surprising, since Ara-C is a cell-cycle-specific agent that selectively inhibits DNA synthesis, and would be expected to be more active when there was a low tumor cell burden and a higher proliferative rate (remission) than when the tumor cell number was greater and more cells were resting (relapse). This apparent resistance during remission may be due in part to a narrow therapeutic index for Ara-C, i.e., relative nonselectivity. That this must be one of the factors is supported by the clinical observation that in order to achieve complete remission in ANLL, one usually must continue therapy until the marrow has become markedly hypoplastic, virtually devoid of normal as well as malignant cells. Since most maintenance programs are not so aggressive, resistance in some patients may be more apparent than real. This possibility is supported by the further observation that some patients who relapse during maintenance may again achieve remission when treated aggressively with the same agents as were used during maintenance.

Metabolic phosphorylation of Ara-C was shown by Chu and Fischer (1962) to be a necessary prerequisite for Ara-C to inhibit cellular proliferation. Comparative studies of leukemia cells sensitive and resistant to Ara-C found resistant cells to be deficient in conversion of Ara-C and deoxycytidine to the corresponding 5'-phosphate esters. Studies in a variety of experimental mouse tumors have shown a good correlation between Ara-C phosphorylation *in vitro* and increased survival of animals treated with Ara-C (Kessel and Hall, 1967). The capacity for phosphorylation of Ara-C *in vitro* also appears to have a correlation with response in human leukemia, although this kind of testing has not been used to any extent to predict subsequent response to drug (Kessel *et al.*, 1969).

Biochemical resistance to Ara-C in murine tumors has been attributed to several mechanisms, including a decrease in deoxycytidine/Ara-C kinase, the Ara-C-activating enzyme (Drahovsky and Kreis, 1969; Schrecker, 1970); increased pool sizes of deoxycytidine nucleotides, which compete with Ara-CTP for DNA polymerase (Momparler *et al.*, 1968); and a change in the affinity of DNA polymerase for Ara-CTP (Bach, 1969).

Steuart and Burke (1971) reported that the inactivating enzyme cytidine deaminase was higher in those who subsequently were nonresponders, and in those with initial response, increased progressively with successive courses of therapy until even transient therapeutic responses to Ara-C were no longer noted. Whether this represented selection of a resistant clone or "induced" enzyme could only be speculated on. Tattersall *et al.* (1974) agreed that cytidine deaminase activity was high in resistant cells, but did not find the difference from responsive cells to be significant. They did find that deoxycytidine kinase activity was either below normal or in the low normal range in all patients with resistant ANLL, and although there was some overlap, the mean level of enzyme activity was significantly lower in cells from resistant patients.

Coleman *et al.* (1975*a, b*) pointed out two problems in the studies described above, which were carried out using crude cell extracts to determine enzyme activity. The first problem is that a high level of cytidine deaminase, if uninhibited, consumes available substrate needed for the deoxycytidine kinase assay, leading to a falsely low apparent kinase level. The assay is further confounded if the product of deamination, deoxyuridine, is converted to dUMP by thymidine kinase; it will then be counted as radioactive nucleotide, leading to a spuriously high apparent level of deoxycytidine kinase. They suggest avoidance of this problem by conducting the assay in the presence of tetrahydrouridine, a potent competitive inhibitor of deaminase. The second problem in the determination of kinase and deaminase activities results from the striking increase in deaminase activity with granulocyte maturation. Thus, crude cell extracts with a relatively high admixture of mature cells could lead to falsely elevated deaminase levels. The current work of these authors (Coleman *et al.*, 1975*a, b*) using purified myeloblasts will attempt to determine whether accurate predictions of Ara-C sensitivity/resistance can be made on the basis of biochemical findings prior to therapy.

3.3. Methotrexate

3.3.1. General Statements and Introduction

Methotrexate (MTX) and a few of its companion analogues of folic acid have been used in the treatment of several types of tumors. While the antitumor activity of these compounds has varied widely from one tumor type to another and among individual patients, they remain as useful agents, particularly in combination with other anticancer drugs, in the treatment of a number of neoplasms. The factors responsible for the resistance of tumors in man to the action of MTX are not well understood. Considerable knowledge has been accumulated, however, about mechanisms of resistance in animal tumor models. That knowledge provides a useful framework around which we may begin to make speculations relevant to humans.

MTX has as its primary mechanism of action the inhibition of dihydrofolate reductase (Osborn *et al.*, 1958; Bertino and Johns, 1972). This enzyme catalyzes the reduction of dihydrofolate to tetrahydrofolate, which in turn serves as a one-carbon donor in a number of critical steps in DNA biosynthesis. These steps

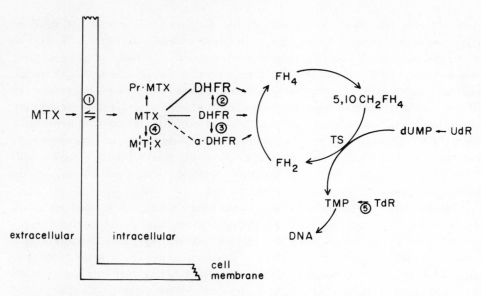

FIGURE 1. Possible mechanisms of resistance to methotrexate: (1) decreased transport; (2) increased DHFR; (3) altered DHFR; (4) metabolism of MTX to inactive compound; (5) increase in thymidine (and purine and serine) from salvage pathways. (MTX) methotrexate; (DHFR) dihydrofolate reductase; $(5,10 \, CH_2FH_4)$ N^5,N^{10}-methylene tetrahydrofolate; (TS) thymidylate synthetase; (UdR) deoxyuridine; (dUMP) deoxyuridine monophosphate; (TdR) thymidine; (TMP) thymidine monophosphate; (FH_2) dihydrofolate; (FH_4) tetrahydrofolate.

include the conversion of deoxyuridylate to deoxythymidylate and two points in the *de novo* biosynthesis of purines. The mechanism of action of this drug, as well as potential sites of resistance, are illustrated in Fig. 1. Starting in the extracellular space, the drug must traverse the cell membrane via an active uptake process that may be altered or deleted in resistant cells. Once inside the cell, the drug faces possible metabolism to inactive forms before it can combine with the target enzyme. The interaction of the antifolate with the reductase itself is influenced by pH, the concentration of the drug, the amount of enzyme, and the affinity of the drug-binding site on the enzyme. Finally, partial circumventions of the action of these drugs can be accomplished by the utilization of so-called "salvage pathways," such as the conversion of preformed thymidine to thymidine monophosphate. The roles that these sites play in the tumors studied will now be considered in greater detail.

3.3.2. Altered Transport

Studies from a number of laboratories have demonstrated that MTX is actively taken into cells by a pathway that is shared by the naturally occurring folates (Jacquez, 1966; Divekar *et al.*, 1967; Goldman *et al.*, 1968; Goldman, 1969; Sirotnak and Donsback, 1974). This generalization appears to be correct in the number of animal tumor models studied, as well as in normal host tissues (Bobzien and Goldman, 1972; Chello *et al.*, 1976; Horne *et al.*, 1976). The significance of transport as a mechanism of resistance to MTX is apparent in both natural and acquired resistant states.

Kessel *et al.* (1965) reported a correlation between the *in vitro* uptake of labeled MTX and the *in vivo* resistance to MTX treatment of a number of rodent tumors. In those tumors that transported MTX poorly (L1210/MTX and P288/MTX), there was a less than 20% increase in survival of animals bearing those tumors when treated with MTX. In contrast, tumors transporting the drug at significantly higher rates (P388 and P815/VLB) were quite sensitive to treatment, with increased survivals being greater than 100% over that of the controls.

Correlations of MTX uptake and natural resistance in man have been made in a few cases using *in vitro* assay systems. Skeel *et al.* (1976) showed that the increased uptake of MTX in human leukemia leukocytes *in vitro* is correlated with the greatest suppression of DNA biosynthesis as measured by the incorporation of [^{3}H]UdR into acid-insoluble material. Unfortunately, there is little correlation between *in vitro* uptake of the drug and clinical response.

Acquired resistance to MTX via transport alterations has also been observed in animal tumor models after exposure to the drug (Fischer, 1962; Sirotnak *et al.*, 1968). The nature of the alteration in the murine L1210 XVI$_4$ resistant line was studied by Sirotnak *et al.* (1968), who found that the rate of transport of MTX was one-fourth that of the sensitive parent line, and that there was an increase in the Michaelis constant (K_m) over that of the parent. The evidence would suggest an alteration in the affinity of the carrier protein for MTX, which in turn results in less efficient transport.

The importance of transport mutants in clinical resistance is not clear. Kessel *et al.* (1968*a*) reported that patients with acute leukemias resistant to MTX had leukocytes that tended not to take up the drug *in vitro* as rapidly as did those from patients who were clinically sensitive to MTX. Unfortunately, such observations also reveal many patients whose leukocytes appear to transport the drug "normally," and yet they are clinically resistant. Thus, it would appear that in the human leukemias, *in vitro* testing of drug uptake is not terribly helpful in predicting a clinical response to MTX (Hryniuk and Bertino, 1969).

3.3.3. Increased Amounts of Dihydrofolate Reductase

The phenomenon of increased enzyme activity following exposure to MTX and accompanied by drug resistance is well characterized in some animal tumor models (Fischer, 1961; Hillcoat *et al.*, 1967). In the murine L1210 tumor, exposure to sublethal doses of MTX has led to the emergence of resistant clones that have 10 or more times the amount of folate reductase than do the sensitive lines. Moreover, the reductase isolated from the resistant line appears to be identical with that of the sensitive line with respect to affinity for the naturally occurring folate substrates as well as for the inhibitor. Similar observations have been made with respect to the sarcoma 180 tumor by Shimpke (personal communication) and his colleagues, who have gone on to demonstrate that an increased amount of mRNA coding for the reductase precedes the appearance of resistance.

A number of investigators have reported a similar phenomenon of increasing amounts of reductase after MTX treatment in the leukocytes and erythrocytes of patients with leukemia (Bertino *et al.*, 1962, 1963). Hryniuk and Bertino (1969) found, in correlating biochemical properties of leukemic blast cells with response to MTX therapy, that those cells that displayed increased amounts of reductase were from the tumors nonresponsive to therapy, while no rise was noted in those tumors responsive to therapy.

The increase in enzyme levels in humans, however, probably does not reflect the total explanation of resistance in those patients. At least a part of the increased enzyme levels is due to the stabilization of the enzyme to degradative steps when it is complexed with MTX (Bertino *et al.*, 1963). Hryniuk and Bertino (1969) go on to suggest that such resistance may be the resultant of both partial stabilization of the enzyme and a more rapid turnover of the enzyme, an endogenous characteristic of some resistant cell populations.

3.3.4. Altered Enzyme

The binding of MTX to mammalian DHFR is both stoichiometric and tight (Osborn *et al.*, 1958). The high affinity of the enzyme for the drug allows for significant inhibition of activity when the drug concentrations are comparable to that of the enzyme. Some correlations have been made between the dissociation constants of the DHFR–MTX complex and the source cell line's intrinsic resistance to MTX. Jackson *et al.* (1976) studied four cultured mammalian cell lines the intrinsic MTX resistance of which covered a 70-fold range of concentration. All the cell types were able to transport extracellular MTX across the cell membrane efficiently and at comparable rates. A kinetic study of highly purified reductase from the four sources, however, revealed large differences in the K_i values for MTX among the four cell lines. These dissociation constants differed by 25-fold between the lowest and the highest, and correlated with each cell type's degree of resistance to MTX in culture.

Altered enzyme has also been implicated as a mechanism of acquired resistance in mouse tumor models (Blumenthal and Greenberg, 1970; Biedler *et al.*, 1972). The data to support such a mechanism in humans, however, are only suggestive. Bertino and Skeel (1973) reported a patient who developed MTX resistance and whose reductase from leukemic blasts was significantly less sensitive to MTX than other human leukemic enzymes or that from the L1210 cell line. A more careful characterization of such apparently altered enzymes was limited by the amount of material available.

3.3.5. Host Metabolism of the Drug

In humans, the metabolism of MTX does not appear to be significant, with most of the drug being excreted unchanged in the urine. Dichloromethotrexate (DCM) is, however, metabolized by the liver to the 7-hydroxy form of DCM. The enzyme responsible for this conversion in some rodents appears to be hepatic aldehyde oxidase (Davidson and Oliverio, 1965), and it probably effects the conversion in humans as well. Attempts have been made to circumvent this "host resistance" to DCM by synthesizing 7-methyl derivatives of DCM that resist hydroxylation by the oxidase. Those synthesized to date, however, are not good inhibitors of DHFR (Rosowsky and Chen, 1974).

3.3.6. Low Growth Function

Since the primary mechanism of action of MTX is to deplete the reduced folate coenzymes necessary for the biosynthesis of DNA, it might be expected that the drug would be most effective against those cell populations that are actively dividing. Conversely, tumors that have large numbers of cells in "resting" phase (G_0), or those with long generation times, would be expected to be relatively resistant to the antimetabolite.

Hryniuk et al. (1969) demonstrated that the rate of kill of log culture L5178Y cells by 10^6 M MTX is nearly 7 times that of the cells from the resting culture. Although the reasons for the heightened sensitivity of the log cells may be biochemical as well as kinetic, it is clear that in animal models, cellular kinetics can greatly influence curability (Skipper, 1968; Schabel, 1968), and undoubtedly play an important role in the response of human tumors as well.

3.3.7. Multiple Sites of Resistance

Combination mutants resistant to MTX via transport deficiencies and elevated reductase levels in mammalian tumor models have been reported (Sirotnak et al., 1967). In the resistant L1210RR subline, reductase levels are elevated over 100 times that of the parent sensitive line, and the active transport of MTX is apparently lacking (Lindquist et al., unpublished data). Whether or not such combinations occur in human tumors is not known. Certainly the potential for this or other combination mutants exists, and further study is warranted.

3.4. Daunorubicin and Adriamycin

Daunorubicin and adriamycin are both effective agents in the treatment of acute leukemia. They have been most important in the management of ANLL, and along with Ara-C, have become part of many treatment programs. While they are effective for remission induction, their utility in maintenance is limited not only by the development of resistance of the leukemia cell, but also by dose-limiting cumulative myocardial degeneration. It would thus be particularly advantageous to be able to detect sensitivity/resistance in order to select patients who might be more likely to respond to treatment.

Uptake and retention of daunorubicin (fluorometrically determined) has been correlated with survival of mice bearing different transplanted tumors, although separation of daunorubicin from metabolites was not done (Kessel et al., 1968b). Chinese hamster cells, made more than 800-fold resistant to daunorubicin by exposure to the drug, incorporate [^{3}H]daunorubicin poorly in comparison with sensitive parent cells (Riehm and Biedler, 1971). Other studies have supported the relationship between uptake of the drug and inhibition of DNA synthesis in tumor cells (Rusconi and DiMarco, 1969).

Resistance to anthracyclines in animals appears to confer cross-resistance to other drugs of the same group, and often to unrelated agents such as vinca alkaloids (Skovsgaard, 1975) and actinomycin D (Riehm and Biedler, 1971).

Clinical response to daunorubicin in adult ANLL has been correlated with daunorubicin reductase activity in the leukemia myeloblasts expressed as a ratio of myeloblast activity to erythrocyte activity (Huffman and Bachur, 1972; Greene *et al.*, 1972). Patients with a high enzyme level responded favorably to daunorubicin therapy, while those with a lower level had no response or died during therapy. Since poorer responders were also older (as is usually the case in ANLL), a comparison was made between age and reductase activity. A significant inverse correlation was found for the leukemia patients, although no such correlation was seen among normal controls.

In vitro survival of leukemia marrow blast cells in short-term cell culture with daunorubicin, alone or with vincristine, has been correlated with *in vivo* tumoricidal effect in children with ALL (7) and ANLL (1) (Laurie and Willoughby, 1969). In a small number of cases, there was a complete separation of responsive and nonresponsive patients, and the authors suggest that this test has practical value for selecting drug therapy. We studied the inhibition of DNA and RNA synthesis by daunorubicin *in vitro* in a patient with ANLL before and after clinical resistance developed. Before treatment, incorporation of [^{3}H]thymidine into DNA and [^{3}H]uridine into RNA by leukemia blast cell suspensions was inhibited 89% and 80%, respectively, by 5 μg daunorubicin/ml; after the patient became resistant, these values fell to 58% and 41% (Skeel *et al.*, 1970).

Cross-resistance between daunorubicin and adriamycin has generally been found (Whitehouse *et al.*, 1972; Mathé *et al.*, 1970), although at least one study has found that patients refractory to daunorubicin (and Ara-C) responded to subsequent adriamycin (and Ara-C) (Smith and McElwain, 1974). Since the relative dose of adriamycin in this latter study was higher than the previous daunorubicin, however, the beneficial effect may have been largely a dose-dependent phenomenon.

3.5. L-Asparaginase

L-Asparaginase is a bacterial protein of about 130,000 mol. wt. that catalyzes the hydrolysis of L-asparagine into L-aspartic acid and ammonia. Its action appears to be dependent on the requirement of cells that are sensitive to L-asparaginase for exogenous L-asparagine. When the enzyme depletes the exogenous source, the tumor cell cannot survive. Resistance to L-asparaginase develops for reasons related and unrelated to the mechanism of action.

Broome and Schwartz (1967) showed that cells from mouse lymphoma 6C₃HED, which was resistant to L-asparaginase, were able to synthesize and liberate more than 8 times more L-asparaginase than sensitive cells. This ability was associated with a retained capacity for protein synthesis by the resistant cells in the presence of low levels of L-asparagine in *in vitro* incubations. These authors further postulated that there might be a linkage between sites of asparagine synthesis and utilization that allows preferential use of the amino acid before equilibration with the whole cell pool (Broome, 1968). Asparagine synthetase activity was found to be low or absent in a wide variety of asparaginase-sensitive murine leukemias, while leukemias insensitive to L-asparaginase had substantial to very high synthetase activity (Horowitz *et al.*, 1968). Prager and Bachynsky (1968) further observed that administration of L-asparaginase to resistant tumor–bearing mice resulted in a large increase (5–19 fold) in asparagine synthetase activity, while susceptible tumor responded only transiently. Normal mouse tissues showed moderate increases in asparagine synthetase activity with L-asparaginase treatment, equivalent to that found in the guinea pig, which normally has asparaginase in its circulation.

Asparagine synthetase levels have been determined in patients with leukemia, before and during or after treatment. Prior to therapy, asparagine synthetase is nearly undetectable, regardless of subsequent response to L-asparaginase treatment. In patients in whom there is an antileukemic effect, no change in synthetase occurs with therapy, while there is a 7-fold increase in those patients who are unresponsive to therapy (Haskell and Canellos, 1969; Haskell *et al.*, 1970). It thus seems clear that in acute leukemia, as in murine tumors, derepression of asparagine synthetase or reduced product inhibition, or both, play an important if not exclusive role in the cellular resistance to L-asparaginase. *In vitro* sensitivity measured by the inhibition of incorporation of [^{3}H]uridine into RNA and [^{14}C]valine into protein by L-asparaginase has shown no correlation with the response to L-asparaginase therapy in humans (Capizzi *et al.*, 1971), thus ruling out these simple incubations to determine cell sensitivity/resistance.

A second mode of resistance to L-asparaginase is immunologic, which often results in anaphylaxis in both animals and humans (Schein *et al.*, 1969; Peterson *et al.*, 1971; Capizzi *et al.*, 1971). Antibodies to L-asparaginase, detectable by passive hemagglutination, are detectable in most but not all patients prior to the development of severe allergic reactions (Peterson *et al.*, 1970; Capizzi *et al.*, 1971; Mitchell, personal communication). Precipitating antibodies and specific reagin antibodies are detectable only occasionally. In addition to causing severe host reaction, the antibodies result in extremely rapid clearance of L-asparaginase from the circulation in mice (Baechtel and Prager, 1973) and humans (Capizzi *et al.*, 1971).

A third type of resistance to L-asparaginase therapy has been found in the L5178Y murine leukemia, for which the liver is a sanctuary during treatment (Fulkerson and Handschumacher, personal communication). The liver has been found to be important in homeostasis of plasma L-asparagine, balancing the level between 30 and 40 μM by asparagine synthesis or catabolism (Woods and Handschumacher, 1971). It is thought that the liver's abundant capacity to synthesize asparagine serves to supply leukemia cells, resident in the reticuloendothelial

127

CLINICAL
ASPECTS OF
RESISTANCE TO
ANTINEOPLASTIC
AGENTS

system of the liver, with sufficient local asparagine, through diffusion processes, to survive plasma depletion. The degree to which this mechanism might pertain to human leukemia has not been determined.

3.6. Corticosteroids

Glucocorticosteroids have a remarkable ability to cause lymphoid destruction in the normal thymic cortex and some peripheral marrow-derived cells of mice, hamsters, rats, and rabbits. Normal lymphocytes from guinea pigs, monkeys, and humans, on the other hand, are relatively resistant to this lymphocyte-depleting action (Claman, 1972). It is somewhat surprising, therefore, that corticosteroids have such a dramatic effect in acute lymphocytic leukemia, resulting in complete remission in 50–60% of children with the disease.

High-affinity glucocorticoid receptors have recently been found in mouse lymphoma cells (Baxter et al., 1971). Studies of steroid binding by these cells have shown a direct correlation between cortisol binding in the cytoplasm and nucleus and sensitivity to killing by cortisol. In human ALL, the level of steroid binding corresponded directly to the inhibition of [^{3}H]thymidine uptake in leukemia blasts (Lippman et al., 1973). In glucocorticoid-resistant cells, steroid-binding protein was not detectable. Steroid-binding protein was found to be present in cells from patients who subsequently responded to combinations of drugs including glucocorticoids. When they became clinically unresponsive, steroid-binding protein was no longer detectable.

Specific glucocorticoid-binding proteins have also been found in myeloblasts of patients with untreated ANLL. As with ALL, glucocorticoid-binding activity was positively correlated with inhibition of macromolecular synthesis in vitro (Lippman et al., 1975). It has been proposed that this relationship can provide assistance in planning chemotherapeutic regimens.

4. Drug Resistance in Cancers Other than Leukemia

4.1. Alkylating Agents

On the basis of what was known at that time, Wheeler (1963) suggested that altered cell permeability or deactivation of drug by combination with nonprotein sulfhydryl groups was the most plausible mechanism for resistance to alkylating agents. While the extent of in vivo fixation of various ^{14}C-labeled alkylating agents did not correlate with tumor-inhibitory activities in sensitive vs. resistant cells (Wheeler and Alexander, 1964), subsequent studies of the uptake of [^{14}C]nitrogen mustard showed that sensitive cells accumulated more drug than resistant cells in Ehrlich ascites tumor (Rutman et al., 1968; Wolpert and Ruddon, 1969), L5178Y lymphoblasts (Goldenberg et al., 1970), and Yoshida sarcoma (Inaba, 1973). Nitrogen mustard transport was found to be an active process mediated by the naturally occurring transport carrier for choline (Goldenberg et al., 1971). Uptake is inhibited by choline, hydrolyzed nitrogen mustard, and the monofunctional analogue dimethyl 2-chlorethylamine, but not by other structural analogues such as chlorambucil and cyclophosphamide (Goldenberg *et al.*, 1970). The K_m was greater and the V_{max} lower for resistant than for sensitive cells, suggesting a decreased affinity and carrying capacity in resistant cells. Correspondingly less [^{14}C]nitrogen mustard was bound to DNA, RNA, and protein of resistant lymphoblasts than of sensitive cells, in contrast to the studies of Wheeler and Alexander (1964).

Detailed studies of cross-resistance have shown that L5178Y cells that were 18-fold more resistant to nitrogen mustard than sensitive parent cells were just 2–3 fold more resistant to other alkylating agents (chlorambucil, melphalan, BCNU) (Goldenberg, 1975). Since transport of nitrogen mustard is not inhibited by these compounds, it was concluded that: (1) cross-resistance may involve nontransport factors, and (2) a major part of resistance to nitrogen mustard might be bypassed by using these drugs.

Resistance to cyclophosphamide has been studied in leukemia L1210 (DeWys, 1973) and PARA-adenovirus 7 transformed cells (Laux and Lausch, 1974). In the former study, an analysis of dose–response curves suggested a difference either in cell uptake or in intracellular handling of drug as mechanisms of resistance. Laux and Lausch (1974) evaluated the development of resistance during drug treatment in individual animals. They observed that: (1) cyclophosphamide was activated normally in the resistant host; (2) during treatment, animals became immunosuppressed, and this contributed to the ability of cells to grow; and (3) isolated tumor cells were less susceptible to the cytotoxic reaction of the drug *in vitro*.

Transport of hydrolyzed nitrogen mustard into normal and leukemic human cells has been found to have two components, a low-affinity, high-capacity system at high drug concentrations, and a high-affinity, low-capacity system that appears to be shared with choline at low drug concentrations (Lyons and Goldenberg, 1972). Morphine and cocaine stimulate transport of the hydrolyzed nitrogen mustard and choline into these same cells (Goldenberg, 1976). The clinical relevance for active (nonhydrolyzed) nitrogen mustard is unclear, since choline uptake was stimulated more in leukemic than normal cells, while the reverse was true for the uptake of hydrolyzed nitrogen mustard. Similar evaluation of nonleukemia tumor cells has not been reported.

Clinical resistance to one alkylating agent does not predict resistance to all other drugs of the same class (Bergsagel and Pruzanski, 1975). This is particularly true if one considers the lack of cross-resistance between classic alkylating agents and the nitrosoureas (DeVita *et al.*, 1965; Lessner, 1968; Tranum *et al.*, 1975) or procarbazine (DeConti, 1971; Spivack, 1974), both of which have some characteristics in common with the mustards, but lack cross-resistance.

4.2. 5-Fluorouracil

5-Fluorouracil (5-FU) is widely used in the treatment of adenocarcinoma of the GI tract and breast. The majority of patients do not respond, even with partial remissions ($>50\%$ decrease in the product of the largest diameters), however, and thus resistance to the drug—used as a single agent—is an important clinical problem.

Heidelberger and co-workers (1960) found that 5-FU and 5-fluoro-2'-deoxyuridine inhibited the incorporation of [^{14}C]formate into DNA to a much greater degree in susceptible than in resistant Ehrlich ascites carcinoma. [^{14}C]Uracil incorporation into DNA was also inhibited by these drugs, whereas there was no inhibition in the resistant cells. Since the nucleotide production in normal and resistant cells was comparable, their results were consistent with a loss of capacity for the active nucleotide to inhibit thymidylate synthetase.

Kasbekar and Greenberg (1963) found that resistant Gardner lymphoma had altered orotic acid metabolism, and had lost the ability to convert 5-FU to fluorouridylic acid. Neither changes in thymidylate synthetase nor permeability differences for 5-FU between the two tumor lines were found. Sköld (1963) found evidence of decreased uridine kinase activity and associated evidence that the stucture of the enzyme was altered during the development of resistance to 5-FU in the Ehrlich ascites tumor. The responsiveness of several other transplantable mouse tumors *in vivo* to 5-fluoro-2'-deoxyuridine was inversely correlated with tumor levels of thymidine kinase (Kessel and Wodinsky, 1970). Since this enzyme transforms the drug into its active nucleotide, the increased levels associated with resistance apparently serve primarily to bypass drug-induced blockade of thymidylate biosynthesis.

Studies on the mechanism of human tumor resistance to 5-FU and fluorodeoxyuridine have also shown several biochemical alterations (Wolberg, 1964, 1969, 1971). Some resistant patients' cells incorporated neither thymidine nor uridine in the absence of drug, and were presumed to have deficiencies in uridine phosphorylase or kinase, or both, and thymidine kinase. Resistance in these patients can be explained by lack of enzymes necessary to convert the drugs to their active nucleotides. Among patients who showed an increased utilization of thymidine during incubation with fluorinated pyrimidines, about one-half responded to treatment. Those patients in whom thymidine and uridine uptake changed but little did not respond, presumably because of an insensitive thymidylate synthetase. All patients in whom the uptake of thymidine was decreased in the presence of the fluorinated pyrimidines, and 2 of 3 whose thymidine uptake was unchanged while uridine uptake decreased responded well to chemotherapy. Wolberg has also found a correlation between *in vitro* incorporation of formate into DNA and clinical response. A good response was associated with greater inhibition of formate incorporation after 5-FU therapy, while resistance was associated with a low initial incorporation less inhibition by 5-FU.

4.3. Sex Hormones and Breast Cancer

The breast is a hormone-sensitive organ in which the risk of development of cancer in humans may well be related to the hormonal milieu (Lemon *et al.*, 1966; Dickenson *et al.*, 1974; B. E. Henderson *et al.*, 1975). It is not surprising, therefore, that there would be cellular determinants of hormonal responsiveness. Chayen *et al.* (1970) found that human breast cancer specimens could be grouped into two distinct classes, depending on their response to estrogen *in vitro*, but did not correlate their studies with *in vivo* response to hormonal manipulation. Jensen *et al.* (1971) correlated estrogen binding by human breast tumors with clinical response. Of 29 patients showing no evidence of estrogen receptor, only 1 had a remission after therapy. In contrast, 10 of 13 patients whose cancer contained estrogen receptor showed objective remission to endocrine therapy. It is generally accepted that 55–60% of estrogen-receptor-positive patients will respond to hormonal therapy, while less than 5% of those without receptor will. More recently, the presence of progesterone receptors has been suggested as an additional discriminant in detecting those who will be responsive/resistant to hormonal therapy (Horowitz *et al.*, 1975). If further correlations confirm this finding, the selection of therapy appropriate to an individual patient may soon be realized.

5. *Ways to Overcome the Problem of Drug Resistance*

Attempts at overcoming drug resistance have been directed at each of the major mechanisms of resistance (Table 3). The dose, schedule, and route of administration have been changed; related and modified drugs have been used; combinations of drugs with each other and with other modes of therapy have been

TABLE 3
Ways to Overcome the Problem of Drug Resistance

A. Change the method of drug administration
   1. Dose
   2. Schedule: frequency and duration
   3. Route

B. Change the drug preparation

C. Use drug combinations and combined modalities
   1. Kinetic reasons
      a. To kill both resting and dividing cells
      b. To synchronize cell populations
      c. To reduce mutant survival
   2. Biochemical reasons
      a. To increase effectiveness of lethal blockade
      b. To "rescue" normal cells
   3. Pharmacological reasons
      a. To increase intracellular accumulation
      b. To reach sanctuary sites
   4. Immunologic reasons

D. Treat earlier in the disease—adjuvant therapy

administered; and disease has been treated earlier in its course. Examples of each of these modes are considered in this section.

5.1. Change the Method of Drug Administration

5.1.1. Dose

Perhaps the best example of changing the dose is the case of MTX. High-dose (up to $1 \, g/M^2$) and very-high-dose (up to $10 \, g/M^2$) treatment has been used with reported success in several tumors, including epidermoid carcinoma of the head and neck (Levitt *et al.*, 1973), carcinoma of the lung (Djerassi *et al.*, 1972), osteogenic sarcoma (Jaffe *et al.*, 1973, 1974), and acute lymphocytic leukemia (Hryniuk and Bertino, 1969; Wang *et al.*, 1976). Whether a high or low dose of drug leads to resistance earlier seems to depend, however, on which drug is used (Schmid and Hutchison, 1972*b*).

5.1.2. Schedule

The scheduling of drug administration, long known to be important in animal tumors (Schabel, 1969; Venditti, 1971; Kline *et al.*, 1972), has also been found important in determining response and toxicity in human tumors (Frei *et al.*, 1969; E. S. Henderson, 1969; Southwest Oncology Group, 1974). The scheduling is important not only because of pharmacokinetic considerations, but also because of kinetic alterations in the cell induced by therapy (Young *et al.*, 1973; Bender and Dedrick, 1975; Myers *et al.*, 1976), and each must be taken into consideration in therapy design.

5.1.3. Route

Changes in the route of drug administration have been successfully used to overcome barriers to drug transport into sanctuary areas such as the CNS (Rieselbach *et al.*, 1963; Rubin *et al.*, 1966; Sullivan *et al.*, 1971; Blasberg *et al.*, 1975), or simply to increase the local tumor drug concentration, e.g., in the liver (Ansfield *et al.*, 1975), or in the head and neck area (Cleveland *et al.*, 1969).

5.2. Change the Drug Preparation

While cross-resistance within a class of drugs or between classes is not infrequently seen (Skipper *et al.*, 1972; Danø, 1972), derivatives and functional analogues may overcome resistance. The clearest case of this is the efficacy of *Erwinia* L-asparaginase in patients who have become immunologically resistant to *E. coli* L-asparaginase (King *et al.*, 1974). Daunorubicin–DNA, adriamycin–DNA, and actinomycin–DNA complexes have been reported to have greater efficacy with less toxicity than the uncomplexed drugs alone (Cornu *et al.*, 1974; Marks and Venditti, 1976). A nonclassic folate antagonist, 2,4-diamino-5-(3',4'-dichlorophenyl)-6-methylpyrimidine (DDMP), was found to be superior to MTX in killing MTX-resistant cells (transport-resistant) (Hill *et al.*, 1973). Further studies with DDMP have shown an additional advantage in that DDMP influx into MTX-sensitive cells was markedly reduced by the simultaneous administration of folinic acid, while in MTX-resistant cells, uptake of DDMP was unaffected (Hill *et al.*, 1975).

133

CLINICAL
ASPECTS OF
RESISTANCE TO
ANTINEOPLASTIC
AGENTS

In tissue culture, cyclic Ara-C monophosphate was more effective in Ara-C-resistant cells than was Ara-C, suggesting that it is hydrolyzed to the 5'-monophosphate intracellularly (Kreis and Wechter, 1972).

5.3. Use Drug Combinations and Combined Modalities

Combination therapy is currently thought to be the most effective way to overcome drug resistance (Skipper, 1974), and one can invoke kinetic, biochemical, pharmacological, and immunologic reasons. Although combinations have in general appeared more effective than single agents, the degree to which this can be ascribed to overcoming any specific kind of resistance has for the most part not been clinically established (DeVita and Schein, 1973; E. S. Henderson and Samaha, 1969).

5.3.1. Kinetic Reasons

Many clinical treatment programs have followed the reasoning proposed by Schabel (1969) by combining cell-cycle-nonspecific agents with cell-cycle-specific ones, either simultaneously or sequentially, in order to kill both resting and actively dividing cells (e.g., Levitt *et al.*, 1972; Skeel *et al.*, 1973; Bodey *et al.*, 1974; Odujinrin *et al.*, 1975; DeLena *et al.*, 1975). Combination therapy has also been used effectively to synchronize tumor cells (Capizzi, 1974, 1975; Klein and Lennartz, 1974). Experimentally, combination therapy prolongs the time to produce resistance, presumably by decreasing the frequency of mutant clone survival (Schmid *et al.*, 1976).

Radiation combined with chemotherapy also appears to be effective, not only for the reason that there is advantage to using cell-cycle-nonspecific and cell-cycle-specific agents, but also because additional treatment can be applied to areas of greatest tumor involvement (Childs *et al.*, 1968; Prosnitz *et al.*, 1973; Moertel *et al.*, 1969), or to reach sanctuary sites (Simone *et al.*, 1972).

5.3.2. Biochemical Reasons

Combinations have also been used for biochemical reasons, to increase effectiveness of lethal blockade (Sartorelli, 1969), and to rescue normal cells (Gee *et al.*, 1969; Capizzi, 1974). Studies with high-dose MTX followed by leucovorin are a special example of this. Thymidine "rescue" after MTX appears effective in the murine leukemia L1210 (Tattersall *et al.*, 1975), and is deserving of clinical trial.

5.3.3. Pharmacological Reasons

Vincristine has been used to increase the intracellular level of MTX. Its effect is apparent both at low and high concentrations of extracellular MTX (Goldman *et al.*, 1976). The lipid-soluble nitrosoureas have been used in combination with other agents in the remission maintenance of meningeal leukemia, but have not been effective (Sullivan *et al.*, 1971), presumably because the leukemia cell itself is not sensitive. The use of intrathecal MTX or cranial/spinal radiation, or both, has been more effective (Simone *et al.*, 1972). Recently, Elias and co-workers (Elias and Brugarolas, 1972; Elias *et al.*, 1975) reported marked improvement in the results of chemotherapy of carcinoma of the lung when patients were anticoagulated with heparin. The mechanism is uncertain, although it is theoretically based on reducing matrix necessary for tumor growth.

5.3.4. Immunologic Reasons

Immunologic tolerance to L-asparaginase may be produced in guinea pigs by using cyclophosphamide together with asparaginase (Ashworth and Maclennan, 1973). Vincristine and prednisone in ALL may reduce the number of hypersensitivity reactions (Land *et al.*, 1972), although the evidence that they do is not great.

5.4. Treat Earlier in the Disease—Adjuvant Therapy

Perhaps the most promising approach to averting resistance in cancer is to treat when there is minimal residual disease, such as immediately after surgical resection of tumor. Clinical results of this kind of "adjuvant" treatment have been encouraging in Wilms tumor (Fleming and Johnson, 1970), breast cancer (Fisher *et al.*, 1975; Bonadonna *et al.*, 1976), and osteogenic sarcoma (Jaffe *et al.*, 1974), although studies thus far in head and neck carcinoma (Tarpley *et al.*, 1975), bronchogenic carcinoma (Shields *et al.*, 1974), and colon cancer (Carter and Friedman, 1974) have not met with success. One can cautiously predict, however, that as we learn better ways to give the drugs, alone or in combination, adjuvant therapy in many additional cancers will result in complete eradication of the neoplastic cells and cure of the patient.

6. Exploitation

Study of drug resistance may be of great value aside from finding ways to delay or prevent it, for if drug resistance is accompanied by specific biochemical change in the cell, this change may be therapeutically exploited in a rational manner.

The phenomenon of collateral sensitivity, which is defined as increased sensitivity of a drug-resistant tumor to another drug, has been well described in model systems (Hutchinson, 1965). Recent evidence from Bonmassar *et al.* (1970), Mihich (1969), and Schmid and Hutchison (1972*a*) suggests that collateral

135

CLINICAL
ASPECTS OF
RESISTANCE TO
ANTINEOPLASTIC
AGENTS

sensitivity may result from increased immunogenicity associated with the drug-resistant tumor, although this is probably not always true, since collateral sensitivity to one drug may be associated with cross-resistance to another (Danø, 1972). Changed immunogenicity is not surprising, however, considering the frequent membrane changes that accompany drug resistance.

Since biochemical drug resistance may result from a mutational event resulting in a cell with a qualitative difference as compared with the sensitive population and with normal host cells, it may be possible to exploit these differences by rational design of new chemotherapeutic agents or immunologic approaches. For example, cells resistant to a drug by virtue of impaired transport may show altered transport of another drug. As mentioned previously, the combination of DDMP and leucovorin takes advantage of a membrane change in MTX-resistant L5178Y cells. The membrane change renders leucovorin ineffective as a competitor for DDMP influx in the resistant cells, as compared with a marked competition of leucovorin for uptake of DDMP in normal cells (Hill *et al.*, 1975). This finding suggests that *in vivo*, the properties of the resistant cell might be exploited to increase its killing while protecting the normal cell.

If resistance is associated with an increased level of a target enzyme, such as DHFR in the case of MTX resistance, analogues may be designed that are substrates for this enzyme that are transformed into substances inhibitory to other enzymes, e.g., thymidylate synthetase (Friedkin, 1967; Mishra and Mead, 1972). If resistance occurs by virtue of an altered enzyme, then new inhibitors may be fabricated with greater affinity for the tumor cell as compared with the normal cell. This kind of approach, based on the observation that increased alkaline phosphatase is one of the mechanisms of resistance to thiopurine, prompted a study of inhibitors of alkaline phosphatase as antitumor agents (Agrawal *et al.*, 1974). Other suggestions, such as use of 5-fluorocytosine in ANLL patients who are resistant to Ara-C by virtue of increased cytidine deaminase, have been made by Tattersall (1973).

7. Conclusion

Clearly, as long as drug resistance continues to be a clinical problem, it will be deserving of study. Although studies in animals have been important, it is imperative that these studies be done in humans as well in order to learn how to: (1) prevent or delay drug resistance; (2) detect drug resistance by *in vitro* testing prior to therapy; and (3) possibly exploit this event for chemotherapeutic advantage.

8. References

AGRAWAL, K. C., LEE, M. H., BOOTH, B. A., MOORE, E. C., AND SARTORELLI, 1974, Potential antitumor agents. 11. Inhibitors of alkaline phosphatase, an enzyme involved in the resistance of neoplastic cells to 6-thiopurines, *J. Med. Chem.* **17**:934.

ASHWORTH, L. A. E., AND MACLENNAN, A. P., 1973, Immunological tolerance to *Erwinia carotovora* L-asparaginase, *Int. Arch. Allergy* **45:**915.

ANSFIELD, F. J., RAMIREZ, G., DAVIS, H. L., WIRTANEN, G. W., JOHNSON, R. O., BRYAN, G. T., MANALO, F. B., BORDEN, E. C., DAVIS, T. E., AND ESMAILI, M., 1975, Further studies with intrahepatic arterial infusion with 5-fluorouracil, *Cancer* **36:**2413.

BACH, M. R., 1969, Biochemical and genetic studies of a mutant strain of mouse leukemia L1210 resistant to 1-β-D-arabinofuranosylcytosine (cytarabine) hydrochloride, *Cancer Res.* **29:**1036.

BAECHTEL, S., AND PRAGER M., 1973, Basis for loss of therapeutic effectiveness of L-asparaginase in sensitized mice, *Cancer Res.* **33:**1966.

BAXTER, J. D., HARRIS, A. W., TOMPKINS, G. M., AND COHN, M., 1971, Glucocorticoid receptors in lymphoma cells in culture: Relationship to glucocorticoid killing activity, *Science* **171:**189.

BENDER, R. A., AND DEDRICK, R. L., 1975, Cytokinetic aspects of clinical drug resistance, *Cancer Chemother. Rep.*, Part I, **59:**805.

BERGSAGEL, D. E., AND PRUZANSKI, W., 1975, Treatment of plasma cell myeloma with cytoxic agents, *Arch. Intern. Med.* **135:**172.

BERTINO, J. R., AND JOHNS, D. G., 1972, Folate antagonists: Cancer chemotherapy II, in: *Twenty-Second Hahnemann Symposium* (I. Brodsky, S. B. Kahn, and J. H. Moyer, eds.), pp. 9–22, Grune & Stratton, New York.

BERTINO, J. R., AND SKEEL, R. T., 1973, Resistance to chemotherapeutic agents: Clinical aspects, in: *Pharmacology and the Future of Man, Proceedings of the 5th International Congress on Pharmacology,* San Francisco 1972, Vol. 3, pp. 376–392, S. Karger, Basel.

BERTINO, J. R., DONOHUE, D. R., GARIO, B. W., SILBER, R., ALENTY, A., MEYER, M., AND HUENNEKENS, F. M., 1962, Increased level of dihydrofolic reductase in leucocytes of patients treated with amethopterin, *Nature (London)* **193:**140.

BERTINO, J. R., DONOHUE, D. M., SIMMONS, B., GABRIO, B. W., SILBER, R., AND HUENNEKENS, F. M., 1963, The "induction" of dihydrofolate reductase activity in leucocytes and erythrocytes of patients treated with amethopterin, *J. Clin. Invest.* **42:**466.

BIEBER, A. L., AND SARTORELLI, A. C., 1964, The metabolism of thioguanine in purine analog–resistant cells, *Cancer Res.* **24:**1210.

BIEDLER, J. L., ALBRECHT, A. M., HUTCHINSON, J. D., AND SPENGLER, B. A., 1972, Drug response, dihydrofolate reductase, and cytogenetics of amethopterin-resistant Chinese hamster cells *in vitro*, *Cancer Res.* **32:**153.

BLASBERG, R. G., PATLAK, C., AND FENSTERMACHER, J. D., 1975, Intrathecal chemotherapy: Brain tissue profiles after ventriculocisternal perfusion, *J. Pharmacol. Exp. Ther.* **195:**73.

BLUMENTHAL, G., AND GREENBERG, D. M., 1970, Evidence for two molecular species of dihydrofolate reductase in amethopterin resistant and sensitive cells of the mouse leukemia L4946, *Oncology* **24:**223.

BOBZIEN, W. F., AND GOLDMAN, I. D., 1972, The mechanism of folate transport in rabbit reticulocytes, *J. Clin. Invest.* **51:**1988.

BODEY, G. P., COLTMAN, C. A., FREIREICH, E. J., BONNET, J. D., GEHAN, E. A., HAUT, A. B., HEWLETT, J. S., MCCREDIE, K. B., SAIKI, J. H., AND WILSON, H. E., 1974, Chemotherapy of acute leukemia: Comparison of cytarabine alone and in combination with vincristine, prednisone, and cyclophosphamide, *Arch. Intern. Med.* **133:**260.

BONADONNA, G., BRUSAMOLINO, E., VALAGUSSA, P., ROSSI, A., BRUGNATELLI, L., BRAMBILLA, C., DELENA, M., TANCINI, G., BAJETTA, E., MUSUMECI, R., AND VERONESI, U., 1976, Combination chemotherapy as an adjuvant treatment in operable breast cancer, *N. Engl. J. Med.* **294:**405.

BONMASSAR, E., BONMASSAR, A., VADLAMUDI, S., AND GOLDIN, A., 1970, Immunological alteration of leukemia cells *in vivo* after treatment with an antitumor drug, *Proc. Natl. Acad. Sci. U.S.A.* **66:**1089.

BRODER, L. E., AND RALL, D. P., 1972, Chemotherapy of brain tumors, *Prog. Exp. Tumor Res.* **17:**373.

BROOME, J. D., 1968, Studies on the mechanisms of tumor inhibition by L-asparaginase. Effects of the enzyme on asparagine levels in the blood, normal tissues, and 6C3HED lymphomas of mice: Differences in asparagine formation and utilization in asparaginase-sensitive and resistant lymphoma cells, *J. Exp. Med.* **127:**1055.

BROOME, J. D., AND SCHWARZ, J. H., 1967, Differences in the production of L-asparagine in asparaginase-sensitive and resistant lymphoma cells, *Biochim. Biophys. Acta* **138:**637.

BRUCE, W. R., AND MEEKER, B. E., 1967, Comparison of the sensitivity of hematopoietic colony-forming cells in different proliferative states to 5-fluorouracil, *J. Natl. Cancer Inst.* **38:**401.

137

CLINICAL
ASPECTS OF
RESISTANCE TO
ANTINEOPLASTIC
AGENTS

BRUCE, W. R., MEEKER, B. E., AND VALERIOTE, F. A., 1966, Comparison of the sensitivity of normal hematopoietic and transplanted lymphoma colony-forming cells to chemotherapeutic agents administered *in vivo*, *J. Natl. Cancer Inst.* **37:**233.

CAPIZZI, R. L., 1974, Schedule-dependent synergism and antagonism between methotrexate and asparaginase, *Biochem. Pharmacol. Suppl.* **2:**151.

CAPIZZI, R. L., 1975, Improvement in the therapeutic index of methotrexate (NSC-740) by L-asparaginase (NSC-109229), *Cancer Chemother. Rep.* **6:**37.

CAPIZZI, R. L., BERTINO, J. R., SKEEL, R. T., CREASEY, W. A., ZANES, R., OLAYON, C., PETERSON, R. G., AND HANDSCHUMACHER, R. E., 1971, L-Asparaginase: Clinical, biochemical, pharmacological, and immunological studies, *Ann. Intern. Med.* **74:**893.

CARTER, S. K., AND FRIEDMAN, M., 1974, Integration of chemotherapy into combined modality treatment of solid tumors. II. Large bowel carcinoma, *Cancer Treatment Rev.* **1:**111.

CASHMORE, A. R., SKEEL, R. T., MAKULU, D. R., GRALLA, E. J., AND BERTINO, J. R., 1975, Pharmacology of a new triazine antifolate in mice, rats, dogs, and monkeys, *Cancer Res.* **35:**17.

CHABNER, B. A., AND YOUNG, R. C., 1973, Threshold methotrexate concentration for *in vivo* inhibition of DNA synthesis in normal and tumorous tissues, *J. Clin. Invest.* **52:**1084.

CHAYEN, J., ALTMAN, F. P., BITENSKY, L., AND DALY, J. R., 1970, Response of human breast cancer tissue to steroid hormones *in vitro*, *Lancet* **1:**868.

CHELLO, P. L., SIROTNAK, F. M., DORICK, D. M., AND HUTCHINSON, D. J., 1976, Specificity of the antifolate transport mechanism of mouse intestinal epithelia versus L1210 leukemia for N^{10} substituents, *Amer. Assoc. Cancer Res.* (Abstract No. 331).

CHILDS, D. S., JR., MOERTEL, C. G., HOLBROOK, M. A., REITMEIER, R. J., AND COLBY, M. Y., JR., 1968, Treatment of unresectable adenocarcinomas of the stomach with a combination of 5-fluorouracil and radiation, *Amer. J. Roentgenol.* **102:**541.

CHU, M. Y., AND FISCHER, G. A., 1962, A proposed mechanism of action of 1-β-D-arabinofuranosylcytosine as an inhibitor of the growth of leukemia cells, *Biochem. Pharmacol.* **11:**423.

CHU, M. Y., AND FISCHER, G. A., 1965, Comparative studies of leukemia cells sensitive and resistant to cytosine arabinoside, *Biochem. Pharmacol.* **14:**333.

CLAMAN, H. N., 1972, Corticosteroids and lymphoid cells, *N. Engl. J. Med.* **287:**388.

CLEVELAND, J. C., JOHNS, D., FARNAM, G., AND BERTINO, J. R., 1969, Arterial infusion of dichloro-methotrexate in cancer of the head and neck: A clinico-pharmacological study, in: *Current Topics in Surgical Research* (G. D. Duidema and D. B. Skinner, eds.), Vol. 1, pp. 113–120, Academic Press, New York.

COLEMAN, C. N., JOHNS, D. G., AND CHABNER, B. A., 1975*a*, Studies on mechanisms of resistance to cytosine arabinoside: Problems in the determination of related enzyme activities in leukemic cells, *Ann. N.Y. Acad. Sci.* **255:**247.

COLEMAN, C. N., STOLLER, R. G., DRAKE, J. C., AND CHABNER, B. A., 1975*b*, Deoxycytidine kinase: Properties of the enzyme from human leukemia granulocytes, *Blood* **46:**791.

CORNU, G., MICHAUX, J.-L., SOKAL, G., AND TROUET, A., 1974, Daunorubicin–DNA: Further clinical trials in acute non-lymphoblastic leukemia, *Eur. J. Cancer* **10:**695.

DANØ, K., 1972, Cross resistance between vinca alkaloids and anthracyclines in Ehrlich ascites tumor *in vivo*, *Cancer Chemother. Rep.* **56:**701.

DAVIDSON, J. D., AND OLIVERIO, V. T., 1965, The physiologic disposition of dichloromethotrexate-Cl^{36} in man, *Clin. Pharmacol. Ther.* **6:**321.

DAVIDSON, J. D., AND WINTER, T. S., 1964, Purine nucleotide pyrophosphorylases in 6-mercaptopurine sensitive and resistant human leukemias, *Cancer Res.* **24:**261.

DECONTI, R. C., 1971, Procarbazine in the management of late Hodgkin's disease, *J. Amer. Med. Assoc.* **215:**927.

DELENA, M., BRAMBILLA, C., MORABITO, A., AND BONADONNA, G., 1975, Adriamycin plus vincristine compared to and combined with cyclophosphamide, methotrexate, and 5-fluorouracil for advanced breast cancer, *Cancer* **35:**1108.

DEVITA, V. T., AND SCHEIN, P. S., 1973, The use of drugs in combination for the treatment of cancer: Rationale and results, *N. Engl. J. Med.* **288:**998.

DEVITA, V. T., CARBONE, P. P., OWENS, A. H., JR., GOLD, G. L., KRANT, M. J., AND EDMONSON, J., 1965, Clinical trials with 1,3-bis(2-chloroethyl)-1-nitrosourea (NSC-409962), *Cancer Res.* **25:**1876.

DEWYS, W. D., 1973, A dose–response study of resistance of leukemia L1210 to cyclophosphamide, *J. Natl. Cancer Inst.* **50:**783.

DICKINSON, L. E., MACMAHON, B., COLE, P., AND BROWN, J. B., 1974, Estrogen profiles of Oriental and Caucasian women in Hawaii, *N. Engl. J. Med.* **291:**1211.

DIVEKAR, A. Y., VAIDYA, N. R., AND BRAGANCA, B. M., 1967, Active transport of aminopterin in Yoshida sarcoma cells, *Biochim. Biophys. Acta* **135:**927.

DJERASSI, I., ROMINGER, L. J., KIM, J. S., TURCHI, J., SUVANSRI, U., AND HUGHS, D., 1972, Phase 1 study of high dose methotrexate with citrovorum factor in patients with lung cancer, *Cancer* **30:**22.

DRAHOVSKY, D., AND KREIS, W., 1970, Studies on drug resistance II. Kinase patterns in P815 neoplasms sensitive and resistant to 1-β-D-arabinofuranosylcytosine, *Biochem. Pharmacol.* **19:**940.

DURIE, B. G. M., AND SALMON, S. E., 1975, A clinical staging system for multiple myeloma: Correlation of measured myeloma cell mass with presenting clinical features, response to treatment, and survival, *Cancer* **36:**842.

ELAIS, E. G., AND BRUGAROLAS, A., 1972, The role of heparin in the chemotherapy of solid tumors: Preliminary clinical trial in carcinoma of the lung, *Cancer Chemother. Rep.* **56:**783.

ELAIS, E. G., SHUKLA, S. K., AND MINK, I. B., 1975, Heparin and chemotherapy in the management of inoperable lung carcinoma, *Cancer* **36:**129.

EMBURY, S. H., HOOD, C. E., GREENBERG, P. K., AND SCHRIER, S. L., 1974, Maintenance chemotherapy: Effect on length of complete remission in acute myelogenous leukemia (AML), *Amer. Soc. Hematol. Abstr.* **18:**157.

EVANS, A. E., AND CRAIG, M., 1964, Central nervous system involvement in children with acute leukemia: A study of 921 patients, *Cancer* **17:**256.

FISCHER, G. A., 1961, Increased levels of folic acid reductase as a mechanism of resistance to amethopterin leukemic cells, *Biochem. Pharmacol.* **7:**75.

FISCHER, G. A., 1962, Defective transport of amethopterin as a mechanism of resistance to the antimetabolite in L5178Y leukemic cells, *Biochem. Pharmacol.* **11:**1233.

FISHER, B., CARBONE, P., ECONOMOU, S. G., FRELICK, R., GLASS, A., LERNER, H., REDMOND, C., AND ZELEN, M., 1975, 1-Phenylalanine mustard (L–PAM) in the management of primary breast cancer, *N. Engl. J. Med.* **292:**117.

FLEMING, I. D., AND JOHNSON, W. D., 1970, Clinical and pathologic staging as a guide in the management of Wilms Tumor, *Cancer* **26:**660.

FREI, E., BICKERS, J. N., HEWLETT, J. S., LANE, M., LEARY, W. V., AND TALLEY, R. W., 1969, Dose schedule and antitumor studies of arabinosyl cytosine (NSC-63878), *Cancer Res.* **29:**1325.

FRIEDKIN, M., 1967, Enzyme studies with new analogues of folic acid and homofolic acid, *J. Biol. Chem.* **242:**1466.

GEE, T. S., YU, K.-P., AND CLARKSON, B. D., 1969, Treatment of adult acute leukemia with arabinosyl-cytosine and thioguanine, *Cancer* **23:**1019.

GOLDENBERG, G. J., 1975, The role of drug transport in resistance to nitrogen mustard and other alkylating agents in L5178Y lymphoblasts, *Cancer Res.* **35:**1687.

GOLDENBERG, G. J., 1976, Drug-induced stimulation of transport of hydrolyzed nitrogen mustard and choline by normal and leukemic human cells *in vitro, Cancer Res.* **36:**978.

GOLDENBERG, G. J., VANSTONE, C. L., ISRAELS, L. G., ILSE, D., AND BIHLER, I., 1970, Evidence for a transport carrier of nitrogen mustard in nitrogen mustard–sensitive and resistant L5178Y lymphoblasts, *Cancer Res.* **30:**2285.

GOLDENBERG, G. J., VANSTONE, C. L., AND BIHLER, I., 1971, Transport of nitrogen mustard on the transport carrier for choline in L5178Y lymphoblasts, *Science* **172:**1148.

GOLDIN, A., VENDITTI, J. M., HUMPHREYS, S. R., AND MANTEL, N., 1956, Modification of treatment schedules in the management of advanced mouse leukemia with amethopterin, *J. Natl. Cancer Inst.* **17:**203.

GOLDMAN, I. D., 1969, Transport energetics of the folic acid analogue MTX in L1210 leukemia cells, *J. Biol. Chem.* **244:**3779.

GOLDMAN, I. D., 1973, Uptake of drugs and resistance, in: *Drug Resistance and Selectivity* (E. Mihich, ed.), pp. 299–358, Academic Press, New York.

GOLDMAN, I. D., LICHTENSTEIN, N. S., AND OLIVERIO, V. T., 1968, Carrier-mediated transport of the folic acid analogue, methotrexate, in the L1210 leukemia cell, *J. Biol. Chem.* **243:**5007.

GOLDMAN, I. D., GUPTA, V., WHITE, J. C., AND LOFTFIELD, S., 1976, Exchangeable intracellular methotrexate levels in the presence and absence of vincristine at extracellular drug concentrations relevant to those achieved in high-dose methotrexate–folinic acid "rescue" protocols, *Cancer Res.* **36:**276.

GREENE, W., HUGGMAN, WIERNIK, P., SCHIMPFF, S., BENJAMIN, R., AND BACHUR, N., 1972, High dose daunorubicin therapy for acute non-lymphocytic leukemia: Correlation of response and toxicity with pharmacokinetics and intracellular daunorubicin reductase activity, *Cancer* **30**:1419.

HASKELL, C. M., AND CANELLOS, G. P., 1969, L-Asparaginase resistance in human leukemia—asparagine synthetase, *Biochem. Pharmacol.* **18**:2578.

HASKELL, C. M., CANELLOS, G. P., COONEY, D. A., AND HANSEN, H. H., 1970, Biochemical and pharmacologic effects of L-asparaginase in man, *J. Lab. Clin. Med.* **75**:763.

HEIDELBERGER, G., GHOLOR, A., BAKER, R. K., AND MUKHERJEE, K. L., 1960, Studies on fluorinated pyrimidines X. *In vivo* studies on tumor resistance, *Cancer Res.* **20**:897.

HENDERSON, B. E., GERKINS, V., ROSARIO, I., CASAGRANDE, J., AND PIKE, M. C., 1975, Elevated serum levels of estrogen and prolactin in daughters of patients with breast cancer, *N. Engl. J. Med.* **293**:790.

HENDERSON, E. S., 1969, Treatment of acute leukemia, *Semin. Hematol.* **6**:271.

HENDERSON, E. S., AND SAMAHA, R. J., 1969, Evidence that drugs in multiple combinations have materially advanced the treatment of human malignancies, *Cancer Res.* **29**:2272.

HILL, B. T., GOLDIE, J. H., AND PRICE, L. A., 1973, Studies concerned with overcoming resistance to methotrexate: A comparison of the effects of methotrexate and 2,4-diamino-5-(3',4'-dichlorophenyl)-6-methylpyrimidine (BW50197) on the colony forming ability of L5178Y cells, *Br. J. Cancer* **28**:262.

HILL, B. T., PRICE, L. A., AND GOLDIE, J. H., 1975, Methotrexate resistance and uptake of DDMP by L5178Y cells: Selective protection with folinic acid, *Eur. J. Cancer* **11**:545.

HILLCOAT, B. L., SWETT, V., AND BERTINO, J. R., 1967, Increase of dihydrofolate reductase activity in cultured mammalian cells after exposure to methotrexate, *Proc. Natl. Acad. Sci. U.S.A.* **58**:1632.

HOBBS, J. R., 1969, Growth rates and responses to treatment in human myelomatosis, *Br. J. Haematol.* **16**:707.

HORNE, D. W., BRIGGS, W. T., AND WAGNER, C., 1976, A functional, active transport system for MTX in freshly isolated hepatocytes, *Biochem. Biophys. Res. Commun.* **68**:70.

HOROWITZ, B., MADRAS, B. K., MEISTER, A., OLD, L. J., BOYSE, E. A., AND STOCKERT, E., 1968, Asparagine synthetase activity of mouse leukemias, *Science* **160**:533.

HORWITZ, K., MCGUIRE, W. L., PEARSON, O. H., AND SEGALOFF, A., 1975, Predicting response to endocrine therapy in human breast cancer: A hypothesis, *Science* **189**:726.

HRYNIUK, W. M., AND BERTINO, J. R., 1969, Treatment of leukemia with large doses of methotrexate and folinic acid: Clinical biochemical correlates, *J. Clin. Invest.* **48**:2140.

HRYNIUK, W. M., FISCHER, G. A., AND BERTINO, J. R., 1969, S-Phase cells of rapidly growing and resting populations: Differences in response to methotrexate, *Mol. Pharmacol.* **5**:557.

HUFFMAN, D. H., AND BACHUR, N. R., 1972, Daunorubicin metabolism in acute myelocytic leukemia, *Blood* **39**:637.

HUTCHINSON, D., 1965, Studies on cross resistance and collateral sensitivity, *Cancer Res.* **25**:1518.

INABA, M., 1973, Mechanism of resistance of Yoshida sarcoma to nitrogen mustard. III. Mechanism of suppressed transport of nitrogen mustard, *Int. J. Cancer* **11**:231.

JACKSON, R. C., HART, L. I., AND HARRUP, K. P., 1976, The intrinsic resistance to methotrexate of cultured mammalian cells in relation to the inhibition kinetics of their dihydrofolate reductase (in press).

JACQUEZ, J. A., 1966, Permeability of Ehrlich ascites cells to folic acid, aminopterin and amethopterin, *Cancer Res.* **26**: 1616.

JAFFE, N., PAED, D., FARBER, S., TRAGGIS, D., GEISER, C., KIM, B. S., DAS, L., FRAUENBERGER, G., DJERASSI, I., AND CASSIDY, J. R., 1973, Response of metastatic osteogenic sarcoma to pulse high-dose methotrexate with citrovorum rescue and radiation therapy, *Cancer* **31**:1367.

JAFFE, N., FREI, E., III, TRAGGIS, D., AND BISHOP, Y., 1974, Adjuvant methotrexate and citrovorum factor treatment of osteogenic sarcoma, *N. Engl. J. Med.* **291**:994.

JENSEN, E. V., BLOCK, G. E., SMITH, S., KYSER, K., AND DESOMBRE, E. R., 1971, Estrogen receptors and breast cancer response to adrenalectomy, *Natl. Cancer Inst. Mongr.* **34**:55.

KASBEKAR, D. K., AND GREENBERG, D. M., 1963, Studies on tumor resistance to 5-fluorouracil, *Cancer Res.* **23**:818.

KESSEL, D., AND BOSMANN, H. B., 1970, On the characteristics of actinomycin D resistance in L5178Y cells, *Cancer Res.* **30**:2695.

KESSEL, D., AND HALL, T. C., 1967, Transport and phosphorylation as factors in the antitumor action of cytosine arabinoside, *Science* **156**:1240.

KESSEL, D., AND HALL, T. C., 1969, Retention of 6-mercaptopurine derivatives by intact cells as an index of drug response in human and murine leukemias, *Cancer Res.* **29:**2116.

KESSEL, D., AND WODINSKY, I., 1970, Thymidine kinase as a determinant of the response to 5-fluorodeoxyuridine in transplantable murine leukemias, *Mol. Pharmacol.* **6:**251.

KESSEL, D., HALL, T. C., ROBERTS, D., AND WODINSKY, I., 1965, Uptake as a determinant of methotrexate response in mouse leukemias, *Science* **150:**752.

KESSEL, D., HALL, T. C., AND ROBERTS, D., 1968a, Modes of uptake of methotrexate by normal and leukemic human leukocytes *in vitro* and their relation to drug response, *Cancer Res.* **28:**564.

KESSEL, D., BOTTERILL, V., AND WODINSKY, I., 1968b, Uptake and retention of daunorubicin by mouse leukemia cells as factors in drug response, *Cancer Res.* **28:**938.

KESSEL, D., HALL, T. C., AND ROSENTHAL, D., 1969, Uptake and phosphorylation of cytosine arabinoside by normal and leukemic human blood cells *in vitro*, *Cancer Res.* **29:**459.

KESSEL, D., AND WODINSKY, I., 1970, Thymidine kinase as a determinant of the response to 5-fluorodeoxyuridine in transplantable murine leukemias, *Mol. Pharmacol.* **6:**251.

KING, O. G., WILBUR, J. R., MUMFORD, D. M., AND SERTOW, W. W., 1974, Therapy with *Erwinia* L-asparaginase in children with acute leukemia after anaphylaxis to *E. coli* L-asparginase, *Cancer* **33:**611.

KLEIN, H. O., AND LENNARTZ, K. J., 1974, Chemotherapy after synchronization of tumor cells, *Semin. Hematol.* **11:**203.

KLINE, I., WOODMAN, R. J., GANG, M., SIRICA, A., VENDITTI, J. M., AND GOLDIN, A., 1972, Influence of the stage of advancement of leukemia L1210 in mice on the optimal schedule of treatment of cytosine arabinoside (NSC-63878), *Cancer Chemother. Rep.* **56:**327.

KREIS, W., AND WECHTER, W. J., 1972, Studies on drug resistance. IV. Synthesis and biological activities of 1-β-D-arabinofuranosylcytosine 3',5'-cyclic monophosphate and a derivative, *Res. Commun. Chem. Pathol. Pharmacol.* **4:**631.

LAMPKIN, B. C., McWILLIAMS, N. B., AND MAUER, A. M., 1972, Cell kinetics and chemotherapy in acute leukemia, *Semin. Hematol.* **9:**211.

LAND, V. J., SUTOW, W. W., FERNBACH, D. J., LANE, D. M., AND WILLIAMS, T. E., 1972, Toxicity of L-amase in children with advanced leukemia, *Cancer* **30:**339.

LAURIE, H. C., AND WILLOUGHBY, M. L. N., 1969, *In vitro* prediction of clinical response to chemotherapy in childhood acute leukemia. I. Combination of daunorubicin, vincristine and prednisolone, *Br. J. Haematol.* **17:**251.

LAUX, D. C., AND LAUSCH, R. N., 1974, Evaluation of factors contributing to tumor resistance to cyclophosphamide, *J. Natl. Cancer Inst.* **52:**863.

LEMON, H. M., WOTIZ, H. H., PARSONS, L., AND MOZDEN, P. J., 1966, Reduced estriol excretion in patients with breast cancer prior to endocrinotherapy, *J. Amer. Med. Assoc.* **196:**1128.

LESSNER, H. E., 1968, BCNU (1,3-bis(2-chloroethyl)-1-nitrosourea). Effects on advanced Hodgkin's disease and other neoplasms, *Cancer* **22:**451.

LEVITT, M., NIXON, P. F., PINCUS, J. H., AND BERTINO, J. R., 1971, Transport characteristics of folates in cerebrospinal fluid; a study utilizing doubly labeled 5-methyltetrahydrofolate and 5-formyltetrahydrofolate, *J. Clin. Invest.* **50:**1301.

LEVITT, M., MARSH, J. C., DeCONTI, R. C., MITCHELL, M. S., SKEEL, R. T., FARBER, L. R., AND BERTINO, J. R., 1972, Combination sequential chemotherapy in advanced reticulum cell sarcoma, *Cancer* **29:**630.

LEVITT, M., MOSHER, M. B., DeCONTI, R. C., FARBER, L. R., SKEEL, R. T., MARSH, J. C., MITCHELL, M. S., PAPAC, R. J., THOMAS, E. D., AND BERTINO, J. R., 1973, Improved therapeutic index of methotrexate with "leucovorin rescue," *Cancer Res.* **33:**1729.

LIPPMAN, M. E., HALTERMAN, R. H., LEVENTHAL, B. G., PERRY, S., AND THOMPSON, E. B., 1973, Glucocorticoid-binding proteins in human acute lymphoblastic leukemic blast cells, *J. Clin. Invest.* **52:**1715.

LIPPMAN, M. E., PERRY, S., AND THOMPSON, E. B., 1975, Glucocorticoid-binding proteins in myeloblasts of acute myelogenous leukemia, *Amer. J. Med.* **59:**224.

LYONS, R. M., AND GOLDENBERG, G. J., 1972, Active transport of nitrogen mustard and choline by normal and leukemic lymphoid cells, *Cancer Res.* **32:**1679.

MARKS, T. A., AND VENDITTI, J. M., 1976, Potentiation of actinomycin D or adriamycin antitumor activity with DNA, *Cancer Res.* **36:**496.

MATHÉ, G., AMIEL, J.-L., VASSAL, F. D., SCHWARZENBERG, L., SCHNEIDER, M., JASMIN, C., AND ROSENFELD, C., 1970, Essai de l'adriamycine dans le traitment des leukémies aiguës, *Presse Med.* **78:**1997.

MAUER, A. M., 1975, Cell kinetics and practical consequences for therapy of acute leukemia, *N. Engl. J. Med.* **293**:389.

MIHICH, E., 1969, Modification of tumor regression by immunologic means, *Cancer Res.* **29**:2345.

MISHRA, L. G., AND MEAD, J. A. R., 1972, Further evaluation of the antitumor activity of hanofolate and its reduced derivatives against methotrexate-resistant tumors, *Chemotherapy* **17**:283.

MOERTEL, C. G., CHILDS, D. S., JR., REITMEIER, R. J., COLBY, M. Y., JR., AND HOLBROOK, M. A., 1969, Combined fluorouracil and supervoltage radiation therapy of locally unresectable gastrointestinal cancer, *Lancet* **2**:865.

MOMPARLER, R. L., CHU., M. Y., AND FISCHER, G. A., 1968, Studies on the new mechanism of resistance of L5178Y murine leukemia cells to cytosine arabinoside, *Biochim. Biophys. Acta (Amsterdam)* **161**:481.

MYERS, C. E., YOUNG, R. C., AND CHABNER, B. A., 1976, Kinetic alterations induced by 5-fluorouracil in bone marrow, intestinal mucosa, and tumor, *Cancer Res.* **36**:1653.

ODUJINRIN, O. O., DECONTI, R. C., AND BERTINO, J. R., 1975, Combination chemotherapy with cyclophosphamide (NSC-26271), cytosine arabinoside (NSC-63878), and methotrexate (NSC-740) in advanced solid tumors, *Cancer Chemother. Rep.* **59**:1091.

OSBORN, M. J., FREEMAN, M., AND HUENNEKENS, F. M., 1958, Inhibition of dihydrofolate reductase by aminopterin and methopterin, *Proc. Soc. Exp. Biol. Med.* **97**:429.

PETERSON, R. G., HANDSCHUMACHER, R. E., AND MITCHELL, M. S., 1970, Immunological responses to L-asparaginase, *J. Clin. Invest.* **50**:1080.

PRAGER, M. D., AND BACHYNSKY, N., 1968, Asparagine synthetase in normal and malignant tissue; correlation with tumor sensitivity to asparaginase, *Arch. Biochem.* **127**:645.

PROSNITZ, L. R., FARBER, L. R., FISCHER, J. J., AND BERTINO, J. R., 1973, Low dose radiation therapy and combination chemotherapy in the treatment of advanced Hodgkin's disease, *Radiology* **107**:187.

RALL, D. P., RIESELBACH, R. E., OLIVERIO, U. T., AND MORSE, E., 1962, Pharmacology of folic acid antagonists as related to brain and cerebrospinal fluid, *Cancer Chemother. Rep.* **16**:187.

RIEHM, H., AND BIEDLER, T. L., 1971, Cellular resistance to daunorubicin in Chinese hamster cells *in vitro*, *Cancer Res.* **31**:409.

RIESELBACH, R. E., MORSE, E. E., RALL, D. P., FREI, E., III, AND FREIREICH, E. J., 1963, Intrathecal aminopterin therapy of meningeal leukemia, *Arch. Int. Med.* **111**:620.

ROSMAN, M., AND WILLIAMS, H. E., 1973, Leukocyte purine phosphoribosyl transferases in human leukemias sensitive and resistant to 6-thiopurines, *Cancer Res.* **33**:1202.

ROSMAN, M., LEE, M. H., CREASEY, W. A., AND SARTORELLI, A. C., 1974, Mechanisms of resistance to 6-thiopurines in human leukemia, *Cancer Res.* **34**:1952.

ROSOWSKY, A., AND CHEN, K. N., 1974, Methotrexate analogs. 4,7-methyl derivative of methotrexate and dichloromethotrexate. A new synthesis and some biological studies, *J. Med. Chem.* **17**:1308.

RUBIN, R. C., OMMAYA, A. K., HENDERSON, E. S., BERING, E. A., AND RALL, D. P., 1966, Cerebrospinal fluid perfusion for central nervous system neoplasms, *Neurology* **16**:680.

RUSCONI, A., AND DIMARCO, A., 1969, Inhibition of nucleic acid synthesis by daunorubicin and its relationship to the uptake of the drug in HeLa cells, *Cancer Res.* **29**:1507.

RUTMAN, R. J., CHUN, E. H. L., AND LEWIS, F. S., 1968, Permeability difference as a source of resistance to alkylating agents in Ehrlich tumor cells, *Biochem. Biophys. Res. Commun.* **32**:650.

SARTORELLI, A. C., 1969, Some approaches to the therapeutic exploitation of metabolic sites of vulnerability of neoplastic cells, *Cancer Res.* **29**:2292.

SCHABEL, F. M., JR., 1968, *In vivo* leukemia cell kill kinetics and "curability" in experimental systems, in: *The Proliferation and Spread of Neoplastic Cells*, pp. 379–409, Williams & Wilkins, Baltimore.

SCHABEL, F. M., JR., 1969, The use of tumor growth kinetics in planning "curative" chemotherapy of advanced solid tumors, *Cancer Res.* **29**:2384.

SCHEIN, P. S., RAKIETEN, N., GORDON, B. M., DAVIS, R. D., AND RALL, D. P., 1969, The toxicity of *Escherichia coli* L-asparaginase, *Cancer Res.* **29**:426.

SCHMID, F. A., AND HUTCHISON, D. J., 1972*a*, Collateral sensitivity of resistant lines of mouse leukemias L1210 and L5178Y, *Cancer Res.* **32**:808.

SCHMID, F. A., AND HUTCHISON, D. J., 1972*b*, Effect of different doses of methotrexate (NSC-740), cytosine arabinoside (NSC-63878), and cyclophosphamide (NSC-26271) on drug resistance in mice with L1210 leukemia, *Cancer Chemother. Rep.* **56**:473.

SCHMID, F. A., HUTCHISON, D. J., OTTER, G. M., AND STOCK, C. C., 1976, Development of resistance to combinations of six antimetabolites in mice with L1210 leukemia, *Cancer Treatment Rep.* **60**:23.

SCHRECKER, A. W., 1970, Metabolism of 1-β-D-arabinofuranosylcytosine in leukemia L1210: Nucleoside and nucleotide kinases in cell free extracts, *Cancer Res.* **30**:632.

141

CLINICAL
ASPECTS OF
RESISTANCE TO
ANTINEOPLASTIC
AGENTS

SCHRECKER, A. W., MEAD, J. A. R., GREENBERG, N. H., AND GOLDIN, A., 1971, Dihydrofolate reductase activity of leukemia L1210 during development of methotrexate resistance, *Biochem. Pharmacol.* **20:**716.

SCHWARTZ, H. S., SODERGREN, J. W., AND AMBAYE, R. Y., 1968, Actinomycin D: Drug concentrations and actions in mouse tissues and tumors, *Cancer Res.* **28:**192.

SHIELDS, T. W., ROBINETTE, C. D., AND KEEHN, R. J., 1974, Bronchial carcinoma treated by adjuvant cancer chemotherapy, *Arch. Surg.* **109:**329.

SIMONE, J., AUR, R. J. A., HUSTU, H. O., AND PINKEL, D., 1972, "Total therapy" studies of acute lymphocytic leukemia in children, *Cancer* **30:**1488.

SIROTNAK, F. M., AND DONSBACK, R. C., 1974, Stereo-chemical characteristics of the folate–antifolate transport mechanism in L1210 leukemia cells, *Cancer Res.* **34:**371.

SIROTNAK, F. M., DURITA, S., SARGENT, M. G., ROBINSON, D. L., AND HUTCHISON, D. J., 1967, Sequential biochemical alterations to antifolate resistance in L1210 leukemia, *Nature (London),* **216:**1236.

SIROTNAK, F. M., DURITA, S., AND HUTCHISON, D. J., 1968, On the nature of a transport alteration determining resistance to amethopterin in the L1210 leukemia, *Cancer Res.* **28:**75.

SKEEL, R. T., BERTINO, J. R., AND CREASEY, W. A., 1970, Clinical and pharmacologic studies with daunorubicin in acute leukemia, *Clin. Res.* **18:**476.

SKEEL, R. T., MARSH, J. C., DeCONTI, R. C., MITCHELL, M. S., HUBBARD, S., AND BERTINO, J. R., 1973, Development of a combination chemotherapy program for adult acute leukemia: CAM and CAM-L, *Cancer* **32:**76.

SKEEL, R. T., SAWICKI, W. L., CASHMORE, A. R., AND BERTINO, J. R., 1976, Inhibition of DNA synthesis in normal and malignant human cells by triazinate (Baker's antifol) and methotrexate, *Cancer Res.* **36:**3659.

SKIPPER, H. E., 1968, Cellular kinetics associated with "curability" of experimental leukemias, in: *Perspectives in Leukemia* (Dameshek and Dutcher, eds.), pp. 187–216, Grune & Stratton, New York.

SKIPPER, H. E., 1974, Thoughts on cancer chemotherapy and combination modality therapy, *J. Amer. Med. Assoc.* **230:**1033.

SKIPPER, H. E., HUTCHISON, D. J., SCHABEL, F. M., JR., SCHMIDT, L. H., GOLDIN, A., BROCKMAN, R. W., VENDITTI, J. M., AND WODINSKY, I., 1972, A quick reference chart on cross resistance between anticancer agents, *Cancer Chemother. Rep.* **56:**493.

SKÖLD, O., 1963, Studies on resistance against 5-fluorouracil. IV. Evidence for an altered uridine kinase in resistant cells, *Biochim. Biophys. Acta* **76:**160.

SKOVSGAARD, T., 1975, Development of resistance to rubidazone (NSC-164011) in Ehrlich ascites tumor *in vivo, Cancer Chemother. Rep.* **59:**301.

SMITH, I. E., AND McELWAIN, T. J., 1974, Adriamycin in acute leukemia, *Lancet* **2:**161.

SOUTHWEST ONCOLOGY GROUP, 1974, Cytarabine for acute leukemia in adults. Effect of schedule on therapeutic response, *Arch. Intern. Med.* **133:**251.

SPIVACK, S. D., 1974, Procarbazine, *Ann. Intern. Med.* **81:**795.

STEUART, C. D., AND BURKE, P. J., 1971, Cytidine deaminase and the development of resistance to Ara-C, *Nature (London) New Biol.* **233:**109.

SULLIVAN, M. P., VIETTI, T. J., HAGGARD, M. E., DONALDSON, M. H., KRALL, J. M., AND GEHAN, E. A., 1971, Remission maintenance therapy for meningeal leukemia: Intrathecal methotrexate vs. intravenous bis-nitrosourea, *Blood* **38:**680.

TARPLEY, J. L., CHRETIEN, P. B., ALEXANDER, J. C., HOYE, R. C., BLOCK, J. B., AND KETCHAM, A. S., 1975, High dose methotrexate as a preoperative adjuvant in the treatment of epidermoid carcinoma of the head and neck, *Amer. J. Surg.* **130:**481.

TATTERSALL, M. H. N., 1973, The emergence of drug resistance in tumors: A characteristic which may be exploited therapeutically, *Br. J. Cancer* **27:**406.

TATTERSALL, M. H. N., GANESHAGURU, K., AND HOFFBRAND, A. V., 1974, Mechanisms of resistance of human leukemia cells to cytosine arabinoside, *Br. J. Haematol.* **27:**39.

TATTERSALL, M. H. N., BROWN, B. L., AND FREI, E., 1975, Methotrexate treatment of murine leukemia, *Ann. N.Y. Acad. Sci.* **255:**261.

TERZ, J. J., CURULCHET, H. P., AND LAWRENCE, W., 1971, Analysis of the cell kinetics of human solid tumors, *Cancer* **28:**1100.

TRANUM, B. L., HAUT, A., RIVKIN, S., WEBER, E., QUAGLIANA, J. M., SHAW, M., TUCKER, W. G., SMITH, F. E., SAMSON, M., AND GOTTLIEB, J., 1975, A phase II study of methyl CCNU in the treatment of solid tumors and lymphomas: A Southwest Oncology Group study, *Cancer* **35:**1148.

VENDITTI, J. M., 1971, Treatment schedule dependency of experimentally active antileukemia (L1210) drugs, *Cancer Chemother. Rep.* **2**:35.

WANG, J. J., FREEMAN, A. I., AND SINKS, L. F., 1976, Treatment of acute lymphocytic leukemia by high-dose intravenous methotrexate, *Cancer Res.* **36**:1441.

WHEELER, G. P., 1963, Studies related to mechanisms of resistance to biological alkylating agents, *Cancer Res.* **23**:1334.

WHEELER, G. P., AND ALEXANDER, J. A., 1964, Studies with mustards. V. *In vivo* fixation of C^{14} of labeled alkylating agents by bilaterally grown sensitive and resistant tumors, *Cancer Res.* **24**:1331.

WHITEHOUSE, J. M. A., CROWTHER, D., BATEMAN, C. J. T., BEARD, M. E. J., AND MALPAS, J. S., 1972, Adriamycin in the treatment of acute leukemia, *Br. Med. J.* **1**:482.

WOHLBERG, W. H., 1964, Studies on the mechanism of human tumor resistance to the fluorinated pyrimidines, *Cancer Res.* **24**:1437.

WOLBERG, W. H., 1969, The effect of 5-fluorouracil on DNA thymine synthesis in human tumors, *Cancer Res.* **29**:2137.

WOLBERG, W. H., 1971, Biochemical approaches to prediction of response in solid tumors, *Natl. Cancer Inst. Monogr.* **34**:189.

WOLPERT, M. K., AND RUDDON, P. W., 1969, A study on the mechanism of resistance to nitrogen mustard (HN2) in Ehrlich ascites tumor cells: Comparison of uptake of HN2-^{14}C into sensitive and resistant cells, *Cancer Res.* **29**:873.

WOODS, J. S., AND HANDSCHUMACHER, R. E., 1971, Hepatic homeostasis of plasma L-asparagine, *Amer. J. Physiol.* **221**:1785.

YOUNG, R. C., GOLDBERG, D., AND SCHEIN, P. S., 1973, Enhanced antitumor effect of cytosine arabinoside given in a schedule dictated by kinetic studies *in vivo*, *Biochem. Pharmacol.* **22**:277.

143

CLINICAL
ASPECTS OF
RESISTANCE TO
ANTINEOPLASTIC
AGENTS

5

Adjunctive Chemotherapy

MICHAEL T. SHAW AND ROBERT D. STEBBINS

1. Introduction

Recent successes achieved in the therapy of various types of cancer have in many instances been attributable to the cytotoxicity of new chemotherapeutic agents. Many of the drugs have been used effectively in hematologic neoplasms, and with their use, complete remission and survival rates in childhood leukemia and in Hodgkin's disease and other lymphomas have increased very significantly. Several of the solid tumors such as sarcomas, breast carcinoma, and testicular cancer have demonstrated sensitivity to single agents and combinations of drugs. Unfortunately, in advanced and metastatic tumors, responses are short-lived, the tumors rapidly become resistant to the drugs, and the patient dies from uncontrollable disease.

It is not surprising that bulky cancers are difficult to eradicate by chemotherapy alone. Although the relationship of the chemotherapeutic response of tumors to cell kinetics is reviewed in detail elsewhere, it is important to reiterate that the growth fraction of a tumor is inversely proportional to the size of the cell population. Since most chemotherapeutic drugs kill cancer cells actively in cell cycle, it stands to reason that the smaller the tumor, the larger its growth fraction and the more likely it is to respond to cytotoxic drugs. Schabel (1975) has pointed out that drug response of the primary tumor may not reliably predict the sensitivity of micrometastases to cell-cycle-specific drugs, and that micrometastases should be more sensitive to antimetabolites than the larger, grossly apparent primary tumor. Most drugs act by first-order kinetics; i.e., they kill a constant fraction or percentage of tumor cells. A drug may kill 99.9% of cancer cells, no matter what their numbers. Thus, in a micrometastasis of 100 cells, all the malignant cells would be destroyed, and the patient would be cured. In a 10-g

MICHAEL T. SHAW AND ROBERT D. STEBBINS ● Section of Medical Oncology, Yale University School of Medicine, New Haven, Connecticut.

metastasis consisting of 10^{10} cells, however, 10 million viable cancer cells would remain (Burchenal, 1976).

A rational approach to the treatment of many cancers is now generally accepted as multimodal therapy. Where possible, bulky tumor masses should be resected surgically or eradicated by radiation therapy. This should be regarded merely as a palliative procedure in those cancers for which the prognosis is poor due to widespread metastatic disease. The medical oncologist's aim is to eradicate micrometastases and to effect a cure. How far it is possible to do so and what the future holds for this approach are described in this chapter.

2. Experimental Evidence from Animal Models

Implants of a single tumor cell of L1210 leukemia in a mouse can result in the death of the animal from the tumor. Similar results have been shown using sarcoma 180 in the mouse, Yoshida sarcoma in the rat, Walker 256 carcinosarcoma in the rat, plasmacytoma in the hamster, and various other tumors (Schabel, 1975). It thus appears that when these tumor models are studied, chemotherapeutic agents must kill every tumor cell to effect a cure. The size of the tumor cell inoculum is important. Schabel (1975) demonstrated that when 10^5 L1210 cells were implanted intraperitoneally into a mouse and a single dose of 6-mercaptopurine was administered 24 hr later, none of 10 animals survived to 45 days. If, however, 10^2 cells were inoculated and followed by the same chemotherapeutic regimen, 9 out of 10 animals survived for this length of time. Burchenal (1976) has pointed out that in mice, the most effective dose of most single agents or combinations of drugs is the maximum tolerated dose, and that decreases in dosage of even 20–33% may seriously compromise the therapeutic effect.

Several studies in animals have demonstrated the potentially beneficial effects of adjuvant chemotherapy. In 1957, McDonald and his colleagues (McDonald *et al.*, 1957), using the Walker rat 256 carcinosarcoma, injected cell suspensions into the portal vein of female Sprague Dawley rats and then treated them with systemic nitrogen mustard or thioTEPA. The percentage of tumor takes was much higher in the control group, which did not receive chemotherapy. Furthermore, those rats that had received 220,000 cells had considerably more "takes" than those that had received only 110,000 cells after injection of the drug. If treatment was delayed for 48 hr after inoculation of the cancer cells, the anticancer agents were not effective in preventing tumor takes. Thus, the number of tumor cells injected, and the timing of drug administration, were the important factors in prevention of tumor formation.

Moore and Kondo (1958) measured the effect of giving actinomycin D intravenously to mice that had been inoculated with 250,000 sarcoma 180 cells given intravenously. There was little difference in the effectiveness of the drug if it was given $\frac{1}{2}$ hr or up to 48 hr after the injection of the tumor cells. It appeared that with a tumor susceptible to a specific agent, some delay in therapy did not reduce

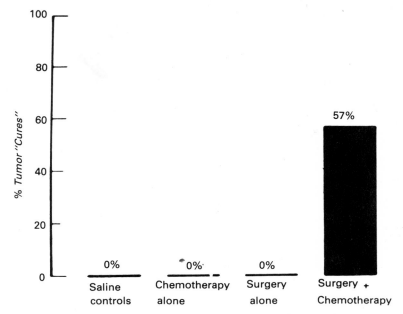

FIGURE 1. Complete regressions obtained from chemotherapy alone, surgery alone, and surgery plus chemotherapy of adenocarcinoma 755 tumors in mice. From Shapiro and Fugmann (1957).

the effectiveness. The authors did point out, however, that if a tumor was less susceptible to the agent, delay in therapy markedly and adversely affected response.

Perhaps the most dramatic experiments were those of Shapiro and Fugmann (1957), who implanted mammary adenocarcinoma 755 into C57BL mice. The tumor was allowed to grow for 15 days, at which time 6-mercaptopurine was administered and produced no cures. Animals receiving saline showed similar results. Another group of animals, undergoing partial surgical excision, demonstrated fatal progression. However, the fourth group of animals, which had a partial surgical excision of the tumor plus administration of 6-mercaptopurine, demonstrated a 57% cure (Fig. 1). Similar results have been seen in C3H mammary carcinoma, Lewis lung carcinoma, and B16 melanoma, with the best results being achieved by full-dose, intensive chemotherapy (Burchenal, 1976).

3. Clinical Applications of Adjuvant Chemotherapy

In the mid 1950s, at about the same time that animal experiments were showing a promising future for adjuvant chemotherapy, a national program to coordinate surgical adjuvant cancer chemotherapy studies was established. Results of the various trials were singularly unimpressive, however, and it is now clear why this was so. First, the number of cytotoxic drugs available was limited. Second, the concept of micrometastases was based on the release of cancer cells into the bloodstream during surgical manipulation. It had been recognized that any form of diagnostic or operative manipulation of a malignant tumor might cause showers of cells to be released into the circulation (L. Long *et al.*, 1960). Cancer cells could be demonstrated by simple techniques in the bloodstream of several patients. Indeed, in one study, on every occasion that free cancer cells were found in the peripheral blood of patients with GI malignancies, the cancer was found to be nonresectable or incurable (Long *et al.*, 1960). Cole and his colleagues (Cole *et al.*, 1954) advocated that venous trunks leading to and from tumors be tied off as early in the operative procedure as was practical, and manipulation of the tumor should be minimal. In initial reports, it was thought that cancer cells were found in the bloodstream only in advanced cases, but it was soon recognized that at least 15% of these positive findings occurred in cases of resectable cancers (Delarue, 1960). Delarue concluded that cancers never implanted themselves on intact epithelial surfaces, but readily engrafted on raw surfaces, and that probably most circulating cancer cells did not form metastases. Salgado *et al.* (1959) reported that the percentage of circulating cancer cells increased in cases in which there was evidence of nodal involvement. The early clinical adjuvant chemotherapy studies were designed to destroy any cancer cells that might be released into the circulation by manipulation of the tumor during the operative procedure. Chemotherapeutic agents were administered for a short time and in quite low doses with little, if any, beneficial effects. It now seems much more likely that the causes of distant recurrences are micrometastases that are present at the time of surgery. The aim of adjuvant therapy is to destroy these micrometastases, to prevent clinical metastases, and to achieve a cure, rather than just delay the appearance of the metastases (Burchenal, 1976).

It was pointed out above that chemotherapy is most effective when the tumor size is small and the growth fraction is high. The following scheme provides a rational approach to adjuvant chemotherapy in the clinical setting.

1. Large, bulky tumor masses should be removed by surgical or radiotherapeutic means or both. Chemotherapeutic agents are least effective against large tumors.

2. Chemotherapy should be commenced as soon as possible after surgery. It is probably advisable to wait until wound healing is adequate.

3. Chemotherapy should be administered as if the tumor were advanced, i.e., in maximally tolerated doses of either a single effective drug or a combination of drugs.

4. Chemotherapy should be continued for a substantial period of time. Although it is impossible to assess accurately the optimum duration of therapy, 1 or 2 years seems to be about the range on which most clinicians agree.

5. Where possible, chemotherapy should be given in an intermittent fashion rather than continuously, as it is likely that immunosuppression will be minimized, and that indeed a recovery with rebound of immunologic competence will be evident.

6. Second-look and even third-look operations are now being undertaken 149
more frequently. This approach is to be encouraged in appropriate situations, ADJUNCTIVE
and may serve as a guide to the duration of chemotherapeutic management. CHEMO-
THERAPY

Most of the experience with adjunctive chemotherapy has been obtained from
trials in breast cancer and lung cancer. More recently, several cooperative groups
have been established, and studies involving adjuvant chemotherapy in carcinoma of the ovary, testis, GI tract, and head and neck cancer are under way.
Malignant tumors of the brain, various sarcomas, melanoma, Wilms's tumor,
and neuroblastoma are also being treated similarly.

3.1. Breast Cancer

Carcinoma of the breast has received a great deal of attention over several decades, but the results of various therapeutic studies have led only to confusion in
evaluating the most efficacious treatment of this disease. Since 1973, when the
American Joint Committee for Cancer Staging and End Results Reporting
published its pamphlet, most clinicians have used the staging system based on the
TNM specifications. The clinical classification is based on the anatomical extent of
cancer that can be detected by examination and radiological and biopsy examination of various sites to demonstrate the presence or absence of metastases. Fisher *et
al.* (1969) showed that the size of the primary lesion and the presence or absence of
axillary node involvement were the most important prognostic indicators of this
neoplasm; these factors are summarized in Table 1. Patients who had positive
nodes had a much higher recurrence rate at 18 months and 5 years than patients
with negative nodes. It is now well recognized that patients with involvement of
axillary nodes are obvious candidates for adjuvant chemotherapy.

Previous trials have been thwarted by lack of agreement as to the most desirable
operation and whether or not postoperative radiation therapy should be administered. At present, most surgeons are doing a modified radical mastectomy (Patey's
operation); however, some surgeons still carry out the classic Halsted radical
mastectomy, while others advocate total mastectomy and even tylectomy (lumpec-
tomy). The disadvantage of the latter two procedures is that the pathological

TABLE 1

*Effect of Primary Tumor Size and Nodal Status on 5-Year
Percentage Recurrence Rate of Breast Cancer*[a]

Axillary node status	Size of lesions (cm)		
	<2	2-4.9	5–6+
Negative	13	16–28	24–34
1–3 Positive	53	51–68	72–84
4+ Positive	65	59–81	86–94

[a] Modified from Fisher *et al.* (1970).

TABLE 2
Single-Agent Activity in Breast Cancer[a]

Drugs	Responses/ Evaluated patients	Response rate (%)
Cyclophosphamide	182/529	34
Methotrexate	120/356	34
5-Fluorouracil	324/1263	26
Adriamycin	67/193	35
Mitomycin C	41/110	37
Vincristine	47/226	20

[a] From Wasserman *et al.* (1975).

status of the axillary nodes is unknown. Postoperative irradiation is administered in many centers. While its effectiveness against local recurrences is not disputed, there is no doubt that distant metastases are not prevented, nor is survival prolonged by this procedure.

It has long been appreciated that many breast cancers are hormone-dependent. Several adjuvant trials were instituted, especially in premenopausal women, involving endocrine manipulative procedures. Prophylactic oophorectomy and ovarian irradiation designed to radically reduce the amount of endogenous estrogen proved to be totally ineffective (Kennedy *et al.*, 1964). Survival was not altered, and differences in recurrence rates, when compared with controls, were not convincing. Similar negative results have been obtained when androgen therapy has been used. It is now generally agreed that endocrine manipulation as a form of prophylaxis in primary breast cancer is of no proven value. Adjuvant chemotherapy trials in breast cancer have been numerous, and, as stated above, the early trials involved short courses of a cytotoxic drug aimed at destroying cancer cells released into the circulation. In addition, many of the agents that have been used have not shown the greatest activity against advanced breast cancer. Until recently, the adjuvant trials have consisted of single-agent therapy only. Table 2 shows cumulative data of the most active drugs in use as single agents. An outline of perioperative and postoperative chemotherapy trials is given below; these studies were well reviewed by Tormey (1975). Perioperative chemotherapy refers to those trials in which chemotherapy was administered for up to 2 months postoperatively. Longer periods of postoperative chemotherapy are called postoperative chemotherapy trials.

3.1.1. Perioperative Chemotherapy Trials

1. National Surgical Adjuvant Breast Project (NSABP) (Fisher *et al.*, 1968). The first protocol randomized patients who had undergone conventional radical mastectomy to thioTEPA and a placebo. ThioTEPA was given in doses of 0.2 mg/kg daily i.v. at the time of operation and for 2 days postoperatively. After 5 years, there was no significant difference in recurrence rates. The only significant finding was that premenopausal patients with four or more positive nodes treated

with thioTEPA had a lower recurrence rate in the 18th–36th postoperative months ($P = 0.05$). In another protocol, the NSABP studied patients following radical mastectomy by randomizing them to 5-fluorouracil, thioTEPA, postoperative radiotherapy, and prophylactic oophorectomy. Again, the thioTEPA-treated patients, who were premenopausal and with four or more positive nodes, showed some beneficial effect. 5-Fluorouracil produced severe toxicity without any beneficial effects.

2. Scandinavian Adjuvant Chemotherapy Study Group (Nissen-Meyer *et al.*, 1971; Nissen-Meyer, 1973). Treated patients received cyclophosphamide, 30 mg/kg i.v. over a 6-day period. After 6 years, there were 201 recurrences in the control group and 155 in the treated group ($P = 0.02$). There was no statistical difference in survival; 135 patients in the control group and 114 in the treated group had died.

3. English trial (Finney, 1971). Most patients underwent simple mastectomy, and all received postoperative radiotherapy for Stages I and II disease. Cyclophosphamide was administered for 5 days beginning 4 days before surgery. After 3 years, the control group demonstrated 25 of 40 patients alive and disease-free, and 18 of 43 cyclophosphamide-treated patients were alive and disease-free.

4. German trial (Rieche *et al.*, 1972). Patients with Stage I to III disease underwent radical mastectomy, and the drug-treated group started cyclophosphamide intravenously on the day of operation for a total dose of 100 mg/kg given over 1–2 months. Although the 3-year local regional recurrence rate was 28.4% in the control group and 12.2% in the cyclophosphamide-treated group, the incidence of distant metastases was the same in both groups.

3.1.2. Postoperative Chemotherapy Trials

1. R. L. Long *et al.* (1969). This trial began in 1962. ThioTEPA was administered intravenously on the day of operation and for 2 days afterward. After discharge from the hospital, patients received 0.2 mg/kg weekly. The study was limited to grade 3 adenocarcinoma or undifferentiated breast cancer, and grade 2 adenocarcinoma with lymph node metastases. In a report after a follow-up period of 24 months, 52.9% of the control group and 20.7% of the treated group had relapsed ($P = 0.03$). More recent data have suggested no statistical difference between the groups with regard to relapse rate and survival.

2. Mrazek (1970). This study, which lasted from 1956 to 1964, involved the administration of nitrogen mustard at the time of a Halsted radical mastectomy, 2 days afterward, and every 3 months until bone marrow intolerance. Three courses was the average number administered. Recurrences occurred in 50% of the control patients and 39.7% of the drug-treated group. The differences were more marked in premenopausal women, especially those without axillary node involvement. Survival in both groups seemed to be similar.

3. NSABP study with phenylalanine mustard (L-PAM) (Fischer *et al.*, 1975). A preliminary report of this study was published in 1975. The study comprised 211 patients. The age limit was 75 years, and all had received conventional modified

radical mastectomy for potentially curable breast cancer, and had one or more axillary nodes proved histologically to contain tumor. Of the total, 103 patients received L-PAM 0.15 mg/kg per day for 5 consecutive days every 6 weeks, and 108 received placebo. Drug therapy was commenced no sooner than 2 weeks and not later than 4 weeks after operation, and was continued until documented evidence of treatment failure or for 2 years, whichever occurred first. Treatment failure occurred in 22% of 108 patients receiving placebo, and in 9.7% of 103 women given L-PAM ($P = 0.01$). A statistically significant difference ($P = 0.02$) existed in favor of L-PAM relative to disease-free interval. Treatment failure occurred in 30% of premenopausal patients receiving placebo, and in 3% of those treated with L-PAM ($P = 0.008$). Although a similar trend was observed in postmenopausal patients, the difference was not statistically significant.

4. Cyclophosphamide, Methotrexate, and 5-Fluorouracil (CMF) Study (Bonadonna et al., 1976). Preliminary reports of this study appeared in 1976. There were 386 patients in the study, and the eligibility criteria were the same as in the L-PAM study. There were 179 controls and 207 who received CMF, which consisted of cyclophosphamide, 100 mg/M^2 p.o. daily for 14 days; methotrexate, 40 mg/M^2 i.v. on days 1 and 8; and 5-fluorouracil, 600 mg/M^2 i.v. on days 1 and 8. The next cycle was started after a 2-week rest period (15th–28th days). Patients received 12 cycles of therapy. Up to 27 months of study, treatment failures occurred in 24% of the control and 5.3% of the drug-treated patients ($P < 10^{-6}$). Those patients with four or more positive axillary nodes had a higher percent of relapses than those with fewer nodes. Toxicity was acceptable.

The L-PAM and CMF studies at first sight appear very impressive. Both should be reviewed with caution, however, since the follow-up time has been comparatively short as seen from previous promising trials. The longer the follow-up, the fewer differences were seen in control vs. treated groups in most studies.

3.2. Lung Cancer

The dismal results that have universally been obtained in the treatment of lung cancer are well known. Histologically, the four main groups that are recognized are: epidermoid, small-cell, large-cell undifferentiated, and adenocarcinoma. Chemotherapy has been most effective in producing responses in the small-cell type, but these responses have been very short-lived. Kinetic studies have indicated labeling indices using tritiated thymidine to be highest in the small-cell and large-cell undifferentiated carcinomas (Muggia, 1974), and it might therefore be expected that these tumors would be most responsive to chemotherapy, especially when given in an adjuvant fashion. It is well recognized, however, that by the time most patients present and are diagnosed as having small-cell carcinoma, the tumor is widely metastatic. For this reason, most surgeons will not contemplate resection for this type of tumor, and therefore chemotherapy is, and will probably continue to be, used as definitive rather than adjunctive therapy.

Several controlled prospective clinical trials using single-agent chemotherapy for all types of lung cancer have been carried out (Selawry, 1974). The drugs used most frequently have been nitrogen mustard and cyclophosphamide. The early studies involved a short-term approach in which the aim was to eradicate circulating tumor cells. Nitrogen mustard was used in this manner in three studies, and did not demonstrate any benefit over the control group. Similar results were obtained when vinblastine was used for 3 months. Cyclophosphamide has been used in short-term and in long-term studies. Very few if any differences in survival have been demonstrated in these studies when compared with the placebo. In one study, survival was worse in the cyclophosphamide-treated group, which suggested that the use of this drug might impair defense mechanisms against tumor cells (Brunner *et al.*, 1973). Recent chemotherapeutic trials have taken into account the different cell types seen in bronchogenic carcinoma. Combination chemotherapy, regimens of which are based on kinetic and animal data, is being used in a more rational manner for each of the cell types. While no dramatic increase in survival has yet been demonstrated, it is probable that use of these regimens in an adjuvant setting and possibly combined with immunotherapy or radiation therapy or both will result in a more favorable outcome.

3.3. Gastrointestinal (GI) Cancer

Medical oncologists have in the past tended to group all these cancers together and to evaluate chemotherapeutic agents on a number of different GI tumors simultaneously. Results have been confusing and disappointing. The drug that has received the most attention as a treatment of this group of tumors has been 5-fluorouracil (5-FU). The overall response rate in advanced disease has been on the order of 20% (Wasserman *et al.*, 1975). Recent work, involving the addition of methyl-CCNU to 5-FU, indicates that the response rate is raised to 30% or perhaps more (Moertel, 1976). It is also possible that mitomycin C may be a useful addition to 5-FU.

Li and Ross (1976) treated 89 patients with Dukes B and C colorectal cancers by surgery plus adjuvant 5-FU therapy. Chemotherapy was administered in two 5-day courses separated by a 4-week interval and beginning 4–6 weeks following surgery. The results were compared with those of 124 historical controls who had surgery without chemotherapy. The 5-year disease-free survival in the chemotherapy-treated Dukes C group was 57.5%, as opposed to 24.3% in matched controls ($P < 0.01$). In patients with Dukes B lesions, the 5-year disease-free survival was 81.6% in the 5-FU-treated group, as opposed to 58.5% in the controls ($P < 0.02$).

Recently, the Gastrointestinal Tumor Study Group has been set up by the National Cancer Institute. Many of their studies have been designed to look into the effects of adjuvant chemotherapy, radiation therapy, and immunotherapy in different GI cancers. Thus, following curative resection of gastric carcinoma, a prospective randomized trial using 5-FU and methyl-CCNU in one group, and no additional therapy in the other, has been started. Similarly, patients who have had a curative resection of rectal carcinoma graded as Dukes B2 or C are randomized to receive no further therapy, radiation therapy alone, 5-FU and methyl-CCNU chemotherapy, or radiation therapy plus 5-FU and methyl-CCNU. In colon cancer, the randomization for Dukes B2 and C lesions comprises a control group, 5-FU and methyl-CCNU, immunotherapy with methanol-extractable residue (MER), and chemoimmunotherapy with MER plus 5-FU and methyl-CCNU. No results have yet been published, as these trials are in their early stages. The use of adjuvant therapy in esophageal and pancreatic carcinomas is probably not yet justified, as no agents have been shown to demonstrate any significant cytotoxic effect.

3.4. Ovarian Cancer

The prognosis in carcinoma of the ovary depends very much on its stage at diagnosis; thus, the 5-year survival ranges from 61% in Stage I disease to 3–5% in Stages III and IV disease. Unfortunately, many patients at presentation demonstrate an advanced stage of the disease. In patients with early-stage ovarian cancer, successful therapy is often accomplished by a combination of surgery and radiation therapy. Most of the studies using chemotherapy have been restricted to patients with advanced disease. Alkylating agents such as melphalan, cyclophosphamide, chlorambucil, and thioTEPA have been shown to have activity, with partial and complete responses around 50% (Wasserman et al., 1975). Adriamycin and hexamethylmelamine are also useful agents, and studies have been set up to evaluate combinations of these two drugs with an alkylating agent. In the M. D. Anderson Hospital, a study was carried out on patients with ovarian cancer Stages I–III following surgery, in whom radiation therapy (whole-abdomen plus pelvic boost) was compared with 12 months of intermittent melphalan therapy (Smith et al., 1975). Two years after beginning treatment, 85% of patients with Stage I cancer who were treated with radiation were without evidence of disease, and 90% of those who received chemotherapy were also without evidence of disease. In Stage II cancer, 55% of the radiation-treated patients and 58% of those who were given chemotherapy were without evidence of disease. At 5 years, however, 63% of those given chemotherapy were without disease, but only 45% of those who were treated with radiation were without evidence of cancer. It is possible that the beneficial effects of adjuvant chemotherapy may be seen at 5 years, and further studies will have to refute or confirm this. The Eastern Cooperative Oncology Group and the Radiotherapy Oncology Group, together with the Gynecologic Oncology Group, have designed a study of patients with Stage II carcinoma of the ovary, in which patients will receive total abdominal hysterectomy, bilateral salpingo-oophorectomy, omentectomy, and evaluation of the undersurface of the diaphragm. They will then be randomized to receive pelvic and abdominal radiation therapy or pelvic radiation and chemotherapy with melphalan. Unfortunately, the study will not include a randomized limb using melphalan without radiation therapy.

3.5. Testicular Cancer

A dramatic improvement in therapeutic response has recently been observed in metastatic nonseminomatous germ-cell tumors of the testicle. This improvement is due to improvement in combination chemotherapy of these cancers. Samuels *et al.* (1975) have demonstrated the effectiveness of combinations of bleomycin and vinblastine. These drugs, with the addition of cyclophosphamide, actinomycin D and dichlorodiamino-*cis*-platinum, have also been shown to be effective by the Memorial Sloan-Kettering group of workers (Cvitkovic *et al.*, 1976). The 10-year survival of patients with Stage IA disease is 80–100%, whereas these figures drop to 30–50% and 7–40% in patients with Stage IB and II disease, respectively (Maier, 1970). Furthermore, the presence of vascular invasion in the primary tumor is associated with a bad prognosis.

Most patients do undergo paraaortic node dissection if they have Stage I or II disease. Thus, bulky disease is removed *en bloc*. Clinical trials involving the use of adjuvant chemotherapy for these groups of patients are urgently needed.

3.6. Head and Neck Cancer

The term *head and neck cancer* is used to describe mostly squamous-cell carcinomas of the oral cavity, pharynx, and larynx. The overall 5-year survival rate is about 60% when surgery and radiotherapy are the modalites used. Carcinomas of the oral cavity have a high incidence of local recurrence. Some tumor regression has been consistently documented in advanced or recurrent disease treated with chemotherapeutic agents. Methotrexate produces a 30–50% response rate; bleomycin and adriamycin, 20–25% response rates (Bertino *et al.*, 1975). Studies in which chemotherapy has been administered together with radiation therapy in advanced disease have not been impressive. On the other hand, there are early encouraging results from methotrexate therapy plus immunotherapy with BCG (R. C. Donaldson, 1973).

The stage has been set for studies involving the use of adjuvant chemotherapy and immunotherapy in protocols with Stages III and IV cancers who have undergone curative surgery or radiation therapy or both. The Eastern Cooperative Oncology Group and Yale University have recently activated such therapeutic protocols.

3.7. Brain Tumors

Malignant brain tumors may be either primary or secondary. Of the primary tumors, malignant gliomas are the most frequent. With the exception of childhood solid low-grade posterior fossa astrocytomas, the prognosis of primary malignant brain tumors is still very poor, despite improvement in surgical and radiotherapeutic techniques. Radical surgery is difficult and seldom leads to cure; radiotherapy is a useful adjunct, but is purely palliative.

Chemotherapy is in its infancy in this setting, and it is doubtful whether increased survival has resulted from the use of single agents or combination chemotherapy for the treatment of gliomas. The only tumor that is sensitive to chemotherapy is medulloblastoma. The desirable characteristic of a useful drug in the treatment of gliomas is a high degree of lipid solubility, which is usually accompanied by a low molecular size and a low degree of ionization. The nitrosoureas have been shown to fulfill these criteria, and have been used extensively in the treatment of various brain tumors. The response rates have varied from 13 to 50%, probably due to the great difficulty in measuring responses in patients with these tumors. Other drugs that may hold promise are procarbazine, dimethyltriazino imidazole carboxamide, bleomycin, and high-dose methotrexate with Leucovorin "rescue" (Wasserman *et al.*, 1975; Rosen *et al.*, 1975b). In addition, vincristine is well known to be active in medulloblastoma. The Brain Tumor Study Group has carried out prospective randomized studies that include postoperative radiation with or without BCNU (Walker, 1975). It is probable that BCNU plus radiation therapy is marginally better in prolonging survival than either alone or no further treatment following surgery. With the advent of new agents and combinations of drugs, more encouraging results may be achieved.

3.8. Osteogenic Sarcoma

Advanced osteogenic sarcoma is a difficult disease to treat effectively with either chemotherapy or radiotherapy. Amputation alone at the time of presentation permits only about a 20% 5-year survival rate, and more than 50% of patients develop pulmonary metastases within 5–9 months after operation.

In 1972, high-dose methotrexate with Leucovorin "rescue," and later adriamycin alone or in combination with methotrexate, were shown to cause some regression of radiologically evident metastatic disease. Treating with radical surgery followed by adjuvant vincristine and high-dose methotrexate and Leucovorin "rescue," Jaffe *et al.* (1974) reported 75% of patients free of disease 13–30 months after surgery. Cortes *et al.* (1975) found no evidence of disease among 27 of 30 patients up to $2\frac{1}{2}$ years after treatment was stopped when maximally tolerated doses of adriamycin were employed. Rosen *et al.* (1975a) utilized preoperative intensive chemotherapy with vincristine, high-dose methotrexate and Leucovorin "rescue," and adriamycin. This treatment was followed by surgical removal of the tumor and replacement of the bone with a metal prosthesis. Postoperative adjuvant chemotherapy with the same drugs plus cyclophosphamide was given for 12 months. Of 14 patients, only 1 had evidence of recurrent disease when observed for a maximum of 17 months. Sutow *et al.* (1975) reported a four-drug adjuvant chemotherapy regimen (CONPADRI-I) utilizing cyclophosphamide, vincristine, melphalan, and adriamycin given at specific intervals over 72 months following operation. Of 18 patients, 10 (55%) remained disease-free 32–47 months after surgery and 16–31 months after discontinuance of adjuvant therapy. These 10 cases may well represent cure of osteogenic sarcoma.

Amputation is a necessary aspect of control of this disease. With subradical operation, Cortes *et al.* (1975) found only 2 of 6 patients remained free of disease, whereas with amputation, 14 of 15 remained disease-free. These results again suggest that chemotherapy of a relatively refractory tumor mass is only palliative, but that treatments of minimal residual tumor may be curative.

3.9. Ewing's Sarcoma

Ewing's sarcoma is a highly anaplastic tumor that in the past has been rapidly and uniformly fatal. In most series, 5-year survival rates range from 5 to 15% whether the patient is treated by surgery or irradiation of the primary tumor site. These poor results reflect the early appearance of clinical metastatic disease, and it is probable that most patients have microscopic metastases at the time of diagnosis.

Chemotherapy together with radiation therapy has yielded increased disease-free survival. This effect was initially shown by Johnson and Humphreys (1969), using cyclophosphamide following radiation, and by Freeman *et al.* (1972) with various chemotherapeutic agents following radiation.

In 1972, a study employing radiation followed by combination chemotherapy with vincristine and cyclophosphamide administered for 1–2 years was reported by Hsutu *et al.* (1972). Of 15 patients, 10 remained continuously free of disease for periods ranging from 4 to 91 months. Johnson and Pomeroy (1975) used actinomycin D, cyclophosphamide, and vincristine plus whole-brain irradiation and intrathecal methotrexate. They observed disease-free intervals of 3–17 months in 11 patients. A review of 66 patients treated since 1964 at the National Cancer Institute with a variety of chemotherapeutic regimens following local irradiation was recently published (Pomeroy and Johnson, 1975). In this review, 43 patients without clinically detectable metastases at diagnosis had a 64% 2-year survival rate and a 52% 5-year survival rate. The current protocol, in which adriamycin is alternated with cyclophosphamide and vincristine plus whole-brain irradiation and intrathecal methotrexate, is reported to provide improved disease-free survival compared with earlier protocols.

Rosen *et al.* (1974) reported 100% disease-free survival in 12 patients over periods from 10 to 37 months when employing a four-drug combination of actinomycin D, adriamycin, vincristine, and cyclophosphamide for 2 years. In this study, however, 2 patients, who received more than 700 mg adriamycin/M^2, developed congestive heart failure after 19 months. Fernandez *et al.* (1974) reported improved disease-free survival in patients receiving cyclophosphamide and vincristine in addition to radiotherapy, compared with radiotherapy alone. Of 19 patients, 6 were disease-free for 12–46 months; the onset of metastases was delayed in those patients receiving chemotherapy in addition to radiation therapy.

Although a small number of patients develop meningeal disease, the value of whole-brain irradiation and intrathecal chemotherapy has not yet been established.

MICHAEL T.
SHAW AND
ROBERT D.
STEBBINS

3.10. Wilms's Tumor

In the treatment of Wilms's tumor, the addition of chemotherapy to standard programs of surgery and radiotherapy has increased survival to more than 80% in localized disease and close to 50% in metastatic disease. Employing surgery and radiotherapy alone, workers have reported cure rates as high as 47% (Wolff, 1975).

In 1966, Farber demonstrated the advantage of adding chemotherapy to the standard treatment of Wilms's tumor (Farber, 1966). In a review of the Boston Children's Medical Center experience from 1957 to 1964, in which actinomycin D was utilized in addition to surgery and radiotherapy, it was shown that 89% of children without metastatic disease were alive and well at 2 years of minimum follow-up. With metastatic disease at diagnosis, 53% of children survived 2 years or more.

In 1968, Childrens Cancer Study Group A reported that the relapse rate following maintenance actinomycin D therapy was lower (14%) than that following a single course of the drug (52%)(Wolff *et al.*, 1968). After further aggressive therapy of patients in relapse, the difference in survival of the two groups in 1974 was approximately the same (80% and 71%, respectively) (Wolff *et al.*, 1974). The use of vincristine as a single agent for treatment of metastatic Wilms's tumor has yielded a 45% 2-year disease-free survival (Sutow, 1965). In localized Wilms's tumor, an 83% disease-free survival during $4\frac{1}{2}$ years has been reported (Wolff, 1975). In 1969, the National Wilms's Tumor Study Group was formed to study various treatment modalities. Accurate tumor staging was developed. Actinomycin D, radiotherapy, and vincristine, either as single agents or in combination, were employed in various treatment protocols. The 2-year actuarial disease-free rates for patients with completely resected tumors was greater than 80%. The 2-year actuarial survival rate was 98% for patients given radiotherapy in addition to surgery and actinomycin D, and 95% for those given surgery and actinomycin D alone (Wolff, 1975). Early experience with adriamycin in treatment of Wilms's tumor has been encouraging, and it is planned to study that drug alone or in combination with actinomycin D and vincristine both as adjuvant and as treatment for advanced tumors.

3.11. Rhabdomyosarcoma

The most common soft-tissue sarcoma in childhood is rhabdomyosarcoma. This tumor may occur in any location in which there is striated muscle, and the most frequent anatomical sites are the head and neck region, trunk, extremities, and GU tract. The three cell types, embryonal, alveolar, and pleomorphic, were once thought to have prognostic significance, but it now appears that survival is the same in patients with tumors of the different cell types. Of patients with rhabdomyosarcoma, 74% develop metastases by 6 months, 83% by 1 year.

Treatment with surgery or radiotherapy alone has been disappointing, with an overall survival rate of 5–10%. Only 20–25% of newly diagnosed tumors can be completely removed surgically. Survival following complete primary tumor resection is approximately 50-60%.

Pratt *et al.* (1972) showed that following surgery and radiotherapy to the primary site, treatment with vincristine, cyclophosphamide, and actinomycin D improved the median duration of survival. Heyn *et al.* (1974) reported the effect of 1 year of therapy with vincristine and actinomycin D after radiotherapy and complete surgical removal of known tumor. Recurrent or metastatic disease occurred in 3 of 17 (18%) of this group. In a control group receiving surgery and radiotherapy only, 8 of 15 (53%) developed further disease. With a follow-up period of 3–6 years, 10 of 11 patients (91%) who had microscopic residual disease at the time of surgery were alive without evidence of disease when treated with chemotherapy and radiotherapy. This disease-free survival rate clearly exceeded that of the group not receiving postoperative chemotherapy. Reporting on rhabdomyosarcoma of the head and neck region, where curative surgery is frequently more difficult, S. S. Donaldson *et al.* (1973) found that combined systemic therapy gave the best chance of cure. These workers used vincristine, actinomycin D, and oral cyclophosphamide following surgery and radiotherapy. Generally, treatment with actinomycin D extended for 15 months, and with cyclophosphamide for 24 months. Of 5 patients with local disease, all showed no evidence of disease at 25–72 months. Of 2 patients with locally invasive disease, both were without evidence of disease at 32 and 33 months.

Ghavmi *et al.* (1976) reported the addition of adriamycin to cyclophosphamide, vincristine, and actinomycin D for the treatment of rhabdomyosarcoma following surgery. Chemotherapy was continued for $1\frac{1}{2}$–2 years unless evidence of disease recurrence appeared. Radiotherapy was administered only to those patients in whom gross or microsopic disease was documented following surgery. Of 60 patients with disease completely removed at surgery, 45 demonstrated disease-free intervals of 4–64 months. No clear benefit has yet been shown, however, from adding adriamycin to the cyclophosphamide–vincristine–actinomycin D regimen, and results obtained from vincristine and actinomycin D alone appear very encouraging. What is clear is that treatment of completely resected rhabdomyosarcoma with radiation therapy and chemotherapy significantly prolongs disease-free survival.

3.12. Neuroblastoma

Neuroblastoma, the most common solid malignant tumor of childhood, accounts for about half of neonatal malignant tumors. Despite the use of several different chemotherapeutic agents, with and without radiation therapy, the survival rate for patients with neuroblastoma has changed little in the last 20 years. Surgery is primary therapy, and many patients have widespread disease at diagnosis. Most patients with localized disease, however, have received no chemotherapy. It may be that, as in Wilms's tumor patients and others treated for microscopic disease, significant benefit from chemotherapy will become evident only when apparently localized disease is treated with adjuvant chemotherapy.

4. Conclusions

MICHAEL T.
SHAW AND
ROBERT D.
STEBBINS

The concept of adjunctive chemotherapy is very attractive, and it is tempting for all and sundry to jump onto the bandwagon. At the time of this writing, the addition of cytotoxic drugs to surgical management of Wilms's tumor and osteogenic sarcoma is acknowledged by most oncologists to be of proven value in preventing metastases and thus in prolonging life. The studies in breast cancer, however, are by no means conclusive as yet. We shall await with much interest the long-term results obtained from the breast cancer adjuvant studies. Much interest will center around the duration of disease-free interval, when compared with groups treated by surgery alone. Even if this interval is significantly prolonged by adjuvant chemotherapy, a truly meaningful result must also include demonstrably prolonged survival. One of the most worrying aspects of adjunctive chemotherapy is the choice of a drug schedule that will not inhibit the immune system for prolonged periods of time. It is probable that immunosuppression will be avoided by ensuring that the drugs are administered on an intermittent basis. It is obvious that therapy must be continued for a length of time that is adequate for total tumor kill and yet as brief as possible. This time period is almost impossible to define or calculate with any accuracy, and will probably have to be based to a large extent on empiricism. More use will be made of "second-look" and even "third-look" operations to evaluate the adequacy of adjuvant therapy.

Before embarking on a long program of adjunctive chemotherapy in various tumors, the potential risks vs. benefits should be weighed carefully in the investigator's mind. Most cytotoxic drugs have significant toxic effects, some of which may be quite intolerable to the patient. Morbidity from infections, resulting from leukopenia and immunosuppression caused by the drugs, may become increasingly frequent. Sterility may become a problem in younger patients. Even if they are able to reproduce, the possibility of the teratogenic effects may have important implications. Recently, the effective chemotherapy of various cancers such as Hodgkin's disease has heralded a new and fearsome aspect, namely, second malignancies. Acute leukemia is being recorded by several observers as a long-term complication of "the cure" of Hodgkin's disease. While it cannot be proved that chemotherapy is a direct cause, it is tempting to believe that it plays a significant role. Alkylating agents, which cause disruption of DNA, have been implicated in carcinogenesis. It would indeed be a tragedy if large numbers of patients entered on adjuvant chemotherapeutic protocols developed second malignancies. Perhaps the avoidance of the use of alkylating agents in this setting would be worthwhile where possible. For the time being, adjunctive chemotherapy remains in an early investigative stage in most instances. It should only be used in well-designed and controlled clinical trials, and should on no account be used lightly or indiscriminately.

5. References

BERTINO, J. G., BOSTON, B., AND CAPIZZI, R. L., 1975, The role of chemotherapy in the management of cancer of the head and neck, *Cancer* **36:**752–758.

BONADONNA, G., BRUSAMOLINO, E., VALAGUSSA, P., *et al.*, 1976, Combination chemotherapy as an adjuvant treatment in operable breast cancer, *N. Engl. J. Med.* **294:**406–410.

BRUNNER, K. W., MARTHALER, T. H., AND MULLER, W., 1973, Effects of long term adjuvant chemotherapy with cyclophosphamide for radically resected bronchogenic carcinoma, *Cancer Chemother. Rep. Part 3* **4:**125–132.

BURCHENAL, J. H., 1976, Adjuvant therapy—theory, practice and potential, *Cancer* **37:**46–57.

COLE, W. H., PACKARD, D., AND SOUTHWICK, H. W., 1954, Carcinoma of the colon with special reference to prevention of recurrence, *J. Amer. Med. Assoc.* **155:**1549–1553.

CORTES, E. P., HOLLAND, J. F., AND WAND, J. J., 1975, Adriamycin in primary osteosarcoma, *Proc. Amer. Soc. Clin. Oncol.* **16:**241 (abstract).

CVITKOVIC, E., HAYES, D., AND GOLBEY, R., 1976, Primary combination chemotherapy (VAB III) for metastatic or unresectable germ cell tumors, *Proc. Amer. Soc. Clin. Oncol.* **17:**296 (abstract).

DELARUE, N. C., 1960, The free cancer cell, *Can. Med. Assoc. J.* **82:**1175–1183.

DONALDSON, R. C., 1973, Chemoimmunotherapy for cancer of the head and neck, *Amer. J. Surg.* **126:**507–512.

DONALDSON, S. S., CASTRO, J. R., WILBUR, J. R., AND JESSE, R. H., JR., 1973, Rhabdomyosarcoma of head and neck in children, *Cancer* **31:**26–35.

FARBER, S., 1966, Chemotherapy in the treatment of leukemia and Wilms's tumor, *J. Amer. Med. Assoc.* **198:**826–836.

FERNANDEZ, C. H., LINDBERG, R. D., SUTOW, W. W., AND SAMUELS, M. L., 1974, Localized Ewing's sarcoma—Treatment and results, *Cancer* **34:**143–148.

FINNEY, R., 1971, Adjuvant chemotherapy in the radical treatment of carcinoma of the breast—a clinical trial, *Amer. J. Roentgenol.* **111:**137–141.

FISHER, B., RAVDIN, R. G., AUSMAN, R. K., *et al.*, 1968, Surgical adjuvant chemotherapy in cancer of the breast: Results of a decade of cooperative investigation, *Ann. Surg.* **168:**337–356.

FISHER, B., SLACK, N. H., BROSS, I. D. J., *et al.*, 1969, Cancer of the breast: Size of neoplasm and prognosis, *Cancer* **24:**1071–1080.

FISHER, B., NELSON, M., SLACK, N. H., CAVANAUGH, P. J., GARDNER, B., RAVDIN, R. G., *et al.*, 1970, Postoperative radiotherapy in the treatment of breast cancer, *Ann. Surg.* **172:**711–732.

FISHER, B., CARBONE, P., ECONOMON, S. G., *et al.*, 1975, L-Phenylalanine mustard (L-PAM) in the management of primary breast cancer. A report of early findings, *N. Engl. J. Med.* **292:**117–122.

FREEMAN, A. I., SACHATELLO, C., GAETA, J., *et al.*, 1972, An analysis of Ewing's tumor in children at Roswell Park Memorial Institute, *Cancer* **29:**1563–1569.

GHAVIMI, F., TEFFT, M., AND MURPHY, M. L., 1976, Further experience with multidisciplinary treatment of embryonal rhabdomyosarcoma, *Proc. Amer. Soc. Clin. Oncol.* **17:**307 (abstract).

HEYN, R. M., HOLLAND, R., NEWTON, W. A., JR., *et al.*, 1974, The role of combined chemotherapy in the treatment of rhabdomyosarcoma in children, *Cancer* **34:**2128–2141.

HSUTU, H. O., PINKEL, D., AND PRATT, C. B., 1972, Treatment of clinically localized Ewing's sarcoma with radiotherapy and combination chemotherapy, *Cancer* **30:**1522–1527.

JAFFE, N., FREI, E., TRAGGIS, D., AND BIHSHOP, Y., 1974, Adjuvant methotrexate and citrovorum-factor treatment of osteogenic sarcoma, *N. Engl. J. Med.* **291:**994–997.

JOHNSON, R., AND HUMPHREYS, S. R., 1969, Past failures and future possibilities in Ewing's sarcoma: Experimental and preliminary clinical results, *Cancer* **23:**161–166.

JOHNSON, R. E., AND POMEROY, T. C., 1975, Evaluation of therapeutic results in Ewing's sarcoma, *Amer. J. Roentgenol.* **123:**583–587.

KENNEDY, B. J., MIELKE, P. W., AND FORTUNY, I. E., 1964, Therapeutic castration versus prophylactic castration in breast cancer, *Surg. Gynecol. Obstet.* **118:**524–540.

LI, M. D., AND ROSS, S. T., 1976, Chemoprophylaxis for patients with colorectal cancer. Prospective study with five-year follow-up, *J. Amer. Med. Assoc.* **235:**2825–2828.

LONG, L., JONASSON, O., ROBERTS, S., McGRATH, R., McGREW, E., AND COLE, W. H., 1960, Cancer cells in blood, *Arch. Surg.* **80:**910–917.

LONG, R. L., DONEGAN, W. L., AND EVANS, A. M., 1969, Extended surgical adjuvant chemotherapy for breast cancer, *Amer. J. Surg.* **117:**701–704.

MAIER, J. G., 1970, Treatment of testicular germ cell malignancies, *J. Amer. Med. Assoc.* **213:**97–98.

McDONALD, G. O., LIVINGSTONE, C., BOYLES, C. F., AND COLE, W. H., 1957, The prophylactic treatment of malignant disease with nitrogen mustard and triethylenethiophosphoramide (Thiotepa), *Ann. Surg.* **145:**624–629.

MOERTEL, C. G., 1976, Gastrointestinal cancer. Treatment with fluorouracil–nitrosourea combinations, *J. Amer. Med. Assoc.* **235:**2135–2136.

MOORE, G. E., AND KONDO, T., 1958, Study of adjuvant cancer chemotherapy by model experiments, *Surgery* **44:**199–209.

MRAZEK, R., 1970, Adjuvant chemotherapy with cancer of the breast at one institution, in: *Chemotherapy of Cancer* (W. H. Cole, ed.), pp. 289–292, Lee and Febiger, Philadelphia.

MUGGIA, F. M., 1974, Cell kinetic studies in patients with lung cancer, *Oncology* **30:**353–361.

NISSEN-MEYER, R., 1973, Cyclophosphamide as adjuvant to the primary surgery for breast cancer—a cooperative controlled clinical trial, presented at the 8th International Congress of Chemotherapy, Athens, Sept. 8–14.

NISSEN-MEYER, R., KJELLGREN, K., AND MANSON, B., 1971, Preliminary report from the Scandinavian Adjuvant Chemotherapy Study Group, *Cancer Chemother. Rep.* **55:**561–566.

POMEROY, T. C., AND JOHNSON, R. E., 1975, Combined modality therapy of Ewing's sarcoma, *Cancer* **35:** 36–47.

PRATT, C. B., HSUTU, H. O., FLEMING, D., AND PINKEL, D., 1972, Coordinated treatment of childhood rhabdomyosarcoma with surgery, radiotherapy, and combination chemotherapy, *Cancer Res.* **32:**606–610.

RIECHE, K., BERNDT, H., AND PROHL, B., 1972, Continuous postoperative treatment with cyclophosphamide in breast carcinoma—a randomized clinical study, *Arch. Geschwulstforsch.* **40:**349–354.

ROSEN, G., WOLLNER, N., TAN, C., et al., 1974, Disease-free survival in children with Ewing's sarcoma treated with radiation therapy and adjuvant four drug sequential chemotherapy, *Cancer* **33:**384–393.

ROSEN, G., MARCOVE, R., BEATTIE, E. J., et al., 1975a, Osteogenic sarcoma: Sequential chemotherapy in 45 consecutive patients, *Proc. Amer. Soc. Clin. Oncol.* **15:**227 (abstract).

ROSEN, G., MEHTA, B. M., GHAVIMI, F., et al., 1975b, Intravenous high dose methotrexate with citrovorum factor "rescue." CNS distribution and therapeutic response of intracranial neoplasms, *Proc. Amer. Assoc. Cancer Res.* **16:**750 (abstract).

SALGADO, I., HOPKIRK, J. F., LONG, R. C., RITCHIE, A. C., RITCHIE, S., AND WEBSTER, D. R., 1959, Tumor cells in the blood, *Can. Med. Assoc. J.* **81:**619–622.

SAMUELS, M. L., JOHNSON, D. E., AND HOLOYE, P. Y., 1975, Continuous intravenous bleomycin (NSC-125066) therapy with vinblastine (NSC-49842) in Stage III testicular neoplasia, *Cancer Chemother. Rep.* **59:**563–570.

SCHABEL, F. M., 1975, Concepts for systemic treatment of micrometastases, *Cancer* **35:**15–24.

SELAWRY, O. S., 1974, The role of chemotherapy in the treatment of lung cancer, *Semin. Oncol.* **1:**259–272.

SHAPIRO, D. M., AND FUGMANN, R. A., 1957, A role for chemotherapy as an adjunct to surgery, *Cancer Res.* **17:**1098–1101.

SMITH, J. P., RUTLEDGE, F. N., AND DELELOS, L., 1975, Results of chemotherapy as an adjunct to surgery in patients with localized ovarian cancer, *Semin. Oncol.* **2:**277–281.

SUTOW, W. W., 1965, Chemotherapy in childhood cancer—an appraisal, *Cancer* **18:**1585–1589.

SUTOW, W. W., SULLIVAN, M. P., FERNBACH, D. J., et al., 1975, Adjuvant chemotherapy in primary treatment of osteogenic sarcoma, *Cancer* **36:**1598–1602.

TORMEY, D. C., 1975, Combined chemotherapy and surgery in breast cancer: A review, *Cancer* **36:**881–892.

WALKER, M. D., 1975, Chemotherapy: Adjuvant to surgery and radiation therapy, *Semin. Oncol.* **2:**69–72.

WASSERMAN, T. H., COMIS, R. L., GOLDSMITH, M., et al., 1975, Tabular analysis of the clinical chemotherapy of solid tumors, *Cancer Chemother. Rep.* **6:**399–419.

WOLFF, J. A., 1975, Advances in the treatment of Wilms's tumor, *Cancer* **35:**901–904.

WOLFF, J. A., KRIVIT, W., NEWTON, W. A., JR., AND D'ANGIO, G. J., 1968, Single versus multiple dose dactinomycin therapy of Wilms's tumor—a controlled cooperative study conducted by the Children's Cancer Study Group A, *N. Engl. J. Med.* **279:**290–299.

WOLFF, J. A., D'ANGIO, G. J., HARTMANN, J., et al., 1974, Long term evaluation of single versus multiple courses of actinomycin-D therapy of Wilms's tumor, *N. Engl. J. Med.* **290:**84–86.

6

Principles of Combination Chemotherapy

L. Wayne Keiser and Robert L. Capizzi

1. Introduction

In 1948, Farber (Farber *et al.*, 1948) reported that the folic acid antagonist aminopterin was able to induce temporary clinical remissions of disease in some children with acute leukemia. Remarkable as these early remissions were, it soon became apparent that with the exception of methotrexate-induced cure of choriocarcinoma (Li *et al.*, 1956) (and later cyclophosphamide-induced cure of Burkitt's lymphoma) (Nkrumah and Perkins, 1976; Ziegler *et al.*, 1973), single-agent chemotherapy yielded only a low percentage of complete responses of relatively short duration. Early studies in the 1960s utilizing combinations of antineoplastic drugs soon demonstrated the superiority of combination chemotherapy over single agents in the treatment of certain tumors. Using the combination of methotrexate, actinomycin D, and chlorambucil for the treatment of advanced testicular carcinoma, Li *et al.* (1960) demonstrated a marked improvement in the response rate as compared with the effect of these agents when used alone. Greenspan (Greenspan *et al.*, 1963; Greenspan, 1966) showed that the objective response rate in metastatic breast carcinoma was more than double the single-agent response rate when thioTEPA and methotrexate were used in combination. When 5-fluorouracil (5-FU) was added to the combination, some patients with hepatic metastases resistant to the drugs used alone showed significant tumor regression. The therapeutic potential of combination chemotherapy became more impressive with the demonstration of the superlative

L. Wayne Keiser and Robert L. Capizzi • Yale University School of Medicine, 333 Cedar Street, New Haven, Connecticut 06510.

effect of five drugs in the treatment of advanced breast cancer (cyclophosphamide, vincristine, methotrexate, prednisone, and 5-FU) (Cooper, 1969). Subsequently, a large number of laboratory and clinical trials against both animal and human tumors followed that utilized empirical combinations of previously known active drugs.

As the number of partially effective single agents increased, the number of possible drug combinations quickly overwhelmed the ability of clinical and laboratory trials to evaluate them. In the absence of any discriminating factors, it has been estimated that there could be 47,905 possible three-drug combinations empirically derived from an available pool of 67 drugs (Lloyd, 1974). To test a five-drug regimen, e.g., the "Cooper regimen" (see above), against breast cancer alone would require 32 separate clinical trials if two dosage levels of each drug were used, and 243 separate trials if three dosage levels were used (Lloyd, 1974). Clearly, it is not possible to test all, or even a small fraction of, the number of available drug combinations. Therefore, it has become useful to develop certain principles of combination chemotherapy to guide us in our selection of potentially synergistic drug combinations, or, at the least, to eliminate combinations not likely to be an improvement over single-drug treatments.

The following discussion is not intended to be an exhaustive review of the laboratory and clinical aspects of combination chemotherapy, but rather a presentation of certain principles that, for the moment, may serve as a guide for the selection of agents to be used in combination.

In combination chemotherapy of neoplastic diseases, the concept of therapeutic synergism has been variously defined, depending on the background of the author. Strictly speaking, synergy represents an end effect that is greater than the effect that would be anticipated from the algebraic sum of the individual effects of the components. Using this definition, true synergy is most easily discerned by the cell biologist or biochemist working with cell cultures or cell-free enzyme systems. When one considers whole-animal studies, however, definitions are not as precise because of the interplay of many factors. These factors include the overall effects of the disease on the host, drug toxicity on normal organs, and the effects of the drugs and the disease on the immune system, as well as the pharmacokinetic and cytokinetic effects of the drugs. Thus, the ultimate observation—host survival or cure—is the result of these interactions, and cannot be simply stated in terms of the effect of the drug(s) on the tumor.

A reasonable use of the word *synergy* in a clinical setting would be a situation in which the percentage of patients responding to a combination or the duration of response, or both, is significantly greater than would be expected from the effects of the individual drugs. Conceivably, the drugs may have acted in an additive fashion, reducing the tumor burden to a level low enough to allow the further elimination of tumor cells through immune means, perhaps stimulated by immune adjuvants. To illustrate this superior effect, the design of the proper clinical trial would include prospectively randomized and stratified patient populations. There is further discussion of these points in the monographs by Venditti and Goldin (1964), Mantel (1974), Carter and Soper (1974), and Valeriote and Lin (1975).

165
PRINCIPLES
OF
COMBINA-
TION
CHEMO-
THERAPY

2. General Principles

2.1. Drugs Individually Effective Against the Tumor

With several possible exceptions, it would seem prudent to restrict the choice of agents for combination to those drugs that have demonstrated efficacy against the tumor when used alone. Arguments against this tenet are that all available drugs have not been individually tested against all tumors (or even the most common tumors) (Livingston and Carter, 1970). In addition, ineffectiveness may be dependent on dose or schedule, or both, and manipulation of either or both may yield significant activity of a heretofore relatively "inactive" agent. Unless dependence on dose or schedule or both has been shown to be a factor and alternate doses or schedules or both can be applied, it makes little sense to reapply an ineffective drug or drugs in the same dose and schedule that had been shown to be ineffective. Illustrative of this point is the randomized study of patients with advanced acute lymphoblastic leukemia (ALL) who were refractory to prednisone and vincristine. Patients were randomly allocated to receive daunomycin alone, in combination with prednisone, or in combination with prednisone and vincristine. There was no difference in the response rate of the three groups; the response of the group treated with daunomycin alone was equivalent to the response of the patients receiving the combinations (Jones et al., 1972). As stated above, however, resistance may be related to dose or schedule, or both. Patients who had relapsed on lower doses and alternate schedules of methotrexate (MTX) may respond to higher doses and alternate schedules and combinations (Capizzi et al., 1974a).

Notable exceptions to the use of ineffective agents in combination chemotherapy for patients exist when laboratory investigations provide a strong rationale for their use. For example, while leucovorin is ineffective as an antitumor agent, its application at an appropriate time interval after MTX was found to improve the therapeutic index of MTX and to lead to a higher curability rate in mice bearing the L1210 leukemia (Goldin et al., 1955). This observation has been effectively applied in clinical studies (Capizzi et al., 1970; Djerassi et al., 1972; Jaffe et al., 1973, 1974).

Tetrahydrouridine (THU) is an effective inhibitor of the enzyme pyrimidine nucleoside deaminase, which metabolizes cytosine arabinoside to the inactive uracil arabinoside. This enzyme exists in high concentration in the intestinal mucosa, thus precluding the oral use of cytosine arabinoside. At doses of THU that have no observable toxicity or intrinsic antitumor activity in mice bearing the L1210 leukemia, the results obtained with the oral combination of THU and cytosine arabinoside are comparable to, or exceed, those achieved with intraperitoneal cytosine arabinoside alone (Neil et al., 1970). This combination awaits clinical trial.

Likewise, recent laboratory studies with adenine arabinoside (Ara-A) in combination with an inhibitor of its catabolic enzyme appear very promising. Mouse leukemia cell lines were found to be resistant to Ara-A because of high concentrations of adenosine deaminase, the drug's catabolic enzyme. The cytotoxic effect of

Ara-A was restored when it was administered in combination with 2′-deoxycoformycin, an effective inhibitor of the deaminase enzyme. 2′-Deoxycoformycin itself has no antitumor effect (Cass and Au-Yeung, 1976; LePage *et al.*, 1976).

An example of the use of two ineffective agents to yield an effective combination is the treatment of a refractory mouse plasmacytoma with an inhibitor of DNA repair in conjunction with an alkylating agent (Stabler, 1971). In this study, the mouse tumor previously refractory to the alkylating agent subsequently responded following the addition of a repair inhibitor.

2.2. Minimal Overlapping Toxicities

Most anticancer drugs in current use possess some degree of toxicity to normal organs (see Chapter 3). By selecting active agents with minimal to no overlapping toxicity, full effective doses of the components can be used with tolerable host toxicity. For example, the use of the combination of cyclophosphamide, vincristine, prednisone, and bleomycin in the treatment of lymphomas, or the use of vinblastine and bleomycin in the treatment of testicular cancer (Samuels *et al.*, 1975*a*, *b*), allows the use of full doses of each drug because the toxicity spectrum for each drug is different. When one is combining agents that may affect the same organ, e.g., bone marrow, the general practice is to decrease the doses of each drug by 25–50%. With appropriate scheduling, agents that do have overlapping toxicity may be used in near-maximal doses when given sequentially. An example is the use of the MOPP [*M*ustargen (nitrogen mustard), *O*ncovin (vincristine), *P*rednisone, and *P*rocarbazine] program for the treatment of Hodgkin's disease. While nitrogen mustard and procarbazine both possess marrow toxic capability, their sequential use (at full doses) has produced enhanced therapeutic effectiveness (DeVita *et al.*, 1970).

Toxic effects of one anticancer drug occurring during the course of therapy may lead to enhanced toxicity by a second agent due to impaired metabolism or excretion. For example, care should be taken if one combines *cis*-diamminedichloroplatinum, a nephrotoxic agent (Higby *et al.*, 1973; Talley *et al.*, 1973), with an agent like MTX, which is predominantly excreted by the kidneys.

2.3. Pharmacological Considerations

2.3.1. Biochemical Mechanism of Action

Most of the currently available anticancer drugs are grouped in a chemical classification indicating their major mechanism of action as currently understood, e.g., alkylating agents, folate antagonists, intercalating agents. Within each category, the toxicity of individual agents is also comparable. Thus, if maximal doses of an alkylating agent such as cyclophosphamide are used, it makes little sense to add another alkylating agent such as chlorambucil or melphalan. Similarly, combining two intercalating agents such as adriamycin and daunorubicin would be of

no value. In addition to the inadvisability of using agents with similar pharmacological classification in combination, natural or acquired resistance to agents
of a given class is sufficiently cross-reacting as to suggest that, say, one alkylating
agent not be substituted for another when clinical resistance is evident. Exceptions
to this rule would be operative if there is sufficient laboratory evidence to suggest
otherwise, as has been shown for MTX and the nonclassic folate antagonist
triazinate. The Walker carcinosarcoma may develop resistance to MTX based on
altered transport capability (see Section 2.3.2). In this MTX-resistant subline,
triazinate has been shown to be effective (Skeel *et al.*, 1973). As a general rule of
thumb, one would be more inclined to combine agents with dissimilar mechanisms
of action. This principle ought not to be applied without further thought,
however, since with certain combinations, one drug may create metabolic and
cytokinetic conditions so as to minimize or completely antagonize the therapeutic
effect of a second agent. These interactions are called *schedule-dependent*.

From a biochemical pharmacological standpoint, understanding of the target
site of action of drugs has suggested certain theoretical considerations that may
serve as a guide to our selection of agents for use in combination. While such
concepts are intellectually appealing, they have not had broad-scale clinical
application. Major problems in using these pharmacological data arise from the
fact that a given drug may not have a single biochemical locus of action, or that the
biochemical pharmacology of the drug may vary with the tumor cell and the dose
and schedule of use.

The terms *sequential, concurrent,* and *complementary inhibition* have been proposed (Sartorelli, 1969; Harrap and Jackson, 1975), and with further study and
drug development, these terms may have wider clinical utility. Potter (1951)
applied the term *sequential inhibition* to the simultaneous action of two inhibitors
acting on different stages of a metabolic pathway. This type of inhibition may be
represented as

$$A \xrightarrow[I_1]{E_1} B \xrightarrow[I_2]{E_2} C$$

where E_1 and E_2 are the enzymes that catalyze the reactions from A to B and from
B to C, and I_1 and I_2 are the inhibitors of these reactions. This concept has found
significant clinical applicability in antibacterial chemotherapy with the design of
the product combination trimethopoim-sulfamethoxazoic, which has been found
to be significantly effective in treating certain bacterial infections as well as the
protozoal infection pneumocystis carinii (Kirby *et al.*, 1971). In these organisms a
sulfa drug (I_1) inhibits the conversion of p-aminobenzoate (A) to dihydrofolate
(B), the further conversion of which to tetrahydrofolate (C) is inhibited by
pyrimethamine (I_2).

A schematic of *concurrent inhibition* (Elion *et al.*, 1954) may be represented as
follows:

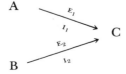

Clinically useful examples of this inhibition are not readily available. It has been suggested, however, that if a potent inhibitor (I_1) of thymidine kinase (E_1) were available, it might be of considerable use in combination with an inhibitor (I_2) of thymidylate synthetase (E_2) such as 5-FU. This combination would provide a concurrent inhibition of the synthesis of thymidylate (Harrap and Jackson, 1975).

Perhaps the most useful model for cancer chemotherapy has been the concept of *complementary inhibition* (Sartorelli, 1969), which involves the use of drugs that act at different loci involved in the formation of certain polymeric molecules. This type of inhibition can be depicted as follows:

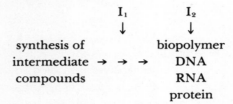

Various inhibitors of precursor or intermediate compounds such as 5-FU, MTX, and cytosine arabinoside have been shown to synergize with agents that attack the polymer directly, such as adriamycin, daunorubicin, and cyclophosphamide. The combination of the intercalating agent daunorubicin (Calendi *et al.*, 1965) with Ara-C has been shown to be synergistic (but highly schedule-dependent) in L1210 murine leukemia (Edelstein *et al.*, 1974). This combination has also been used clinically with encouraging results (Gluckman *et al.*, 1973). In metastatic breast carcinoma, the combination of the alkylating agent cyclophosphamide with the antimetabolites MTX and 5-FU (Canellos *et al.*, 1976) has shown significant improvement over the results obtained using each agent alone (Livingston and Carter, 1970).

2.3.2. Transport

Passage of a drug across cell membranes and entry into the cell is an obvious prerequisite for drug effect in most instances. The only anticancer drug that exerts its effect extracellularly is asparaginase. Drugs that enter the cell via a passive diffusion–concentration–gradient-dependent mechanism are probably of no concern from a combination-chemotherapy standpoint. Some drugs, however, must enter the cell through an active energy-dependent mechanism. Interference with this transport mechanism through the action of a second drug can significantly alter the therapeutic outcome. MTX has been extensively studied in this regard (Goldman, 1971; Nahas *et al.*, 1972). The sensitivity of animal tumor cells to the cellular destructive effect of MTX is clearly an inverse function of the ability of these cells to transport the drug (Kessel *et al.*, 1965; Sirotnak and Donsbach, 1976). Acquired drug resistance to MTX in human leukemia has also been related to impaired active transport ability (Bertino and Skeel, 1973). The very high doses of MTX that are possible with the various leucovorin rescue programs provide very high extracellular concentrations of MTX, which may enter the cell by passive diffusion, thus overcoming the transport deficiency. This mechanism may account for the clinical efficacy of high-dose MTX and leucovorin rescue in osteogenic sarcoma, a disease that is not usually responsive to conventional doses of MTX (Jaffe *et al.*, 1973). The effect of MTX on the cell has been shown to be dependent not only on a sufficient concentration of drug to bind the enzyme dihydrofolate reductase, but also on the presence of free intracellular drug (Goldman, 1975). Vincristine has been shown to impair the flux mechanism for MTX, thus enabling the retention of a higher amount of drug for a longer period of time (Bender, 1975; Fyfe and Goldman, 1973). This retention has been shown to occur in human leukemia cells *in vitro* (Bender, 1975), and could conceivably be of some clinical value.

The protein-synthesis inhibitor L-asparaginase has been shown to inhibit the active transport of MTX in asparagine-requiring mouse (Nahas and Capizzi, 1974) and human leukemia cells (Capizzi, unpublished observation). This is a schedule-dependent phenomenon that occurs within a short time interval after asparaginase administration and is probably related to a membrane effect of asparaginase or its inhibitory effect on protein synthesis. Thus, impaired transport of MTX may account for the attenuated therapeutic results seen with certain schedules of these two drugs (Capizzi, 1974a, b). Other drugs that may be administered to the patient for other reasons may also impair MTX transport, and thus affect therapeutic efficacy (Zager *et al.*, 1973).

Other drug–drug interactions at the transport level may be of future clinical interest. Laboratory studies have indicated amphotericin's potential for facilitating the transport of anticancer drugs (Medoff *et al.*, 1974).

2.3.3. Biotransformation

a. Anabolism. Antineoplastic-drug-induced alteration of the enzymatic activation of a second anticancer drug given concurrently or sequentially has not been demonstrated to be of clinical importance, but remains theoretically possible. The alkylating agent cyclophosphamide requires "activation" by the mixed-function oxidase enzymes present in the hepatic microsomal fraction (Sladek, 1971). The physiologically active metabolite of cyclophosphamide has not been positively identified (Colvin *et al.*, 1973), but phenobarbital (an inducer of the mixed-function oxidases) appears to cause increased activation and therapeutic response to cyclophosphamide in the rat (Sladek, 1971). Phenobarbital has also been shown to cause an increased rate of activation of cyclophosphamide in man, but this increased rate has not resulted in increased toxicity or therapeutic effectiveness (Jao *et al.*, 1972).

b. Catabolism. The decreased catabolic rate of cytosine arabinoside and adenine arabinoside when given concurrently with THU and 2'-deoxycoformycin, respectively, were discussed above.

The xanthine oxidase inhibitor allopurinol inhibits the oxidation of naturally occurring purines and 6-mercaptopurine. Both the toxicity and antineoplastic

activity of 6-mercaptopurine are increased several-fold with concurrent administration of allopurinol (Hitchings, 1963; *Medical Letter*, 1968).

Although current clinical application of the modification of drug catabolism
and excretion is rare, with the exception of prevention of drug toxicity, the
principle is well established and has practical potential. The increasing information on antitumor drug disposition in normal and neoplastic cells will make drug
combinations based on this principle possible.

2.4. Cytokinetic Considerations

In-depth discussion of cell kinetics appears in Chapter 2.

The cell cycle may be defined as the necessary sequence of events that occur in
the growth and division of both normal and neoplastic cells. Since little is known of
the events of cytoplasmic growth and reproduction, the cell cycle has usually been
represented in terms of nuclear events. The length, in time, of the cell cycle
(generation time) may be defined as the time from the midpoint of mitosis of a cell
to the midpoint of the subsequent mitosis in one or both daughter cells (B. T. Hill
and Baserga, 1975). Although few of the molecular events in G_1, the "presynthetic" period, are known, it is generally assumed that at least the end of G_1 contains
preparations for DNA synthesis (Prescott, 1968), primarily in the form of RNA
and protein synthesis (Kishimoto and Lieberman, 1964; Baserga *et al.*, 1965;
Terasima and Yasukawa, 1966). In a given tissue, the variability in the length of
the G_1 period causes the variability in the cell cycle time; $S+G_2+M$ appear to
remain relatively constant (Prescott, 1968).

The S period, or the time when cells are actively undergoing DNA synthesis,
shows a marked difference in duration between tumor cells and normal cells. In
normal cells, S is 11–13 hr long, while benign tumor S periods last 11–17 hr, and
malignant tumor S periods are 18–25 hr (Bleiberg and Galand, 1976; Fabrikant,
1970). The labeling index may be defined as $LI = N_s/N$, where N is the number of
cells in a population, and N_s is the number of cells in that population in DNA
synthesis, as determined by autoradiographic methods. This index, as a measure
of the general proliferative state of a tumor, has been found to correlate with the
responsiveness of the tumor to cycle-active agents (Vogler *et al.*, 1974; Kremer *et
al.*, 1976; Braunschweiger and Schiffer, 1976; Sulkes *et al.*, 1976; Hillen *et al.*,
1975; Skipper and Perry, 1970).

The G_2 period comprises the events that link the end of chromosome replication with chromosome segregation. This involves chromosome condensation,
synthesis, and assembly of the mitotic apparatus, and chromosome alignment,
movement, and separation.

The M_1, or mitosis, period is that time during which cell division actually occurs,
resulting in the formation of two "daughter cells." From this point, the daughter
cells may go into G_1 or G_0. G_0 may be considered to be a prolonged G_1, or "resting
state," from which cells may be induced back into cycle (recruitment) and subsequent multiplication. Also included in G_0 are the cells that will go on to die without
dividing.

Bruce *et al.* (1966) were one of the first groups to explore the kinetics of drug-induced cytotoxicity of normal and malignant tissue. Using the spleen colony-forming assay in the mouse for assessment of normal bone marrow stem cell and AKR lymphoma cell sensitivity to cytotoxic agents, they were able to classify these agents into several groups. Class I, or non-phase-specific, agents appeared to be equally toxic for proliferating and resting (G_0) cells, and showed no difference in toxicity against the normal hematopoietic stem cells and tumor cells. These agents included nitrogen mustard and irradiation. Class II, or "phase-specific," agents killed cells during only a specific part of the cell cycle, and did not appear to affect G_0 cells if exposure time was short. These agents showed increasing cell kill with increasing dose until a plateau was reached, after which there was no further increase in cell kill. These agents included vinblastine, MTX, and azaserine. Class III, or cycle-specific, agents damaged both proliferating and resting cells, but dividing cells were more sensitive than G_0 cells, and were killed throughout the cell cycle. These agents included 5-FU, actinomycin D, and cyclophosphamide. The greater cell kill of tumor cells as opposed to normal marrow stem cells with both phase- and cycle-specific agents was felt to be due to the fact that most stem cells were in a G_0 state, and most tumor cells were actively dividing. Later studies by Valeriote and Bruce (1967) showed increased sensitivity of normal stem cells with increased exposure to drug, and loss of specificity for malignant cells vs. normal stem cells if the stem cells were rapidly proliferating to repair previous marrow damage. Subsequent studies (Bruce *et al.*, 1967, 1969; Valeriote and Tolen, 1972; Van Putten and Lelieveld, 1970, 1971) confirmed and extended these results. Figure 1 summarizes the cell-cycle specificity of many anticancer drugs.

Both phase- and cycle-specific agents are usually given in short, intensive courses using maximally tolerated doses. These doses should be repeated once hematologic recovery has occurred (approximately 2–3 weeks).

The use of small daily doses of phase- and cycle-specific agents should be avoided, since it results in less tumor kill and greater hematologic toxicity. Early studies by Skipper *et al.* (1967) with the L1210 murine leukemia showed that single daily doses of Ara-C reduced survival of leukemic cells by only 50–70%, but that constant infusion of Ara-C over 12–24 hr (one to two doubling times) resulted in 96–99.95% cell kill.

Once an initial threshold value of marrow toxicity has been reached when using a phase-specific agent, further toxicity is not dose-dependent, but is related to the duration of exposure. This allows very high doses of phase-specific agents to be given with relative safety, if exposure time is kept to less than two normal hematopoietic stem cell cycle times.

Combinations of cycle- or phase-specific agents or both given concurrently show additive toxicity; doses should be appropriately reduced, since marrow toxicity will be both time- and dose-dependent. Agents that exert their maximum toxic effects in the same phase may give additive toxicity, but not necessarily additive or synergistic tumor effects. This has been demonstrated both in experimental systems (Grindey and Nichol, 1972; Tattersall and Harrap, 1973) and in

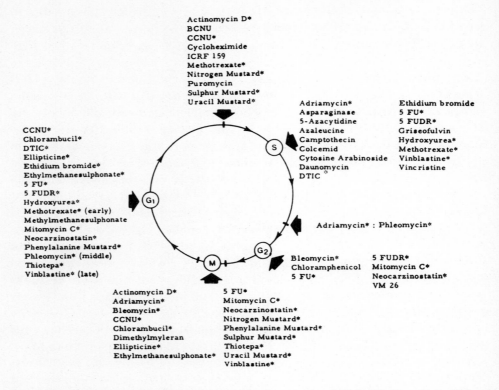

CCNU*
Chlorambucil*
DTIC*
Ellipticine*
Ethidium bromide*
Ethylmethanesulphonate*
5 FU*
5 FUDR*
Hydroxyurea*
Methotrexate* (early)
Methylmethanesulphonate
Mitomycin C*
Neocarzinostatin*
Phenylalanine Mustard*
Phleomycin* (middle)
Thiotepa*
Vinblastine* (late)

Actinomycin D*
BCNU
CCNU*
Cycloheximide
ICRF 159
Methotrexate*
Nitrogen Mustard*
Puromycin
Sulphur Mustard*
Uracil Mustard*

Adriamycin*
Asparaginase
5-Azacytidine
Azaleucine
Camptothecin
Colcemid
Cytosine Arabinoside
Daunomycin
DTIC

Ethidium bromide
5 FU*
5 FUDR*
Griseofulvin
Hydroxyurea*
Methotrexate*
Vinblastine*
Vincristine

Adriamycin* : Phleomycin*

Bleomycin*
Chloramphenicol
5 FU*

5 FUDR*
Mitomycin C*
Neocarzinostatin*
VM 26

Actinomycin D*
Adriamycin*
Bleomycin*
CCNU*
Chlorambucil*
Dimethylmyleran
Ellipticine*
Ethylmethanesulphonate*

5 FU*
Mitomycin C*
Neocarzinostatin*
Nitrogen Mustard*
Phenylalanine Mustard*
Sulphur Mustard*
Thiotepa*
Uracil Mustard*
Vinblastine*

FIGURE 1. Phases of the cell cycle in which antitumor agents exert their lethal effects. From Hill and Baserga 1975. Reprinted by permission of the authors and *Cancer Treatment Reviews*.

human tumors. In a given combination, therefore, agents that exert their maximal effects in different phases of the cell cycle should be chosen.

Effective combinations of drugs may be obtained by using one agent that arrests cells at one stage, followed by an agent that maximally kills cells during that stage immediately succeeding the block. This cell-proliferation arrest may cause a partial synchronization, and therefore, with proper drug scheduling, may result in increased cell kill or even therapeutic synergy, whereas improper scheduling may show no increased kill, or even drug antagonism.

Several attempts have been made at recruitment and synchronization in human acute leukemia (Vogler *et al.*, 1974; Kremer *et al.*, 1976; Lampkin *et al.*, 1971, 1974). In general, if an increase in cycling cells (usually defined by labeling index) could be obtained following a "synchronizing" agent (usually Ara-C), the patient's chances of obtaining a remission were much increased. Evidence is also available in solid tumor systems that the appropriate timing of a phase-specific agent following "synchronization" by a cycle-specific agent (as defined by an increase in the labeling index and growth fraction) results in significant improvement over results obtained with giving the drugs together (Braunschweiger and Schiffer, 1976; Schenken and Hagemann, 1976). This timing may prove to be of significant clinical importance, since it has been shown that the mean pretreatment labeling index of human breast carcinoma is an extremely good predictor of subsequent response to combination chemotherapy (Sulkes *et al.*, 1976).

2.5. Schedule Dependency

Closely allied to cytokinetic considerations is the phenomenon of schedule dependency. Schedule dependency may occur as a result of cytokinetic or biochemical interactions between drugs. For example, when drugs are given sequentially, the first drug may produce a delay in cell-cycle progression such that when the second drug, a cell-cycle or phase-specific agent, is given, the cell may or may not be in a phase of its generative cycle that is sensitive to the second drug. Obviously, the appropriate timing of administration of the second drug is most important. Such a manipulation would produce an improvement in the therapeutic index, provided normal host cells have not been affected in precisely the same way. Alternatively, the first drug may produce sufficient biochemical imbalance within the cell to attenuate the effects of the second. Schedule dependency has been observed with many drug combinations. The following examples are cited to illustrate the problem, and are not intended to be an exhaustive review.

Significant schedule dependency has been shown between L-asparaginase and MTX. In tumor cells that are sensitive to L-asparaginase, protein synthesis is inhibited, and shortly thereafter, there is a profound inhibition of DNA synthesis. This "shutdown" in DNA synthesis, as well as the asparaginase-induced inhibition of MTX transport (Nahas and Capizzi, 1974), greatly attenuates the MTX effect. While the precise mechanism of MTX-induced cell death is unknown, unbalanced growth, i.e., the continued cytoplasmic synthesis of protein and RNA, appears to be a contributing factor. Cessation of protein synthesis has been shown to attenuate or abolish thymineless death in bacteria (Maaloe and Hanawalt, 1961), and to affect MTX cytotoxicity in mammalian cells (Borsa and Whitmore, 1969). Asparaginase pretreatment of asparagine-requiring leukemic cells in culture or *in vivo* has been shown to severely attenuate the cytotoxic effect of MTX (Capizzi, 1974a). By delaying the administration of MTX until there is a postasparaginase recovery of DNA synthesis, however, one may achieve increased cell kill in leukemic mice and humans without an increase in host toxicity (Capizzi, 1974a, 1975; Capizzi *et al.*, 1974a). In certain patients, the increase in DNA synthesis has surpassed the pre-asparaginase values, suggesting some degree of tumor cell synchronization *in vivo* (Capizzi, 1974b).

The interactions between MTX and cytosine arabinoside appear to be very schedule-dependent, although the conclusions drawn by different authors are very divergent. The simultaneous administration of the drugs has been reported to be antagonistic (Grindey and Nichol, 1972; Tattersall and Harrap, 1973) or synergistic (Avery and Roberts, 1974; Edelstein *et al.*, 1975). However, the studies reporting the antagonistic results were carried out in cell culture using inhibition of growth as an endpoint, while the studies reporting synergy used *in vivo* tumor cell kill as an endpoint. Furthermore, the doses of both drugs in the *in vitro* vs. *in vivo* studies varied enormously. Of interest was the observation that the combination producing synergistic tumor cell kill (simultaneous MTX and cytosine arabinoside) produced subadditive cytotoxicity on hematopoietic stem cells, suggesting a possible improvement in the therapeutic index. Authors citing either observation made suggestions regarding the clinical use of this combination. It would be advisable, however, to perform studies in man before making firm clinical recommendations.

Results of studies of the interaction between MTX and 5-FU are also quite divergent. Studies by Tattersall *et al.* (1973) report mutually antagonistic effects whether the drugs are added to a tumor cell suspension simultaneously or in alternate sequences. In contrast, studies reported by Gupta and Bertino (Gupta *et al.*, 1977) indicate synergistic results when MTX precedes 5-FU *in vivo*.

Schedule-dependent synergy has been reported with the combination of cytosine arabinoside and daunorubicin in the treatment of the L1210 murine leukemia, the optimal sequence being cytosine arabinoside followed by daunorubicin (Edelstein *et al.*, 1974). Although this combination has been used clinically in the treatment of acute myelogenous leukemia, schedule dependency has not been investigated, and the clinical results appear additive (Gluckman *et al.*, 1973).

The combination of cytosine arabinoside and 6-thioguanine is one of the more effective regimens for the treatment of acute myelocytic leukemia (Gee *et al.*, 1969). Laboratory studies with L1210 leukemia have shown that certain schedules of this combination are therapeutically synergistic, with an apparent cytosine-arabinoside-induced decrease in 6-thioguanine toxicity (Schmidt *et al.*, 1970).

It is important to suspect schedule-dependent interaction between drugs when agents that possess diverse mechanisms of action and have previously displayed therapeutic activity in treating a disease are found to produce subadditive or antagonistic effects when used in combination. Finally, it may be extremely misleading to directly apply schedule and sequence data derived from animal or cell culture studies to clinical practice—or, for that matter, to apply such data from one human neoplastic disease to another. Optimal schedules for the same drugs have been shown to vary among animal tumors (Tattersall and Harrap, 1973; Edelstein *et al.*, 1975) and between mouse and human leukemia (Capizzi, 1974*a*, *b*).

2.6. Miscellaneous Considerations

2.6.1. Drug Resistance: An Obstacle to Tumor Eradication

As has been stated above, the majority of the responses that occur subsequent to clinical cancer chemotherapy are partial responses, indicating that a significant proportion of the tumor cell population is resistant to the drug(s). It has also been stated that in the responsive tumors, a greater percentage of complete responses is produced with combination chemotherapy than with single agents. It is realized that in patients with advanced, disseminated disease, the tumor cell population is a heterogeneous one with regard to drug sensitivity. Estimates of the total tumor cell burden in patients with acute leukemia in relapse are in the range of 10^{12} cells. While methods are not currently available for the assessment of the proportion of drug-sensitive and -resistant populations in human leukemia, such studies have been done in mouse leukemias. At the time of death, the tumor cell burden in leukemic mice is in the range of 10^9 cells (Capizzi et al., 1974b). Assessment of a number of spontaneously occurring drug-resistant mutants to various antimetabolites occurring in such a population has been in the range of 1 per million cells (10^{-6}) (Fischer, 1971). For two agents that have dissimilar mechanisms of action and that do not appreciably interact with each other, the probability of having a cell that is resistant to both drugs is $10^{-6} \times 10^{-6}$, or 10^{-12}. On a sole basis of biochemical resistance mechanisms, it should be easy to cure advanced mouse leukemia with many two-drug combinations. It is not always easy to do so, however, since there are other factors that contribute to natural drug resistance, including low growth fraction and long generation time of the tumor, and scheduling and dose factors for the drug, which also involve pharmacokinetic and cytokinetic interrelationships. Given a tumor with a high growth fraction, a relatively short generation time, and a high degree of sensitivity and accessibility to several drugs, the proper dose and schedule of these drugs should be curative.

Proper consideration of the kinetics of drug distribution and the distribution of tumor cells in the body has facilitated the design of potentially curative regimens for ALL. Since none of the clinically effective antileukemic agents crosses the blood–brain barrier in effective concentrations, the presence of disease in the CNS serves as a sanctuary of disease unaffected by systemic chemotherapy. Therefore, previous attempts to control the disease with the same drugs and combinations that are used today had failed, not because of innate tumor cell refractoriness to the combination, but because of the inaccessibility of the drugs for the tumor. However, since the introduction of treatment directed toward the CNS disease in ALL—viz, whole-brain irradiation and intrathecal MTX—the durations of complete responses and potential cures have increased appreciably (Simone et al., 1975).

2.6.2. Drug Doses

One of the advantages of combining drugs with nonoverlapping host toxicity is that full doses of the chemotherapeutic agents can be used simultaneously if so desired. If two or more drugs with a similar toxicity spectrum are used, then the doses of each drug must be appropriately attenuated if the drugs are to be used concurrently, or a sufficient time interval must elapse between doses to allow host recovery from the previous drug. For maintenance of remission in childhood ALL, there is good evidence to support the use of maximally tolerated doses of drugs in a combination. Pinkel et al. (1971) conducted a prospectively randomized trial comparing the remission maintenance capability of four drugs given in either full or half dosage. Median durations of complete remission and of hematologic remission were longer in the full-dosage than in the half-dosage group.

Preliminary results in the treatment of malignant melanoma with DTIC alone or in combinations with BCNU, CCNU, VCR, and/or hydroxyurea have shown that if no hematologic toxicity was produced (WBC > 4000/mm^3), the response rate was 8%, and the median survival time was 22 weeks. However, if hematologic toxicity was produced (WBC < 4000/mm^3) by using maximally tolerated doses, the response rate was 35%, and the median survival time was 41 weeks (G. J. Hill *et al.*, 1976).

As other tumors are studied, exceptions to the full-dosage concept may be found. Use of half to two-thirds the conventionally used doses of cyclophosphamide, MTX, and 5-FU for advanced breast cancer was associated with a response rate and a median duration of response comparable to those achieved by the full doses (Creech *et al.*, 1975). It may be that under certain circumstances of innate tumor cell sensitivity to the right combination and schedule of drugs, true pharmacological synergy will be obtained, thus enabling the use of modified dosages. It would be difficult, however, to predict *a priori* that this can be done; it can be proved only through the use of properly randomized and controlled studies. One must also remember that most anticancer drugs are also excellent immunosuppressive agents. Thus, the use of full doses of multiple drugs in a continuous fashion coupled with only marginal tumor-destructive capability can actually allow enhanced tumor growth and a shortening of the survival time.

2.6.3. How Many Drugs Are Enough?

As noted previously, the results of combination chemotherapy are frequently superior to those produced by single agents. There may be great temptation, therefore, to add more and more drugs to an effective combination (as long as host toxicity permits), in the hope that therapeutic effectiveness will be enhanced. In at least two human cancers, there has been no such enhancement. The highest response rate to five-drug therapy in advanced breast cancer has been 90% (Cooper, 1969). Attempts to reproduce this effect have produced responses in the 30–60% range (see Table 5). This degree of response is essentially comparable to that which can be achieved with the three-drug regimen of cyclophosphamide, MTX, and 5-FU (see Table 5). The addition of prednisone or vincristine or both to the three-drug regimen therefore appears to add little, even though they do show some activity when used singly. Similar studies have shown no advantage in adding MTX and 5-FU to the combination of adriamycin and cyclophosphamide in the treatment of advanced breast cancer (Boston *et al.*, 1976). Likewise, a randomized trial conducted in childhood ALL has shown no advantage of a three- or four-drug maintenance regimen over a two-drug regimen (Simone *et al.*, 1975).

2.6.4. Cumulative and Delayed Drug Toxicity

The primary choice of agents for combination is obviously limited by whatever effective drugs are available. But given a reasonable degree of selection, one would obviously also consider the nature of the disease and the potential for serious delayed effects. In aggressive or far-advanced neoplasms, or in tumors that are responsive only to certain agents, use of essentially any effective agent can be justified, despite potential long-term deleterious effects. However, in neoplasms with a naturally long course or prospect of relatively easy control (e.g., nonaggressive chronic lymphocytic leukemia, some types of nodular lymphoma), or in the adjuvant treatment of patients with a fair chance of cure by surgery or irradiation alone, drugs should be selected that cause fewer long-term deleterious effects. Almost all the available alkylating agents have been shown to be carcinogenic in animals or man. While the potential may very well exist, the antimetabolites that affect DNA synthesis indirectly by inhibiting an enzyme system would probably be less mutagenic and carcinogenic than those agents that are directly incorporated into DNA or bind to DNA through intercalation or alkylation. Despite the considerations just expressed, however, the physician should not lose sight of the fact that he or she is dealing, for the most part, with a highly aggressive, debilitating , and fatal group of diseases. Concern over possible long-term effects should not deny the cancer patient significant short-term palliation or the chance of long-term disease control or possible cure.

2.6.5. Chemotherapy–Radiotherapy Interactions

Many cancer patients are treated with both radiotherapy and chemotherapy, either sequentially or concurrently. Early studies (D'Angio *et al.*, 1959, 1962) showed that previous or concurrent therapy with actinomycin D caused increased radiation tissue damage for a given dose, and that the administration of actinomycin D after radiotherapy was completed could "recall" and enhance radiotherapy skin damage. Later studies with adriamycin (Donaldson *et al.*, 1974; Haskell *et al.*, 1974; Cassady *et al.*, 1975; Etcubanas and Wilbur, 1974), bleomycin (Samuels *et al.*, 1976), and combination chemotherapy with MOPP for Hodgkin's disease (Lamoureux, 1974) demonstrated similar radiotherapeutic enhancement and recall reactions in skin and other tissues. The phenomenon of a flare of radiation pneumonitis in previously irradiated Hodgkin's disease patients while the prednisone of the first and fourth cycles is being tapered has also been reported (Castellino *et al.*, 1974). Enhanced cardiotoxicity of adriamycin at the same or lower doses in patients with previous cardiac irradiation has also been noted (Eltringham *et al.*, 1975; Gilladoga *et al.*, 1974; Merrill *et al.*, 1975). Evaluation of the combined effects of radiotherapy and chemotherapy in mice has shown that enhancement of effect is not only drug-specific, but also organ-specific (Phillips *et al.*, 1975).

It is clear that in the patient being treated with radiotherapy and chemotherapy, appropriate dosage modification in one or both modalities should be made. A schedule for dosage modification for lung irradiation following previous actinomycin D chemotherapy has been suggested (Wara *et al.*, 1973), but in general, few guidelines exist for the administration of chemotherapy following radiotherapy. The prudent physician should reduce dosage (e.g., to one-half or two-thirds) in this situation, and escalate dosage only with close observation and as patient tolerance permits.

2.6.6. Chemoimmunotherapy

A more complete discussion of the rationale of chemoimmunotherapy can be found elsewhere in this volume.

The addition of immunotherapy to maintenance chemotherapy for AML has been shown to be of significant value. In a study comparing chemotherapy alone (Ara-C, TG, cyclophosphamide, CCNU, daunomycin) and the same chemotherapy plus MER (*M*ethanol *E*xtractable *R*esidue of BCG) for remission maintenance in AML, Cuttner *et al.* (1976) reported a median duration of remission of 3.5 months for the chemotherapy-alone group vs. 18 months for the chemotherapy–immunotherapy group. In a similar study of remission mainte-nance in AML, Bekesi *et al.* (1976) reported a median duration of remission of 20 weeks for the chemotherapy-alone group vs. more than 78 weeks for the immunotherapy–chemotherapy group. The immunotherapy in this study was neuraminidase-treated allogeneic myeloblasts with or without MER. Powles (1976) reports in his study of AML remission maintenance that median duration of remission is 195 days for chemotherapy alone vs. 305 days for chemotherapy plus immunotherapy (BCG plus irradiated myeloblasts) and 252 days for immunotherapy alone. The treatment of many other tumors with the combina-tion of chemotherapy and immunotherapy is currently being studied extensively, with most evaluations not yet completed. However, it can be stated that for at least some human malignancies, the combination of chemotherapy and immuno-therapy is significantly better than chemotherapy alone.

2.7. Combination vs. Single-Agent Chemotherapy: Selected Examples

For certain tumors, combinations of drugs have produced results clearly superior to those obtained with the use of single agents. Not only is the percentage of complete remissions increased, but also the probability of long-term disease-free survival and cure appears to be a reality for certain patients with widespread disseminated disease. These effects are the result of the ability to achieve a complete remission, i.e., the absence of all clinically detectable disease. With single-agent chemotherapy, the percentages of complete remissions, even with the responsive tumors, were low. The attainment of a partial remission is usually associated with a modest or no significant prolongation of life, which is usually of variable quality. The major emphasis of modern programs, therefore, is an attempt to achieve a complete remission with aggressive combination chemotherapy, at times combined with surgery or irradiation or both.

2.7.1. Acute Lymphatic Leukemia in Childhood

Beginning with the demonstration by Farber *et al.* (1948) that aminopterin produced some temporary remissions in childhood ALL, steady progress was made with single agents in the treatment of this disease. Table 1 illustrates that it was not until the successful use of drug combinations that the majority of children

179

PRINCIPLES
OF
COMBINA-
TION
CHEMO-
THERAPY

TABLE 1

Percentage of Complete Bone Marrow Remissions Induced by Active Drugs Used Singly or in Combination in Acute Lymphatic Leukemia[a]

Treatment	Recent complete bone marrow remissions
Methotrexate (MTX)	22
6-Mercaptopurine (MP)	27
Prednisone (P)	63
Cyclophosphamide (CTX)	40
Vincristine (VCR)	57
Daunorubicin (D)	38
Asparaginase (A)	67
P, VCR	90
VAMP (VCR, P, MTX, MP)	88
POMP (VCR, P, MTX, MP)	94
P, VCR, D	97
P, VCR, D	100

[a] Modified from DeVita *et al.* (1975*b*); references in original article.

could be expected to achieve a complete remission. As can be seen from Table 2, once complete remission is achieved, drug combinations also maintain remission better than single agents.

In 1956, the median survival of patients treated with single agents for childhood ALL was 6 months (Burchenal, 1970). Of 35 patients who began combination

TABLE 2

Length of Remission and Survival in Acute Lymphatic Leukemia—Effect of Consolidation Treatment After Remission[a]

Treatment program		Duration of treatment during remission (months)	Duration of subsequent remission (months)	Overall survival (months)
Induction therapy	Consolidation therapy			
Prednisone	None	—	1.3	
Vincristine	None	—	2.0	
V + P	None	—	2.0	20
	MTX	1.5	3.3	
	MP	1.5	3.0	
	CTX	1.5	2.0	
	MTX + MP + CTX	1.5	3.5	
	MTX + MP + CTX + BCNU	2.0	5.3	
BIKE (V + P)	MTX + MP + CTX	5.0	4.7	24
VAMP	VAMP	5.0	4.7	25
POMP	POMP	14.0	8.0	33

[a] Modified from DeVita *et al.* (1975*b*); references in original article.

chemotherapy in 1968, 18 were in continuous complete remission for 63–70 months, and had been off all therapy for 27–41 months (Simone *et al.*, 1975). Today, the median survival of children with ALL is approaching 5 years. Despite the improvement in supportive care and the development of additional effective agents in childhood ALL, most of this increase is due to the use of effective drug combinations.

2.7.2. Hodgkin's Disease

It can be seen from Table 3 that until the first use of combination chemotherapy in 1963 (DeVita *et al.*, 1965), the percentage of complete remissions was low, and the median duration of complete remissions was short. Use of the four-drug combination MOPP [*m*ustargen (nitrogen mustard), *o*ncovin, *p*rocarbazine, and *p*rednisone] produced an increase in the percentage of complete remissions, with a median duration of 36 months (DeVita *et al.*, 1970). Once such superiority has been demonstrated, it often becomes difficult, if not impossible, to compare a single agent to a combination in a randomized prospective study. One such study (Huguley *et al.*, 1975) comparing MOPP with nitrogen mustard has been done, however, and is the last study listed in Table 3. Each group was treated intensively for six cycles to hematologic tolerance. Of significance again is that once complete remission is obtained with either treatment, remission duration and overall survival are the same, but the combination produces a 4-fold increase in the number of complete remissions over the single agent.

TABLE 3

Percentage Complete Remissions and Remission Duration for Single and Reported Combination Drug Programs in the Treatment of Hodgkin's Disease[a]

Treatment program	Complete remissions (%)	Median duration of complete remission (months)
Prednisone (P)	<5	—
Nitrogen mustard (HN$_2$)	20	2.5
Cyclophosphamide (CTX)	20	3.0
Vinblastine (VLB)	27	3.0
Vincristine (VCR)	<10	—
Procarbazine (PCZ)	<10	—
BCNU	<5	—
VLB+chlorambucil	40	—
VCR+CTX+MTX+P	80	—
MOPP		
VCR+P+HN$_2$+PCZ	81	36
MVPP		
VLB+HN$_2$+P+PCZ	71	—
Nitrogen mustard (HN$_2$)	13	12
MOPP	48	15

[a] Modified from DeVita *et al.* (1975*b*); references in original article.

Further exciting results in advanced Hodgkin's disease stages III-B and IV have been achieved with the use of a five-drug combination plus supplemental irradiation to all sites of disease. This program has produced a 75% complete remission rate, with only a 10% relapse rate; the median duration of remission will be in excess of 5 years (Prosnitz *et al.*, 1976).

2.7.3. Diffuse Histiocytic Lymphoma

Of the non-Hodgkin's lymphomas, diffuse histiocytic lymphoma is the most aggressive and has the worst prognosis (Schein *et al.*, 1974; S. E. Jones *et al.*, 1972). Treatment of stage III or IV disease with single agents is usually not associated with any survivors beyond 24 months (S.E. Jones *et al.*, 1972). In marked contrast, DeVita *et al.* (1975*a*) reported a median survival of 42+ months for those patients who sustained a complete response when treated with cyclophosphamide, vincristine, prednisone, and procarbazine. They also noted that the median survival in the group of partial and nonresponders was 6 months with a maximum of 11 months, except for one patient who survived for 24 months. Berd *et al.* (1975) reported that following treatment with cyclophosphamide, vincristine, methotrexate, and Ara-C, 6 of 8 patients achieved complete remission, and the median time free of disease following completion of therapy was 43+ months. Thus, achievement of complete remission status is again seen to be extremely important. Furthermore, a disease that is minimally responsive to single-agent therapy can be brought under long-term control and possibly cured by the vigorous use of combination chemotherapy.

2.7.4. Testicular Carcinoma

Single-agent chemotherapy has produced regression, but few complete responses lasting beyond 1 yr, in metastatic (i.e., stage III or IV) testicular carcinoma (MacKenzie, 1966; Merrin and Murphy, 1974; Samuels and Howe, 1970). In one large series, the "Li regimen" (Li *et al.*, 1960), utilizing actinomycin D, MTX, and chlorambucil, has been shown to produce a 50% response rate, but only 11/90 complete responses, and only 5/11 survived beyond 1 year in remission (MacKenzie, 1966). Significant improvement over these results has been seen with the use of other drug combinations. Using vinblastine and intermittent bleomycin with or without cyclophosphamide, vincristine, MTX, and 5-FU, Samuels *et al.* (1975*a*) reported 22/70 patients with complete response and 31/70 partial responses. Figure 2 shows the dramatic difference in survival between complete and partial or nonresponders, and emphasizes the need for achieving complete remission. The combination using intermittent bleomycin yields a low complete remission rate for the subclasses of advanced abdominal (12%) or pulmonary (19%) disease. By using the bleomycin as a continuous infusion, overall complete response rate in these subclasses can be increased to 40% (Samuels *et al.*, 1975*b*). In 20 patients with advanced pulmonary metastases, Einhorn *et al.* (1976) reported 15 complete responders and 5 partial responders, using *cis*-platinum, vinblastine, and bleomycin in combination. At the time of report, 13 of the 15 complete responses were

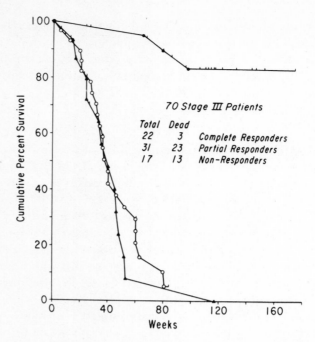

FIGURE 2. Survival as related to response in stage III testicular cancer. There is a significant difference between complete responders (●) vs. the partial (○) and nonresponders (▲) ($P < 0.01$, modified Wilcoxin test). (|) Still alive. From Samuels *et al.*, 1975*a*. Reprinted by permission of the authors and *Cancer*.

disease-free from 6 to 18 months, with a median of 9 months. Therefore, although the reports of combinations utilizing new agents such as bleomycin and *cis*-platinum are preliminary, with the median duration of response not yet clear, it does appear that combination chemotherapy is clearly superior to single-agent therapy for remission induction in metastatic testicular carcinoma.

2.7.5. Breast Carcinoma

As can be seen from Table 4, advanced breast carcinoma has been one of the most responsive solid tumors, with the percentage responses to single agents ranging from 5 to 38%. "Responses" are not divided into complete and partial response in Table 4, however, because most studies using single-agent chemotherapy for breast carcinoma have failed to make this distinction. Remission durations with the most commonly used single agents, cyclophosphamide, 5-FU, and MTX, range between 5 and 10 months (Talley *et al.*, 1965; Johnson *et al.*, 1973; Vogler *et al.*, 1968). Patient populations vary among studies, but in general, response to the drug confers a survival time of 2–3 times that of the nonresponder.

Following the encouraging early reports of Greenspan and co-workers (Greenspan *et al.*, 1963; Greenspan, 1966) and Cooper (1969), several prospective randomized trials have been performed or are ongoing, and are summarized in Table 5. Patterns of response are remarkably similar among studies. From 5 to 20% of patients achieve a complete response, and in regimens with cyclophos-

183

PRINCIPLES
OF
COMBINA-
TION
CHEMO-
THERAPY

TABLE 4

Single-Agent Therapy in Advanced Breast Carcinoma[a]

Drug	Patients evaluable	Patients responding	Response (%)
Alkylating agents			
Cyclophosphamide	529	182	34
Nitrogen mustard	92	32	35
Phenylalanine mustard	86	20	23
Chlorambucil	54	11	20
ThioTEPA	162	48	30
Antimetabolites			
5-Fluorouracil	1236	324	26
Methotrexate	356	120	34
6-Mercaptopurine	44	6	14
Cytosine arabinoside	64	6	9
Hydroxyurea	16	2	12
Mitotic inhibitors			
Vincristine	226	47	21
Vinblastine	95	19	20
Antitumor antibiotics			
Adriamycin	221	81	37
Mitomycin	60	23	38
Other antibiotics (actinomycin D, mithramycin, streptonigrin, bleomycin, daunomycin)	99	13	13
Random synthetics[b]			
BCNU	76	16	21
CCNU	155	18	12
MCCNU	33	2	6
Hexamethylmelamine	39	11	28
Imidazole carboxamide	29	2	7
Dibromodulcitol	22	6	27
Procarbazine	21	1	5

[a] Modified from Broder and Tormey (1974); references in original article.
[b] Abbreviations: CCNU: 1-(2-chloroethyl)-3-cyclohexyl-1-nitrosourea; MCCNU: 1-(2-chloroethyl)-3-(4-methyl-cyclohexyl)-1-nitrosourea.

phamide, MTX, and 5-FU, or adriamycin and cyclophosphamide, approximately 40–60% of patients achieve a good partial remission. Median duration of remission is about 6–10 months, and median duration of survival is approximately 12–24 months. With the exception of the studies by Irwin (reported in Broder and Tormey, 1974) and Otis and Armentrout (1975), median durations of remission and survival are given for the combined complete and partial response groups, making it impossible to tell whether a complete remission confers a longer survival or remission duration than a partial remission. In the study by Irwin, the median survival was 11.2 months for the complete responders, and 5.7 months for the partial responders. In contrast to previously mentioned tumors, there also appears to be a group of "no change, minimal response, or stable disease" patients

TABLE 5

Combination Chemotherapy of Advanced Breast Cancer

Study No.	Treatment program	PR	CR	Median duration of remission (months)	Median duration of survival (months)	References
1	CTX/MTX/5-FU	45%	11%		22	Brambilla
	ADM/VCR	44%	8%		24	*et al.* (1976)
2	CTX/MTX/5-FU	47%	20%		18	Canellos *et al.* (1976)
3	CTX/CLB	16%	4%			Brunner
	CTX/MTX	13%	5%	5.6	12.7	*et al.* (1975)
	CTX/MTX/VCR	26%	7%	7.9	18.5	
	CTX/MTX/Pred	38%	6%			
	CTX/MTX/Pred	39%	4%	7.3	15.4	
	CTX/MTX/VCR/5-FU/Pred	42%	7%	8.0	16.0	
4	CTX/VCR/5-FU/Pred	46%		8.0		Ahmann
	CTX/5-FU/Pred	59%		9.0		*et al.* (1975)
5	CTX/(BCNU)/MTX/5-FU low dose	14%	43%	15 PR 9 CR	15 PR 12 CR	Otis and Armentrout (1975)
6	CTX/VCR/MTX/5-FU/Pred	62%			13	Ramirez
	CTX/VCR/MTX/5-FU	44%			13.5	*et al.* (1975)
7	CTX/VCR/MTX/5-FU/Pred	34%	8%	5–6	12.0	Broder and
	VCR/5-FU/Pred	29%	7%	5–6	8.0	Tormey (1974)
	CTX/MTX/5-FU/VCR/Pred	42%	15%	10.0		
	CTX/MTX/5-FU/VCR/Pred high-dose	43%	8%	10.0		
	ADM	53%	4%	4.0		
	CTX/MTX/5-FU/Pred	28%				
	CTX/MTX/5-FU/Pred/VCR	30%				
	CTX/MTX/5-FU/Pred/T$_3$	24%	32%	11.2 CR 5.7 PR	6.8+	
	Single agent sequential at disease progression					
	5-FU	4%	23%	3.9 CR 4 PR	3.3+	
	CTX	4%	24%	4 PR 2.5 PR		
	Pred	6%	0			
	MTX		7%			
8	ADM/CTX	68%	12%	22+ CR 10 PR	22+ 16	S. E. Jones *et al.* (1975)

in several studies (Brunner *et al.*, 1975; Otis and Armentrout, 1975) who may do as
well as those patients who sustain a complete or partial response. Whether this
unique group of patients will be seen in most evaluations of drug combinations
against advanced breast carcinoma remains to be seen.

185

PRINCIPLES
OF
COMBINA-
TION
CHEMO-
THERAPY

3. References

AHMANN, D. L., BISEL, H. F., HAHN, R. G., EAGAN, R. T., EDMONSON, J. H., STEINFELD, J. L., TORMEY, D. C., AND TAYLOR, W. F., 1975, An analysis of a multiple-drug program in the treatment of patients with advanced breast cancer utilizing 5-fluorouracil, cyclophosphamide, and prednisone with or without vincristine, *Cancer* **36**:1925–1935.

AVERY, T. L., AND ROBERTS, D., 1974, Dose-related synergism of cytosine arabinoside and methotrexate against murine leukemia L1210, *Eur. J. Cancer* **10**:425–429.

BASERGA, R., ESTENSEN, R. D., AND PETERSEN, R. O., 1965, Inhibition of DNA synthesis in Ehrlich ascites cells by actinomycin D, II. The presynthetic block in the cell cycle, *Pathology* **54**:1141–1147.

BEKESI, J. G., HOLLAND, J. F., CUTTNER, J., SILVER, R., COLEMAN, M., JAROWSKI, C., AND VINCEGUERRA, V., 1976, Immunotherapy in acute myelocytic leukemia (AML) with neuraminidase (N'Ase) treated allogeneic myeloblasts with or without MER, *Proc. Amer. Assoc. Cancer Res.* **17**:184.

BENDER, R. A., 1975, Membrane transport of methotrexate (NSC-740) in human neoplastic cells, *Cancer Chemother. Rep. Part 3* **6**:73–82.

BERD, D., CORNOG, J., DeCONTI, R. C., LEVITT, M., AND BERTINO, J. R., 1975, Long-term remission in diffuse histiocytic lymphoma treated with combination sequential chemotherapy, *Cancer* **35**:1050–1054.

BERTINO, J. R., AND SKEEL, R. T., 1973, Resistance to chemotherapeutic agents, clinical aspects, in: *Pharmacology and the Future of Man, Proceedings of the 5th International Congress of Pharmacology, San Francisco, 1972*, Vol. 3, pp. 376–392, Karger, Basel.

BLEIBERG, R., AND GALAND, P., 1976, *In vitro* autoradiographic determination of cell kinetic parameters in adenocarcinomas and adjacent healthy mucosa of the human colon and rectum, *Cancer Res.* **36**:325–328.

BORSA, J., AND WHITMORE, G. F., 1969, Cell killing studies on the mode of action of methotrexate on L-cells *in vitro*, *Cancer Res.* **29**:737–744.

BOSTON, B., MITCHELL, M., FARBER, L., AND BERTINO, J., 1976, Combination vs. combination–sequential non-hormonal chemotherapy in advanced breast cancer, *Proc. Amer. Assoc. Cancer Res.* **17**:247.

BRAMBILLA, C., DE LENA, M., ROSSI, A., VALAGUSSA, A., AND BONADONNA, G., 1976, Response and survival in advanced breast cancer after two non-cross-resistant combinations, *Br. Med. J.* **1**:801–804.

BRAUNSCHWEIGER, P. G., AND SCHIFFER, L. M., 1976, Cell kinetics as a basis for chemotherapy scheduling in solid tumors, *Proc. Amer. Assoc. Cancer Res.* **17**:57.

BRODER, L. E., AND TORMEY, D. C., 1974, Combination chemotherapy of carcinoma of the breast, *Cancer Treatment Rev.* **1**:183–203.

BRUCE, W. R., MEEKER, B. E., AND VALERIOTE, F. A., 1966, Comparison of the sensitivity of normal hematopoietic and transplanted lymphoma colony-forming cells to chemotherapeutic agents administered *in vivo*, *J. Natl. Cancer Inst.* **37**:233–245.

BRUCE, W. R., VALERIOTE, F. A., AND MEEKER, B. E., 1967, Survival of mice bearing a transplanted syngeneic lymphoma following treatment with cyclophosphamide, 5-fluorouracil, or 1,3-bis(2-chloroethyl)-1-nitrosourea, *J. Natl. Cancer Inst.* **39**:257–266.

BRUCE, W. R., MEEKER, B. E., POWERS, W. E., AND VALERIOTE, F. A., 1969, Comparison of the dose- and time-survival curves for normal hematopoietic and lymphoma colony-forming cells exposed to vinblastine, vincristine, arabinosylcytosine, and amethopterin, *J. Natl. Cancer Inst.* **42**:1015–1025.

BRUNNER, K. W., SONNTAG, R. W., MARTZ, G., SENN, H. J., OBRECHT, P., AND ALBERTO, P., 1975, A controlled study in the use of combined drug therapy for metastatic breast cancer, *Cancer* **35**:1208–1219.

BURCHENAL, J. H., 1970, Long term survivors in acute leukemia, *Recent Results Cancer Res.* **30**:167–170.

CALENDI, E., DI MARCO, A., REGGIANI, M., SCARPINATO, B., AND VALENTINI, L., 1965, On physico-chemical interactions between daunomycin and nucleic acids, *Biochim. Biophys. Acta* **103**:25–49.

CANELLOS, G. P., DEVITA, V. T., GOLD, G. L., CHABNER, B. A., SCHEIN, P. S., AND YOUNG, R. C., 1976, Combination chemotherapy for advanced breast cancer: Response and effect on survival, *Ann. Intern. Med.* **84**:389–392.

CAPIZZI, R. L., 1974a, Schedule-dependent synergism and antagonism between methotrexate and asparaginase, *Biochem. Pharmacol.* Suppl. 2, pp. 151–161.

CAPIZZI, R. L., 1974b, Biochemical interaction between asparaginase (A'ase) and methotrexate (MTX) in leukemia cells, *Proc. Amer. Assoc. Cancer Res.* **15**:77.

CAPIZZI, R. L., 1975, Improvement in the therapeutic index of methotrexate (NSC-740) by L-asparaginase (NSC-109229), *Cancer Chemother. Rep. Part 3* **6**:37–41.

CAPIZZI, R. L., DECONTI, R. C., MARSH, J. C., AND BERTINO, J. R., 1970, Methotrexate therapy of head and neck cancer: Improvement in therapeutic index by the use of leucovorin "rescue," *Cancer Res.* **30**:1782–1788.

CAPIZZI, R., CASTRO, O., ASPNES, G., BOBROW, S., BERTINO, J., FINCH, S., AND PEARSON, H., 1974a, Treatment of acute lymphocytic leukemia (ALL) with intermittent high dose methotrexate and asparaginase (A'Ase), *Proc. Amer. Assoc. Cancer Res.* **15**:182.

CAPIZZI, R. L., PAPIRMEISTER, B., MULLINS, J. M., AND CHENG, E., 1974b, The detection of chemical mutagens using the L5178Y/Asn murine leukemia *in vitro* and in a host-mediated assay, *Cancer Res.* **34**:3073–3082.

CARTER, S. K., AND SOPER, W. T., 1974, Integration of chemotherapy into combined modality treatment of solid tumors: 1. The overall strategy, *Cancer Treatment Rev.* **1**:1–13.

CASS, C. E., AND AU-YEUNG, T. H., 1976, Enhancement of 9-β-D-arabinofuranosyladenine cytotoxicity to mouse leukemia L1210 *in vitro* by 2'-deoxycoformycin, *Cancer Res.* **36**:1483–1491.

CASSADY, J. R., RICHTER, M. P., PIRO, A. J., AND JAFFE, N., 1975, Radiation–adriamycin interactions: Preliminary clinical observations, *Cancer* **36**:946–949.

CASTELLINO, R. A., GLATSTEIN, E., TURBOW, M. M., ROSENBERG, S., AND KAPLAN, H. S., 1974, Latent radiation injury of lungs or heart activated by steroid withdrawal, *Ann. Intern. Med.* **80**:593–599.

COLVIN, M., PADGETT, C. A., AND FENSELAU, C., 1973, A biologically active metabolite of cyclophosphamide, *Cancer Res.* **33**:915–918.

COOPER, R. G., 1969, Combination chemotherapy in hormone resistant breast cancer, *Proc. Amer. Assoc. Cancer Res.* **10**:15.

CREECH, R. H., CATALANO, R. B., MASTRANGELO, M. J., AND ENGSTROM, P. F., 1975, An effective low-dose intermittent cyclophosphamide, methotrexate and 5-fluorouracil treatment regimen for metastatic breast cancer, *Cancer* **35**:1101–1107.

CUTTNER, J., BEKESI, J. G., AND HOLLAND, J. F., 1976, Chemoimmunotherapy of acute leukemia using MER, *Proc. Amer. Assoc. Cancer Res.* **17**:196.

D'ANGIO, G. J., 1962, Clinical and biological studies of actinomycin D and roentgen irradiation, *Amer. J. Roentgenol.* **87**:106–109.

D'ANGIO, G. J., FARBER, S., AND MADDOCK, C. L., 1959, Potentiation of x-ray effects by actinomycin-D, *Radiology* **73**:175–177.

DEVITA, V. T., JR., MOXLEY, J. H., III, BRACE, K. C., AND FREI, E., III, 1965, Intensive combination chemotherapy and x-irradiation in the treatment of Hodgkin's disease, *Proc. Amer. Assoc. Cancer Res.* **6**:15.

DEVITA, V. T., JR., SERPICK, A. A., AND CARBONE, P. P., 1970, Combination chemotherapy in the treatment of advanced Hodgkin's disease, *Ann. Intern. Med.* **73**:881–895.

DEVITA, V. T., CANELLOS, G. P., CHABNER, B., SCHEIN, P., HUBBARD, S., AND YOUNG, R. C., 1975a, Advanced diffuse histiocytic lymphoma, a potentially curable disease; results with combination chemotherapy, *Lancet* **(7901)**:248–250.

DEVITA, V. T., JR., YOUNG, R. C., AND CANELLOS, G. P., 1975b, Combination versus single agent chemotherapy: a review of the basis for selection of drug treatment of cancer, *Cancer* **35**:98–110.

DJERASSI, I., ROMINGER, C. J., KIM, J. S., TURCHI, J., SUVANSRI, U., AND HUGHES, D., 1972, Phase I study of high doses of methotrexate with citrovorum factor in patients with lung cancer, *Cancer* **30**:22–30.

DONALDSON, S. S., GLICK, J. M., AND WILBUR, J. R., 1974, Letter: Adriamycin activating a recall phenomenon after radiation therapy, *Ann. Intern. Med.* **81**:407, 408.

EDELSTEIN, M., VIETTI, T., AND VALERIOTE, F., 1974, Schedule-dependent synergism for the combination of 1-β-D-arabinofuranosylcytosine and daunorubicin, *Cancer Res.* **34**:293–297.

EDELSTEIN, M., VIETTI, T., AND VALERIOTE, F., 1975, The enhanced cytotoxicity of combinations of 1-β-D-arabinofuranosylcytosine and methotrexate, *Cancer Res.* **35**:1555–1558.

EINHORN, L. H., FURNAS, B. E., POWELL, N., 1976, Combination chemotherapy of disseminated testicular carcinoma with *cis*-platinum diamminedichloride (CPDD), vinblastine (VLB) and bleomycin (Bleo), *Proc. Amer. Assoc. Cancer Res.* **17**:240.

ELION, G. B., SINGER, S., AND HITCHINGS, H. G., 1954, Antagonists of nucleic acid derivatives. VIII. Synergism in combinations of biochemically related antimetabolites, *J. Biol. Chem.* **208**:477–488.

ELTRINGHAM, J. R., FAJARDO, L. F., AND STEWART, J. R., 1975, Adriamycin cardiomyopathy: Enhanced cardiac damage in rabbits with combined drug and cardiac irradiation, *Radiology* **115**:471, 472.

ETCUBANAS, E., AND WILBUR, J. R., 1974, Letter: Uncommon side effects of adriamycin (NSC-123127), *Cancer Chemother. Rep. Part 1* **58**:757, 758.

FABRIKANT, J. I., 1970, The kinetics of cellular proliferation in human tissues; determination of duration of DNA synthesis using double labeling autoradiography, *Br. J. Cancer* **24**:122–127.

FARBER, S., DIAMOND, L. K., MERCER, R. D., SYLVESTER, R. F., JR., AND WOLFF, J. A., 1948, Temporary remissions in acute leukemia in children produced by folic acid antagonist, 4-aminopteroyl-glutamic acid (aminopterin), *N. Engl. J. Med.* **238**:787–793.

FISCHER, G. A., 1971, Predictive tests in culture of drug-resistant mutants selected *in vivo*, in: Hall, *Prediction of Response in Cancer Therapy, Natl. Cancer Inst. Monogr.* **34**:131–134.

FYFE, M. J., AND GOLDMAN, I. D., 1973, Characteristics of the vincristine-induced augmentation of methotrexate uptake in Ehrlich ascites tumor cells, *J. Biol. Chem.* **248**:5067–5073.

GEE, T. S., YU, K.-P., AND CLARKSON, B. D., 1969, Treatment of adult acute leukemia with arabinosyl-cytosine and thioguanine, *Cancer* **23**:1019–1032.

GILLADOGA, A. C., TAN, C. T., PHILIPS, F. S., STERNBERG, S. S., TANG, C., WOLLNER, N., AND MURPHY, M. L., 1974, Cardiac status of 40 children receiving adriamycin (Adr) over 495 mg/M² and animal studies, *Proc. Amer. Assoc. Cancer Res.* **15**:107.

GLUCKMAN, E., BASCH, A., VARET, B., AND DREYFUS, B., 1973, Combination chemotherapy with cytosine arabinoside and rubidomycin in 30 cases of acute granulocytic leukemia, *Cancer* **31**:487–491.

GOLDIN, A., VENDITTI, J. M., HUMPHREYS, S. R., DENNIS, D., MANTEL, N., AND GREENHOUSE, S. W., 1955, Factors influencing the specificity of action of an antileukemic agent (aminopterin). Multiple treatment schedules plus delayed administration of citrovorum factor, *Cancer Res.* **15**:57–61.

GOLDMAN, I. D., 1971, The characteristics of the membrane transport of amethopterin and the naturally occurring folates, *Ann. N.Y. Acad. Sci.* **186**:400–422.

GOLDMAN, I. D., 1975, Membrane transport of methotrexate (NSC-740) and other folate compounds: Relevance to rescue protocols, *Cancer Chemother. Rep. Part 3* **6**:63–72.

GREENSPAN, E. M., 1966, Combination cytotoxic chemotherapy in advanced disseminated breast carcinoma, *J. Mt. Sinai Hosp.* **33**:1–27.

GREENSPAN, E. M., FIEBER, M., LESNICK, G., AND EDELMAN, S., 1963, Response of advanced breast carcinoma to the combination of the anti-metabolite, methotrexate, and the alkylating agent, thio-TEPA, *J. Mt. Sinai Hosp.* **30**:246–267.

GRINDEY, G. B., AND NICHOL, C. A., 1972, Interaction of drugs inhibiting different steps in the synthesis of DNA, *Cancer Res.* **32**:527–531.

GUPTA, V., LINDQUIST, C., SAWICKI, W., AND BERTINO, J. R., 1977, Schedule dependent antitumor effects of methotrexate and 5-fluorouracil (in press).

HARRAP, K. R., AND JACKSON, R. C., 1975, Enzyme kinetics and combination chemotherapy: An appraisal of current concepts, *Adv. Enzyme Res.* **13**:77–96.

HASKELL, C. M., SILVERSTEIN, M. J., RANGEL, D. M., HUNT, J. S., SPARKS, F. C., AND MORTON, D. L., 1974, Multimodality cancer therapy in man: A pilot study of adriamycin by arterial infusion, *Cancer* **33**:1485–1490.

HIGBY, D. J., WALLACE, H. J., AND HOLLAND, J. F., 1973, *cis*-Diamminedichloroplatinum (NSC-119875): A Phase I study, *Cancer Chemother. Rep.* **57**:459–463.

HILL, B. T., AND BASERGA, R., 1975, The cell cycle and its significance for cancer treatment, *Cancer Treatment Rev.* **2**:159–175.

HILL, G. J., METTER, G. E., MOSS, S., KREMENTZ, E., FLETCHER, W., MINTON, J., AND GOLOMB, F., 1976, DTIC therapy for melanoma: Correlation of toxicity with response and longevity in 742 patients, *Proc. Amer. Assoc. Cancer Res.* **17**:244.

HILLEN, H., WESSELS, J., AND HAANEN, C., 1975, Bone-marrow-proliferation patterns in acute myeloblastic leukaemia determined by pulse cytophotometry, *Lancet* **(7907)**:609–611.

187

PRINCIPLES
OF
COMBINA-
TION
CHEMO-
THERAPY

HITCHINGS, G. H., 1963, Summary of informal discussion on the role of purine antagonists, *Cancer Res.* **23:**1218–1225.

HUGULEY, C. M., JR., DURANT, J. R., MOORES, R. R., CHAN, Y. C., DORFMAN, R. F., AND JOHNSON, L., 1975, A comparison of nitrogen mustard, vincristine, procarbazine and prednisone (MOPP) vs. nitrogen mustard in advanced Hodgkin's disease, *Cancer* **36:**1227–1240.

JAFFE, N., PAED, D., FARBER, S., TRAGGIS, D , GEISER, C., KIM, B. S., DAS, L. D., FRAUENBERGER, G., DJERASSI, I., AND CASSADY, J. R., 1973, Favorable response of metastatic osteogenic sarcoma to pulse high dose methotrexate with citrovorum rescue and radiation therapy, *Cancer* 31:1267–1373.

JAFFE, N., FREI, E., III, TRAGGIS, D., AND BISHOP, Y., 1974, Adjuvant methotrexate and citrovorum-factor treatment of osteogenic sarcoma, *N. Engl. J. Med.* **291:**994–997.

JAO, J. Y., JUSKO, W. J., AND COHEN, J. L., 1972, Phenobarbital effects on cyclophosphamide pharmacokinetics in man, *Cancer Res.* **32:**2761–2764.

JOHNSON, E. C., ANSFIELD, F. J., RAMIREZ, G., AND DAVIS, H. L., JR., 1973, Further clinical studies of 5-fluorouracil (5-FU; NSC-19893) given by the multiple daily dose method in disseminated breast cancer, *Cancer Chemother. Rep. Part 1* **57:**59–63.

JONES, B., CUTTNER, J., LEVY, R. N., PATTERSON, R. B., KUNG, F., PLEUSS, H. J., FALKSON, G., TREAT, C. L., HAURANI, F., BURGERT, E. O., JR., ROSNER, F., CAREY, R. W., LUKENS, J., BLOM, J., DEGNAN, T. J., WOHL, H., GLIDEWELL, O., AND HOLLAND, J. F., 1972, Daunorubicin (NSC-83142) versus daunorubicin plus prednisone (NSC-10023) versus daunorubicin plus vincristine (NSC-67574) plus prednisone in advanced childhood acute lymphocytic leukemia, *Cancer Chemother. Rep. Part 1* **56:**729–737.

JONES, S. E., ROSENBERG, S. A., KAPLAN, H. S., KADIN, M. E., AND DORFMAN, R. F., 1972, Non-Hodgkin's lymphomas. II. Single agent chemotherapy, *Cancer* **30:**31–38.

JONES, S. E., DURIE, B. G. M., AND SALMON, S. E., 1975, Combination chemotherapy with adriamycin and cyclophosphamide for advanced breast cancer, *Cancer* **36:**90–97.

KESSEL, D., HALL, T. C., ROBERTS, D., AND WODINSKY, I., 1965, Uptake as a determination of methotrexate response in mouse leukemias, *Science* **150:**752, 753.

KIRBY, H. B., KENAMORE, B., AND GUCKIAN, J. C., 1971, *Pneumocystis carini* pneumonia treated with pyrimethamine and sulfadiazine, *Ann. Intern. Med.* **75:**505–509.

KISHIMOTO, S., AND LIEBERMAN, I., 1964, Synthesis of RNA and protein required for the mitosis of mammalian cells, *Exp. Cell. Res.* **36:**92–101.

KREMER, W. B., VOGLER, W. R., AND CHAN, Y. I., 1976, An attempt at synchronization of marrow cells in actue leukemia, *Cancer* **37:**390–403.

LAMOUREUX, K. B., 1974, Increased clinically symptomatic pulmonary radiation reactions with adjuvant chemotherapy, *Cancer Chemother. Rep. Part 1* **58:**705–708.

LAMPKIN, B. C., NAGAO, T., AND MAUER, A. M., 1971, Synchronization and recruitment in acute leukemia, *J. Clin. Invest.* **50:**2204–2214.

LAMPKIN, B. C., MCWILLIAMS, N. B., MAUER, A. M., FLESSA, H. C., HAKE D. A., AND FISCHER, V. L., 1974, Manipulation of the mitotic cycle in treatment of acute myeloblastic leukemia (AML), *Proc. Amer. Soc. Hematol.* **17:**930 (in Blood **44:**930).

LEPAGE, G. A., WORTH, L. S., AND KIMBALL, A. P., 1976, Enhancement of the antitumor activity of arabinofuranosyladenine by 2'-deoxycoformycin, *Cancer Res.* **36:**1481–1485.

LI, M. C., HERTZ, R., AND SPENCER, D. B., 1956, Effect of methotrexate therapy upon choriocarcinoma and chorioadenoma (22757), *Proc. Soc. Exp. Biol. Med.* **93:**361–366.

LI, M. C., WHITMORE, W. F., GOLBEY, R., AND GRABSTALD, N., 1960, Effects of combined drug therapy on metastatic cancer of the testis, *J. Amer. Med. Assoc.* **174:**1291–1299.

LIVINGSTON, R. B., AND CARTER, S. K., 1970, *Single Agents in Cancer Chemotherapy,* IFI/Plenum Press, New York.

LLOYD, H. H., 1974, Combination chemotherapy: Considerations for design and analysis, *Cancer Chemother. Rep. Part 2* **4:**157–165.

MAALOE, O., AND HANAWALT, P. C., 1961, Thymine deficiency and the normal DNA replication cycle, *J. Mol. Biol.* **3:**144–155.

MACKENZIE, A. R., 1966, Chemotherapy of metastatic testis cancer, *Cancer* **19:**1369–1376.

MANTEL, N., 1974, Therapeutic synergism, *Cancer Chemother. Rep. Part 2* **4:**147–149.

MEDICAL LETTER, 1968, Allopurinol and the control of hyperuricemia in neoplastic disease, *Med. Lett., Drugs Ther.* **10:**103, 104.

MEDOFF, G., VALERIOTE, F., LYNCH, R. G., SCHLESSINGER, D., AND KOBAYASHI, G. S., 1974, Synergistic effect of amphotericin B and 1,3-bis(2-chloroethyl)-1 nitrosourea against a transplantable AKR leukemia, *Cancer Res.* **34:**947–978.

MERRILL, J., GRECO, F. A., ZIMBLER, R. H., BERETON, H. D., LAMBERG, J. D., AND POMEROY, T. C., 1975, Letter: Adriamycin and radiation: Synergistic cardiotoxicity, *Ann. Intern. Med.* **82:**122, 123.

MERRIN, C. E., AND MURPHY, G. P., 1974, Metastatic testicular carcinoma. Single agent chemotherapy (actinomycin-D) in treatment, *N. Y. State J. Med.* **74:**654–657.

NAHAS, A., AND CAPIZZI, R. L., 1974, Effect of *in vivo* treatment with L-asparaginase on the *in vitro* uptake and phosphorylation of some antileukemic agents, *Cancer Res.* **34:**2689–2693.

NAHAS, A., NIXON, P. F., AND BERTINO, J. R., 1972, Uptake and metabolism of N^5-formyltetrahydrofolate by L1210 leukemia cells, *Cancer Res.* **32:**1416–1421.

NEIL, G. L., MOXLEY, T. E., AND MANAK, R. C., 1970, Enhancement by tetrahydrouridine of 1-β-D-arabinofuranosylcytosine (cytarabine) oral activity in L1210 leukemic mice, *Cancer Res.* **30:**2166–2172.

NKRUMAH, F. K., AND PERKINS, I. V., 1976, Burkitt's lymphoma. A clinical study of 110 patients, *Cancer* **37:**671–676.

OTIS, P. T., AND ARMENTROUT, S. A., 1975, Combination chemotherapy in metastatic carcinoma of the breast. Results with a three-drug combination, *Cancer* **36:**311–317.

PHILLIPS, T. L., WHARAM, M. D., AND MARGOLIS, L. W., 1975, Modification of radiation injury to normal tissues by chemotherapeutic agents, *Cancer* **35:**1678–1684.

PINKEL, D., HERNANDEZ, K., BORELLA, L., HOLTON, C., AUR, R., SAMOY, G., AND PRATT, C., 1971, Drug dosage and remission duration in childhood lymphocytic leukemia, *Cancer* **27:**247–256.

POTTER, V. R., 1951, Sequential blocking of metabolic pathways *in vivo*, *Proc. Soc. Exp. Biol. Med.* **76:**41–46.

POWLES, R. L., 1976, Immunotherapy in the management of acute leukemia, *Br. J. Haematol.* **32:**145–148.

PRESCOTT, D. M., 1968, Regulation of cell reproduction, *Cancer Res.* **28:**1815–1820.

PROSNITZ, L. R., FARBER, L. R., FISCHER, J. J., BERTINO, R. J., AND FISCHER, D. B., 1976, Long term remissions with combined modality therapy for advanced Hodgkin's disease, *Cancer* **37:**2826–2833.

RAMIREZ, G., KLOTZ, J., STRAWITZ, J. G., WILSON, W. L., CORNELL, G. N., MADDEN, R. E., MINTON, J. P., AND THE CENTRAL ONCOLOGY GROUP, 1975, Combination chemotherapy in breast cancer. A randomized study of 4 versus 5 drugs, *Oncology* **32:**101–108.

SAMUELS, M. L., AND HOWE, C. D., 1970, Vinblastine in the management of testicular cancer, *Cancer* **25:**1009–1017.

SAMUELS, M. L., HOLOYE, P. Y., AND JOHNSON, D. E., 1975a, Bleomycin chemotherapy in the management of testicular neoplasia, *Cancer* **36:**318–326.

SAMUELS, M. L., JOHNSON, D. E., AND HOLOYE, P. Y., 1975b, Continuous intravenous bleomycin (NSC-125066) therapy with vinblastine (NSC-49842) in stage III testicular neoplasia, *Cancer Chemother. Rep.* **59:**563–570.

SAMUELS, M. L., JOHNSON, D. E., HOLOYE, P. Y., AND LANZOTTI, V. J., 1976, Large dose bleomycin therapy and pulmonary toxicity: A possible role of prior radiotherapy, *J. Amer. Med. Assoc.* **235:**1117–1120.

SARTORELLI, A. C., 1969, Some approaches to therapeutic exploitation of metabolic sites of vulnerability of neoplastic cells, *Cancer Res.* **29:**2292–2299.

SCHEIN, P. S., CHABNER, B. A., CANELLOS, G. P., YOUNG, R. C., BERARD, C., AND DEVITA, V. T., 1974, Potential for prolonged disease-free survival following combination chemotherapy of non-Hodgkin's lymphoma, *Blood* **43:**181–189.

SCHENKEN, L. L., AND HAGEMANN, R. F., 1976, Recruitment oncotherapy schedules for enhanced efficacy of cycle active agents, *Proc. Amer. Assoc. Cancer Res.* **17:**88.

SCHMIDT, L. H., MONTGOMERY, J. A., LASTER, W. R., JR., AND SCHABEL, F. M., JR., 1970, Combination therapy with arabinosylcytosine and thioguanine, *Proc. Amer. Assoc. Cancer Res.* **11:**70.

SIMONE, J. V., AUR, R. J. A., HUSTU, H. O., VERZOSA, M., AND PINKEL, D., 1975, Combined modality therapy of acute lymphocytic leukemia, *Cancer* **35:**25–35.

SIROTNAK, F. M., AND DONSBACH, R. C., 1976, Kinetic correlates of methotrexate transport and therapeutic responsiveness in murine tumors, *Cancer Res.* **36:**1151–1158.

SKEEL, R. T., SAWICKI, W. L., CASHMORE, A. R., AND BERTINO, J. R., 1973, The basis for the disparate sensitivity of L1210 leukemia and Walker 256 carcinoma to a new triazine folate antagonist, *Cancer Res.* **33:**2972–2976.

SKIPPER, H. E., AND PERRY, S., 1970, Kinetics of normal and leukemic leukocyte populations and relevance to chemotherapy, *Cancer Res.* **30:**1883–1897.

SKIPPER, H. E., SCHABEL, F. M., JR., AND WILCOX, W. S., 1967, Experimental evaluation of potential anticancer agents. XXI. Scheduling of arabinocytosine to take advantage of its S-phase specificity against leukemia cells, *Cancer Chemother. Rep.* **51:**125–165.

189

PRINCIPLES
OF
COMBINA-
TION
CHEMO-
THERAPY

190

L. WAYNE
KEISER AND
ROBERT L.
CAPIZZI

SLADEK, N. E., 1971, Metabolism of cyclophosphamide by rat hepatic microsomes, *Cancer Res.* **31**:901–908.

STABLER, A., JR., 1971, Effects of the DNA repair inhibitor chloroquine on the therapeutic response of Cytoxan sensitive plasmacytomas and host toxicity to treatment with Cytoxan, *Ala. J. Med. Sci.* **8**:184.

SULKES, A., LIVINGSTON, R., AND TAYLOR, G., 1976, Pre-treatment labeling index (LI%) in breast carcinoma patients as a predictor of response to combination chemotherapy, *Proc. Amer. Assoc. Cancer Res.* **17**:59.

TALLEY, R. W., VAITKEVICIUS, V. K., AND LEIGHTON, G. A., 1965, Comparison of cyclophosphamide and 5-fluorouracil in the treatment of patients with metastatic breast cancer, *Clin. Pharmacol. Ther.* **6**:740–748.

TALLEY, R. W., O'BRYAN, R. M., GUTTERMAN, J. U., BROWNLEE, R. W., AND MCCREDIE, K. B., 1973, Clinical evaluation of toxic effects of *cis*-diamminedichloroplatinum (NSC-119875)—Phase 1 clinical study, *Cancer Chemother. Rep.* **57**:465–471.

TATTERSALL, M. H. N., AND HARRAP, K. R., 1973, Combination chemotherapy: The antagonism of methotrexate and cytosine arabinoside, *Eur. J. Cancer* **9**:229–232.

TATTERSALL, M. H. N., JACKSON, R. C., CONNORS, T. A., AND HARRAP, K. R., 1973, Combination chemotherapy: The interaction of methotrexate and 5-fluorouracil, *Eur. J. Cancer* **9**:733–739.

TERASIMA, T., AND YASUKAWA, M., 1966, Synthesis of G1 protein preceding DNA synthesis in cultured mammalian cells, *Exp. Cell Res.* **44**:669–672.

VALERIOTE, F. A., AND BRUCE, W. R., 1967, Comparison of the sensitivity of hematopoietic colony-forming cells in different proliferative states to vinblastine, *J. Natl. Cancer Inst.* **38**:393–399.

VALERIOTE, F., AND LIN, H., 1975, Synergistic interaction of anticancer agents: A cellular perspective, *Cancer Chemother. Rep.* **59**:895–900.

VALERIOTE, F. A., AND TOLEN, S. J., 1972, Survival of hematopoietic and lymphoma colony-forming cells *in vivo* following the administration of a variety of alkylating agents, *Cancer Res.* **32**:470–476.

VAN PUTTEN, L. M., AND LELIEVELD, P., 1970, Factors determining cell killing by chemotherapeutic agents *in vivo*. I. Cyclophosphamide, *Eur. J. Cancer* **6**:313–321.

VAN PUTTEN, L. M., AND LELIEVELD, P., 1971, Factors determining cell killing by chemotherapeutic agents *in vivo*. II. Melphalan, chlorambucil and nitrogen mustard, *Eur. J. Cancer* **7**:11–16.

VENDITTI, J. M., AND GOLDIN, A., 1964, Drug synergism in antineoplastic chemotherapy, *Adv. Chemother.* **1**:397–498.

VOGLER, W. R., FURTADO, V. P., AND HUGULEY, C. M., JR., 1968, Methotrexate for advanced cancer of the breast, *Cancer* **21**:26–30.

VOGLER, W. R., COOPER, L. E., AND GROTH, D. P., 1974, Correlation of cytosine arabinoside–induced increment in growth fraction of leukemic blast cells with clinical response, *Cancer* **33**:603–610.

WARA, W. M., PHILLIPS, T. L., MARGOLIS, L. W., AND SMITH, V., 1973, Radiation pneumonitis: A new approach to the derivation of time dose factors, *Cancer* **32**:547–552.

ZAGER, R. F., FRESBY, S. A., AND OLIVIERIO, V. T., 1973, The effects of antibiotics and cancer chemotherapeutic agents on the cellular transport and antitumor activity of methotrexate in L1210 murine leukemia, *Cancer Res.* **33**:1670–1676.

ZIEGLER, J. L., BLUMING, A. Z., FASS, L., MORROW, R. H., JR., AND IVERSEN, O. H., 1973, *Bibl. Haematol.* **39**:1046–1052 (R. M. Dutcher and L. Chieco-Bianchi, eds.), Karger, Basel.

7

Intraarterial Chemotherapy

W. Bruce Lundberg

1. Introduction and History

Malignant disease, even when metastatic, frequently produces symptoms and causes death by growth in relatively localized areas. Local therapy by the judicious use of surgery and irradiation (external beam and isotope implantation) has traditionally occupied an important place in the systematic management of patients with advanced malignancy. Systemic chemotherapy can also be used to treat predominantly regional disease, and the intraarterial delivery of chemotherapeutic agents can provide a greater degree of selectivity. When drugs are administered intraarterially, the local concentrations and infusion durations are greater than when the same agents are administered intravenously. At the same time, systemic toxicity is frequently reduced because of the absorption or inactivation, or both, of the drug on passage through the arterial bed. Although the procedure is technically more difficult, effluent drug-containing blood has been diverted from the systemic circulation or prevented from reaching sensitive normal tissues during the drug infusion.

The serendipitous observation of localized skin toxicity that followed an inadvertent intraarterial injection of nitrogen mustard (HN_2) led to the initial experimental use of intraarterial drug therapy in the clinic (Klopp *et al.*, 1950). Following the impetus of these workers, investigators directed their research toward increasingly complex methods to isolate the vascular supply of the tumor and *perfuse* with high doses of alkylating agents (Creech *et al.*, 1958). The techniques employed high local concentrations of drugs administered over short ($\frac{1}{2}$–2 hr) time periods. Systemic toxicity was monitored by measuring leakage of the perfused blood

W. Bruce Lundberg ● Section of Medical Oncology, Yale University School of Medicine, New Haven, Connecticut.

back into the patient's circulation. Major surgical manipulation, which varied in the areas perfused, and extracorporeal oxygenation of the isolated areas were required (Creech *et al.*, 1959). In an effort to reduce surgical morbidity, complex regional tourniquets (Lawrence *et al.*, 1961) or intraarterial balloons (Watkins *et al.*, 1960) were used to divert blood from sensitive normal tissues. Even autologous bone marrow rescue was employed following "total-body" perfusion (Creech *et al.*, 1959). At times, dramatic tumor responses were attained, and systemic toxicity was reduced. However, the surgical morbidity and high incidence of local toxicity have led to the virtual abandonment of these techniques in intrathoracic and abdominal tumors. Isolation–perfusion remains a viable investigative approach in the treatment of extremity tumors, principally melanoma (Stehlin *et al.*, 1965; McBride, 1970). Extremity perfusion (most frequently with L-phenylalanine mustard) has been used to treat locally advanced melanoma and as an adjuvant to primary surgical treatment for poor-risk lesions. Responses have been obtained with perfusion of advanced melanoma that have reduced morbidity and at times prevented amputations. Perfusion used as a surgical adjuvant decreased the frequency of local recurrences. Simpler intraarterial infusion without isolation with a more active drug (DTIC) may prove to be as effective (Savlov *et al.*, 1971).

Sullivan *et al.* (1959) piloted the use of chemotherapy by prolonged intraarterial *infusion.* They treated head and neck tumors with intraarterial methotrexate (MTX) and systemic leucovorin rescue, and obtained some dramatic tumor regressions. They reasoned that prolonged exposure to cell-cycle-active antimetabolites was required in slow-growing solid tumors, and that more of the drug would reach the tumor with less systemic toxicity by the intraarterial route. Using the fluorinated pyrimidines, this approach was then applied to intrahepatic tumors (Clarkson *et al.*, 1962; Sullivan *et al.*, 1964), again with objective tumor responses. The two approaches that are presently being investigated, predominantly in hepatic tumors, employ long-term continuous infusion over weeks to months (usually with surgical catheter placement) or short-term intermittent infusions over days to weeks (usually by percutaneous catheter placement). Neither method has produced clearly better results. Objective responses have consistently been reported at 2–3 times those obtained with conventional systemic therapy. The patients who are considered to have responded have lived longer than either those who did not respond or those from retrospective series. In a large study employing 5-fluorouracil (5-FU) by intermittent intraarterial infusion to metastasis in the liver, Ansfield *et al.* (1975) obtained objective responses in 55% of 293 patients studied. The significance of this result is enhanced by the fact that three-fourths of those patients had already progressed on intravenous 5-FU. The responding patients lived on the average an additional 7 months.

2. Pharmacology

The ideal pharmacological properties of an antitumor drug for intraarterial infusion were recognized by Klopp *et al.* (1950). The drug should have high antitumor activity and specificity, with minimal toxicity to local normal tissues. In order to avoid systemic toxicity, the drug should be inactivated, metabolized, or absorbed on a single passage through the capillary bed fed by the infused artery. In order to exploit these pharmacological properties, it must be technically feasible to cannulate an artery that supplies the entire tumor and maintain that catheter in the appropriate location.

The ideal drug or drug combination has yet to be found. However, intraarterial infusion has resulted in higher local drug concentrations and longer infusion durations than are attainable by ordinary systemic drug administration. These results are achieved without an attendant increase, and frequently with a decrease, in systemic toxicity. Drugs that have been demonstrated to have activity when used systemically have also proved to be the most useful when administered intraarterially. It is conceivable, however, that some drugs that have not shown promise in routine phase II screening may have activity when administered intraarterially because of differences in dose and schedule attainable by this route. There is precedent for this pharmacological principle. An example is the responsiveness of osteogenic sarcoma to high-dose MTX after the drug was found to be useless in treating this tumor in conventional doses (Jaffe et al., 1968).

The local arterial infusion allows one to exploit unique pharmacological properties of particular chemotherapeutic agents. In liver infusions, drugs sensitive to hepatic metabolic enzymes may be inactivated before entering the vena cava. Alternatively, a drug with a short biological half-life may "self-destruct" on passage through the tumor bed. Alkylating agents with shorter and shorter half-lives were specifically synthesized for this purpose (Witten et al., 1962a, b; Seligman et al., 1962; Schilling et al., 1963; Goodman et al., 1962, 1965; Ulfohn et al., 1968; Bakal et al., 1971). This approach was combined with extremity tourniquets (Conrad and Crosby, 1960; Schilling et al., 1963; Meyza and Cobb, 1971). This technique afforded some hematopoietic protection in children who have sufficient long bone marrow. Because the rapidly hydrolyzed mustards required inert solvents, ester-linked alkylators susceptible to ubiquitous catabolic enzymes were also synthesized. This approach was scientifically reasonable, and some tumor regressions were obtained (Ulfohn et al., 1968). Local toxicity was severe, however, and these drugs have not proved to be practically useful.

The use of antimetabolites has met with more success. Sullivan et al. (1959) used high local concentrations of MTX. They prevented systemic toxicity with leucovorin. The MTX analogue dichloromethotrexate (DCM) is metabolized by microsomal enzymes in the liver. Its use in intrahepatic arterial infusion for hepatoma has resulted in tumor regressions (Harrison et al., 1973). Systemic toxicity was minimal. Incomplete drug metabolism is a risk with this type of approach. For example, patients with underlying liver disease treated with DCM developed systemic toxicity, presumably because of incomplete metabolism by the diseased liver (Cleveland et al., 1969). Fluorodeoxyuridine (FUDR) and 5-FU can be infused safely into the hepatic artery in higher doses and over longer intervals than can be given when these drugs are used intravenously. In this case, the combination of the extraction (Mukherjee et al., 1963) and the metabolism

(Sullivan *et al.*, 1963) of the drug leads to a decrease in the amount of the active metabolite reaching the marrow and sensitive gastrointestinal mucosa. Cytosine arabinoside is also metabolized in the liver. Its use by intrasplenic arterial infusion to treat splenomegaly in chronic myelogenous leukemia has resulted in reduced systematic toxicity (Canellos, personal communication). Hepatic deactivation occurs after the drug is delivered to the portal system.

The antitumor antibiotics have been used by intraarterial infusion. Streptozotocin given intraarterially for islet cell tumors metastatic to the liver has produced tumor regressions. In addition, blood levels and renal excretion of this nephrotoxic agent were reduced with intraarterial infusion when compared with intravenous administration (Kahn *et al.*, 1975). The authors attributed these reductions to extraction of the drug by the tumor. Adriamycin is partially metabolized in the liver and largely excreted in the bile (Bachur, 1975). Although systemic toxicity of the drug does not appear to be diminished following intraarterial infusion in the extremities, the use of adriamycin by hepatic artery infusion has pharmacological rationale and deserves further investigation (Owleny and McIntire, 1974; Haskell *et al.*, 1975; Bern *et al.*, 1976).

Extreme caution must be exercised in intraarterial administration of drugs at doses that are higher than those tolerated by the systemic route. Alterations in enzymatic or excretory functions, differences in drug extraction by different tissues and tumors, and problems with arteriovenous shunting and catheter dislodgment may all result in enhanced systemic drug levels. Careful monitoring for signs of toxicity and, when available, measurement of levels of drug in peripheral blood will help avert disastrous complications.

Many drugs require *in vivo* anabolic activation. This requirement is also a consideration when selecting a drug for intraarterial use. As an example, cyclophosphamide is activated predominantly in the liver. There would be no advantage gained, therefore, in infusing this drug into an extremity or the head and neck region. Although tumor responses were obtained in 2 of 6 patients treated with intraarterial infusions of DTIC for advanced melanoma in an extremity (Savlov *et al.*, 1971), DTIC may require hepatic microsomal alteration to a more active metabolite for maximal activity (Skibba *et al.*, 1970). This requirement could have bearing on the frequency of tumor responses following the intraarterial administration of this drug.

3. Technical Considerations and Complications

As a result of the cannulization of any vessel, a significant number of both minor and major complications can arise. Cannulas can be placed surgically by direct arterotomy of the isolated vessel (Watkins *et al.*, 1970), or by selective percutaneous catheterization of the femoral or brachial artery (Wirtanen, 1973). Surgical hepatic arterial catheterization generally requires a separate laparotomy, although the catheter can be placed at the time of primary surgery. Direct

catheterization provides maximal assessment of disease status and vascular
anatomy, ensures secure catheter placement, and allows patient mobility after
surgical recovery. Anatomical alteration of the vascular supply to ensure perfusion of the entire liver is feasible in the patients (about 35%) with aberrant right or
left hepatic artery takeoff (Cady, 1973). The advantages, however, are often
outweighed by the surgical morbidity in a patient whose life, even with a response,
will generally be prolonged less than a year. The surgical approach requires
selection of patients to avoid the high operative mortality (liver failure) associated
with massive hepatomegaly and ascites (Cady and Oberfield, 1974b), and therefore biases treatment results in its favor.

Percutaneous catheter placement is technically feasible in most patients, but is
more frequently associated with catheter-tip displacement or incomplete tumor-
bed perfusion because of the complexity of the vascular anatomy. Dual arterial
supply can be dealt with by using two catheters (Ansfield et al., 1975; Goldman et
al., 1975; Suzuki et al., 1972). Unfortunately, this approach results in increased
morbidity to the patient. Brachial artery catheterization has the advantage of
greater patient mobility. The short-term infusions can be accomplished with
closed sterile plastic bags put under pressure (300 mm Hg) with a Fenwal blood
pump (Ansfield et al., 1971). For the prolonged infusions, a "chronometric"
infusion pump has been devised (Oberfield, 1974), and new devices are being
developed (Alza Corporation).

The complications of the isolation–perfusion techniques were both frequent
and severe because of the extensive surgery required and high doses of drugs
used. Complications were most often the result of massive local necrosis. Paradoxically, good tumor responses resulted in perforations, fistulas, and hemorrhages.
Systemic toxicity that accompanied massive tumor necrosis included fever,
metabolic acidosis, and death (Hurley et al., 1961). Skin sloughs and long-term
vascular injury with ischemia sometimes resulted. In the head and neck tumors,
carotid hemorrhages or cutaneous and brain fistulas, or both, were produced. In
the mediastinum, bronchial and esophageal fistulas, perforations, and major-
vessel bleeding resulted. Bowel perforations and vesico- and rectovaginal fistulas
resulted from abdominal and pelvic perfusions.

A different set of complications have been associated with the longer-duration
arterial infusions. These complications can be grouped into problems at the
percutaneous site of entry into the artery, problems at the catheter tip, and
complications resulting from the systemic toxicity of the drugs. They are summarized in Table 1.

Infection at the percutaneous insertion site can be reduced to 5% or less by
meticulous care of the entry site (Wirtanen, 1973; Goldman et al., 1975). Infectious problems are increased by the manipulations required when the catheter tip
displaces, however, and in a large study, infections occurred in one-third of the
patients (Ansfield et al., 1975). Treatment of infection with catheter removal, local
measures, and systemic antibiotics is generally successful. It is not advisable to
attempt to treat infections without catheter removal, since doing so has resulted in
mycotic aneurysms and septic embolization (Labelle et al., 1968). Cracks, leaks,

TABLE 1
Complications of Intraarterial Infusions

Percutaneous puncture site
  Infection—local and systemic
  Leakage and cracks
  Hemorrhage
  Thrombosis—embolism

Catheter tip
  Dislodgment
  Blockage
  Thrombosis—arterial occlusion; retrograde propagation
  Embolization
  Bleeding
  Migration of catheter tip and perforation

Systemic toxicity
  Catheter dislodgment
  Incomplete drug absorption or inactivation

and local hemorrhage all require manipulation, and hence increase the incidence of infection. Thromboses have developed at the entry site, but rarely. When they occur, ischemic symptoms are more frequent in the brachial than in the femoral artery. Downstream embolization, especially when the catheter is pulled out, occurs more frequently than is clinically evident, since 40% of the catheters develop angiographically demonstrable fibrin sheaths (Goldman *et al.*, 1975). Pulse losses and cerebral ischemic symptoms (brachial and carotid artery infusions) are usually transient, but in some instances, embolectomy has been required. During the placement procedure, extravasation of angiographic dye and arterial dissections are risks.

The most frequent complication that occurs at the tip of the catheter is displacement and, consequently, inadequate or improper infusion. Tip placement should be checked by X ray at least twice weekly when the catheter has been placed percutaneously. This procedure may require a small angiographic dye injection. When 5-FU is being infused, the selective development of nausea or diarrhea suggests catheter-tip displacement in the arterial distribution of the stomach or large bowel, respectively (Ansfield *et al.*, 1975). Thrombosis at the catheter tip, which has a reported occurrence of 3% (Wirtanen, 1973) to 28% (Goldman *et al.*, 1975), results in catheter blockage, vessel occlusion, and downstream embolization. Hepatic artery occlusion is generally asymptomatic, and occurred in almost one-third of the patients treated with prolonged infusions (Cady, 1973). Abdominal ischemic symptoms have occurred from coeliac axis and superior mesenteric arterial thrombosis. Gastrointestinal bleeding resulting from ischemia and mucosal drug toxicity is rare. This complication is enhanced, however, by a prior history of acid-peptic disease (Cady, 1973) and systemic heparinization (Goldman *et al.*, 1975). Catheter-tip migration and erosion through vessels into other intraabdominal structures has been seen with the prolonged infusions (Cady, 1973). Any of these complications can be severe, and they have resulted in the death of some patients.

Systemic toxicity is the same as that resulting from the usual route of administration of the drug. Some degree of systemic toxicity is the rule in order to assure the infusion of a maximum amount of drug.

4. Results of Infusions in Specific Locations

4.1. Liver

A greater number of intrahepatic tumors, both primary and metastatic, have been treated by intraarterial infusion than tumors in any other location. The majority of these tumors have been of primary colonic origin.

Considerable theoretical rationale exists for hepatic artery infusion. The normal hepatocyte has a low mitotic rate and is nourished by a dual vascular supply (portal vein and hepatic artery). Metastatic disease in the liver should theoretically have higher mitotic activity than the hepatic parenchyma. In addition, the hepatic artery has been shown to provide the predominant blood supply of metastatic tumors in the livers of both animals and humans in both postmortem (Breedis and Young, 1954) and *in vivo* angiographic injection studies (Bierman *et al.*, 1951). This has been shown to be true experimentally in rats whether tumor cells were introduced into the hepatic artery or the portal vein (Fisher *et al.*, 1961). In support of this thesis, some patients with hepatic metastasis have benefited from hepatic artery ligation (Sparks *et al.*, 1975; Fortner *et al.*, 1973). The concept has been disputed, however, since the pattern of metastatic spread within the liver is highly variable, and many tumors are relatively avascular (Healey, 1965). For this reason, portal vein infusions have been attempted with catheter placement at surgery. It is possible that selection of this route of infusion may be determined by angiographic demonstration of portal blood supply of the tumor. Another factor that encourages the use of infusion therapy to the liver is that tumor growth can occur here without gross evidence of spread to other organs. In patients with colon carcinoma, death often results from hepatic metastasis without evidence of compromise to other organs. Therefore, tumor regression resulting from arterial drug infusion could result in prolonged survival, even though there are micrometastases to other areas. Finally, the liver is rich in microsomal drug-metabolizing enzymes that can inactivate chemotherapeutic agents and help prevent their systemic toxicity (see Section 2).

Decreased liver size and improved liver chemistries, scans, and angiograms have been followed as objective parameters of tumor response. Overall clinical improvement of the patient has also been considered as evidence of a response (Cady and Oberfield, 1974b). Studies of infusion therapy have reported the frequency of objective tumor responses and the length of survival of the treated patients compared with retrospective controls. About 10% of patients with colon carcinoma are found to have metastatic liver disease at the time of their initial surgery (Galante *et al.*, 1967; Cady *et al.*, 1970). The average survival of these patients is 5–6 months (Jaffe *et al.*, 1968; Bengmark and Hafström, 1969). There is a significant tail to this survival curve, and a few patients live for 5 or more years

TABLE 2

Reported Results in Selected Studies of the Use of the Fluorinated Pyrimidines by Intrahepatic Arterial Infusion

Reference	Catheter placement method[a]	Drug	Dose and duration	Patients evaluable	Response			Comments
					Rate	Median survival of responders (months)	In colorectal	
Sullivan and Zurek (1965)	IO	5-FU FUDR	5.0–7.5 mg/kg · day or 0.3 mg/kg · day	73	58%	9.4	61%	
Rochlin and Smart (1966)	IO+PC	5-FU	10 mg/kg · day × 2 wk	51	44%	6.0	50%	
Burrows et al. (1967)	PC	5-FU 5-FU FUDR	40 mg/kg × 5 or 20 mg/kg × 10 days 1 mg/kg × 10–40 days	29 39 22	58% 73% 25%	6.2	59%	
Labelle et al. (1968)	IO+PC	5-FU FUDR	10–40 mg/kg × "months" 0.1–0.7 mg/kg × "months"	66	47%	?	60%	
Donegan et al. (1969)	IO	5-FU	500 mg × 14 days or more	13	39%	7.7	50%	No response; portal vein
Massey et al. (1971)	PC	5-FU	15–30 mg/kg × less than 21 days	38	60%	10.8	60%	
Tandon et al. (1973)	PC	5-FU	25–30 mg/kg × 7–9 days	95	64%	?	67%	Prior Rx c̄ 5-FU
Cady and Oberfield (1974b)	IO	FUDR	0.1–0.3 mg/kg · day for 6–9 months	51	71%	16	71%	
Fortuny et al. (1975)	PC	5-FU	25 mg/kg × 12 days	12	84%	12.5	84%	Mitomycin C 46%
Ansfield et al. (1975)	PC	5-FU	20–30 mg/kg × 4 days; then 15 mg/kg × 17 days	293	55%	7.3	55%	Prior Rx c̄ 5-FU

[a] IO: intraoperative; PC: percutaneous.

without therapy; they represented as many as 5% of the patients in one series (Galante *et al.*, 1967). Gastrointestinal adenocarcinomas other than colon and colon carcinomas with extensive hepatic and extrahepatic involvement have a considerably worse prognosis. Patients who develop metachronous hepatic metastasis after primary tumor resection survive longer, on the average 10 months (Jaffe *et al.*, 1968). These patients, therefore, represent a somewhat more favorable group. There has been no reported randomized study comparing the survival of a group of patients treated with intraarterial chemotherapy with the survival of a simultaneous control group treated with systemic chemotherapy or not treated beyond surgery.

5-FU and FUDR are the most frequently used drugs in hepatic arterial therapy. Neither drug, nor any particular dose and schedule, has emerged as clearly superior. It is difficult, however, to compare the drugs on the basis of the reported studies. Consistent from study to study has been a greater than 50% response rate measured by objective criteria in patients with colorectal primary tumors (Table 2). This rate represents an obvious improvement over that achieved with systemically administered 5-FU (about 20%). The average survival of the responding patients has also been consistently improved when compared with retrospective controls. The survival of the nonresponding patients, however, has been worse than untreated comparison patients, a result that dampens the overall results of the studies. A patient can be expected to live an additional 6–16 months if an objective response is attained. In two of the studies (Tandon *et al.*, 1973; Ansfield *et al.*, 1975), objective tumor responses were obtained in patients who had progressed while receiving systemic 5-FU. Additional benefit on top of any that may have been obtained with systemic 5-FU was therefore possible. This observation lends clinical support to a pharmacological advantage of this route of drug administration. Responses in patients who had previously responded to systemic 5-FU were unfortunately not specifically tabulated. Although the reported results of intraarterial infusion in the liver have been encouraging, considerable room for improvement remains. The infusions require additional in-hospital time. Morbidity is significant, and prolongation of life remains short. Relatively few patients have been treated by arterial infusion, and the results reported by researchers in this area will have to be confirmed by those less enthusiastic about its use.

Hepatoma has also been treated by arterial infusion. Responses have been reported using MTX (Geddes and Falkson, 1970), DCM (Harrison *et al.*, 1973), and FUDR (Cady and Oberfield, 1974*a*). The survival of responding patients has been prolonged. APUD tumors in the liver have been treated with intraarterial infusion of 5-FU (Rochlin and Smart, 1966) and streptozotocin (Kahn *et al.*, 1975; Stadil *et al.*, 1976). Objective responses were obtained in carcinoid tumors and some hormone-producing islet-cell tumors.

4.2. Head and Neck

Because head and neck tumors tend to invade locally and frequently cause death without distant spread, they are good candidates for intraarterial infusion. It was anticipated that higher concentrations of drugs locally would improve responses, and at the same time decrease systemic toxicity. Significant problems have resulted from infusion therapy to this area. Because of the complications, the results have fallen short of the desired goals. In the head and neck area, it is technically difficult to infuse the entire tumor, which is frequently poorly vascularized. The adjacent mucous membranes receive as much drug as the tumor. The normal mucosa, often damaged by prior radiation, has proved to be as sensitive to the chemotherapeutic agents as the neoplastic tissue, possibly because of similar cell cycle times. Therefore, mucositis is common, and limits the amount of drug that can be given. Cerebrovascular accidents resulting from the indwelling catheters have been common. The occurrence of strokes has been decreased by open placement of the catheter in the superficial temporal artery, but the risk remains significant.

Drugs that have been used by intraarterial infusion in head and neck tumors are MTX with leucovorin and the fluorinated pyrimidines (Oberfield *et al.*, 1973), and bleomycin (Huntington *et al.*, 1973; Berdal *et al.*, 1973). To exploit the radiosensitizing properties of the drugs, infusion therapy has been coupled with irradiation (Friedman and Daly, 1963; Jesse *et al.*, 1969; Goffinet *et al.*, 1972; Goepfer *et al.*, 1973). To this combined approach, surgical ablation has been added in an effort to eliminate all residual disease (Sato *et al.*, 1970; Cruz *et al.*, 1974). Direct tumor measurements and rebiopsy of the treated area can provide objective parameters of a response. Dramatic tumor regressions have resulted from regional infusions in some patients. By employing prolonged antimetabolite infusions in 94 patients, Oberfield *et al.* (1973) achieved a reduction of greater than 50% in tumor size in half their patients. More impressive, complete responses were achieved in one-fourth of the patients. Survival was prolonged to over 1 year in half these complete responders. These responses were accomplished at the cost of severe local toxicity in one-third and severe systemic toxicity in one-half of the patients. There was a 9% incident of stroke.

Arterial drug infusion remains an investigative procedure in head and neck tumors. With the existing technology, it is difficult to foresee a significant place for this therapy in the treatment of advanced disease. But as an adjunct to surgery and radiation in the patient with a high probability of recurrence at the time of initial presentation, infusion therapy may well prove to be useful for tumors of the head and neck.

4.3. Other Sites

Lung tumors have been treated by intraarterial infusion of the bronchial arteries. While the pulmonary parenchyma is nourished by a dual blood supply, lung tumors are predominantly supplied by brachial artery blood (Henderson and Maddock, 1963). Objective tumor regressions have been reported following therapy with MTX (Miller *et al.*, 1964), HN_2 (Clifton, 1969), and mitomycin C (Neyazaki *et al.*, 1969). However, it is difficult to see any advantage of this treatment over external irradiation at this time.

Intraarterial infusion of primary and metastatic brain tumors is attractive, considering the low mitotic activity of the brain parenchyma and relatively rapid growth of many brain tumors. An additional advantage could be obtained from the radiosensitizing properties of the infused drug (Goffinet *et al.*, 1972). Complications resulting from brain infusions have been frequent and severe (Aronson *et al.*, 1963; Oberfield, 1974), and the approach remains experimental.

Local chest wall recurrences of breast cancer have been treated with arterial chemotherapy. Regressions were obtained in one study (Koyama *et al.*, 1975), but were difficult to interpret, since other treatment modalities were employed simultaneously. Here again, the advantage of this approach over radiation or systemic chemotherapy, except possibly in some selected patients, is not obvious.

5. Future Considerations

Much of the essential ground work on intraarterial infusion chemotherapy has been completed. With the present technology, patients with tumors of the extremities and in the liver may benefit from this approach. Some of the pharmacological advantages of the intraarterial route of drug administration have been realized in these two areas. Successes with this technique have been restrained by the limitations of the drugs available, the technical difficulties inherent in indwelling catheters, and the basic underlying systemic nature of the disease being treated. More effective and less toxic drugs are always being sought. A very active drug for a specific tumor may, however, eliminate the need for the intraarterial approach. Combination drug treatment has met with success in systemic treatment programs. Combinations of drugs could possibly increase the response rates in arterial infusions as well (Fortner *et al.*, 1976). Problems will always result from indwelling catheters, but advances in catheter and infusion system technology may significantly reduce these complications. That the disease being treated is systemic does not eliminate potential benefits that may be gained from local therapy. Combined modality approaches, including surgery, radiation, immunotherapy, and both local and systemic chemotherapy, may be judiciously combined with both palliative and curative intent. Radioactive isotopes have also been given by the intraarterial approach (Ariel and Pack, 1967; Simon *et al.*, 1968). Intraarterial chemotherapy remains experimental, and should be employed under clinical research circumstances.

6. References

ANSFIELD, F. J., RAMIREZ, G., SKIBBA, J. L., BRYAN, G. T., DAVIS, H. L., JR., AND WIRTANEN, G. W., 1971, Intrahepatic arterial infusion with 5-fluorouracil, *Cancer* **28**:1147.

ANSFIELD, F. J., RAMIREZ, G., DAVIS, H. L. JR., WIRTANEN, G. W., JOHNSON, R. O., BRYAN, G. T., MANALO, F. B., BORDEN, E. C., DAVIS, T. E., AND ESMAILI, M., 1975, Further clinical studies with intrahepatic arterial infusion with 5-fluorouracil, *Cancer* **36**:2413.

ARIEL, I. M., AND PACK, G. T., 1967, Treatment of inoperable cancer of the liver by intra-arterial radioactive isotopes and chemotherapy, *Cancer* **20**:793.

ARONSON, H. A., FLANIGEN, S., AND MARK, J. B. D., 1963, Chemotherapy of malignant brain tumors using regional perfusion: I. Technic and patient selection, *Ann. Surg.* **157**:394.

BACHUR, N. R., 1975, Adriamycin (NSC-123127) pharmacology, *Cancer Chemother. Rep. Part 3* **6**:153.

BAKAL, D., GOODMAN, L. E., ULFOHN, A., MAMARIL, A. G., CAPLAN, Y. H., CALLE, S., BHAGAVAN, B. S., WITTEN, B., WILLIAMSON, C. E., SASS, S., AND SELIGMAN, A. M., 1971, Enzyme alterable alkylating agents. XI. Clinical trials of an esterase-susceptible water-soluble agent (S-73) for regional chemotherapy, *J. Surg. Res.* **11**:217.

BENGMARK, S., AND HAFSTRÖM, L., 1969, The natural history of primary and secondary malignant tumors of the liver. I. The prognosis for patients with hepatic metastases from colonic and rectal carcinoma by laparotomy, *Cancer* **23**:198.

BERDAL, P., EKROLL, T., IVERSEN, O. H., AND WEYDE, R., 1973, Treatment of squamous cell carcinomas in head and neck with bleomycin and with combined bleomycin and x-rays, *Acta Otolaryngol.* **75**:318.

BERN, M., PARKER, L., OBERFIELD, R., CADY, B., MCDERMOTT, W., CLOUSE, M., TREY, C., AND FREI, E., III, 1976, Adriamycin therapy by hepatic artery infusion: Clinical and pharmacologic study, *Proc. Amer. Assoc. Cancer Res. Amer. Soc. Clin. Oncol.: Amer. Soc. Clin. Oncol. Abstr.*, p. 272.

BIERMAN, H. R., BYRON, R. L., KELLEY, K. H., AND GRADY, A., 1951, Studies on the blood supply of tumors in man. III. Vascular patterns of the liver by hepatic arteriography *in vivo*, *J. Natl. Cancer Inst.* **12**:107.

BREEDIS, C., AND YOUNG, G., 1954, The blood supply of neoplasms in the liver, *Amer. J. Pathol.* **30**:969.

BURROWS, J. H., TALLEY, R. W., DRAKE, E. H., SAN DIEGO, E. L., AND TUCKER, W. G., 1967, Infusion of fluorinated pyrimidines into hepatic artery for treatment of metastatic carcinoma of liver, *Cancer* **20**:1886.

CADY, B., 1973, Hepatic arterial patency and complications after catheterization for infusion chemotherapy, *Ann. Surg.* **178(2)**:156.

CADY, B., AND OBERFIELD, R. A., 1974a, Arterial infusion chemotherapy of hepatoma, *Surg. Gynecol. Obstet.* **138**:381.

CADY, B., AND OBERFIELD, R. A., 1974b, Regional infusion chemotherapy of hepatic metastases from carcinoma of the colon, *Amer. J. Surg.* **127**:220.

CADY, B., MONSON, D. O., AND SWINTON, N. W., 1970, Survival of patients after colonic resection for carcinoma with simultaneous liver metastases, *Surg. Gynecol. Obstet.* **131**:697.

CLARKSON, B., YOUNG, C., DIERICH, W., KUEHN, P., KIM, M., BLARETT, A., CLAPP, P., AND LAWRENCE, W., JR., 1962, Effects of continuous hepatic artery infusion of antimetabolites on primary and metastatic cancer of the liver, *Cancer* **15**:472.

CLEVELAND, J. C., JOHNS, D. G., FARNHAN, G., AND BERTINO, J. R., 1969, Arterial infusion of dichloromethotrexate in cancer of the head and neck: A clinico-pharmacologic study, *Curr. Top. Surg. Res.* **1**:113.

CLIFFTON, E. E., 1969, Bronchial artery perfusion for treatment of advanced lung cancer, *Cancer* **23**:1151.

CONRAD, M. E., AND CROSBY, W. H., 1960, Massive nitrogen mustard therapy in Hodgkin's disease with protection of bone marrow by tourniquets, *Blood* **16**:1089.

CREECH, O., JR., KREMENTZ, E. T., RYAN, R. F., AND WINBLAD, J. N., 1958, Chemotherapy of cancer: Regional perfusion utilizing an extracorporeal circuit, *Ann. Surg.* **148**:616.

CREECH, O., JR., KREMENTZ, E. T., RYAN, R. F., REEMTSMA, K., AND WINBLAD, J. N., 1959, Experiences with isolation–perfusion technics in the treatment of cancer, *Ann. Surg.* **149**:627.

CRUZ, A. B., JR., MCINNIS, W. D., AND AUST, J. B., 1974, Triple drug intra-arterial infusion combined with x-ray therapy and surgery for head and neck cancer, *Amer. J. Surg.* **128**:573.

DONEGAN, W. L., HARRIS, H. S., AND SPRATT, J. S., JR., 1969, Prolonged continuous hepatic infusion. Results with fluorouracil for primary and metastatic cancer in the liver, *Arch. Surg.* **99**:149.

FISHER, B., FISHER, E. R., AND LEE, S. H., 1961, The effect of alteration of liver blood flow upon experimental hepatic metastases, *Surg. Gynecol. Obstet.* **112**:11.

FORTNER, J. G., MULCARE, R. J., SOLIS, A., WATSON, R. C., AND GOLBEY, R. B., 1973, Treatment of primary and secondary liver cancer by hepatic artery ligation and infusion chemotherapy, *Ann. Surg.* **178(2)**:162.

FORTNER, J. G., KIM, D. K., BARETT, M. K., AND GOLBEY, R. B., 1976, Intrahepatic infusional chemotherapy using multiple agents for cancer in the liver, *Proc. Amer. Assoc. Cancer Res. Amer. Soc. Clin. Oncol.: Amer. Soc. Clin. Oncol. Abstr.*, p. 293.

FORTUNY, I. E., THEOLOGIDES, A., AND KENNEDY, B. J., 1975, Hepatic arterial infusion for liver metastases from colon cancer: Comparison of mitomycin C (NSC-26980) and 5-fluorouracil (NSC-19893), *Cancer Chemother. Rep.* **59**:401.

FRIEDMAN, M., AND DALY, J. F., 1963, Combined irradiation and chemotherapy in the treatment of squamous cell carcinoma of the head and neck, *Amer. J. Roentgenol.* **90**:246.

GALANTE, M., DUNPHY, J. E., AND FLETCHER, W. S., 1967, Cancer of the colon, *Ann. Surg.* **165**:732.

GEDDES, E. W., AND FALKSON, G., 1970, Malignant hepatoma in the Bantu, *Cancer* **25**:1271.

GOEPFERT, H., JESSE, R. H., AND LINDBERG, R. D., 1973, Arterial infusion and radiation therapy in the treatment of advanced cancer of the nasal cavity and paranasal sinuses, *Amer. J. Surg.* **126**:464.

GOFFINET, D. R., BROWN, J. M., BAGSHAW, M. A., AND KAPLAN, H. S., 1972, Prolonged carotid arterial radiosensitizer infusion and radiation therapy of mouse gliomas, *Amer. J. Roentgenol.* **114**:7.

GOLDMAN, M. L., BILBAO, M. K., RÖSCH, J., AND DOTTER, C. T., 1975, Complications of indwelling chemotherapy catheters, *Cancer* **36**:1983.

GOODMAN, L. E., KRAMER, S. P., GABY, S. D., BAKAL, D., SOLOMON, R. D., WILLIAMSON, C. E., MILLER, J. I., SASS, S., WITTEN, B., AND SELIGMAN, A. M., 1962, Enzyme alterable alkylating agents. II. Clinical evaluation of N,N'-bis[(2-chloroethylthio)acetyl]-1,2-ethylenediamine (S-46), *Cancer* **15**:1056.

GOODMAN, L. E., ULFOHN, A., KRAMER, S. P., CENDANA, E. H., FLORES, A. B., BAKAL, D., ABRAMS, S. J., HIRSCHFELD, R. L., CALLE, S., WILLIAMSON, C. E., SASS, S., WITTEN, B., AND SELIGMAN, A. M., 1965, Enzyme alterable alkylating agents: VIII. Clinical trials with intra-arterial infusion of an alkylating agent with a half-life of 0.2 second, *Ann. Surg.* **162**:663.

HARRISON, N. W., DHRU, D., PRIMACK, A., BHANA, D., AND KYALWAZI, S. K., 1973, The surgical management of primary hepatocellular carcinoma in Uganda, *Br. J. Surg.* **60**:565.

HASKELL, C. M., EILBER, F. R., AND MORTON, D. L., 1975, Adriamycin (NSC-123127) by arterial infusion, *Cancer Chemother. Rep.* **6**:187.

HEALEY, J. E., JR., 1965, Vascular patterns in human metastatic liver tumors, *Surg. Gynecol. Obstet.* **120**:1187.

HENDERSON, I. W. D., AND MADDOCK, C. I., 1963, Chemotherapeutic approach to inoperable pulmonary lesions, *Cancer* **16**:708.

HUNTINGTON, M. C., DUPRIEST, R. W., AND FLETCHER, W. S., 1973, Intra-arterial bleomycin therapy in inoperable squamous cell carcinomas, *Cancer* **31**:153.

HURLEY, J. D., WALL, T., WORMAN, L. W., AND SCHULTE, W. J., 1961, Experiences with pelvic perfusion for carcinoma, *Arch. Surg.* **83**:127.

JAFFE, B. M., DONEGAN, W. L., WATSON, F., AND SPRATT, J. S., JR., 1968, Factors influencing survival in patients with untreated hepatic metastases, *Surg. Gynecol. Obstet.* **127**:1.

JESSE, R. H., GOEPFERT, H., LINDBERG, R. D., AND JOHNSON, R. H., 1969, Combined intra-arterial infusion and radiotherapy for the treatment of advanced cancer of the head and neck, *Amer. J. Roentgenol.* **105**:20.

KAHN, C. R., LEVY, A. G., GARDNER, J. D., MILLER, J. V., GORDEN, P., AND SCHEIN, P. S., 1975, Pancreatic cholera: Beneficial effects of treatment with streptozotocin, *N. Engl. J. Med.* **292**:941.

KLOPP, C. T., ALFORD, T. C., BATEMAN, J., BERRY, G. N., AND WINSHIP, T., 1950, Fractionated intra-arterial cancer. Chemotherapy with methyl bis amine hydrochloride; a preliminary report, *Ann. Surg.* **132**:811.

KOYAMA, H., WADA, T., TAKAHASHI, Y., IWANAGA, T., AOKI, Y., WADA, A., TERAZAWA, T., AND KOSAKI, G., 1975, Intra-arterial infusion chemotherapy as a pre-operative treatment of locally advanced breast cancer, *Cancer* **36**:1603.

LABELLE, J. J., LUCAS, R. J., EISENSTEIN, B., REED, M. D., VAITKEVICIUS, V. K., AND WILSON, G. S., 1968, Hepatic artery catheterization for chemotherapy, *Arch. Surg.* **96**:683.

LAWRENCE, W., JR., KUEHN, P., MASLE, E. T., AND MILLER, D. G., 1961, An abdominal tourniquet for regional chemotherapy, *J. Surg. Res.* **1**:142.

MASSEY, W. H., FLETCHER, W. S., JUDKINS, M. P., AND DENNIS, D. L., 1971, Hepatic artery infusion for metastatic malignancy using percutaneously placed catheters, *Amer. J. Surg.* **121**:160.

MCBRIDE, C. M., 1970, Advanced melanoma of the extremities, *Arch. Surg.* **101**:122.

MEYZA, J., AND COBB, L. M., 1971, The clinical trial of an alkylating agent with a short half-life designed for intra-arterial chemotherapy, *Cancer* **27**:369.

MILLER, B. J., TALSANIA, S. J., AND CONNOLLY, J. M., JR., 1964, An improved method of intra-arterial infusion in the treatment of solid tumors by metabolite–anti-metabolite therapy, *Surg. Gynecol. Obstet.* **118**:555.

MUKHERJEE, K. L., CURRERI, A. R., JAVID, M., AND HEIDELBERG, C., 1963, Studies on fluorinated pyrimidines. XVI. Metabolism of 5-fluorouracil-2-C^{14} and 5-fluoro-2'-deoxyuridine-2-C^{14} in cancer patients, *Cancer Res.* **23**:67.

NEYAZAKA, T., IKEDA, M., SEKI, Y., EGAWA, N., AND SUZUKI, C., 1969, Bronchial artery infusion therapy for lung cancer, *Cancer* **24**:912.

OBERFIELD, R. A., 1974, Current status of regional arterial infusion chemotherapy, *Med. Clin. North Amer.* **59**:411.

OBERFIELD, R. A., CADY, B., AND BOOTH, J. C., 1973, Regional arterial chemotherapy for advanced carcinoma of the head and neck. A ten-year review, *Cancer* **32**:82.

OWLENY, C. L. M., AND MCINTIRE, K. R., 1974, Treatment of hepatocellular carcinoma (hc) with adriamycin, *Clin. Res.* **22**:494 (abstract).

ROCHLIN, D. B., AND SMART, C. R., 1966, An evaluation of 51 patients with hepatic artery infusion, *Surg. Gynecol. Obstet.* **123**:535.

SATO, Y., MORITA, M., TAKAHASHI, H., WATANABE, N., AND KIRIKAE, I., 1970, Combined surgery, radiotherapy, and regional chemotherapy in carcinoma of the paranasal sinuses, *Cancer* **25**:571.

SAVLOV, E. D., HALL, T. C., AND OBERFIELD, R. A., 1971, Intra-arterial therapy of melanoma with dimethyl triazeno imidazole carboxamide (NSC-45388), *Cancer* **28**:1161.

SCHILLING, A., ULFOHN, A., AYBAR, O., MILLER, S., KRAVITZ, S. C., GOODMAN, L. E., GABY, S. E., BAKAL, D., KRAMER, S. P., WILLIAMSON, C. E., SASS, S., MILLER, J. I., WITTEN, B., AND SELIGMAN, A. M., 1963, Enzyme-alterable alkylating agents. IV. Treatment of cancer in children with repetitive massive doses of S-46, protecting the extremity marrow by tourniquets, *Cancer* **16**:727.

SELIGMAN, A. M., ULFOHN, A., GABY, S. E., GOODMAN, L. E., AYBAR, O., KRAMER, S. P., BAKAL, D., HABER, S., WILLIAMSON, C. E., MILLER, J. I., SASS, S., AND WITTEN, B., 1962, Enzyme-alterable alkylating agents: A new approach to regional chemotherapy by intra-arterial infusion of new short-lived alkylating agents, *Ann. Surg.* **156**:429.

SIMON, N., WARNER, R. P. R., BARON, M. G., AND RUDAVSKY, A. Z., 1968, Intra-arterial irradiation of carcinoid tumors of the liver, *Amer. J. Roentgenol.* **102**:552.

SKIBBA, J. L., BEAL, D. D., RAMIREZ, G., AND BRYAN, G. T., 1970, N-Demethylation of the antineoplastic agent 4(5)-(3,3-dimethyl-1-triazeno)imidazole-5(4)-carboxamide by rats and man, *Cancer Res.* **30**:147.

SPARKS, F. C., MOSHER, M. B., HALLAUER, W. C., SILVERSTEIN, M. J., RANGEL, D., PASSARO, E., JR., AND MORTON, D. L., 1975, Hepatic artery ligation and postoperative chemotherapy for hepatic metastases: Clinical and pathophysiological results, *Cancer* **35**:1074.

STADIL, F., STAGE, G., REHFELD, J. F., EFSEN, F., AND FISCHERMAN, K., 1976, Treatment of Zollinger-Ellison syndrome with streptozotocin, *N. Engl. J. Med.* **294**:1440.

STEHLIN, J. S., JR., AND CLARK, R. L., 1965, Melanoma of the extremities. Experiences with conventional treatment and perfusion in 339 cases, *Amer. J. Surg.* **110**:366.

SULLIVAN, R. D., AND ZUREK, W. Z., 1965, Chemotherapy for liver cancer by protracted ambulatory infusion, *J. Amer. Med. Assoc.* **194**:93.

SULLIVAN, R. D., MILLER, E., AND SIKES, M. P., 1959, Antimetabolite–metabolite combination cancer chemotherapy. Effects of intra-arterial methotrexate–intramuscular citrovorum factor therapy in human cancer, *Cancer* **12**:1248.

SULLIVAN, R. D., WATKINS, E., JR., RODRIGUEZ, F. R., MILLER, E., AND NORCROSS, J. W., 1963, Continuous arterial infusion chemotherapy of human liver cancer using 5-fluoro-2'-deoxyuridine: Autodetoxification studies and clinical effects, *Proc. Amer. Assoc. Cancer Res.* **4**:66.

SULLIVAN, R. D., NORCROSS, J. W., AND WATKINS, E., JR., 1964, Chemotherapy of metastatic liver cancer by prolonged hepatic-artery infusion, *N. Engl. J. Med.* **270**:321.

SUZUKI, T., KAWABE, K., IMAMURA, M., ASAKUMA, R., AND HONJO, I., 1972, Percutaneous double catheter infusion technique for the treatment of carcinoma in the abdomen, *Surg. Gynecol. Obstet.* **134**:403.

TANDON, R. N., BUNNELL, I. L., AND COOPER, R. G., 1973, The treatment of metastatic carcinoma of the liver by the percutaneous selective hepatic artery infusion of 5-fluorouracil, *Surgery* **73**:118.

ULFOHN, A., KRAMER, S. P., CALLE, S., SASS, S., WILLIAMSON, C. E., WITTEN, B., AND SELIGMAN, A. M., 1968, Enzyme alterable alkylating agents. X. Experimental study of an esterase-susceptible water-soluble agent (S-73) for regional chemotherapy, *J. Surg. Res.* **8**:345.

WATKINS, E., JR., HERING, A. C., LUNA, R., AND ADAMS, H. D., 1960, The use of intravascular balloon catheters for isolation of the pelvic vascular bed during pump-oxygenator perfusion of cancer chemotherapeutic agents, *Surg. Gynecol. Obstet.* **111**:464.

WATKINS, E., JR., KHAZEI, A. M., AND NAHRA, K. S., 1970, Surgical basis for arterial infusion chemotherapy of disseminated carcinoma of the liver, *Surg. Gynecol. Obstet.* **130**:581.

WIRTANEN, G. W., 1973, Percutaneous transbrachial artery infusion catheter techniques, *Amer. J. Roentgenol.* **117**:696.

WITTEN, B., WILLIAMSON, C. E., SASS, S., MILLER, J. I., BEST, R., WICKS, G. E., JR., KRAMER, S. P., WEINBERG, T., SOLOMON, R. D., GOODMAN, L. E., AND SELIGMAN, A. M., 1962a, Enzyme-alterable alkylating agents. I. Synthesis, chemical properties and toxicities of sulfur mustards containing enzyme-susceptible amide bonds, *Cancer* **15:**1041.

WITTEN, B., SASS, S., MILLER, J. I., WILLIAMSON, C. E., GUERRERO, H. G., KRAMER, S. P., SOLOMON, R. D., GOODMAN, L. E., AND SELIGMAN, A. M., 1962b, Enzyme-alterable alkylating agents. III. Synthesis, chemical properties, and toxicities of mustards containing enzyme-susceptible ester bonds, *Cancer* **15:**1062.

8

Treatment of Malignant Disease in Closed Spaces

R. J. PAPAC

1. Malignant Pleural Effusions

Pleural effusion is a frequent complication in the course of disseminated neoplastic disease, and its development poses a variety of important problems in management. Its occurrence, while a manifestation of systemic disease, does not bear a relationship to prognosis, except perhaps in malignant lymphoma. While removal may be necessary for symptomatic relief, repeated thoracentesis may have significant complications. For this reason, ideal treatment should prevent fluid accumulation.

1.1. Pathogenesis

There are several mechanisms by which malignant pleural effusions develop. Most commonly, serosal nodules may exfoliate cells into the pleural space. The circulation of free tumor cells within the pleural space, without tumor nodules, may also give rise to effusion. A third mechanism is the obstruction of lymphatics of the mediastinal or hilar area, with an acellular transudate. This mechanism is most frequent in patients with malignant lymphoma, and may be associated with thoracic duct obstruction and chylous effusion. Table 1 shows the neoplastic

R. J. PAPAC • Yale University School of Medicine, New Haven, Connecticut, and West Haven Veterans Administration Hospital, West Haven, Connecticut.

TABLE 1

Most Frequent Types of Neoplasms in Malignant Pleural Effusions in Order of Decreasing Incidence[a]

1. Carcinoma of breast	6. Carcinoma arising in GI tract
2. Carcinoma of lung	7. Mesothelioma
3. Malignant lymphoma or leukemia	8. Carcinoma of uterus
4. Carcinoma of ovary	9. Carcinoma of kidney
5. Unknown primary	10. Sarcoma

[a] Based on data from the following 12 collected series: Izbick *et al.* (1975), Lambert *et al.* (1967), Dybicki *et al.* (1959). Bonte *et al.* (1956), Jones (1969), Adler and Rappole (1967), Camishion *et al.* (1962), Suhrland and Weisberger (1965), Anderson *et al* (1974), Ultmann *et al.* (1957), Jensik *et al.* (1963), and Leininger *et al.* (1969).

diseases most frequently associated with malignant pleural effusions. Carcinoma of the lung and breast occur with very nearly equal frequency as the cause of malignant effusion.

Since not all effusions in the course of a malignant disease are on a neoplastic basis, evaluation of the effusion is mandatory. Pulmonary infarcts, granulomatous pleuritis, tuberculosis, congestive failure, pancreatitis, and pulmonary infarctions must be excluded.

1.2. Diagnosis

Diagnostic evaluation of the fluid allows for gross inspection, determination of glucose, protein, complement, amylase, specific gravity, cultures, lactic dehydrogenase (LDH), and cytology. In addition to cytology, which identifies neoplastic cells in 50–75% of patients with malignant effusion, pleural biopsy yields a positive diagnosis in 50–55% of cases (Salyer *et al.*, 1975; VonHoff and Livolsi, 1975). Both procedures result in detection of malignancy in 90% of neoplastic effusions.

Malignant effusions may be serous or serosanguinous in appearance, and are generally exudates. The glucose content may be low, with high protein content (Clarkson, 1964). Lowered glucose concentration occurs not only with neoplasia, but also with tuberculosis and in rheumatoid arthritis (Gelenger and Wiggers, 1949; Lellington *et al.*, 1971). In rheumatoid arthritis and in lupus erythematosus, however, pleural fluid complement may be low (Hunder *et al.*, 1972). If the protein concentration is more than 3 g/dl, the fluid may be classified as an exudate (Carr and Power, 1958). A more accurate means of classifying exudates is to determine the ratio of protein in pleural fluid to serum and the ratio of LDH in pleural fluid to that in serum (Light *et al.*, 1972). In most exudates, the ratio of pleural fluid protein to serum protein is greater than 0.5, and the ratio of pleural fluid LDH to serum LDH is greater than 0.6.

If the pleural fluid does not appear grossly chylous, cholesterol concentration of 400 mg/dl fluid suggests chylothorax, as does a positive Sudan black stain (Roy *et al.*, 1967). Levels of heavy metals have been examined in patients with malignant effusion and found not to be helpful in differentiating benign from malignant effusions (Dines *et al.*, 1974). A positive regression curve of serum copper on pleural fluid copper was noted, with the best association in lymphoma.

Cytogenetic studies indicate abnormal chromosomes in all cases studied with neoplastic cells (Benedict and Porter, 1972). Some cases without neoplastic cells, however, showed chromosomal abnormalities on cytology.

1.3. Therapy

After a careful analysis of the effusion to exclude causes other than malignant disease, assessment of the underlying neoplastic disease must be made. In a patient whose disease requires systemic therapy, a trial of drainage of the chest fluid seems reasonable, combined with appropriate systemic treatment. Thoracentesis alone is known to be associated with frequent recurrence, generally symptomatic. Repeated thoracenteses increase the risk of pneumothorax, infection, and loculation of fluid, so that thoracentesis is not a recommended mode of management.

In a trial of pleural drainage alone (using a large thoracostomy tube), as compared with pleural drainage with the addition of radioactive phosphorus, pleural drainage controlled the effusion (no recurrence) in 17 of 39 episodes, as compared with 17 of 30 given the isotope in addition (Izbick *et al.*, 1975). Earlier studies demonstrated that tube drainage alone controlled the effusion with less morbidity and shorter hospitalization than instillational therapy (Lambert *et al.*, 1967).

Since it appears that tube drainage is almost as effective as instillational therapy, tube drainage would appear to be the most desirable initial approach. Should the fluid recur or systemic therapy fail, however, a trial of instillation therapy should be attempted.

The mechanism by which instillational agents are effective is presumed to be the local irritant action, causing adhesive pleuritis (Thorsnud, 1965). Antitumor effects locally are possible, but probably contribute little to effectiveness, since tumor types that are usually unresponsive to the cytotoxic agents used may show excellent response to intrapleural treatment. Systemic absorption may contribute somewhat to effectiveness in tumor types that are responsive to agents used.

In terms of specific instillational material, several types of agents have been employed. These agents include radioactive isotopes such as gold, phosphorus, yttrium, and yttrium–gold combination (Dybicki *et al.*, 1959; Bonte *et al.*, 1956; Jacobs, 1954; Card *et al.*, 1960). Sclerosing materials such as talc, quinacrine, and tetracycline have been tried (Jones, 1969; Adler and Rappole, 1967; Camishion *et al.*, 1962; Dollinger *et al.*, 1967; Borja and Pugh, 1973; Rubinson and Bolooki, 1972). Antineoplastic drugs such as 5-fluorouracil, nitrogen mustard, thioTEPA, and cytoxan have also been utilized (Bonte *et al.*, 1956; Suhrland and Weisberger, 1964; Ultmann *et al.*, 1957; Anderson *et al.*, 1974; Fracchia *et al.*, 1970; Rosato *et al.*, 1974; Leininger *et al.*, 1969).

Clinical studies with isotopes indicate, in rather small series, that about half the patients have no recurrence following administration of the isotope. The disadvantage of the use of the isotopes is that special precautions and facilities for handling the material are necessary. Radioactive chromic phosphate is preferred because it produces only beta particles; gold emits gamma and beta particles, necessitating isolation of patients for short periods.

There has been a 20-year experience with the use of chemotherapeutic agents in the control of malignant effusions by instillation into serous cavities. Nitrogen mustard has had extensive use, and on comparison with radioactive colloidal gold, is equally effective (Bonte *et al.*, 1956). There is some nausea and vomiting, as well as rather mild hematopoetic depression, associated with its use. The dosage for intrapleural use is the full systemic dose, 0.4 mg/kg. Other alkylating agents, notably thioTEPA and cyclophosphamide, are also effective agents in the control of malignant pleural effusions. They tend to cause less severe nausea, with diminished risk of necrosis on cutaneous contact. Alopecia can follow intrapleural use of cyclophosphamide.

The method of instillation is important. A chest tube should be inserted with a water seal drainage and the effusion drained off with the patient in a supine position. The agent to be used is then inserted and the chest tube clamped. Over an interval of 30 min to several hours, the position of the patient is varied to allow contact with a large area of pleural surface. The chest tube is reconnected to the drainage, and the tube drainage is observed. When fluid accumulation ceases, the tube is removed.

5-Fluorouracil compares favorably with other agents used in the management of neoplastic effusions. Recurrence developed in 34 of the initial series of 55 cases (Anderson *et al.*, 1974). Side effects are minimal (slight nausea and mild leukopenia), without reactive recurrence. A single injection of 500 or 1000 mg is used.

Sclerosing agents such as talc are also effective in controlling malignant pleural effusion. Talc is considered by some authors as the best agent, having been used in the treatment of spontaneous pneumothorax initially, and also having been shown to be effective when intrapleural antineoplastic agents have failed (Jones, 1969; Adler and Rappole, 1967; Camishion *et al.*, 1962). The results obtained with the use of talc indicate that few cases have recurrence of effusion. The disadvantage of talc is that it produces a painful pleuritis, and occasional cases of empyema have complicated its use. Additionally, it necessitates an insufflation technique or thoracostomy.

Quinacrine as a sclerosing agent is capable of inhibiting reoccurrence of effusion in about half the cases. Administration of 100–200 mg daily for 3–5 days is recommended, with careful monitoring of the effusion for infection and cell count (Dollinger *et al.*, 1967). Single doses are also employed with similar response, in terms of recurrence, while toxicity seems greater with the larger doses in both incidence and severity (Borja and Pugh, 1973). Side effects include local pain, fever in almost all cases to 103–104°F, occasional changes in skin pigmentation, and, rarely, hypertension and convulsions.

Tetracycline has not been reported in large series, but is clearly an effective means of controlling malignant pleural effusions (Rubinson and Bolooki, 1972). In the majority of cases, 500–100 mg given intrapleurally controls the effusion. Local discomfort is the only significant associated side effect.

Alternatives to instillational therapy, besides thoracostomy drainage, include pleurectomy with or without decortication (Jensik *et al.*, 1963; Martini *et al.*, 1975), hemithoracic irradiation (Strober *et al.*, 1973; Weick *et al.*, 1973), and the use of diuretics (Weeth and Segaloff, 1962).

Pleurectomy with or without decortication is often successful in carefully selected cases. Indications are failure to control the effusion by tube drainage and instillational agents, presence of trapped lung, and malignant effusion at thoracostomy (Martini *et al.*, 1975). The morbidity due to the procedure makes it necessary to be highly selective in patients whose life expectancy is limited, and whose general condition may not be good. Operative mortality of 6–27% is cited, with the lowest mortality associated with breast cancer cases (Jensik *et al.*, 1963; Martini *et al.*, 1975).

Irradiation is the treatment of choice when the effusion is a transudate related to large mediastinal masses (Strober *et al.*, 1973). If parenchymal or pleural involvement with lymphoma is associated with an effusion, and without extrathoracic disease, hemithoracic irradiation is the treatment recommended (Weick *et al.*, 1973). Intrapleural therapy has not been very successful in the management of effusions in patients with malignant lymphoma, unless combined with systemic treatment.

Hemithoracic irradiation is also useful, however, in the control of nonlymphomatous malignant effusions. About half the patients with recurrent effusions demonstrate control of such effusions (Jensik *et al.*, 1963).

There are instances of failure with two or more therapeutic attempts, and other means of controlling rapid accumulation of fluid must then be attempted. A trial with diuretics may be worthwhile, although there are no data available regarding relative efficacy. Beneficial results are reported with the combination of thiazide and spironolactone (Weeth and Segaloff, 1962).

There are remarkably few convincing studies to define optimal therapy for malignant pleural effusion, a frequent and troublesome complication of neoplastic disease. Considerations in management include whether it is a recurrent effusion, since tube thoracostomy is often successful in initial management; whether the systemic disease is in need of therapy and responsive to it; and whether the patient's general condition indicates the ability to withstand the contemplated procedures. It appears that the three types of instillational therapy discussed—sclerosing agents, radioactive isotopes, and cytotoxic agents—are almost equally effective in managing recurrent effusion. The least morbidity and greatest ease of administration appear to be associated with use of tetracycline, 5-fluorouracil, and alkylating agents. Should this method of treatment fail, hemithoracic irradiation (the treatment of choice for effusions in malignant lymphoma), pleurectomy, or diurectic therapy may be employed.

2. Malignant Peritoneal Effusions

R. J. PAPAC

Ascites in the course of malignant disease is often a distressing complication. Repeated removal of the fluid is symptomatically distressing to patients, and may result in depletion of protein.

2.1. Pathogenesis

The mechanisms by which effusion of the peritoneum occurs in malignant disease are predominantly seeding of the peritoneal surface by tumor or as a response to free-floating tumor cells. With regard to the distribution of intraabdominal malignant seeding, a recent study demonstrates the predominant sites to be dependent on the natural flow of ascites, occurring in preferential areas (Meyers, 1973). Chylous effusions may occur with damage to the cisterna chyli, but obstruction of lymphatic flow is an uncommon cause of ascites. Chylous ascites to the abdomen may also occur as a consequence of radiation therapy (Murray and Massey, 1974; Weinstein *et al.*, 1969).

Table 2 shows the types of neoplasms most frequently associated with malignant peritoneal effusions.

2.2. Diagnosis

Diagnostic study of ascitic fluid is essential to exclude nonmalignant causes. Renal disease, myxedema, cirrhosis, constrictive pericarditis, tuberculosis, and congestive heart failure must all be considered in the differential diagnosis. Additionally, ascites has followed radiation therapy for intraabdominal malignancy.

The diagnosis of ascites due to malignancy is based on cytological examination of the peritoneal fluid, reported as positive in about 50% of cases (Rosata *et al.*, 1974). Both smears and paraffin block of the centrifuged sediment should be examined. When the cytology is repeatedly negative, and the index of suspicion for carcinomatous ascites is high, peritoneoscopy or limited laparotomy may be indicated.

Another parameter suggested to differentiate benign from malignant ascites is determination of coagulation factors and fibrinolytic components of the ascitic

TABLE 2

Most Frequent Types of Neoplasms Causing Malignant Peritoneal Effusions in Order of Decreasing Incidence[a]

1. Ovary	5. Breast
2. Stomach	6. Lymphoma
3. Uterus	7. Mesothelioma
4. Unknown	

[a] Based on data from Dybicki *et al.* (1959), Bonte *et al.* (1956), Ultmann *et al.* (1957), Suhrland *et al.* (1965), Borja and Pugh (1973), and Pollack (1975).

fluid. In patients with ovarian carcinoma, large amounts of fibrin split products are found in ascitic fluid, as contrasted with cirrhosis and benign tumors (Svanberg and Astedt, 1975).

2.3. Therapy

Therapy of malignant effusions in the peritoneal cavity poses more problems than the management of pleural effusions; similarly, the data regarding efficacy of modalities used are sparse.

It appears that the best management is primary treatment of the specific neoplastic disease—radiation or chemotherapy, or both. Should fluid accumulation remain troublesome, diuretics or combinations thereof may be helpful, with careful monitoring of electrolytes (Weeth and Segaloff, 1962).

If the ascites is resistant to this type of management, instillational therapy could be attempted. Instillational therapy for recurrent ascites of neoplastic origin consists of the radioisotopes used to control pleural effusions, namely, gold, chromic phosphate, and yttrium (Dybicki *et al.*, 1959; Bonte *et al.*, 1956), alkylating agents (Bonte *et al.*, 1956; Ultmann *et al.*, 1957), 5-fluorouracil (Suhrland, 1965), and quinacrine (Borja and Pugh, 1973). Most reported series are small, and agents have been instilled often after the initial paracentesis. Criteria for benefit are not uniform but benefit is reported in about half the cases treated with alkylating agents and radioisotopes. Interestingly, the best results are reported in patients with ovarian carcinoma, suggesting that direct cytotoxicity plays a role in the effectiveness of peritoneal instillational agents (Ultmann *et al.*, 1957; Borja and Pugh, 1973). With 5-fluorouracil, in a group of 17 cases given intraperitoneal therapy, only 6 were improved (Suhrland and Weisberger, 1965). Quinacrine intraperitoneally controlled ascites in 1 of 4 trials, the 1 patient having a mesothelioma (Borja and Pugh, 1973). As a last resort, repeated trocar drainage may be necessary.

Instillational therapy into the peritoneal cavity seems less successful than intrapleural therapy. Complications are of greater significance with an increased tendency for loculation of fluid to occur. Adhesive peritonitis may result in episodes of bowel obstruction.

A surgical approach to malignant ascites, by draining the fluid through a one-way valve into a central vein, has been reported (Pollock, 1975). In a small series, long-term control of ascites developed in 5 of 10 cases, of whom 2 died before evaluation was possible. One patient who failed this treatment was felt to have developed obstruction to the valve by particulate matter.

In patients whose chylous ascites develops following radiation treatment (whole-abdomen) for carcinoma, a diet of medium-chain triglyceride and a diet with low fat has controlled the ascites (Murray and Massey, 1974; Weinstein *et al.*, 1969).

In summary, malignant ascites is best managed by systemic therapy of the underlying disease. If this therapy proves ineffective, instillational therapy with radiosiotopes or alkylating agents may be beneficial. Limited experience with a surgical approach suggests that this is an additional alternative for some cases.

3. Malignant Pericardial Effusions

Malignant pericardial effusions are of particular importance because of their life-threatening potential. Their occurrence may be insidious, or an effusion may develop as an abrupt fulminant episode.

3.1. Pathogenesis

The pathogenesis of pericardial effusions involves several mechanisms. Tumor implantation on serosal surfaces is probably the most frequent, although lymphatic obstruction by mediastinal or hilar masses is documented experimentally as a cause of pericardial transudation (Lokich, 1973).

When pericardial effusion develops in the course of, or following, mediastinal irradiation, the pathogenetic mechanisms involve pericardial lymphatic obstruction, probably on an inflammatory basis (Buckdeschel *et al.*, 1975).

Table 3 shows the types of neoplasms most frequently associated with malignant pericardial effusions.

3.2. Diagnosis

Diagnostic approaches to pericardial effusion involve initially those studies that define the presence of effusion. The classic signs may be subtle, so that specific techniques may be helpful. The echocardiogram is the preferred method of establishing the diagnosis, detecting an ultrasound echo from the pericardium distinct from that produced by the posterior heart border (Soulen *et al.*, 1966). Ancillary procedures include simultaneous cardiac and lung scans to demonstrate an increased space between the heart and lungs or liver (Charkes and Skalroff, 1963), intravenous injection of carbon dioxide to form a radiolucent interface along the inner right heart border (Shuford *et al.*, 1966), and cardiac catheterization with angiography.

TABLE 3
Most Frequent Types of Neoplasms Causing Pericardial Effusions in Decreasing Order of Incidence[a]

1. Leukemia, lymphoma	2. Breast	3. Lung

[a] Data based on Terry and Kligerman (1970) and Bachman *et al.* (1954).

Pericardiocentesis is important to establish the presence of malignant effusion cytologically (Lokich, 1973). Simultaneous injection of air, after removal of fluid, may outline irregularities of pericardial contour due to tumor implants. As in other types of effusions suspected of being malignant, cultures should be obtained, as well as protein, LDH, and glucose, to exclude nonmalignant causes.

3.3. Therapy

The therapeutic approaches to the management of malignant pericardial effusion are similar to those of effusion in other serous cavities. If possible and when indicated, systemic treatment for the disseminated neoplastic disease is the initial attempt. When systemic therapy is proved to be of little benefit (i.e., malignant melanoma, carcinoma of the lung), local therapy is appropriate if the fluid recurs following pericardiocentesis. This therapy may consist in radiation, intracavity therapy, or surgery.

In rapidly progressive malignant pericardial effusions, radiotherapy consisting of 2000–4000 rads delivered to the cardiac and lower mediastinal region successfully controls about half the effusions. It is initiated promptly following diagnostic pericardiocentesis and establishment of the malignant etiology (Lokich, 1973). In the control of effusions with lymphoma and leukemia, radiotherapy is particularly effective, although the number of cited cases is small (Terry and Kligerman, 1970; Smith et al., 1974).

In patients whose earlier treatment includes radiotherapy to the mediastinum with the likelihood of inclusion of the pericardium in the area of treatment, other forms of treatment must be employed.

Intracavity therapy has been reported in relatively small numbers of reported cases. The agents used are the radioactive isotopes (primarily gold[198]) (Bachman et al., 1954; Dollinger et al., 1967), 5-fluorouracil (Dollinger et al., 1967), alkylating agents (Bachman et al., 1954; Dollinger et al., 1967), and quinacrine (Smith et al., 1974; Dollinger et al., 1967).

With the use of intracavitary gold, occasional instances of control are cited. In the few reported cases, it seems less effective than in the management of pleural effusion; that is, benefits consisted of control of effusion for several weeks or months, followed by recurrence.

5-Fluorouracil, which, again, is reported in very few cases, is considered advantageous because reactive effusions following instillation with alkylating agents did not occur, and side effects are minimal.

The surgical approach to the palliation of malignant pericardial effusions involves establishing a pleural pericardial window or stripping the pericardium. A surgical attempt is recommended when systemic or intracavitary treatment, or both, fails to control the recurrent effusions, and when cardiac tamponade is a consequence of the recurrent effusion (Fredriksen et al., 1971; Hill and Cohen, 1970).

Involvement of the meningeal space by neoplastic disease presents interesting problems of detection and management. Certain malignant diseases appear to have a predilection to involve this space, but there is also an increasing frequency of this complication in diseases that in the past have only rarely been reported to involve the leptomeninges (Griffin *et al.*, 1971; Wolk *et al.*, 1974; Bunn *et al.*, 1976). This increasing frequency may be a natural consequence of longer survival in these diseases, enabling foci of cells to proliferate in an area in which optimal amounts of systemic therapy may not permeate the blood–brain barrier.

Cerebrospinal involvement by lymphoblastic leukemia in childhood is a well-recognized entity (Moore *et al.*, 1960; Evans *et al.*, 1970; West *et al.*, 1972). Recent reports suggest that a greater percentage of adults with acute leukemia demonstrate evidence of CNS leukemia; the improved remission rates may be responsible for the increasing frequency of this complication (Wolk *et al.*, 1974). The incidence of clinically evident and autopsy-evident leukemic involvement in acute lymphoblastic leukemia in adults is almost identical (Wolk *et al.*, 1974). There is, however, a disparity between clinically evident and autopsy-observed incidence in acute myelocytic and blast crisis of chronic granulocytic leukemia, with much higher autopsy findings (McKee and Collins, 1974). Of acute myelocytic leukemia cases, 19% had evidence of leukemic CNS involvement at autopsy, and only 6.5% clinically; 39% of blast crisis cases at postmortem showed leukemic CNS involvement, with 3.5% clinically significant (Wolk *et al.*, 1974). In chronic leukemias, it is exceptional to find clinical complications associated with leukemic infiltrations, although there is often pathological evidence for them (Wolk *et al.*, 1974).

Leptomeningeal involvement in patients with malignant lymphoma is considered rare, but recent studies suggest an increasing incidence of this complication in diffuse hystiocytic lymphoma and diffuse undifferentiated lymphoma (Griffin *et al.*, 1971; Bunn *et al.*, 1976).

Patients with the American form of Burkitt's lymphoma tend to show involvement of the dura and leptomeninges more frequently than patients with other forms of lymphocytic lymphoma (Banks *et al.*, 1975). Leptomeningeal syndromes rarely occur in mycosis fungoides and multiple myeloma (Hauch *et al.*, 1975; Afifi, 1974).

Carcinomatous meningitis is probably more frequent than suspected. The spectrum of clinical findings is wider than generally appreciated, and it has been reported with virtually all types of solid tumors.

4.1. Pathogenesis

Increased survival of patients with acute lymphoblastic leukemia is presumed to be related to CNS involvement (Evans *et al.*, 1970; Moore *et al.*, 1960; West *et al.*, 1972). Systemic disease may be controlled, while the CNS is a "sanctuary" for malignant cell proliferation. In patients with leukemia, it is suggested that malignant cells spread from the medullary cavity through the dura and into the arachnoid space, which is in continuity with the perivascular space, as reported by Thomas, and confirmed by others (Thomas, 1965; Price and Johnson, 1973). Such seeding produces neurological deficit by direct infiltration of cortex, cranial, and spinal nerves, and may cause obstruction of CSF pathways.

Lymphomatous leptomeningitis shows a consistent correlation of bone marrow tumor with CNS disease. In patients with diffuse histiocytic lymphoma and Burkitt's lymphoma, the pathological findings are identical to those observed in leukemia (Bunn *et al.*, 1976; Banks *et al.*, 1975). For this reason, the method of spread is presumed to be similar.

Metastases of carcinoma to the leptomeninges appear to be unrelated to cortical or ventricular lesions, although extension occurs, particularly into the spinal column (Little *et al.*, 1974).

4.2. Diagnosis

The signs and symptoms of meningeal involvement in leukemia are primarily those of increased intracranial pressure. Headache, lethargy, and vomiting may occur, and examination may show papilledema and nuchal rigidity. Meningeal involvement, however, can be detected in asymptomatic patients, and in those with blood and marrow remission of disease (Wolk *et al.*, 1974).

The diagnosis is based on the spinal fluid findings. Spinal fluid cytology may be difficult, so that careful morphological study is essential. This study may involve a membrane filtration technique concentrating the cells, resuspension in serum, or use of the cytocentrifuge. The actual cell number may not be high (Aaronson *et al.*, 1975). The protein content of the spinal fluid is usually elevated and the sugar content decreased, in inverse relationship to the spinal fluid pleocytosis. Opening pressures may be elevated.

The differential diagnosis includes subarachnoid hemorrhage, and bacterial, fungal, and viral meningitis or encephalitis. Cultures are essential, as well as India ink preparations. Occasionally, leptomeningial involvement and infectious meningitis coexist (Morganroth *et al.*, 1972).

In general, the signs and symptoms of lymphomatous involvement of the meninges are similar to those observed with leukemic involvement. Alterations in mental status are common, as well as cranial nerve palsies, meningismus, papilledema, and headaches.

CSF examination yields positive cytology in almost all cases; the protein content is generally elevated, with concentrations up to 2 g/100 ml; glucose concentrations are decreased in about one-third to one-half the patients (Griffin *et al.*, 1971; Bunn *et al.*, 1976). Cell counts tend to be in excess of 30 cells/mm^3, with positive cytology.

In carcinomatous meningitis, the presenting signs are more commonly headache and extremity and back pain. Cranial nerve palsies and altered mental status are late manifestations. The CSF examination more frequently (three-fourths of cases) shows decreased glucose and increased protein content (Little *et al.*, 1974). Cytological examination may require several sequential examinations because of difficulty in identification of cell type, but the majority of cases show positive cytology. Other procedures such as brain scan, EEG, and angiography are useful only in excluding other neurological lesions.

4.3. Therapy

Because of the frequency of CNS involvement in acute lymphoblastic leukemia in childhood, attempts have been made to eradicate undetectable cells by preventive therapy. The preventive value of CNS irradiation was demonstrated early when CNS leukemia terminated remissions in one-half the children who did not receive it, compared with fewer than 3% of those who did (Aur *et al.*, 1972). Studies have employed craniospinal irradiation simultaneously with intrathecal methotrexate (MTX) and craniospinal irradiation alone at varying dose levels (Simone *et al.*, 1975).

Present conclusions regarding effective prophylaxis of CNS leukemia are that craniospinal irradiation of 2400 rads is as effective as 2400 rads cranial combined with intrathecal MTX (Aur *et al.*, 1973). MTX is administered on the 2nd and 3rd days as 12 mg/M^2 repeated every 3 days for a total of 5 injections. For children aged 1–2 years, the dose of cranial vault irradiation is 2000 rads, and for those under 1 year, 1500 rads. Pyrimithamine is also reported to be an effective agent for prophylaxis of CNS leukemia (Hamers *et al.*, 1974).

Should CNS leukemia develop following prophylactic treatment, intrathecal MTX may be used. Indeed, it appears that intrathecal MTX (15 mg/M^2 every 2 or 3 days until abnormal cells disappear from the CSF) is as effective as 2400 rads to the cranial vault with MTX (Duttera *et al.*, 1973). Intrathecal MTX is effective even when systemic resistance to the drug has developed. Adding spinal irradiation to the cranial therapy offers therapeutic advantage, however (Willoughby, 1974).

If severe toxic reactions to MTX occur, or if MTX becomes ineffective, cytosine arabinoside may be useful (Band *et al.*, 1973). It appears to be well tolerated in doses of 48–384/mg/M^2. Systemic nitrosourea therapy has also been tried in cases of meningeal leukemia, but is not yet adequately evaluated (Wolk *et al.*, 1974).

In patients with leptomeningeal lymphoma, therapy has not been uniform in an adequate number of cases to draw firm conclusions regarding optimal management. Radiation is usually employed, in doses of 3000 rads to the craniospinal region (Griffin *et al.*, 1971; Bunn *et al.*, 1976). Intrathecal drugs, MTX, 12–15 mg/M^2 twice weekly, or cytosine arabinoside, 30 mg/M^2 twice weekly, are continued until the CSF is normal. In one series, 7 of 14 cases responded to drugs with irradiation; 3 patients had no residual meningeal tumor at the autopsy. All patients responded to either drugs or radiotherapy (Bunn *et al.*, 1976). Since leptomeningeal involvement tends to occur in the context of generalized systemic involvement, the impact of craniospinal irradiation and intrathecal MTX on marrow reserve may be considerable, in patients receiving systemic treatment. For this reason, citrovorum factor is often used with MTX to protect marrow reserve.

Treatment of meningeal carcinomatosis is generally considered unsatisfactory. Isolated reports cite benefit from irradiation and intrathecal MTX. A patient with breast carcinoma and another with adenocarcinoma of the lung showed disappearance of symptoms and abnormal CSF cytology with intrathecal MTX (Bender, 1974; McKelvey, 1968). Of 37 cases from the Memorial Hospital, 14 improved with radiotherapy, and 4 of 25 given intrathecal MTX were benefited (Posner, 1971).

Because of the difficulty of repeated lumbar punctures in the management of leukemic and carcinomatous meningitis, a ventricular cannula, an Ommaya device, is employed in some centers (Galicich and Guido, 1974). This device assures distribution and diffusion of drugs within the ventricular system, in the event that lumbar or subdural trapping occurs. Contraindications to the use of the device are severe thrombopenia and granulopenia.

There are some reports of serious complications from intrathecal instillation of MTX (McIntosh et al., 1976; Duttera et al., 1973; Rubinstein et al., 1975). Arachnoiditis, encephalopathy, and demyelination can occur. A postirradiation syndrome with fever, somnabulance, and EEG abnormalities is recognized (Garwicz et al., 1975). Prospective studies will yield data regarding the long-term effects of CNS therapy on intellectual performance, behavior patterns, and sensory or motor effects (Soni et al., 1975).

In summary, the principles invoked in management of malignant disease invading the meningeal area involve both prophylactic and therapeutic approaches. In diseases with a known predilection for this complication, namely, acute lymphoblastic leukemia, prophylactic treatment is shown to be beneficial. Trial of agents known to cross the blood–brain barrier, and development of newer agents with this capability, should provide a potentially useful approach for the future.

With increasing survival of patients with acute nonlymphocytic leukemia, it may be worthwhile to investigate the benefit of prophylactic CNS therapy in long-term survivors.

In patients with diffuse histiocytic and diffuse undifferentiated lymphoma, and with the American form of Burkitt's lymphoma, documentation of bone marrow involvement should stimulate a careful examination of the CNS, because of the correlation of the occurrence in these two sites. In asymptomatic cases with cytological evidence of involvement, prophylactic treatment should be investigated.

Therapeutic approaches to leptomeningeal involvement with neoplastic disease are primarily craniospinal irradiation and intrathecal instillation of cytotoxic agents.

5. References

AARONSON, A. G., HAJDU, S. I., AND MELAMED, M. R., 1975, Spinal fluid cytology during chemotherapy of leukemia of the central nervous system in children, Amer. J. Clin. Pathol. **63**:528.

ADLER, R. H., AND RAPPOLE, B. W., 1967, Recurrent malignant pleural effusions and talc powder aerosol treatment, Surgery **62** (6):1000.

AFIFI, A. M., 1974, Myeloma cells in the cerebrospinal fluid in plasma cell neoplasia, *J. Neurol Neurosurg. Psychiatry* **37**:1162.

ANDERSON, C. B., PHILPOTT, G. W., AND FERGUSON, T. B., 1974, The treatment of malignant pleural effusions, *Cancer* **33**:916.

AUR, R. J. A., SIMONE, J. V., HUSTU, H. O., AND VERZOSA, M. S., 1972, A comparative study of central nervous sytem irradiation and intensive chemotherapy early in remission of childhood acute lymphocytic leukemia, *Cancer* **29**:381.

AUR, R. J. A., HUSTU, H. O., VERZOSA, M. S., WOOD, A., AND SIMONE, J. V., 1973, Comparison of two methods of preventing central nervous system leukemia, *Blood* **42**:349.

BACHMAN, K. P., FOSTER, C. G., JACKSON, M. A., SHERSHIN, P. H., AND OARD, H. C., 1954, Radioactive gold instilled intrapericardially: Report of a case, *Ann. Intern. Med.* **40**:811.

BAND, P. R., HOLLAND, J. F., BERNARD, J., WEIL, M., WALKER, M., AND RALL, D., 1973, Treatment of central nervous system leukemia with intrathecal cytosine arabinoside, *Cancer* **32**(4):744.

BANKS, P. M., ARSENEAU, J. C., GRALNICK, H. R., CANELLOS, G. P., DEVITA, V. T., JR., AND BERARD, C. W., 1975, American Burkitt's lymphoma: A clinicopathologic study of 30 cases, II. Pathologic correlations, *Amer. J. Med.* **58**:322.

BENDER, R. A., 1974, Meningeal carcinomatosis: Treatment with intrathecal methotrexate, *Oncology* **30**:328.

BENEDICT, W. F., AND PORTER, I. A., 1972, Cytogenic studies of malignancy in effusion, *Acta Cytol.* **16**:304.

BONTE, F. J., STORAASLI, J. P., AND WEISBERGER, A. S., 1956, Comparative evaluation of radioactive colloidal gold and nitrogen mustard in the treatment of serous effusions of neoplastic origin, *Radiology* **67**:63.

BORJA, E. R., AND PUGH, R. P., 1973, Single-dose quinacrine (atabrine) and thoracostomy in the control of pleural effusions in patients with neoplastic diseases, *Cancer* **31**:899.

BUCKDESCHEL, J. C., CHANG, P., MARTIN, R. G., BYHARDT, R. W., O'CONNEL, M. J., SUTHERLAND, J. C., AND WIERNIK, P. H., 1975, Radiation-related pericardial effusions in patients with Hodgkin's disease, *Medicine* **54**(3):245.

BUNN, P. A., JR., SCHEIN, P. S., BANKS, P. M., AND DEVITA, V. T., JR., 1976, Central nervous system complications in patients with diffuse histiocytic and undifferentiated lymphoma: Leukemia revisited, *Blood* **47**(1):3.

CAMISHION, R. C., GIBBON, J. H., JR., AND NEALON, T. F., JR., 1962, Talc poudrage in the treatment of pleural effusion due to cancer, *Surg. Clin. N. Amer.* **42**:1521.

CARD, R. Y., COLE, D. R., AND HENSCKKE, U. K., 1960, Summary of ten years of the use of radioactive colloids in intracavitary therapy, *J. Med.* **1**:195.

CARR, D. T., AND POWER, M. H., 1958, Clinical value of measurements of concentration of protein in pleural fluid, *N. Engl. J. Med.* **259**:926.

CHARKES, N. D., AND SKLAROFF, D. M., 1963, Radioisotope photoscanning as a diagnostic aid in cardiovascular disease, *J. Amer. Med. Assoc.* **186**:920.

CLARKSON, B., 1964, Relationship between cell type, glucose concentration, and response to treatment in neoplastic effusions, *Cancer* **17**:914.

DINES, D. E., ELVEBACK, L. A., AND McCALL, J. T., 1974, Zinc, copper and iron contents of pleural fluid in benign and neoplastic disease, *Mayo Clin. Proc.* **49**:102.

DOLLINGER, M. R., KRAKOFF, I. H., AND KARNOFSKY, D. A., 1967, Quinacrine (atabrine) in the treatment of neoplastic effusions, *Ann. Intern. Med.* **66**(2):249.

DUTTERA, M. J., BLEYER, W. A., POMEROY, T. C., LEVENTHAL, C. M., AND LEVENTHAL, B., 1973, Irradiation, methotrexate toxicity, and the treatment of meningeal leukaemia, *Lancet* **2**:703.

DYBICKI, J., BALCHUM, O. J., AND MENEELY, G. R., 1959, Treatment of pleural and peritoneal effusion with intracavitary colloidal radiogold (Au[198]), *Arch. Intern. Med.* **104**:802.

EVANS, A. E., GILBERT, E. S., AND ZANDSTRA, R., 1970, The increasing incidence of central nervous system leukemia in children, *Cancer* **26**:404.

FRACCHIA, A. A., KNAPPER, W. H., CAREY, J. T., AND FARROW, J. H., 1970, Intrapleural chemotherapy for effusion from metastatic breast carcinoma, *Cancer* **26**:626.

FREDRIKSEN, R. T., COHEN, L. S., AND MULLINS, C. B., 1971, Pericardial windows or pericardiocentesis for pericardial effusions, *Amer. Heart J.* **82**(2):158.

GALICICH, J. H., AND GUIDO, L. J., 1974, Ommaya device in carcinomatous and leukemic meningitis. Surgical experience in 45 cases, *Symp. Surg. Oncol.* **54**(4):915.

GARWICZ, S., ARONSON, A. S., ELMQVIST, D., AND LANDBERG, T., 1975, Postirradiation syndrome and EEG findings in children with acute lymphoblastic leukaemia, *Acta Paediatr. Scand.* **64**:399.

GELENGER, S. M., AND WIGGERS, R. F., 1949, Relationship of the pleural fluid sugar to pulmonary tuberculosis, *Dis. Chest.* **15**:325.

GRIFFIN, J. W., THOMPSON, R. W., MITCHINSON, M. J., DE KIEWIET, J. C., AND WELLAND, F. H., 1971, Lymphomatous leptomeningitis, *Amer. J. Med.* **51**:200.

HAMERS, J., VAN HOVE, W., AND BAELE, G., 1974, Pyrimethamine in prophylaxis of meningeal leukaemia, *Lancet* **1**:310.

HAUCH, T. W., SHELBOURNE, J. D., COHEN, H. J., MASON, D., AND KREMER, W. B., 1975, Meningeal mycosis fungoides: Clinical and cellular characteristics, *Ann. Intern. Med.* **82**:499.

HILL, G. J., II, AND COHEN, B. I., 1970, Pleural pericardial window for palliation of cardiac tamponade due to cancer, *Cancer* **26**(1):81.

HUNDER, G. G., MCDUFFIE, F. C., AND HEPPER, N. G. G., 1972, Pleural fluid complement in systemic lupus erythematosus and rheumatoid arthritis, *Ann. Intern. Med.* **76**:357.

IZBICK, R., WEYHING, B. T., BAKER, L., CAVILI, E. M., VAITKEVICIUS, V. K., AND CAOILI, E., 1975, Pleural effusion in cancer patients, *Cancer* **36**:1511.

JACOBS, M. L., 1954, Use of radioactive chromic phosphate in pleural effusions, *Calif. Med.* **81**:268.

JENSIK, R., CAGLE J., JR., MILLOY, F., PERLIA, C., TAYLOR, S., KOFMAN, S., AND BEATTIE, E. J., JR., 1963, Pleurectomy in the treatment of pleural effusion due to metastatic malignancy, *J. Thorac. Cardiovasc. Surg.* **46**(3):322.

JONES, G. R., 1969, Treatment of recurrent malignant pleural effusion by iodized talc pleurodesis, *Thorax* **24**:69.

LAMBERT, C. J., SHAH, H. H., URSCHEL, H. C., JR., AND PAULSON, D. L., 1967, The treatment of malignant pleural effusions by closed trocar tube drainage, *Ann. Thorac. Surg.* **3**(1):1.

LEININGER, B. J., BARKER, W. L., AND LANGSTON, H. T., 1969, A simplified method for management of malignant pleural effusion, *J. Thorac. Cardiovasc. Surg.* **58**(5):758.

LELLINGTON, G. A., CARR, B. T., AND MAYNE, J. G., 1971, Rheumatoid pleurisy with effusion, *Arch. Intern. Med.* **128**:764.

LIGHT, R. W., MACGREGOR, M. I., LUCHSINGER, P. C., AND BALL, W. C., JR., 1972, Pleural effusions: The diagnostic separation of transudates and exudates, *Ann. Intern. Med.* **77**:507.

LITTLE, J. R., DALE, A. J. D., AND OKAZAKI, H., 1974, Meningeal carcinomatosis, *Arch. Neurol.* **30**:138.

LOKICH, J. J., 1973, The management of malignant pericardial effusions, *J. Amer. Med. Assoc.* **224**(10):1401.

MARTINI, N., BAINS, M. S., AND BEATLIE, E. T., JR., 1975, Indications for pleurectomy in malignant effusion, *Cancer* **35**:734.

MCINTOSH, S., KLATSKIN, E. H., O'BRIAN, R. T., ASPNES, G. T., KAMERER, B. L., SNEAD, C., KALAVSKY, S. M., AND PEARSON, H. A., 1976, Chronic neurologic disturbance in childhood leukemia, *Cancer* **37**:853.

MCKEE, L. C., JR., AND COLLINS, R. D., 1974, Intravascular leukocyte thrombi and aggregates as a cause of morbidity and mortality in leukemia, *Medicine* **53**(6):463.

MCKELVEY, E. M., 1968, Meningeal involvement with metastatic carcinoma of the breast treated with intrathecal methotrexate, *Cancer* **22**(3):576.

MEYERS, M. A., 1973, Distribution of intra-abdominal malignant seeding: Dependency on dynamics of flow of ascitic fluid, *Amer. J. Roentgenol. Radium Ther. Nucl. Med.* **119**:198.

MOORE, E. W., THOMAS, L. B., SHAW, R. K., AND FREIREICH, E. J., 1960, The central nervous system in acute leukemia, *Arch. Intern. Med.* **105**:451.

MORGANROTH, J., DEISSEROTH, A., WINOKUR, S., AND SCHEIN, P., 1972, Differentiation of carcinomatous and bacterial meningitis, *Neurology* **22**:1240.

MURRAY, J. M., AND MASSEY, F. M., 1974, Chylous ascites after radiation therapy for ovarian cancer, *Obstet. Gynecol.* **44**(5):749.

POLLOCK, A. V., 1975, The treatment of resistant malignant ascites by insertion of a peritoneo-atrial holter valve, *Br. J. Surg.* **62**:104.

POSNER, J. B., 1971, Leptominingeal metastasis from systemic cancer, *Trans. Amer. Neurol. Assoc.* **96**:291.

PRICE, R. A., AND JOHNSON, W. W., 1973, The central nervous system in childhood leukemia. I. The arachnoid, *Cancer* **31**:520.

ROSATO, F. E., WALLACH, M. W., AND ROSATO, E. F., 1974, The management of malignant effusions from breast cancer, *J. Surg. Oncol.* **6**(5):357.

ROY, P. H., CARR, B. T., AND PAYNE, P. S., 1967, The problem of chylothorax, *Mayo Clin. Proc.* **42**:457.

RUBINSON, R., AND BOLOOKI, H., 1972, Intrapleural tetracycline for control of malignant pleural effusion, *South. Med. J.* **65**:847.

RUBINSTEIN, L. J., HERMAN, M. M., LONG, T. F., AND WILBUR, R., JR., 1975, Disseminated necrotizing leukoencephalopathy: A complication of treated central nervous system leukemia and lymphoma, *Cancer* **35**:291.

SALYER, W. R., EGGLESTON, J. C., AND EROZAN, Y. S., 1975, Efficacy of pleural needle biopsy and pleural fluid cytopathology in the diagnosis of malignant neoplasm involving the pleura, *Chest* **67**(5):536.

SHUFORD, W. H., SYBERS, R. G., ACKER, J. J., AND WEENS, H. S., 1966, A comparison of carbon dioxide and radiopaque angiocardiographic methods in the diagnosis of pericardial effusion, *Radiology* **86**:1064.

SIMONE, J. V., AUR, R. J. A., HUSTU, H. O., AND VERZOSA, M., 1975, Acute lymphocytic leukemia in children, *Cancer* **36**:770.

SMITH, F. E., LANE, M., AND HUDGINS, P. T., 1974, Conservative management of malignant pericardial effusion, *Cancer* **33**(1):47.

SONI, S. S., MARTEN, G. W., PITNER, S. E., DUENAS, D. A., AND POWAZEK, M., 1975, Effects of central-nervous-system irradiation on neuropsychologic functioning of children with acute lymphocytic leukemia, *N. Engl. J. Med.* **293**(3):113.

SOULEN, R. L., LAPAYOWKER, M. S., AND GIMENEZ, T. L., 1966, Echocardiography in the diagnosis of pericardial effusion, *Radiology* **86**:1047.

STROBER, S. J., KLOTZ, E., KUPERMAN, A., AND GHOSSEIN, N. A., 1973, Malignant pleural disease. A radiotherapeutic approach to the problem, *J. Amer. Med. Assoc.* **226**(3):296.

SUHRLAND, L. G., AND WEISBERGER, A. S., 1965, Intracavitary 5-fluorouracil in malignant effusions, *Arch. Intern. Med.* **116**:431.

SVANBERG, L., AND ASTEDT, B., 1975, Coagulative and fibrinolytic properties of ascitic fluid associated with ovarian tumors, *Cancer* **35**:1382.

TERRY, L. N., JR., AND KLIGERMAN, M. M., 1970, Pericardial and myocardial involvement by lymphomas and leukemias; the role of radiotherapy, *Cancer* **25**:1003.

THOMAS, L. B., 1965, Pathology of leukemia in the brain and meninges—postmortem studies of patients with acute leukemia and of mice liver inoculations of L1210 leukemia, *Cancer Res.* **25**:1555.

THORSNUD, G. K., 1965, Pleural reactions to irritants, *Acta Chir. Scand. Suppl.* **335**:1.

ULTMANN, J. E., HYMAN, G. A., CRANDALL, C., NAUJOKS, H., AND GELLHORN, A., 1957, Triethylenethiophosphoramide (thioTEPA) in the treatment of neoplastic disease, *Cancer* **10**:902.

VONHOFF, D. D., AND LIVOLSI, V., 1975, Diagnostic reliability of needle biopsy of the parietal pleura. A review of 272 biopsies, *Amer. J. Clin. Pathol.* **64**:200.

WEETH, J. B., AND SEGALOFF, A., 1962, Diuretic therapy for malignant effusion, *J. Amer. Med. Assoc.* **181**(3):258.

WEICK, J. K., KIELY, J. M., HARRISON, E. G., JR., CARR, D. T., AND SCANLON, P. W., 1973, Pleural effusion in lymphoma, *Cancer* **31**:848.

WEINSTEIN, L. D., SCANLON, G. T., AND HERSH, T., 1969, Chylous ascites, *Amer. J. Dig. Dis.* **14**(7):500.

WEST, R. J., GRAHAM-POLE, J., HARDISTY, R. M., AND PIKE, M. C., 1972, Factors in pathogenesis of central-nervous-system leukemia, *Br. Med. J.*, **3**:311.

WILLOUGHBY, M. L. N., 1974, Treatment of overt meningeal leukaemia, *Lancet* **1**:363.

WOLK, R. W., MASSE, S. R., CONKLIN, R., AND FREIREICH, E. J., 1974, The incidence of central nervous system leukemia in adults with acute leukemia, *Cancer* **33**(3):863.

9

Supportive Care in the Cancer Patient

WILLIAM H. GREENE

1. Introduction

"Supportive care," as the term is currently used, embraces a large and diverse group of medical and paramedical specialties, of which the common bond is the minimization or prevention of the common complications of cancer and its therapy. Although not unique to those with malignancy, the art and science of caring for their social, psychological, and somatic distress have become more highly developed than for perhaps any other single patient group. There have been a number of recent reviews of all or parts of this field (Holland and Frei, 1973; Goepp and Hammond, 1975).

The interest that has been focused on supportive care in the cancer patient is heightened by the ubiquity and proximity of death. Nowhere is the confrontation with death more vivid than in the control of bleeding and infection, which together account for more than 90% of mortality in patients with hematologic malignancy and perhaps one-third to one-half that in patients with solid tumors (Bodey, 1975; H. Chang *et al.*, 1976). In contrast to psychosocial support workers, who attempt to ease the pain and fear of ultimate debilitation and death, at a time when effective therapy has been exhausted, supportive care in the management of infection and hemorrhage is concerned primarily with the avoidance of death, at a time when effective therapy has not yet been applied or applied only in part. Because infection and bleeding so often terminate life before potentially adequate tumor control can be administered, strenuous efforts at their prophylaxis and therapy have been undertaken. Advances in the rate of remission and duration of

WILLIAM H. GREENE • Department of Internal Medicine, Yale University School of Medicine, New Haven, Connecticut.

survival of patients with hematologic malignancy may well be due, in part, to advances in supportive care coincident with progress in antitumor therapy.

This chapter will deal with the causes and management of red cell loss and infectious complications in cancer patients, with attention to recent advances in the field. The reader is referred elsewhere for reviews of other aspects of supportive care (Holland and Frei, 1973; Goepp and Hammond, 1975).

2. Blood Loss

2.1. General Aspects

If "blood loss" is used broadly to mean any loss of a normally produced red cell mass, diverse clinical situations in cancer patients may cause such loss. These situations are summarized in Table 1. Prophylaxis and management of red blood

TABLE 1
Causes of Blood Loss Associated with Cancer

Mechanism of blood loss	Major clinical situations
I. Nonhemorrhagic	
A. Hemolytic	
1. Intravascular	
a. Immunologic	
i. Cold-reacting antibody	Malignant lymphoma
ii. ABO-incompatible transfusion	
b. Microangiopathic	Disseminated intravascular coagulation
	Vascular tumors (hemangiomas)
	Disseminated carcinoma
c. Septic	*Clostridum perfringens* sepsis
	(GI, GU malignancy)
2. Extravascular	
a. Immunologic	Lymphoproliferative, ovarian neoplasia
i. Warm-reacting antibody	Chronic lymphocytic leukemia
ii. Cold-reacting antibody	Malignant lymphoma
B. Sequestration	
1. Hypersplenism	Hematologic malignancy
	Chronic leukemia, malignant lymphoma
2. Erythrophagocytosis	Histiocytic medullary reticulosis
3. Anemia of chronic disease	Duration of disease >2 months
II. Hemorrhagic	
A. Loss of vascular integrity	
1. Tumor proliferation	
a. Erosion	GI, GU,
	head and neck malignancy
b. Vascular plugging	
i. Tumor emboli	To lung—hypernephroma
	To arteries—cardiac myxomas, lung
	carcinoma
ii. Leukocyte thrombi	Acute leukemia

TABLE 1—*continued*

225

SUPPORTIVE
CARE
IN THE
CANCER
PATIENT

Mechanism of blood loss	Major clinical situations
II. Hemorrhagic (*continued*)	
2. Thrombocytopenia	
3. Drug-induced	Corticosteroids
4. Infection	*Pseudomonas aeruginosa*
	Aspergillus and *Mucor* infection
5. Other	Inanition, amyloid
B. Abnormalities of clotting	
1. Decreased synthesis	Vitamin K deficiency; hepatic disease
2. Increased consumption	
a. Disseminated intravascular coagulation (DIC)	
i. Tumor-associated	Acute progranulocytic leukemia
	Rapid cell lysis
ii. Infection-associated	Gram-negative sepsis
b. Circulating anticoagulant	Lymphoproliferative disease; paraproteinemias
C. Abnormalities of platelets	
1. Quantitative	
a. Thrombocytopenia	
i. Decreased production	Marrow infiltration, drug effect
ii. Sequestration	Hypersplenism
iii. Increased utilization	"Idiopathic" thrombocytopenic purpura; DIC
b. Thrombocytosis	Myeloproliferative disease
2. Qualitative	
a. Tumor-associated	Myeloproliferative disease; multiple myeloma
b. Drug-induced	Carbenicillin, aspirin, others
c. Metabolic dysfunction	Uremia, hepatic disease
D. Miscellaneous	
1. Mucosal ulcerations	
a. Stress-induced	"Stress" ulcers
b. Tumor-induced	
c. Drug-induced	Corticosteroids, cytotoxic agents
d. Infection-induced	
2. Marantic endocarditis	
3. Vascular tumors	
4. Hyperviscosity	Paraproteinemias

cell (RBC) depletion must be predicated on a knowledge of the mechanisms by which the depletion occurs. The following discussion distinguishes the diminution of red cell mass by whether or not there is evidence of hemorrhage (Holland and Frei, 1973).

2.2. Nonhemorrhagic Red Cell Loss

As indicated in Table 1, this form of loss can be subdivided into loss that is a result of sequestration of an excess of essentially normal RBCs, usually in reticuloendothelial tissue, and loss that is secondary to destruction or removal of RBCs because they are damaged, i.e., the hemolytic disorders. Because bleeding is not evident in these situations, the diagnosis of accelerated blood loss, if not considered, may go unrecognized, particularly when the bone marrow has sufficient proliferative capacity to compensate for the RBC destruction. In the cancer patient, the diagnosis of cancer will usually be followed by a therapeutic modality, i.e., surgery, radiation therapy, or chemotherapy, or some combination thereof, that will have a marrow-depressive effect. In the face of increased RBC removal, the resulting fall in peripheral blood hematocrit may be rapid and even precipitous. Not only does this pose its own physiological threat, but the rapidity of fall may suggest hemorrhage. The patient with malignancy, especially the patient with a hematologic neoplasm, deserves to have an early evaluation of nonhemorrhagic red cell loss, including a reticulocyte count and direct Coombs' test.

2.2.1. Hemolytic Disease

Hemolysis may be "intravascular," with hemoglobin release into plasma and urine and hemosiderin in urine, or "extravascular," but within the reticuloendothelial system (RES). The predominant mode of hemolysis, in general and among cancer patients specifically, is of the latter type.

   a. Intravascular Hemolysis. Except for hemolytic transfusion reactions, usually secondary to ABO-incompatibility (when significant intravascular hemolysis is present; Masouredis, 1972), immune hemolysis with clinically apparent release of free hemoglobin is an uncommon event more often associated with cold-reacting antibody than with the warm-reacting variety. These conditions will be further discussed below.

   In microangiopathic hemolytic disorders, which are uncommon, red cell fragmentation is due to the physical trauma of passage through small vessels altered by disease. In the most severe forms, there is evidence of hemoglobinemia and hemoglobinuria, but the hallmark of these states is the presence of markedly fragmented RBCs, or schistocytes, in the circulation. Among patients with neoplasia, several mechanisms for microangiopathy have been invoked, among which are: (1) widespread tumor emboli (Wintrobe, 1974b); (2) tortuosity or local coagulation or both in the neoplastic blood vessels of giant hemangiomas and hepatic hemangioendotheliomas (Alpert and Benisch, 1970); (3) disseminated intravascular coagulation (DIC) (Whitecar, 1973). The first two mechanisms are present occasionally, but DIC is much more common, occurring as a result of the liberation into the bloodstream of thromboplastic substances derived either from infection, especially gram-negative septicemia (Yoshikawa *et al.*, 1971), or from the malignancy itself, particularly in acute progranulocytic leukemia (less often in other forms of hematologic malignancy), after chemotherapy-induced rapid cell lysis (Brodsky *et al.*, 1976), and in disseminated carcinoma, notably mucin-secreting adenocarcinomas (Brain *et al.*, 1970) of the stomach, colon, prostate, and other sites (Forshaw and Harwood, 1966). Although hemolysis is a frequent part of DIC, it is rarely life-threatening, and further discussion will be reserved for Section 2.3.

Although hemolysis has been reported as a part of many infections (Wintrobe, 1974a; Beutler, 1972), in cancer patients, only *Clostridium perfringens* sepsis seems to occur in excess incidence, particularly among those with extensive GI involvement or ulceration. In a minority of instances, *C. perfringens* sepsis is accompanied by massive intravascular hemolysis, probably due to the red-cell-membrane active exotoxin α-lecithinase elaborated by the organism. In such instances, hemolysis may proceed with extraordinary rapidity, and death may supervene prior to adequate antibiotic control. There is an association between hemolysis and *Salmonella* spp. infections, but the hemolysis appears to predispose to the infection, not vice versa.

b. Extravascular Hemolysis. "Extravascular hemolysis" is a misnomer, but generally refers to removal and destruction of RBCs occurring in the RES, particularly the spleen, largely because of changes in the cells' morphology or surface characteristics. As such, the removal is a normal function, a way of "weeding out" senescent or inefficient cells. What is pathological is the mechanism by which the cells have become altered. Apart from the isoimmune hemolysis of a mismatched transfusion, which may yield a transiently positive Coombs' test, the autoimmune hemolytic disorders in cancer patients are largely confined to those with hematologic malignancy, especially chronic lymphocytic leukemia (CLL) (in which the incidence has been estimated at 10–20%), Hodgkin's disease (HD), and non-Hodgkin's lymphoma (Pirofsky, 1968; Kremer and Laszlo, 1973). Rarely, these disorders are seen in patients with solid tumors, of which benign and occasionally malignant ovarian neoplasms are most frequent (Dawson *et al.*, 1971).

These "secondary" autoimmune hemolytic anemias (AIHA) can be categorized into two types by the kind of antibody found on the RBC surface: the more common warm-reacting (maximally active at 37°C) and the infrequent cold-reacting (maximally active at 2–4°C). The former are almost always IgG in type, are usually directed against the Rh substance, and are the typical finding in CLL (Wintrobe, 1974c); the latter are IgM, are largely anti-I or i, and are noted most commonly in patients with malignant lymphoma (Wintrobe, 1974c). Although fixation of some complement components occurs, it rarely proceeds to intravascular red cell lysis, particularly with warm-reacting antibodies. Rather, the coated RBCs, probably as a result of F_c and complement receptors on tissue macrophages, are removed from the circulation on passage through the spleen and other reticuloendothelial organs. When clinically evident intravascular hemolysis does occur, it is usually in cold agglutinin disease, in which in cooler areas of the body, IgM antibodies fix complement and lead to lysis (Swisher, 1972).

Clinically, in addition to the splenomegaly, anemia, reticulocytosis, marrow erythroid hyperplasia, and elevated (largely indirect) bilirubin of most hemolytic anemias, the two forms of antibody can often be distinguished by the presence of extensive spherocytosis in the warm-reacting variety and autoagglutination and acrocyanosis in the cold-antibody form (Swisher, 1972). The hallmark of this disease, however, is the positive direct Coombs' test using Coombs' reagent (antiserum to whole human serum), which is capable of detecting on the surface of the red cell not only immunoglobulins, but also complement components. Using monospecific antisera, and performing the test at both 4°C and 37°C, it is possible to characterize with certainty the form of autoantibody that has been elaborated.

The management of this complication of malignancy is based, in the warm-reacting type, on the use of corticosteroids, and in both forms, on the treatment of the underlying disease, the exacerbations of which may be paralleled by the severity of hemolysis. Occasionally, splenectomy will be necessary to control the hemolysis, and some evidence has been developed that patients who sequester ^{51}Cr-labeled RBCs preferentially in the spleen compared with the liver will respond better to splenectomy (Wintrobe, 1974c).

A diagnostic dilemma occurs in those occasional patients with clinical and laboratory evidence of hemolytic disease, but without demonstrable anti-RBC antibodies on Coombs' testing. Some of these patients have been shown, with the use of more sensitive techniques, to have smaller quantities of antibody on the RBC surface than the Coombs'-positive cases, but to be otherwise similar (Gilliland et al., 1971). Others in this group are often placed in the diffuse category of "hypersplenism," particularly when splenomegaly is present.

2.2.2. Sequestration

In contrast to hemolysis, sequestration is the pathological removal by reticuloendothelial cells of largely normal RBCs. As in hemolysis, the development of anemia will be dependent on the capacity of bone marrow to respond to such removal with erythroid hyperplasia.

The anemia of chronic disease is the most common form of loss of RBC mass seen in cancer patients. Usually occurring 1–2 months after the onset of chronic illness, it is mentioned here because of its ubiquity, and because one component of this anemia is a shortened life span for endogenous RBCs, which when transfused into normal subjects have a normal survival (Hyman et al., 1956). That this modest decrease in RBC survival is not the sole defect is evident from the fact that a moderate anemia develops with only a mild reticulocytosis, suggesting that there is impaired erythropoiesis as well. This form of anemia, in contrast to that due to iron deficiency, is characterized by a depressed serum transferrin level and an even lower serum iron, the percentage of saturated transferrin thus being decreased. Despite this decrease, tissue and bone marrow iron stores are plentiful. Some workers have explained this paradox by documentation of abnormalities of iron reutilization in this disorder (Haurani et al., 1963). Others (Zucker and Lysik, 1976) have suggested subnormal responses of bone marrow to erythropoietin. The mechanism of accelerated RBC removal has been attributed to stimulation of the RES, especially the spleen (Kremer and Laszlo, 1973), but the source of this stimulation is uncertain. While the anemia of chronic disease is rarely of sufficient severity to require transfusion, its recognition is important so as to forestall the adoption of more serious diagnoses and their therapeutic imperatives.

Generally accepted criteria for "hypersplenism" have included: (1) cytopenia of one or more formed elements of the blood; (2) a cellular bone marrow; (3)

229
SUPPORTIVE
CARE
IN THE
CANCER
PATIENT

splenomegaly; and (4) improvement of the cytopenia after splenectomy (Wintrobe, 1974*d*). In patients with cancer, "secondary" hypersplenism, i.e., hypersplenism in association with another disease, is largely confined to patients with hematologic malignancy, notably CLL and chronic myelocytic leukemia, and HD and non-Hodgkin's lymphoma (Jacob, 1972). Complicating the diagnosis of hypersplenism in these patients, however, is the fact that the presence or absence of one or more criteria, e.g., splenomegaly, cytopenia, or a cellular bone marrow, may be attributed to the malignancy, its therapy, or both. To assist in establishing the diagnosis and in predicting the response to therapeutic maneuvers, a number of tests have been devised making use of radiopharmaceuticals and radiolabeling of cells to measure splenic size, cell uptake, and persistence. These tests have recently been reviewed (Wintrobe, 1974*d*). They are particularly useful in the evaluation of anemia, as would perhaps be expected from our understanding of the deleterious effects of sequestration and stasis on red cell viability (Jacob, 1972). The splenic contributions to thrombopenia and neutropenia are less easily assessed and the prediction of response to splenic irradiation or splenectomy less reliably made (Wintrobe, 1974*d*). Some data are suggestive of the utility of splenectomy in managing patients with hematologic malignancy and cytopenia, regardless of the presence or absence of other criteria (Nies and Creger, 1967; Adler *et al.*, 1975; Lowenbraun *et al.*, 1971). It is also important to remember that splenomegaly and cytopenia may occasionally represent the presenting manifestations of infection, including tuberculosis and candidiasis (Bodey *et al.*, 1969*a*).

Erythrophagocytosis is not specific to histiocytic medullary reticulosis, a rapidly fatal form of malignant proliferation of histiocytes, but the ingestion of normal RBCs by neoplastic macrophages is thought to represent one mechanism for the rapid development of anemia in this disorder.

2.3. Hemorrhage

Among patients with acute leukemia and lymphoma, thrombocytopenia, disease- and drug-induced, is by far the most frequent cause of hemorrhage; for patients with solid tumors, one must also consider invasion of blood vessels by the tumor and the appearance of stress ulceration in the gastric mucosa as major elements of the differential diagnosis. Cancer-associated hemorrhage is subdivided below into hemorrhage due primarily to (1) vascular, (2) clotting, and (3) platelet abnormalities, and (4) a diverse group of causes of GI and GU ulceration. A battery of simple tests, including the performance of a bleeding time, a platelet count, a prothrombin time (PT), and a partial thromboplastin time (PTT), will usually be sufficient, along with an adequate history and physical, to narrow possibilities to one of the major classes discussed below.

2.3.1. Loss of Vascular Integrity

This condition is marked by normal to slightly prolonged bleeding time; other tests are normal.

Recognized loss of connective tissue support for blood vessels is largely confined to disease states such as scurvy, "senile purpura," and the purpura of chronic corticosteroid administration, but it is likely that in many instances, purpuric lesions in patients with advanced malignancy are due to starvation and wasting. Of related etiology are the hemorrhagic and purpuric lesions of amyloidosis, most commonly seen in multiple myeloma, in which amyloid is deposited in perivascular and subcutaneous tissues, thereby increasing vascular fragility (Kyle and Bayrd, 1975). Data from microscopic studies have also suggested that platelets, in addition to their role in thrombogenesis, may play an important part in preserving endothelial integrity, and that this function may require smaller numbers than those necessary to stop thrombopenic hemorrhage (Roy and Djerassi, 1972). This may explain the seemingly paradoxical findings that low-dose platelet transfusions given prophylactically to thrombopenic patients have virtually as great a protective effect as higher doses (Roy et al., 1973).

The most direct effect of tumor growth on vascular structure is invasion of vessel walls, of particular consequence in those with solid tumors of the head and neck and the GI and GU tracts. Corresponding to this in the leukemias is the situation encountered when patients with acute leukemia and chronic myelogenous leukemia in "blast" crisis have more than 100,000 blasts per cubic millimeter of peripheral blood. When counts are this high, leukostasis in small vessels occurs, leading to the proliferation and formation of leukemic nodules in vessel walls, with consequent weakening and hemorrhage. Prevention of catastrophic hemorrhage in the CNS can be largely accomplished by a rapid reduction in the circulating blast count using chemotherapy or, recently, the cell separator for massive leukophoresis; some also administer prophylactic cranial irradiation (Pochedly, 1975; McKee and Collins, 1974). Rarely, clinically recognizable hemorrhagic infarction will occur due to embolization of fragments of solid tumor, an event most commonly seen in the lungs secondary to hypernephroma, and in the arterial circulation from left-sided myxomas and from primary lung tumors that have invaded the pulmonary vein (Greene et al., 1974c).

Although many infections may be associated with nonthrombocytopenic petechiae and purpura, such as subacute bacterial endocarditis, viral exanthems, and rickettsial diseases, only a few organisms have a special association with both cancer patients and blood vessels. Most frequent of these is *Pseudomonas aeruginosa*, an aerobic gram-negative bacillus, which is a particularly frequent cause of perirectal abscess, pneumonia, and sepsis in granulopenic, especially leukemic, patients. In 5–10% of septic episodes, there occurs a virtually pathognomonic skin lesion, ecthyma gangrenosum, that is due to the proliferation of the organism in the walls of small vessels, with resultant thrombosis, necrosis, and sometimes hemorrhage into the area supplied by the vessel (Bodey, 1975; Whitecar et al., 1970).

In the GI tract, bleeding may be due to erosion of candidal gastroenteritis or colitis into a blood vessel, in some instances a fatal event. In the pulmonary parenchyma, two other fungi, *Aspergillus* and *Mucor*, when they occur, are commonly associated with hemorrhagic infarction because the fungus grows across tissue planes, including arterial and venous walls, with subsequent thrombosis. Among viral infections, measles pneumonia and exanthem may be hemorrhagic, and *Herpes simplex* meningoencephalitis commonly results in RBCs in the spinal fluid. In each of these instances, of course, the presence of other factors, such as thrombocytopenia, may worsen the hemorrhagic propensity.

231

SUPPORTIVE
CARE
IN THE
CANCER
PATIENT

2.3.2. Abnormalities of the Clotting Cascade

In these abnormalities, platelet count and bleeding time are normal (except in DIC); the PTT is prolonged; and the PT is normal when the abnormality is in the intrinsic coagulation pathway, and abnormal when it is in the common pathway.

Clotting abnormalities in cancer patients are acquired disorders of decreased synthesis or increased consumption. The two major causes of the former are: (1) vitamin K deficiency and (2) severe liver disease. It is unusual for either a decreased dietary source or an altered endogenous source (e.g., GI sterilization or surgery) to result in deficiencies of such degree as to produce depressions in the K-dependent clotting factors prothrombin, VII, IX, and X, unless they occur together. Correction of clotting abnormalities due to vitamin K deficiency occurs within 24–48 hr of 10–20 mg parenteral vitamin K administration, provided hepatic synthetic function is not impaired. A failure to correct with vitamin K should suggest the latter possibility. Hepatic dysfunction sufficient to cause clotting abnormalities is unusual with malignancy alone, and is more likely to be seen as a result of transfusion or drug-induced hepatitis. There is little information on the effects of antineoplastic drugs on synthesis of coagulation factors, although L-asparaginase has been reported to interfere with such synthesis, as well as to be associated with low-grade DIC (Capizzi and Handschumacher, 1973).

Increased consumption is due largely to DIC or to circulating anticoagulants. The appearance of DIC is due to the liberation of thromboplastic substances into the bloodstream, with resultant activation of the clotting cascade, and consumption of clotting factors, platelets, and fibrinogen. The diagnosis of DIC can be made and confirmed in three ways: (1) the clinical picture; (2) the laboratory abnormalities of hemostasis; and (3) the pathology on biopsy or autopsy. Clinically, one can often distinguish between acute DIC and chronic DIC, for, in the acute form, the rapidity of consumption leads to hemorrhage and to thrombosis, notably in the kidney, and to microangiopathic hemolysis. In the chronic form, coagulation proceeds more slowly, and hemorrhage, although present, is less severe, and thromboembolic phenomena in the kidney, GI tract, adrenals, lungs, and CNS may dominate. Laboratory diagnosis is dependent on demonstration of thrombocytopenia; prolongation of PT, PTT, and thrombin times; and fibrinogenopenia, often with associated circulating fibrin degradation products due to secondary fibrinolysis (Kwaan, 1972; Whitecar, 1973; Yoshikawa *et al.*, 1971).

In the setting of neoplasia, both the etiologies and differential diagnosis of DIC are more limited than in the general medical setting. The neoplastic causes of DIC have been previously noted, and may often be of the chronic variety. The sudden appearance of DIC-related extensive bleeding in a patient previously free of it may be associated with progression of underlying disease, chemotherapy-induced lysis of tumor cells, or the onset of infection. Most frequent of the latter in cancer patients is gram-negative bacterial sepsis, but endotoxin-deficient gram-positive bacteria are also capable of inducing DIC, perhaps as a result of circulating antigen–antibody complexes, as suggested in recent reports of overwhelming pneumococcal sepsis (Coonrod and Leach, 1976). These or other mechanisms, including reticuloendothelial blockade, tissue damage with release of thrombo-plastins, or induction of platelet aggregation and degranulation, may explain the occasional occurrence of DIC in sepsis due to Group-A β-hemolytic streptococci, *Staphylococcus aureus, Clostridia* spp., exanthematous viruses and arboviruses, and rickettsia (Yoshikawa *et al.*, 1971).

In considering therapy, the essential elements are (1) establishing the presence of DIC, (2) estimating the risk, and (3) knowing the etiology. When the characteristic laboratory abnormalities are present, there are few alternatives to the diagnosis, with the exception of liver failure and primary fibrinogenolysis. Each of these abnormalities is quite uncommon in patients with cancer, but, if necessary, the former can often be distinguished by a normal level of factor VIII, which is not synthesized in the liver but is consumed in DIC, and the latter by a normal platelet count and absence of microangiopathic hemolysis. In the presence of chronic DIC, compensatory mechanisms may obscure the accelerated turnover of clotting factors and platelets, and distinctions may be uncertain. If DIC has been established, treatment is probably necessary only if there is evidence of hemorrhage, serious hemolysis, or thromboembolic events, all of which may be absent. In any case, the underlying cause of the DIC must also be treated. Eradication of sepsis with appropriate antibiotics will remove the stimulus to DIC, and may obviate its treatment; similarly, rapid lysis of cells by therapy, as in acute progranulocytic leukemia, will often result in only a transient induction of DIC until tumor cell burden is reduced.

When therapy is required, the generally accepted agent is heparin, which inhibits thrombin and other coagulation steps, terminating clotting and consumption. This effect is usually evidenced by a rise in 24–48 hr of fibrinogen level and platelet count. Where DIC is tumor-induced and subacute or chronic, heparin therapy is effective. Its efficacy in improving prognosis in the acute DIC of sepsis is less clear, probably because of the overwhelming influence of shock and persistent bacteremia on eventual outcome (Yoshikawa *et al.*, 1971; Gralnick *et al.*, 1972*a, b,* Goldman; 1974).

The vast majority of patients with circulating anticoagulants, which are usually immunoglobulins with antibody activity against one of the clotting factors, have hemophilia or a connective tissue dissorder. Rare cases of multiple myeloma and malignant lymphoma have been reported in which the monoclonal protein has displayed anti–factor VIII antibody, with a resultant hemophilia-like syndrome (Wenz and Friedman, 1974). Factor XI deficiency in amyloidosis and multiple clotting and platelet abnormalities in paraprotein-associated states have been described, but their relationship to clinical bleeding is uncertain (Wintrobe, 1974*e*).

2.3.3. Platelet Abnormalities

233

SUPPORTIVE
CARE
IN THE
CANCER
PATIENT

a. Quantitative Platelet Abnormalities. The causes of thrombocytopenia can be divided into three groups, although in any one patient, more than one mechanism may be operative. These groups are: (1) decreased production, (2) increased utilization, and (3) increased sequestration. In the setting of patients with malignancy, it is common for hematologic abnormalities to be attributed to the underlying disease or its therapy. However, the appearance of thrombocytopenia should also initiate a consideration of the role of infection and of drug toxicity. In the former, even without DIC, thrombocytopenia may be an early sign of bacterial sepsis or viral or other infection (Riedler *et al.*, 1971). In the latter, many drugs, on an immune basis or from bone marrow toxicity, find frequent use clinically and have been implicated in the causation of thrombocytopenia, including digitoxin, thiazide diuretics, and sulfonamides (Aster, 1972).

Among cancer patients, decreased platelet production, secondary to marrow replacement by neoplasia or ablation by drug or radiation therapy, is the most common cause of both minor and severe bleeding. At a given level of platelets, bleeding is more common in the presence of fever and infection, when drugs interfering with platelet function are present and when the count is falling rather than stable or rising, which may be related to the fact that young platelets function better than old ones (Harker and Slichter, 1972). Nevertheless, there is a rough quantitative correlation between the platelet count and frequency of hemorrhage. In patients with leukemia, bleeding of any sort is quite uncommon with levels of more than 50,000/mm^3, and life-threatening pulmonary, GI, intracerebral, or subarachnoid hemorrhage is unusual with counts of more than 20,000/mm^3 (Gaydos *et al.*, 1962).

The success of replacement therapy for thrombocytopenic hemorrhage has been documented in many retrospective studies that demonstrate that since 1960, when platelet transfusions were first routinely instituted, the frequency of severe hemorrhage as a cause of death among patients with leukemia has declined dramatically, from 63 to 15% in one study (Han *et al.*, 1966), and from 67 to 37% in another (Hersh *et al.*, 1965). There is no disagreement about the use of platelet transfusions for thrombocytopenic patients who are already bleeding, but their use prophylactically, while widespread, has been tempered by the fact that repeated random donor platelet transfusions result in sensitization and refractoriness to further transfusion (Grumet and Yankee, 1970), and sometimes in prolonged leukopenia (R. H. Herzig *et al.*, 1974). Nevertheless, most workers regard it as desirable to use prophylactic platelets to keep the count above 20,000/mm^3 in acute leukemia patients. Recently, this policy was corroborated in a controlled prospective trial in childhood leukemia of "prophylactic" transfusions, to keep the platelet count above 20,000/mm^3, vs. transfusions given only for bleeding, which demonstrated a significant decrease in serious bleeding episodes and a trend toward increased survival in the "prophylactic transfusion" group (Murphy *et al.*, 1976). Prophylactic platelets should be avoided in conditions of chronic bone marrow suppression, such as aplastic anemia, and of excessive utilization, as in ITP syndromes or splenic pooling, because in the former, sensitization will inevitably occur, and in the latter, desired increments will not be reached without massive doses.

In an effort to prevent sensitization and improve the efficiency of platelet transfusion, several lines of research have been pursued: (1) decreasing the antigenicity of platelet transfusions, (2) defining an effective prophylactic dose, and (3) improving the storage and survival of platelets prior to transfusion. Yankee *et al.*, (1969) demonstrated that platelets from *HLA* compatible siblings would survive well in patients with aplastic anemia refractory to random donor platelets, and this finding was extended by the same workers to include unrelated *HLA* identical donors (Yankee *et al.*, 1973). Recently, it was found that highly alloimmunized recipients refractory to even matched donors could be made responsive by centrifugation and removal of contaminating leukocytes (R. H. Herzig *et al.*, 1975). These leukocytes were postulated to be causing leukocyte–antileukocyte antibody reactions that destroyed platelets in an "innocent-bystander" mechanism. Where *HLA* matching is unavailable, a clinical trial of siblings as donors, with careful attention to posttransfusion increments at 1 and 20 hr, will usually reveal the most nearly histocompatible person. Some studies suggest that *in vitro* (besides *HLA*) matching tests may also predict response to platelet transfusions (Wu *et al.*, 1976; Creech, 1976).

The definition of a minimal dose of prophylactic platelets that is still effective will reduce the number of donors to which the recipient need be exposed. Some studies have been done along these lines (Roy *et al.*, 1973), and further work may succeed in defining a dose or schedule that minimizes platelet sensitization without sacrificing hemostasis.

The optimum storage conditions for maintaining platelets between collection and transfusion are unknown. Freezing of platelets results in poor recovery posttransfusion, although technical improvements such as freezing in 5% DMSO–5% polyvinylpyrrolidone (Wybran *et al.*, 1972) may make this more feasible, and allow platelet autotransfusion. Currently, platelets are stored at room temperature if it is expected that they will be used within 24 hr; longer storage at 22°C may result in poorer hemostatic function than platelets stored at 4°C. Part of this decrement in function may be due to a drop in pH to less than 6.3 during storage (Kunicki *et al.*, 1975; Murphy and Gardner, 1975).

Accelerated removal of platelets from the circulation can be separated into states of immunologic injury to platelets and states of increased consumption. Among the latter, except for the rare case of thrombotic thrombocytopenic purpura reported in association with widespread carcinoma (Brook and Konwaler, 1965), virtually all others are part of the DIC syndrome (see above). Immunologic injury to platelets can be seen in: (1) idiopathic thrombocytopenic purpuralike (ITP) syndromes; (2) posttransfusion purpura; and (3) drug-induced purpura. In ITP, a chronic disease of adults, thrombocytopenia is caused by accelerated removal of platelets by the spleen and other reticuloendothelial organs, due in most instances to coating of the platelet by an autoantibody. The bone marrow shows normal or increased numbers of megakaryocytes. Although ITP, by definition, refers to thrombocytopenia without apparent etiology, the presence of thrombocytopenic purpura, a normal bone marrow, and minimal, if any, splenomegaly, and the absence of alternate etiology in some patients with lymphoproliferative disease and disseminated carcinoma, have resulted in reports of ITP "in association with" malignancy, particularly chronic lymphocytic leukemia (Ebbe et al., 1962; Rudders et al., 1972).

235
SUPPORTIVE
CARE
IN THE
CANCER
PATIENT

More recently, the development of sophisticated "immunoinjury" techniques for the detection of antiplatelet antibodies (Karpatkin et al., 1972) has shown that the pathophysiology of true ITP and that of "secondary" ITP are similar. The management of this complication is predicated on treatment of the underlying disease, and, if that is unsuccessful, on the standard measures of use in true ITP, viz., corticosteroids and, if necessary, splenectomy, sometimes followed by corticosteroids or immunosuppressants if remission still does not occur. Platelet transfusions should be avoided except in the management of acute bleeding episodes.

Posttransfusion purpura and drug-induced immunologic injury to platelets are very uncommon, and can be reviewed elsewhere (Abramson et al., 1974; Zeigler et al., 1975; Weiss, 1975).

Isolated thrombocytopenia can be one manifestation of hypersplenic sequestration, but the thrombopenia is rarely of sufficient degree, in the presence of adequate marrow function, to cause serious bleeding (Jacob, 1972). In patients with lymphoma, splenic sequestration beyond the usual one-third of the platelet mass may occur along with bone marrow involvement, resulting in levels of platelets that may cause hemorrhage and that limit adequate chemotherapy. Under these circumstances, splenic irradiation or splenectomy may resolve these problems (Abrahamsen, 1972; Crosby, 1972; Adler et al., 1975).

Elevations in the circulating platelet count are not uncommon as secondary phenomena, i.e., in reaction to other processes such as postsplenectomy, after hemorrhage, in acute and chronic infections, or in association with nonmarrow malignancies, such as carcinoma or Hodgkin's disease (Williams, 1972; Kremer and Laszlo, 1973). However, bleeding with excessive platelets is largely confined to the myeloproliferative syndromes, in which thrombosis may occur concomitantly. The cause of hemorrhage is uncertain, but there have been a number of reports of abnormal platelet function in these disorders (McClure et al., 1966). Clinically, bleeding may vary from easy bruisability to epistaxis and GI hemorrhage and sometimes severe blood loss with even minor surgery. Therapy consists of lowering the platelet count by use of P^{32} or antineoplastic drugs or, more acutely, plateletpheresis.

b. Qualitative Platelet Abnormalities. The acquired platelet function disorders do not alone often result in significant bleeding, but their occurrence may initiate hemorrhage when other hemostatic controls are already compromised. The acquired disorders consist of those due to (1) the underlying malignancy; (2) organ function abnormalities; and (3) drugs. Myeloproliferative disorders (and some lymphoproliferative diseases) have been shown to have various defects, including a decrease in initial aggregation to ADP, epinephrine, thrombin, and collagen, absence of a second wave of aggregation to ADP and epinephrine, decreased release of adenine nucleotides, and decreased availability of platelet factor 3 (Cowan and Haut, 1972; Sultan and Caen, 1972; Weiss, 1972; Kremer and Laszlo, 1973). Not all patients with the same myeloproliferative disorder show the same defects, however, and remission of the disease does not necessarily result in complete correction of the dysfunction (Cowan and Haut, 1972). Similar defects have been reported in patients with macroglobulinemia and some with multiple myeloma, and these defects, along with hyperviscosity and an interaction with fibrinogen in clot formation, may contribute to the moderate bleeding diathesis seen. It is likely that the paraprotein, by adsorption to platelet and other surfaces, is responsible for this since correction can often be obtained by plasmapheresis (Weiss, 1972).

The appearance of uremia, hepatic failure, and fibrinogenolysis may all confer functional abnormalities on platelets, with particular effects on aggregation and platelet factor 3 availability (Weiss, 1972, 1975). In each instance, the elaboration of substances into plasma is implicated—in uremia, the substance(s) is known to be dialyzable; in hepatic failure and fibrinogenolysis, fibrin degradation products may be of importance (Weiss, 1972).

There are many drugs that can interfere with platelet function, of which aspirin is well known. Most are unlikely to find use in patients with cancer for other reasons, but some of those that may are phenothiazines, tricyclic amine antidepressants, diphenhydramine, and, of particular importance because of its frequent use in patients with acute leukemia, carbenicillin, which has been implicated not only in dysfunction, but also in actual bleeding episodes (Waisbren *et al.*, 1971; Weiss, 1972; Brown *et al.*, 1974).

The assessment of platelet function by the various *in vitro* tests is often unavailable, and, when available, of uncertain relationship to *in vivo* phenomena. Recently, a careful study (Harker and Slichter, 1972) documented the value of the standardized template bleeding time, a modification of the Ivy bleeding time, to measure the effect of platelet dysfunction as well as platelet levels on prolongation of bleeding time. Performance of this test, particularly serially in a given patient, may be useful in guiding clinical judgment about plasmapheresis in hyperviscosity states, dialysis in azotemic patients, and drug administration.

2.3.4. Miscellaneous Causes of Hemorrhage

Table 1 lists some miscellaneous causes of hemorrhage, of which most are uncommon, rarely life-threatening, and not difficult to diagnose. One cause deserves comment. A recent review of upper GI hemorrhage among cancer patients (Klein *et al.*, 1973) revealed that 16 (32%) of 49 with significant blood loss had acute mucosal ("stress") erosions, the single most common cause. Other factors contributing to such erosions included active cancer chemotherapy, corticosteroids, sepsis [an association often noted previously (Altemeier *et al.*, 1972)], and previous surgery. Probably because of these factors of comorbidity, the mortaliy rate was 100%. Of interest was the fact that of 44 patients for whom a source for the bleeding was found, only 6 were directly bleeding from tumor.

237

SUPPORTIVE
CARE
IN THE
CANCER
PATIENT

2.4. Approach to the Patient with Blood Loss

A broad evaluation of loss of RBC mass in the patient with cancer should include, in addition to a full history and physical examination and a stool guaiac, a complete blood count, a blood smear, platelet count, reticulocyte count, indirect Coombs' test, bleeding time, prothrombin time (PT), partial thromboplastin time (PTT), and, as a baseline, a fibrinogen level. In the patient with known bone marrow disease, without evidence of hemorrhage or occult blood loss, anemia is likely to be due to decreased erythropoiesis, which can be confirmed by an examination of the marrow and an absence of reticulocytosis. Where the anemia seems out of proportion to erythroid hypoplasia, however, or where the rapidity of fall of hematocrit or hemoglobin exceeds the usual, serious consideration should be given to nonhemorrhagic red cell loss, particularly among patients with splenomegaly, lymphoproliferative disorders, or ovarian carcinoma, in whom hypersplenism and immune hemolytic anemia are most frequent.

Among patients without evident bone marrow involvement, moderate anemia is often the anemia of chronic disease, but confirmation of this diagnosis should be attempted by viewing the blood smear, by measurement of the serum iron and transferrin levels, and by an examination of bone marrow for stainable iron. If the anemia is severe, alternate or additional diagnoses are likely, such as occult bleeding or nonhemorrhagic red cell destruction. If bleeding is evident, of primary importance is the measurement of the platelet count, PTT, PT, and fibrinogen level. If these are all normal, then local factors such as vascular injury, tumor erosion, and, if bleeding is of GI origin, mucosal ulcerations become likely. When the clotting and fibrinogen studies are normal, but thrombopenia is present, the likelihood that the latter is responsible for bleeding is small if the count is greater than 50,000, unless drugs, azotemia, or liver disease are contributing to platelet dysfunction, and the latter possibility should be examined with a template bleeding time. The absence of petechiae or purpura also mitigates against thrombocytopenic bleeding. When platelet depression is more severe, particularly if fever or infection or both are present, bleeding on this basis alone is more common.

When the platelet count, PT, and fibrinogen are normal, but the PTT is abnormal, consideration should be given to a circulating anticoagulant, particularly among patients with lymphoproliferative disease. A normal platelet count, PT, and PTT and a decreased fibrinogen raise the unusual possibility of primary fibrinogenolysis. When the PT and PTT are both abnormal, and if fibrinogen or platelet count is decreased or even low normal, two major diagnoses should be considered—severe liver dysfunction or disseminated intravascular coagulation. When the former is already present, distinguishing the onset of DIC may be difficult, as previously discussed, but the clinical setting usually allows ready differentiation. DIC is particularly likely in the setting of severe infection or rapid dissolution of tumor, or among patients with acute progranulocytic leukemia or mucin-secreting adenocarcinoma.

A final diagnostic caution should be raised: Progressive anemia in the hospitalized cancer patient, without any obvious explanation, may be iatrogenic in origin. The blood-drawing of modern medicine may result in the withdrawal of 50–150 ml per day—sufficient, particularly when marrow reserve is limited, to resemble low grade hemolysis or bleeding.

3. Infection

3.1. General Comments

Since 1960, when prophylactic and therapeutic platelet transfusions made possible the control of life-threatening hemorrhage in patients with acute leukemia, the nature of infection and its predominance as a cause of death in this disease and other malignant diseases have received increasing attention. The purpose of this review is to consider some aspects of factors predisposing to such infections in cancer patients, and their prophylaxis, diagnosis, and therapy. No attempt will be made to describe in detail the clinical syndromes associated with each of the many pathogens, for which there are ample and recent reviews (Bodey, 1975; Levine *et al.*, 1974; Sutnick and Engstrom, 1976).

3.2. Oncology and the Infectious Disease Service

Despite the necessity for a close relationship between a medical oncology and an infectious disease service, remarkably little has been written about the nature of that relationship. In some major cancer centers, a separate infectious disease subsection has been established that relates primarily or exclusively to cancer patients. At the other extreme, no formal ties are in existence, and infectious disease consultation is conducted on an *ad hoc* basis. A number of considerations make this haphazard approach to infection in the cancer patient undesirable:

1. Many infections are preventable by proper attention to minimizing predisposing factors.
2. Crucial elements of management often arise within the first 24–48 hr of onset of infection, at a time when consultation is rarely initiated.
3. Specialized knowledge may be essential to a favorable outcome, as in:
   a. Distinguishing among tumor, tumor therapy, and infection as causes of the observed signs and symptoms.
   b. Utilizing limited data to narrow diagnostic choices within a group of potential pathogens both unusual in their presentation and infrequent in the noncancer patient.
   c. Performing special services, such as serologic studies, useful in diagnosis and therapy.

4. Initial approaches to management, prior to diagnosis, often require a data base of infectious problems obtainable only by retrospective chart review and prospective surveillance on the oncology unit.

5. Clinical research on the prophylaxis, diagnosis, and therapy of opportunistic infections in cancer patients is making use of unusual and time-consuming modalities, such as laminar air-flow rooms and granulocyte transfusions, and are best conducted in concert with infectious disease specialists.

6. A failure to formulate "protocol" studies of measures of infectious disease supportive care, in major medical centers, is a loss of opportunity and clinical resources equivalent to the failure to study the underlying disease.

239

SUPPORTIVE
CARE
IN THE
CANCER
PATIENT

Some of these considerations are also applicable to other groups of patients without cancer, but apart from situations also involving extensive host compromise such as transplants or burns, the distinguishing aspect of the patient with cancer, especially with hematologic malignancy, is the regularity with which infection occurs and the impact such infection has on anticipated survival. Since the greatest period of risk corresponds to the most intensive radiation and chemotherapy, infection may supervene prior to the desirable effects of such agents. The more responsive such tumors are, the greater the tragedy should life be ended during induction remission. The increasing application of adjuvant and combination drug and radiation therapy makes mandatory a formalized link between infectious disease specialists and the oncology service. This relationship should be expected to result in four broad areas of mutual endeavor:

1. Epidemiology of Infectious Disease. The organisms responsible for nosocomial and opportunistic infection and their antibiotic susceptibilities vary from institution to institution. The factors responsible for the development of infection will be dependent, in part, on the kinds of malignancies being treated by the oncology section, on the drugs used and the manner in which they are used, and on the patterns of care and traffic to which the patient is exposed. The rational formulation of "empirical" antibacterial therapy, the likely alternatives when nonbacterial infection seems most probable, the decision as to what elements of supportive care can be subjected to study, the outcome of previous modes of diagnosis and therapy—all must extend from some knowledge of what has gone before within the given institution. A retrospective chart review of these elements must be undertaken, and it should be the product of cooperation between the oncologist and the infectious disease (ID) specialist.

2. Infection Surveillance. In addition to a retrospective review, one must initiate prospective surveillance of infection. Ideally, the oncology ward should have its own nurse epidemiologist, trained in the kinds of drugs, radiation, and surgery utilized in cancer patients and charged with collecting data relevant not only to the hospital infection control committee, but also to the interaction between malignancy and infection. Such collected data should be tabulated and easily retrievable, and periodic summaries should be made available to the clinical staff.

3. Infectious Disease Consultation. Many infections and infectious deaths in cancer patients are preventable or treatable. What is lacking is not the necessary tools, but rather the application of such tools *at the right time.* ID consultation in the setting of leukemia and lymphoma should in reality begin on admission, and the patient should be followed until death or discharge. The rigorous invocation of prophylactic measures early in the course of hospitalization, the prompt participation of the ID consultant in the planning of diagnostic measures and therapy, and the invaluable aid of "knowing the patient" when asked to render judgment on a putative infection can only improve present results. Furthermore, longitudinal participation will allow the ID consultant and the oncologist each to become familiar with the clinical practice of the other—to appreciate, for example, that daunorubicin may cause fever and pharyngitis.

4. Protocol Studies. When the oncology and ID services work closely, the major problems plaguing the former in the field of the latter will suggest clinical and laboratory studies to solve those problems. In particular, the design of prospective studies of infection control must be cognizant of the antitumor treatment plan, and accrual of patients to the study must depend on the oncologist's awareness that the study exists and that the patient is eligible. In short, it must be planned together.

In summary, a cancer center must incorporate an ID section of its own or must formalize ties to an external section in such a way that recent advances of supportive care can be applied throughout hospitalization, and not solely, as is so often the case, when the patient is already severely infected.

3.3. Predisposing Factors to Infection

Cancer patients vary as to the kinds of infections to which they are predisposed. The reason such variation occurs is that cancer, *per se*, does not lead to infection— it is the effect of that cancer and its therapy on the systems of host defense that determines the frequency and nature of complicating infection. Such defenses against microbial invasion can be divided into four systems, each of which interacts with the others: (1) mucocutaneous barriers, (2) the inflammatory response, (3) the humoral immune system, and (4) the cellular immune system. Modifications of these component parts may derive from the malignancy itself, from the antitumor therapy, or from other non-tumor-directed iatrogenic intervention.

3.3.1. Mucocutaneous Barriers

Man interacts with two microbial environments, one external, the other internal, and each is populated by "normal flora" that vary by geographic location and by body site. The interface at which this interaction occurs is the skin and mucous membranes, and the factors responsible for preventing the flora from being altered or from invading or both are only beginning to be understood. Alterations of one or more components of this system are responsible in whole or in part for the vast majority of infections afflicting cancer patients, especially those with lymphomas and solid tumors, among whom granulocytopenia is less common, until terminal stages, than in patients with leukemia.

241

SUPPORTIVE
CARE
IN THE
CANCER
PATIENT

At least four elements of this system that play essential roles can be identified: (1) exposure to nonindigenous flora, (2) mechanical barriers to invasion, (3) interbacterial inhibition, and (4) secretory immunoglobulin A.

Invasion by microorganisms cannot occur without prior exposure. In a study of patients with acute nonlymphocytic leukemia (Schimpff *et al.*, 1972*a*), in whom serial "surveillance" cultures of multiple body sites were performed, isolation of an offending organism from these cultures preceded infection with the organism in 75/87 (86%) instances. In almost half, these organisms were not part of the patient's flora on admission; i.e. the organism, predominantly gram-negative bacilli, had been acquired in the hospital. Many sources of nosocomial acquisition of pathogens have been identified, the most prominent of which is probably hand carriage by medical personnel, a subject recently reviewed (Steere and Mallison, 1975). Other modes of exposure have included food (Shooter *et al.*, 1971), particularly uncooked food, such as salads and fruits and vegetables; medical instruments, such as respirators (Rhoades *et al.*, 1971; Matsen, 1973; Phillips *et al.*, 1974), endoscopes (F. M. Chang *et al.*, 1973), and ECG electrode pads (Lockey *et al.*, 1973); disinfectants, particularly quaternary ammonium compounds (Hardy *et al.*, 1970); and medications, including live virus vaccines, which should be avoided in those with lymphoproliferative disorders or receiving corticosteroids.

In the intact host, mere exposure to these organisms often would be insufficient to result in invasion, and perhaps not even more than transient colonization. But the simultaneous breaching of the mechanical barriers of skin and mucous membranes allows resident flora to become pathogenic and some nosocomial flora to bypass colonization entirely. Among cancer patients, the association of solid tumors of the colon, lung, and GU tract with anaerobic, gram-negative aerobic, and mixed bacterial infections reflects the predominance of this flora in these areas and the local effects of mucosal ulceration and obstruction-induced stasis (Keusch, 1974). In contrast, anaerobic infection is much less common in leukemia patients, despite their evident compromise, because disease-induced ulceration and obstruction are not as prominent (Felner and Dowell, 1971; Kagnoff *et al.*, 1972). Some have suggested that another factor contributing to the frequency of anaerobic bacteremia, in which *Bacteroides fragilis* and *Clostridia* spp., particularly *Clostridia septicum* (Alpern and Dowell, 1969), are often isolated is the anaerobic environment within and around the growing and necrotic tumor, which allows such bacteria to proliferate.

Antitumor therapy causing devitalization of tissue or breaching mechanical barriers will have similar effects. In one report of bacteroides bacteremia from a cancer center (Kagnoff *et al.*, 1972), only 11% of the patients had even moderate leukopenia, but 58% had had recent surgery, with sepsis arising from postoperative anastomotic leaks and incision sites, as well as tumor progression. Other complications of therapy such as radiation-induced bowel necrosis or enteritis, or chemotherapy-induced ulceration of the oral mucosa, by methotrexate or daunorubicin, or of the colonic mucosa, by 5-fluorouracil, have also resulted in local and blood-borne bacterial infection (Kagnoff *et al.*, 1972; McLaughlin *et al.*, 1973).

An interesting association, frequently documented, is that of *Salmonella* infection and leukemia, lymphoma, and solid tumors of the colon and pelvis (Han *et al.*. 1967; Sinkovics and Smith, 1969; Wolfe *et al.*, 1971). Speculation about the predisposing factors has included discussions of hemolysis and resultant reticuloendothelial blockade, the protected nature of necrotic tumors from the usual antibacterial mechanisms, cellular anergy, and the influence of iatrogenic factors, such as surgery, antibiotics, and hospitalization, which have been associated with salmonellosis in patients without malignancy (Black *et al.*, 1960).

Perhaps most common, and yet most subject to favorable manipulation, are the non-tumor-directed iatrogenic breaches. In most instances, the well-recognized infectious complications of intravenous catheters, urethral catheters, tracheostomies, and endoscopy can be traced to colonizing bacteria, endogenous or hospital-acquired, which follow the artificial pathway created to cause, respectively, cellulitis and sepsis, cystitis, pyelonephritis and prostatitis, pneumonia, and bacteremia (Feingold, 1970; Matsen, 1973; Davis *et al.*, 1975). Less commonly, these paths serve to cause introduction of microorganisms associated with the vehicle itself, rather than the host, and some of these microorganisms have caused death or profound debilitation. In a patient with sepsis and an intravenous line in place, it should be remembered that intravenous solutions, blood transfusions, and platelet transfusions can be and have been contaminated with bacteria (Buchholz *et al.*, 1971; Duma *et al.*, 1971; Rhame *et al.*, 1973); that blood cell transfusions have been implicated in the transmission of toxoplasmosis and malaria (Siegel *et al.*, 1971; Tapper and Armstrong, 1976); that blood products are probably the most common source of nosocomial viral infections in the transmission of cytomegalovirus (Prince *et al.*, 1971) and the agents of viral hepatitis; and that hyperalimentation fluids have frequently been associated with candidal and bacterial sepsis (Ryan *et al.*, 1974). In addition, the "disinfectant" of urethral catheterization sets (Hardy *et al.*, 1970) and the humidifiers and respiratory medications, usually from multiple-dose vials, of patients with endotracheal tubes and tracheostomies have delivered directly to target organs bacteria that did not have to encounter any of the barriers designed to prevent their entry. Recently, we reported (Greene *et al.*, 1974*b*) several instances in which an esophagoscope served not only to induce bacteremia in two patients with acute leukemia—a phenomenon documented with many endoscopic and invasive procedures, including peroral biopsy (Petty and Wenger, 1970), kidney biopsy (Samellas, 1964), and endoscopic retrograde cholangiopancreatography (Davis *et al.*, 1975)—but also clinical sepsis with an organism (*P. aeruginosa*) introduced into the patient by the instrument. This infection arose because the endoscope had not been properly decontaminated from previous sessions, and had not been handled in a clean, if not sterile, manner.

The mode by which the normal floras on mucocutaneous surfaces inhibit the proliferation of one another as well as nonindigenous organisms is largely unknown. Postulated mechanisms have included competition for essential nutrients, elaboration of compounds toxic to other strains of the same genera and species (bacteriocins) or other genera, and "lag times" before entry into a growth phase by bacteria new to the particular microenvironment (Freter, 1974).

243
SUPPORTIVE
CARE
IN THE
CANCER
PATIENT

Secretory IgA has been shown to be protective against viral infections that require mucosal penetration, but the precise role of the humoral immune system and of secretory IgA in regulating bacterial numbers and invasion is uncertain. There is some evidence in experimental animals that indigenous bacteria are less immunogenic in their host, and therefore less likely to be eradicated, than "foreign" organisms. Since IgA does not fix complement and phagocytic cells do not have F_c receptors for IgA, a mechanism by which secretory IgA could lead to inhibition or killing of bacteria has been lacking. More recently, several studies (Freter, 1970; Fubara and Freter, 1973) have suggested that such antibody-mediated inhibition of growth can occur, and, in addition, that bacteria coated by secretory immunoglobulin could be prevented from attaching to mucosal cells. More recent studies (Shedlofsky and Freter, 1974) in an experimental *Vibrio cholera* model in germ-free mice have also demonstrated that interbacterial inhibition and local immunity may be synergistic in their actions, the effectiveness of the latter in the cecum being considerably greater in reducing bacterial numbers when a competing flora had previously been introduced.

In human disease states, alterations of cutaneous and pharyngeal mucosal flora toward predominantly gram-negative organisms have been amply demonstrated to be proportional, in a rough way, to the seriousness of illness (Johanson *et al.*, 1969), but mechanisms responsible for this proportionality have not been elucidated. Although IgA deficiency has been implicated in the pathogenesis of recurrent or unusual gastroenteric, respiratory, and sinus infections (Tomasi, 1972), and has been associated with some forms of cancer, particularly lymphomas, it is doubtful that most malignancies and most forms of tumor therapy induce significant IgA alterations. While the host may be responsible for some shifts in normal flora, the most important single factor in such changes is the use of antibacterial antibiotics.

In 1954, Weinstein and co-workers (Weinstein *et al.*, 1954) demonstrated the association between the administration of broad-spectrum antibiotics and the appearance of resistant gram-negative colonization and superinfection, and this association has been confirmed many times since, for both topically and systemically applied antibiotics (Stone and Kolb, 1971; Pollack *et al.*, 1972). In recent years, there has been a considerable increase in nonbacterial, especially fungal, infections among cancer patients, particularly those with leukemia and lymphoma (Bodey, 1966; Levine *et al.*, 1974). Our own studies (Greene *et al.*, 1973a) and those of others (Goodall and Vosti, 1975) have demonstrated a direct relationship between the duration of broad-spectrum antibiotic therapy and the frequency of superinfection, predominantly fungal in our study (Table 2), such that after 12 or

TABLE 2

Relationship of Duration of Carbenicillin/Gentamicin/Cephalothin Therapy to the Rate of Superinfection[a]

Group	Duration of therapy (days)			TOTALS
	1–7	8–11	12 or more	
Superinfected	20 (16.6%)	11 (36.7%)	15 (55.5%)	46
Not superinfected	100 (83.4%)	19 (63.3%)	12 (44.5%)	131
TOTALS:	120	30	27	177

[a] From Greene *et al.* (1973*a*).

more days of continuous antibiotics, more than 50% of granulopenic patients had developed superinfection, usually candidal.

3.3.2. The Inflammatory Response

This complex mechanism involves at least the following major steps: (1) generation of chemotactic factors that promote the entry of inflammatory cells into an area of infection; (2) a vascular supply capable of bringing such inflammatory cells; (3) an adequate number of phagocytes with normal: (a) responsiveness to chemotactic factors, (b) mobility, (c) phagocytosis, and (d) intracellular killing. Promoting phagocytosis are (4) opsonins, which derive primarily from the humoral immune system and complement components. Each of these areas has recently been reviewed (Klebanoff, 1975; Senn and Jungi, 1975; Stossel, 1975; Winkelstein, 1973).

As the details of granulocyte (PMN) function have become known, methods by which to assess these functions have been applied to many disease states, especially the hematologic malignancies. In acute myelogenous leukemia in relapse, defects demonstrated have included decreases in migration into skin abrasions (Senn and Jungi, 1975), in adhesiveness and phagocytosis (Penny and Galton, 1966; Rosner *et al.*, 1970), in intracellular killing by granulocytes (Quie, 1975) and by mononuclear phagocytes (Quie, 1975), in myeloperoxidase content and killing (Cline, 1974), and in the ability to form and to promote leukocyte colonies in soft agar *in vitro* (Greenberg *et al.*, 1971). In ALL in relapse, colony formation and stimulation have been abnormal (Ragab *et al.*, 1974), as well as candidacidal activity (Rosner *et al.*, 1970), and, in some, a transient defect in microbicidal activity in children receiving prophylactic CNS radiation (Quie, 1975). Patients with chronic myelogenous leukemia have reportedly had defects in killing when the WBC count was more than 90,000 (Odeberg *et al.*, 1975), and diminished adhesiveness and phagocytosis (Penny and Galton, 1966). Other deficiencies have been variably reported for patients with chronic lymphocytic leukemia, multiple myeloma and macroglobulinemia, Hodgkin's disease, and non-Hodgkin's lymphoma (Penny and Galton, 1966; Senn and Jungi, 1975; Ward and Berenberg, 1974); in the former two, the deficiencies were apparently related to lack of opsonins and presence of M-protein, respectively (Penny and Galton, 1966; Sbarra *et al.*, 1964). Studies of this sort have been largely lacking in patients with solid tumors, although a recent report documented the presence of a serum inhibitor of chemotaxis in 75% of patients tested (Ward *et al.*, 1976). Some drugs used in cancer patients are also known to compromise PMN function, particularly the effect of corticosteroids (Peters *et al.*, 1972), vincristine (Quie, 1975), vinblastine (Edelson and Fudenberg, 1973), and colchicine (Baehner, 1972) on chemotaxis, and of sulfonamides on PMN candidacidal activity (Quie, 1975).

245

SUPPORTIVE
CARE
IN THE
CANCER
PATIENT

Despite these investigations, there is little evidence to suggest that functional defects or abnormal complement synthesis or metabolism is of great importance in predisposing cancer patients to infection compared with the role of granulocytopenia. Bodey's study of neutropenia (Bodey *et al.*, 1966) in 52 patients with acute leukemia demonstrated a clear increase in the frequency of all infections and of severe infections with progressively lower PMN counts, beginning at approximately 1000/mm^3 and accelerating with levels of less than 500/mm^3. In this study, infection was present on approximately 55% of all patient days spent at a granulocyte level of less than 100/mm^3. The duration of granulocytopenia is also important. After 3 weeks of less than 100 PMNs/mm^3, 100% of patients were infected, and approximately 75% had severe infection; for counts of less than 1000, the figures were approximately 60% and 50%, respectively. In addition, several studies have demonstrated (Middleman *et al.*, 1972; Valdivieso *et al.*, 1974) that the outcome of bacterial infection in the granulocytopenic host is dependent on the ability of the patient to raise his neutrophil count, with death in 60–80% of episodes in which such a rise was absent.

The etiology of granulopenia is usually obvious and related to the underlying malignancy, its therapy, or both. It is useful to remember, however, that even patients receiving chemotherapy or radiation therapy may have iatrogenic causes of neutropenia other than the usual toxic agents, including such drugs as carbenicillin (Reyes *et al.*, 1973), methicillin, sulfonamides, and phenothiazines (Quie, 1975). R. H. Herzig *et al.* (1974) have also reported incompatible platelet transfusions as a cause of persistent neutropenia.

Among patients with severe neutropenia, pneumonia, septicemia, skin, perirectal, and pharyngeal bacterial infections are particularly frequent, and bacteremia complicates localized infection far more commonly than those with normal counts (Sickles *et al.*, 1975). Ordinarily nonpathogenic microorganisms become invasive, so that in addition to *Staphylococcus aureus*, infections are caused by gram-negative enteric bacilli, especially *P. aeruginosa*, *Escherichia coli*, and *Klebsiella* spp., and, often as superinfections after successful eradication of bacterial disease, by fungi such as *Candida*, *Aspergillus*, and *Mucor*, all of which carry a very high mortality (Bodey, 1975).

3.3.3. The Humoral Immune System

Antibodies, primarily IgG and IgM, carry out two major functions in combating infection: (1) the neutralization of the organism directly, and (2) the opsonization of the pathogen for subsequent phagocytosis. IgM, a large molecule confined to the intravascular space, is efficient in fixing complement and in promoting aggregation, but it can promote phagocytosis only through the attachment of complement components because the major phagocytic cells, the monocyte and PMN, have receptors only for complement and for the F_c fragment of IgG. IgG, however, can leave the vascular space, and it promotes phagocytosis in tissue spaces by opsonization directly or through complement fixation (Roitt, 1974).

In viral illness and in diseases due to the elaboration of bacterial toxins, such as diphtheria and tetanus, antibodies directed against the organism or the toxin are correlated with resistance to infection and to disease (Winkelstein, 1973; Roitt, 1974). In bacterial infections, their role is less clear. For some organisms coated with capsules or envelopes that inhibit phagocytosis, opsonization appears to be essential to adequate eradication of the infection, and immunization with the capsule as antigen is associated with protection against disease. Thus, pneumococci, streptococci, meningococci, and *Hemophilus influenzae* have been particularly common pathogens among hosts whose compromise has been primarily hypogammaglobulinemia (Salmon *et al.*, 1967; Meyers *et al.*, 1972; Gold, 1974). Gram-negative enteric organisms have also caused infection with regularity in such patients, and until recently, little has been known about the role of antibody in prevention or eradication of these pathogens. Recent animal studies have suggested that opsonization for gram-negative bacteria is carried out much more efficiently by IgG molecules than by IgM (A. B. Bjornson and Michael, 1970), and clinical studies suggest a direct correlation between high titers of IgG antibody, but not of IgM antibody, to the somatic antigen of an organism causing bacteremia and the absence of shock and death (McCabe *et al.*, 1972; Zinner and McCabe, 1976).

Among cancer patients, hypogammaglobulinemia as an accompaniment of early disease is primarily in patients with chronic lymphocytic leukemia and multiple myeloma (MM), both diseases of the "B" cell system. The etiology of the hypogammaglobulinemia has been uncertain, with theories of "crowding" out and feedback inhibition by the monoclonal protein predominating. In some patients with MM, hypercatabolism of IgG has also been implicated (Salmon *et al.*, 1967). Recently, Waldmann's laboratory (Broder *et al.*, 1975) demonstrated that the macrophages of some patients with MM actively inhibit the secretion of immunoglobulins by circulating B cells. Patients with advanced Hodgkin's disease and non-Hodgkin's lymphoma may also have antibody deficiency, but patients with acute leukemia, chronic myelogenous leukemia, and solid tumors usually have normal immunoglobulins (Harris and Copeland, 1974). Chemotherapy may depress antibody responses, but the effect is usually transient, and much greater depression of the primary than of secondary or anamnestic responses is seen (Hersh *et al.*, 1966).

In patients with hypogammaglobulinemia, encapsulated gram-positive organisms and gram-negative aerobic bacilli predominate as pathogens, with the latter playing an increasing role (Meyers *et al.*, 1972), due primarily to the advent of chemotherapy and other iatrogenic and nosocomial exposures.

3.3.4. The Cellular Immune Response

247
SUPPORTIVE
CARE
IN THE
CANCER
PATIENT

Cell-mediated immunity (CMI) has classically been measured by the extent of induration to intradermal skin-testing with tuberculin and other "recall" antigens. The identification of the circulating small lymphocyte as a thymus-derived (T) cell vested with this capacity to express "delayed hypersensitivity" has revolutionized modern immunology. Experiments of nature and of man have demonstrated many functions of the T cell, which are generally acknowledged to include: (1) graft rejection, (2) contact dermatitis, (3) cooperation with B cells for antibody synthesis to most antigens, (4) suppression or regulation of other humoral or cellular immune responses, (5) antitumor immunity, and (6) defense against some infections (Roitt, 1974). It is beyond the scope of this chapter to review the enormous recent literature that has grown up concerning the expression of CMI in patients with malignancy. The elucidation of the steps between exposure of T cells to antigen and the production of an effector cell response has brought with it multiple ways by which to measure the extent of impairment of CMI, ranging from *in vivo* skin-testing (with recall or "new" antigens) (Catalona *et al.*, 1975) and counting of T and B lymphocytes in peripheral blood (Harris *et al.*, 1975) to more sophisticated, but possibly less relevant, *in vitro* assays of lymphocyte proliferation to mitogenic and antigenic stimulation (R. C. Young *et al.*, 1973), production of soluble "lymphokines" (Lawrence, 1973), and effector actions, such as cytotoxicity (Herberman and Oldham, 1975) and macrophage activation (Borges and Johnson, 1975).

In the context of defense against infection, perhaps the most accurate guide to whether CMI is impaired to a clinically significant degree in a given tumor diagnosis is to identify whether infection occurs with organisms for which CMI is felt to be important. Such organisms are those for which an intracellular residence and proliferation provide protection from the PMN inflammatory and humoral immune responses, and include intracellular bacteria, such as *Salmonella* and *Brucella*; mycobacteria; fungi, notably *Cryptococcus, Candida, Aspergillus,* and *Mucor*; protozoa, particularly *Toxoplasma* and *Pneumocystis*; and viruses, especially the herpes viruses (cytomegalovirus, herpes simplex, varicella-zoster virus), measles, and vaccinia (Gold, 1974; Levine *et al.*, 1974; Bodey, 1975).

The prototypic malignancy associated with cellular anergy is Hodgkin's disease, in which unresponsiveness on skin-testing and in *in vitro* stimulation of circulating lymphocytes by the plant mitogen phytohemagglutinin (PHA) has been correlated with a later stage of disease, a lymphocyte-depleted and mixed-cellularity histology, systemic symptoms, and a low absolute peripheral lymphocyte count (Young *et al.*, 1973; Harris and Copeland, 1974). There is general agreement that among patients with localized disease, the CMI is not often abnormal as gauged by any test, and in patients with extensive and active disease, CMI is very often depressed. Similar generalizations can be made for patients with non-Hodgkin's lymphoma, but there are fewer such studies available (Harris and Copeland, 1974). In contrast to the frequent hypogammaglobulinemia of chronic lymphocytic leukemia and multiple myeloma, T-cell function is relatively intact in these diseases (Harris and Bagai, 1972). Patients with acute leukemia and with chronic myelogenous leukemia in some studies have shown decreased reactivity on skin-testing and with PHA stimulation (Hersh *et al.*, 1971), but this finding has not been confirmed in other studies (Greene *et al.*, 1974*a*), and where evident, the defect has been a mild one. Solid-tumor patients also generally display normal cell-mediated immunity, *in vivo* and *in vitro*, but advanced or metastatic disease often leads to lymphocytopenia and cellular anergy (Harris and Copeland, 1974). It should be noted that many of these studies have been performed in the context of the role of CMI in preventing the development or progression of malignancy, and that abnormalities of one measure or another of CMI have usually been related to overall prognosis, and not to infection. Thus, the importance of these findings in regard to infectious risk is not well assessed.

Clinical studies demonstrate that the risk of nonbacterial infection is largely confined to patients with leukemia and, to a lesser extent, lymphoma. A recent review of infection in cancer patients (Bodey, 1975) showed that of the 70% of acute leukemias dying from infection, one-third had nonbacterial disease, almost all fungal; 13% of the lymphoma patients and only 6% of the solid tumor patients dying from infection had a fungal etiology. Protozoal and viral infections accounted for less than one-tenth that due to fungi. These data agree with our own (Greene *et al.*, 1972) in a 3-year review of autopsied patients with cancer. These figures mislead, however, for they (1) refer to infection at death, and do not give any indication of whether these infections occurred early in the course of disease or only after the exhaustion of useful therapy and survival; and (2) reflect, not the susceptibility of the disease state alone, but in addition the impact of immunosuppressive therapy.

In regard to the first consideration, the primary disease in which survival is curtailed by nonbacterial infection is acute myelogenous leukemia, for only about 50% of such patients achieve complete remission, and of those who don't, 70–90% die from infection (Levine *et al.*, 1974; H. Chang *et al.*, 1976). In contrast, nonbacterial infection in acute lymphocytic leukemia (ALL) is found in more advanced disease or in remission. Among 100 previously untreated patients with ALL studied at St. Jude's, during remission induction therapy, only 7 had severe infection, of which 1 was nonbacterial; only 3 patients failed induction remission because of infection (Hughes and Smith, 1973). Also at St. Jude's, however, among 199 patients dying with childhood leukemia (Hughes, 1971*a*), 155 had infection, in 89 of whom it was the primary cause of death. Of these, fungal disease involved 52 patients, in 17 it was disseminated, and all these patients were in relapse. In patients dying in remission, *Pneumocystis carinii* was most often responsible. In large part, the absence of serious fungal disease early in ALL, and in non-Hodgkin's lymphoma and other malignancies as well, is attributable to the use of nonmyelosuppressive therapy or cyclic therapy with periods of recovery, which leaves CMI intact or only intermittently depressed. A corollary to this is that the underlying diseases, particularly acute leukemias, multiple myeloma, and solid tumors, do not in themselves contribute to susceptibility to infection with intracellular organisms. In acute myelogenous leukemia, the major defect is granulocytopenia, and in the years prior to effective chemotherapy and broad-spectrum antibiotics, nonbacterial infection as a cause of death was rare (Keye and Magee, 1956; Baker, 1962). Progressive Hodgkin's disease, in contrast, with its clear association with anergy, was so commonly associated in the past with an intracellular infection, tuberculosis, that at one time *Mycobacterium tuberculosis* itself was considered as an etiologic agent for the neoplasm (Kaplan *et al.*, 1974; Feld *et al.*, 1976). The decline in exposure to tuberculosis from the general population and the advent of more severe endogenous and iatrogenic immunosuppression in advanced Hodgkin's disease has shifted the spectrum of illness to fungi, protozoans, and viruses. This same shift has been noted among other patients with severe host compromise, such as those with extensive burns, in whom fungal infections have become increasingly common (Nash *et al.*, 1971).

Two iatrogenic interventions occupy special roles in the induction of nonbacterial infections. Among patients with acute leukemia, broad-spectrum antibiotics, as previously discussed, when administered for a prolonged period, are associated with a high incidence of fungal superinfection (Greene *et al.*, 1973*a*; Seelig, 1966). In addition, in all cancer patients, the administration of corticosteroids, a potent suppressor of both inflammation and CMI, appears to broaden greatly the range of potential pathogens, with a special predisposition to *Pneumocystis carinii* and *Nocardia*, as well as fungal infections (Bodey, 1966; L. S. Young *et al.*, 1971).

The propensity to develop infection with fungi does not extend to all mycologic genera. Zimmerman (1955), in some early work, classified the mycoses into two groups: (1) those found in increased frequency among patients with underlying diseases, and (2) those not more frequent in patients with a primary disease. In the latter, he included actinomycosis, nocardiosis, sporotrichosis, blastomycosis, chromoblastomycosis, coccidioidomycosis, and maduromycosis. Among the former, he distinguished between those responsible for a rise in reported instances of largely malignancy-related mycoses, which included candidiasis, aspergillosis, and mucormycosis, and those found more commonly in patients with leukemia and lymphoma, but not in a progressively increasing incidence, cryptococcosis and histoplasmosis. These distinctions are not without exception; e.g., nocardiosis (not a true mycosis) is clearly more common among patients receiving steroids (L. S. Young *et al.*, 1971; Palmer *et al.*, 1974), and some reports suggest that dissemination of sporotrichosis (Lynch *et al.*, 1970) and coccidioidomycosis (Roberts *et al.*, 1968) is related to host compromise. Nevertheless, these distinctions remain valuable, and approximately correct, 20 years later. Nearly all fungal infections in patients with leukemia are caused by species of *Candida*, *Aspergillus*, and *Mucor*, most often *Candida albicans*, followed by *Aspergillus* (Levine *et al.*, 1974; Armstrong *et al.*, 1971). In some centers, aspergillosis has become much more frequent in recent years (Meyer *et al.*, 1973; Mirsky and Cuttner, 1972), even surpassing candidiasis; in others, *Torulopsis glabrata* has been increasingly seen (Marks *et al.*, 1970; Pankey and Daloviso, 1973). Thus, there are

249

SUPPORTIVE
CARE
IN THE
CANCER
PATIENT

sufficient regional and nosocomial differences so that it is incumbent on each institution to determine its own pattern of nonbacterial, as well as bacterial, infection.

3.4. Prophylaxis of Infection

3.4.1. General Comments

Prevention of opportunistic infection is the ultimate goal of those dealing with cancer patients, not solely to avoid the mortality of the infectious episode itself, but also because the occurrence of infection exposes the patient to modes of diagnosis and therapy that in themselves contribute to further infection, to debility with loss of muscle mass, appetite, and a sense of well-being that may compromise the quality of remaining life, and to the restructuring of schedules and doses of antineoplastic therapy that may compromise the adequacy of that therapy, and hence the duration of survival. It is in the setting of acute leukemia that the most persistent and expensive efforts at prophylaxis have been conducted, and these efforts will therefore receive the bulk of attention herein. An understanding of the factors predisposing to infection allows rational efforts at prophylaxis, and this section will follow the same overall outline as the preceding one.

3.4.2. Decreased Exposure

Because colonization precedes invasion, a major goal has been to decrease the frequency with which patients are exposed to potential pathogens, deriving from either the endogenous or the exogenous (nosocomial) microflora. Most attention has been directed at the GI tract as the primary respository of endogenous flora. Prophylaxis has taken two major forms: (1) alteration of the flora toward non-pathogens, or (2) suppression of the existing flora. Only the latter has been subjected to extensive clinical trial, using oral, nonabsorbable antibiotics (ONAs), and this form of prophylaxis will be summarized below in the discussion of reverse isolation, with which it has often been associated. Several other methods of gut flora suppression have also been tried, involving the use, singly or in combination, of oral, absorbable antibiotics (Bodey, 1972), systemic antibiotics (Freireich et al., 1975), and elemental diets (Winitz et al., 1970a). In most instances, such methods have been investigated microbiologically, but without careful evaluation of their clinical utility in preventing infection. Bodey (1972) described the use of oral, absorbable chloramphenicol, tetracycline, and ampicillin for gut flora suppression, but found an unacceptably high rate of development of bacterial resistance to the antibiotics used, and did not recommend their use alone for infection prophylaxis.

One approach that has received only limited attention is the use of elemental (amino acid) diets to reduce the bulk and bacterial content of the stool and to improve gut tissue nutrition. These diets have been reported to provide adequate nutritional support while decreasing the frequency and bulk of the stool (Winitz et al., 1970a, b) and the number and variety of bacteria per gram wet weight of stool (Winitz et al., 1970a). That they effect the latter has been denied

(Dickman *et al.*, 1975). Among patients with severe granulocytopenia, in whom perirectal abscesses and bacteremias of GI origin are frequent, a diminution in bacterial numbers and stool bulk might reduce the frequency of such infection, but the relative unpalatibility of these diets has made long-term administration a difficult task, thus far. Bounous and co-workers (Bounous *et al.*, 1971*a*, *b*; Hugon and Bounous, 1972) have reported that the ingestion of an elemental diet prior to and during exposure to 5-fluorouracil, in rat and man, and to radiation, in the mouse, will protect against the induction of enteritis and colitis, perhaps by allowing faster regeneration of the damaged epithelium. If confirmed, such prophylaxis might reduce the frequency of bacterial invasion through denuded mucosa.

No attempts have been made to alter the quality but not the quantity of bacteria in cancer patients. In newborn nurseries, repopulation of the nasal passages of medical personnel carrying *Staphylococcus aureus* with nonpathogenic *S. epidermidis* has proved successful in aborting carriage and transmission of the virulent strain. In the GI tract, the establishment of new strains is a very difficult task, and attempts to do so with *E. coli* and *Lactobacillus* given orally have been unsuccessful. Experiments with germ-free animals subsequently associated with bacteria under controlled conditions may further delineate factors responsible for control of microbial growth that might be subject to clinical manipulation.

From the vantage of infection control, the hospital is perhaps the worst environment in which to care for the compromised host. The proximity of other patients, many with infections; the sharing of medical personnel and equipment among patients; the dependency and limitations on physical activity imposed by hospital regulations—all contribute to the development of nosocomial infection. Where possible, cancer therapy should be administered on an outpatient basis, including the use of nearby hotels or intermediate care facilities for the housing of ambulatory patients who must travel long distances or who require daily drug or radiation therapy.

When hospitalization cannot be avoided, the following suggestions may reduce potential exposure:

1. The patient with active disease, or undergoing cancer therapy, should be in a single-bed room.
2. For those in whom significant prolonged granulocytopenia (<1000 PMNs/mm^3) is anticipated, the diet should be restricted to cooked food, with vitamin supplements. The omission of fresh fruits and vegetables, and their replacement by canned or cooked items, does not usually render a great hardship, and there is little doubt from multiple studies by Shooter and co-workers (Shooter *et al.*, 1969, 1971) that such items represent frequent sources of exposure to gram-negative aerobic bacilli. Similarly, the direct handling of plants and flowers by such patients should be avoided.
3. Most important, and worth emphasis, is the practice of washing one's hands. There is evidence that the predominant mode of spread of both gram-positive and gram-negative organisms is by direct contact, particularly by the

hands of medical personnel and, sometimes, visitors (Rammelkamp *et al.*, 1964; Salzman *et al.*, 1967; Burke *et al.*, 1971). The subject of hand-washing has recently been reviewed and recommendations have been made (Steere and Mallison, 1975). In caring for the usual patient with cancer, hand-washing with soap and water, before and after contact with the patient, would seem sufficient for removal of transient flora and reduction of resident flora. In the severely granulopenic patient, however, the wearing of gloves or the use of an iodophor antiseptic is warranted. The major impediment to interdicting hand-carriage of nosocomial organisms is not disagreement over the technical aspects, but inertia. Physicians and nurses must be repeatedly reminded of the importance of hand-washing, and provision must be made for ready access to soap and water, iodophors, or gloves, at the bedside or at the entrance to the room. A private sink in the patient's room with soap and iodophor alongside it, in dispensers rather than packets, will expedite the process and assure its observance. Because of splashing and dripping, the area around the sink should be clear and easily cleanable.

4. Medical instrumentation, particularly nondisposable equipment, has the potential for transmission of nosocomial organisms. In patients with severe granulocytopenia, when it is necessary to use equipment, such as endoscopes and inhalation and respiratory therapy apparatus, and such mundane items as stethoscopes, blood pressure cuffs, and tongue depressors, it is particularly incumbent upon medical staff to minimize cross-contamination. The measures taken should include gas-sterilization or soaking in iodophors for endoscopes (F. M. Chang *et al.*, 1973) and the placing in the patient's room of a single blood pressure cuff, stethoscope, and other pieces of everyday equipment for the duration of the patient's stay, with regular cleaning.

That patients with acute leukemia, especially acute myelogenous leukemia, have been dying of bacterial infection before chemotherapy has had an opportunity to induce remission has led in the past decade to efforts (Levitan and Perry, 1967, 1968; Preisler *et al.*, 1970; Bodey *et al.*, 1969*b*) to prevent exposure to both exogenous and endogenous organisms by (1) decreasing endogenous flora with ONAs, topical antibiotic ointments, and antibiotic sprays; and (2) minimizing contact with hospital bacteria by instituting barrier isolation facilities. It has long been known that germ-free animals were capable of surviving doses of radiation and chemotherapy that cause death in conventional animals (Pollard and Sharon, 1970; White and Claflin, 1963). It was also realized that the use of reverse isolation alone would not prevent colonization of the patient's environment or direct invasion by endogenous microorganisms. After what can only be considered anecdotal reports of the success of "gut decontamination" or reverse isolation or both in infection prevention in acute leukemia (Levitan and Perry, 1967; Preisler *et al.*, 1970), several controlled clinical trials were begun in the late 1960s and 1970 to evaluate the separate and combined contributions of each of these modalities on (1) the incidence and severity of infection, and (2) remission rate and survival.

The results of these studies have recently been published and reviewed [Levine *et al.*, 1973 (NCI); Yates and Holland, 1973 (RPMI); Schimpff *et al.*, 1975 (BCRC)]. A number of other retrospectively controlled or uncontrolled studies have purported to show the utility of gut decontamination or one or another form of reverse isolation, but will not be further discussed (see Preisler and Bjornsson, 1975, and the discussion in Schimpff *et al.*, 1975).

The three prospectively controlled trials were conducted at the Baltimore Cancer Research Center (BCRC), at the National Cancer Institute (NCI) in Bethesda, and at the Roswell Park Memorial Institute (RPMI) in Buffalo, New York. All used a "laminar air flow" (LAF) room with a bank of high-efficiency particulate air (HEPA) filters through which was blown a sterile, unidirectional flow of air from the head to the foot of the room. As demonstrated by air-sampling and environmental cultures in all studies, the stream of air bathing the patients was virtually sterile, and the surfaces within the LAF room were very clean. The first two studies (BCRC and NCI) randomly assigned patients with acute leukemia to one of three arms: care on a conventional ward; care on the same ward receiving ONAs; and care in an LAF facility receiving ONAs. The RPMI study added a fourth arm, LAF without ONAs, and housed the non-LAF patients taking ONAs in private rooms under reverse isolation, not on an open ward or in a multibed room. Although within each study the patients in each arm appeared comparable for factors of risk for infection and remission, among studies there were some important differences, which involved the number of previous remission induction attempts, the presence of infection at the time of admission, the use of orificial or topical antibiotics, and the criteria for terminating study. Nevertheless, the impact of these differences on the overall findings is uncertain, and they do not fully explain the varying conclusions.

The studies agree that patients receiving ONAs within an LAF facility experience one-half to two-thirds fewer overall infections, severe infections, and infectious deaths; in particular, there are fewer pneumonias and septicemias. Unfortunately, the three studies did not agree as to whether the LAFs or the ONAs or both were crucial elements in this prophylaxis. Thus, in the BCRC study, patients receiving ONAs alone experienced a significant reduction in severe infections, especially bacteremias and pneumonias, and some decrease in infectious deaths from that seen in the ward group alone. Similarly, in the RPMI study, there appeared to be a decrease in infectious deaths among patients receiving ONAs alone, as well as in the group in the LAF taking ONAs. In the NCI study, however, no contribution of ONAs in a ward setting can be discerned, while patients in an LAF receiving gut prophylaxis had a marked reduction in frequency of infection, and no infectious death whatever.

The issue of whether infection is prevented by these measures is an important one. But it is not the only one. The purchase and the maintenance of LAFs, in terms of added personnel, sterile supplies, dietary alterations, and other factors, are expensive in time, effort, and money. ONAs are very expensive, not very pleasant to take every 4 hr, and productive of several days of nausea and diarrhea. The cost of this program has been estimated to be $200–300 per day above

253

SUPPORTIVE
CARE
IN THE
CANCER
PATIENT

conventional care (Esterhay *et al.*, 1975). Added to this cost must be some consideration, less easily quantified, of the restrictions imposed on the patients housed in the LAF during what for many are the last days of life. Ultimately, the allocation of scarce resources must justify itself in terms of a change in the prognosis for remission or survival. Measured by these criteria, only the BCRC study demonstrated an improved remission rate and survival, and this was seen in both the LAF and ONA and the ward plus ONA arms. In contrast, despite the absence of infection in the NCI study, a higher remission rate was not observed, without explanation. In the RPMI study, a decreased infectious mortality in the groups taking ONAs was offset by an increase in hemorrhagic deaths, a problem not encountered by other studies nor among the RPMI patients placed in the LAF but without ONAs, thus giving the latter group the best survival. Remission rates, however, were not increased.

More recent studies have not helped in explaining these discrepancies. A report from the BCRC, in abstract form, by Hahn *et al.* (1975) noted a decrease in gram-negative infections and showed that the use of ONAs in a ward setting continued to be associated with a decreased infection rate, but controls were retrospective or not truly comparable, while in another study using prospective randomized controls, the addition of ordinary reverse isolation or air filtration confined to the bed area only did not enhance the prophylactic effect of ONAs (Schimpff *et al.*, 1976). In each of these studies, as in the full BCRC LAF trial (Schimpff *et al.*, 1975, 1976; Hahn *et al.*, 1975), patients discontinuing gut prophylaxis while still granulopenic had a significantly increased infection rate compared with when the ONAs were being ingested. The factors leading to noncompliance by the patient in taking the ONAs may, however, also predispose to further infection. Hence, the reliability of these observations is uncertain. Other studies have not noted this problem. Freireich *et al.* (1975), in a major program involving some 100 adult patients with acute leukemia (both ALL and AML) at the M. D. Anderson Hospital, described a prospective trial of protected environments (LAFs) plus either prophylactic oral antibiotics (PAs) or systemic antibiotics (SAs) compared with PAs or SAs administered outside an LAF. This very complicated study showed major advantages for the LAFs, both in decreasing infection rate and in increasing remission rate and survival, but the import of these data must await publication of the full study.

In summary, the value of an LAF and/or ONA program in patients with acute leukemia remains uncertain, and it must be considered investigational. Resolution of the differences would require a multicenter cooperative trial, along lines similar to the RPMI study, with uniform modes of antileukemia and antiinfection therapy and careful criteria for infection. Nevertheless, it is possible that several factors will obviate the necessity or desirability of a prophylaxis program of this sort: (1) Other prophylactic and therapeutic measures for infection in patients with acute leukemia may lower infectious mortality significantly. (2) Antileukemic therapy may progress, as in Hodgkin's disease or childhood ALL, to the point where marrow toxicity is small and remissions prompt and frequent. (3) Further investigation may reveal that gut flora suppression alters the pharmacokinetics or absorption, or both, of antineoplastic therapy (Scheline, 1968; Dubos and Schaedler, 1962), accounting perhaps for the lack of improvement in remission rates in the NCI and RPMI studies despite reductions in infectious deaths, or, in the BCRC trial, the observation that an improved remission rate was seen only in those patients treated with daunorubicin alone, in either of two schedules. (4) Finally, it is possible that adult acute leukemics are the wrong patients to house in LAFs and to give ONAs. Rather, it may be that patients not so massively or continuously compromised might benefit more from these prophylactic measures, which are of only marginal or moderate effect in adult leukemics.

255

SUPPORTIVE
CARE
IN THE
CANCER
PATIENT

Antibiotic prophylaxis has been most effective when directed against a single organism the antibiotic resistance of which changes slowly, if at all, as in the penicillin prophylaxis of rheumatic fever. Such prophylaxis has not been attempted for specific bacterial invaders in cancer patients because: (1) there are many such pathogens, usually gram-negative; (2) the antibiotics to which they are susceptible are often toxic; and (3) gram-negative organisms frequently develop resistance to antibiotics after prolonged exposure. Such a complication was reported by the author several years ago in connection with the use of gentamicin orally in the LAF program at the BCRC (Greene et al., 1973c).

Some advances have been made in preventing clinical infection in nonbacterial disease. Among viral illnesses, two drugs have been found useful as prophylactic agents. Amantidine, when given during the incubation period, is clearly effective in reducing the frequency of clinical illness after exposure to influenza A_2 virus, and may ameliorate symptoms even when given early in the course of disease (Wingfield et al., 1969; Galbraith et al., 1971). It should be used in the unvaccinated cancer patient exposed to the virus, particularly if immunosuppressive agents are being used, or there is underlying cardiac or respiratory disease. Still experimental, and infrequently used, is methisazone, which may prevent smallpox if given after exposure but before clinical illness (Goldstein et al., 1975). Its use as *therapy* in complications of vaccinia immunization will be discussed below.

The value of isoniazid as a "prophylactic agent" in the patient with evidence of previous contact with tuberculosis is well known. Recently, the recognition of the hepatic toxicity of this drug, especially in older patients, has shifted the balance of benefit and risk, so that its use is primarily among patients less than 35–40 years of age (Johnston and Wildrick, 1974). However, in any patients undergoing immunosuppressive therapy, particularly with corticosteroids, the risk of developing clinical tuberculosis increases, and the benefit of using isoniazid may outweigh the risk even in older age groups.

Finally, an exciting development recently reported from St. Jude's has been the use of a combination of trimethoprim–sulfamethoxazole (T/S) in children with acute lymphocytic leukemia (ALL) undergoing chemotherapy to prevent *P. carinii* infection and death. As noted previously, this protozoan accounts for a major portion of infectious deaths among children with ALL in remission. With the success of T/S therapeutically in this illness (Hughes et al., 1975) (see Section 3.5.2) and in animal studies of prophylaxis in the steroid-treated rat (Hughes et al., 1974b), a prospective, double-blind, randomized controlled trial of prophylaxis was begun in ALL children. The preliminary results of this trial have been extremely encouraging (Simone, 1976), with marked reductions in frequency of disease with minimal side effects.

3.4.3. Improved Host Defenses

The preceding section detailed methods of preventing exposure to or illness caused by pathogens in patients already compromised in their ability to ward off infection. More likely to succeed in preventing infection are measures designed to minimize or repair the host defect, which itself leads to undue susceptibility. This section will review such "host-oriented" prophylaxis. To the extent that compromise of defenses against infection is tumor-induced, such as granulocytopenia in acute leukemia or bronchial obstruction in carcinoma of the lung, prompt therapy may alleviate the threat of infection. More often, the administration of drug and radiation therapy increases the risk of infection, though perhaps transiently. The search for improved dosage schedules of chemotherapy and radiation to increase the therapeutic ratio is a traditional part of oncology, but recently, several studies have demonstrated the ability of a second agent or modality to specifically lessen toxicity. Most widely applied is the use of folinic acid to improve the therapeutic index of methotrexate (Levitt *et al.*, 1973). Capizzi has described the clinical use of L-asparaginase sequentially with methotrexate to accomplish the same purpose (Capizzi, 1975). Animal experiments suggest that cycloheximide, like L-asparaginase a protein-synthesis inhibitor, can lessen the bone marrow toxicity of cytosine arabinoside and, to a lesser extent, nitrogen mustard (Ben-Ishay and Farber, 1975). Similarly, there are laboratory (Houchens *et al.*, 1974) and anecdotal clinical observations that antitumor immunotherapy may also be capable of lessening the effect of alkylating agents on hematopoiesis.

Other tentative approaches to lessening the systemic toxicity of antineoplastic drugs are the binding of these agents to molecules, such as antibodies (Hurwitz *et al.*, 1975) and hormones that are specific for the tumor, thereby directing the drug to the tumor bed, or identifying clinical situations likely to result in excessive drug toxicity (Medical Research Council, 1975; Rosenoff *et al.*, 1975). Whether these approaches will be of major significance in cancer therapy awaits further investigation.

a. Mucocutaneous Barriers. Intravenous catheters should be avoided because of the high rate of phlebitis and bacteremia associated with their use, and scalp vein needles employed in their place, with appropriate cleansing of the skin with iodophors and alcohol beforehand and use of antibiotic ointments at the puncture site afterward. Scalp vein needles should be removed after 48 hr, and the tubing and connections should be replaced every 24 hr, particularly after use of blood products. In most instances, intravenous hyperalimentation should be avoided in patients with hematologic malignancy, and when employed, the catheter should not be used for other purposes, such as blood-drawing or drug administration. A single person or small group of people should be responsible for maintaining the catheter site and checking it daily. The appearance of fever in patients with catheters in place should prompt cultures of blood, and the documentation of blood-borne infection, particularly with *Candida*, should require removal of the catheter and culture of its tip.

257
SUPPORTIVE
CARE
IN THE
CANCER
PATIENT

Urethral catheters should be employed only as a last resort for bladder drainage, and when inserted should use a closed drainage system (Stamm, 1975). The necessity for sterile handling of tracheostomy tubes is well recognized, though often ignored. Skin care is an essential component of prophylaxis. Avoidance of both excessive drying and maceration of the skin will prevent breaks in continuity that would favor invasion. Decubitus ulcers are well established as the source of a significant percentage of bacteremias, particularly anaerobic sepsis, and their prevention by frequent rotation, protection of bony prominences, avoidance of continuous corticosteroid use, and maintenance of adequate diet is far simpler than attempts to manage them once they occur. Once developed, vigorous debridement, both surgical and enzymatic, of dead and infected tissue is essential.

In patients with profound granulocytopenia, particularly acute leukemics, the perirectal area is a frequent site of infection, with ensuing sepsis and death, accounting for as much as 10–25% of severe infections (Levine *et al.*, 1974; Schimpff *et al.*, 1972c). These infections occur with particular frequency in patients with a history of hemorrhoids and rectal or anal fissures. In these settings, the anal region must be kept particularly clean and free from irritation. To accomplish this, both constipation, with the necessary straining at stool, and diarrhea, with its frequent soiling and irritation, should be prevented or treated promptly. The use of stool softeners is to be recommended. Another very useful adjunct is the prophylactic sitz bath. It is an accepted form of therapy for thrombosed hemorrhoids and perirectal fissures, and we have found it useful, once or twice daily, to prevent their occurrence and to keep the perineal and perianal region clean.

Previous discussion has stressed the importance of the normal bacterial flora to the inhibition of appearance of nosocomial pathogens. In order to maintain such flora, prolonged "blind" antibiotic usage should be avoided. As will be noted subsequently, in the febrile granulopenic patient, broad-spectrum antibiotics should be begun promptly, after physical examination and culturing, if there is a clinical suspicion of infection. But if no clinical response or infectious source is evident after 4–5 days of therapy, the antibiotics should be as promptly discontinued. Some fraction of patients may display evidence of infection after discontinuation of antibiotics (Rodriguez *et al.*, 1973; S. Bjornsson and Preisler, 1976). However, prompt reinstitution of therapy in this minority of subjects minimizes the inherent risk of such a policy (Rodriguez *et al.*, 1973), which is, in any event, outweighed by the avoidance of superinfection, particularly fungal superinfection. This complication is likely to occur in as many as one-half of patients treated continuously for 12 days or more with carbenicillin, gentamicin, and cephalothin (Greene *et al.*, 1973a). Recent reports have confirmed these findings, and have made similar recommendations (Levine *et al.*, 1974; Goodall and Vosti, 1975). It is also necessary to remember that even unusual predisposing factors, such as prostatic obstruction of urinary outflow (Mitch and Serpick, 1970) or respiratory obstruction (Morris and Shaw, 1974), may arise as a result of neoplastic infiltration, not only by solid tumors and lymphoma, but also by leukemic cells. If thought of, local measures such as radiotherapy may prevent infection from occurring or allow more rapid resolution of existing infection.

b. The Inflammatory Response. Definable abnormalities of inflammation in cancer patients can usually be traced to one of two factors: (1) granulocytopenia, or (2) drug-, especially corticosteroid-, induced PMN dysfunction. Recent advances have suggested modes of prophylaxis. The increasing availability of granulocyte transfusions, the recent demonstration in well-controlled trials of their efficacy in therapeutic situations (see Section 3.5.2), and the realization that prophylactic reconstitution makes sense have spurred clinical trials of prophylactic PMN transfusions in several centers. Cooper *et al.* (1975) reported favorable preliminary results of such a program several years ago, and early reports of their use in Seattle in a randomized trial during the phase of pancytopenia following bone marrow transplantation are also encouraging (Thomas, 1976). In acute leukemic patients with granulocyte counts of less than $500/mm^3$, the data of Bodey (1966) suggest that a small increment of $100-300/mm^3$ in the average daily circulating PMN level might dramatically decrease the frequency of infection. Transient, usually subclinical bacterial invasion of mucosal surfaces is undoubtedly a common daily event. Such microscopic foci would seem much more amenable to eradication by small numbers of granulocytes than an infection that has become of sufficient size to reach clinical awareness. Although still early in the investigational stages, this approach to infection prevention in granulocytopenic patients holds promise of being one of the most rewarding.

Recent work by Dale, Fauci, and co-workers (Dale *et al.*, 1974a; Fauci and Dale, 1975) has confirmed earlier studies that the use of alternate-day schedules of prednisone in patients requiring long-term corticosteroids is associated with significant decreases in the metabolic, cutaneous, and infectious complications seen with daily therapy. Furthermore, their studies suggest that even short courses of daily corticosteroids will be associated with significant impairment of the neutrophilic and monocytic inflammatory response (Dale *et al.*, 1974a). Their recommendation that alternate-day programs be instituted whenever steroid treatment is warranted (Dale *et al.*, 1974a) should be considered when long-term prednisone is to be used, and should be extended to comparative clinical trials of daily vs. alternate-day steroids in cyclic chemotherapeutic regimens to be certain that antineoplastic effectiveness is not being sacrificed. Similar considerations pertain to the intriguing finding in a well-controlled study (Peters *et al.*, 1972) that the fluorinated steroid analogues, such as dexamethasone, impair the neutrophilic inflammatory response far less than the prednisone–prednisolone congeners. If dexamethasone retains antineoplastic activity and is indeed less compromising, its substitution for other steroids may also be a useful prophylactic maneuver.

The study of pharmacological stimulation of granulocyte function is in its early phases. An exception is the assessment of bone marrow granulocyte reserve among cancer patients as a guide to subsequent tolerance of chemotherapy or radiation therapy, employing the steroid etiocholanolone (Godwin *et al.*, 1968) or the *Pseudomonas* lipopolysaccharide Piromen® (Korbitz *et al.*, 1969). In these tests the failure to increase the absolute level of PMNs by at least 2600–2800/mm^3 8–18 hr after parenteral injection indicates a decreased marrow reserve, and may presage undue myelopoietic toxicity following therapy. Early reports suggest that other PMN functions may be augmented, e.g., with clofazimine (Brandt, 1971) or levamisole (G. W. Fisher *et al.*, 1974), but clinical application seems some years off.

259

SUPPORTIVE
CARE
IN THE
CANCER
PATIENT

c. Humoral Immunity. Attempts at prophylaxis in cancer patients have included both active and passive immunization, and replacement therapy for those who were hypogammaglobulinemic. The latter include primarily patients with multiple myeloma and chronic lymphocytic leukemia, and to a lesser degree other lymphoproliferative disorders. The usefulness of gamma globulin (GG) in children with inherited disorders of antibody production has not been comparably established in adults with neoplasia. Salmon *et al.* (1967) investigated this area and conducted a prospective randomized trial of GG in a series of patients with multiple myeloma, and found no difference in frequency of infection between the group receiving GG and those not receiving it. In part, this result was explained by the hypercatabolism of GG seen in patients with IgG myeloma, resulting in rapid loss of circulating levels of exogenous IgG beyond the ability to administer it intramuscularly. However, in patients with other forms of cancer or among those with myeloma in whom the half-life of GG is not markedly shortened, a clinical trial of prophylactic GG may be warranted when infections are frequently recurrent. Further well-controlled studies are needed in this field.

Other forms of passive immunization have involved the administration of globulins of high titer against specific pathogens to susceptible patients at special risk for infection with these organisms. Most useful is zoster immune globulin (ZIG), a biological prepared from plasma of postzoster patients and available from the Center for Disease Control (CDC) for the prophylaxis of varicella in immunosuppressed children and adolescents exposed to varicella or zoster (Geiser *et al.*, 1975; Wilfert, 1975). The studies of Gershon and Brunell and their co-workers (Brunell and Gershon, 1973; Gershon *et al.*, 1974) have demonstrated that the presence of antibody appears to play little protective role in the development or dissemination of herpes zoster. ZIG would not be expected to be useful in adult zoster, because in most instances, zoster is a cell-to-cell reactivation of the primary varicella infection acquired in childhood, dormant since then in the CNS (Brunell and Gershon, 1973), and not susceptible to extracellular defenses. In contrast, ZIG, when administered within 72 hr of exposure in a dose of 0.2–0.4 ml/kg, completely prevents or significantly ameliorates the severity of varicella (Wilfert, 1975; Geiser *et al.*, 1975), lessening the risk of disseminated varicella, a frequently fatal complication in immunosuppressed patients. Once the disease manifests itself, ZIG is no longer of value. Because of the difficulty in obtaining ZIG and its increasing use, the indications outlined above are rigidly adhered to by the CDC. Vaccinia immune globulin (VIG) is also available from the CDC, and is of value in the management of the immunosuppressed patient inadvertently vaccinated for smallpox. The abandonment of routine smallpox immunization in the United States has decreased the likelihood of this problem occurring, but should it occur, VIG should be used in patients with lymphoproliferative malignancy or receiving steroids to prevent disseminated vaccinia or vaccinia necrosum (Goldstein *et al.*, 1975). Immune serum globulin is useful in the child with no prior history of measles to prevent severe rubeola or rubeola pneumonia, an often fatal complication, if exposure has taken place (Levine *et al.*, 1974; Hughes *et al.*, 1974*a*). Such prophylaxis will usually be unnecessary in adults.

Two other immune globulins warrant particular mention. The frequency of hepatitis B (HB) infection among leukemic patients, found to be about 20% in two recent studies (Steinberg *et al.*, 1975; Wands *et al.*, 1974; *Morbidity and Mortality Weekly Report*, 1976), and the risk of transmission to staff and family provide a rationale for the use of HB immune globulin in these populations. This globulin has been shown in recent carefully controlled trials to be an effective form of prophylaxis (Surgenor *et al.*, 1975; Prince *et al.*, 1975; Grady and Lee, 1975), but guidelines for its use have not yet been formulated, since it remains at present a limited and investigational product. *Pseudomonas* hyperimmune globulin has been tried in selected groups of patients particularly susceptible to *Pseudomonas* infections. Among patients with acute leukemia it has not been found to be effective.

Active immunization against both bacterial and nonbacterial pathogens is enjoying a renaissance of interest. In the cancer patient, and especially the patient with hematologic malignancy, who is most susceptible to infection, a cardinal rule is the avoidance of live virus vaccines. Influenza vaccine as a killed virus preparation is effective, and should be used routinely in cancer patients, not solely to prevent the viral illness, but also to prevent the postviral bacterial complications which form a major part of mortality to influenza.

Other vaccines of special relevance to cancer patients are experimental. One that has received extensive clinical trial is a polyvalent *Pseudomonas* vaccine comprised of killed preparations of the seven immunotypes of M. W. Fisher *et al.* (1969). In burn patients, using historical controls, this vaccine has reportedly been effective in decreasing the frequency and mortality of *Pseudomonas* infection (Alexander *et al.*, 1971). In a well-controlled study in cancer patients (L. S. Young *et al.*, 1973), the vaccine reduced *Pseudomonas*-associated deaths only moderately, and bacteremic death was not significantly decreased. In addition, 92% of vaccinees had significant local or systemic reaction to the vaccine. Thus, its use at present is very limited, as confirmed in another study (Haghbin *et al.*, 1973).

Other experimental vaccines include a modified preparation of hepatitis B antigen, which has been shown effective in clinical trial (Krugman and Giles, 1973), and a vaccine prepared from a mutant *E. coli*, which, because of deficiency of an enzyme, epimerase, exposes on its surface an antigen shared by many gram-negative bacilli, including *E. coli*, *Klebsiella*, and *Pseudomonas* (Ziegler *et al.*, 1973). Experiments in normal and granulopenic animals have demonstrated excellent protection against challenge with gram-negative bacteria (Ziegler *et al.*, 1975). A prospective controlled double-blind clinical trial in cancer patients is currently evaluating this vaccine.

Theoretically, the efficacy of these attempts to provide opsonins for common bacterial pathogens would be enhanced greatly by also supplying phagocytes in the form of prophylactic granulocyte transfusions. Combined trials of this sort have not yet been done.

261

SUPPORTIVE
CARE
IN THE
CANCER
PATIENT

d. Cellular Immunity. Despite the importance of the intact cellular immune response in preventing invasion by many intracellular organisms, our ability to manipulate this response to the patient's benefit is limited. Presently, one can suggest avoidance of continuously immunosuppressive regimens by the use of cyclic chemotherapy with rest periods (Hersh *et al.*, 1966) or alternate-day corticosteroids (Dale *et al.*, 1974*a*; Fauci and Dale, 1975). Inadequate nutrition and intercurrent viral infections also appear capable of inducing anergy, and other stresses of cell-mediated immunity (CMI) should be postponed, if possible, until adequate food intake has been restored and viral infection resolved.

The active administration of agents to enhance the immune response has been investigated largely to achieve antitumor immunity, using bacillus Calmette-Guérin (BCG), *Corynebacterium parvum*, MER (an extract of BCG), polyribonucleotides, and levamisole, an antihelminthic agent (Bluming, 1975). There are experimental and clinical data that show enhancement of CMI responses with these agents, and some data suggest a lessening of the infectious complications and myelosuppressive effects of chemotherapy in immunotherapy-treated patients (Jordan and Merigan, 1975), but no specific application or trial relevant to infection prophylaxis has been mounted. Cell products, such as interferon and transfer factor, have been receiving extensive trial as therapeutic agents in nonbacterial infections (Stevens *et al.*, 1974; Levine *et al.*, 1974), with some promising results for the latter in chronic mucocutaneous candidiasis and coccidioidomycosis (Valdimarsson *et al.*, 1972; Graybill *et al.*, 1973). A recent trial of interferon in patients with osteogenic sarcoma also suggested a reduced frequency of infectious complications compared with an untreated control group (Strander *et al.*, 1976). At present, however, none of these agents can be recommended for infection prophylaxis.

3.5. Management of Infection

3.5.1. Diagnosis of Infection

The appearance of fever is the usual stimulus for initiating a search for infection in the patient with cancer. Until proved otherwise, one must assume that infection is the cause. Nevertheless, it is recognized that the frequency with which infection can be documented as the source of fever varies with each tumor type. Among patients with acute leukemia, 60–70% of febrile episodes are due to infection (Boggs and Frei, 1960); in chronic lymphocytic leukemia, it is virtually 100%; while in patients with lymphomas, especially Hodgkin's disease, only 25% may be secondary to infection (Boggs and Frei, 1960). Patients with solid tumors rarely have fever ascribable solely to the tumor—5% of all febrile episodes in one study

(Browder *et al.*, 1961)—although metastatic disease and certain types of neoplasia, such as hypernephroma, appear to increase this percentage. The diagnostic process must start with a thorough physical examination that encompasses the areas known to be frequently involved. In leukemic patients, attention must especially be paid to the fundi, gingiva, pharynx, lungs, urinary tract, perirectal area, and skin. Both the fundi and the skin may develop lesions in disseminated infection that may be the sole clue to etiology. The characteristic appearance of fungal endophthalmitis, which occurs in 5–10% of patients with disseminated candidiasis (Greene and Wiernik, 1972), and sporadically in other generalized fungal diseases (McLean, 1963), may allow presumptive diagnosis. Skin lesions, such as ecthyma gangrenosum, may be present in 20–60% of those with *Pseudomonas* bacteremia (Fishman and Armstrong, 1972), in a smaller percentage of patients with disseminated candidal infections (Bodey and Luna, 1974), and in generalized viral disease, especially atypical forms of herpes zoster (Schimpff *et al.*, 1972*b*). Rapid identification of these lesions may facilitate early diagnosis and therapy. Hence, the appearance of cutaneous lesions in the febrile patient should prompt aspiration, biopsy, and culture.

Equally as important as the recognition of positive evidence of infection is the realization that the absence of signs or symptoms in a given organ system, especially in the patient with severe granulocytopenia or receiving corticosteroids, does not eliminate infection in that area. In a recent study (Sickles *et al.*, 1975), severe granulocytopenia (less than $100/mm^3$) was associated with a marked reduction in such "hard" signs as exudate, fluctuance, ulceration, or fissure, necessitating reliance on erythema, tenderness, and pain to localize and follow the course of infection. As an example, anorectal infections in the patients with PMN counts of less than 100 were accompanied by exudate in 15%, fluctuance or fissure in 31%, and bacteremia in 46%, while pain and erythema were always present; patients with PMN counts of more than 100 also had pain and erythema, but 87% had fluctuance or fissure, and a similar percentage had an exudate, while bacteremia was present in only 12%. This diminution of objective findings necessitates even greater reliance on ancillary diagnostic aids, of which culture techniques and radiography are most often useful.

A review of X-ray diagnosis of infection is beyond the scope of this chapter, but two special situations require comment. In the compromised, especially neutropenic, host with pneumonia, the chest X-ray is often the most reliable guide in diagnosis and management (Sickles *et al.*, 1973). Because of the inadequacies of physical examination in granulocytopenic patients, it is recommended that chest X rays be taken at least once weekly as a routine, and more often, as much as daily, if fever of unknown etiology persists or if pulmonary infection is established. Discerning the etiology of pneumonia in the noncancer patient is the result of combination of culture results, interpretation of chest X-rays, and knowledge of epidemiology of lung infection. In the cancer patient, one undergoes the same process, but the spectrum of possible etiologic organisms becomes greater, and with it the alternative therapies. The chest X-ray pattern—diffuse vs. nodular, segmental vs. multilobar, interstitial vs. alveolar, etc.—may be a valuable guide to the likely range of causative organisms. This subject has been summarized recently (Blank *et al.*, 1973; Bragg and Janis, 1973). In the neutropenic patient, the initial pulmonary infection is usually bacterial, but nonbacterial pneumonia becomes more likely if the patient has been receiving corticosteroids or prolonged broad-spectrum antiobiotic therapy, the former causing a special predisposition to *P. carinii, Nocardia*, and fungi, and the latter to fungi. Within the classes of pathogens, however, the chest radiograph only infrequently allows definitive diagnosis, for which histology or culture must serve. One increasingly common clinical circumstance in which radiography may define an etiology is candidal esophagitis (Levine *et al.*, 1974), and a barium "swallow" should be performed in any patient complaining of substernal pain or dysphagia to look for the characteristic disruption of motility or mucosal architecture or both (Eras *et al.*, 1972; Holt, 1968). Since disseminated candidiasis often originates from the GI tract (Eras *et al.*, 1972) prompt therapy may forestall more serious illness. Occasionally, other organisms or the underlying disease may cause esophagitis indistinguishable from *Candida* (Gildenhorn *et al.*, 1962).

Adequate culturing is the basic laboratory test of infection. In the neutropenic patient, blood cultures, which are more often positive than in the usual patient, may be the only means by which to identify an etiologic agent. A recent review of this subject (Washington, 1975) recommends, in suspected septicemia, 3 separate sets of blood cultures of at least 10 ml each, taken at intervals to be determined by clinical circumstances. Washington (1975) also suggests that these cultures consist of a trypticase soy broth and a Columbia broth bottle with added sodium polyanetholesulfonate, an antiphagocytic, anticomplementary polyanionic anticoagulant that has been shown to increase the recovery of bacteria from blood cultures. R. C. Young *et al.* (1974) recently reviewed the experience with fungemia at the National Cancer Institute, and formulated several guidelines for the interpretation of a positive fungal blood culture. There is some evidence that "surveillance" cultures will often help in defining the range of likely organisms causing bacterial infection (Schimpf *et al.*, 1972*a*), with positive nasal cultures for *Aspergillus* spp. (Steere *et al.*, 1975) and multiple sites positive for *P. aeruginosa* (Schimpff *et al.*, 1970) perhaps presaging infection with these organisms. The recovery of anaerobic organisms from sites of infection will be of particular importance, as previously noted, among patients with bronchial or intestinal obstruction or abscess formation. Where abscess fluid can be obtained, it will serve as an excellent carrying medium to the laboratory. If only swabs are available, care must be taken either to plate them promptly on appropriate media or to transport them in a moistened state in an oxygen-free environment.

The recovery of pulmonary pathogens from expectorated sputum is notoriously difficult, even for bacterial pneumonias. When sputum is nonpurulent, as in granulocytopenic subjects, or the organism nonbacterial, its identification is more unlikely. This has led to a number of invasive methods of obtaining samples of pulmonary tissue for culture or histology or both, including transtracheal aspiration, flexible bronchoscopy, bronchial brushing, transbronchoscopic biopsy, percutaneous needle aspiration or biopsy, and, of course, open lung biopsy (Bode *et al.*, 1974). A recent retrospective study (Greenman *et al.*, 1975) of the latter three methods in diagnosing diffuse lung disease demonstrated the utility and safety of lung biopsy in the compromised host, even when the platelet count was less than 100,000, provided coagulation studies were normal. Open lung biopsy established a specific diagnosis on 65% of the occasions it was performed, but only marginally improved the yield of the other two procedures in diagnosing infection. Of importance was the finding that establishment of a specific etiology was associated with an improved outcome. This study did not examine transbronchial biopsy, but recent results (Joyner and Scheinhorn, 1975) suggest an efficacy similar to that of open biopsy. The actual choice of procedure will obviously vary with the skill of the bronchoscopist, radiologist, and surgeon, but where hemostasis is of concern, open biopsy probably offers greater opportunities for control.

In the patient in whom localized infection is suspected, cultures of the site are, of course, mandatory. Even minimal symptoms referable to the CNS should prompt lumbar puncture, since there appears to be an increasing frequency of such infections (Chernik *et al.*, 1973). As a routine in the asymptomatic patient, however, CSF and bone marrow aspirate cultures are unrewarding (Greene *et al.*, 1973*b*). In contrast, among patients in whom infection with an intracellular organism is suspected, such as tuberculosis, histoplasma, cryptococcosis, *Toxoplasma*, or *Salmonella*, examination of the bone marrow aspirate may occasionally yield the diagnosis, either microscopically or by culture (Hughes, 1971*b*), even when blood cultures are negative.

Other diagnostic aids of general use include radioactive scans, ultrasound examination (Sandweiss *et al.*, 1975), and the technique of computerized axial tomography, with and without contrast, each of which may outline distortions of architecture or fluid collections that represent infectious sources. Radioactive gallium scanning takes advantage of the fact that this isotope is taken up by cytoplasmic granules of phagocytic cells, especially neutrophils (Arseneau *et al.*, 1974), collections of which can then be imaged. This method has been most extensively applied to the detection of abscesses, particularly intraabdominal (Silva and Harvey, 1974). Nevertheless, gallium has successfully demonstrated infectious processes in patients with acute leukemia and aplastic anemia, despite severe neutropenia (Oster *et al.*, 1975; Milder *et al.*, 1973). The gallium scan may also demonstrate areas of involvement by such malignancies as lymphomas, leukemias, carcinoma of the lung, and melanomas, clouding to some extent the interpretation of the positive scan in patients with such tumors (Milder *et al.*, 1973). Despite this, gallium imaging of infectious lesions is a valuable diagnostic adjunct.

Infection by specific agents, particularly viral, has been diagnosed by serologic means for many years. Recently, detection of changes in antibody titers and of the presence of antigen has been applied to bacterial and fungal infections as well. Among patients with cancer, tests for cryptococcal antigen in CSF (Goodman *et al.*, 1971) and *Pseudomonas* antigens in sera (Bartram *et al.*, 1974) have particular relevance, but only the former test is widely available. Detection of antigen has the advantage over antibody determinations of not requiring the inherent delay of acute and convalescent phase sera for changes in titer. In subacute, nonviral infections, antibody determinations have been of value in the diagnosis of cryptococcosis (Bindschadler and Bennett, 1968), aspergillosis (Coleman and Kaufman, 1972), histoplasmosis, and coccidioidomycosis, as well as toxoplasmosis (Ruskin and Remington, 1976). The reliability of precipitin detection and complement fixation for diagnosis of candidiasis and cytomegalovirus, respectively, is less certain (Dee and Rytel, 1975; Preisler *et al.*, 1971; Weller, 1971). Serologic studies are currently unavailable for establishing the etiology of infections due to *P. carinii*, *Nocardia*, and *Mucor*. Because of the value of serology and the frequent lack of a "baseline" serum from which to measure titer changes, among patients undergoing extensive chemotherapy, some centers currently have a frozen "serum bank," into which serial, routine serum specimens are placed for possible use subsequently, should the patient become infected.

265

SUPPORTIVE
CARE
IN THE
CANCER
PATIENT

3.5.2. *Therapy of Infection*

This section will deal with some guidelines for therapy of presumed bacterial infection in the neutropenic patient ($<1000/mm^3$). In addition, brief discussions will deal broadly with infections caused by fungi, protozoa, and viruses.

Several principles underlie the approach to therapy of the febrile granulocytopenic patient. First, about 70% of febrile episodes in these patients not clearly related to drug or blood product administration will be due to infection (Atkinson *et al.*, 1974). Second, the recognition of the sources of infection by localizing signs and symptoms will be hampered by severe granulocytopenia, while the likelihood that sepsis accompanies the infection is increased (Sickles *et al.*, 1975). Third, untreated gram-negative sepsis in these patients will result in approximately 50% mortality within 2–3 days (Schimpff *et al.*, 1973), i.e., often before the results of cultures have returned. These considerations have led to the widespread use of "empirical" broad-spectrum antibiotic therapy instituted promptly after the onset of fever in the neutropenic subject, though not before a careful physical examination and adequate cultures have been taken, as outlined in the preceding section. The choice of the particular combination of antibiotics of greatest efficacy for this purpose has been intensively studied, using both prospective randomized comparative trials (Klastersky *et al.*, 1974, 1975) and retrospective comparisons (Bloomfield and Kennedy, 1974; Tattersall *et al.*, 1973) of two or more of the aminoglycosides, cephalosporins, and carbenicillin-like agents. Many of these data can be summarized as follows: (1) Carbenicillin is superior to gentamicin for the treatment of *P. aeruginosa* infections in the granulocytopenic patient (Schimpff *et al.*, 1973). (2) The combination of gentamicin and cephalothin probably results in some excess of renal toxicity compared with gentamicin and carbenicillin (Klastersky *et al.*, 1975), and may occasionally be associated with acute renal failure (Bobrow *et al.*, 1972). (3) There is little evidence that combinations of three or more antibiotics are more efficacious than carbenicillin and gentamicin or tobramycin. (4) Carbenicillin in doses of 30 g/day is effective anaerobic therapy, including most strains of *Bacteroides fragilis*. As a result, it is the opinion of the author that empirical therapy should be initiated with carbenicillin, 500 mg/kg per day to a maximum of 30 g/day, in divided doses every 4 hr i.v., and gentamicin or tobramycin, 5 mg/kg per day, in divided doses i.v. every 6–8 hr. Although gentamicin is probably an adequate antistaphylococcal agent (Richards *et al.*, 1971), at least initially, many would add a semisynthetic penicillin, such as oxacillin or nafcillin, in doses of 100–150 mg/kg per day, given i.v. every 4 hr.

After the initiation of these antibiotics, there are several possible subsequent courses. If an organism is isolated as a pathogen, antibiotic therapy should be tailored to the susceptibilities of the isolate, using carbenicillin and gentamicin for *P. aeruginosa*, *Enterobacter* spp., and *E. coli*, and gentamicin or gentamicin plus cephalothin for *Klebsiella* strains. Gram-positive organisms, including *S. aureus*, respond well to an appropriate penicillin or cephalosporin, without combination therapy.

If no organism is identified, but a site of infection is known, such as the perirectal area, lung, or pharynx, then continuation of the initial regimen is recommended. "Surveillance" cultures of the nose, throat, skin (axilla), and rectal area may serve to identify unusual organisms or susceptibility patterns that might require further therapeutic agents. If the patient should fail to respond or responds and then relapses while on broad-spectrum agents, and no organism has been isolated, serious consideration should be given to the possibility that a nonbacterial infection or mixed infection was present initially, or has been induced as a superinfection.

If neither a site nor an organism is known, but the patient has: (1) a clinical response to therapy, with a decrease in fever and an improvement in well-being, antibiotics should be continued for 7–10 days and for at least 3–5 days after the patient's symptoms have returned to baseline; (2) no response to therapy after 4–5 days of antibiotics, then a difficult choice must be made as to whether to continue antibiotics. Because of the high rate of fungal superinfection (Greene *et al.*, 1973*a*) with prolonged antibiotics in granulopenic subjects, as well as the toxicity of these agents, it is felt that antibiotics should be discontinued after no more than 4–7 days of unavailing therapy. Reculturing should be performed within 24 hr of discontinuation, and, should clinical worsening follow cessation of antibiotics, they should be restarted promptly.

The administration of aminoglycoside antibiotics on a milligram-per-kilogram basis results in highly variable serum levels. In addition to renal function, both fever and anemia, through increases in renal clearance, will affect the serum concentration of gentamicin. Hence, it is essential that serum levels of gentamicin, or other aminoglycosides in use, be measured directly at both peak and trough and dosage adjusted accordingly. Recently, tobramycin has become generally available as an alternative to gentamicin. There is *in vitro* evidence that tobramycin is 2–4 times more active against *P. aeruginosa* than gentamicin, and approximately equivalently active against other gram-negative bacilli (Rosenthal, 1975). However, there are no comparable data for *in vivo* efficacy. In addition to the potential advantage of tobramycin in the treatment of *P. aeruginosa* infections, some strains of organisms resistant to gentamicin are susceptible to tobramycin. Amikacin, a kanamycin derivative that is also active against *P. aeruginosa*, has recently been marketed, and displays even greater lack of cross-resistance with gentamicin than does tobramycin, and may eventually find more widespread use (Tally *et al.*, 1975).

267

SUPPORTIVE
CARE
IN THE
CANCER
PATIENT

An adjunctive form of therapy in the granulopenic patient for the past decade has been the use of granulocyte transfusions. The short biological half-life and the low circulating numbers of peripheral granulocytes made the practical use of granulocyte transfusion for supportive care lag considerably behind its theoretical conception. Freireich *et al.* (1964) exploited the high circulating counts of chronic myelogenous leukemia donors and transfused leukocyte-rich preparations into 40 granulopenic subjects, of whom 35 were leukemic. Their encouraging results (Morse *et al.*, 1966), though uncontrolled and largely anecdotal, led in turn to the development of the IBM Blood Cell Separator for the harvesting of granulocytes from normal donors by a process that "skimmed" the leukocytes from whole blood during continuous-flow centrifugation. Despite initial enthusiasm for the instrument, yields of granulocytes have not been great, the process remains time-consuming and technically difficult, and the equipment is expensive.

More recently, Djerassi *et al.* (1971) introduced the use of nylon-fiber filters (Leukopak® for the selective trapping of granulocytes present in whole blood and pumped through the filter by continuous flow. This filtration leukopheresis (FL) has greatly increased the efficiency of collection, and thus the yield for a given donation, and has decreased the duration and complexity of the collection process. Low-cost and efficient equipment now exists using this method (Buchholz *et al.*, 1975). The *in vivo* recovery of transfused FL granulocytes is not as good as that of PMNs harvested by the centrifugation method (Graw *et al.*, 1972), and granulocyte function appears to be slightly impaired when compared with normal leukocytes (G.P. Herzig *et al.*, 1973; Wright *et al.*, 1975). This defect may be correctable by decreasing adherence to and time on the nylon filter (Wright *et al.*, 1975). The large number of cells that can be collected by FL may more than compensate for a slight reduction in *in vitro* function and *in vivo* recovery.

Experimental models have been developed to demonstrate the effectiveness of granulocyte transfusion in treating infection in granulocytopenic dogs. In 1953, Brecher *et al.* (1953) used sedimented white cells ($4–9 \times 10^9$) to treat lethally irradiated dogs, and demonstrated granulocytes that were not present in untransfused control dogs in sites of infection. Dale *et al.* (1974b) produced leukopenia in dogs by irradiation and induced *Pseudomonas* pneumonia. Therapy consisted of gentamicin compared with gentamicin and granulocytes. Dogs transfused with granulocytes (12×10^9) survived longer, cleared *Pseudomonas* from the lung, were prevented from developing endotoxemia, and localized transfused granulocytes at the site of pneumonia. These studies have been expanded in a controlled fashion (Dale *et al.*, 1976). Epstein *et al.* (1974) challenged leukopenic dogs with intravenous *Pseudomonas*, and showed a transient decrease in the number of circulating organisms following granulocyte transfusion ($2–15 \times 10^9$). Similar observations have been confirmed in rats (Tobias *et al.*, 1976).

In the past several years, a number of supportive care groups have published or reported their experience with the use of therapeutic granulocyte transfusions in man (Schwarzenberg *et al.*, 1967; McCredie *et al.*, 1973; Djerassi *et al.*, 1975; Vallejos *et al.*, 1975; Lowenthal *et al.*, 1975; Schiffer *et al.*, 1975), and the subject has been reviewed (Boggs, 1974; Higby *et al.*, 1975*b*). Six studies have been controlled (Graw *et al.*, 1972; Higby *et al.*, 1975*a*; Fortuny *et al.*, 1975; Vogler and Winton, 1976; R. H. Herzig *et al.*, 1976; Alavi *et al.*, 1976). Their overall conclusion is that granulocytes can be effective in treating infection in selected granulocytopenic patients. The optimal method of harvest, time of initiation and scheduling of transfusion, numbers of granulocytes needed, and the method of infusion with the least morbidity have not yet been determined. The patients that seem to benefit most from these transfusions are those with prolonged granulocytopenia, but at present, such patients cannot be defined prospectively. The overall impact of this therapeutic maneuver on the outcome of cancer chemotherapy has yet to be determined, but it can be recommended that, where available, granulocyte transfusions should be instituted in the patient with documented infection, particularly if antibiotic therapy appears to be failing. Such transfusions should be ABO matched, but it is unclear whether *HLA* matching has any bearing on the therapeutic effect. Once initiated, transfusions should probably be continued until either the granulopenia or the infection has resolved. There is no *in vitro* method presently available to reliably predict the likelihood of constitutional reactions of fever, chills, or dyspnea and wheezing. The occurrence of dyspnea and wheezing during transfusion is increased among patients with active pneumonia, and should prompt interruption of transfusion. Unless severe, fever and chills does not necessarily warrant such interruption. Further studies are necessary to define optimal treatment schedules, as well as to devise *in vitro* methods of "matching" granulocytes for maximal posttransfusion life.

The antibiotic treatment of infection in the patient with a normal granulocyte count is similar to that for the granulopenic patient, except that the necessity for carbenicillin therapy of *Pseudomonas* infection is diminished. Thus, cephalothin and gentamicin (or tobramycin), oxacillin and gentamicin or, if anaerobic infection with *B. fragilis* is suspected, clindamycin and gentamicin are alternative regimens with broad coverage.

In fungal infections, the basis for therapy of invasive disease is amphotericin B (Bennett, 1974). Localized infection, such as thrush, candidal esophagitis, and candidal cystitis, may be treated topically with amphotericin B, nystatin, or clotrimazole, but failure to respond to such treatment in severe local disease or the presence of parenchymal involvement by fungus calls for the use of parenteral amphotericin B. Among patients with subacute or indolent disease, a 1-mg test dose is followed by daily increments of 5 mg until therapeutic levels are achieved, assuming an absence of severe pyrexia or hypotension with drug administration. When fungal illness is acute and progressive, the 1-mg test dose should be followed by a dose more likely to be therapeutic, of approximately 0.3 mg/kg (Bennett, 1974), often necessitating concomitant corticosteroid administration (25–50 mg hydrocortisone) to lessen constitutional reactions. Subsequent daily doses should be increased to approximately 0.5–0.6 mg/kg, and then gradually switched over to 1.0–1.2 mg/kg on alternate days.

The limiting toxicity of amphotericin B is azotemia, which is dose-dependent. A number of approaches to ameliorating this toxicity have been tried, and have centered on: (1) lower doses of amphotericin B, (2) simultaneous addition of other agents to prevent renal toxicity, (3) lower doses of amphotericin B combined with other antifungal agents, and (4) pharmacological modification of the drug. Medoff *et al.* (1972*a*) reported that some candidal infections will respond to daily doses of amphotericin B of far less than the 0.5–0.6 mg/kg per day usually used for serious fungal disease. Our own experience has been favorable with doses of 10–20 mg/day for severe mucosal disease, less so with parenchymal invasion. Both intravenous mannitol (Hellebusch *et al.*, 1972) and sodium bicarbonate (Gouge and Andriole, 1971) orally have been suggested as being capable of lessening the renal injury secondary to amphotericin B. The former, however, was not found to be of value in a controlled, randomized prospective study by Bullock *et al.* (1975). The use of urinary alkalinization for this purpose remains untested. Recently, Medoff and co-workers (Medoff *et al.* 1972*b*; Kitahara *et al.*, 1976) reported that amphotericin B, because of its action on the fungal cell membrane, allows entry into the fungus of other agents, such as rifampin or 5-fluorocytosine (5-FC), which then display synergistic antifungal activity. Clinically, trials of combination antifungal chemotherapy are in their infancy, although a recent report (Utz *et al.*, 1975) of combined amphotericin B–5-FC treatment of cryptococcal dissemination was encouraging, making use of a relatively low dose of amphotericin B with attendant reduction in renal toxicity. Amphotericin B-methyl ester is a derivative of amphotericin reported to be less renotoxic (but more water-soluble) when administered in doses with fungal activity equal to that of the parent compound, but further experience is necessary with this agent, as it is for miconazole, which has been used in chronic coccidioidomycosis with reported success (Stevens *et al.*, 1976).

In the patient with cancer and invasive parenchymal fungal disease, amphotericin in full dosage remains the therapy of choice. In the absence of reversal of the underlying predisposition (see above), the outcome of therapy is usually poor, particularly when diagnosis is delayed or the etiologic organism is *Aspergillus* or *Mucor*. If the patient is failing to respond to amphotericin alone, several additional modes of therapy may be tried, all largely unproven: combined therapy with rifampin or 5-FC, leukocyte transfusions (Lowenthal *et al.*, 1975), or transfer factor (Valdimarsson *et al.*, 1972).

The treatment of *P. carinii* infection with a fixed combination of trimethoprim–sulfamethoxazole (T/S) has been demonstrated to be equally efficacious (60–70% response rate) but much less toxic than the former standard, pentamidine (Hughes *et al.*, 1975). The recommended dosage for *P. carinii* infection is 100 mg/kg per day sulfamethoxazole and 20 mg/kg per day trimethoprim in 4 divided doses for 14 days. Failure to respond to T/S does not preclude subsequent response to pentamidine, and the latter should be begun if stabilization or improvement has not been noted within 3–4 days of T/S therapy. In contrast, T/S is not adequate therapy for toxoplasmosis, since trimethoprim is inactive against this protozoan. The accepted therapy is pyrimethamine and sulfadiazine, which appears to be quite effective (80% response rate) when the diagnosis is considered,

269

SUPPORTIVE
CARE
IN THE
CANCER
PATIENT

and confirmed by serologic or histologic means (Ruskin and Remington, 1976). A possible alternative to pyrimethamine and sulfadiazine in the treatment of disseminated toxoplasmosis is clindamycin, but this remains investigational.

Among the viral infections afflicting cancer patients, modest progress has been made in therapy, of which some has been reviewed in Section 3.4. In the herpes virus infections, adenine arabinoside has been reported to be capable of ameliorating the course of herpes zoster (Whitley *et al.*, 1976), and is effective against herpes keratitis in several clinical trials. Topical phototherapy with dyes such as neutral red or proflavine for herpes simplex infections of the mouth or genitalia has received extensive clinical testing, with conflicting results (Myers *et al.*, 1975). The potential carcinogenicity of this form of therapy is less of a contraindication in the patient with malignancy already, but efficacy is uncertain, and its use remains controversial. The treatment of cytomegaloviral disease with either adenine or cytosine arabinoside has been disappointing, in both the congenital and adult forms of disease. The subject of antiviral therapy has been very recently reviewed (*Journal of Infectious Diseases*, Vol. 133, June 1976, Supplement).

ACKNOWLEDGMENTS

The author would like to express his appreciation for the extraordinary secretarial assistance of Ms. Susan Proto, Mrs. Carol Dauer, and, in particular, that of Ms. Betsy Zickler, without whom this chapter would not have been possible.

4. References

ABRAHAMSEN, A. F., 1972, Effects of an enlarged splenic platelet pool in Hodgkin's disease, *Scand. J. Haematol.* **9**:153.

ABRAMSON, N., EISENBERG, P. D., AND ASTER, R. H., 1974, Post-transfusion purpura: Immunologic aspects and therapy, *N. Engl. J. Med.* **291**:1163.

ADLER, S., STUTZMAN, L., SOKAL, J. E., AND MITTLEMAN, A., 1975, Splenectomy for hematologic depression in lymphocytic lymphoma and leukemia, *Cancer* **35**:521.

ALAVI, J. B., ROOT, R. K., EVANS, A. E., DJERASSI, I., GUERRY, D., SCHREIBER, A. D., SHAW, J., AND COOPER, R. A., 1976, Granulocyte transfusions in acute leukemia, *Clin. Res.* **24**:373A.

ALEXANDER, J. W., FISHER, M. W., AND MACMILLAN, B. G., 1971, Immunological control of *Pseudomonas* infection in burn patients: A clinical evaluation, *Arch. Surg.* **102**:31.

ALPERN, R. J., AND DOWELL, V. R., 1969, *Clostridium septicum* infections and malignancy, *J. Amer. Med. Assoc.* **209**:385.

ALPERT, L. I., AND BENISCH, B., 1970, Hemangioendothelioma of the liver associated with microangiopathic hemolytic anemia, *Amer. J. Med.* **48**:624.

ALTEMEIER, W. A., FULLEN, W. D., AND MCDONOUGH, J. J., 1972, Sepsis and gastrointestinal bleeding, *Ann. Surg.* **175**:759.

ARMSTRONG, D., YOUNG, L. S., MEYER, R. D., AND BLEVINS, A. H., 1971, Infectious complications of neoplastic disease, *Med. Clin. North Amer.* **55**:729.

ARSENEAU, J. C., AAMODT, R., JOHNSTON, G. S., AND CANELLOS, G. P., 1974, Evidence for granulocytic incorporation of [67]gallium in chronic granulocytic leukemia, *J. Lab. Clin. Med.* **83**:496.

271
SUPPORTIVE
CARE
IN THE
CANCER
PATIENT

ASTER, R. H., 1972, Disorders of hemostasis—quantitative platelet disorders, in: *Hematology* (W. J. Williams, ed.), p. 1124, McGraw-Hill, New York.

ATKINSON, K., KAY, H. E. M., AND MCELWAIN, T. J., 1974, Fever in the neutropenic patient, *Br. Med. J.* **3**:160.

BAEHNER, R. L., 1972, Disorders of leukocytes leading to recurrent infection, *Pediatr. Clin. North Amer.* **19**:935.

BAKER, R. D., 1962, Leukopenia and therapy in leukemia as factors predisposing to fatal mycoses, *Amer. J. Clin. Pathol.* **37**:358.

BARTRAM, C. E., CROWDER, J. G., BEELER, B., AND WHITE, A., 1974, Diagnosis of bacterial diseases by detection of serum antigens by counterimmunoelectrophoresis, sensitivity, and specificity of detecting *Pseudomonas* and pneumococcal antigens, *J. Lab. Clin. Med.* **83**:591.

BEN-ISHAY, Z., AND FARBER, E., 1975, Protective effects of an inhibitor of protein synthesis, cyclohex-imide, on bone marrow damage induced by cytosine arabinoside or nitrogen mustard, *Lab. Invest.* **33**:478.

BENNETT, J. E., 1974, Chemotherapy of systemic mycoses (first of two parts), *N. Engl. J. Med.* **290**:30.

BEUTLER, E., 1972, Hemolytic anemia due to infections with microorganisms, in: *Hematology* (W. J. Williams, ed.), p. 483, McGraw-Hill, New York.

BINDSCHADLER, D. D., AND BENNETT, J. E., 1968, Serology of human cryptococcosis, *Ann. Intern. Med.* **69**:45.

BJORNSON, A. B., AND MICHAEL, J. G., 1970, Biological activities of rabbit immunoglobulin M and immunoglobulin G antibodies to *Pseudomonas aeruginosa*, *Infect. Immun.* **2**:453.

BJORNSSON, S., AND PREISLER, H. D., 1976, Combination antibiotic therapy for FUO in neutropenic cancer patients, *Proc. Amer. Soc. Clin. Oncol.* (abstract C-193).

BLACK, P. H., KUNZ, L. J., AND SWARTZ, M. N., 1960, Salmonellosis—a review of some unusual aspects, *N. Engl. J. Med.* **262**:811, 864, 921.

BLANK, N., CASTELLINO, R. A., AND SHAH, V., 1973, Radiographic aspects of pulmonary infection in patients with altered immunity, *Radiol. Clin. North Amer.* **11**:175.

BLOOMFIELD, C., AND KENNEDY, B. J., 1974, Cephalothin, carbenicillin, and gentamicin combination therapy for febrile patients with acute non-lymphocytic leukemia, *Cancer* **34**:431.

BLUMING, A. Z., 1975, Current status of clinical immunotherapy, *Cancer Chemother. Rep. Part 1* **59**:901.

BOBROW, S. N., JAFFE, E., AND YOUNG, R. C., 1972, Anuria and acute tubular necrosis associated with gentamicin and cephalothin, *J. Amer. Med. Assoc.* **222**:1546.

BODE, F. R., PARE, J. A. P., AND FRASER, R. G., 1974, Pulmonary diseases in the compromised host, *Medicine* **53**:255.

BODEY, G. P., 1966, Fungal infections complicating acute leukemia, *J. Chron. Dis.* **19**:667.

BODEY, G. P., 1972, Oral antibiotic prophylaxis in protected environment units: Effect of nonabsorba-ble and absorbable antibiotics on the fecal flora, *Antimicrob. Agents Chemother.* **1**:343.

BODEY, G. P., 1975, Infections in cancer patients, *Cancer Treatment Rev.* **2**:89.

BODEY, G. P., AND LUNA, M., 1974, Skin lesions associated with disseminated candidiasis, *J. Amer. Med. Assoc.*, **229**:1466.

BODEY, G. P., BUCKLEY, M., SATHE, Y. S., AND FREIREICH, E. J., 1966, Quantitative relationships between circulating leukocytes and infection in patients with acute leukemia, *Ann. Intern. Med.* **64**:328.

BODEY, G. P., DEJONGH, D., ISASSI, A., AND FREIREICH, E. J., 1969a, Hypersplenism due to disseminated candidiasis in a patient with acute leukemia, *Cancer* **24**:417.

BODEY, G. P., FREIREICH, E. J., AND FREI, E., 1969b, Studies of patients in a laminar air flow unit, *Cancer* **24**:972.

BOGGS, D. R., 1974, Transfusion of neutrophils as prevention or treatment of infection in patients with neutropenia, *N. Engl. J. Med.* **290**:1055.

BOGGS, D. R., AND FREI, E., 1960, Clinical studies of fever and infection in cancer, *Cancer* **13**:1240.

BORGES, J. S., AND JOHNSON, W. D., 1975, Inhibition of multiplication of *Toxoplasma gondii* by human monocytes exposed to T-lymphocyte products, *J. Exp. Med.* **141**:483.

BOUNOUS, G., HUGON, J., AND GENTILE, J. M., 1971a, Elemental diet in the management of the intestinal lesion produced by 5-fluorouracil in the rat, *Can. J. Surg.* **14**:298.

BOUNOUS, G., GENTILE, J. M., AND HUGON, J., 1971b, Elemental diet in the management of the intestinal lesion produced by 5-fluorouracil in man, *Can. J. Surg.* **14**:312.

BRAGG, D. G., AND JANIS, B., 1973, The radiographic presentation of pulmonary opportunistic inflammatory disease, *Radiol. Clin. North. Amer.* **11**:357.

BRAIN, M. C., AZZAPARDI, J. G., BAKER, L. R. I., PINEO, G. F., ROBERTS, P. D., AND DACIE, J. V., 1970, Microangiopathic haemolytic anemia and mucin-forming adenocarcinoma, *Br. J. Haematol.* **18**:183.

BRANDT, L., 1971, Phagocytosis-promoting effect of clofazimine (B 663) in patients with subnormal granulocyte function, *Scand. J. Haematol.* **8**:400.

BRECHER, G., WILBUR, K. M., AND CRONKITE, F. P., 1953, Transfusion of separated leukocytes into irradiated dogs with aplastic marrows, *Proc. Soc. Exp. Biol. Med.* **84**:54.

BRODER, S., HUMPHREY, R., DURM, M., BLACKMAN, M., MEADE, B., GOLDMAN, C., STROBER, W., AND WALDMANN, T., 1975, Impaired synthesis of polyclonal immunoglobulins in myeloma, *N. Engl. J. Med.* **293**:887.

BRODSKY, I., FUSCALDO, A., AND FUSCALDO, K. E., 1976, Hemostasis and cancer, in: *Oncologic Medicine* (A. I. Sutnick and P. F. Engstrom, eds.), p. 247, University Park Press, Baltimore.

BROOK, J., AND KONWALER, B. E., 1965, Thrombotic thrombocytopenic purpura. Association with metastatic gastric carcinoma and a possible autoimmune disorder, *Calif. Med.* **102**:222.

BROWDER, A. A., HUFF, J. W., AND PETERSDORF, R. G., 1961, The significance of fever in neoplastic disease, *Ann. Intern. Med.* **55**:932.

BROWN, C. H., NATELSON, E. A., BRADSHAW, M. W., WILLIAMS, T. W., AND ALFREY, C. P., 1974, The hemostatic defect produced by carbenicillin, *N. Engl. J. Med.* **291**:265.

BRUNELL, P. A., AND GERSHON, A. A., 1973, Passive immunization against varicella-zoster infections and other modes of therapy, *J. Infect. Dis.* **127**:415.

BUCHHOLZ, D. H., YOUNG, V. M., FRIEDMAN, N. R., REILLY, J. A., AND MARDINEY, M. 1971, Bacterial proliferation in platelet products stored at room temperature, *N. Engl. J. Med.* **285**:429.

BUCHHOLZ, D. H., SCHIFFER, C. A., WIERNIK, P. H., BETTS, S. W., AND REILLY, J. A., 1975, Granulocyte transfusion: A low cost method for filtration leukapheresis, in: *Proceedings of the International Symposium on Leukocyte Separation and Transfusion*, London, Sept. 9–11, 1974 (R. M. Lowenthal and J. M. Goldman, eds.), p. 137, Academic Press, New York.

BULLOCK, W. E., LUKE, R. G., NUTALL, C. E., AND BHATHENA, D., 1976, Can mannitol reduce amphotericin B nephrotoxicity? *Antimicrob. Agents Chemother.* **10**:555.

BURKE, J. P., INGALL, D., KLEIN, J. O., GEZON, H. M., AND FINLAND, M., 1971, *Proteus mirabilis* infections in a hospital nursery traced to a human carrier, *N. Engl. J. Med.* **284**:115.

CAPIZZI, R. L., 1975, Improvement in the therapeutic index of methotrexate by asparaginase, *Cancer Chemother. Rep., Part 3* **6**:37.

CAPIZZI, R. L., AND HANDSCHUMACHER, R. E., 1973, Asparaginase, in: *Cancer Medicine* (J. F. Holland and E. Frei, eds.), p. 850, Lea and Febiger, Philadelphia.

CATALONA, W. J., TARPLEY, J. L., POTVIN, C., AND CHRETIEN, P. B., 1975, Correlations among cutaneous reactivity to DNCB, PHA-induced lymphocyte blastogenesis and peripheral blood E rosettes, *Clin. Exp. Immunol.* **19**:327.

CHANG, F. M., SAKAI, Y., AND ASHIZAWA, S., 1973, Bacterial pollution and disinfection of the colonofiberscope, *Amer. J. Digestive Dis.* **18**:946.

CHANG, H., RODRIGUEZ, V., NARBONI, G., BODEY, G. P., LUNA, M. A., AND FREIREICH, E. J., 1976, Causes of death in adults with acute leukemia, *Medicine* **55**:259.

CHERNIK, N. L., ARMSTRONG, D., AND POSNER, J. B., 1973, Central nervous system infections in patients with cancer, *Medicine* **52**:563.

CLINE, M. J., 1974, Granulocytes in human disease, *Ann. Intern. Med.* **81**:801.

COLEMAN, R. M., AND KAUFMAN, L., 1972, Use of the immunodiffusion test in the serodiagnosis of aspergillosis, *Appl. Microbiol.* **23**:301.

COONROD, J. D., AND LEACH, R. P., 1976, Antigenemia in fulminant pneumococcemia, *Ann. Intern. Med.* **84**:561.

COOPER, M. R., HEESE, E., RICHARDS, F., KAUFMANN, J., AND SPURR, C. L., 1975, A prospective study of histocompatible leukocyte and platelet transfusions during chemotherapeutic induction of acute myeloblastic leukaemia, in: *Proceedings of the International Symposium on Leukocyte Separation and Transfusion*, London, September 9–11, 1974 (R. M. Lowenthal and J. M. Goldman, eds.), p. 436, Academic Press, New York.

COWAN, D. H., AND HAUT, M. J., 1972, Platelet function in acute leukemia, *J. Lab. Clin. Med.* **79**:893.

CREECH, R. H., 1976, Management of acute leukemia, in: *Oncologic Medicine* (A. I. Sutnick and P. F. Engstrom, eds.), p. 173, University Park Press, Baltimore.

CROSBY, W. H., 1972, Splenectomy in hematologic disorders, *N. Engl. J. Med.* **286**:1252.

DALE, D. C., FAUCI, A. S., AND WOLFF, S. M., 1974a, Alternate-day prednisone, *N. Engl. J. Med.* **291**:1154.

DALE, D. C., REYNOLDS, H. Y., PENNINGTON, J. F., ELIN, R. J., PITTS, T. W., AND GRAW, R. G., 1974b, Granulocyte transfusion therapy of experimental *Pseudomonas* pneumonia, *J. Clin. Invest.* **54**:664.

273

SUPPORTIVE
CARE
IN THE
CANCER
PATIENT

DALE, D. C., REYNOLDS, H. Y., PENNINGTON, J. E., ELIN, R. J., AND HERZIG, G. P., 1976, Experimental *Pseudomonas* pneumonia in leukopenic dogs: Comparison of therapy with antibiotics and granulocyte transfusions, *Blood* **47**:869.

DAVIS, J. L., MILLIGAN, F. D., AND CAMERON, J. L., 1975, Septic complications following endoscopic retrograde cholangiopancreatography, *Surg. Gynecol. Obstet.* **140**:365.

DAWSON, M. A., TALBERT, W., AND YARBRO, J. W., 1971, Hemolytic anemia associated with an ovarian tumor, *Amer. J. Med.* **50**:552.

DEE, T. H., AND RYTEL, M. W., 1975, Clinical application of counterimmunoelectrophoresis in detection of candida serum precipitins, *J. Lab. Clin. Med.* **85**:161.

DICKMAN, M. D., CHAPPELKA, A. R., AND SCHAEDLER, R. W., 1975, Evaluation of gut microflora during administration of an elemental diet in a patient with an ileoproctostomy, *Amer. J. Digestive Dis.* **20**:377.

DJERASSI, I., KIM, J., AND SUVANSRI, U., 1971, Filtration-leukopheresis for separation and transfusion of large amounts of granulocytes from single normal donors, *Proc. Amer. Assoc. Cancer Res.* **12**:28.

DJERASSI, I., KIM, J. S., SUVANSRI, U., CIESIELKA, W., AND LOHRKE, J., 1975, Filtration leukopheresis: Principles and techniques of harvesting and transfusion of filtered granulocytes and monocytes, in: *Proceedings of the International Symposium on Leukocyte Separation and Transfusions*, London, Sept. 9–11, 1974 (R. M. Lowenthal and J. M. Goldman, eds.), p. 123, Academic Press, New York.

DUBOS, R., AND SCHAEDLER, R. W., 1962, Some biological effects of the digestive flora, *Amer. J. Med. Sci.* **244**:265.

DUMA, R. J., WARNER, J. F., AND DALTON, H. P., 1971, Septicemia from intravenous infusions, *N. Engl. J. Med.* **284**:257.

EBBE, S., WITTELS, B., AND DAMESHEK, W., 1962, Autoimmune thrombocytopenic purpura ("ITP" type) with chronic lymphocytic leukemia, *Blood* **19**:23.

EDELSON, P. J., AND FUDENBERG, H. F., 1973, Effect of vinblastine on the chemotactic responsiveness of normal human neutrophils, *Infect. Immun.* **8**:127.

EPSTEIN, R. B., WAXMAN, F. J., BENNETT, B. T., AND ANDERSON, B. R., 1974, *Pseudomonas* septicemia in neutropenic dogs I. Treatment with granulocyte transfusions, *Transfusion* **14**:51.

ERAS, P., GOLDSTEIN, M. J., AND SHERLOCK, P., 1972, *Candida* infection of the gastrointestinal tract, *Medicine* **51**:367.

ESTERHAY, R. J., VOGEL, V. G., FORTNER, C. L., AND SHAPIRO, H. M., 1975, Cost-analysis of leukemia treatment: A problem-oriented approach, *Proceedings of the American Society of Clinical Oncology*, Abstract 1067, p. 237.

FAUCI, A. S., AND DALE D. C., 1975, Alternate-day prednisone therapy and human lymphocyte subpopulations, *J. Clin. Invest.* **55**:22.

FEINGOLD, D. S., 1970, Hospital-acquired infections, *N. Engl. J. Med.* **283**:1384.

FELD, R., BODEY, G. P., AND GROSCHEL, D., 1976, Mycobacteriosis in patients with malignant disease, *Arch. Intern. Med.* **136**:67.

FELNER, J. M., AND DOWELL, V. R., 1971, "Bacteroides" bacteremia, *Amer. J. Med.* **50**:787.

FISHER, M. W., DEVLIN, H. B., AND GNABASIK, F. J., 1969, New immunotype schema for *Pseudomonas aeruginosa* based on protective antigens, *J. Bacteriol.* **98**:835.

FISHER, G. W., OI, V. T., KELLEY, J. L., PODGORE, J. K., BASS, J. W., WAGNER, F. S., AND GORDON, B. L., 1974, Enhancement of host defense mechanisms against gram-positive pyogenic coccal infections with levo-tetramisole (levamisole) in neonatal rats, *Ann. Allergy* **33**:193.

FISHMAN, L. S., AND ARMSTRONG, D., 1972, *Pseudomonas aeruginosa* bacteremia in patients with neoplastic disease, *Cancer* **30**:764.

FORSHAW, J., AND HARWOOD, L., 1966, Poikilocytosis associated with carcinoma, *Arch. Intern. Med.* **117**:203.

FORTUNY, I. E., BLOOMFIELD, C. D., HADLOCK, D. C., GOLDMAN, A., KENNEDY, B. J., AND McCULLOUGH, J. J., 1975, Granulocyte transfusion—a controlled study of patients with acute nonlymphocytic leukemia, *Transfusion* **15**:548.

FREIREICH, E. J., LEVIN, R. H., WHANG, J., CARBONE, P. P., BRONSON, W., AND MORSE, E. E., 1964, The function and fate of transfused leukocytes from donors with chronic myelocytic leukemia in leukopenic recipients, *Ann. N. Y. Acad. Sci.* **113**:1081.

FREIREICH, E. J., RODRIGUEZ, V., GEHAN, E., SMITH, T., AND BODEY, G. P., 1975, A controlled clinical trial to evaluate a protected environment prophylactic antibiotic program in the treatment of adult acute leukemia, *Trans. Am. Assoc. Phys.*

FRETER, R., 1970, Mechanism of action of intestinal antibody in experimental cholera. II. Antibody-mediated antibacterial reaction at the mucosal surface, *Infect. Immun.* **2**:556.

FRETER, R., 1974, Interactions between mechanisms controlling the intestinal microflora, *Amer. J. Clin. Nutr.* **27**:1409.

FUBARA, E. S., AND FRETER, R., 1973, Protection against enteric bacterial infection by secretory IgA antibodies, *J. Immunol.* **111**:395.

GALBRAITH, A. W., OXFORD, J. S., SCHILD, G. C., POTTER, C. W., AND WATSON, G. I., 1971, Therapeutic effect of L-adamantadine hydrochloride in naturally occurring influenza A₂/Hong Kong infection. A controlled double blind study, *Lancet* **2**:113.

GAYDOS, L. A., FREIREICH, E. J., AND MANTEL, N., 1962, The quantitative relation between platelet count and hemorrhage in patients with acute leukemia, *N. Engl. J. Med.* **266**:905.

GEISER, C. F., BISHOP, Y., MYERS, M., JAFFE, N., AND YANKEE, R., 1975, Prophylaxis of varicella in children with neoplastic disease: Comparative results with zoster immune plasma and gamma globulin, *Cancer* **35**:1027.

GERSHON, A. A., STEINBERG, S., AND BRUNELL, P. A., 1974, Zoster immune globulin, *N. Engl. J. Med.* **290**:243.

GILDENHORN, H. L., FAHEY, J. L., AND SOLOMON, R. D., 1962, Functional esophageal obstruction due to leukemic infiltration, *Amer. J. Radiol.* **88**:736.

GILLILAND, B. C., BAXTER, E., AND EVANS, R. S., 1971, Red-cell antibodies in acquired hemolytic anemia with negative antiglobulin serum tests, *N. Engl. J. Med.* **285**:252.

GODWIN, H. A., ZIMMERMAN, T. S., KIMBALL, H. R., WOLFF, S. M., AND PERRY, S., 1968, Correlation of granulocyte mobilization with etiocholanolone and the subsequent development of myelosuppression in patients with acute leukemia receiving therapy, *Blood* **31**:580.

GOEPP, C. E., AND HAMMOND, W. (eds.), 1975, Supportive care of the cancer patient, *Semin. Oncol.* **2**:283.

GOLD, E., 1974, Infections associated with immunologic deficiency diseases, *Med. Clin. North Amer.* **58**:649.

GOLDMAN, J. M., 1974, Acute promyelocytic leukaemia, *Br. Med. J.* **1**:380.

GOLDSTEIN, J. A., NEFF, J. M., LANE, J. M., AND KOPLAN, J. P., 1975, Smallpox vaccination reactions, prophylaxis, and therapy of complications, *Pediatrics* **55**:342.

GOODALL, P. T., AND VOSTI, K. L., 1975, Fever in acute myelogenous leukemia, *Arch. Intern. Med.* **135**:1197.

GOODMAN, J. S., KAUFMAN, L., AND KOENIG, M. G., 1971, Diagnosis of crytococcal meningitis: Value of immunologic detection of cryptococcal antigen, *N. Engl. J. Med.* **285**:343.

GOUGE, T. H., AND ANDRIOLE, V. T., 1971, An experimental model of amphotericin B nephrotoxicity with renal tubular acidosis, *J. Lab. Clin. Med.* **78**:713.

GRADY, G. F., AND LEE, V. A., 1975, Prevention of hepatitis from accidental exposure among medical workers, *N. Engl. J. Med.* **293**:1067.

GRALNICK, H. R., MARCHESI, S., AND GIVELBER, H., 1972*a*, Intravascular coagulation in acute leukemia: Clinical and subclinical abnormalities, *Blood* **40**:709.

GRALNICK, H. R., BAGLEY, J., AND ABRELL, E., 1972*b*, Heparin treatment for the hemorrhagic diathesis of acute promyelocytic leukemia, *Amer. J. Med.* **52**:167.

GRAW, R. G., HERZIG, G., PERRY, S., AND HENDERSON, E. S., 1972, Normal granulocyte transfusion therapy: Treatment of septicemia due to gram-negative bacteria, *N. Engl. J. Med.* **287**:367.

GRAYBILL, J. R., SILVA, J., ALFORD, R. H., AND THOR, D. E., 1973, Immunologic and clinical improvement of progressive coccidioidomycosis following administration of transfer factor, *Cell. Immunol.* **8**:120.

GREENBERG, P. L., NICHOLS, W. C., AND SCHRIER, S. L., 1971, Granulopoiesis in acute myeloid leukemia and preleukemia, *N. Engl. J. Med.* **284**:1225.

GREENE, W. H., AND WIERNIK, P. H., 1972, *Candida* endophthalmitis. Successful treatment in a patient with acute leukemia, *Amer. J. Ophthalmol.* **74**:1100.

GREENE, W. H., SCHIMPFF, S., YOUNG, V. M., AND GLUSMAN, S., 1972, Non-bacterial infections at autopsy in cancer patients, *Clin. Res.* **20**:529.

GREENE, W. H., SCHIMPFF, S. C., YOUNG, V. M., AND WIERNIK, P., 1973*a*, Empiric carbenicillin, gentamicin, and cephalothin therapy for presumed infection, *Ann. Intern. Med.* **78**:825.

GREENE, W. H., SCHIMPFF, S. C., VERMEULEN, G. D., YOUNG, V. M., AND WIERNIK, P., 1973*b*, The value of routine bone marrow and cerebrospinal fluid cultures in patients with cancer—a negative report, *Amer. J. Clin. Pathol.* **60**:404.

GREENE, W. H., MOODY, M., SCHIMPFF, S., YOUNG, V. M., AND WIERNIK, P. H., 1973*c*, *Pseudomonas aeruginosa* resistant to carbenicillin and gentamicin, *Ann. Intern. Med.* **79**:684.

275

SUPPORTIVE
CARE
IN THE
CANCER
PATIENT

GREENE, W. H., SCHIMPFF, S. C., AND WIERNIK, P. H., 1974a, Cell-mediated immunity in acute nonlymphocytic leukemia: Relationship to host factors, therapy, and prognosis, *Blood* **43**:1.

GREENE, W. H., MOODY, M., HARTLEY, R., YOUNG, V. M., EFFMAN, E., AISNER, J., AND WIERNIK, P. H., 1974b, Esophagoscopy as a source of *Pseudomonas aeruginosa* sepsis in patients with acute leukemia, *Gastroenterology* **67**:912.

GREENE, W. H., BENJAMIN, R. S., GLUSMAN, S., WARD, S., AND WIERNIK, P. H., 1974c, Arterial embolism of tumor causing fatal organ infarction, *Arch. Intern. Med.* **134**:545.

GREENMAN, R. L., GOODALL, P. T., AND KING, D., 1975, Lung biopsy in immunocompromised hosts, *Amer. J. Med.* **59**:488.

GRUMET, F. C., AND YANKEE, R. A., 1970, Long-term support of patients with aplastic anemia—effect of splenectomy and steroid therapy, *Ann. Intern. Med.* **73**:1.

HAGHBIN, M., ARMSTRONG, D., AND MURPHY, M. L., 1973, Controlled prospective trial of *Pseudomonas aeruginosa* vaccine in children with acute leukemia, *Cancer* **32**:761.

HAHN, D., SCHIMPFF, S., FORTNER, C., SMYTH, A., LANDESMAN, S., YOUNG, V., AND WIERNIK, P., 1975, Changing spectrum of infection in acute leukemia patients receiving oral nonabsorbable antibiotic prophylaxis, *ICAAC* (24–26 Sept., Washington, D. C.), Abstract No. 49.

HAN, T., STUTZMAN, L., COHEN, E., AND KIM, U., 1966, Effect of platelet transfusion on hemorrhage in patients with acute leukemia, *Cancer* **19**:1937.

HAN, T., SOKAL, J. E., AND NETER, E., 1967, Salmonellosis in disseminated malignant diseases, *N. Engl. J. Med.* **276**:1045.

HARDY, P. C., EDERER, G. M., AND MATSEN, J. M., 1970, Contamination of commercially packaged urinary catheter kits, *N. Engl. J. Med.* **282**:33.

HARKER, L. A., AND SLICHTER, S. J., 1972, The bleeding time as a screening test for evaluation of platelet function, *N. Engl. J. Med.* **287**:155.

HARRIS, J., AND BAGAI, R., 1972, Immune deficiency states associated with malignant disease in man, *Med. Clin. North Amer.* **56**:501.

HARRIS, J., AND COPELAND, D., 1974, Impaired immunoresponsiveness in tumor patients, *Ann. N.Y. Acad. Sci.*, **230**:56.

HARRIS, J., STEWART, T., SENGAR, D. P. S., AND HYSLOP, D., 1975, Quantitation of T-and B-lymphocytes in peripheral blood of patients with solid tumors I. Relation to other parameters of *in vivo* and *in vitro* immune competence, *Can. Med. Assoc. J.* **112**:948.

HAURANI, F. I., YOUNG, K., AND TOCANTINS, L. M., 1963, Reutilization of iron in anemia complicating malignant neoplasms, *Blood* **22**:73.

HELLEBUSCH, A. A., SALAMA, F., AND EADIE, E., 1972, The use of mannitol to reduce the nephrotoxicity of amphotericin B, *Surg. Gynecol. Obstet.* **134**:241.

HERBERMAN, R. B., AND OLDHAM, R. K., 1975, Problems associated with study of cell-mediated immunity to human tumors by microcytotoxicity assays, *J. Natl. Cancer Inst.* **55**:749.

HERSH, E. M., BODEY, G. P., NIES, B. A., AND FREIREICH, E. J., 1965, Causes of death in acute leukemia, *J. Amer. Med. Assoc.* **193**:105.

HERSH, E. M., CARBONE, P. P., AND FREIREICH, E. J., 1966, Recovery of immune responsiveness after drug suppression in man, *J. Lab. Clin. Med.* **67**:566.

HERSH, E. M., WHITECAR, J. P., McCREDIE, K. B., BODEY, G. P., AND FREIREICH, E. J., 1971, Chemotherapy, immunocompetence, immunosuppression and prognosis in acute leukemia, *N. Engl. J. Med.* **285**:1211.

HERZIG, G. P., ROOT, R. K., AND GRAW, R. G., 1973, Granulocyte collection by continuous flow filtration leukapheresis, *Blood* **39**:554.

HERZIG, R. H., POPLACK, D. G., AND YANKEE, R. A., 1974, Prolonged granulocytopenia from incompatible platelet transfusions, *N. Engl. J. Med.* **290**:1220.

HERZIG, R. H., HERZIG, G. P., BULL, M. I., DECTER, J. A., LOHRMANN, H.-P., STOUT, F. G., YANKEE, R. A., AND GRAW, R., 1975, Correction of poor platelet transfusion responses with leukocyte-poor *HL-A*-matched platelet concentrates, *Blood* **46**:743.

HERZIG, R. H., HERZIG, G. P., BULL, M., RAY, K., DECTER, J., KAUFFMANN, J., ALOIS, G., APPELBAUM, F., FAY, J., ZOHRMANN, H., AND GRAW, R., 1976, Efficacy of granulocyte transfusion therapy for gram negative sepsis: A prospectively randomized controlled study, *Proc. Amer. Soc. Clin. Oncol.* **17**:253.

HIGBY, D. J., YATES, J. W., HENDERSON, E. S., AND HOLLAND, J. F., 1975a, Filtration leukopheresis for granulocyte transfusion therapy: Clinical and laboratory studies, *N. Engl. J. Med.* **292**:761.

HIGBY, D. J., AND HENDERSON, E. S., 1975b, Granulocyte transfusions for infection during neutropenia, *Semin. Oncol.* **2**:361.

HOLLAND, J. F., AND FREI, E. (eds.), 1973, *Cancer Medicine*, Lea and Febiger, Philadelphia.

HOLT, J. M., 1968, *Candida* infection of the oesophagus, *Gut.* **9**:227.

HOUCHENS, D. P., GASTON, M. R., KINNEY, Y., AND GOLDIN, A., 1974, Prevention of cyclophosphamide (NSC-26271) immunosuppression by bacillus Calmette-Guerin, *Cancer Chemother. Rep. Part 1*, **58**:931.

HUGHES, W. T., 1971*a*, Fatal infections in childhood leukemia, *Amer. J. Dis. Child.* **122**:283.

HUGHES, W. T., 1971*b*, Leukemia monitoring with fungal bone marrow cultures, *J. Amer. Med. Assoc.* **218**:441.

HUGHES, W. T., AND SMITH, D. R., 1973, Infection during induction of remission in acute lymphocytic leukemia, *Cancer* **31**:1008.

HUGHES, W. T., FELDMAN, S., AND COX, 1974*a*, Infectious diseases in children with cancer, *Pediatr. Clin. North Amer.* **21**:583.

HUGHES, W. T., MCNABB, P. C., MAKRES, T. D., AND FELDMAN, S., 1974*b*, Efficacy of trimethoprim and sulfamethoxazole in the prevention and treatment of·*Pneumocystis carinii* pneumonitis, *Antimicrob. Agents. Chemother.* **5**:289.

HUGHES, W. T., FELDMAN, S., AND SANYAL, S. K., 1975, Treatment of *Pneumocystis carinii* pneumonitis with trimethoprimsulfamethokazole, *Can. Med. Assoc. J.* **112**:1475.

HUGON, J. S., AND BOUNOUS, G., 1972, Elemental diet in the management of the intestinal lesions produced by radiation in the mouse, *Can. J. Surg.* **15**:18.

HURWITZ, E., LEVY, R., MARON, R., WILCHEK, M., ARNON, R., AND SELA, M., 1975, The covalent binding of daunomycin and adriamycin to antibodies with retention of both drug and antibody activities, *Cancer Res.* **35**:1175.

HYMAN, G. A., GELLHORN, A., AND HARVEY, J. L., 1956, Studies on the anemia of disseminated malignant neoplastic disease. II. Study of the life span of the erythrocyte, *Blood* **11**:618.

JACOB, H. S., 1972, Hypersplenism, in: *Hematology* (W. J. Williams, ed.), p. 1308, McGraw-Hill, New York.

JOHANSON, W. G., PIERCE, A. K., AND SANFORD, J. P., 1969, Changing pharyngeal bacterial flora of hospitalized patients, *N. Engl. J. Med.* **281**:1137.

JOHNSTON, R. F., AND WILDRICK, K. H., 1974, "State of the art" review. The impact of chemotherapy on the care of patients with tuberculosis, *Amer. Rev. Respir. Dis.* **109**:636.

JORDAN, G. W., AND MERIGAN, T. C., 1975, Enhancement of host defense mechanisms by pharmacological agents, *Annu. Rev. Med.* **26**:157.

JOYNER, L. R., AND SCHEINHORN, D. J., 1975, Transbronchial lung biopsy through the fiberoptic bronchoscope in diffuse lung disease, *Ann. Otol. Rhinol. Laryngol.* **84**:596.

KAGNOFF, M. F., ARMSTRONG, D., AND BLEVINS, A., 1972, Bacteroides bacteremia, *Cancer* **29**:245.

KAPLAN, M. H., ARMSTRONG, D., AND ROSEN, P., 1974, Tuberculosis complicating neoplastic disease, *Cancer* **33**:850.

KARPATKIN, S., STRICK, N., KARPATKIN, M. B., AND SISKIND, G. W., 1972, Cumulative experience in the detection of antiplatelet antibody in 234 patients with idiopathic thrombocytopenic purpura, systemic lupus erythematosus and other clinical disorders, *Amer. J. Med.* **52**:776.

KEUSCH, G. T., 1974, Opportunistic infections in colon carcinoma, *Amer. J. Clin. Nutr.* **27**:1481.

KEYE, J. D., AND MAGEE, W. E., 1956, Fungal diseases in a general hospital—a study of 88 patients, *Amer. J. Clin. Pathol.* **26**:1235.

KITAHARA, M., SETH, V. K., MEDOFF, G., AND KOBAYASHI, G. S., 1976, Activity of amphotericin B, 5-fluorocytosine, and rifampin against six clinical isolates of *Aspergillus*, *Antimicrob. Agents Chemother.* **9**:915.

KLEBANOFF, S. J., 1975, Antimicrobial mechanisms in neutrophilic polymorphonuclear leukocytes, *Semin. Hematol.* **12**:117.

KLEIN, M. S., ENNIS, F., SHERLOCK, P., AND WINAWER, S. J., 1973, Stress erosions, *Amer. J. Digestive Dis.* **18**:167.

KLASTERSKY, J., HENRI, A., HENSGENS, C., AND DANEAU, D., 1974, Gram-negative infections in cancer, *J. Amer. Med. Assoc.*, **227**:45.

KLASTERSKY, J., HENSGENS, C., AND DEBUSSCHER, L., 1975, Empiric therapy for cancer patients: Comparative study of ticarcillin–tobramycin, ticarcillin–cephalothin, and cephalothin–tobramycin, *Antimicrob. Agents Chemother.* **7**:640.

KORBITZ, B. C., TOREN, F. A., DAVIS, H. L., RAMIREZ, G., AND ANSFIELD, F. J., 1969, The piromen test: A useful assay of bone marrow granulocyte reserves, *Curr. Ther. Res.* **11**:491.

KREMER, W. B., AND LASZLO, J., 1973, Hematologic effects of cancer, in: *Cancer Medicine* (J. F. Holland and E. Frei, eds.), p. 1085, Lea and Febiger, Philadelphia.

277

SUPPORTIVE
CARE
IN THE
CANCER
PATIENT

KRUGMAN, S., AND GILES, J. P., 1973, Viral hepatitis, Type B (MS-2-Strain), *N. Engl. J. Med.*, **288**:755.

KUNICKI, T. J., TUCCELLI, M., BECKER, G. A., AND ASTER, R. H., 1975, A study of variables affecting the quality of platelets stored at "room temperature," *Transfusion* **15**:414.

KWAAN, H. C., 1972, Disseminated intravascular coagulation, *Med. Clin. North Amer.* **56**:177.

KYLE, R. A., AND BAYRD, E. D., 1975, Amyloidosis: Review of 236 cases, *Medicine* **54**:271.

LAWRENCE, H. S., 1973, Mediators of cellular immunity, *Transplant. Proc.* **5**(March):49.

LEVINE, A. S., SIEGEL, S. E., SCHREIBER, A. D., HAUSER, J., PREISLER, H., GOLDSTEIN, I. M., SEIDLER, F., SIMON, R., PERRY, S., BENNETT, J. E., AND HENDERSON, E. S., 1973, Protected environments and prophylactic antibiotics. A prospective controlled study of their utility in the therapy of acute leukemia, *N. Engl. J. Med.* **288**:477.

LEVINE, A. S., SCHIMPFF, S. C., GRAW, R. G., JR., AND YOUNG, R. C., 1974, Hematologic malignancies and other marrow failure states: Progress in the management of complicating infections, *Semin. Hematol.* **11**:141.

LEVITAN, A. A., AND PERRY, S., 1967, Infectious complications of chemotherapy in a protected environment, *N. Engl. J. Med.* **276**:881.

LEVITAN, A. A., AND PERRY, S., 1968, The use of an isolator system in cancer chemotherapy, *Amer. J. Med.* **44**:234.

LEVITT, M., MOSHER, M. B., DeCONTI, R. C., FARBER, L. R., SKEEL, R. T., MARSH, J. C., MITCHELL, M. S., PAPAC, R. J., THOMAS, E. D., AND BERTINO, J. R., 1973, Improved therapeutic index of methotrexate with "leucovorin rescue," *Cancer Res.* **33**:1729.

LOCKEY, E., PARKER, J., AND CASEWELL, M. W., 1973, Contamination of ECG electrode pads with *Klebsiella* and *Pseudomonas* species, *Br. Med. J.* **2**:400.

LOWENBRAUN, S., RAMSEY, H. E., AND SERPICK, A. A., 1971, Splenectomy in Hodgkin's disease for splenomegaly, cytopenias and intolerance to myelosuppressive chemotherapy, *Amer. J. Med.* **50**:49.

LOWENTHAL, R. M., GOLDMAN, J. M., BUSKARD, N. A., MURPHY, B. C., GROSSMAN, L., STORRING, R. A., PARK, D. S., SPIERS, A. S. D., AND GALTON, D. A. G., 1975, Granulocyte transfusions in treatment of infections in patients with acute leukemia and aplastic anemia, *Lancet* **1**:353.

LYNCH, P. J., VOORHEES, J. J., AND HARRELL, E. R., 1970, Systemic sporotrichosis, *Ann. Intern. Med.* **73**:23.

MARKS, M. I., LANGSTON, C., AND EICKHOFF, T. C., 1970, *Torulopsis glabrata*—an opportunistic pathogen in man, *N. Engl. J. Med.* **283**:1131.

MASOUREDIS, S. P., 1972, Clinical use of blood and blood products, in: *Hematology* (W. J. Williams, ed.), p. 1308, McGraw-Hill, New York.

MATSEN, J. M., 1973, The sources of hospital infection, *Medicine* **52**:271.

MCCABE, W. R., KREGER, B. E., AND JOHNS, M., 1972, Type-specific and cross-reactive antibodies in Gram-negative bacteremia, *N. Engl. J. Med.* **287**:261.

MCCLURE, P. D., INGRAM, G. I. C., STACY, R. S., GLASS, U. H., MATCHETT, M. O., 1966, Platelet function test in thrombocythaemia and thrombocytosis, *Br. J. Haematol.* **12**:478.

MCCREDIE, K. B., FREIREICH, E. J., HESTER, J. P., AND VALLEJOS, C., 1973, Leukocyte transfusion therapy for patients with host-defense failure, *Transplant. Proc.* **5**:1285.

MCKEE, L. C., JR., AND COLLINS, R. D., 1974, Intravascular leukocyte thrombi and aggregates as a cause of morbidity and mortality in leukemia, *Medicine* **53**:463.

MCLAUGHLIN, P., MEBAN, S., AND THOMPSON, W. G., 1973, Anaerobic liver abscess complicating radiation enteritis, *Can. Med. Assoc. J.* **108**:353.

MCLEAN, J. M., 1963, Oculomycosis, *Amer. J. Ophthalmol.* **56**:537.

MEDICAL, RESEARCH COUNCIL, 1975, Analysis of treatment in childhood leukaemia. I.—Predisposition to methotrexate-induced neutropenia after craniospinal irradiation, *Br. Med. J.* **3**:563.

MEDOFF, G., DISMUKES, W. E., MEADE, R. H., III, AND MOSES, J. M., 1972a, A new therapeutic approach to *Candida* infections, *Arch. Intern. Med.* **130**:241.

MEDOFF, G., KOBAYASHI, G. S., KWAN, C. N., SCHLESSINGER, D., AND VENKOV, P., 1972b, Potentiation of rifampicin and 5-fluorocytosine as antifungal antibiotics by amphotericin B, *Proc. Natl. Acad. Sci. U.S.A.* **69**:196.

MEYER, R. D., YOUNG, L. S., ARMSTRONG, D., AND YU, B., 1973, Aspergillosis complicating neoplastic disease, *Amer. J. Med.* **54**:6.

MEYERS, B. R., HIRSCHMAN, S. Z., AND AXELROD, J. A., 1972, Current patterns of infection in multiple myeloma, *Amer. J. Med.* **52**:87.

MIDDLEMAN, E. L., WATANABE, A., KAIZER, H., AND BODEY, G. P., 1972, Antibiotic combinations for infections in neutropenic patients, *Cancer* **30**:573.

MILDER, M. S., GLICK, J. H., HENDERSON, E. S., AND JOHNSTON, G. S., 1973, ^{67}Ga scintigraphy in acute leukemia, *Cancer* **32**:803.

MIRSKY, H. S., AND CUTTNER, J., 1972, Fungal infection in acute leukemia, *Cancer* **30**:348.

MITCH, W. E., AND SERPICK, A. A., 1970, Leukemic infiltration of the prostate: a reversible form of urinary obstruction, *Cancer* **26**:1361.

MORBIDITY AND MORTALITY WEEKLY REPORT (SUPPLEMENT), 1976, Perspectives on the control of viral hepatitis, Type B, **25**:1.

MORRIS, P., AND SHAW, E. A., 1974, Acute upper respiratory tract obstruction complicating childhood leukaemia, *Br. Med. J.* **2**:703.

MORSE, E. E., FREIREICH, E. J., CARBONE, P. P., BRONSON, W., AND FREI, E., III, 1966, The transfusion of leukocytes from donors with chronic myelocytic leukemia to patients with leukopenia, *Transfusion* **6**:183.

MURPHY, S., AND GARDNER, F. H., 1975, Platelet storage at 22°C: Role of gas transport across plastic containers in maintenance of viability, *Blood* **46**:209.

MURPHY, S., KOCH, P. A., AND EVANS, A. E., 1976, Randomized trial of prophylactic versus therapeutic platelet transfusion in childhood acute leukemia, *Clin. Res.* **24**:379A.

MYERS, M, G., OXMAN, M. N., CLARK, J. E., AND ARNDT, K. A., 1975, Failure of neutral-red photodynamic inactivation in recurrent *Herpes simplex* virus infections, *N. Engl. J. Med.* **293**:945.

NASH, G., FOLEY, F. D., GOODWIN, M. N., JR., BRUCK, H. M., GREENWALD, K. A., AND PRUITT, B. A., JR., 1971, Fungal burn wound infection, *J. Amer. Med. Assoc.* **215**:1664.

NIES, B. A., AND CREGER, W. P., 1967, Tolerance of chemotherapy following splenectomy for leukopenia or thrombocytopenia in patients with malignant lymphomas, *Cancer* **20**:558.

ODEBERG, H., OLOFSSON, T., AND OLSSON, I., 1975, Granulocyte function in chronic granulocytic leukaemia, *Br. J. Haematol.* **29**:427.

OSTER, M. W., GELRUD, L. G., LOTZ, M. J., HERZIG, G. P., AND JOHNSTON, G. S., 1975, Psoas abscess localization by gallium scan in aplastic anemia, *J. Amer. Med. Assoc.* **232**:377.

PALMER, D. L., HARVEY, R. L., AND WHEELER, J. K., 1974, Diagnostic and therapeutic considerations in *Nocardia asteroides* infection, *Medicine* **53**:391.

PANKEY, G. A., AND DALOVISO, J. R., 1973, Fungemia caused by *Torulopsis glabrata*, *Medicine* **52**:395.

PENNEY, R., AND GALTON, D. A. G., 1966, Studies on neutrophil function. II. Pathological aspects, *Br. J. Haematol.* **12**:633.

PETERS, W. P., HOLLAND, J. F., SENN, H., RHOMBERG, W., AND BANERJEE, T., 1972, Corticosteroid administration and localized leukocyte mobilization in man, *N. Engl. J. Med.* **286**:342.

PETTY, A. M., AND WENGER, J., 1970, Bacteremia following peroral biopsy of the small intestine, *Gastroenterology* **59**:140.

PHILLIPS, I., JENKINS, S., KING, A., AND SPENCER, G., 1974, Control of respirator-associated infection due to *Pseudomonas aeruginosa*, *Lancet* **3**:871.

PIROFSKY, B., 1968, Autoimmune hemolytic anemia and neoplasia of the reticuloendothelium, *Ann. Intern. Med.* **68**:109.

POCHEDLY, C., 1975, Neurologic manifestations in acute leukemia, *N.Y. State J. Med.* **75**:575, 715, 878.

POLLACK, M., NIEMAN, R. E., REINHARDT, J. A., CHARACHE, P., JETT, M. P., AND HARDY, P. H., JR., 1972, Factors influencing colonisation and antibiotic-resistance patterns of Gram-negative bacteria in hospital patients, *Lancet* **2**:668.

POLLARD, M., AND SHARON, N., 1970, Chemotherapy of spontaneous leukemia in germ-free AKR mice, *J. Natl. Cancer Inst.* **45**:677.

PREISLER, H. D., AND BJORNSSON, S., 1975, Protected environment units in the treatment of acute leukemia, *Semin. Oncol.* **2**:369.

PREISLER, H. D., GOLDSTEIN, I. M., AND HENDERSON, E. S., 1970, Gastrointestinal "sterilization" in the treatment of patients with acute leukemia, *Cancer* **26**:1076.

PREISLER, H. D., HASENCLEVER, H. F., AND HENDERSON, E. S., 1971, Anti-*Candida* antibodies in patients with acute leukemia. A prospective study, *Amer. J. Med.* **51**:352.

PRINCE, A. M., SZMUNESS, W., MILLIAN, S. J., AND DAVID, D. S., 1971, A serologic study of cytomegalovirus infections associated with blood transfusions, *N. Engl. J. Med.* **284**:1125.

PRINCE, A. M., SZMUNESS, W., MANN, M. K., VYAS, G. N., GRADY, G. F., SHAPIRO, F. L., SUKI, W. N., FRIEDMAN, E. A., AND STENZEL, K. H., 1975, Efficacy of prophylactic HBIG against dialysis-associated hepatitis, *N. Engl. J. Med.* **293**:1063.

QUIE, P., 1975, Pathology of bactericidal power of neutrophils, *Semin. Hematol.* **12**:143.

RAGAB, A. H., GILKERSON, E. S., AND MYERS, M. L., 1974, Granulopoiesis in childhood leukemia, *Cancer* **33**:791.

RAMMELKAMP, C. H., MORTIMER, E. A., JR., AND WOLINSKY, E., 1964, Transmission of streptococcal and staphylococcal infections, *Ann. Intern. Med.* **60:**753.

REYES, M. P., PALUTKE, M., AND LERNER, A. M., 1973, Granulocytopenia associated with carbenicillin, *Amer. J. Med.* **54:**413.

RHAME, F. S., ROOT, R. K., MACLOWRY, J. D., DADISMAN, T. A., AND BENNETT, J. V., 1973, Salmonella septicemia from platelet transfusions, *Ann. Intern. Med.* **78:**633.

RHOADES, E. R., RINGROSE, R., MOHR, J. A., BROOKS, L., MCKOWN, B. A., AND FELTON, F., 1971, Contamination of ultrasonic nebulization equipment with Gram-negative bacteria, *Arch. Intern. Med.* **127:**228.

RICHARDS, F., MCCALL, C., AND COX, C., 1971, Gentamicin treatment of staphylococcal infections, *J. Amer. Med. Assoc.* **215:**1297.

RIEDLER, G. F., STRAUB, P. W., AND FRICK, P. G., 1971, Thrombocytopenia in septicemia, *Helv. Med. Acta* **36**(Fasc. 1):23.

ROBERTS, P. I., KNEPSHIELD, J. H., AND WELLS, R. F., 1968, Coccidioides as an opportunist, *Arch. Intern. Med.* **121:**568.

RODRIGUEZ, V., BURGESS, M., AND BODEY, G. P., 1973, Management of fever of unknown origin in patients with neoplasms and neutropenia, *Cancer* **32:**1007.

ROITT, I., 1974a, in: *Essential Immunology*, pp. 148–180, Blackwell Scientific Publications, Oxford.

ROSENOFF, S. H., BOSTICK, F., AND YOUNG, R. C., 1975, Recovery of normal hematopoietic tissue and tumor following chemotherapeutic injury from cyclophosphamide: Comparative analysis of biochemical and clinical techniques, *Blood* **45:**465.

ROSENTHAL, S. L., 1975, Aminoglycoside antibiotics, *N. Y. State J. Med.* **75:**535.

ROSNER, F., VALMONT, I., KOZINN, P. J., AND CAROLINE, L., 1970, Leukocyte function in patients with leukemia, *Cancer* **25:**835.

ROY, A. J., AND DJERASSI, I., 1972, Effects of platelet transfusions: Plug formation and maintenance of vascular integrity, *Proc. Soc. Exp. Biol. Med.* **139:**137.

ROY, A. J., JAFFE, N., AND DJERASSI, I., 1973, Prophylactic platelet transfusions in children with acute leukemia; a dose–response study, *Transfusion* **13:**283.

RUDDERS, R. A., AISENBERG, A. C., AND SCHILLER, A. L., 1972, Hodgkin's disease presenting as "idiopathic" thrombocytopenic purpura, *Cancer* **30:**220.

RUSKIN, J., AND REMINGTON, J. S., 1976, Toxoplasmosis in the compromised host, *Ann. Intern. Med.* **84:**193.

RYAN, J. A., ABEL, R. M., ABBOTT, W. M., HOPKINS, C. C. CHESNEY, T. McC., COLLEY, R., PHILLIPS, K., AND FISCHER, J. E., 1974, Catheter complications of total parenteral nutrition, *N. Engl. J. Med.* **290:**757.

SALMON, S. E., SAMAL, B. A., HAYES, D. M., HOSLEY, H., MILLER, S. P., AND SCHILLING, A., 1967, Role of gamma globulin for immunoprophylaxis in multiple myeloma, *N. Engl. J. Med.* **277:**1336.

SALZMAN, T. C., CLARK, J. J., AND KLEMM, L., 1967, Hand contamination of personnel as a mechanism of cross-infection in nosocomial infections with antibiotic-resistant *Escherichia coli* and *Klebsiella–Aerobacter*, *Antimicrob. Agents. Chemother.*, p. 97.

SAMELLAS, W., 1964, Death due to septicemia following percutaneous needle biopsy of the kidney, *J. Urol.* **91:**317.

SANDWEISS, D. A., HANSON, J. C., GOSINK, B. B., AND MOSER, K. M., 1975, Ultrasound in diagnosis, localization, and treatment of loculated pleural empyema, *Ann. Intern. Med.* **82:**50.

SBARRA, A. J., SHIRLEY, W., SELVARAJ, R. J., OUCHI, E., AND ROSENBAUM, E., 1964, The role of the phagocyte in host–parasite interactions. I. The phagocytic capabilities of leukocytes from lymphoproliferative disorders, *Cancer Res.* **24:**1958.

SCHELINE, R. R., 1968, Drug metabolism by intestinal microorganisms, *J. Pharm. Sci.* **57:**2021.

SCHIFFER, C. A., BUCHHOLZ, D. H., AISNER, J., BETTS, S. W., AND WIERNIK, P. H., 1975, Clinical experience with transfusion of granulocytes obtained by continuous flow filtration leukopheresis, *Amer. J. Med.* **58:**373.

SCHIMPFF, S. C., MOODY, M., AND YOUNG, V. M., 1970, Relationship of colonization with *Pseudomonas aeruginosa* to development of *Pseudomonas* bacteremia in cancer patients, *Antimicrob. Agent Chemother.*, p. 240.

SCHIMPFF, S. C., YOUNG, V. M., GREENE, W. H., VERMEULEN, G., MOODY, M., AND WIERNIK, P., 1972a, Origin of infection in acute nonlymphocytic leukemia, *Ann. Intern. Med.* **77:**707.

SCHIMPFF, S. C., SERPICK, A., STOLER, B., RUMACK, B., MELLIN, H., JOSEPH, J. M., AND BLOCK, J., 1972b, Varicella-zoster infection in patients with cancer, *Ann. Intern. Med.* **76:**241.

SCHIMPFF, S. C., BLOCK, J. B., AND WIERNIK, P. H., 1972c, Rectal abscesses in cancer patients, *Lancet* **2:**844.

SCHIMPFF, S. C., GREENE, W. H., YOUNG, V. M., AND WIERNIK, P. H., 1973, *Pseudomonas* septicemia: Incidence, epidemiology, prevention and therapy in patients with advanced cancer, *Eur. J. Cancer* **9**:449.

SCHIMPFF, S. C., GREENE, W. H., YOUNG, V. M., FORTNER, C. L., JEPSEN, L., CUSACK, N., BLOCK, J. B., AND WIERNIK, P. H., 1975, Infection prevention in acute nonlymphocytic leukemia. Laminar air flow room reverse isolation with oral nonabsorbable antibiotic prophylaxis, *Ann. Intern. Med.* **82**:351.

SCHIMPFF, S. C., YOUNG, V. M., AND HAHN, D., 1976, Infection prevention in acute leukemia. Comparison of oral nonabsorbable antibiotics alone, with reverse isolation, or with reverse isolation plus air filtration in standard hospital rooms, *Proceedings of the Annual Meeting of the American Society of Clinical Oncology,* Abstract C-96.

SCHWARZENBERG, L., MATHÉ, G., AMIEL, J. L., CATTAN, A., SCHNEIDER, M., AND SCHLUMBERGER, J. R., 1967, Study of factors determining the usefulness and complications of leukocyte transfusions, *Amer. J. Med.* **43**:206.

SEELIG, M. S., 1966, The role of antibiotics in the pathogenesis of *Candida* infections, *Amer. J. Med.* **40**:887.

SENN, H. J., AND JUNGI, W. F., 1975, Neutrophil migration in health and disease, *Semin. Hematol.* **12**:27.

SHEDLOFSKY, S., AND FRETER, R., 1974, Synergism between ecologic and immunologic control mechanisms of intestinal flora, *J. Infect. Dis.* **129**:296.

SHOOTER, R. A., GAYA, H., COOKE, E. M., KUMAR, P., PATEL, N., PARKER, M. T., THOM, B. T., AND FRANCE, D. R., 1969, Food and medicaments as possible sources of hospital strains of *Pseudomonas aeruginosa,* *Lancet* **1**:1227.

SHOOTER, R. A., FAIERS, M. C., COOKE, E. M., BREADEN, A. L., AND O'FARRELL, S. M., 1971, Isolation of *Escherichia coli, Pseudomonas aeruginosa,* and *Klebsiella* from food in hospitals, canteens, and schools, *Lancet* **2**:390.

SICKLES, E. A., YOUNG, V. M., GREENE, W. H., AND WIERNIK, P. H., 1973, Pneumonia in acute leukemia, *Ann. Intern. Med.* **79**:528.

SICKLES, E. A., GREENE, W. H., AND WIERNIK, P. H., 1975, Clinical presentation of infection in granulocytopenic patients, *Arch. Int. Med.* **135**:715.

SIEGEL, S. E., LUNDE, M. N., GELDERMAN, A. H., HALTERMAN, R. H., BROWN, J. A. LEVINE, A. S., AND GRAW, R. G., JR., 1971, Transmission of toxoplasmosis by leukocyte transfusion, *Blood* **37**:388.

SILVA, J., JR., AND HARVEY, W. C., 1974, Detection of infections with gallium-67 and scintigraphic imaging, *J. Infect. Dis.* **130**:125.

SIMONE, J., 1976, delivered at a symposium on The Management of Leukemia, Yale School of Medicine, New Haven, Connecticut.

SINKOVICS, J. G., AND SMITH, J. P., 1969, Salmonellosis complicating neoplastic diseases, *Cancer* **24**:631.

STAMM, W. E., 1975, Guidelines for prevention of catheter-associated urinary tract infections, *Ann. Intern. Med.* **82**:386.

STERRE, A. C., AND MALLINSON, G. F., 1975, Handwashing practices for the prevention of nosocomial infections, *Ann. Intern. Med.* **83**:683.

STEERE, A. C., AISNER, J., ANDERSON, R. L., BENNETT, J. V., AND SCHIMPFF, S. C., 1975, The predictive value of nose cultures in the diagnosis of aspergillosis, *Program of the 15th Interscience Conference on Antimicrobial Agents and Chemotherapy,* Abstract 207.

STEINBERG, S. C., ALTER, H. J., AND LEVENTHAL, B. G., 1975, The risk of hepatitis transmission to family contacts of leukemia patients, *J. Pediatr.* **87**:753.

STEVENS, D. A., PAPPAGIANIS, D., MARINKOVICH, V. A., AND WADDELL, T. F., 1974, Immunotherapy in recurrent coccidioidomycosis, *Cell. Immunol.* **12**:37.

STEVENS, D. A., LEVINE, H. B., AND DERESINSKI, S. C., 1976, Miconazole in coccidioidomycosis. II. Therapeutic and pharmacologic studies in man, *Amer. J. Med.* **60**:191.

STONE, H. H., AND KOLB, L. D., 1971, The evolution and spread of gentamicin-resistant pseudomonads, *J. Trauma* **11**:586.

STOSSEL, T. P., 1975, Phagocytosis: Recognition and ingestion, *Semin. Hematol.* **12**:83.

STRANDER, H., CANTELL, K., CARLSTROM, G., INGIMARSSON, S., JAKOBSSON, P., AND NILSONNE, U., 1976, Acute infections in interferon-treated patients with osteosarcoma: Preliminary report of a comparative study, *J. Infect. Dis.* **133S**:A245.

SULTAN, Y., AND CAEN, J. P., 1972, Platelet dysfunction in preleukemic states and in various types of leukemia, *Ann. N. Y. Acad. Sci.* **201**:300.

SURGENOR, D. M., CHALMERS, T. C., CONRAD, M. E., FRIEDEWALD, W. T., GRADY, G. F., HAMILTON, M., MOSLEY, J. W., PRINCE, A. M., AND STENGLE, J. M., 1975, Clinical trials of hepatitis B immune globulin in the prevention of hepatitis, *N. Engl. J. Med.* **293**:1060.

SUTNICK, A. I., AND ENGSTROM, P. F. (eds.), 1976, *Oncologic Medicine*, University Park Press, Baltimore.

SWISHER, S. N., 1972, Cryopathic hemolytic syndromes, in: *Hematology* (W. J. Williams, ed.), p. 498, McGraw-Hill, New York.

TALLY, F. P., LOUIE, T. J., WEINSTEIN, W. M., BARTLETT, J. G., AND GORBACH, S. L., 1975, Amikacin therapy for severe gram-negative sepsis, *Ann. Intern. Med.* **83**:484.

TAPPER, M. L., AND ARMSTRONG, D., 1976, Malaria complicating neoplastic disease, *Arch. Intern. Med.* **136**:807.

TATTERSALL, M. H. N., HUTCHINSON, R. M., GAYA, H., AND SPIERS, A. S. D., 1973, Empirical antibiotic therapy in febrile patients with neutropenia and malignant disease, *Eur. J. Cancer* **9**:417.

THOMAS, E. D., 1976, delivered at a symposium on the Management of Leukemia, Yale School of Medicine, New Haven, Connecticut.

TOBIAS, J. S., BROWN, B. L., BRIVKALNS, A., AND YANKEE, R. A., 1976, Prophylactic granulocyte support in experimental septicemia, *Blood* **47**:473.

TOMASI, T. B., 1972, Secretory immunoglobulins, *N. Engl. J. Med.* **287**:500.

UTZ, J. P., GARRIQUES, I. L., SANDE, M. A, WARNER, J. F., MANDELL, G. L., McGEHEE, R. F., DUMA, R., AND SHADOMY, S., 1975, Therapy of cryptococcosis with a combination of flucytosine and amphotericin B, *J. Infect. Dis.* **132**:368.

VALDIVIESO, M., HORIKOSHI, N., RODRIGUEZ, V., AND BODEY, G. P., 1974, Therapeutic trials with tobramycin, *Amer. J. Med. Sci.* **268**:149.

VALDIMARSSON, H., WOOD, C. B. S., HOBBS, J. R., AND HOLT, P. J. L., 1972, Immunological features in a case of chronic granulomatous candidiasis and its treatment with transfer factor, *Clin. Exp. Immunol.* **11**:151.

VALLEJOS, C., McCREDIE, K. B., BODEY, G. P., HESTER, J. P., AND FREIREICH, E. J., 1975, White blood cell transfusions for control of infections in neutropenic patients, *Transfusion* **15**:28.

VOGLER, W. R., AND WINTON, E. F., 1976, The efficacy of granulocyte transfusions in neutropenic patients, *Proc. Amer. Soc. Clin. Oncology* **17**:252.

WAISBREN, B. A., EVANI, S. V., AND ZIEBERT, A. P., 1971, Carbenicillin and bleeding, *J. Amer. Med. Assoc.* **217**:1243.

WANDS, J. R., WALKER, J. A., DAVIS, T. T., WATERBURY, L. A., OWENS, A. H., AND CARPENTER, C. C. J., 1974, Hepatitis B in an oncology unit, *N. Engl. J. Med.* **291**:1371.

WARD, P. A., AND BERENBERG, J. L., 1974, Defective regulation of inflammatory mediators in Hodgkin's disease, *N. Engl. J. Med.* **290**:76.

WARD, P. A., ANTON, T., AND MADERAZO, E., 1976, Defective leukotaxis in cancer patients, *Clin. Res.* **24**:463A.

WASHINGTON, J. A., 1975, Blood cultures: Principles and techniques, *Mayo Clin. Proc.* **50**:91.

WEINSTEIN, L., GOLDFIELD, M., AND CHANG, T.-W., 1954, Infections occurring during chemotherapy, *N. Engl. J. Med.* **251**:247.

WEISS, H. J., 1972, Acquired qualitative platelet disorders, in: *Hematology* (W. J. Williams, ed.), p. 1171, McGraw-Hill, New York.

WEISS, H. J., 1975, Platelets: Physiology and abnormalities of function, *N. Engl. J. Med.* **293**:531.

WELLER, T. H., 1971, The cytomegaloviruses, *N. Engl. J. Med.* **285**:203.

WENZ, B., AND FRIEDMAN, G., 1974, Acquired factor VIII inhibitor in a patient with malignant lymphoma, *Amer. J. Med. Sci.* **268**:295.

WHITE, L. P., AND CLAFLIN, E. F., 1963, Nitrogen mustard: Diminution of toxicity in axenic mice, *Science* **140**:1400.

WHITECAR, J., 1973, Disseminated intravascular coagulation, in: *Cancer Medicine* (J. F. Holland and E. Frei, eds.), pp. 1129–1133, Lea and Febiger, Philadelphia.

WHITECAR, J. P., LUNA, M., AND BODEY, G. P., 1970, *Pseudomonas* bacteremia in patients with malignant diseases, *Amer. J. Med. Sci.* **260**:216.

WHITLEY, R. J., CH'IEN, L. T., DOLIN, R., GALASSO, G. J., ALFORD, C. A., (eds.), AND THE COLLABORATIVE STUDY GROUP, 1976, Adenine arabinoside therapy of *herpes zoster* in the immunosuppressed, *N. Engl. J. Med.* **294**:1193.

281

SUPPORTIVE
CARE
IN THE
CANCER
PATIENT

WILFERT, C. M., 1975, Priorities in preventing varicella-zoster, *Drug Therapy*, October, p. 150.

WILLIAMS, W. J., (ed.), 1972, Thrombocytosis, in: *Hematology*, p. 1162, McGraw-Hill, New York.

WINGFIELD, W. L., POLLACK, D., AND GRUNERT, R., 1969, Therapeutic efficacy of amantadine HCl and rimantadine HCl in naturally occurring influenza A_2 respiratory illness in man, *N. Engl. J. Med.* 281:579.

WINITZ, M., SEEDMAN, D. A., AND GRAFF, J., 1970*a*, Studies in metabolic nutrition employing chemically defined diets, *Amer. J. Clin. Nutr.* 23:525.

WINITZ, M., ADAMS, R. F., SEEDMAN, D. A., DAVIS, P. N., JAYKO, L. G., AND HAMILTON, J. A., 1970*b*, Studies in metabolic nutrition employing chemically defined diets, *Amer. J. Clin. Nutr.* 23:546.

WINKELSTEIN, J. A., 1973, Opsonins: Their function, identity, and clinical significance, *J. Pediatr.* 82:747.

WINTROBE, M. M. (ed.), 1974*a*, in: *Clinical Hematology*, p. 717, Lea and Febiger, Philadelphia.

WINTROBE, M. M. (ed.), 1974*b*, in: *Clinical Hematology*, p. 934, Lea and Febiger, Philadelphia.

WINTROBE, M. M. (ed.), 1974*c*, in: *Clinical Hematology*, p. 891, Lea and Febiger, Philadelphia.

WINTROBE, M. M. (ed), 1974*d*, in: *Clinical Hematology*, p. 1405, Lea and Febiger, Philadelphia.

WINTROBE, M. M. (ed.), 1974*e*, in: *Clinical Hematology*, p. 1201, Lea and Febiger, Philadelphia.

WOLFE, M. S., ARMSTRONG, D., LOURIA, D. B., AND BLEVINS, A., 1971, Salmonellosis in patients with neoplastic disease, *Arch. Intern. Med.* 128:546.

WRIGHT, D. G., KAUFFMANN, J. C., CHUSID, M. J., HERZIG, G. P., AND GALLIN, J. I., 1975, Functional abnormalities of human neutrophils collected by continuous flow filtration leukopheresis, *Blood* 46:901.

WU, K. K., HOAK, J. C., THOMPSON, J. S., AND KOEPKE, J. A., 1976, Platelet transfusion refractoriness and donor selection, *Clin. Res.* 24:323A,

WYBRAN, J., STACQUEZ, C., AND GOVAERTS, A. E., 1972, Storage of human platelets in liquid nitrogen–isotopic studies, *Transfusion* 12:413.

YANKEE, R. A., GRUMET, F. C., AND ROGENTINE, G. N., 1969, Platelet transfusion therapy: The selection of compatible platelet donors for refractory patients by lymphocyte *HL-A* typing, *N. Engl. J. Med.* 281:1208.

YANKEE, R. A., GRAFF, K. S., DOWLING, R., AND HENDERSON, E. S., 1973, Selection of unrelated compatible platelet donors by lymphocyte *HL-A* matching, *N. Engl. J. Med.* 288:760.

YATES, J. W., AND HOLLAND, J. F., 1973, A controlled study of isolation and endogenous microbial suppression in acute myelocytic leukemia, *Cancer* 32:1490.

YOSHIKAWA, T., TANAKA, K. R., AND GUZE, L. B., 1971, Infection and disseminated intravascular coagulation, *Medicine* 50:237.

YOUNG, L. S., ARMSTRONG, D., BLEVINS, A., AND LIEBERMAN, P., 1971, *Nocardia asteroides* infection complicating neoplastic disease, *Amer. J. Med.* 50:356.

YOUNG, L. S., MEYER, R. D., AND ARMSTRONG, D., 1973, Controlled prospective trial of *Pseudomonas aeruginosa* vaccine in cancer patients, *Ann. Intern. Med.* 79:518.

YOUNG, R. C., CORDER, M. P., BERARD, C. W., AND DEVITA, V. T., 1973, Immune alterations in Hodgkin's disease, *Arch. Intern. Med.* 131:446.

YOUNG, R. C., BENNETT, J. E., GEELHOED, G. W., AND LEVINE, A. S., 1974, Fungemia with compromised host resistance, *Ann. Intern. Med.* 80:605.

ZEIGLER, Z., MURPHY, S., AND GARDNER, F. H., 1975, Post-transfusion purpura: A heterogeneous syndrome, *Blood* 45:529.

ZIEGLER, E. J., DOUGLAS, H., SHERMAN, J. E., DAVIS, C. E., AND BRAUDE, A. I., 1973, Treatment of *E. coli* and *Klebsiella* bacteremia in agranulocytic animals with antiserum to a UDP-GAL epimerase-deficient mutant, *J. Immunol.* 111:433.

ZIEGLER, E. J., DOUGLAS, H., AND BRAUDE, A. I., 1975, Prevention of lethal *Pseudomonas* bacteremia with epimerase-deficient *E. coli* antiserum, *Clin. Res.* 23:445A.

ZIMMERMAN, L. E., 1955, Fatal fungus infections complicating other diseases, *Amer. J. Clin. Pathol.* 25:46.

ZINNER, S. H., AND MCCABE, W. R., 1976, Effects of IgM and IgG antibody in patients with bacteremia due to Gram-negative bacilli, *J. Infect. Dis.* 133:37.

ZUCKER, S., AND LYSIK, R. M., 1976, Anemia in cancer, in: *Oncologic Medicine* (A. I. Sutnick and P. F. Engstrom, eds.), p. 261, University Park Press, Baltimore.

Chemotherapeutic Agents

10

Alkylating Agents and the Nitrosoureas

David B. Ludlum

1. Introduction

1.1. History

The alkylating agents as a group have long held the interest of both practical cancer chemotherapists and experimental pharmacologists. They have assumed this position of importance because they were among the first clinical agents of recognized value, and because their study has increased our understanding of cancer chemotherapy in general. At a molecular level, interest in alkylating agents has led to studies of alterations in DNA structure, and to investigations of the repair of chemically induced damage to DNA. Interest in cyclophosphamide has led to important studies of drug metabolism, while interest in the distribution of alkylating agents has led to investigations of drug transport. Besides these and other contributions in the area of cancer chemotherapy, studies of alkylating agents have also increased our understanding of mutagenesis and chemical carcinogenesis.

Many of the alkylating agents are related to mustard gas, first used for chemical warfare in World War I. At that time, it was noted that limited exposure to this agent caused bone marrow suppression somewhat similar to that produced by radiation. Following this observation, a group at Yale University tried a nitrogen mustard, *tris* chloroethylamine, for the treatment of certain marrow-related malignancies. These studies, which were undertaken during World War II and described afterward by Gilman (1963), not only established the clinical usefulness

DAVID B. LUDLUM ● Department of Pharmacology and Experimental Therapeutics, Albany Medical College, Albany, New York 12208.

of the mustards, but also demonstrated their chief disadvantages: toxicity to the host and development of resistance by the tumor.

The impact of these studies cannot be overestimated: they were the first clear indication that chemotherapy had something definite to offer the cancer patient. Consequently, a wide search was initiated for new and more selective alkylating agents and for other, structurally unrelated compounds with antitumor activity.

A large number of alkylating agents have been synthesized, including many mustards and compounds with other functional groups. Most of these agents have been tested against animal tumors, and a smaller number against human malignancies. Studies undertaken prior to 1965 were summarized in a special supplement to *Cancer Chemotherapy Reports* (Schmidt *et al.*, 1965).

In the last decade or so, there has been somewhat less emphasis on alkylating agents than on other classes of compounds, possibly because of a feeling that all the alkylating agents are rather similar. Although there may be some truth in this point of view, some extremely important differences have emerged, and it seems entirely possible that these differences can be exploited further.

1.2. Classification of Alkylating Agents and Nitrosoureas

Representative agents are shown in Fig. 1, arranged according to the nature of their alkylating groups. Sulfur mustard is too reactive for clinical use, but many nitrogen mustards have been synthesized, and the last three, chlorambucil, phenylalanine mustard, and cyclophosphamide, are all in common use.

Nitrogen mustards contain the grouping $-N(CH_2CH_2Cl)_2$, which undergoes internal cyclization in aqueous media to form aziridinium ions. These, in turn, attack electron-rich regions in cellular macromolecules, as discussed below. Since all tissues are subject to this attack, there have been numerous efforts to devise a mustard that would be activated by the tumor itself.

Cyclophosphamide was developed with this rationale in mind. The electron-withdrawing group attached to the mustard prevents cyclization and activation until the ring structure is metabolized. Although it is now recognized that this metabolism occurs at least partially in the liver, and an activated species is transported to the tumor, the concept of a tumor-activated agent is valid, and this area is still being investigated.

Methyl methanesulfonate and ethyl methanesulfonate have been employed extensively in the laboratory as model alkylating agents. One member of the series, busulfan, has been rather widely used in the treatment of chronic myelogenous leukemia, but these agents have not been particularly useful against solid tumors.

The ethylenimines resemble the active, cyclized form of the nitrogen mustards. They are active by the oral route, but absorption appears to be somewhat variable. Although triethylenemelamine and triethylenethiophosphoramide contain three functional groups, the cross-linking activity of these agents has not been studied in detail. Clinically, they are less widely used than the other agents mentioned above.

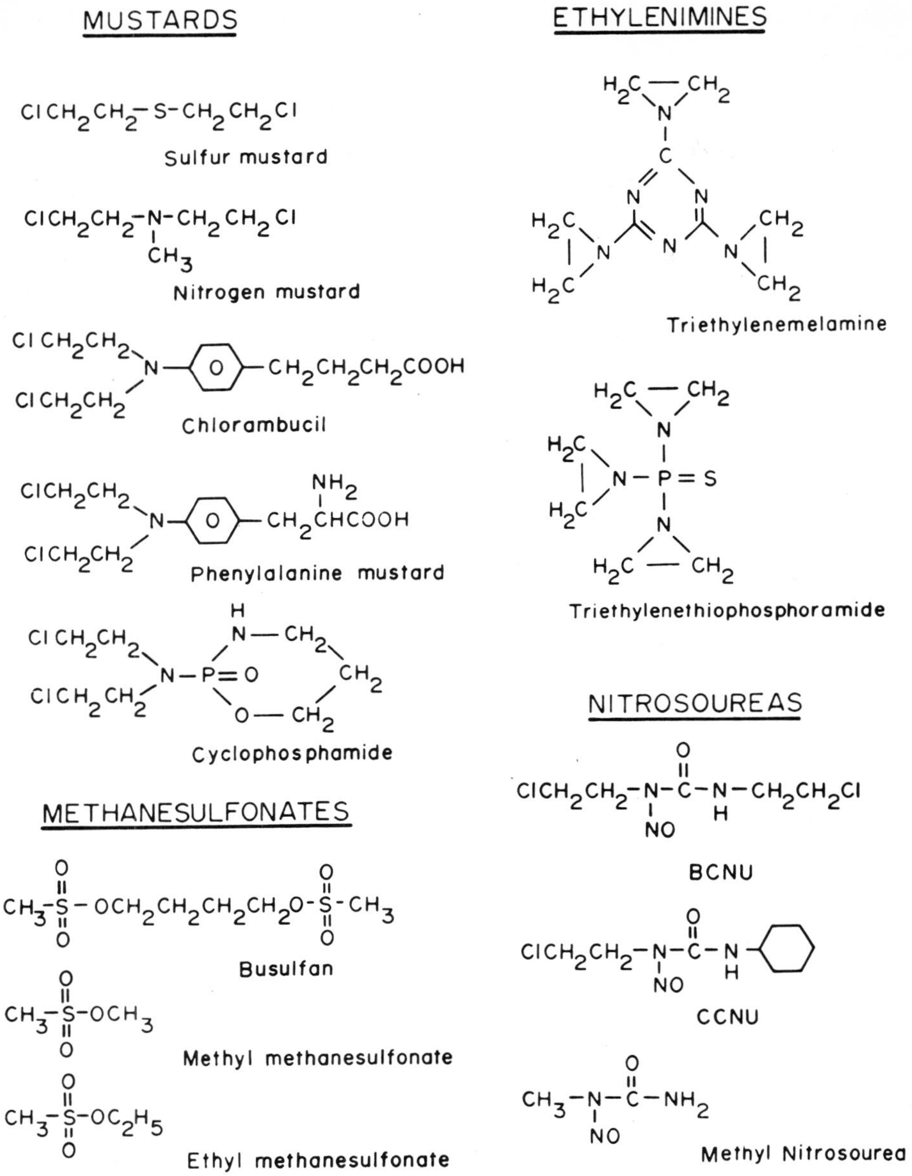

MUSTARDS

$ClCH_2CH_2-S-CH_2CH_2Cl$

Sulfur mustard

$ClCH_2CH_2-N-CH_2CH_2Cl$
$\quad\quad\quad\;\; | $
$\quad\quad\quad CH_3$

Nitrogen mustard

Chlorambucil

Phenylalanine mustard

Cyclophosphamide

METHANESULFONATES

Busulfan

Methyl methanesulfonate

Ethyl methanesulfonate

ETHYLENIMINES

Triethylenemelamine

Triethylenethiophosphoramide

NITROSOUREAS

BCNU

CCNU

Methyl Nitrosourea

FIGURE 1. Chemical structures of the alkylating agents and nitrosoureas. Although most of these compounds are used clinically, sulfur mustard, methyl methanesulfonate, ethyl methanesulfonate, and methyl nitrosourea are of theoretical interest only.

The final class of compounds discussed here, the nitrosoureas, are of very great practical and theoretical interest. Methyl nitrosourea and the closely related compound, methyl nitro nitrosoguanidine, have long been recognized as mutagenic agents. Following the observation that these compounds were active against L1210 leukemia, many substituted nitrosoureas were synthesized and tested in animal systems (Johnston *et al.*, 1963, 1966). Of these, *bis* chloroethyl nitrosourea (BCNU) and chloroethyl cyclohexyl nitrosourea (CCNU) were chosen for further study because of their activity against L1210 cells. A newer agent, chloroethyl methylcyclohexyl nitrosourea (methyl-CCNU), is especially active against Lewis lung tumor. Consequently, this compound is being tested clinically against solid tumors.

The nitrosoureas undoubtedly possess alkylating activity, as defined by their reaction with nitrobenzylpyridine (Wheeler and Chumley, 1967). However, tumors that are resistant to nitrogen mustards are sometimes sensitive to the nitrosoureas. Thus, they are frequently considered in a somewhat separate class from the older agents. As more differences are recognized among the individual alkylating agents, however, they may fit clinically into the broad spectrum of such compounds.

1.3. Purpose of This Review

The literature on alkylating agents is already extensive, and several reviews are available that cover the areas indicated by their titles in the reference section (Connors, 1975a, b; Fox, 1975; Lawley, 1966; Loveless, 1966; Ludlum, 1975; Ochoa and Hirschberg, 1967; Price, 1975; Ross, 1962, 1975; Singer, 1975; Van Duuren, 1969; Wheeler, 1975). The purpose of this chapter is twofold: to outline our knowledge of the alkylating agents, and to present certain areas of active research in greater detail. Inevitably, these areas will reflect the author's interest, but particular attention will be paid to those investigations that modify previous concepts and that may lead to new progress in this field.

2. Mechanism of Action

2.1. Biological Effects of Alkylating Agents and Nitrosoureas

The alkylating agents and nitrosoureas are important because of their ability to destroy neoplastic tissue, but their specificity for malignant cells is far from complete, and they exhibit a wide range of toxicities when administered to whole animals. These include bone marrow suppression, nausea and vomiting, alopecia, interference with spermatogenesis, and other less frequently encountered toxicities. These side effects appear to represent the increased cytotoxicity of these agents for rapidly proliferating tissue, and they can be explained in terms of an attack on DNA, as described below. In general, sensitivity to alkylating agents and nitrosoureas is related to the fraction of cells that are in an active phase of cell division, although some resting (G_0) cells may also be affected. Sections on cell kinetics in previous volumes of this work, and Chapter 2 of this volume, may be consulted for details of this process.

When alkylating agents and nitrosoureas are administered to the pregnant female at an early state of embryo development, there is frequently a teratogenic outcome. This biological effect is important for two reasons: it is an obvious consideration in the clinical use of these drugs, and it draws attention to the action of these agents on genetic material.

Studies at the unicellular level emphasize this action, since alkylating agents and nitrosoureas are mutagenic to a wide range of viruses and bacteria. The molecular biology in this area has been reviewed recently by several authors (Drake, 1970; Lawley, 1974; Loveless, 1966; Singer, 1975; Yanofsky *et al.*, 1966), and the particular DNA modifications that are most likely to be mutagenic are discussed in Section 5.3.

One other effect of these agents is important from both a practical and a theoretical point of view. Most alkylating agents and nitrosoureas have now been shown to be carcinogenic under appropriate test conditions (Fishbein *et al.*, 1970; WHO monograph, 1975). Clearly, this is a major concern when these agents are administered to patients with significant long-term survival. Again, in view of the somatic mutation theory of carcinogenesis, this action focuses attention on the genetic effects produced by these drugs.

2.2. *Chemistry of Alkylation*

Alkylating agents are either electrophiles or generate electrophiles *in vivo*, producing active species that may be carbonium ions or polarized molecules with positively charged regions. As electrophiles, these agents attack the electron-rich regions of nearly all cellular molecules, adding alkyl groups to oxygen, nitrogen, or sulfur atoms.

Because these compounds have an active role in modifying DNA, it is perhaps natural to view them as electrophilic agents that attack other molecules. However, it is the electrons in the electron-rich regions of the cellular molecules that shift to form chemical bonds. Substitution reactions are therefore frequently considered from the reverse point of view, and we speak of the alkylating agents themselves as undergoing nucleophilic attack by cellular molecules.

From this point of view, a distinction has been drawn between S_N1 and S_N2 reactions. In the former, substitution takes place in two steps: a relatively slow, rate-limiting generation of a carbonium ion, and a relatively rapid attack on this carbonium ion by a nucleophilic site. In the sequence of reactions 1a and b below, this nucleophilic site is represented by the anion, Z^-:

$$RX \rightarrow R^+ + :\ddot{X}:^- \quad \text{(slow)} \tag{1a}$$

$$:\ddot{Z}:^- + R^+ \rightarrow RZ \quad \text{(fast)} \tag{1b}$$

S_N2 reactions, on the other hand, involve a simultaneous attack by the nucleophile, Z^-, on the alkylating agent, RX, with the departure of the leaving group, X^-. This is shown in reaction 2:

$$:\ddot{Z}:^- + RX \rightarrow RZ + :\ddot{X}:^- \tag{2}$$

The terminology for the S_N1 and S_N2 reactions was developed from the fact that the first type of nucleophilic substitution followed first-order kinetics, with the rate depending solely on the concentration of alkylating agent, while the second type followed second-order kinetics, with dependence on both the alkylating agent and nucleophile concentrations. The situation is usually more complex than this simple representation would imply, but the distinction is still useful, because the nucleophilic sites that are substituted seem to depend somewhat on the tendency of the alkylating agent to undergo an S_N1 type of reaction. Thus, agents that follow an S_N1 type of reaction tend to substitute 0 atoms in DNA and to esterify the phosphate groups in the sugarphosphate backbone (Lawley, 1972, 1974; Lawley *et al.*, 1971–1972; Kuśmierek and Singer, 1976*b*). It is important to note in this regard that the nitrosoureas may tend more toward the S_N1 mechanism.

A further point, which will be emphasized in Section 3, is that the alkylating agent is often converted *in vivo* into an entirely different species that is involved in the actual alkylation step.

2.3. DNA as the Primary Target of Alkylation

Clearly, there are many nucleophilic sites in a living cell, and alkylating agents have been shown to react with a wide range of cellular components. Thus, cellular proteins and nucleic acids are alkylated, as well as most of the low-molecular-weight compounds. A major question, therefore, is which of these many reactions is instrumental in causing the cytotoxic action of the alkylating agents.

Many lines of evidence support the hypothesis that DNA is the primary target of alkylation. That alkylating agents are mutagenic, teratogenic, and carcinogenic, as well as cytotoxic, certainly directs attention to the genetic material. Furthermore, DNA is unique and essential for replication. A cell may have many duplicates of low-molecular-weight compounds, but there is usually only one copy of the basic genetic material. Aside from these general considerations, however, there is also some direct evidence that DNA is the most sensitive target of alkylation.

Several investigators have looked at the response of various cellular processes to gradually increasing concentrations of alkylating agents. Although most metabolic processes are affected at high enough concentrations, DNA synthesis is usually affected first. Wheeler and Alexander (1969) have summarized much of this information.

Other lines of evidence also point to a primary action on DNA. In some bacteriophage systems, there is a fairly close relationship between the number of DNA lesions and lethality (Loveless, 1966; Verly and Brakier, 1969; Brakier and Verly, 1970). There is also evidence that cells that can repair lesions in DNA are less sensitive to the effects of alkylating agents. Thus, the hypothesis that DNA is the primary target of alkylation is widely accepted, and much of the recent work in this field has been concerned with the action of these agents on DNA. This chapter will therefore deal primarily with this hypothesis. The possibility that other reactions are also important should always be kept in mind, however.

3. Formation of the Alkylating Species

3.1. General

Identification of the actual alkylating species is important in understanding the distribution and delivery of the cytotoxic agent, and in determining the nature of the DNA lesion that it produces. Some modifications are relatively simple; for example, nitrogen mustards undergo a spontaneous cyclization in aqueous solutions to form aziridinium ions:

$$\begin{array}{c} R_1 \\ \diagdown \\ N-CH_2CH_2Cl \\ \diagup \\ R_2 \end{array} \rightarrow \begin{array}{c} R_1 \quad CH_2^+ \\ \diagdown \diagup \\ N \\ \diagup \diagdown \\ R_2 \quad CH_2 \end{array} + Cl^- \qquad (3)$$

The rate at which this cyclization occurs depends on the nature of R_1 and R_2. In the special case where R_1 and R_2 are both ethyl groups, Price $et\ al.$ (1969) used nuclear magnetic resonance measurements to show that cyclization is rapid, and that the product is quite stable. Nucleophilic attack under these circumstances is still second-order, with a dependence on both the alkylating agent and nucleophile concentrations. When cyclization is the rate-limiting step, however, the kinetics may become first-order. Since this does not imply any real change in the step involving nucleophilic attack, this situation is different from that of a classic S_N1 reaction. That is, preliminary steps that generate the alkylating species do not affect the sites of alkylation.

Colvin $et\ al.$ (1976b) used deuterium-labeled compounds to show that alkylation proceeds through the cyclic aziridinium form. They synthesized nornitrogen mustard and cyclophosphamide mustard with deuterium atoms on the β (chlorine-substituted) carbon. Alkylation by direct displacement of the chlorine atom would leave the deuterium-labeled carbon attached to the nucleophile, whereas the other carbon would be attached just as often if alkylation occurred through the cyclized form. In fact, it was found that the nucleophile attacked the two carbons equally, indicating that alkylation proceeds through the aziridinium ion.

In many cases, alkylating agents undergo complicated spontaneous or enzymatic alterations that generate the active alkylating species. Transformations of cyclophosphamide and the nitrosoureas are considered in the following sections.

3.2. Cyclophosphamide

As administered in its unmetabolized form, cyclophosphamide has no activity as an alkylating agent. Although it was originally thought that the compound might be selectively activated by phosphoramidases in tumor tissue, it was soon discovered that metabolism occurs in the liver (Brock and Hohorst, 1963; Cohen and Jao, 1970). A scheme for this metabolism is shown in Fig. 2.

Cyclophosphamide (I), shown in the upper left of the figure, is excreted in the urine primarily as the oxidized product, 2-carboxyethyl-*N,N-bis* (2-chloroethyl)phosphorodiamidate or carboxyphosphamide (V) (Struck *et al.*, 1971). 4-Ketocyclophosphamide (III) has also been identified by the same workers. Since neither of these metabolites has much cytotoxicity, it must be assumed that an intermediate compound produces the sought-for effect.

The hepatic mixed-function oxidases apparently produce 4-hydroxycyclophosphamide (II) as the initial oxidation product (Hill *et al.*, 1972), although this compound has not been identified *in vivo*. 4-Hydroxycyclophosphamide and its ring-opened tautomer, aldophosphamide (IV), with which it would be in equilibrium, are both cytotoxic. They decompose spontaneously to generate acrolein, first identified by Alarcon and Meienhofer (1971), and phosphoramide mustard (VII), identified as a product of microsomal metabolism by Colvin *et al.* (1973). Phosphoramide mustard is cytotoxic, and breaks down to produce another cytotoxic compound, nornitrogen mustard (VIII). However, nornitrogen mustard is considerably less cytotoxic than phosphoramide mustard, perhaps because its lower pK inhibits aziridinium ion formation. Present evidence would therefore support the hypothesis that phosphoramide mustard is the active species (Colvin *et al.*, 1976*b*).

Thus, we have a situation in which cyclophosphamide is activated by the liver to produce a circulating intermediate that may be 4-hydroxycyclophosphamide. From this, the final alkylating species, most probably phosphoramide mustard, is generated intracellularly.

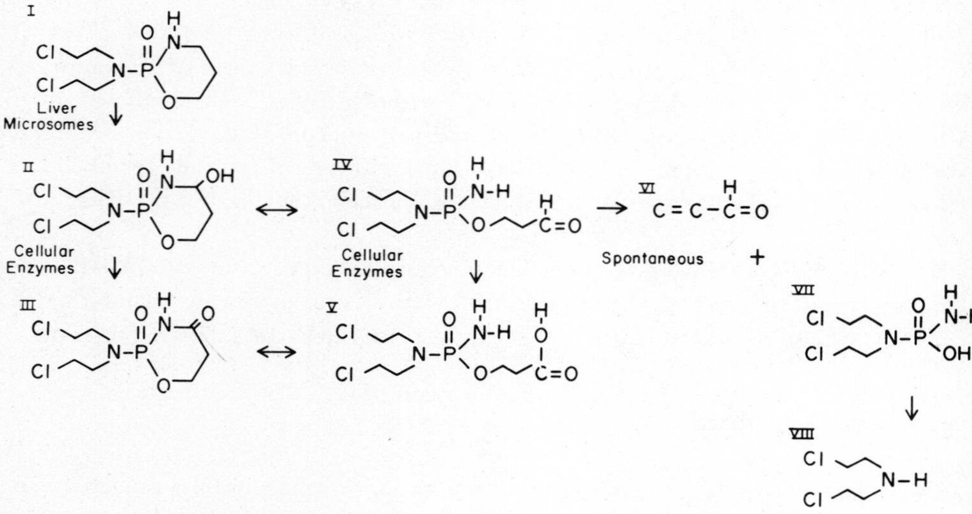

FIGURE 2. Metabolic transformation and decomposition of cyclophosphamide (I). Hydroxycyclophosphamide (II), aldophosphamide (IV), and phosphoramide mustard (VII) are cytotoxic in *in vitro* assays. Cyclophosphamide itself, ketocyclophosphamide (III), and carboxyphosphamide (V) have little or no *in vitro* activity.

Connors *et al.* (1974) and Connors (1975*a*) used this scheme to explain why cyclophosphamide has a relatively higher toxicity for tumor than normal tissue. They suggest that normal tissue detoxifies the circulating species enzymatically to ketocyclophosphamide and carboxyphosphamide, but that tumor tissue may be relatively deficient in these enzymes. Spontaneous decomposition of 4-hydroxy-cyclophosphamide to phosphoramide mustard in the tumor would then lead to a cytotoxic outcome. This scheme also suggests a mechanism for the development of tumor resistance, since tumors could become resistant by developing higher levels of detoxifying enzymes.

3.3. Nitrosoureas

The nitrosoureas undergo rapid spontaneous decomposition in aqueous solution at a rate that is affected by the buffer, pH, and temperature. Loo *et al.* (1966) found that the half-life of BCNU was approximately 15 min in plasma at 37°C. As pointed out by Garrett *et al.* (1965), this decomposition leads to the formation of an isocyanate that can carbamoylate cellular proteins, the possible importance of which will be discussed later.

Wheeler and Chumley (1967) showed that the nitrosoureas generate an alkylating species, as demonstrated by a positive reaction with nitrobenzylpyridine. Montgomery *et al.* (1967) studied several nitrosoureas and found some variations in the mode of decomposition. They suggested that BCNU produced primarily vinyl carbonium ions, while *bis* fluoroethyl nitrosourea (BFNU) produced fluoroethyl carbonium ions. This difference in products was attributed to the greater stability of the carbon–fluorine bond.

More recently, we have reexamined this decomposition in a search for the origin of several unusual nucleotide derivatives, which are described in Section 5. Our results (Colvin *et al.*, 1974, 1976*a*) suggest that the major mode of decomposition of both BCNU and BFNU at neutral pH results in the generation of a haloethyl carbonium ion.

At the same time, Reed and his co-workers (Reed and May, 1975; Reed *et al.*, 1975; May *et al.*, 1975) made a careful and detailed study of the decomposition of CCNU and methyl-CCNU. Their data show that both these nitrosoureas generate chloroethyl carbonium ions at neutral pH. These investigators have also shown that the hepatic drug-metabolizing system hydroxylates the cyclohexyl ring of CCNU to produce a mixture of 3- and 4-hydroxycyclohexyl derivatives.

Montgomery *et al.* (1975) reexamined the decomposition of BCNU, CCNU, BFNU, and several other nitrosoureas in a variety of aqueous and mixed solvents. Their data show a marked dependence of the spectrum of decomposition products on pH. At low pH, BCNU generates considerable acetaldehyde and relatively little chloroethanol, a set of products that could be explained by decomposition to a vinyl carbonium ion. At neutral pH, however, more chloroethanol is formed, which would suggest a chloroethyl carbonium ion intermediate. BFNU seems to decompose to the fluoroethyl carbonium ion at all pHs.

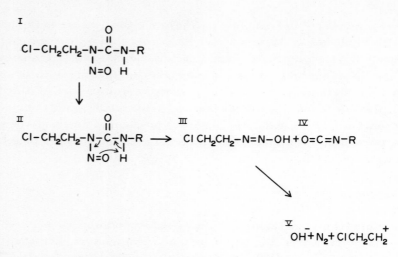

FIGURE 3. Spontaneous decomposition of a 3-substituted 1-chloroethyl-1-nitrosourea. The chloroethyl carbonium ion (V) is believed to be the active alkylating species.

Thus, at neutral pH, all the data would seem to support the decomposition scheme shown in Fig. 3, although it would be hard to rule out some decomposition by another route. This scheme, with the generation of chloroethyl carbonium ions, would explain the finding of the nucleotide derivatives described in Section 5.1.

4. Distribution and Cellular Uptake of Agents

It is apparent from the information presented above that many of the alkylating agents and their metabolites are charged, and are consequently not very permeable to the usual biological membranes. However, the nitrosoureas are much more lipid-soluble, and are able to cross cellular membranes including the blood–brain barrier with ease (Schabel *et al.*, 1963). This property has led to their use in the treatment of CNS tumors, as will be discussed in Section 6.

The ability of compounds to penetrate biological membranes frequently parallels their octanol/water coefficients. Hansch *et al.* (1972) published these values for a variety of nitrosoureas. More recently, Wheeler *et al.* (1974) studied the effect of this parameter, as well as that of alkylating and carbamoylating activity, on the effectiveness of the nitrosoureas against intraperitoneally injected mouse L1210 cells.

Their data clearly demonstrate the importance of lipid solubility. Whole-animal toxicity increased with increasing octanol/water distribution coefficient, and correlated closely with this parameter alone. When therapeutic ratio was considered, it was found that the most effective compounds had high octanol/water distribution coefficients. Thus, the ability of the agent to get to the target tissue was of primary importance. Since toxicity was associated with high carbamoylating activity, optimal therapeutic properties were found in compounds with high lipid solubility, high alkylating activity, and low carbamoylating activity. This finding would, of course, be consistent with the hypothesis that DNA alkylation is important for the nitrosoureas, as well as for the alkylating agents.

Although the nitrosoureas probably penetrate cells by passive diffusion, there is considerable evidence that the classic mustards are transported across cellular membranes by a carrier mechanism. Goldenberg and his colleagues have published a series of papers on the transport of nitrogen mustard itself (Goldenberg *et al.*, 1970, 1971; Lyons and Goldenberg, 1972; Goldenberg, 1975), and of cyclophosphamide (Goldenberg *et al.*, 1974).

These investigators have found that nitrogen mustard is transported into L5178Y cells by a mechanism that is saturable and that can be blocked completely by the hydrolysis product of nitrogen mustard, *bis* hydroxyethyl methyl amine. Interestingly enough, the system that transports nitrogen mustard is apparently the same as the one that transports choline in these cells, so that uptake can also be blocked by choline and hemicholinium. Other alkylating agents, including chlorambucil, melphalan, and cyclophosphamide, do not block uptake of nitrogen mustard, however, so it is apparent that different agents are transported differently.

Cyclophosphamide is transported by two separate carrier systems, only one of which is saturable at low doses. Transport is not inhibited by other alkylating agents, choline, or any other naturally occurring substance that was tested. Both systems demonstrated a temperature and sodium ion dependence that would suggest that they were carrier-mediated.

Thus, it appears that the cellular uptake of alkylating agents is very complex. Differences between normal and tumor cells, if they are found, could be exploited to improve therapeutic indices. On the other hand, loss of carrier mechanisms can lead to the development of tumor resistance.

5. Modifications of DNA

5.1. Sites of Reaction

If we accept the hypothesis that an attack on DNA is basic to the action of the alkylating agents and nitrosoureas, then a first step in understanding these agents is determining what changes actually occur. Particular modifications may render the DNA inactive, alter the informational content of the macromolecule, or lead to further spontaneous or enzyme-mediated structural changes.

The various types of reactions that are known to occur with DNA are shown in Table 1. Primary substitution occurs on the nucleic acid bases and phosphate groups. Since all the clinically useful alkylating agents are bifunctional, the initial substitution reaction attaches to the DNA a group that can react further. Similarly, substitution by a haloethyl carbonium ion from a nitrosourea also attaches a highly

TABLE 1
Reactions of Alkylating Agents with DNA

1. Substitution reactions
   a. Alkylation of bases
   b. Esterification of phosphate groups
2. Cross-linking reactions
   a. Intrastrand cross-linking reactions
   b. Interstrand cross-linking reactions
3. Strand-breaking reactions
   a. Single-strand breaks
   b. Double-strand breaks

reactive group. The secondary reactions that follow can lead to either inter- or intrastrand cross-links.

On the other hand, certain substitutions lead to single- or double-strand chain scissions. These scissions can be either spontaneous, as in the case of phosphate esterification, or the result of enzymatic action, as in the case of base substitution.

Viewing DNA as a whole, one might expect that the phosphate groups would be particularly active nucleophiles. They are negatively charged and uniformly distributed along the DNA helix in an unhindered location. Nevertheless, there has been considerable difficulty in obtaining convincing evidence that phosphates are, in fact, alkylated.

Lett *et al.* (1962) published light-scattering and viscosity data that indicated that internucleotide phosphates in DNA were alkylated by esters of methanesulfonic acid, but their data were hard to interpret because of the high molecular weight of the DNA that was used. Later, taking advantage of the fact that precise light-scattering data can be obtained on synthetic polyribonucleotides, we showed that reaction with nitrogen mustard and ethylmethanesulfonate led to chain scission (Ludlum, 1967, 1969). This change in molecular weight occurred when there was little or no detectable base alkylation. Thus, we concluded that chain scission was evidence for attack on the phosphate groups with subsequent breakdown of phosphotriesters.

Rhaese and Freese (1969) studied the reaction of dideoxynucleotides with ethyl methanesulfonate and methyl methanesulfonate, separating the reaction products by column chromatography. In this way, they demonstrated the formation of new compounds that evidently arose from alkylation of phosphate groups. Finally, Bannon and Verly (1972) published convincing evidence for phosphate esterification in DNA with ethyl methanesulfonate, and less, but still significant, esterification with methyl methanesulfonate. Their experiments utilized radiolabeled alkylating agents, and showed clearly that the residual radioactivity remaining in DNA after the alkylated bases were removed was attached to phosphate groups. Other investigators have shown that phosphate alkylation occurs with methyl nitrosourea (Lawley, 1973); with ethyl methanesulfonate, isopropyl methanesulfonate, and ethyl nitrosourea (Shooter *et al.*, 1974); with ethyl methanesulfonate, dimethyl sulfate, and ethyl nitrosourea (Singer and

Fraenkel-Conrat, 1975); and *in vivo* with dimethylnitrosamine (O'Connor *et al.*, 1975).

The significance of phosphate alkylation still remains to be determined. If it leads to chain scission, as it did in our work, one can expect significant effects, including cytotoxicity and antitumor activity. Alterations in base structure are cytotoxic if they interfere with the proper function of DNA, as cross-links undoubtedly do, and are probably even more important than phosphate alkylations in causing mutagenesis and carcinogenesis.

The sites of primary base alkylation are shown in Fig. 4. Classic alkylating agents attack the 7 position of guanosine selectively, and this frequently accounts for 90% or more of the total base substitution. Considerable attention is now being paid to reactions at other positions, and it appears that all the nitrogens and oxygens can be substituted under certain conditions. Much of this work has been done with model alkylating agents, e.g., dimethyl sulfate, diethyl sulfate, methyl methanesulfonate, or ethyl methanesulfonate. Similarly, methyl nitrosourea and ethyl nitrosourea, simple nitrosoureas that were chosen because of their importance in chemical carcinogenesis, have been studied almost exclusively. It is not certain how these data relate to the sites of attack by the more complicated agents in clinical use, but they certainly indicate where reaction can occur. Surprisingly few of the nucleoside derivatives that result from reaction of clinically useful agents have been studied. However, we can expect to see further advances in this area as more sophisticated methods of structure determination, especially mass spectroscopy, are applied to this problem.

Intensive efforts by Brookes and Lawley (1961), Lawley and Brookes (1963), Lawley (1966), and other investigators established that substitution of the 7 position of guanosine was the major reaction for most alkylating agents in neutral aqueous solution. The 1 position of guanosine, the 1, 3, and 7 positions of adenosine, and the 3 position of cytosine were also identified as reactive sites.

More recently, considerable attention has been focused on minor products of alkylation. Much of this work has been initiated by investigators primarily interested in mutagenesis and carcinogenesis, but the results are relevant to antitumor therapy for two reasons. First, any alteration in DNA structure may be

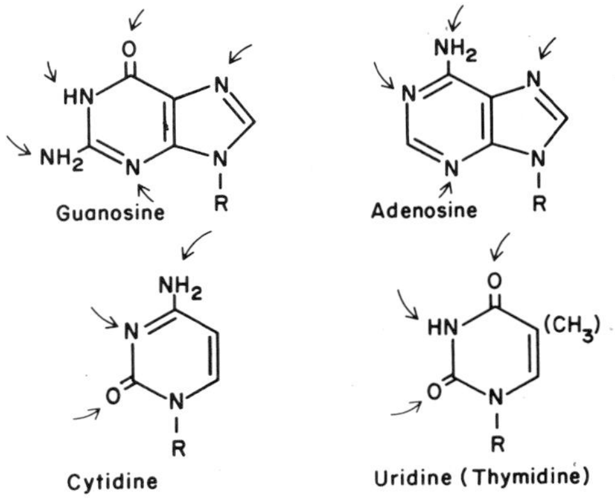

FIGURE 4. Sites on nucleic acid bases that are subject to initial attack by alkylating agents. These sites vary greatly in reactivity, depending on the agent and nature of the nucleic acid. Although the 7 position of guanosine is by far the most reactive under most conditions, other sites may be of equal biological importance.

important in causing cytotoxicity, and second, carcinogenesis is a possible side effect that must be considered in the treatment of cancer.

Loveless (1969) gave a major impetus to this area by calling attention to the possible importance of the reaction of nitrosamines and nitrosamides with the O–6 position of guanosine. Lawley $et\ al.$ (1971–1972, 1973) then described alkylation at the N-3 position of guanosine and the O–4 position of thymidine. Singer, in an intensive series of investigations, has described reaction at the O–2 position of cytidine (Singer, 1976); the O–2, N-3, O–4, $2'$–O and phosphate groups of uridylic acid in poly U (Kuśmierek and Singer, 1976b); the $2'$–O position of all ribonucleotides of TMV RNA (Singer and Kuśmierek, 1976); and, finally, all nucleotide oxygens in TMV RNA and M 13 DNA (Singer, private communication).

Thus, there is evidence for reaction of model compounds with all the nucleophilic sites of nucleic acids. It is becoming increasingly evident that different agents may produce somewhat different spectra of minor alkylation products (Singer and Fraenkel-Conrat, 1969, 1975; Lawley and Thatcher, 1970). For example, methylating agents react differently from ethylating agents, and $S_N 2$ agents in general react differently from $S_N 1$ agents. It will be important to determine whether different agents in clinical use, particularly those with somewhat different properties, react differently.

Lawley and Brookes (1963) have shown that the secondary structure of DNA influences the sites of alkylation. Ludlum (1965) and others have shown that this influence is very marked indeed in studies on polynucleotides that form helical structures. Changes in secondary structure that occur during replication of DNA may well explain the increased sensitivity of dividing cells to alkylation (Ludlum, 1965; Cerdá-Olmeda $et\ al.$, 1968); enhancement of this difference could increase the effectiveness of these agents.

The sites of attack mentioned above represent the initial points of substitution by the alkylating agents. Bifunctional agents are then free to react a second time with a nucleoprotein or another nucleoside. Interstrand links can be formed between the two strands in a helical DNA, or intrastrand links can be formed within a single strand of DNA. Lawley and Brookes (1963) have identified derivatives consisting of two guanines linked by the residue of an alkylating agent in DNA hydrolysates, suggesting that most of the cross-links are between neighboring guanines.

Some similarities and differences are beginning to appear between classic alkylating agents and nitrosoureas in their interaction with DNA. The alkylating activities of nitrosoureas were noted by Wheeler and Chumley (1967). Cheng $et\ al.$ (1972) reported that a radioactive label in the chloroethyl group of CCNU was bound to DNA, RNA, and synthetic polyribonucleotides. BCNU was also found to react with synthetic polynucleotides (Kramer $et\ al.$, 1974; Ludlum $et\ al.$, 1975), and hydrolysates of these polymers were used to identify modified nucleosides.

Cytidine and guanosine were the most reactive nucleosides under the conditions studied, and two derivatives of cytidine and one of guanosine were isolated. The structure of these derivatives has been rigorously established by a combina-

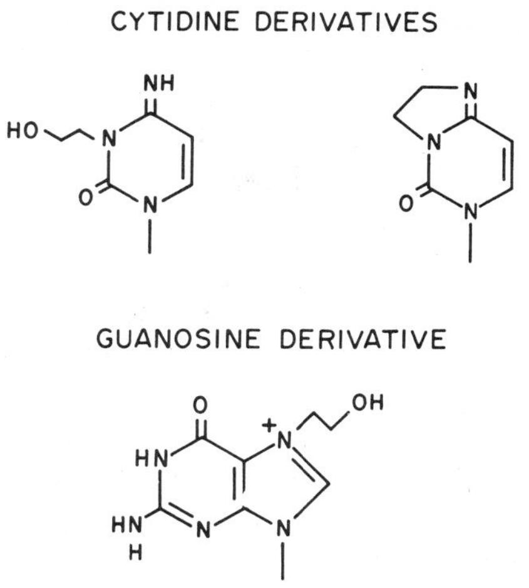

CYTIDINE DERIVATIVES

GUANOSINE DERIVATIVE

FIGURE 5. Nucleoside derivatives that are formed when synthetic polynucleotides are reacted with BCNU.

tion of chemical, ultraviolet, and mass spectral data (Kramer *et al.*, 1974; Ludlum *et al.*, 1975). These structures are shown in Fig. 5.

The identity of these derivatives stimulated our investigation of the aqueous decomposition of BCNU mentioned above, and it appears that they arise from attack by a chloroethyl carbonium ion on the *N*-3 position of cytidine or the *N*-7 position of guanosine. In the first cytidine derivative and the guanosine derivative, the chlorine has evidently been hydrolyzed, but in the cyclic 3,*N*-4 ethanocytidine, an intramolecular condensation has occurred. This, in a way, represents the simplest possible intrastrand cross-link. Ewig and Kohn (1976) now have evidence for interstrand cross-linking reactions. Thus, although the details of substitution are entirely different, it appears that there are elements of similarity with the classic alkylating agents at a molecular level.

5.2. Amplification and Repair of Damage

Many of the lesions in DNA that are described above are known to be modified further by chemical or enzymatic action. The occurrence of secondary cross-linking reactions following attack by a bifunctional agent and of chain scission following phosphate esterification have already been mentioned. Spontaneous chemical change can also result in the loss of alkylated purines (Lawley *et al.*, 1969; Brakier and Verly, 1970; Lindahl and Nyberg, 1972) and pyrimidines (Lindahl and Karlström, 1973). Of the various substituted bases, *N*-3 alkyl adenines and *N*-7 alkyl guanines are lost especially rapidly.

There is good evidence that some purines are removed by enzymatic action as well. Strauss *et al.* (1969) described the degradation of methylated DNA by an enzyme system that seemed to attack some, but not all, methylated sites. Endonuclease II has been purified from *E. coli* and found to degrade alkylated and depurinated DNA (Friedberg and Goldthwait, 1969; Hadi and Goldthwait, 1971). Some lesions evidently lead to more rapid degradation than others; for example, Papirmeister *et al.* (1970) found that the DNA of T_1 bacteriophage was sensitized to attack by adenine alkylation, rather than the more prevalent guanine alkylation. 3-Methyl adenine and O–6-methyl guanine are released more readily than 7-methyl guanine by intact *E. coli* (Lawley and Orr, 1970) and by purified Endonuclease II (Kirtikar and Goldthwait, 1974).

Since apurinic DNA is also a substrate for endonuclease attack, it becomes somewhat difficult to separate spontaneous loss of an alkylated base followed by endonuclease action from a combined enzymatic depurination and degradation by two enzymes or two activities in one enzyme. In any case, once alkylated purines are released, the apurinic DNA is subject to attack by other enzymes. Thus, Verly and Paquette (1972) described an endonuclease from *E. coli* that degrades DNA at apurinic sites. This enzyme was purified (Paquette *et al.*, 1972) and found to be specific for these sites, having no activity toward normal or alkylated DNA.

The action of these enzymes may amplify the original damage to DNA or be the initial step in repairing the damage. DNA repair is a rapidly developing field, with at least one mechanism, the excision-repair process, well established. Other major references (Altmann and Schattauer, 1972; Hanawalt and Setlow, 1975) should be consulted for details of the repair mechanisms.

The point to be emphasized here is that repair is an important process that could explain the development of resistance, for example. Once the most significant lesions in DNA are identified, and the activities that magnify or repair them are understood, we will be much closer to explaining the biological effects of alkylation on a chemical basis.

Finally, it should be noted that the possibility of repair would explain why cells that have just completed the S phase of the cell cycle are less sensitive to alkylation that those in G_1 or S. If DNA replication has occurred, the cell can presumably proceed to G_2 or M. Damage to DNA that occurs during G_2 or M could be repaired before the next synthetic phase.

5.3. Significance of DNA Modifications

According to the hypothesis adopted here, alkylating agents and nitrosoureas produce their cytotoxicity and antitumor effect by damaging cellular DNA. Ultimately, this damage must be expressed as interference with replication or transcription, or both. A fragmented template would probably lead to an inactive product during replication or transcription, while a cross-link might block these processes altogether. It is somewhat less clear, however, how a slightly damaged DNA—e.g., one with a single modified base— would function. Such a lesion could be cytotoxic if it interfered with the production of a key substance, or if it resulted in a malfunctioning product.

The information imparted by a modified base can be determined with synthetic polynucleotide templates in the systems shown in Table 2. For each of these systems, information from the template at the left is used to produce the product strand at the right. A template that contains a single modified base can be compared with an unmodified template to determine the effect of that particular modification.

TABLE 2
Systems for Testing the Effects of Base Modifications

Process	Enzyme or system
DNA → DNA	DNA polymerase
DNA → RNA	RNA polymerase
RNA → RNA	RNA polymerase
RNA → protein	Cell extract

The author suggested this approach, and has used it with his colleagues to study several base modifications. The first studies of this kind used synthetic messenger RNA to produce a polypeptide product. 7-Methylguanine was introduced into a messenger strand by direct alkylation, and amino acid incorporation was sought that would correspond to a misreading of 7-methylguanine as adenine (Wilhelm and Ludlum, 1966). No such misincorporation was found, although the total level of incorporation was diminished, perhaps because of decreased binding of the modified template to the ribosomes.

Much more effort has been expended on a system that uses RNA polymerase of bacterial origin to copy an RNA template. Although this is a somewhat artificial system, it seems probable that the same base-pairing properties will be revealed between two RNA strands as between two DNA strands, or between one DNA and one RNA strand.

Using this system, we have shown that 7-methylguanine still base-pairs like guanine, making it somewhat unlikely that this lesion is cytotoxic or mutagenic without further modification (Ludlum, 1970a). However, the presence of 3-methylcytidine (Ludlum and Wilhelm, 1968; Ludlum, 1970b; Singer and Fraenkel-Conrat, 1969, 1970) or of O–6 methylguanine (Gerchman and Ludlum, 1973) leads to extensive misincorporation. Both these lesions interfere with base-pairing positions in the nucleosides, and may prove to be particularly significant from a biological standpoint. Clearly, more work needs to be done in this area to determine the effect of other lesions, especially those produced by clinical agents.

6. Role of Alkylating Agents and Nitrosoureas in Chemotherapy

The clinical applications of alkylating agents and nitrosoureas will be summarized briefly in this section, noting the range of diseases to which they have been applied and some of the differences that have been observed among them. Differences are of potential importance in that they may lead the way to a better understanding of the various agents, and to subsequent improvements in their properties.

Alkylating agents and nitrosoureas have been tested against a variety of malignancies, and remain primary choices for the treatment of several of them, either alone or in combination with other drugs. Cyclophosphamide, chlorambucil, and nitrogen mustard are all effective against Hodgkin's disease; nitrogen mustard is, in fact, the "M" in the well-known MOPP regimen [Mustargen (nitrogen mustard), Oncovin (viscristine), procarbazine, and prednisone]. The nitrosoureas, especially BCNU, have also been used effectively against this disease.

Cyclophosphamide is used in combinations for the treatment of acute lymphocytic leukemia and acute myelocytic leukemia. Busulfan is particularly effective in chronic myelocytic leukemia, and chlorambucil is widely used in chronic lymphocytic leukemia. Cyclophosphamide and phenylalanine mustard, as well as the nitrosoureas, are effective against multiple myeloma.

Cross-resistance may develop among the different alkylating agents, but its development is not absolute, and multiple myeloma frequently responds to high-dose cyclophosphamide when it fails to respond to phenylalanine mustard (Bergsagel *et al.*, 1972). Several groups have also noted that Hodgkin's disease may respond to a nitrosourea after resistance has developed to an alkylating agent.

Cyclophosphamide is the first choice, and is a surprisingly effective drug, for the treatment of Burkitt's lymphoma. Results with intermittent high doses are superior to those obtained with more continuous administration. Again, Burkitt's lymphoma has also responded to BCNU.

Several solid tumors may be treated with the alkylating agents, and some success has evidently been achieved in treating micrometastases from breast cancer with phenylalanine mustard (Fisher *et al.*, 1975) and with a multiple-drug regimen that includes cyclophosphamide (Bonadonna *et al.*, 1976).

Bronchogenic carcinoma has responded somewhat to treatment with alkylating agents. Interestingly enough, it has been reported that squamous-cell carcinoma responds better to nitrogen mustard than to cyclophosphamide, while undifferentiated carcinoma responds better to cyclophosphamide, again suggesting some differences in these agents (Green *et al.*, 1969). Other solid tumors frequently show some response to the alkylating agents, particularly cyclophosphamide.

Nitrosoureas are especially effective in the treatment of CNS tumors (Walker, 1973), presumably because they pass the blood–brain barrier, while classic alkylating agents do not. A naturally occurring nitrosourea, streptozotocin, has been used effectively against malignant insulinomas, in which it is superior to other agents. Again, this probably represents a distribution phenomenon, with concentration of this agent in these cells.

Both the alkylating agents and the nitrosoureas usually exhibit bone marrow depression as a limiting clinical toxicity. There is an interesting difference in the time relationships between drug administration and minimum white count, however. This minimum is usually reached in about a week with the classic alkylating agents, whereas it may take 3 or 4 weeks with the nitrosoureas. It is possible that part of this delayed toxicity is related to the carbamoylating activity of the nitrosoureas.

There are other important clinical toxicities, of which nausea and vomiting are probably the most general. There are also some specific toxicities that probably reflect differences in drug distribution; for example, cyclophosphamide causes alopecia and hemorrhagic cystitis. The latter may be a serious immediate clinical problem. Furthermore, to make the theoretical relationship between the alkylating carcinogens and antineoplastic agents more significant, there have been some reports of bladder tumors associated with cyclophosphamide therapy (Wall and Clausen, 1975).

7. Summary

The literature on alkylating agents and nitrosoureas is very extensive, partly because of their wide range of clinical applications and partly because of their basic scientific interest. It is tempting to try to pull the maximum number of these observations together in some theoretical framework, and we have done this here by focusing on DNA as the primary target for both the alkylating agents and the nitrosoureas.

There are differences in the actions of these agents, but there are also differences in their metabolism and distribution, and in their reaction with DNA. Furthermore, cellular enzymes can magnify or repair some of the lesions in DNA. Thus, it would seem that there is enough flexibility in this model to explain most of the diverse biological effects of the alkylating agents and nitrosoureas. Further correlations will necessarily depend on a deeper understanding of the DNA modifications produced under various treatment conditions. As this information develops, it seems likely that these agents can be made even more effective.

ACKNOWLEDGMENT

This work was supported by Grants No. CA 20129 and No. CA 20292 from the National Cancer Institute, Department of Health, Education and Welfare.

8. References

ALARCON, R. A., AND MEIENHOFER, J., 1971, Formation of the cytotoxic aldehyde acrolein during the *in vitro* degradation of cyclophosphamide, *Nature (London) New Biol.* **233**:250.

ALTMANN, H., AND SCHATTAUER, F., (eds.), 1972, *DNA Repair Mechanisms*, Schattauer, Stuttgart–New York.

BANNON, P., AND VERLY, W., 1972, Alkylation of phosphates and stability of phosphate triesters in DNA, *Eur. J. Biochem.* **31**:103.

BERGSAGEL, D. E., COWAN, D. H., AND HASSELBACK, R., 1972, Plasma cell myeloma: Response of melphalan-resistant patients to high-dose intermittent cyclophosphamide, *Can. Med. Assoc. J.* **107**:851.

BONADONNA, G., BRUSAMOLINO, E., VALAGUSSA, P., ROSSI, A., BRUGNATELLI, L., BRAMBILLA, DELENA, M., TANCINI, G., BAJETTA, E., MUSUMECI, R., AND VERONESI, U., 1976, Combination chemotherapy as an adjuvant treatment in operable breast cancer, *N. Engl. J. Med.* **294**:405.

BRAKIER, L., AND VERLY, W. G., 1970, The lethal action of ethyl methanesulfonate, nitrogen mustard, and Myleran on the T₇ coliphage, *Biochim. Biophys. Acta* **213**:296.

BROCK, N., AND HOHORST, N. J., 1963, Über die Aktivierung von Cyclophosphamid *in vivo* und *in vitro*, *Arzneim.-Forsch.* **13**:1021.

BROOKES, P., AND LAWLEY, P. D., 1961, The reaction of mono- and difunctional alkylating agents with nucleic acids, *Biochem. J.* **80**:495.

CERDÁ-OLMEDA, E., HANAWALT, P. C., AND GUEROLA, N., 1968, Mutagenesis of the replication point by nitrosoguanidine: Map and patterns of replication of the *Escherichia coli* chromosome, J. Mol. Biol. **33**:705.

CHENG, C. J., FUJIMURA, S, GRUNBERGER, D., AND WEINSTEIN, I. B., 1972, Interaction of 1-(2-chloroethyl)-3-cyclohexyl-1-nitrosourea (NSC 79037) with nucleic acids and proteins *in vivo* and *in vitro*, *Cancer Res.* **32**:22.

COHEN, J. L., AND JAO, J. Y., 1970, Enzymatic basis of cyclophosphamide activation by hepatic microsomes of the rat, *J. Pharmacol. Exp. Ther.* **174**:206.

COLVIN, M., PADGETT, C. A., AND FENSELAU, C., 1973, A biologically active metabolite of cyclophosphamide, *Cancer Res.* **33**:915.

COLVIN, M., COWENS, J. W., BRUNDRETT, R. B., KRAMER, B. S., AND LUDLUM, D. B., 1974, Decomposition of BCNU [1,3-*bis*(2-chloroethyl)-1-nitrosourea] in aqueous solution, *Biochem. Biophys. Res. Commun.* **60**:515.

COLVIN, M., BRUNDRETT, R. B., COWENS, W., JARDINE, I., AND LUDLUM, D. B., 1976a, A chemical basis for the antitumor activity of chloroethylnitrosoureas, *Biochem. Pharmacol.* **25**:695.

COLVIN, M., BRUNDRETT, R. B., KAN, M. N., JARDINE, I., AND FENSELAU, C., 1976b, Alkylating properties of phosphoramide mustard, *Cancer Res.* **36**:1121.

CONNORS, T. A., 1975a, Alkylating agents, *Top. Curr. Chem.* **52**:141.

CONNORS, T. A., 1975b, Mechanism of action of 2-chloroethylamine derivatives, sulfur mustards, epoxides, and aziridines, in: *Handbook of Experimental Pharmacology*, Vol. XXXVIII/2 (A. C. Sartorelli and D. G. Johns, eds.), pp. 18–34, Springer-Verlag, Berlin.

CONNORS, T. A., COX, P. J., FARMER, P. B., FOSTER, A. B., AND JARMAN, M., 1974, Some studies of the active intermediates formed in the microsomal metabolism of cyclophosphamide and isophosphamide, *Biochem. Pharmacol.* **23**:115.

DRAKE, J. W., 1970, *The Molecular Basis of Mutation*, Holden-Day, San Francisco.

EWIG, R. A. G., AND KOHN, K. W., 1976, Crosslinking of DNA in L1210 cells by *bis*-chloroethylnitrosourea (BCNU). Difference between BCNU and nitrogen mustard (HN₂), *Proc. Amer. Assoc. Cancer Res.* **17**:147.

FISHBEIN, L., FLAMM, W. G., AND FOLK, H. L., 1970, *Chemical Mutagens: Environmental Effects on Biological Systems*, Academic Press, New York.

FISHER, B., CARBONE, P., ECONOMOU, S. G., FRELICK, R., GLASS, A., LERNER, H., REDMOND, C., ZELEN, M. BAND, P., KATRYCH, D. L., WOLMARK, N., AND FISHER, E. R., 1975, L-Phenylalanine mustard in the management of primary breast cancer, *N. Engl. J. Med.* **292**:117.

FOX, B. W., 1975, Mechanism of action of methanesulfonates, in: *Handbook of Experimental Pharmacology*, Vol. XXVII/2 (A. C. Sartonelli and D. G. Johns, eds.), pp. 35–46, Springer-Verlag, Berlin.

FRIEDBERG, E. C., AND GOLDTHWAIT, D. A., 1969, Endonuclease II of *E. coli*, I. Isolation and purification, *Proc. Natl. Acad. Sci. U.S.A.* **62**:934.

GARRETT, E. R., GOTO, S., AND STUBBINS, J. F., 1965, Kinetics of solvolysis of various *N*-alkyl-*N*-nitrosoureas in neutral and alkaline solution, *J. Pharm. Sci.* **54**:119.

GERCHMAN, L. L., AND LUDLUM, D. B., 1973, The properties of *O*–6 methylguanine in templates for RNA polymerase, *Biochim. Biophys. Acta* **308**:310.

GILMAN, A., 1963, The initial clinical trial of nitrogen mustard, *Amer. J. Surg.* **105**:574.

GOLDENBERG, G. J., 1975, The role of drug transport in resistance to nitrogen mustard and other alkylating agents in L5178 Y lymphoblasts, *Cancer Res.* **35**:1687.

GOLDENBERG, G. J., VANSTONE, C. L., ISRAELS, L. G., ILSE, D., AND BIHLER, I., 1970, Evidence for a transport carrier of nitrogen mustard in nitrogen mustard-sensitive and -resistant L5178 Y lymphoblasts, *Cancer Res.* **30**:2285.

GOLDENBERG, G. J., LYONS, R. M., LEPP, J. A., AND VANSTONE, C. L., 1971, Sensitivity to nitrogen mustard as a function of transport activity and proliferative rate in L5178 Y lymphoblasts, *Cancer Res.* **31**:1616.

GOLDENBERG, G. J., LAND, H. B., AND CORMACK, D. V., 1974, Mechanism of cyclophosphamide transport by L5178 Y lymphoblasts *in vitro*, *Cancer Res.* **34**:3274.

GREEN, R. A., HUMPHREY, E., CLOSE, H., AND PATNO, M. E., 1969, Alkylating agents in bronchogenic carcinoma, *Amer. J. Med.* **46**:516.

HADI, S. M., AND GOLDTHWAIT, D. A., 1971, Endonuclease II of *Escherichia coli*. Degradation of partially depurinated deoxyribonucleic acid, *Biochemistry* **10**:4986.

HANAWALT, P. C., AND SETLOW, R. B. (eds.), 1975, *Molecular Mechanisms for Repair of DNA*, Plenum Press, New York.

HANSCH, C., SMITH, N., ENGLE, R., AND WOOD, H., 1972, Quantitative structure–activity relationships of antineoplastic drugs: Nitrosoureas and triazeno-imidazoles, *Cancer Chemother. Rep. Part 1* **56**:442.

HILL, D. L., LASTER, W. R., JR., AND STRUCK, R. F., 1972, Enzymatic metabolism of cyclophosphamide and nicotine and production of a toxic cyclophosphamide metabolite, *Cancer Res.* **32**:658.

JOHNSTON, T. P., McCALEB, G. S., AND MONTGOMERY, J. A., 1963, The synthesis of antineoplastic agents, XXXII. *N*-Nitrosoureas I, *J. Med. Chem.* **6**:669.

JOHNSTON, T. P., McCALEB, G. S., OPLIGER, P. S., AND MONTGOMERY, J. A., 1966, The synthesis of potential anticancer agents, XXXVI. *N*-Nitrosoureas II. Haloalkyl derivatives, *J. Med. Chem.* **9**:892.

KIRTIKAR, D. M., AND GOLDTHWAIT, D. A., 1974, The enzymatic release of O^6-methylguanine and 3-methyladenine from DNA reacted with the carcinogen, N-methyl-N-nitrosourea, *Proc. Natl. Acad. Sci. U.S.A.* **71**:2022.

KRAMER, B. S., FENSELAU, C. C., AND LUDLUM, D. B., 1974, Reaction of BCNU [1,3-*bis*(2-chloroethyl)-1-nitrosourea] with polycytidylic acid. Substitution of the cytosine ring, *Biochem. Biophys. Res. Commun.* **56**:783.

KUŚMIEREK, J. T., AND SINGER, B., 1976a, Reaction of diazoalkanes with 1-substituted 2,4-dioxopyrimidines. Formation of O^2, N-3 and O^4-alkyl products, *Nucleic Acids Res.* **3**:989.

KUŚMIEREK, J. T., AND SINGER, B., 1976b, Sites of alkylation of poly U by agents of varying carcinogenicity and stability of products, *Biochim. Biophys. Acta* **442**:420.

LAWLEY, P. D., 1966, Effects of some chemical mutagens and carcinogens on nucleic acids, *Prog. Nucleic Acid Res. Mol. Biol.* **5**:89.

LAWLEY, P. D., 1972, The action of alkylating mutagens and carcinogens on nucleic acids: *N*-Methyl-*N*-nitroso compounds as methylating agents, in: *Topics in Chemical Carcinogenesis* (W. Nakahara, S. Takayama, T. Sugimura, and S. Odashima, eds.), pp. 237–258, University Park Press, Baltimore.

LAWLEY, P. D., 1973, Reaction of *N*-methyl-*N*-nitrosoureas with ^{32}P-labelled DNA: Evidence for formation of phosphotriesters, *Chem.–Biol. Interact.* **7**:127.

LAWLEY, P. D., 1974, Some chemical aspects of dose–response relationships in alkylation mutagenesis, *Mutat. Res.* **23**:283.

LAWLEY, P. D., AND BROOKES, P., 1963, Further studies on the alkylation of nucleic acids and their constituent nucleotides, *Biochem. J.* **89**:127.

LAWLEY, P. D., AND ORR, D. J., 1970, Specific excision of methylation products from DNA of *Escherichia coli* treated with *N*-methyl-*N'*-nitro-*N*-nitrosoguanidine, *Chem.–Biol. Interact.* **2**:154.

LAWLEY, P. D., AND THATCHER, C. J., 1970, Methylation of deoxyribonucleic acid in cultured mammalian cells by *N*-methyl-*N'*-nitro-*N*-nitrosoguanidine, *Biochem. J.* **116**:693.

LAWLEY, P. D., LETHBRIDGE, J. H., EDWARDS, P. A., AND SHOOTER, K. V., 1969, Inactivation of bacteriophage T$_7$ by mono- and difunctional sulphur mustards in relation to cross-linking and depurination of bacteriophage DNA, *J. Mol. Biol.* **39**:181.

LAWLEY, P. D., ORR, D. J., AND SHAH, S. A., 1971–1972, Reaction of alkylating mutagens and carcinogens with nucleic acids: *N*-3 of guanine as a site of alkylation by *N*-methyl-*N*-nitrosourea and dimethyl sulphate, *Chem.–Biol. Interact.* **4**:431.

LAWLEY, P. D., ORR, D. J., SHAH, S. A., FARMER, P. B., AND JARMAN, M., 1973, Reaction products from *N*-methyl-*N*-nitrosourea and deoxyribonucleic acid containing thymidine residues. Synthesis and identification of a new methylation product, O^4-methylthymidine, *Biochem. J.* **135**:193.

LETT, J. T., PARKINS, G. M., AND ALEXANDER, P., 1962, Physiochemical changes produced in DNA after alkylation, *Arch. Biochem. Biophys.* **97**:80.

LINDAHL, T., AND KARLSTRÖM, O., 1973, Heat-induced depyrimidination of deoxyribonucleic acid in neutral solution, *Biochemistry* **12**:5151.

LINDAHL, T., AND NYBERG, B., 1972, Rate of depurination of native deoxyribonucleic acid, *Biochemistry* **11**:3618.

LOO, T. L., DION, R. L., DIXON, R. L., AND RALL, D. P., 1966, The antitumor agent, 1,3-*bis*(2-chloroethyl)-1-nitrosourea, *J. Pharm. Sci.* **55**:487.

LOVELESS, A., 1966, *Genetic and Allied Effects of Alkylating Agents*, Pennsylvania State University Press, University Park and London.

LOVELESS, A., 1969, Possible relevance of O–6 alkylation of deoxyguanosine to the mutagenicity and carcinogenicity of nitrosamines and nitrosamides, *Nature (London)* **223**:206.

LUDLUM, D. B., 1965, Alkylation of polynucleotide complexes, *Biochim. Biophys. Acta* **95**:674.

LUDLUM, D. B., 1967, Reaction of nitrogen mustard with synthetic polynucleotides, *Biochim. Biophys. Acta* **142**:282.

LUDLUM, D. B., 1969, Ethylation of polyadenylic acid, *Biochim. Biophys. Acta* **174:**773.

LUDLUM, D. B., 1970*a*, The properties of 7-methylguanine-containing templates for ribonucleic acid polymerase, *J. Biol. Chem.* **245:**477.

LUDLUM, D. B., 1970*b*, Alkylated polycytidylic acid templates for RNA polymerase, *Biochim. Biophys. Acta* **213:**142.

LUDLUM, D. B., 1975, Molecular biology of alkylation: An overview, in: *Handbook of Experimental Pharmacology*, Vol. XXXVIII/2 (A. C. Sartorelli and D. G. Johns, eds.), pp. 6–17, Springer-Verlag, Berlin.

LUDLUM, D. B., AND WILHELM, R. C., 1968, Ribonucleic acid polymerase reactions with methylated polycytidylic acid templates, *J. Biol. Chem.* **243:**2750.

LUDLUM, D. B., KRAMER, B. S., WANG, J., AND FENSELAU, C., 1975, Reaction of 1,3-*bis*(2-chloroethyl)-1-nitrosourea with synthetic polynucleotides, *Biochemistry* **14:**5480.

LYONS, R. M., AND GOLDENBERG, G. J., 1972, Active transport of nitrogen mustard and choline by normal and leukemic human lymphoid cells, *Cancer Res.* **32:**1679.

MAY, H. E., BOOSE, R., AND REED, D. J., 1975, Microsomal monooxygenation of the carcinostatic 1-(2-chloroethyl)-3-cyclohexyl-1-nitrosourea. Synthesis and identification of *cis* and *trans* monohydroxylated products, *Biochemistry* **14:**4723.

MONTGOMERY, J. A., JAMES, R., MCCALEB, G. S., AND JOHNSTON, T. P., 1967, The modes of decomposition of 1,3-*bis*(2-chloroethyl)-1-nitrosourea and related compounds, *J. Med. Chem.* **10:**668.

MONTGOMERY, J. A., JAMES, R., MCCALEB, G. S., KIRK, M. C., AND JOHNSTON, T. P., 1975, Decomposition of *N*-(2-chloroethyl)-*N*-nitrosoureas in aqueous media, *J. Med. Chem.* **18:**568.

OCHOA, M., JR., AND HIRSCHBERG, E., 1967, Alkylating agents, in: *Experimental Chemotherapy*, Vol. 5, pp. 1–132, Academic Press, New York and London.

O'CONNOR, P. J., MARGISON, G. P., AND CRAIG, A. W., 1975, Phosphotriesters in rat liver deoxyribonucleic acid after the administration of the carcinogen, *N,N*-dimethylnitrosamine *in vivo*, *Biochem. J.* **145:**475.

PAPIRMEISTER, B., DORSEY, J. K., DAVIDSON, C. L., AND GROSS, C. L., 1970, Sensitization of DNA to endonuclease by adenine alkylation and its biological significance, *Fed. Proc. Fed. Amer. Soc. Exp. Biol.* **29:**726.

PAQUETTE, Y., CRINE, P., AND VERLY, W. G., 1972, Properties of the endonuclease for depurinated DNA from *Escherichia coli*, *Can. J. Biochem.* **50:**1199.

PRICE, C. C., 1975, Chemistry of alkylation, in: *Handbook of Experimental Pharmacology*, Vol. XXXVIII/2 (A. C. Sartorelli and D. G. Johns, eds.), pp. 1–5, Springer-Verlag, Berlin.

PRICE, C. C., GAUCHER, G. M., KONERU, P., SHIBAKAWA, R., SOWA, J. R., AND YOMAGUCHI, M., 1969, Mechanism of action of alkylating agents, *Ann. N. Y. Acad. Sci.* **163:**593.

REED, D. J., AND MAY, H. E., 1975, Alkylation and carbamoylation intermediates from the carcinostatic 1-(2-chloroethyl)-3-cyclohexyl-1-nitrosourea (CCNU), *Life Sci.* **16:**1263.

REED, D. J., MAY, H. E., BOOSE, R. B., GREGORY, K. M., AND BEILSTEIN, M. A., 1975, 2-Chloroethanol formation as evidence for a 2-chloroethyl alkylating intermediate during chemical degradations of 1-(2-chloroethyl)-3-cyclohexyl-1-nitrosourea and 1-(2-chloroethyl)-3-(*trans*-4-methylcyclohexyl)-1-nitrosourea, *Cancer Res.* **35:**568.

RHAESE, H. J., AND FREEZE, E., 1969, Chemical analysis of DNA alterations. IV. Reactions of oligodeoxynucleotides with monofunctional alkylating agents leading to backbone breakage, *Biochim. Biophys. Acta* **190:**418.

ROSS, W. C. J., 1962, *Biological Alkylating Agents*, Butterworths, London.

ROSS, W. C. J., 1975, Rational design of alkylating agents, in: *Handbook of Experimental Pharmacology*, Vol. XXXVIII/1 (A. C. Sartorelli and D. G. Johns, eds.), pp. 33–51, Springer-Verlag, Berlin.

SCHABEL, F. M., JR., JOHNSTON, T. P., MCCALEB, G. S., MONTGOMERY, J. A., LASTER, W. R., AND SKIPPER, H. E., 1963, Experimental evaluation of potential anticancer agents. VIII. Effects of certain nitrosoureas on intracerebral L1210 leukemia, *Cancer Res.* **23:**725.

SCHMIDT, L. H., FRADKIN, R., SULLIVAN, R., AND FLOWERS, A., 1965, Comparative pharmacology of alkylating agents, *Cancer Chemother. Rep. Suppl.* **2:**1.

SHOOTER, K. V., HOWSE, R., AND MERRIFIELD, R. K., 1974, The reaction of alkylating agents with bacteriophage R$_{17}$. Biological effects of phosphotriester formation, *Biochem. J.* **137:**313.

SINGER, B., 1975, The chemical effects of nucleic acid alkylation and their relation to mutagenesis and carcinogenesis, *Prog. Nucleic Acid Res. Mol. Biol.* **15:**219.

SINGER, B., 1976, A new major product of neutral aqueous reaction of cytidine with carbinogens, *FEBS Lett.* **63:**85.

SINGER, B., AND FRAENKEL-CONRAT, H., 1969, Chemical modifications of viral ribonucleic acid. VII. The action of methylating agents and nitrosoguanidine on polynucleotides including tobacco mosaic virus ribonucleic acid, *Biochemistry* **8**:3260.

SINGER, B., AND FRAENKEL-CONRAT, H., 1970, Messenger and template activities of chemically modified polynucleotides, *Biochemistry* **9**:3694.

SINGER, B., AND FRAENKEL-CONRAT, H., 1975, The specificity of different classes of ethylating agents toward various sites in RNA, *Biochemistry* **14**:772.

SINGER, B., AND KUŚMIEREK, J. T., 1976, Alkylation of ribose in RNA reacted with ethynitrosourea at neutrality, *Biochemistry* **15**:5052.

STRAUSS, B., COYLE, M., AND ROBBINS, M., 1969, Consequences of alkylation for the behavior of DNA, *Ann. N. Y. Acad. Sci.* **163**:765.

STRUCK, R. F., KIRK, M. C., MELLETT, L. B., EL DAREER, S., AND HILL, D. L., 1971, Urinary metabolites of the antitumour agent cyclophosphamide *Mol. Pharmacol.* **7**:519.

VAN DUUREN, B. L. (ed.), 1969, Biological effects of alkylating agents, *Ann. N. Y. Acad. Sci.* **163**:589.

VERLY, W. G., AND BRAKIER, L., 1969, The lethal action of monofunctional and bifunctional alkylating agents on T$_7$ coliphage, *Biochim. Biophys. Acta* **174**:674.

VERLY, W. G., AND PAQUETTE, Y., 1972, An endonuclease for depurinated DNA in *Escherichia coli* B, *Can. J. Biochem.* **50**:217.

WALKER, M. D., 1973, Nitrosoureas in central nervous system tumors, *Cancer Chemother. Rep. Suppl.* **4**:21.

WALL, R. L., AND CLAUSEN, K. P., 1975, Carcinoma of the urinary bladder in patients receiving cyclophosphamide, *N. Engl. J. Med.* **293**:271.

WHEELER, G. P., 1975, Mechanism of action of nitrosoureas, in *Handbook of Experimental Pharmacology*, Vol. XXXVIII/2 (A. C. Sartorelli and D. G. Johns, eds.), pp. 65–84, Springer-Verlag, Berlin.

WHEELER, G. P., AND ALEXANDER, J. A., 1969, Effects of nitrogen mustard and cyclophosphamide upon the synthesis of DNA *in vivo* and in cell-free preparations, *Cancer Res.* **29**:98.

WHEELER, D. G., AND CHUMLEY, S., 1967, Alkylating activity of 1,3-*bis*(2-chloroethyl)-1-nitrosoureas and related compounds, *J. Med. Chem.* **10**:259.

WHEELER, G. P., BOWDEN, B. J., GRIMSLEY, J. A., AND LLOYD, H. H., 1974, Interrelationships of some chemical, physicochemical, and biological activities of several 1-(2-haloethyl)-1-nitrosoureas, *Cancer Res.* **34**:194.

WILHELM, R. C., AND LUDLUM, D. B., 1966, Coding properties of 7-methylguanine, *Science* **153**:1403.

WHO, 1975, *IRAC* (*Int. Agency Res. Cancer*) *Sci. Publ. Evaluation of Carcinogenic Risk of Chemicals to Man*, **9**, Lyon, France.

YANOFSKY, C., ITO, J., AND HORN, V., 1966, Amino acid replacement and the genetic code, *Cold Spring Harbor Symp. Quant. Biol.* **31**:151.

11

Purine Antagonists

G. A. LePage

1. Introduction

Since purines are essential components of the RNA, DNA, and coenzymes that must be synthesized in the proliferation of cancer cells, it has long seemed logical to use purine antagonists as potentially active agents for cancer therapy. Mammalian cells have, to varying extents, the capacity to either use preformed purines or make them *de novo*. It is therefore expedient in this discussion to include agents capable of inhibiting either process.

Studies of purine antagonists as agents for use against cancers were initiated in 1949 with the findings concerning the activity of 8-azaguanine (Kidder *et al.*, 1949). However, 8-azaguanine did not achieve lasting interest. It showed some undesirable side effects, lacked sustained activity, and was soon eclipsed by the emergence of other purine analogues (Parks and Agarwal, 1975). In 1953 and 1954, both the purinethiols, 6-mercaptopurine (6-MP) and 6-thioguanine (6-TG), and the glutamine antagonists able to inhibit synthesis of purines *de novo* became available. Attention was then focused on these drugs. They underwent clinical trials and sustained basic studies. The purinethiols have retained great clinical interest. Many derivatives have been made and tested. They therefore deserve the most attention in a discussion of examples of purine antagonists as useful drugs.

2. 6-Mercaptopurine

2.1. History

An analogue of hypoxanthine, 6-mercaptopurine (6-MP, NSC-755), was synthesized by Hitchings and Elion (1954), who reported a practical synthesis in 1954.

G. A. LePage ● McEachern Laboratory, University of Alberta, Edmonton, Canada.

This relatively simple change in the chemical structure of a natural purine (Fig. 1) resulted in a compound with almost unrivaled clinical and basic scientific interest. It was first tested as an antileukemic agent by Burchenal *et al.* (1953).

2.2. Chemistry

6-MP is readily crystallized as a monohydrate, with a molecular weight of 170. In solution, except at alkaline pH, it is probably present in keto form. In alkaline solution, however, it would be present largely as an anion. It has relatively low solubility in water at neutral pH, but this solubility is greatly increased in alkaline solutions. Stability to oxidation is poor in alkaline solutions, however, and such alkaline solutions should therefore be stored at low temperature or made up shortly before use. It is insoluble in lipids.

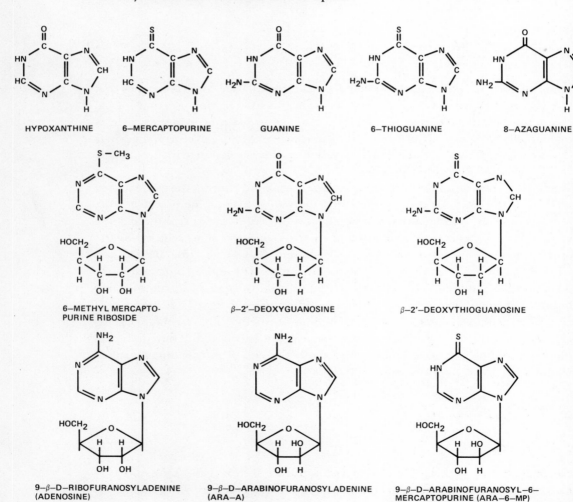

FIGURE 1. Purine structures.

2.3. Pharmacology

6-MP is most commonly given orally in tablet form. The absorption after an oral dose is incomplete and variable. The oral dosage required is therefore about twice that required by intravenous injection. The usual dosage, orally, is 75–95 mg/M^2 or 2.0–2.5 mg/kg daily. Use of intravenous injection is still an experimental procedure, and for this, 6-MP would be prepared as a sodium salt. After intravenous injection, plasma half-time is 20–45 min. At the concentrations attained in plasma, about 20% is bound to protein. About 20% of a parenteral dose is excreted in 6 hr (Loo *et al.*, 1968). Penetration of the blood–brain barrier is minimal.

2.4. Metabolism and Metabolic Effects

In both experimental animals and man, 6-MP is extensively metabolized to thioxanthine, thiouric acid, and 6-methylthiopurine (Fig. 2). This metabolism has been studied by Elion *et al.* (1954, 1963*a, b*) and Hamilton and Elion (1954). The *in vivo* oxidation of 6-MP is apparently a function of xanthine oxidase, and it can be greatly reduced by simultaneous treatment with the xanthine oxidase inhibitor allopurinol (Elion *et al.*, 1963). This is not commonly done, however, because there is no practical advantage. One is only reducing the requirement for 6-MP by adding allopurinol, with the added uncertainty of using two drugs instead of one. When this combination is used, the excretion pattern is shifted from thiouric acid to thioxanthine.

The anabolism of 6-MP is to ribonucleotide by reaction with phosphoribosyl-pyrophosphate, catalyzed by the enzyme hypoxanthine-guanine phosphoribosyl-transferase. As the ribonucleotide, 6-MP acts as a negative feedback inhibitor of

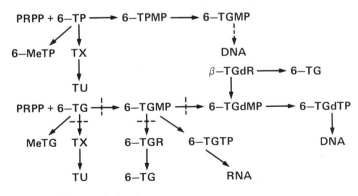

--- Resistance Mechanisms

FIGURE 2. Thiopurine interconversions. 6-TP, 6-thiopurine; 6-TG, 6-thioguanine; PRPP, phophoribosyl pyrophosphate; TPMP, thiopurine (riboside) monophosphate; MeTG, methyl thioguanine; β-TGdR, β-2′-deoxythioguanine.

purine synthesis *de novo* by its effects on the initial step of purine synthesis, the conversion of phosphoribosylpyrophosphate to phosphoribosylamine (Brockman, 1963). In addition, the ribonucleotide of 6-MP inhibits the conversion of inosinic acid to xanthylic acid and the conversion of inosinic acid to adenylic acid via adenylosuccinate. The inhibitor constants would indicate greatest sensitivity of the reaction involving inosinic dehydrogenase (Elion, 1967). Additionally, LePage and Jones (1961*a*) showed that a similar extent of inhibition of purine synthesis *de novo* (feedback) occurred in both sensitive and resistant tumor cells *in vivo*, indicating that feedback inhibition of purine synthesis by 6-MP is not limiting to growth.

More recently, observations of Tidd and Paterson (1974) indicate that delayed cytotoxic effects of 6-MP on mouse leukemic cells in culture correlated with incorporation of 6-MP into cellular DNA, which when isolated was found to be present in the DNA as thioguanine deoxynucleotide. Thus, a conversion of 6-MP to 6-TG was involved. These observations leave unexplained a singular finding of Scannell and Hitchings (1966) that a mouse ascites tumor line, Ad755, sensitive to 6-MP did not incorporate as much 6-MP into DNA as a 6-MP-resistant cell line. The resistant line was found to have 6-TG present in DNA in deoxynucleotide linkage. Therefore, after over 20 years of study, we are unable to categorically state what the mechanism of action of 6-MP is. The conversion to 6-TG and incorporation into DNA is an attractive way to explain some other observations. For example, it would account for a ratio of some 25 to 1 in the toxicities and therapeutic doses of 6-MP and 6-TG in rodents. It would imply that interconversion must be much more efficient in humans, in whom the effective dosages of the two thiols are very similar.

Resistance to 6-MP provided the initial indication that nucleotide formation was necessary for activation. Brockman (1960) showed that bacterial and mammalian cells selected for resistance by treatment with 6-MP had lost the hypoxanthine-guanine phosphoribosyltransferase (HGPRT) enzyme, and that this loss prevented formation of 6-MP nucleotides. However, subsequent studies (Davidson and Winter, 1964; Rosman and Williams, 1973) have indicated that this is not a common mechanism of resistance to 6-MP in cancer patients. Ability to degrade 6-MP nucleotides with alkaline phosphatases appears to be one mechanism involved in such patients (Rosman *et al.*, 1974).

2.5. Derivatives

The ribonucleoside of 6-MP (6-MPR, NSC4911) has received some study, since its activation would involve a kinase, rather than the HGPRT enzyme. It might have potential for the treatment of neoplastic cells resistant to 6-MP by reason of the deletion of the HGPRT enzyme. However, it is relatively rapidly cleaved to 6-MP by a nucleoside phosphorylase (Paterson and Sutherland, 1964). It does, however, exhibit some activity against some experimental neoplasms resistant to 6-MP (Skipper *et al.*, 1959).

Another 6-MP derivative that has achieved prominence and utility is 6-[(1-methyl-4-nitro-5-imidazolyl)thio]purine (azathioprine, imuran, NSC-39084). Imuran acts as a "depot form" of 6-MP. It is converted to 6-MP at a moderate rate. It has activity against some experimental neoplasms, but has not been widely accepted as a substitute for 6-MP in cancer therapy. Instead, it has superseded 6-MP as an immune suppressor (Hitchings and Elion, 1969), and is commonly used for this property in patients who have received organ grafts (Markinodan *et al.*, 1970) to prevent rejection of the graft. It can be given at 60 mg/M^2 per day for at least 12 weeks without serious toxic effects (Maibach and Epstein, 1965).

Another structural analogue of 6-MP made in an effort to bypass resistance mechanisms was 6-methylthiopurine riboside (MMPR, NSC40774). Unlike 6-MPR, MMPR is not cleaved by nucleoside phosphorylases. It is readily phosphorylated by the ubiquitous enzyme adenosine kinase. It is not readily converted to di- and triphosphate, but as the monophosphate, it is a potent feedback inhibitor of the initial step in purine synthesis *de novo*. It is indeed effective against some experimental tumors resistant to 6-MP (Bennett *et al.*, 1965). A cell line resistant to MMPR was found to lack adenosine kinase (Caldwell *et al.*, 1976). MMPR is readily absorbed after oral administration. It is rapidly taken up and phosphorylated in tissues, including the red blood cells, and retained for a relatively long period in the latter. 6-MP and MMPR have been shown to be synergistic in some rodent tumors, probably because MMPR inhibits phosphoribosylpyrophosphate utilization for purine synthesis, and thereby makes more available for conversion of 6-MP to ribonucleotide (Paterson and Moriwaki, 1969). Clinical tests have indicated no activity for MMPR·alone (Freireich *et al.*, 1967). Unlike 6-MP, MMPR exhibited toxicity to the GI tract that was more limiting than myelosuppression (Luce *et al.*, 1967).

Treatment with a combination of 6-MP and MMPR produced complete hemotologic remissions in 4 of 10 acute granulocytic leukemias (Bodey *et al.*, 1968). No further studies appear to have been reported.

3. 6-Thioguanine

3.1. History

6-Thioguanine (6-TG, NSC752) was synthesized by Elion and Hitchings (1955), and reports of its biological effects were made along with those of 6-MP (Hitchings and Elion, 1954). The early results suggested that 6-TG had the same metabolic effects as 6-MP, because the remission rates were the same for leukemias treated with either drug, and experimental tumors resistant to one were cross-resistant to the other. Experimental tumor lines were found, however, that responded better to combinations of the two than to any dose of either drug alone (Henderson and Junga, 1960), and a 6-TG-resistant tumor cell line was not cross-resistant to 6-MP (LePage and Jones, 1961*b*). Subsequent studies of mechanisms involved in the resistance to the two drugs show why the initial tests of cross-resistance were positive (deletion of the HGPRT enzyme), and show some differences (see Fig. 2).

3.2. Chemistry

6-TG in the pure state is a white or slightly yellow powder. In the dry state, it is relatively stable, but slowly oxidizes, and should therefore be held at low temperatures if it is to be stored for prolonged periods. It can be readily dissolved in water to 10–15 mg/ml by the addition of 1–2 equivalents of NaOH (mol. wt. 167). On neutralization, about 0.5 mg/ml remains in solution. Such solutions can be freeze-dried and stored for reconstitution in water, but alkaline solutions oxidize relatively rapidly. Alkaline solutions made with 1.2 equivalents NaOH can be held up to 8 days at 2–4°C before significant deterioration occurs (LePage and Whitecar, 1971).

3.3. Pharmacology

The absorption, distribution, metabolism, and excretions of 6-TG have been studied in mice (Moore and LePage, 1958) and in man (LePage and Whitecar, 1971). On parenteral administration, 6-TG was rapidly removed from the plasma by tissues and rapidly excreted in the urine, with thiouric acid the major metabolite. The metabolism and excretion in mice and man were in contrast after oral and parenteral dosage. The oral dosage was not well absorbed in either case. In man, as contrasted with mouse, one chief metabolite after an oral dose was a methylated derivative in an amount about equal to that of thiouric acid. The plasma half-time in man with intravenous 6-TG was about 80 min (LePage and Whitecar, 1971). The urinary excretion was about 75% in 24 hr.

3.4. Metabolism and Metabolic Effects

Most of the 6-TG given to animals or man found in the tissues was in nucleotide form, including mono-, di-, and triphosphates. Incorporation occurred into both RNA and DNA (E. C. Moore and LePage, 1958; LePage and Whitecar, 1971). Inbred mice given otherwise lethal doses of 6-TG could be saved by injecting them 48 hr later with infusions of compatible bone marrow cells (Sartorelli and LePage, 1957). Unlike 6-MP, 6-TG showed cumulative toxicity when repeated doses were given, and this cumulative toxicity was clearly related to dosage schedules (LePage, 1964). Bone marrow has a metabolism geared to use of preformed purines (salvage). It is vulnerable to an antimetabolite incorporated into DNA. It is therefore not surprising that 6-TG appears to exert its host toxicity by damaging bone marrow. The other most vulnerable tissues, GI mucosa and skin, are apparently protected because they possess relatively higher levels of an enzyme (guanase) that deaminates and therefore inactivates 6-TG.

In vitro and *in vivo* studies of metabolism in experimental tumors have shown that 6-TG produced several metabolic effects, those also observed for 6-MP (Sartorelli and LePage, 1958*b*). These effects included inhibition of preformed guanine (competitive), feedback inhibition of purine synthesis *de novo*, and interconversion of purines (hypoxanthine, adenine, guanine). In addition, the incorporation into both DNA and RNA of susceptible tumors and normal tissues was observed (LePage, 1960; LePage and Jones, 1961*a*). Incorporation into RNA occurred in some cell lines unresponsive to 6-TG, indicating that this incorporation was not damaging or could be repaired. It also indicated that an attempt by Miech *et al.* (1967) to account for the cell lethality of 6-TG on the basis of a combination of the effects of 6-TG described above is without validity. All data to date support a correlation between the incorporation of 6-TG into DNA and cell lethality, except an isolated and strange finding of Scannell and Hitchings (1966) for two Ad755 tumor lines in mice. A 6-MP-resistant line incorporated 6-MP into its DNA, as 6-TG deoxynucleotide, to a level twice that observed in the 6-MP-sensitive counterpart. The level of incorporation was at 1 6-TG nucleotide per 1500 DNA-nucleotides, a level below that found by LePage and Jones (1961*a*) and by Adams (1964) to be lethal; in their studies, 1 nucleotide per 1000 seemed to be a threshold of lethality. The latter provided indirect evidence of DNA repair when sublethal incorporation had occurred. Various other support has accumulated for the concept that incorporation of 6-TG into DNA is necessary for its lethal effects. Schmidt *et al.* (1970) and LePage and White (1973) demonstrated that simultaneous administration of arabinosylcytosine inhibited DNA synthesis in mouse bone marrow, and prevented both incorporation of 6-TG into DNA and the lethal effects of 6-TG. Recently, Nelson *et al.* (1975) concluded that a series of their experiments supported the concept that the lethal effects of 6-MP and 6-TG were due to incorporation of 6-TG into DNA.

3.5. Derivatives

As a result of the indications that 6-TG had to be incorporated into DNA for lethal effect on the cell, and in view of the resistance mechanisms (see Fig. 2)—i.e., (1) guanase in tumors degrading the drug, (2) deletion of the HGPRT enzyme involved in nucleotide formations, (3) phosphohydrolase activity cleaving 6-TG riboside, and (4) inability to convert 6-TG ribotide to deoxyribotide—it seemed appropriate to synthesize β-2'-deoxythioguanosine. Both α- and β-anomers (α-TGdR, NSC71851; β-TGdR, NSC71261) were obtained (Iwamoto *et al.*, 1963). Phosphorylation of β-TGdR, if it occurred, would provide a direct precursor for incorporation into DNA and bypass at least three of four resistance mechanisms found for 6-TG (Ellis and LePage, 1963). To a reasonable extent, this was achieved (LePage *et al.*, 1964), except for cell lines having high levels of nucleoside phosphorylase and therefore rapid cleavage to 6-TG (see Fig. 2). Some evidence has been obtained in humans that β-TGdR acts as such, and not after conversion to 6-TG (LePage and Gottlieb, 1973). β-TGdR has been tested in a Phase II clinical study and found to produce some remissions in leukemias refractory to 6-TG (Omura, 1975). α-TGdR is under study in a Phase I, II clinical protocol, in which it has shown no toxic effects at doses as high as 1500 mg/M^2. The interest in α-TGdR stems from the findings that it is not appreciably cleaved to 6-TG, is not phosphorylated to nucleotide in normal tissues—and therefore is not toxic—but is phosphorylated in some cancers (Peery and LePage, 1969) and produces responses in some experimental neoplasms (LePage et al., 1964; LePage, 1968). α-TGdR is incorporated into the DNA of cancer cells having the necessary phosphorylating enzyme and produces chain-termination, with accumulation of short DNA chains in the cell resulting (Tamaoki and LePage, 1975).

3.6. Clinical Uses

6-TG alone produces about a 15% remission rate in acute leukemias. β-TGdR showed activity in leukemias refractory to 6-MP or 6-TG therapy, and perhaps should replace 6-TG (Omura, 1975). 6-TG showed some activity against colorectal cancer (Horton et al., 1975). In combination with arabinosylcytosine, 6-TG is perhaps as good as any therapy for remission induction in acute myelocytic leukemia of adults (Ellison, 1973). It should undoubtedly be used in combination therapy with other agents for a variety of neoplastic diseases.

4. Allopurinol

Allopurinol [4-hydroxypyrazolo(3,4-d)pyrimidine, NSC1390] is not a carcinostatic agent (Skipper et al., 1957). It is useful clinically, however, because of its ability to inhibit xanthine oxidase and therefore reduce uric acid formation in patients with chronic gout. In leukemia and lymphoma patients under treatment with carcinolytic agents, it can be used to prevent urate nephropathy. It is relatively innocuous at effective doses (e.g., 600–800 mg/day for 2–3 days), but should be monitored carefully, particularly in regard to adequate liver function, if it is used for longer periods.

5. Arabinosyl-6-Mercaptopurine

A considerable range of basic studies was conducted on arabinosyl-6-mercaptopurine (Ara-6-MP, NSC406021) by Kimball et al. (1964, 1966, 1967). The drug, though a purine analogue, had no effect on purine metabolism, but produced 65–80% inhibition of cytidylate reductase (part of the activity of ribonucleotide reductase), and as a consequence an incomplete inhibition of DNA synthesis (Hersh and LePage, 1971). Unlike most other such antimetabolites, it is not converted to nucleotide (LePage et al., 1969), and was active as nucleoside, probably by reason of occupation of an allosteric site on the enzyme. It was effective against experimental neoplasms resistant to 6-MP. Little or no host toxicity was observed at high doses. This differential toxicity to tumor and not host may result from an incomplete inhibition of the target enzyme in a situation in which the enzyme level is growth-limiting in tumor cells, but present in excess in normal cells. It is relatively rapidly excreted, at about the same rate by mouse, dog, and man, mostly as unchanged drug (Loo *et al.*, 1970). In Phase I testing, it was administered to patients at up to 13 g/M² without toxicity. Phase II trials have not been performed, however, and the observation in mice that in combination with low-dose glutamine antagonists such as azaserine it was effective at 1/50 of the dose effect alone was not extended to humans. Sequential inhibition of cytidine nucleotide and then the reductase is assumed to be the reason for this drug interaction, since the glutamine antagonists reduced pool sizes of cytidine nucleotides.

6. Arabinosyladenine

6.1. History

9-β-D-Arabinofuranosyladenine (Ara-A, NSC404241) was synthesized chemically (Lee *et al.*, 1960; Reist *et al.*, 1962) in a program directed at finding carcinostatic agents. It has more recently been produced by a fermentation process (Parke-Davis and Company, 1967*) with *Streptomyces antiboticus*. This latter method now appears to be by far the more economical source.

The biological properties of Ara-A were first studied by Hubert-Habart and Cohen (1962) in *E. coli*, in which it was inhibitory. Ara-A was deaminated to arabinosylhypoxanthine (Ara-H), or converted to nucleotide.

Ara-A has been studied extensively both as an antiviral agent and as an anticancer agent. It is now evident that this nucleoside has considerable potential in both these categories. It has efficacy in the treatment of infections with DNA viruses. That it does has been extensively documented by Ch'ien *et al.* (1973) and Pavan-Langston *et al.* (1975), and will not be discussed in further detail here.

6.2. Chemistry

Ara-A should probably be regarded as an analogue of deoxyadenosine (see Fig. 1). Ara-A is relatively stable in water solution at pHs near neutrality, and such solutions can be stored for at least several days at room temperature or below, if sterile. The solubility exhibits a steep rise with temperature. Solutions at neutral pH can be made 1.0 mg/ml at 37°C or 0.5 mg/ml at room temperature. The dry powder is stable indefinitely.

* Belgian Pat. No. 671557.

6.3. Metabolism and Metabolic Effects

Ara-A was found to inhibit the growth of several experimental tumors of mice (Brink and LePage, 1964a, b; 1965). Catabolism was by deamination to arabinosylhypoxanthine (Ara-H), and excretion in the urine was 87% in 4 hr. This deamination was by adenosine deaminase, which is widely distributed in tissues. Alternatively, Ara-A was converted to nucleotides, mainly Ara-ATP. The latter was demonstrated by York and LePage (1966), in crude extracts of murine tumor, to be the actual active form and an inhibitor of DNA polymerase. That it is was confirmed by Furth and Cohen (1967) with purified DNA polymerase from bovine lymphosarcoma, though a DNA polymerase from E. coli was unresponsive. The latter result, in view of findings with Ara-C (Reddy et al., 1971), probably results from testing of E. coli DNA polymerase I, rather than the DNA polymerase II, which was discovered subsequent to the tests with Ara-ATP. Furth and Cohen (1968) showed that while Ara-ATP inhibited both DNA polymerase and ribonucleotide reductase, the former was the more sensitive site of inhibition. LePage (1969) showed that experimental neoplasms with low or moderate levels of adenosine deaminase are quite responsive to treatment with Ara-A. Lack of toxicity to the host animals, particularly lack of immunosuppression, can be explained on the basis that these normal tissues are protected by relatively high levels of the deaminase. One experimental neoplasm that was manifestly unresponsive, L1210, has a very high deaminase level. Inhibition of this tumor became quite profound when Ara-A was used in combination with an inhibitor of the deaminase (LePage et al., 1976).

6.4. Pharmacology

Studies have been made of the tissue distribution and excretion of Ara-A in mice (Brink and LePage, 1964b). Both the studies of Ara-A as an antiviral agent (Pavan-Langston et al., 1975) and those of it as an anticancer agent (LePage et al., 1973) have led to generation of data on the distribution and excretion in humans. In the latter case, intravenous and intramuscular administrations were compared. Absorption was poor in the latter. Excretion was relatively rapid after intravenous injection, indicating that optimum therapy would require continuous intravenous infusions. Short intravenous infusions were essentially completely cleared by urinary excretion in the 24-hr period. Excretion was almost all as Ara-H in the first few hours. Later excretion was not completely recovered as Ara-H, indicating some further catabolism.

6.5. Derivatives

The findings of relatively rapid degradation and excretion of Ara-A, together with the low solubility, led to work with the 5'-monophosphate of Ara-A. This derivative is much more soluble, is not a substrate for adenosine deaminase, and would be expected to be largely confined to the plasma space on intravenous injection. Only as it was cleaved by phosphohydrolases would it disperse into tissues and become rephosphorylated to active form. Investigations with this derivative, Ara-A-5'-phosphate (LePage *et al.*, 1972, 1975) have demonstrated that at doses equivalent to Ara-A at 500–1000 mg/M^2 i.v. as a single injection, the nucleotide maintains Ara-A concentrations of 4–10 μM in plasma throughout the 24-hr period. Tests on cell lines in culture (Cass and Au-Yeung, 1976) indicate that this concentration is adequate to kill cancer cells.

6.6. Clinical Uses

Ara-A has already undergone Phase I clinical testing (Bodey *et al.*, 1974), and a Phase II clinical trial with the 5'-phosphate of Ara-A in chronic myelogenous leukemia is in progress. In the Phase I testing, some encouraging therapeutic effects were obtained. At the highest and most sustained dosages, some myelosuppressive effects were obtained, but none has been seen in several patients given equally high doses (1300 mg/M^2 for 10 days) of Ara-A-5'-phosphate. Since this derivative moderates the peak levels of Ara-A in plasma (LePage *et al.*, 1975), this may be a sustained finding.

7. Glutamine Antagonists

7.1. History

The initial step in the synthesis of purines *de novo* requires glutamine, as does one of the subsequent steps. Since cancer cells can to varying degrees use preformed purines or make them *de novo* (Henderson and LePage, 1959), antagonists of glutamine are inhibitors of purine synthesis. Several antibiotics have been found that are glutamine antagonists. The first of these described was azaserine (*O*-diazoacetyl-L-serine, NSC742), which was found in cultures of a *Streptomyces* (Bartz *et al.*, 1954) and quickly found to be an inhibitor of some experimental neoplasms (Stock *et al.*, 1954). Thereafter, screening of *Streptomyces* cultures led to the discovery of several similar agents, notably 6-diazo-5-oxo-L-norleucine (DON, NSC7365), which was found by Ehrlich *et al.* (1956). Duazomycin (*N*-acetyl DON) and azotomycin (DON triglutamate, NSC56654) are active only after conversion in tissues to DON.

7.2. Chemistry

Azaserine and DON are highly soluble in water and relatively stable in neutral solutions. However, they are very unstable at pHs divergent in either direction from neutrality. They are analogues of glutamine, but are also alkylating agents, and so are very reactive. Their structures, along with that of glutamine, are

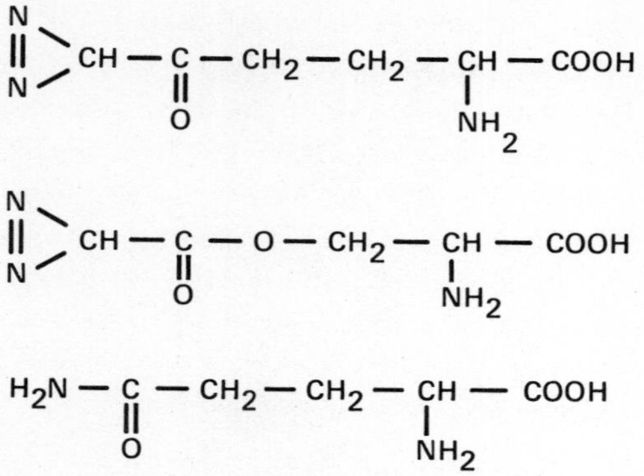

$$\text{N} = \text{N} > \text{CH} - \underset{\overset{\|}{O}}{\text{C}} - \text{CH}_2 - \text{CH}_2 - \underset{\overset{|}{NH_2}}{\text{CH}} - \text{COOH} \qquad \text{DON}$$

$$\text{N} = \text{N} > \text{CH} - \underset{\overset{\|}{O}}{\text{C}} - \text{O} - \text{CH}_2 - \underset{\overset{|}{NH_2}}{\text{CH}} - \text{COOH} \qquad \text{AZASERINE}$$

$$\text{H}_2\text{N} - \underset{\overset{\|}{O}}{\text{C}} - \text{CH}_2 - \text{CH}_2 - \underset{\overset{|}{NH_2}}{\text{CH}} - \text{COOH} \qquad \text{L-GLUTAMINE}$$

FIGURE 3. Structures of glutamine and glutamine antagonists.

illustrated in Fig. 3. They have been stored in the dry state at low temperatures (e.g., $-20°C$) with no detectable deterioration for a period of several years. Both agents have been synthesized chemically (J. A. Moore *et al.*, 1954; Dewald and Moore, 1956).

7.3. Pharmacology

The toxicology of azaserine in mice, rats, and dogs has been reported (Sternberg and Philips, 1957). At toxic doses, the rodents were found to have a great variety of lesions, including pancreatitis, hepatitis, necrotizing nephrosis, bone marrow hypoplasia, and erosion of the intestinal epithelium. In dogs treated with doses that were more nearly therapeutic levels, the toxic effects were largely restricted to the GI mucosa. At the dose levels effective against experimental neoplasms, mice do not show overt signs of toxicity. Side effects in patients treated with azaserine are chiefly related to GI toxicity (nausea, vomiting, diarrhea, stomatitis). Blood levels of azaserine were determined in mice and humans at intervals after parenteral treatment with azaserine (Henderson *et al.*, 1957). The blood levels were detectable in mice for 20–60 min periods only, even after 6–20 mg/kg doses. Humans, in contrast, had measurable blood levels for up to 4 hr, even after doses of only 0.4–1.25 mg/kg. The blood levels and rate of excretion of DON were also studied in humans (Magill *et al.*, 1957). Patients could tolerate only 0.1–0.3 mg/kg parenterally, but higher doses were necessary orally to achieve the same effects, presumably due to the sensitivity of the drug to gastric acidity. Therapeutic doses of DON gave appreciable blood levels for about 4 hr. Higher doses maintained blood levels for 8 hr or more. Very little DON was detected in the urine of patients (<1% of dose).

7.4. Metabolism and Metabolic Effects

Azaserine and DON are both amino acid analogues and alkylating agents. Particularly in microbial systems, they have shown a multitude of effects, many related to the reactivity, others to concentration by the amino acid transport system of cells and competition for this by amino acids. A comprehensive discussion of these biological effects is available (Bennett, 1975). This discussion will be limited to factors directly concerned with their carcinostatic properties. Azaserine is degraded by an enzymatic deamination *in vivo*. The activity is by far the greatest in liver (Jacquez and Sherman, 1962). In contrast, DON has not been shown to be destroyed enzymatically. It probably undergoes chemical degradation.

Shortly after its isolation, azaserine was shown to be an inhibitor of purine synthesis (Skipper *et al.*, 1954; Bennett *et al.*, 1956). LePage and Sartorelli (1957) showed that at therapeutic levels, azaserine inhibited the amidation of formyl-glycinamide ribotide to the amidine by irreversibly combining with the enzyme. DON also combined with the first enzyme of purine synthesis (Hartman, 1963). There was an initial period when there were competitive effects, then an irreversible reaction. Glutamine could partially prevent the effect, but not reverse it. There were distinct differences in the susceptibility of tissues to azaserine and DON (E. C. Moore and LePage, 1957).

At least two forms of resistance to azaserine and DON were found in experimental neoplasms. A plasma cell tumor, 70429, in C3H mice was very sensitive to azaserine, DON, and *N*-methylformamide. A line of cells resistant to all three agents was readily obtained, by drug treatment, in one transplant generation. This line has been studied, but its resistance mechanism was not readily explained. It did not have any change in transport or degradative capacity for azaserine (Anderson and Jacquez, 1962). In contrast, an azaserine-resistant line of the TA3 mouse mammary adenocarcinoma was obtained only after many transplant generations in drug-treated mice. Again, there was cross-resistance to DON and *N*-methylformamide. Evidence was obtained (Sartorelli and LePage, 1958a) that the sensitive and resistant lines were both inhibited equally, but that the cells of the resistant line recovered more rapidly, perhaps by enzyme resynthesis.

DON is effective at doses that are 1/20 to 1/40 those required for azaserine. It is not entirely clear whether this greater effectiveness reflects the rate of degradation of azaserine by enzymatic deamination, or whether DON is a better structural analogue. Azaserine may be the more desirable drug for pharmacological reasons. Both react irreversibly with the two enzymes for the amidation reactions of purine synthesis. Tissues quite evidently differ in sensitivity, and the experimental tumors are more sensitive than normal mouse tissues (E. C. Moore and LePage, 1957). In such a situation, it would be best to have the agent present in body fluids only long enough to "titrate" the key enzyme in the sensitive neoplastic cells. To have it present for longer would lead to "titration" of normal cells, and unacceptable toxicity. To have an agent destroyed in a reasonable time is thus desirable. Azaserine appears to answer these requirements better than DON, and at therapeutically effective doses, inhibits only one enzymatic step. The GI mucosa is a tissue that exhibits rapid growth and has considerable dependence on synthesis of purines *de novo*. It is the most sensitive normal tissue. From the human pharmacology (Henderson *et al.*, 1957), one probably should give azaserine in doses of about 0.4 mg/kg only, and combination with other agents is indicated.

Several clinical tests of these agents have been performed. In one (Ellison *et al.*, 1954), 56 cancer patients were given azaserine at 8–10 mg/kg per day p.o. Toxicity appeared in 5–20 days, and first involved the GI mucosa, with jaundice and depressed leukocyte counts later in some instances. Bone marrow depression may result from the high doses, which would also inhibit pyrimidine synthesis (Kammen and Hurlbert, 1959). Azaserine was tested orally in the treatment of multiple myeloma without benefit (Holland *et al.*, 1961). Azaserine was used in combination with thioguanine, both given intravenously (Schroeder *et al.*, 1964). Of 7 breast carcinoma patients, 4 showed improvement; 1 with squamous-cell carcinoma showed improvement, and 11 were unresponsive.

The pharmacological effects of azaserine and DON were not taken into account in the early clinical trials. It seems quite possible that if they were to be used with regard to their mechanism of action, they have a place in combination chemotherapy that has not been appropriately exploited.

8. References

ADAMS, D. H., 1964, Further studies on the chemotherapy of adenocarcinoma 755 with 6-thioguanine, *Cancer Res.* **24**:250.

ANDERSON, E. P., AND JACQUEZ, J. A., 1962, Azaserine resistance in a plasma-cell neoplasm without change in active transport of the inhibitor, *Cancer Res.* **22**:27.

BARTZ, Q. R., ELDER, C. C., FROHARDT, R. P., FUSAI, S. A., HASKELL, T. H., JOHANNESSEN, D. W., AND RYDER, A., 1954, Isolation and characterization of azaserine, *Nature (London)* **173**:71.

BENNETT, L. L., JR., 1975, Glutamine antagonists, in: *Antineoplastic and Immunosuppressive Agents II* (A. C. Sartorelli and D. G. Johns, eds.), pp. 484–511, Springer-Verlag, New York.

BENNETT, L. L., JR., SCHABEL, F. M., JR., AND SKIPPER, H. E., 1956, Studies on the mode of action of azaserine, *Arch. Biochem. Biophys.* **64**:423.

BENNETT, L. L., JR., BROCKMAN, R. W., SCHNEBLI, R. W., CHUMLEY, H. P., CHUMLEY, S., DIXON, G. J., SCHABEL, F. M., JR., DULMADGE, E. A., SKIPPER, H. E., MONTGOMERY, J. A., AND THOMAS, H. J., 1965, Activity and mechanism of action of 6-methylthiopurine ribonucleoside in cancer cells resistant to 6-mercaptopurine, *Nature (London)* **205**:1276.

BODEY, G. P., BRODOVSKY, H. S., ISSASI, A. A., SAMUELS, M. L., AND FREIREICH, E. J., 1968, Studies of combination 6-mercaptopurine (NSC-755) and 6-methylmercaptopurine riboside (NSC-40774) in patients with acute leukemia and metastatic cancer, *Cancer Chemother. Rep.* **52**:315.

BODEY, G. P., GOTTLIEB, J., McCREDIE, K. B., AND FREIREICH, E. J., 1974, Arabinosyl adenine (Ara-A) as an antitumor agent, *Proc. Am. Assoc. Cancer Res.* **15**:129.

BRINK, J. J., AND LePAGE, G. A., 1964a, Metabolic effects of 9-arabinosylpurines in ascites tumor cells, *Cancer Res.* **24**:312.

BRINK, J. J., AND LePAGE, G. A., 1964b, Metabolism and distribution of 9-β-D-arabinofuranosyladenine in mouse tissues, *Cancer Res.* **24**:1042.

BRINK, J. J., AND LePAGE, G. A., 1965, 9-β-D-Arabinofuranosyladenine as an inhibitor of metabolism in normal and neoplastic cells, *Can. J. Biochem.* **43**:1.

BROCKMAN, R. W., 1960, A mechanism of resistance to 6-mercaptopurine: Metabolism of hypoxanthine and 6-mercaptopurine by sensitive and resistant neoplasms, *Cancer Res.* **20**:63.

BROCKMAN, R. W., 1963, Biochemical aspects of mercaptopurine inhibition and resistance, *Cancer Res.* **23**:1191.

BURCHENAL, J. H., MURPHY, M. L., ELLISON, R. R., SYKES, M. P., TAN, T. C., LEONE, L. A., KARNOFSKY, D. A., CRAVER, L. F., DARGEON, H. W., AND RHOADS, C. P., 1953, Clinical evaluation of a new antimetabolite, 6-mercaptopurine, in the treatment of leukemia and allied diseases, *Blood* 8:965.

CALDWELL, I. C., HENDERSON, J. F., AND PATERSON, A. R. P., 1967, Resistance to purine ribonucleoside analogues in an ascites tumor, *Can. J. Biochem.* 45:735.

CASS, C. E., AND AU-YEUNG, T., 1976, Enhancement of 9-β-D-arabinofuranosyladenine cytotoxicity to mouse leukemia L1210 cells *in vitro* by 2'-deoxycoformycin, *Cancer Res.* 36:1508.

CH'IEN, T., SCHABEL, F. M., JR., AND ALFORD, C. A., JR., 1973, Arabinosyl nucleosides and nucleotides, in: *Selective Inhibitors of Viral Functions* (W. A. Carter, ed.), pp. 227–258, CRC Press, Cleveland, Ohio.

DAVIDSON, J. D., AND WINTER, T. S., 1964, Purine nucleoside pyrophosphorylases in 6-mercaptopurine-sensitive and -resistant human leukemias, *Cancer Res.* 24:261.

DEWALD, H. A., AND MOORE, A. M., 1956, 6-Diazo-5-oxo-L-norleucine, a new tumor-inhibitory substance. Preparation of L (D and L) forms, American Chemical Society, 129th meeting, Abstract 13–14M.

EHRLICH, J., COFFEY, G. L., FISHER, M. W., HILLEGAS, A. B., KOHBERGER, D. L., MACHAMER, H. E., RIGHTSEL, W. A., AND ROEGNER, F. R., 1956, 6-Diazo-5-oxo-L-norleucine, a new tumor-inhibitory substance. I. Biologic studies, *Antibiot. Chemother.* 6:487.

ELION, G. B., 1967, Biochemistry and pharmacology of purine analogues, *Fed. Proc. Fed. Amer. Soc. Exp. Biol.* 26:898.

ELION, G. B., AND HITCHINGS, G. H., 1955, The synthesis of 6-thioguanine, *J. Amer. Chem. Soc.* 77:1676.

ELION, G. B., BIEBER, S., AND HITCHINGS, G. H., 1954, The fate of 6-mercaptopurine in mice, *Ann. N. Y. Acad. Sci.* 60:297.

ELION, G. B., CALLAHAN, S., RUNDLES, R. W., AND HITCHINGS, G. H., 1963a, Relationship between metabolic fates and antitumor activities of thiopurines, *Cancer Res.* 23:1207.

ELION, G. B., CALLAHAN, S., NATHAN, H., BIEBER, S., RUNDLES, R. W., AND HITCHINGS, G. H., 1963b, Potentiation by inhibition of drug degradation: 6-Substituted purines and xanthine oxidase, *Biochem. Pharmacol.* 12:85.

ELLIS, D. B., AND LEPAGE, G. A., 1963, Biochemical studies of resistance to 6-thioguanine, *Cancer Res.* 23:436.

ELLISON, R. R., 1973, Acute myelocytic leukemia, in: *Cancer Medicine* (J. F. Holland and E. Frie, eds.), pp. 1199–1234, Lea and Febiger, Philadelphia.

ELLISON, R. R., KARNOFSKY, D. A., STERNBERG, S. S., MURPHY, M. L., AND BURCHENAL, J. H., 1954, Clinical trials of O-diazoacetyl-L-serine (azaserine) in neoplastic disease, *Cancer* 7:801.

FREIREICH, E. J., BODEY, G. P., HARRIS, J. E., AND HART, J. S., 1967, Therapy for acute granulocytic leukemia, *Cancer Res.* 27:2573.

FURTH, J. J., AND COHEN, S. S., 1967, Inhibition of mammalian DNA polymerase by the 5'-triphosphate of 9-β-D-arabinofuranosyladenine, *Cancer Res.* 27:1528.

FURTH, J. J., AND COHEN, S. S., 1968, Inhibition of mammalian DNA polymerase by the 5'-triphosphate of 1-β-D-arabinofuranosylcytosine and the 5'-triphosphate of 9-β-D-arabinofuranosyladenine, *Cancer Res.* 28:2061.

HAMILTON, L., AND ELION, G. B., 1954, The fate of 6-mercaptopurine in man, *Ann. N. Y. Acad. Sci.* 60:304.

HARTMAN, S. C., 1963, The interaction of 6-diazo-5-oxo-L-norleucine with phosphoribosyl-pyrophosphate amidotransferase, *J. Biol. Chem.* 238:3036.

HENDERSON, J. F., AND JUNGA, I. G., 1960, Potentiation of carcinostasis by combinations of thioguanine and 6-mercaptopurine, *Biochem. Pharmacol.* 5:167.

HENDERSON, J. F., AND LEPAGE, G. A., 1959, Utilization of host purines by transplanted tumors, *Cancer Res.* 19:67.

HENDERSON, J. F., LEPAGE, G. A., AND McIVOR, F. A., 1957, Observations on the action of azaserine in mammalian tissues, *Cancer Res.* 17:609.

HERSH, E. M., AND LEPAGE, G. A., 1971, Effect of arabinosyl-6-mercaptopurine on the blastogenic responses *in vitro* of human lymphocytes to mitogenic agents, *Biochem. Pharmacol.* 20:2459.

HITCHINGS, G. H., AND ELION, G. B., 1954, The chemistry and biochemistry of purine analogs, *Ann. N. Y. Acad. Sci.* 60:195.

HITCHINGS, G. H., AND ELION, G. B., 1969, The role of antimetabolites in immuno-suppression and transplantation, *Acc. Chem. Res.* 2:202.

HOLLAND, J. F., GEHAN, E. A., BRINDLEY, C. O., DEDRICK, M. M., OWENS, A. H., JR., SNIDER, B. J., TAYLOR, R., FREI, E., III, SELAWREY, O. S., REGELSON, W., AND HALL, T. C., 1961, A comparative study of optional medical care with and without azaserine in multiple myeloma, *Clin. Pharmacol. Ther.* **2**:22.

HORTON, J., MITTELMAN, A., TAYLOR, S. G., III, JURKOWITZ, L., BENNETT, J. M., EZDINLI, E., COLSKY, J., AND HANLEY, J. A., 1975, Phase II trials with procarbazine (NSC 77213), streptozotocin (NSC85998), 6-thioguanine (NSC 752) and CCNU (NSC79037) in patients with metastatic cancer of the large bowel, *Cancer Chemother. Rep.* **59**:333.

HUBERT-HABART, M., AND COHEN, S. S., 1962, The toxicity of 9-β-D-arabinofuranosyl-adenine to purine-requiring *Escherichia coli*, *Biochim. Biophys. Acta* **59**:468.

IWAMOTO, R. H., ACTON, E. M., AND GOODMAN, L., 1963, 2'-Deoxythioguanosine and related nucleosides, *J. Med. Chem.* **6**:684.

JACQUEZ, J. A., AND SHERMAN, J. H., 1962, Enzymatic degradation of azaserine, *Cancer Res.* **22**:56.

KAMMEN, H. O., AND HURLBERT, R. B., 1959, The formation of cytidine nucleotides and RNA cytosine from orotic acid by the Novikoff tumor *in vitro*, *Cancer Res.* **19**:654.

KIDDER, G. W., DEWEY, V. C., PARKS, R. E., JR., AND WOODSIDE, G. L., 1949, Purine metabolism in Tetrahymena and its relation to malignant cells in mice, *Science* **109**:511.

KIMBALL, A. P., LEPAGE, G. A., AND BOWMAN, B., 1964, The metabolism of 9-arabinosyl-6-mercaptopurine in normal and neoplastic tissues, *Can. J. Biochem.* **42**:1753.

KIMBALL, A. P., BOWMAN, B., BUSH, P. S., HERRIOT, J., AND LEPAGE, G. A., 1966, Inhibitory effects of the arabinosides of 6-mercaptopurine and cytosine on purine and pyrimidine metabolism, *Cancer Res.* **26**:337.

KIMBALL, A. P., LEPAGE, G. A., AND ALLINSON, P. S., 1967, Further studies on the metabolic effects of 9-β-D-arabinofuranosyl-9-*H*-purine-6-thiol, *Cancer Res.* **27**:106.

LEE, W. W., BENITEZ, A., GOODMAN, L., AND BAKER, B. R., 1960, Potential anticancer agents. XL. Synthesis of the β-anomer of 9-(D-arabinofuranosyl) adenine, *J. Amer. Chem. Soc.* **82**:2648.

LEPAGE, G. A., 1960, Incorporation of 6-thioguanine into nucleic acids, *Cancer Res.* **20**:403.

LEPAGE, G. A., 1964, Basic biochemical effects and mechanism of action of 6-thioguanine, *Cancer Res.* **23**:1202.

LEPAGE, G. A., 1968, The metabolism of α-2'-deoxythioguanosine in murine tumor cells, *Can. J. Biochem.* **46**:655.

LEPAGE, G. A., 1969, Alterations in enzyme activity in tumors and the implications for chemotherapy, in: *Advances in Enzyme Regulation* (G. Weber, ed.), pp. 321–332, Pergamon Press, London.

LEPAGE, G. A., AND GOTTLIEB, J. A., 1973, Deoxythioguanosine and thioguanine, *Clin. Pharmacol. Ther.* **14**:966.

LEPAGE, G. A., AND JONES, M., 1961a, Purinethiols as feedback inhibitors of purine synthesis in ascites tumor cells. *Cancer Res.* **21**:642.

LEPAGE, G. A., AND JONES, M. 1961b, Further studies on the mechanism of action of 6-thioguanine, *Cancer Res.* **21**:1590.

LEPAGE, G. A., AND SARTORELLI, A. C., 1957, Purine synthesis in ascites tumor cells, *Tex. Rep. Biol. Med.* **15**:169.

LEPAGE, G. A., AND WHITE, S. C., 1973, Scheduling of arabinosylcytosine and 6-thioguanine therapy, *Cancer Res.* **33**:946.

LEPAGE, G. A., AND WHITECAR, J. P., JR., 1971, Pharmacology of 6-thioguanine in man, *Cancer Res.* **31**:1627.

LEPAGE, G. A., JUNGA, I. G., AND BOWMAN, B., 1964, Biochemical and carcinostatic effects of 2'-deoxythioguanosine, *Cancer Res.* **24**:835.

LEPAGE, G. A., BELL, J. P., AND WILSON, M. J., 1969, Arabinosyl-6-mercaptopurine and arabinosyl-6-mercaptopurine-5'-phosphate: Comparison of their metabolic effects, *Proc. Soc. Exp. Biol. Med.* **131**:1038.

LEPAGE, G. A., LIN, Y. T., ORTH, R. E., AND GOTTLIEB, J. A., 1972, 5'-Nucleotides as potential formulations for administering nucleoside analogs in man, *Cancer Res.* **32**:2441.

LEPAGE, G. A., KHALIQ, A., AND GOTTLIEB, J. A., 1973, Studies of 9-β-D-arabinofuranosyladenine in man, *Drug Metab. Dispos.* **1**:756.

LEPAGE, G. A., NAIK, S. R., KATAKKAR, S. B., AND KHALIQ, A., 1975, 9-β-D-Arabinofuranosyladenine-5'-phosphate metabolism and excretion in humans, *Cancer Res.* **35**:3036.

LEPAGE, G. A., WORTH, L. S., AND KIMBALL, A. P., 1976, Enhancement of the antitumor activity of arabinofuranosyladenine by 2'-deoxycoformycin, *Cancer Res.* **36**:1481.

Loo, T. L., Luce, J. K., Sullivan, M. P., and Frei, E., III, 1968, Clinical pharmacological observations on 6-mercaptopurine and 6-methylmercaptopurine ribonucleoside, *Clin. Pharmacol. Ther.* **9:**180.

Loo, T. L., Lu, K., Richards, M. T., and LePage, G. A., 1970, Pharmacologic disposition of arabinosyl-6-mercaptopurine and β-deoxythioguanosine, *Pharmacologist* **12:**555.

Luce, J. K., Frenkel, E. P., Vietta, T. J., Issasi, A. A., Hernandes, K. W., and Howard, J. P., 1967, Clinical studies of 6-methylmercaptopurine riboside (NSC40774) in acute leukemia, *Cancer Chemother. Rep.* **51:**535.

Magill, G. B., Myers, W. P. L., Rheilly, H. C., Putman, R. C., Magill, J. W., Sykes, M. P., Escher, G. C., Karnofsky, D. A., and Burchenal, J. H., 1957, Pharmacological and initial therapeutic observations on 6-diazo-5-oxo-l-norleucine (DON) in human neoplastic disease, *Cancer* **10:**1138.

Maibach, H. I., and Epstein, W. L., 1965, Immune response of healthy volunteers receiving azathioprine (Imuran), *Int. Arch. Allergy* **27:**102.

Markinodan, T., Santos, G. W., and Quin, R. P., 1970, Immunosuppressive drugs, *Pharmacol. Rev.* **22:**189.

Miech, R. P., Parks, R. E., Jr., Anderson, J. H., Jr., and Sartorelli, A. C., 1967, An hypothesis on the mechanism of action of 6-thioguanine, *Biochem. Pharmacol.* **16:**2222.

Moore, E. C., and LePage, G. A., 1957, *In vivo* sensitivity of normal and neoplastic mouse tissues to azaserine, *Cancer Res.* **17:**804.

Moore, E. C., and LePage, G. A., 1958, The metabolism of 6-thioguanine in normal and neoplastic tissues, *Cancer Res.* **18:**1075.

Moore, J. A., Dice, J. R., Nicolaides, E. D., Westland, R. D., and Wittle, E. L., 1954, Azaserine, synthetic studies, I, *J. Amer. Chem. Soc.* **76:**2884.

Nelson, J. A., Carpenter, J. W., Rose, L. M., and Adamson, D. J., 1975, Mechanisms of action of 6-thioguanine, 6-mercaptopurine and 8-azaguanine, *Cancer Res.* **35:**2872.

Omura, G. A., 1975, Phase II trial of beta-deoxythioguanosine (β-TGdR, NSC 71261) in refractory adult acute leukemia, *Proc. Amer. Assoc. Cancer Res.* **16:**140.

Parks, R. E., Jr., and Agarwal, K. C., 1975, 8-Azaguanine, in: *Antineoplastic and Immunosuppressive Agents* (A. C. Sartorelli and D. G. Johns, eds.), pp. 458–467, Springer-Verlag, New York.

Paterson, A. R. P., and Moriwaki, A., 1969, Combination chemotherapy: Synergistic inhibition of lymphoma L5178Y cells in culture and *in vivo* with 6-mercaptopurine and 6(methylmercapto)purine ribonucleoside, *Cancer Res.* **29:**681.

Paterson, A. R. P., and Sutherland, A., 1964, Metabolism of 6-mercaptopurine ribonucleoside by Ehrlich ascites carcinoma cells, *Can. J. Biochem.* **42:**1415.

Pavan-Langston, D., Buchanan, R. A., and Alford, C. A., Jr. (eds.), 1975, *Adenine Arabinoside: An Antiviral Agent*, Raven Press, New York.

Peery, A., and LePage, G. A., 1969, Formation of nucleotides from α,β-2′-deoxythioguanosine in extracts of murine and human tissues, *Cancer Res.* **29:**617.

Reddy, G. V. R., Goulian, M., and Hendler, S., 1971, Inhibition of *Escherichia coli* DNA polymerase II by Ara-CTP, *Nature (London) New Biol.* **234:**286.

Reist, E. J., Benitez, A., Goodman, L., Baker, B. R., and Lee, W. W., 1962, Potential anti-cancer agents LXXVI. Synthesis of purine nucleosides of β-arabinofuranose, *J. Org. Chem.* **27:**3274.

Rosman, M., and Williams, H. E., 1973, Leukocyte purine phosphoribosyltransferases in human leukemias sensitive and resistant to 6-thiopurines, *Cancer Res.* **33:**1202.

Rosman, M., Lee, M. H., Creasey, W. A., and Sartorelli, A. C., 1974, Mechanism of resistance to 6-thiopurines in human leukemia, *Cancer Res.* **34:**1952.

Sartorelli, A. C., and LePage, G. A., 1957, Modification of thioguanine toxicity in tumor-bearing mice with bone marrow transplants, *Proc. Amer. Assoc. Cancer Res.* **2:**246.

Sartorelli, A. C., and LePage, G. A., 1958a, The development and biochemical characterization of resistance to azaserine in a TA3 ascites carcinoma, *Cancer Res.* **18:**457.

Sartorelli, A. C., and LePage, G. A., 1958b, Metabolic effects of thioguanine II. *In vivo* and *in vitro* biosynthesis of nucleic acid purines, *Cancer Res.* **18:**1329.

Scannell, J. P., and Hitchings, G. H., 1966, Thioguanine in deoxyribonucleic acid from tumors of 6-mercaptopurine-treated mice, *Proc. Soc. Exp. Biol. Med.* **122:**627.

Schmidt, L. H., Montgomery, J. A., Laster, W. R., and Schabel, F. M., Jr., 1970, Combination therapy with arabinosyl cytosine and thioguanine, *Proc. Am. Assoc. Cancer Res.* **11:**70.

Schroeder, J. M., Ansfield, F. J., Curreri, A. R., and LePage, G. A., 1964, Toxicity and clinical trial of azaserine and 6-thioguanine in advanced solid malignant neoplasms, *Br. J. Cancer* **18:**449.

SKIPPER, H. E., SCHABEL, F. M., JR., AND BENNETT, L. L., JR., 1954, Mechanism of action of azaserine, *Fed. Proc. Fed. Amer. Soc. Exp. Biol.* **13**:298.

SKIPPER, H. E., ROBINS, R. K., THOMSON, J. R., CHENG, C. C., BROCKMAN, R. W., AND SCHABEL, F. M., JR., 1957, Structure–activity relationships observed on screening a series of pyrazolopyrimidines against experimental neoplasms, *Cancer Res.* **17**:579.

SKIPPER, H. E., MONTGOMERY, J. A., THOMSON, J. R., AND SCHABEL, F. M., JR., 1959, Structure–activity relationships and cross-resistance observed on evaluation of a series of purine analogs against experimental neoplasms, *Cancer Res.* **19**:425.

STERNBERG, S. S., AND PHILIPS, F. S., 1957, Azaserine: Pathological and pharmacological studies, *Cancer* **19**:889.

STOCK, C. C., REILLY, H. C., BUCKLEY, S. M., CLARKE, D. A., AND RHOADS, C. P., 1954, Azaserine, a new tumor-inhibitory substance, *Nature (London)* **173**:72.

TAMAOKI, T., AND LEPAGE, G. A., 1975, Inhibition of DNA chain growth by α-2′-deoxythioguanosine, *Cancer Res.* **35**:1015.

TIDD, D. M., AND PATERSON, A. R. P., 1974, A biochemical mechanism for the delayed cytotoxic reaction of 6-mercaptopurine, *Cancer Res.* **34**:738.

YORK, J. L., AND LEPAGE, G. A., 1966, A proposed mechanism for the action of 9-β-O-arabinofuranosyladenine as an inhibitor of the growth of some ascites cells, *Can. J. Biochem.* **44**:19.

12

Pyrimidine Antagonists

FRANK MALEY

1. Introduction

1.1. Logic Behind the Development and Use of Metabolic Antagonists

In order for any pathological state to be treated successfully by chemotherapy, an exploitable biochemical difference must exist between the host and its unwelcome visitor. While this approach has been eminently successful in the case of bacterial, fungal, and, to some extent, parasitic infections, less impressive results, unfortunately, have been obtained with neoplastic disease. The reasons for this dichotomy become obvious when metabolic and structural differences between the host and the invading organisms are enumerated, differences that may be exploited with metabolic antagonists that are selectively toxic to the offending cells, but do little or no damage to the host. The rationale for this fact has been amply documented in the case of the microbial antibiotics, and has become the key to successful chemotherapy. Thus, the peptidoglycan component of the bacterial cell wall, a material completely foreign to animal cells, is impaired at specific steps in its synthesis by penicillin and bacitracin with little detriment to the host (Strominger, 1968–1969; Storm and Strominger, 1974). In a similar vein, the cell wall of fungi is damaged by the polyene antibiotics (Novak, 1971).

Another area in which metabolic antagonists have been successfully employed is in the realm of bacterial nutrition. Because most microorganisms must synthesize their vitamins *de novo* in order to survive, a feature foreign to animal nutrition, any drug that impairs an organism's capacity to synthesize a vitamin selectively destroys its ability to survive in an animal host. An early example of this atavistic approach to chemotherapy utilized the antagonism between sulfanilamide and *p*-aminobenzoic acid (Woods, 1940), in which the latter was eventually shown to be

FRANK MALEY ● Division of Laboratories and Research, New York State Department of Health, Albany, New York 12201.

a precursor of folic acid. Since the animal host's requirement for folic acid is satisfied by its dietary supply, it is not placed at the same disadvantage as a bacterium that can neither synthesize its own nor utilize the host's source of folic acid.

Selective toxicity can also be achieved by exploiting the differential sensitivity to inhibitors of enzymes common to two species. This technique has been rather impressively employed with dihydrofolate reductase (Hitchings, 1973), the enzyme from bacteria having been shown to be about 10^4 times more sensitive to trimethoprim than that from animal tissue. By combining this drug with another that prevents folic acid synthesis, such as sulfamethoxazole, a two-pronged assault on a bacterium's capacity to synthesize and to utilize an essential component in its metabolism is effected.

The examples above are presented to illustrate what is hoped for in a rational approach to chemotherapy.

1.2. Why Logic Can Fail

Because a high degree of success in the treatment of microbial disease has been achieved, due in large measure to the logical extension of information gathered on microbial metabolism, it was anticipated that this approach, when applied to the treatment of neoplastic disease, would yield comparable dividends. Unfortunately, except for a few isolated instances, such has not been the experience for the following reasons:

1. The metabolic pathways and nutritional requirements of normal and neoplastic cells are in most cases basically identical. Because of this similarity, antimetabolites directed against the latter cells are also toxic to the former, requiring extreme care in the administration of these agents. This lack of selectivity often manifests itself in the extremely dangerous states of immunosuppression and bone marrow depletion.
2. The structural organization and organelle composition of normal and neoplastic cells are not dissimilar enough to exploit.
3. A significant differential sensitivity of vital enzymes to metabolic antagonists has not yet become apparent.
4. In those cases in which some degree of selective toxicity has been obtained, resistance to the cytotoxic agent often develops.

Despite these limitations, which cannot help but provide an adverse climate for chemotherapy, significant enough advances have been made in some areas of treatment to warrant further development and study. It is the purpose of this chapter to explore those pyrimidine antagonists that have shown promise, to discuss why they are of limited utility, and to review what has been done recently to improve their effectiveness. In addition, their future prospects in the treatment of cancer will be considered.

A rational approach to the design of pyrimidine antagonists requires that detailed information on the biosynthesis and metabolism of pyrimidines be available, with particular emphasis on those sites that, because of their location, are sensitive to attack. Since an adequate description of the biosynthesis and utilization of pyrimidine nucleotides has been documented in several reviews (Reichard, 1959b; Crosbie, 1960; Henderson and Paterson, 1973), this subject will not be elaborated on further. For purposes of discussion, however, schematics describing the known pathways for pyrimidine biosynthesis (Fig. 1) and deoxynucleotide interconversion (Fig. 2) are presented. The structures of most of the antagonists discussed in this article are indicated in Fig. 3.

2.1. Cytosine Arabinoside

2.1.1. Background

The story of the nucleoside arabinosides provides an excellent example of the way scientific endeavor in one area may be useful in another. Little was it realized at the time of their discovery in the sponge, *Cryptotethia crypta* (Bergmann and Feeney,

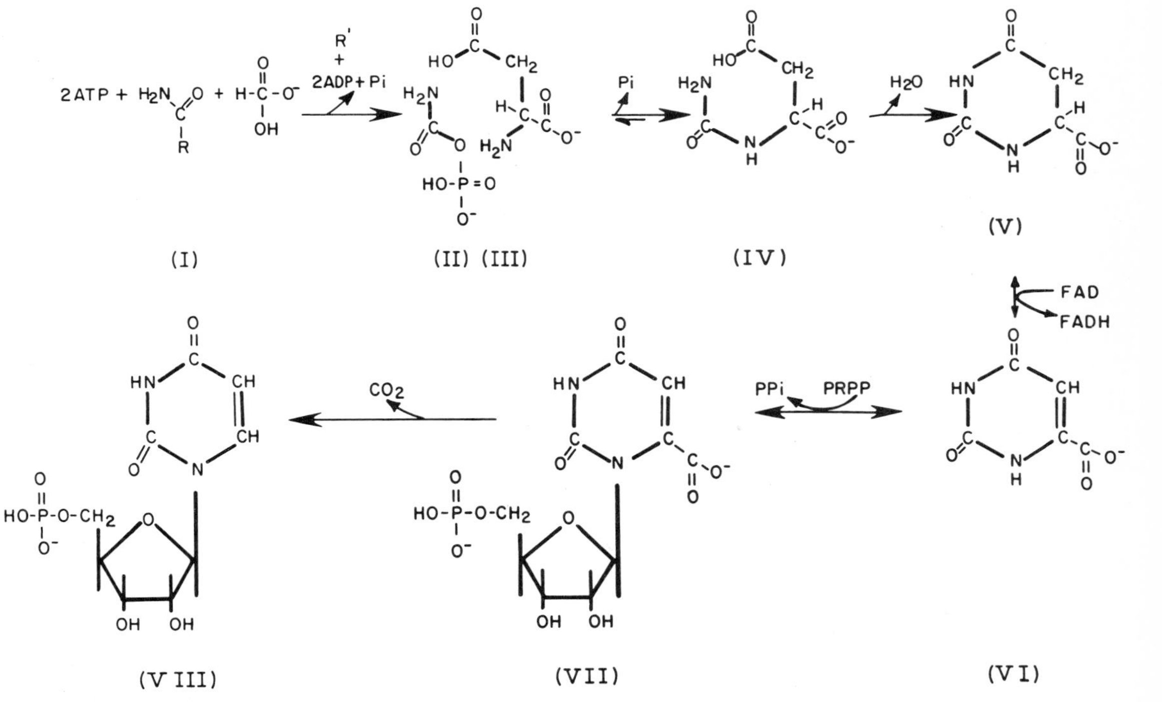

FIGURE 1. Biosynthesis *de novo* of UMP. (I) Glutamine; (II) carbamylphosphate; (III) aspartic acid; (IV) carbamyl aspartic acid; (V) dihydroorotic acid; (VI) orotic acid; (VII) orotidylic acid; (VIII) UMP; (PRPP) 5-phosphoribosyl pyrophosphate.

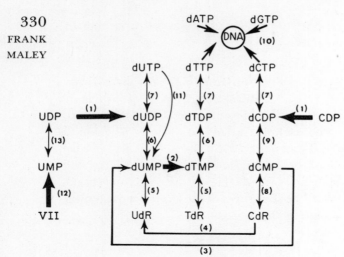

FIGURE 2. Ribo- and deoxyribonucleotide interconversions. (1) Ribonucleotide reductase; (2) thymidylate synthetase; (3) deoxycytidylate deaminase; (4) cytidine-deoxycytidine deaminase; (5) deoxyuridine-thymidine kinase; (6) thymidylate kinase; (7) nucleoside diphosphate kinase; (8) deoxycytidine kinase; (9) deoxycytidylate kinase; (10) DNA polymerase; (11) deoxyuridine triphosphatase; (12) orotidylate decarboxylase; (13) nucleoside monophosphate kinase. The heavy arrows indicate those sites against which the drugs have been developed.

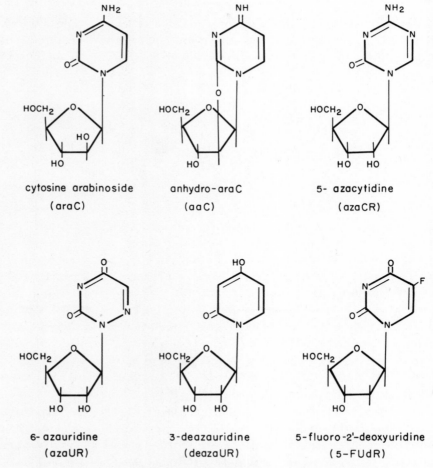

FIGURE 3. Structures of pyrimidine antagonists discussed in this chapter.

1950), that the arabinosides of uracil and thymine would lead to the application of analogues of these compounds to the therapy of specific tumors in man. Strangely enough, the first studies with these compounds were concerned with their role as potential intermediates in the biosynthesis of the pyrimidine deoxyribonucleoside (Pizer and Cohen, 1960; Reichard, 1959a). Shortly thereafter, a synthetic derivative (Walwick et al., 1959) of the naturally occurring arabinosides, cytosine arabinoside (1-β-D-arabinofuranosyl cytosine; cytarabine), was found to be an effective inhibitor of such mouse tumors as Ehrlich ascites cells, sarcoma 180, and L1210 leukemia (Evans et al., 1961). For more detailed presentations of the history, chemistry, and biochemistry of these fascinating compounds, earlier excellent reviews on this subject should be consulted (Suhadolnik, 1970a; Cohen, 1966).

2.1.2. *Metabolism*

Information relating to the metabolic interconversions of cytosine arabinoside is attributable to several groups, and follows essentially those routes described for CdR in Fig. 2 and below.

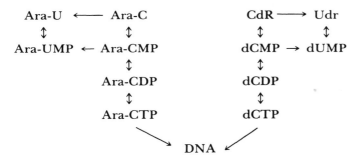

Despite the presence of hydroxyl at the 2′ position in place of the H of CdR, Ara-C is either phosphorylated by deoxycytidine kinase (Schrecker and Urshel, 1968; Kessel, 1968; Durham and Ives, 1968; Momparler and Fisher, 1968) or deaminated to Ara-U (Camiener and Smith, 1965). The enzyme effecting the deamination is referred to as a cytidine deaminase because its affinity for CR is greater than that for CdR.

In most tissues studied so far, the K_m of dexoycytidine kinase for CdR is from 5 to 10 times lower than that for Ara-C (Kessel, 1968; Durham and Ives, 1968; Momparler and Fisher, 1968), which in effect explains why the toxic effects of Ara-C can be reversed so easily. Because the deamination of Ara-C destroys its potency (Wilkoff et al., 1972), the effectiveness of Ara-C as a cytotoxic agent is determined by the outcome of the competition for this compound by deoxycytidine kinase and cytidine deaminase. This point becomes extremely important in attempting to maximize the efficiency of the drug and will be elaborated on further in Section 2.1.4. Ara-C can also be detoxified by deoxycytidylate deaminase, an enzyme that is elevated in mitotically active tissue (F. Maley and Maley, 1972), and is reported to convert Ara-CMP to Ara-UMP (Rossi et al., 1970). It is doubtful, though, that this enzyme is as effective as cytidine deaminase in inactivating Ara-C, but the two enzymes together, under the appropriate conditions, can protect mitotically active normal cells from the debilitating effects of this drug. It is this balance of deamination vs. phosphorylation in normal and neoplastic cells that determines where Ara-C can be used safely and effectively.

Following the phosphorylation of Ara-C to Ara-CMP, a specific phosphotransferase, deoxycytidylate kinase, converts the monophosphate to a diphosphate (Sugino *et al.*, 1966), which in turn is acted on by a nonspecific nucleoside diphosphate kinase (Nakamura and Sugino, 1966) to yield Ara-CTP.

2.1.3. Mechanism of Action

An early explanation for the effectiveness of Ara-C, which was based on the ability of CdR to reverse the toxicity of Ara-C, was that the drug prevented the synthesis of deoxycytidine nucleotides by inhibiting ribonucleotide reductase (Chu and Fischer, 1962). Although this explanation was a logical interpretation of the data at the time, one based on the same type of toxicity attributed to both AdR (G. F. Maley and Maley, 1960; Klenow, 1962) and TdR (Morse and Potter, 1965), more recent studies with purified ribonucleotide reductase (Moore and Cohen, 1967) appear to have eliminated this mechanism from serious consideration. A more likely explanation for the ability of CdR to reverse the inhibitory effects of Ara-C appears to reside in the favored status of CdR as a substrate for deoxycytidine kinase, an effect possibly enhanced additionally at the nucleotide level by competition from the natural nucleotides for the enzymes deoxycytidylate kinase, deoxycytidylate deaminase, and DNA polymerase. In the latter case, both dCTP and Ara-CTP appear to compete equally for the enzyme (Momparler, 1972).

Although there is still some uncertainty regarding the site most responsible for the cytotoxicity exhibited by Ara-C, it appears now that Ara-C is incorporated into both RNA (Chu, 1971) and DNA (Momparler, 1972; Graham and Whitmore, 1970), in support of the somewhat controversial early studies (Silagi, 1965; Chu and Fischer, 1968) on this subject. The incorporation into DNA would explain, in part, why Ara-C is an S-phase-cell-cycle-inhibitor, particularly if, as found in *in vitro* studies (Young and Fischer, 1968; Karon and Shirakawa, 1969), Ara-CMP, when incorporated on the 3'-terminal ends of DNA, prevents strand elongation. *In vivo* studies, however, demonstrating the incorporation of Ara-CMP into internal regions of DNA (Graham and Whitmore, 1970), and also those purporting to show that the lethal effects of Ara-C correlate with its incorporation into RNA (Chu, 1971), complicate this picture still further. Nonetheless, recent studies in both bacterial (Masker and Hanawalt, 1974) and animal (Steinstrom *et al.*, 1974) systems indicate that semiconservative replication is far more sensitive to inhibition by Ara-C than repair synthesis. Because the latter is subject to inhibition at more toxic levels of Ara-CTP, however, an explanation may be provided for why Ara-C inhibition eventually becomes irreversible and is associated with lethal chromatid breaks (Karon *et al.*, 1972).

It is fair to say at present that while the most probable site associated with the

cytotoxic effects of Ara-C is at the level of DNA, a completely satisfactory
explanation is wanting.

2.1.4. Effectiveness

Despite the severe toxicity exerted by Ara-C against the marrow, immune system, and intestinal mucosa, it is still the most effective drug used today for the treatment of acute myelogenous leukemia (Ellison *et al.*, 1968; Bodey *et al.*, 1969). Due to its extremely short half-life of about 15 min (Borsa *et al.*, 1969; Baguley and Falkenhaug, 1971; Ho and Frei, 1972; Mulligan and Mellett, 1968), a consequence of its rapid deamination and its limited site of action (the S phase), it must be given in judicious doses and at specific times to derive maximal benefit and minimal toxicity.

Because of these limitations, the drug must be administered by infusion according to a protocol that maintains a maximum number of leukemic cells in the dividing state, where they can be exposed to an optimal dose of Ara-C. As determined by several groups (Skipper *et al.*, 1967; Neil and Homan, 1973; Bhuyan *et al.*, 1973), the intervals between infusions should be short enough to prevent those cells in the G_1 phase from passing through the S phase of the cell cycle without being exposed to Ara-C, but long enough for those cells in G_2 to pass through M and G_1 and be exposed once again in the S phase to a lethal dose of Ara-C. Since the S phase in human leukemic cells is about 10 hr, and the therapeutic effectiveness of Ara-C is a function of the interval between doses, it has been estimated that this interval should be somewhat less than S (Momparler, 1974). With this protocol, it should be possible to trap an optimum number of leukemic cells in the S phase, as diagrammatically presented for L1210 cells in Fig. 4. By applying this technique of optimal scheduling, which has been so effective in treating L1210 mouse leukemia (Neil and Homan, 1973), to a patient who was unresponsive to conventional therapy, a 99% reduction in leukemic blast cells was achieved (Momparler, 1974).

The success of this type of protocol is based on the supposition that the drug does not trap cells in a specific phase for a considerable length of time following removal of the drug and that large enough doses can be given to destroy potentially resistant cells. Unfortunately, the use of such doses may be counterproductive, since it has been claimed that leukemic cells can be trapped in G_1 by Ara-C for several days (Yataganas *et al.*, 1974).

Despite the greatly improved remission rates obtained through the use of optimal scheduling techniques and single-drug protocols, the impressive cure rates obtained with L1210 mouse leukemia are still to be approached. This problem is invariably encountered in transposing drugs from the model animal system to the patient. One possible reason appears to be related to metabolic differences between the two, particularly the much higher cytidine deaminase levels encountered in man (Camiener and Smith, 1965; Ho, 1973). Another

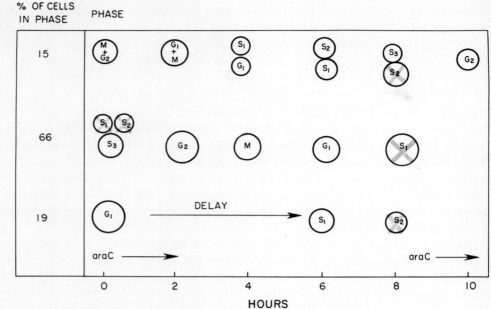

FIGURE 4. Effect of Ara-C on various events in the L1210 cell cycle. The stippled Xs indicate cells that are killed by Ara-C. The arrow shows the delay that may be effected by Ara-C as a result of cells being trapped in a specific phase for prolonged periods.

reason may be associated with the length of time that the model cell resides in the S phase relative to the total cell cycle, which in the case of L1210 is about 66%. This factor alone enables a rapid course of treatment to eliminate most of the leukemic cells, if not all. A similar type of treatment of human leukemia is rather severely compromised by the fact that the cells spend only about 25% or less of their time in the S phase (Momparler, 1974), making it much more difficult to achieve the desired optimum schedule of drug administration.

Another explanation considered responsible for the gradual loss in responsiveness of leukemic cells to Ara-C is the development of resistance. Primarily, this consists of the repopulation of the host with cells (normally 1 cell in 10^6) containing higher levels of cytidine deaminase (Stewart and Burke, 1971) or lower levels of deoxycytidine kinase (Tattersall *et al.*, 1974), the enzyme essential for the uptake of Ara-C. If both properties were incorporated in a resistant line, an even more difficult situation would obtain.

The problem of resistance based on enzyme levels has become even more difficult to interpret, since it has been found that the ratio of kinase to deaminase is determined by the maturity of the lymphoid line in question. By fractionating lymphoid cells on a ficoll-gradient (Coleman *et al.*, 1975), it was shown that the more mature the cell type, the higher the deaminase level, indicating that an elevated deaminase level in an unfractionated cell population may be related more to the proportion of granulocytes than to resistant cells. This consideration is extremely important when it is seen that the kinase:deaminase ratio can vary from 9.4×10^{-3} with unfractionated cells from a patient with acute myelogenous leukemia to 1.2×10^{-3} from one with chronic myelogenous leukemia, which compares with 0.5×10^{-3} from a normal marrow population.

Thus, while an elevated cytidine deaminase level is a logical explanation for the development of resistance to treatment with Ara-C, this situation is complicated, as discussed above, by the association of considerably higher levels of deaminase with mature cells and the report that decreased deoxycytidine kinase levels are associated with poor responses to Ara-C therapy. It would appear, therefore, that the nature of resistance is still to be clearly defined in human leukemia.

The rapid deamination of Ara-C has stimulated a search for methods to limit this hydrolysis. One such method has been to employ cyclocytidine, 2,2'-anhydro-1-β-D-arabinosyl-cytosine, a compound that is not deaminated until the anhydro ring is opened. With this compound as a reservoir of Ara-C, longer-lasting protective effects were obtained in the treatment of L1210 leukemia (Vendetti *et al.*, 1972). Because cyclocytidine appears to be an effective nontoxic reservoir of Ara-C, it has been proposed as a potential replacement for the continuous-infusion techniques now employed to maintain Ara-C levels in the bloodstream (Ho, 1974). Still another compound that acts as a reservoir of Ara-C is its 5'-*O*-adamantate (Gray, 1975), which, although inactive and insoluble, provides a slow, sustained release of Ara-C as it is hydrolyzed by serum esterases.

An alternate means of reducing the rate of deamination of Ara-C is through the simultaneous administration of a deaminase inhibitor. One such compound, believed to be a transition state analogue associated with the enzymic deamination of cytidine (Wentworth and Wolfenden, 1975), is produced on hydrogenating CR in the presence of a Rh–Al catalyst (Hanze, 1967). This compound, tetrahydroUR (H_4UR), possesses an affinity for cytidine deaminase that is 7000 times greater than that of the substrate. Studies in mice have revealed H_4UR to enhance the therapeutic effectiveness of Ara-C (Neil *et al.*, 1970), primarily by preventing the deamination of this compound.

H_4UR is probably phosphorylated *in vivo* by uridine kinase, and has been found to inhibit deoxycytidylate deaminase, but with about 1/100 the effectiveness of H_4dCMP (F. Maley and Maley, 1971). Thus, H_4UdR might be even more effective than H_4UR in maintaining Ara-C levels, since the deoxynucleoside analogue also inhibits cytidine deaminase, and because H_4dUMP is a much more potent inhibitor of deoxydytidylate deaminase than H_4UMP, deamination at both the nucleoside and nucleotide levels should be limited.

Another concept that has evolved in recent years in an effort to potentiate the therapeutic effectiveness of Ara-C is that of combination drug therapy, since it has become rather obvious that no one antimetabolite can eradicate a stubborn population of cancer cells. Its principle is based on the use of several drugs which attack at diverse sites rather than at a single site. This topic will be explored further in Section 3.

Recent interest in Ara-C as an immunosuppressive agent stems from observations that indicate that this compound also possesses antiviral activity against the herpes viruses (Gray, 1975). The clinical significance of a compound that possesses both immunosuppressive and antiviral properties is rather obvious, but unfortunately, clinically unfavorable responses in addition to the favorable ones have been obtained, and more work will have to be done in this area.

2.2. 6-Azauracil and Azauridine

2.2.1. Background

As in the case of most potential antimetabolites and antineoplastic agents, these symmetrical triazines and their derivatives, azathymine, azaorotic acid, and azacytosine, were first recognized for their antibiotic properties in studies with microbial systems. Application of these compounds to studies on tumor growth yielded encouraging results at first, but this encouragement was soon dispelled when azauracil (Aza-U) was found to cause neurological problems, and its antitumor activity appeared to be more carcinostatic than cytotoxic. These early studies have been extensively reviewed (Handschumacher and Welch, 1960; Škoda, 1963), and it appears that the 6-azapyrimidines as such are of little value clinically.

The nucleoside derivative, azauridine (Aza-UR), appeared to have a more promising future, since it was even more of an antimetabolite than Aza-U and possessed the added dividend of being nontoxic in animal studies, even at extremely high levels. The reason for the latter phenomenon will become apparent in the following review of the metabolism of this compound.

2.2.2. Metabolism and Mechanism of Action

The following scheme for the utilization of Aza-U was developed from studies with bacterial and animal systems, both of which indicated that a block is imposed by a derivative of Aza-U somewhere early in the pyrimidine biosynthetic pathway. This suggestion was derived from the observation that Aza-UR was considerably more effective than Aza-U against sarcoma 180 and the Ehrlich ascites tumor (Schindler and Welch, 1958). The nature of the site affected by the drug was implicated by the finding of orotidine in tumors and in the urine of animals treated with Aza-U (Habermann and Šorm, 1958; Handschumacher and Pasternak, 1958). Similarly, orotic acid and OMP were isolated from cultures of *E. coli* inhibited by Aza-U (Handschumacher, 1958). *In vitro* studies with a partially purified enzyme system clearly revealed that Aza-UMP formed from Aza-U, as indicated below, competitively inhibited orotidylic decarboxylase (Pasternak

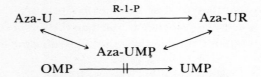

and Handschumacher, 1959). Of significance is the fact that once Aza-U is converted to Aza-UR, the latter cannot be hydrolyzed back to Aza-U. The irreversibility of this reaction accounts for some of the properties of Aza-UR described below.

In addition to being only marginally effective relative to other chemotherapeutic agents, Aza-U can pass the blood–brain barrier and, in some unknown manner, causes severe neurological symptoms (Handschumacher *et al.*, 1962). This problem can be obviated, however, by administering Aza-UR intravenously, since the latter cannot be hydrolyzed to Aza-U once it is in the bloodstream. By comparison with Aza-U, Aza-UR is essentially nontoxic, as judged by the fact that 40 g/kg per day can be given to patients by the intravenous route, with no noticeable symptoms (Cardoso *et al.*, 1961; Fallon *et al.*, 1961). Due to its rapid excretion, the maintenance of high levels of this drug was essential for effecting remissions.

To circumvent this problem, a compound was sought that could be administered intravenously or orally and would serve as a reservoir for the slow release of Aza-UR. This compound was found in 2',3',5'-tri-*O*-acetyl Aza-UR (azaribine), which when given orally is efficiently absorbed, in contrast to Aza-UR (Calabresi *et al.*, 1975). Unfortunately, the antineoplastic properties of this compound were not striking, and the small degree of hydrolysis to Aza-U that occurred in the intestine was cause for concern.

Although of little value against neoplasms, due possibly to compensatory mechanisms for producing higher intracellular levels of uridine nucleotides, azaribine yielded a bonus in being extremely effective against the noncancerous proliferative disorder of the epidermis, psoriasis (Calabresi *et al.*, 1975). The drug appears less toxic than methotrexate, which is also used to treat this disorder, and in cases in which such symptoms as anemia or neurotoxicity arise, they can be easily reversed with uridine.

2.3. *5-Azacytidine*

2.3.1. *Background*

Unlike 6-Aza-UR, this asymmetrical triazine is considerably more stable and more effective as an antimetabolite and antineoplastic agent. For a more extensive discussion of its chemical, biological, and clinical properties, earlier reviews should be consulted (Suhadolnik, 1970*b*; Heidelberger, 1973; Čihak, 1975).

Although first obtained by a synthetic procedure (Pískala and Šorm, 1964), Aza-CR was subsequently found as an antibiotic in cultural filtrates from *Streptoverticillum ladakanus* (Hanka *et al.*, 1966). In addition to its antibiotic properties, the compound was found soon after its synthesis to be cytotoxic to proliferating animal cells, particularly mouse embryo (Seifertová *et al.*, 1968), leukemia (Hanka *et al.*, 1966; Šorm and Veselý, 1964), and Ehrlich ascites cells (Šorm *et al.*, 1964). A precise reason for the cytotoxicity of Aza-CR is still not apparent, but a discussion of its metabolism may provide an explanation.

2.3.2. *Metabolism*

Most of the early studies with Aza-CR did not really clarify its metabolic interconversions, except to indicate that it was converted to nucleotides and incorporated into both RNA and DNA (Pačes *et al.*, 1968; Li *et al.*, 1970*a, b*). This incorporation was associated with a profound inhibition of protein synthesis (Doskočil *et al.*, 1967) by a mechanism that is not completely understood, but that occurs in conjunction with polyribosome dissociation (Levitan and Webb, 1969). Based on the information available, the following metabolic route has been assigned to Aza-CR, but since many of the individual steps have not been carefully investigated, much of it is conjecture (indicated by the broken lines).

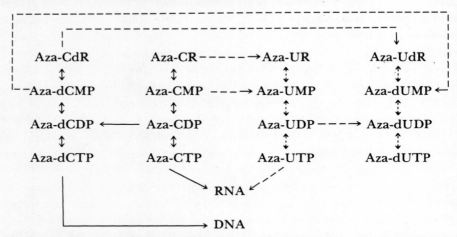

This scheme is based on studies with *E. coli* and leukemic mouse tissue in addition to extracts from normal tissue (Suhadolnik, 1970*b*; Čihak, 1975), using ^{14}C-labeled Aza-CR and Aza-CdR. Aside from being used as a metabolite, Aza-CR inhibited DNA synthesis to a greater extent than RNA synthesis in L1210 leukemia cells (Li *et al.*, 1970*a*), and appeared to inhibit *de novo* pyrimidine nucleotide biosynthesis (Rǎska *et al.*, 1965) in a manner similar to that of Aza-UR, although not as effectively. Thus, Aza-CMP was shown to inhibit OMP decarboxylase (Veselŷ *et al.*, 1967), but another potential inhibitor, 5-Aza-UMP, was not tested.

Little attention has been given to the contribution of the deamination products of Aza-CR metabolism to the observed cytotoxic effects, despite the finding that the inhibition of protein synthesis by Aza-CR was virtually eliminated in a cytidine deaminase-less mutant of *E. coli* (Doskočil and Šorm, 1970). The consequences of this deamination in animal tissues, which are known to contain a cytidine deaminase, do not appear to have been clearly delineated.

Regardless of the nature of the products of Aza-CR metabolism incorporated into the nucleic acids, particularly RNA, there is a dramatic inhibition of net protein synthesis, with variable effects on the activities of specific enzymes. Thus, induced enzyme synthesis is prevented in bacteria (Doskočil and Šorm, 1970), as is the hormone induction of tryptophan pyrrolase (Čihak *et al.*, 1967), serine dehydrase, and tyrosine aminotransferase (Čihak *et al.*, 1972). Explanations for these effects have ranged from an alteration in enzyme-specific mRNA (Čihak and Veselŷ, 1969) to defects in an RNA required for the proper initiation of translation (Reichman and Penman, 1973).

The effects of Aza-CR, when administered immediately after partial hepatectomy, are if anything cytostatic, since regeneration is not prevented but merely delayed, as evidenced by the delay in the synthesis of DNA (Čihak and Veselý, 1972) and the appearance of enzymes that normally increase after partial hepatectomy, i.e., ornithine decarboxylase (Cavia and Webb, 1972), thymidine kinase, and thymidylate kinase (Čihak and Veselý, 1972). These effects are apparently associated with an alteration in the state of the liver polysomes, which is eventually corrected with time, enabling the mRNAs associated with liver regeneration to be translated.

In contrast to the restrictions on enzyme synthesis indicated above, the synthesis of uridine kinase in rat liver is enhanced 4–5 fold by Aza-CR (Čihak and Veselý, 1973). This enzyme was suggested from earlier studies with Aza-CR-resistant leukemia cells to be involved in the initial uptake of Aza-CR (Veselý et al., 1967). It is of interest to note that while the uridine kinase was reduced considerably in the resistant line, the uptake of Aza-CdR was not impaired, indicating that deoxycytidine kinase was responsible for its utilization. Subsequent studies (Keefer et al., 1975) revealed that the resistant enzyme was somewhat altered in properties and associated with two isozymic forms, each increasing in response to Aza-CR, but to different degrees.

The enzyme that phosphorylates Aza-CR to Aza-CMP has been purified (Lee et al., 1974) 300-fold from calf thymus and clearly shown to be uridine-cytidine kinase. Its affinity for Aza-CR is only about a quarter of that for UR and CR, and the apparent K_m for Aza-CR in situ is probably much less, due to competition from the natural substrates. This limiting feature must be taken into account in maintaining effective tissue levels of Aza-CR during the course of treatment.

2.3.3. Mechanism of Action

As indicated above, several studies have shown the polyribosome content of cells to be diminished by Aza-CR, an effect believed to be in some way reponsible for the inhibition of protein synthesis. The molecular level at which this impairment may occur is in the processing of 45s RNA for ribosomal RNA, as first shown in HeLa cells (Reichman et al., 1973) and verified in Novikoff hepatoma cells (Čihak et al., 1974). Extension of these studies to nucleolar RNA (Weiss and Pitot, 1975) has revealed that the 45s RNA is processed to 32s, but that further conversion to the normal 28s and 18s ribosomal RNAs was blocked. Associated with this impairment in ribosomal RNA maturation was an incorporation of Aza-CR to the extent of 37% into the 45s and 32s ribosomal RNA precursors. The secondary structure of these RNAs relative to normal 45s and 32s RNA was apparently altered by the incorporation of Aza-CR, as judged by their comparative electrophoretic mobilities in acrylamide gel. Recognition of the altered RNAs by the appropriate processing enzymes could be affected and might explain the apparent defect in ribosomal maturation that results from the incorporation of Aza-CR.

Unfortunately, it is not clear whether the impairment in ribosomal processing is affecting protein synthesis, or whether continued protein synthesis is required for processing to take place.

2.3.4. Effectiveness

Aza-CR can be cytotoxic or nontoxic, depending on the conditions employed. These properties are clearly seen with growing L1210 leukemia cells, exposure of which for 24 hr to a concentration of 0.1–0.3 μg/ml reduced their viability by 90%, but under conditions in which the cells were dormant, Aza-CR was relatively inert (Lloyd et al., 1972). As indicated in Section 2.3.2, regenerating liver is relatively unaffected, except for a delay in the time that regeneration is initiated. It appears that Aza-CR, like Ara-C, is an S-phase drug, but because of the diverse number of metabolic sites affected by Aza-CR, it is difficult to establish the site most responsible for the loss in cell viability. It is possible that a combination of events may be contributory, but because the cell is most sensitive to Aza-CR in its S phase, the DNA synthesis site is a likely candidate. Supporting evidence comes from the findings that cell death is associated with chromosomal breaks (Li et al., 1970b) and that the viability of nondividing cells is unaffected (Lloyd et al., 1972). From the amount of Aza-CR required for a lethal effect, it appears that only a minor degree of incorporation is required to affect viability. The mechanism whereby this is affected can be direct or indirect; i.e., the replication of DNA is inhibited, or the transcription of essential mRNAs is impaired. The contribution of ribosomal RNA processing is questionable at present, since the concentrations of Aza-CR necessary to impair this process are much higher than those required to affect cell viability.

The potent toxicity of Aza-CR to mouse leukemias and to human acute myelogenous leukemia (Karon et al., 1973; McCredie et al., 1973) has made it a potentially useful drug for effecting remissions, particularly where Ara-C resistance has developed. This response to Aza-CR is possibly a consequence of Ara-C requiring deoxycytidine kinase for its phosphorylation and Aza-CR, uridine-cytidine kinase. The remissions effected by Aza-CR did not last as long as hoped for, which may reflect a decrease in the level of uridine kinase. Direct administration of Ara-C and Aza-CR simultaneously yielded an antagonistic response, but effective responses could be obtained when the antimetabolites were given several hours apart (Momparler et al., 1975).

Since Aza-CR has many undesired side effects, such as diarrhea, nausea, leukopenia, and hepatotoxicity, a means of limiting the quantities of this drug required for remission would be desirable. The necessity for such large quantities results from the rapid excretion of Aza-CR, and possibly from its competition in situ with CR and UR. Perhaps by the prior administration of 6-Aza-UR, the levels of the natural nucleosides could be reduced to a point at which lower doses of Aza-CR would be effective.

2.4. 3-Deazauridine

2.4.1. Background

In contrast to pyrimidine analogues containing three nitrogens, replacement of N_3 of the pyrimidine ring with a carbon atom (Robbins and Currie, 1968) yielded a molecule that inhibited the growth of microorganisms and tumor cells in culture (Wang and Bloch, 1972). One of the compound's most interesting properties is its ability to inhibit the growth of an Ara-C-resistant subline of L1210 leukemia cells. The manner in which this inhibition occurs is considered below.

2.4.2. Metabolism and Mechanism of Action

Unlike most nucleoside analogues, with the possible exception of Aza-UR, deAza-UR and its corresponding cytidine analogue are not hydrolyzed by nucleoside phosphorylase, a property much desired in nucleoside antagonists. These compounds are phosphorylated, though, and while the nucleotides inhibit nucleic acid synthesis, neither analogue is incorporated into RNA or DNA. Despite the impairment of nucleic acid synthesis (Wang and Bloch, 1972), protein synthesis is unaffected. The major block, as indicated below, appears to result from the

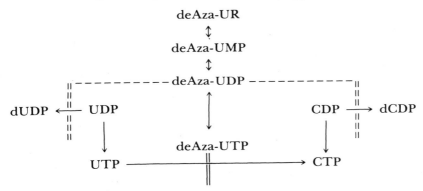

inhibition *de novo* of cytidine nucleotide synthesis, with deAza-UDP also acting as a competitive inhibitor of ribonucleotide reductase (Brockman *et al.*, 1975). Although some conversion of the deazauridine nucleotides to deoxynucleotides takes place, neither deAza-UTP nor its corresponding deoxy analogue is a substrate for RNA or DNA polymerase, respectively, which explains the apparent lack of deAza-UR incorporation in the *in vivo* studies.

2.4.3. Effectiveness

In a limited series, the drug was found to prolong the life span of animals with L1210/Ara-C from 2.2 to 9.2 days. Although of questionable utility alone, deAza-UR might be useful in enhancing the effectiveness of other drugs, such as 5-FU or Ara-C, by reducing the size of the CdR pool.

2.5. 5-Fluorouracil, 5-Fluorodeoxyuridine, and 5-Fluorouridine

2.5.1. Background

The rationale behind the development of 5-fluorouracil (5-FU), its biochemistry, and its use as a chemotherapeutic agent in animals and man have been extensively reviewed (Heidelberger, 1965, 1970, 1973).

While this drug and its various derivatives have proved to be more effective against specific mouse tumors than as a therapeutic agent in man, it has served as an extremely valuable model for the synthesis and study of other pyrimidine analogues. The chemical synthesis of 5-FU was stimulated by the finding that uracil was more efficiently and rapidly used by tumor cells than by normal tissue (Rutman *et al.*, 1954; Heidelberger *et al.*, 1957), and in an attempt to impair this utilization, fluorine, a known toxic element, was substituted for an H at the 5 position of uracil (Duschinsky *et al.*, 1975). Since this position is also occupied by the methyl group of thymine, it was reasoned that DNA synthesis might be inhibited. Not only did this early approach to chemotherapy work better than anticipated, but also a new era in the development of therapeutic pyrimidine antagonists was stimulated, an era that after two decades continues unabated today. Some of the mysteries of the mechanism of action of 5-FU are still being unraveled at the cellular and molecular level, and will be expanded on in Section 2.5.3.

2.5.2. Metabolism

From the numerous studies on 5-FU and FUdR anabolism, there is little doubt that these compounds follow the respective metabolic paths of U and UdR. As indicated below, 5-FU is converted to FUMP directly through the mediation of a phosphoribosyl transferase and PRPP (Reyes, 1969), or indirectly by the sequential action of nucleoside phosphorylase and R-1-P to yield FUR, followed by uridine kinase and ATP (Heidelberger, 1965, 1970):

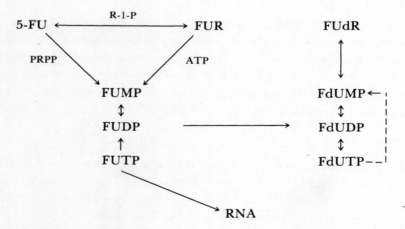

Additional phosphorylations to the di- and triphosphates (as indicated also for uracil and UR in Figs. 2 and 3) enables 5-FU to be incorporated into RNA. The deoxyribonucleotides of FUR are provided by ribonucleotide reductase (Kent and Heidelberger, 1972), or via the direct phosphorylation of FUdR by thymidine kinase. FdUTP is probably synthesized, but similar to dUTP, it is rapidly converted to the monophosphate by the action of a specific pyrophosphatase (broken line), which is normally elevated in proliferating tissue (Bertani *et al.*,

1963; Labow and Maley, 1967). It may be for this reason that neither UdR nor FUdR is found in DNA, but since dTTP is not a substrate for this enzyme, TdR is readily incorporated *in vivo*. The presence of a deoxynucleoside triphosphatase that restricts the incorporation of potentially detrimental nucleotides into DNA is not without precedence in biological systems, as evidenced by the deoxycytidine triphosphatase induced by the T-even bacteriophage (Wu and Geiduscheck, 1975; Kutter *et al.*, 1975). The evolutionary advantages of the enzyme to the phage are obvious from recent studies that indicate that the incorporation of deoxycytidine into the phage DNA in place of 5-hydroxymethyl deoxycytidine impairs the late stages of maturation of this organism in infected *E. coli*. The presence of a deoxyuridine triphosphatase in animal systems suggests that this enzyme plays an analogous protective role.

Similar to uracil, 5-FU is rapidly catabolized to CO_2, a metabolic route that is normally lower in dividing cells than in mitotically inert cells (Heidelberger, 1965, 1970, 1973; Weber *et al.*, 1970). Because of this catabolic process, higher levels of drug must be administered than would be necessary if FUdR and FUR were not hydrolyzed to 5-FU. The greater toxicity of FUdR relative to 5-FU can be rationalized on the basis of the former compound's slower rate of catabolism. For this reason, it is unfortunate that 3-deAza-FUdR has been found to be inactive as an antimetabolite (Nesnow *et al.*, 1973), since 3-deazanucleosides are not hydrolyzed by nucleoside phosphorylase.

2.5.3. Mechanism of Action

It was noted soon after the synthesis of 5-FU that the drug prevents the incorporation of labeled formate into the thymidine methyl group of Ehrlich ascites cell suspensions (Bosch *et al.*, 1958). Once the role of thymidylate synthetase in the formation of the methyl group was revealed (Friedkin and Kornberg, 1957; Friedkin, 1973), it became only a matter of time before FdUMP was discovered to be the inhibitor (Cohen *et al.*, 1958). The enzyme has since been purified to homogeneity from several sources (Dunlap *et al.*, 1971; Leary and Kisliuk, 1971; Fridland *et al.*, 1971; Horinishi and Greenberg, 1972; Galivan *et al.*, 1974), and found to react almost stoichiometrically and irreversibly with FdUMP, provided the methyl donor, $5,10\text{-}CH_2H_4$-folate, is also present (Santi and McHenry, 1972; Danenberg *et al.*, 1974; Santi *et al.*, 1974; Aull *et al.*, 1974). If the natural substrate, dUMP, is added simultaneously with FdUMP, the inhibition is less effective and competitive (Mathews and Cohen, 1963; Lorenson *et al.*, 1967). The overall reaction, as indicated below, requires a one-carbon donor in the form of serine, or a formate donor subject to reduction to the formaldehyde level, to convert H_4-folate to its active state, $5,10\text{-}CH_2H_4$-folate. The latter then reacts with dUMP in the presence of the synthetase to form a transient ternary complex (Danenberg *et al.*, 1974; Santi *et al.*, 1974), which dissociates rapidly, providing both the necessary reducing equivalents from the 6 position of the pteridine ring (Lorenson *et al.*, 1967) and the 5,10-methylene group to the 5 position of dUMP, to yield the products dTMP and H_2 folate. Any compound that either prevents the

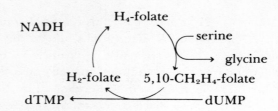

reduction of H_2 folate (i.e., methotrexate) or inhibits thymidylate synthetase directly (i.e., FdUMP) will impair DNA synthesis.

The mechanism of the synthetase reaction and its inhibition by FdUMP is currently under intensive investigation, and it appears that during the course of the inhibition, 2 moles of FdUMP become bound per mole of enzyme (Santi *et al.*, 1974; Galivan *et al.*, 1976). It has been proposed on the basis of model reactions (Santi and Brewer, 1973; Santi and Sakai, 1971) that a nucleophile from the enzyme adds across the 5,6 double bond of the pyrimidine ring to form a stable ternary complex composed of enzyme, FdUMP, and $5,10\text{-}CH_2H_4\text{-}folate$. The nature of this nucleophile has been investigated, and while preliminary evidence suggested it to be cysteine (Sommer and Santi, 1974), the latter could not be detected in a stable FdUMP-containing peptide from thymidylate synthetase. More recent studies (Bellisario *et al.*, 1976) on an FdUMP-nonapeptide isolated from a cyanogen bromide fragment of *Lactobacillus casei* thymidylate synthetase, however, implicate cysteine, as evidenced by the following sequence:

Ala-Leu-Pro-Pro-Cys-His-Thr-Leu-Tyr-
|
FdUMP

Verification of these findings has been obtained recently (Pogolotti *et al.*, 1976), completely erasing doubts that were raised regarding the involvement of cysteine (McHenry and Santi, 1974).

Although most of the evidence suggests that the inhibition of thymidylate synthetase is the most probable explanation for the cytotoxicity of 5-FU, not all of the existing tumor inhibition data can be explained on this basis. Thus, in some instances, the inhibitory action of 5-FU on cell cultures cannot be completely reversed by thymidine, and may be related to the ability of 5-FU to impair the maturation of ribosomal RNA (Wilkinson *et al.*, 1975), as was described for Aza-CR (Reichman *et al.*, 1973; Čihak *et al.*, 1974; Weiss and Pitot, 1975). This effect can in turn impair the orderly sequence of events in the cell that culminates eventually in DNA synthesis. Cell death appears to correlate with chromosomal breaks (Taylor *et al.*, 1962), but whether this effect is due to "thymineless death" (Barner and Cohen, 1957), a consequence of dTMP depletion, is not known.

In addition, it has been shown in microbial systems that the incorporation of 5-FU into messenger RNA can alter the latter's coding properties to the extent of providing aberrant proteins (Heidelberger, 1965; Mandel, 1969). It is possible, though not yet proved, that 5-FU can have a similar mutagenic effect on animal proteins.

Unlike Ara-C, which directs its cytotoxicity at the S phase of the cell cycle, 5-FU, while active mainly against dividing cells, has been claimed to kill cells at any stage of the cell cycle (Bruce and Meeker, 1967). The most sensitive phases, though, appear to be G_1 and S (Kovacs *et al.*, 1975). By selecting an inhibitor, such as vinblastine, that impairs the mitotic part of the cell cycle and an appropriate scheduling procedure, the inhibitory capacity of both drugs may be enhanced without incurring an increase in toxicity (Frankfurt, 1973). Similar results may be obtained with adriamycin, a drug with a fair degree of effectiveness against both dividing and nondividing cells (Barranco and Novak, 1974).

2.5.4. Effectiveness

Because the initial trials with 5-FU were directed against a tumor (sarcoma 180) that was very susceptible to the drug and could be eradicated with little toxicity to the animal host, there were great hopes that a comparable experience would be obtained with human neoplasms. Unfortunately, as has been the case too often when model systems are applied to man, results consistent with expectations were not realized. While probably the most effective drug in general use today against GI and breast cancer and tumors of the head and neck, 5-FU is more palliative than curative. This statement should be tempered, however, as a result of recent findings that indicate that the effectiveness of 5-FU against colorectal cancer can be greatly improved with radiation (Vongtama *et al.*, 1975), as can the treatment of breast cancer by combining cyclophosphamide and methotrexate with 5-FU (Bonadonna *et al.*, 1976).

Since 5-FU and its derivatives cannot discriminate between normal proliferating cells and cancer cells, these antagonists are extremely toxic to mucosal cells of the intestine and oral cavity, in addition to being very effective as myelosuppressive agents. Such adverse effects as leukopenia, anorexia, stomatitis, diarrhea, nausea, and vomiting are not uncommon in patients receiving the drug.

Recent studies with FUR, a compound initially reported to be more toxic and less effective than 5-FU, have indicated that this drug may be useful against leukemias and osteogenic sarcomas that have become resistant to methotrexate and vincristine (Burchenal *et al.*, 1975).

As with most other drugs, continued treatment results in resistance to 5-FU, which is usually associated with an alteration of the activity of enzymes necessary for the potentiation of the drug's effectiveness. In the case of 5-FU and FUdR, several enzymes have been implicated in the development of resistance through (1) a decrease in uridine kinase activity (Reichard *et al.*, 1962), (2) a decrease in phosphoribosyltransferase activity (Reyes, 1969), or (3) a resistant form of thymidylate synthetase (Heidelberger *et al.*, 1960). More recently, an 8-fold increase in thymidylate synthetase was found to be associated with a 2000-fold increase in resistance to FUdR by a line of mouse neuroblastoma cells (Baskin *et al.*, 1975). Unfortunately, an adequate explanation for the lack of correlation between the increase in enzyme activity and resistance was not found. Similarly, few examples of altered enzyme levels from 5-FU-resistant human tumors have been provided. In general, it has been difficult, even in model animal systems, to correlate the degree of resistance with an alteration in activity of a specific enzyme believed to be responsible for the resistance, since *in vitro* studies may not present a true measure of the enzyme's activity *in vivo*.

It is conceivable that in making assessments about resistance, intracellular levels of substrates relative to inhibitor should also be taken into account. The importance of such levels was emphasized recently (Myers *et al.*, 1974) in findings that suggest that the degree of thymidylate synthetase inhibition sustained in a cell and its capacity to recover from this inhibition are directly related to the FdUMP/dUMP ratio in that cell. Although the pool size of dTMP decreased markedly in response to 5-FU, the dUMP level increased to the point at which it could compete effectively enough with the synthetase for FdUMP to permit the reinitiation of DNA synthesis. The latter situation would prevail when FdUMP levels are diminishing, as in the case of the cessation of treatment. Also to be considered are salvage mechanisms that enable UdR and TdR to be converted more readily to their respective monophosphates as a result of the depletion of dTTP, a feedback inhibitor of thymidine kinase (Ives *et al.*, 1963). In any event, if the most effective antimetabolite effects are to be obtained, consideration must be given to the flux of intracellular substrates that may reduce the effectiveness of an inhibitor. Thus, in the case of 5-FU, conditions should be sought to reduce the level of UdR *in situ* with compounds that inhibit ribonucleotide reductase. In at least one instance (Ockey and Allen, 1975), the effectiveness of 5-FU was shown to be enhanced by hydroxyurea, a drug believed to promote this type of inhibition. Other compounds known to be ribonucleotide reductase inhibitors, such as the 2-formylpyridine thiosemicarbazones (Sartorelli *et al.*, 1971), should also be tested in this regard.

2.6. Other 5-Alkyl Pyrimidines

2.6.1. Ftorafur

A compound that has received considerable attention because it has been reported to be less toxic and more effective than 5-FU in the treatment of breast and colon cancer is the *N*-3 furanyl derivative of 5-FU, ftorafur [N_1-(2'-tetrahydrofuryl)-5-fluorouracil] (Smart *et al.*, 1975). The active component is still 5-FU, but because it is released only slowly from the ftorafur reservoir, results comparable to the prolonged intravenous administration of 5-FU, a technique that is normally used to lessen the toxicity of 5-FU, have been obtained. Ftorafur is currently undergoing more intensive clinical studies, although some of the earlier Russian work has been confirmed (Karev, 1972). It is of interest that the compound is completely inert with Ehrlich ascites cells in culture (Fujimoto *et al.*, 1976), indicating that the furanyl moiety is released by the liver or some other organ in the body.

2.6.2. Anhydro-ara-fluorocytosine

Because of the rapid deamination of Ara-C to an inactive product, anhydro-ara-fluorocytosine (2,2'-anhydro-1-β-D-arabinosyl-5-fluorocytosine) was prepared in an effort to circumvent this problem. It was reasoned that if Ara-FU was as inhibitory as its precursor, Ara-FC, a double-edged antagonist would be provided. Initial studies (Fox *et al.*, 1972) with intraperitoneally and intracerebrally inoculated L1210 leukemia indicated Ara-FC to be effective against both, probably by inhibition of DNA synthesis at the polymerase level, through Ara-FCTP and also thymidylate synthetase, via Ara-FdUMP. More recent studies (Kreis *et al.*, 1975) indicate that the anhydro derivatives of both Ara-C and Ara-FC are excreted rapidly, releasing insufficient amounts of Ara-C and Ara-FC to be effective against the leukemic cells. Unless more effective ways are found to enhance the levels of the active components of the anhydro compounds, it is questionable that they will become clinically important.

2.6.3. Trifluoromethylthymidine

a. Background and Metabolism. Originally designed as a second-generation pyrimidine substitute for FUdR, trifluoromethylthymidine (F_3TdR; 5-trifluoromethyl-2′-deoxyuridine) was found in clinical trials to be no more useful than either 5-FU or FUdR. However, because it is metabolized somewhat differently than FUdR, it may be very useful in the treatment of certain DNA virus infections.

A detailed analysis of F_3TdR catabolism and anabolism has been presented (Heidelberger, 1970, 1973), and briefly, this compound, unlike 5-FU, is completely ineffective as the free base; as such, it is catabolized to 5-carboxymethyluracil in animal cells. F_3TdR is, however, converted by thymidine kinase to F_3dTMP, and then to the triphosphate in the same manner as dTMP, where it is incorporated into DNA.

$$F_3TdR \rightarrow F_3dTMP \rightarrow F_3dTDP \rightarrow F_3dTTP$$
$$dUMP \not\Rightarrow dTMP \qquad\qquad DNA$$

As indicated above, F_3dTMP is also an inhibitor of thymidylate synthetase; however, not only are the kinetics of inhibition different, but its K_i is also about an order of magnitude higher than that for FdUMP, still a potent degree of inhibition (Reyes and Heidelberger, 1965). The nucleotide appears to bind slowly and irreversibly to the enzyme, but since the early studies were conducted with crude extracts, more definitive studies with pure enzyme are needed.

b. Mechanism of Action and Effectiveness. The most significant aspect of F_3TdR metabolism is its incorporation into DNA, which occurs most probably because F_3dTTP cannot be hydrolyzed by deoxyuridine triphosphatase (Bertani *et al.*, 1963; Labow and Maley, 1967). When incorporation does occur, DNA synthesis is disrupted, and mutagenic events are initiated (Heidelberger, 1975). One of the most exciting properties of F_3TdR is its effectiveness in the treatment of herpes simplex keratitis, in which it was shown to be 50–100 times more potent than other antiviral drugs, such as Ara-C, IUdR, and BUdR (Heidelberger, 1975).

Studies on the mechanism of action of F_3TdR at the molecular level have revealed that replacement of as little as 1.4% of the thymidine of vaccinia virus DNA inactivates the virus (Fujiwara and Heidelberger, 1970). Not only does this incorporation prevent a single round of cell division, which is usually permitted by BUdR and IUdR, but also the DNA and RNA transcripts were about 30% smaller than normal (Dexter *et al.*, 1973). In studies with the DNA polymerases from uninfected HeLa cells and from vaccinia virus, it was found that a greater degree of incorporation of F_3dTTP was supported by the enzyme from the latter source than that from the former, which in effect may explain the selectivity of the antiviral effect (Heidelberger, 1975).

2.6.4. 5-Mercapto-2′-deoxyuridine

This compound, like the other 5-substituted uracil derivatives, is an active antimicrobial and antitumor agent (Baranski *et al.*, 1969). Its main site of action appears to be thymidylate synthetase, where the 5′-phosphate derivative has been shown to be a competitive inhibitor, with an apparent K_i of 4×10^{-8} M (Kalman and Bardos, 1970; Bardos *et al.*, 1975).

2.6.5. 5-Vinyl-2′-deoxyuridine

Although few studies have been conducted with this compound, it is presented to indicate the versatility of 5-substituted UdR derivatives. In this case, the compound inhibits the growth of Ehrlich ascites cells (Langen and Bärwolff, 1975), apparently by being incorporated into DNA, similar to its 5-ethyl derivative (Swierkowska *et al.*, 1973). The effect of 5-vinyl dUMP on thymidylate synthetase was not indicated, but since most 5-substituted derivatives of dUMP inhibit the synthetase, it would be surprising if it did not do so too.

2.6.6. 5-Iodo-2′-deoxyuridine

The history of this compound's antimicrobial and antitumor activity has been thoroughly reviewed (Heidelberger, 1970; Prusoff, 1963). Like F_3TdR, it is not considered an effective antitumor agent, but on incorporation into DNA, it can disrupt the infectivity of such DNA viruses as herpes and vaccinia (Goz and Prusoff, 1970).

IUdR is metabolized like TdR and F_3TdR, and similarly to these compounds, it is incorporated into DNA, most probably because IdUTP cannot be hydrolyzed by deoxyuridine triphosphatase (Bertani *et al.*, 1963; Labow and Maley, 1967). Thymidine kinase, thymidylate kinase, and thymidylate synthetase are inhibited by derivatives of IUdR, but IUdR probably contributes its primary lesion to cellular metabolism by permitting only one round of semiconservative replication when incorporated into DNA.

A recent exciting development has occurred with the synthesis of the 5′-amino analogue of IUdR, which was shown to selectively inhibit viral DNA replication (Cheng *et al.*, 1975a, b). While it was apparently less potent than F_3TdR, its therapeutic index was greater, and unlike IUdR, Ara-C, and Ara-A, this com-

pound does not appear to exhibit any cytotoxicity. The latter effect results from
the apparent inability of this compound to be incorporated into the host's DNA
while being selectively incorporated to a lethal extent into the DNA of the virus
(Chen *et al.*, 1976).

349
PYRIMIDINE
ANTAGONISTS

3. Improving the Effectiveness of the Pyrimidine Antagonists by Combination Therapy

In retrospect, the original assumption that a single antagonist would be as effective
in the control if not the cure of cancer in man as in rodents was naive. It was for this
reason, coupled with the extraordinary clinical experience obtained with antibiotics, that so much was expected, so quickly, from cancer chemotherapy. To add to
the dilemma, which was encouraged in part by an excessive zeal for the all-too-
available research funds, results were slow in coming. Thus, the unbridled
optimism of the 1960s, encouraged by both scientists and the press, has culmi-
nated in disillusionment on the part of the public and their representatives, with
increasing demands for reasons for the apparent lack of progress.

We now have a better perspective on the cancer problem and can comprehend
many of the reasons for our past failures and the magnitude of the challenge
facing us. Whether these problems can be circumvented remains to be seen, but
they are just as monumental now as they were in the past. Let us look briefly at the
nature of some of these problems:

1. It was initially assumed that an exploitable metabolic or structural difference
   between normal and cancer cells would be found, as it had been for bacterial
   systems. Unfortunately, this assumption has not been validated, except in
   the case of leukemic cells and lymphomas, which have shown a greater
   requirement for folic acid (Heinle and Welch, 1948; Farber *et al.*, 1948) and
   asparagine (Broome, 1963). Even in this case, only limited success has been
   obtained in single-agent therapy with methotrexate and asparaginase. More
   recently, it has been reported that some neoplasms lack the capacity to
   synthesize methionine, making them candidates for high-dose methotrexate
   treatment and 5-methyltetrahydrofolate rescue, in place of leucovorin
   "rescue" (Halpern *et al.*, 1975).
2. The assumption that the growth patterns of normal dividing and neoplastic
   cells would be sufficiently different to enable the latter to be impaired with a
   minimum of damage to the former has been verified to only a very limited
   extent. In most instances, antagonists of DNA synthesis, particularly those
   that affect *de novo* synthesis, invariably damage both normal and neoplastic
   cells and are usually found to be immunosuppressive, toxic to mucosal and
   hemopoietic cells, teratogenic, mutagenic, and even oncogenic under certain
   circumstances, as recently described for 5-FU (Jones *et al.*, 1976) and Ara-C
   (Kouri *et al.*, 1975). In those cases in which cancer cells are more sensitive to

antagonists than normal cells, it is because of differences in growth synchrony and rates of cell division.

3. The degree to which neoplastic cells would become refractory to treatment was not anticipated. Although model animal systems have to some extent provided an explanation for the gradual evolution of resistant cell lines following treatment, this problem has still not been carefully evaluated in the human.

For these reasons and others, it became apparent soon after the introduction of single-agent chemotherapy that limiting the activity of a single critical enzyme is usually not effective enough to damage a cell irreversibly. This is particularly true in those instances in which "salvage" pathways are available to bypass the block imposed by a metabolic antagonist. Where effective drugs are available—such as methotrexate or 5-FU, compounds that bind almost stoichiometrically to critical enzymes involved in the synthesis of an essential DNA precursor—cells could be damaged irreversibly, but with indiscriminate selectivity. Even assuming that a population of cells could be selectively depleted without irretrievably affecting the normal dividing mucosal and marrow cells, resistant cells might evolve before the sensitive line is completely eliminated.

For dividing cells to be effectively assaulted, several factors must be considered (Sartorelli, 1969):

1. More than one site in a pathway should be hit, preferably in sequence, which in effect requires more than one agent. Thus, to impair purine synthesis, azaserine and 6-mercaptopurine should be administered simultaneously.

2. If two pathways meet concurrently to provide a common product, as in the case of purines and pyrimidines to yield DNA, specific sites in each should be blocked. The simultaneous use of 6-mercaptopurine and 5-FU would be indicated in this instance.

3. Complementary inhibition at the metabolite and final product level (DNA) should be more successful than inhibiting either step alone. An example would be the combined use of Ara-C and hydroxyurea or 1,3-*bis*(2-chloroethyl)-1-nitrosourea (BCNU) and 5-FU. Another example for which evidence of a marked synergistic response has been obtained is with the combination of Ara-C and Aza-UR (Brenkman *et al.*, 1973).

4. The inhibition must be effective enough at several sites to prevent resistance at one from impairing cell destruction.

The methodology currently employed in chemotherapy is therefore based on the logic that a combination of drugs directed against specific target sites involved in DNA synthesis, and also against the DNA itself, will optimize efforts to prevent DNA replication. Drugs such as adriamycin, daunomycin, BCNU, vincristine, Ara-C, and thioguanine are used in the latter case, while Ara-C and thioguanine may be used with 5-FU, hydroxyurea, asparaginase, and methotrexate to impair metabolite synthesis.

In addition, the precise scheduling of optimal doses has become of prime importance in maximizing effective responses, since it has been shown that high doses may impair the transition from one cell phase to another and complicate the administration of phase-specific drugs. Thus, Ara-C, a very effective synchronizing agent, potentiates the action of Aza-CR (Momparler *et al.*, 1975), as it does daunorubicin (Edelstein *et al.*, 1974), and requires that they be administered in an appropriate temporal sequence, and not simultaneously. High doses of Ara-C can cause cells to accumulate for prolonged periods in the G_1–S stage, while bleomycin effects cell synchrony at the S–G_2 boundary (Barranco *et al.*, 1973; Desai *et al.*, 1974), and hydroxyurea blocks cells in G_1 (Sinclair, 1967). With this information, not only can appropriate scheduling be undertaken, but also drugs can be deployed to specifically attack cells trapped in a specific phase, such as vincristine, which kills cells in the M phase (Valierote *et al.*, 1966), and daunomycin, which kills cells that are in G_1 (Silvestrini *et al.*, 1970). Unfortunately, the actual schedules and nature of drugs used are determined initially in model systems, and must finally be derived in a rather empirical manner, since there is a large margin for error in extrapolating from L1210 cells in culture to the human.

However, by accumulating and interfacing the information gained from the long-drawn-out procedure of clinical trial and mistrial, extremely effective protocols can be derived, as evidenced by that for the treatment of childhood acute lymphocytic leukemia (ALL) (Haghbin *et al.*, 1975). One such protocol requires a 24-week treatment period consisting of an induction phase of vincristine, prednisone, and daunorubicin, followed by a consolidation phase of Ara-C and thioguanine, and finally a maintenance phase of thioguanine, cyclophosphamide, hydroxyurea, daunorubicin, methotrexate, BCNU, Ara-C, and vincristine. Also required is a procedure to eliminate CNS leukemia by means of intrathecal methotrexate, cranial radiation, or a combination of both. With this schedule or variations of it (Simone *et al.*, 1975), remission rates of 90–100% and projected cures of up to 50% have been obtained.

It is obvious that we have come a long way from the initial promise of single-agent therapy to an extremely complex regimen of multiple drugs, precise doses, and appropriate timing. It is little wonder that results were so slow in coming, and they will, unfortunately, continue to come in this manner unless some dramatic breakthrough is achieved. For a more detailed account of the degree to which combination therapy has improved the treatment of various neoplastic diseases, a recent review (DeVita *et al.*, 1975) is available.

The accomplishments described above are not meant to detract from the successes achieved with single-agent therapy in certain cases. This success is evidenced by the results obtained in the treatment of choriocarcinoma with methotrexate, Burkitt's lymphoma with cyclophosphamide, and islet-cell tumors with streptozotocin (DeVita *et al.*, 1975). But the overwhelming evidence to date indicates that combination therapy is far superior to any single agent in both the *number* and *duration* of remissions. For example, the median survival for single-agent treatment of ALL was 6 months in 1956; by 1965, this survival was increased to 3 years through combination drug therapy, and with the current programs, a

50% potential cure rate (Simone *et al.*, 1975; DeVita *et al.*, 1975) has been projected. In the case of Hodgkin's disease, the median survival time has been increased from 2.5 years with single-agent therapy to more than 8 years with combination therapy (DeVita *et al.*, 1975).

More recently, the response rate for the treatment of breast cancer has been shown to be increased from 23% with 5-FU alone to about 60% with 5-FU combined with methotrexate, cyclophosphamide, vincristine, and prednisone (DeVita *et al.*, 1975). With the combination of 5-FU with radiation, greater than 5-year survivals have been reported for the treatment of colorectal cancer (Vongtama *et al.*, 1975). Even in the treatment of acute myelogenous leukemia, which has been extremely resistant to treatment, a 20% complete and partial remission rate with Ara-C alone has been increased to about 48% with a combination of Ara-C and thioguanine, or Ara-C and daunorubicin (Clarkson *et al.*, 1975; Carey *et al.*, 1975).

4. Prospects for the Future

While the pyrimidine antagonists were originally designed to impair specific steps in the *de novo* pyrimidine biosynthetic pathway, in the hope that nucleic acid synthesis would be prevented (see Fig. 1), they often accomplished more than was intended for them. If this were not the case, the use of these antagonists would be severely restricted. As it now stands, only a few, such as Ara-C, 5-FU, and Aza-CR, are of use clinically.

Where they are most effective, the antagonists both limit the synthesis of a specific metabolite and are incorporated into DNA. It is this latter property that is most responsible for the utility and effectiveness of the pyrimidine antagonists, particularly against the DNA viruses. An outstanding example of this incorporation is seen with Ara-C, which by being incorporated into nucleic acids kills cells in the S phase and, in the process, synchronizes the remaining cells to attack by other phase-specific reagents. It is apparent, therefore, that to be truly antagonistic to a cell, a pyrimidine analogue should possess properties similar to those of Ara-C.

Where metabolite limitation may be important is in those cases in which the normal supply of nucleotides may compete effectively with the analogue under consideration. Thus, reducing the *in situ* levels of CdR may be useful in promoting the effectiveness of Ara-C; in a similar vein, reducing the levels of deoxynucleotides, in particular dUMP, might enable a lower concentration of 5-FU or FUdR to elicit a desired response.

The pyrimidine antagonists, like most other anticancer agents, are basically nonselective in their action, although, as indicated above, some selectivity may be achieved in the treatment of acute lymphocytic leukemias and lymphomas. But, since these treatable types of neoplastic disease represent only about 7% of the total, one cannot accept this hard-won battle as a victory. No explanation is available at present for the lack of success in the treatment of acute myelogenous

leukemia in children and adults, or lymphocytic leukemia in adults (Clarkson *et*
al., 1975). Meanwhile, 52% of the cancers detected are too disseminated to be
reasonably treated, as the dose of chemotherapeutic agents necessary to reduce
the tumor to a manageable level would be too toxic to the patient. Before
chemotherapy can be useful in these cases, a more effective means of early
detection is essential.

One problem that has greatly limited the capacity to achieve optimally effective
responses with the pyrimidine antagonists, as with other chemotherapeutic
agents, results from our lack of knowledge about tumor cell metabolism. Even
with model animal systems, little is really known concerning the reasons for drug
resistance, and in the case of human tumors, even less information is available. If
definitive reasons could be established for the resistance of one type of leukemia to
treatment as compared with another, or even acceptable reasons for the evolution
of resistance during the course of treatment, perhaps better treatment schedules
and drugs might be perfected.

For the future, it appears that studies on the development of pyrimidine
antagonists will probably be restricted to improving those drugs and combinations
of them that are most effective at present, developing methods for limiting the
metabolic inactivation of drugs, and increasing their potential for virus inactivation.

5. References

AULL, J. L., LYON, J. A., AND DUNLAP, R. B., 1974, Separation, identification and stoichiometry of the
ternary complexes of thymidylate synthetase, *Arch. Biochem. Biophys.* **165**:805.
BAGULEY, B. D., AMD FALKENHAUG, E. M., 1971, Plasma half-life of cytosine arabinoside (NSC-63878)
in patients treated for acute myeloblastic leukemia, *Cancer Chemother. Rep.* **55**:291.
BARANSKI, K., BARDOS, T. J., BLOCH, A., AND KALMAN, T. I., 1969, 5-Mercaptodeoxyuridine—its
enzymatic synthesis and mode of action in microbial systems, *Biochem. Pharmacol.* **18**:347.
BARDOS, T. J., ARADI, J., HO, Y. K., AND KALMAN, T. I., 1975, Biochemical properties of 5-sulfur-
substituted pyrimidine nucleosides and nucleotides, *Ann. N. Y. Acad. Sci.* **255**:522.
BARNER, H. D., AND COHEN, S. S., 1957, The isolation and properties of amino acid requiring mutants
of a thymineless bacterium, *J. Bacteriol.* **74**:350.
BARRANCO, S. C., AND NOVAK, S. C., 1974, Survival responses of dividing and non-dividing mammalian
cells after treatment with hydroxyurea arabinosyl cytosine or adriamycin, *Cancer Res.* **34**:1616.
BARRANCO, S. C., LUCE, J. K., ROMSDAHL, M. M., AND HUMPHREY, R. M., 1973, Bleomycin as a possible
synchronizing agent for human tumor cells *in vivo*, *Cancer Res.* **33**:882.
BASKIN, F., CARLIN, S. C., KRAUS, P., FRIEDKIN, M., AND ROSENBERG, R. N., 1975, Experimental
chemotherapy of neuroblastoma, II. Increased thymidylate synthetase activity in a 5-
fluorodeoxyuridine resistant variant of mouse neuroblastoma, *Mol. Pharmacol.* **11**:105.
BELLISARIO, R. L., MALEY, G. F., GALIVAN, J. H., AND MALEY, F., 1976, The amino acid sequence at the
FdUMP binding site of thymidylate synthetase, *Proc. Natl. Acad. Sci.* **73**:1848.
BERGMANN, W., AND FEENEY, R. J., 1950, The isolation of a new thymine pentoside from sponges, *J.
Amer. Chem. Soc.* **72**:2809.
BERTANI, L. E., HÄGGMARK, A., AND REICHARD, P., 1963, Enzymatic synthesis of deoxyribonucleotides,
II. Formation and interconversion of deoxyuridinephosphates, *J. Biol. Chem.* **238**:3407.
BHUYAN, B. K., FRASER, T. J., GRAY, L. G., KUENTZEL, S. L., AND NEIL, G. L., 1973, Cell-kill kinetics of
several S-phase-specific drugs, *Cancer Res.* **33**:888.

BODEY, G. P., FREIREICH, E. J., MONTO, R. W., AND HEWLETT, J. S., 1969, Cytosine arabinoside (NSC-63878) therapy for acute leukemia in adults, *Cancer Chemother. Rep.* **53**:59.

BONADONNA, G., BRUSAMOLINO, E., VALAGUSSA, P., ROSSI, A., BRUGANTELLI, L., BRAMBILLA, C., DE LENA, M., TANCINI, G., BAJETTA, E., MUSUMECI, R., AND VERONESI, U., 1976, Combination chemotherapy as an adjuvant treatment in operable breast cancer, *N. Engl. J. Med.* **294**:405.

BORSA, J., WHITMORE, G. F., VALERIOTE, F. A., COLLINS, P., AND BRUCE, W. R., 1969, Studies on the persistance of methotrexate, cytosine arabinoside, and leukovorin in serum of mice, *J. Natl. Cancer Inst.* **42**:235.

BOSCH, L., HABERS, E., AND HEIDELBERGER, C., 1958, Studies on fluorinated pyrimidines, V. Effects on nucleic acid metabolism *in vitro*, *Cancer Res.* **18**:335.

BRENKMAN, W. D., JR., CHU, M.-Y., AND FISCHER, G. A., 1973, Schedule dependence of the lethal effects of 6-azauridine and cytosine arabinoside in murine leukemia cells (L51784) in culture, *Biochem. Biophys. Res. Commun.* **52**:1368.

BROCKMAN, R. W., SHADDIX, S. C., WILLIAMS, M., NELSON, J. A., ROSE, L. M., AND SCHABEL, F. M., JR., 1975, The mechanism of action of 3-deazauridine in tumor cells sensitive and resistant to arabinosyl cytosine, *Ann. N. Y. Acad. Sci.* **225**:501.

BROOME, J. D., 1963, Evidence that the L-asparaginase of guinea pig serum is responsible for its antilymphoma effects. I. Properties of the L-asparaginase of guinea pig serum in relation to those of the antilymphoma substance, *J. Exp. Med.* **118**:99.

BRUCE, W. R., AND MEEKER, W. R., 1967, Comparison of the sensitivity of hematopoetic colony forming cells in different proliferative states to 5-fluorouracil, *J. Natl. Cancer Inst.* **38**:401.

BURCHENAL, J. H., CURRIE, V. E., DOWLING, M. D., FOX, J. J., AND KRAKOFF, I. H., 1975, Experimental and clinical studies on nucleoside analogs as antitumor agents, *Ann. N.Y. Acad. Sci.* **255**:202.

CALABRESI, P., DOOLITTLE, C. H., III, HEPPNER, G. H., AND MCDONALD, C. J., 1975, Nucleoside analogs in the treatment of nonneoplastic diseases, *Ann. N. Y. Acad. Sci.* **255**:190.

CAMIENER, G. W., AND SMITH, G. G., 1965, Studies on the enzymatic deamination of cytosine arabinoside. I. Enzymatic distribution and species specificity, *Biochem. Pharmacol.* **14**:1405.

CARDOSO, S. S., CALABRESI, P., AND HANDSCHUMACHER, R. E., 1961, Alterations in human pyrimidine metabolism as a result of therapy with 6-azauridine, *Cancer Res.* **21**:1551.

CAREY, R. W., RIBAS-MUNDO, M., ELLISON, R. R., GLIDEWELL, O., LEE. S. T., CUTTNER, J., LEVY, R. N., SILVER, R., BLOM, J., HAURANI, F., SPURR, C. L., HARLEY, J. B., KYLE, R., MOON, J. H., EAGAN, R. T., AND HOLLAND, J. F., 1975, Comparative study of cytosine arabinoside therapy alone and combined with thioguanine, mercaptopurine, or daunorubicin in acute myelocytic leukemia, *Cancer* **36**:1560.

CAVIA, E., AND WEBB, T. E., 1972, Modified induction of ornithine decarboxylase by factors which affect liver regeneration, *Biochim. Biophys. Acta* **262**:546.

CHEN, M. S., WARD, D. C., AND PRUSOFF, W. H., 1976, Specific herpes simplex virus induced incorporation of 5-iodo-5'-amino-2',5'-dideoxyuridine into deoxyribonucleic acid, *J. Biol. Chem.* **251**:4833.

CHENG, Y. C., GOZ, B., NEENAN, J. P., WARD, D. C., AND PRUSOFF, W. H., 1975a, Selective inhibition of herpes simplex virus by 5-amino-2',5'-dideoxy-5-iodouridine, *J. Virol.* **15**:1284.

CHENG, Y.-C., NEENAN, J. P., GOZ, B., WARD, D. C., AND PRUSOFF, W. H., 1975b, Synthesis and biological activity of some novel analogs of thymidine, *Ann. N. Y. Acad. Sci.* **255**:332.

CHU, M. Y., 1971, Incorporation of arabinosyl cytosine into 27 S ribonucleic acid and cell death, *Biochem. Pharmacol.* **20**:2057.

CHU, M. Y., AND FISCHER, G. A., 1962, A proposed mechanism of 1-β-D-arabinofuranosyl-cytosine as an inhibitor of the growth of leukemic cells, *Biochem. Pharmacol.* **11**:423.

CHU, M. Y., AND FISCHER, G. A., 1968, The incorporation of ^{3}H-cytosine arabinoside and its effects on murine leukemic cells (L5178Y), *Biochem. Pharmacol.* **17**:753.

ČIHAK, A., 1975, Biological effects of 5-azacytidine in eukaryotes, a review, *Oncology* **30**:405.

ČIHAK, A., AND VESELÝ, J., 1969, Altered liver regeneration in partially hepatectomized rats following 5-azacytidine treatment, *Collect. Czech. Chem. Commun.* **34**:910.

ČIHAK, A., AND VESELÝ, J., 1972, Prolongation of the lag period preceding the enhancement of thymidine and thymidylate kinase activity in regenerating rat liver by 5-azacytidine, *Biochem. Pharmacol.* **21**:3257.

ČIHAK, A., AND VESELÝ, J., 1973, Enhanced uridine kinase in rat liver following 5-azacytidine administration, *J. Biol Chem.* **248**:1307.

ČIHAK, A., VESELÝ, J., AND ŠORM, F., 1967, Differences in the inhibition of hormone and substrate induction of rat liver tryptophan pyrrolase by 5-azacytidine, *Collect. Czech. Chem. Commun.* **32**:3427.

ČIHAK, A., VESELÝ, J., INOUE, H., AND PITOT, H. C., 1972, Effect of 5-azacytidine on dietary and hormone induction of serine dehydrase and tyrosine aminotransferase, *Biochem. Pharmacol.* **21**:2545.

ČIHAK, A., WEISS, J. W., AND PITOT, H. C., 1974, Characterization of polyribosomes and maturation of ribosomal RNA in hepatoma cells treated with 5-azacytidine, *Cancer Res.* **34**:3003.

CLARKSON, B. D., DOWLING, M. D., GEE, T. S., CUNNINGHAM, I. B., AND BURCHENAL, J. H., 1975, Treatment of acute leukemia in adults, *Cancer* **36**:775.

COHEN, S. S., 1966, Introduction to the biochemistry of the D-arabinosyl nucleosides, in: *Progress in Nucleic Acid Research and Molecular Biology* (J. N. Davidson and W. E. Cohen, eds.), pp. 1–88, Academic Press, New York.

COHEN, S. S., FLAKS, J. G., BARNER, H. D., LOEB, M. R., AND LICHTENSTEIN, J., 1958, The mode of action of 5-fluorouracil and its derivatives, *Proc. Natl. Acad. Sci. U.S.A.*, **44**:1004.

COLEMAN, C., JOHNS, D. G., AND CHABNER, B. A., 1975, Studies on the mechanism of resistance to cytosine arabinoside; problems in the determination of related enzyme activities in leukemic cells, *Ann. N. Y. Acad. Sci.* **255**:247.

CROSBIE, G. W., 1960, Biosynthesis of pyrimidine nucleotides, in: *The Nucleic Acids*, Vol. III (E. Chargaff and J. N. Davidson, eds.), pp. 323–348, Academic Press, New York.

DANENBERG, P. V., LANGENBACH, R. J., AND HEIDELBERGER, C., 1974, Structures of reversible and irreversible complexes of thymidylate synthetase and fluorinated pyrimidine nucleotides, *Biochemistry* **13**:927.

DESAI, I. S., KRISHNAN, A., AND FOLEY, G. E., 1974, Effects of bleomycin on cells in culture: A quantitative cytochemical study, *Cancer* **34**:1873.

DEVITA, V. T., JR., YOUNG, R. C., AND CANELLOS, G. P., 1975, Combination vs. single agent chemotherapy: A review of the basis of drug treatment of cancer, *Cancer* **35**:98.

DEXTER, D. L., OKI, T., AND HEIDELBERGER, C., 1973, Fluorinated pyrimidines. XLII. Effect of 5-trifluoromethyl-2′-deoxyuridine on transcription of vaccinia viral messenger ribonucleic acid, *Mol. Pharmacol.* **9**:283.

DOSKOČIL, J., AND ŠORM, F., 1970, The effects of 5-azacytidine and 5-azauridine on protein synthesis in *Escherichia coli*, *Biochem. Biophys. Res. Commun.* **38**:569.

DOSKOČIL, J., PASČES, AND ŠORM, F., 1967, Inhibition of protein synthesis by 5-azacytidine in *E. coli*, *Biochim. Biophys. Acta* **145**:771.

DUNLAP, R. B., HARDING, N. G. L., AND HUENNEKENS, F. M., 1971, Thymidylate synthetase from amethopterin-resistant *Lactobacillus casei*, *Biochemistry* **10**:88.

DURHAM, J. P., AND IVES, D. H., 1968, Deoxycytidine kinase I. Distribution in normal and neoplastic tissues and interrelations of deoxycytidine and 1-β-D-arabinofuranosylcytosine phosphorylation, *Mol. Pharmacol.* **5**:358.

DUSCHINSKY, R., PLEVEN, E., AND HEIDELBERGER, C., 1975, The synthesis of 5-fluoropyrimidines, *J. Amer. Chem. Soc.* **79**:4559.

EDELSTEIN, M., VIETTI, T., AND VALERIOTE, F., 1974, Schedule-dependent synergism for the combination of 1-β-D-arabinofuranosylcytosine and daunorubicin, *Cancer Res.* **34**:293.

ELLISON, R. R., HOLLAND, J. F., WEIL, M., JACQUILLAT, C., BOIRON, M., BERNARD, J., SAWITSKY, A., ROSNER, F., GUSSOFF, B., SILVER, R. T., KARANAS, A., CUTTNER, J., SPURR, C. L., HAYES, D. M., BLOM, J., LEONE, L. A., HAURANI, F., KYLE, R., HUTCHINSON, J. L., FORCIER, R. J., AND MOON, J. H., 1968, Arabinosylcytosine: A useful agent in the treatment of acute leukemia in adults, *Blood* **32**:507.

EVANS, J. S., MUSSER, E. A., MENGEL, G. D., FORSBLAD, K. R., AND HUNTER, J. H., 1961, Antitumor activity of 1-β-D-arabinofuranosyl cytosine hydrochloride (26335), *Proc. Soc. Exp. Biol. Med.* **106**:350.

FALLON, H. I., FREI, E., BLOCK, J., AND SEEGMILLER, J. E., 1961, The uricosuria and orotic aciduria induced by 6-azauridine, *J. Clin. Invest.* **49**:1906.

FARBER, S., DIAMOND, L. K., MERCER, R. D., SYLVESTER, R. F., JR., AND WOLFF, J. A., 1948, Temporary remissions in acute leukemia in children produced by folic acid antagonist, 4-aminopteroyl-glutamic acid (aminopterin), *N. Engl. J. Med.* **238**:787.

FOX, J. J., FALCO, E. A., WEMPEN, I., POMEROY, D., DOWLING, M. D., AND BURCHENAL, J. H., 1972, Oral and parenteral activity of 2,2′-anhydro-1-β-D-arabinofuranosyl-5-fluorocytosine against both intraperitoneally and intracerebrally inoculated mouse leukemia, *Cancer Res.* **32**:2269.

FRANKFURT, O. S., 1972, Enhancement of the antitumor activity of 5-fluorouracil by drug combinations, *Cancer Res.* **33**:1043.

FRIDLAND, A., LANGENBACH, R. J., AND HEIDELBERGER, C., 1971, Purification of thymidylate synthetase from Ehrlich ascites carcinoma cells, *J. Biol Chem.* **246**:7110.

FRIEDKIN, M., 1973, Thymidylate synthetase, in: *Advances in Enzymology* (A. Meister, ed.), pp. 235–292, John Wiley and Sons, New York,

FRIEDKIN, M., AND KORNBERG, A., 1957, The enzymatic conversion of deoxyuridylic acid to thymidylic acid and the participation of tetrahydrofolic acid, in: *The Chemical Basis of Heredity* (W. D. McElroy and B. Glass, eds.), pp. 609–614, The Johns Hopkins Press, Baltimore.

FUJIMOTO, S., AKAO, T., ITOH, B., KOSHIZUKA, I., KOYANU, K., KITSUKAWA, Y., TAKAHASHI, M., MINAMANI, T., ISHIGAMI, H., NOMURA, Y., AND ITOH, K., 1976, Effect of N_1-(2'-tetrahydrofuryl)-5-fluorouracil and 5-fluorouracil on nucleic acid and protein biosynthesis in Ehrlich ascites cells, *Cancer Res.* **36**:33.

FUJIWARA, Y., AND HEIDELBERGER, C., 1970, Fluorinated pyrimidines, XXXVIII. The incorporation of 5-trifluoromethyl-2'-deoxyuridine into the deoxyribonucleic acid of vaccinia virus, *Mol. Pharmacol.* **6**:281.

GALIVAN, J., MALEY, G. F., AND MALEY, F., 1974, Purification and properties of T2 bacteriophage-induced thymidylate synthetase, *Biochemistry* **13**:2282.

GALIVAN, J. H., MALEY, G. F., AND MALEY, F., 1976, Factors affecting substrate binding in *Lactobacillus casei* thymidylate synthetase as studied by equilibrium dialysis, *Biochemistry* **15**:356.

GOZ, B., AND PRUSOFF, W. H., 1970, Pharmacology of viruses, *Annu. Rev. Pharmacol.* **10**:143.

GRAHAM, F. L., AND WHITMORE, G. F., 1970, Studies in mouse L-cells on the incorporation of DNA polymerase by 1-β-D-arabinofuranosylcytosine 5'-triphosphate, *Cancer Res.* **30**:2636.

GRAY, G. D., 1975, Ara-C and derivatives as examples of immuno-suppressive nucleoside analogs, *Ann. N. Y. Acad. Sci.* **225**:372.

HABERMANN, V., AND ŠORM, F., 1958, Mechanism of the cancerostatic action of 6-azauracil and riboside, *Collect. Czech. Chem. Commun.* **23**:2201.

HAGHBIN, M., TAN, C. T. C., CLARKSON, B. D., MIKE, V., BURCHENAL, J. H., AND MURPHY, M. L., 1975, Treatment of acute lymphoblastic leukemia in children with "prophylactic" intrathecal methotrexate and intensive systemic chemotherapy, *Cancer Res.* **35**:807.

HALPERN, R. M., HALPERN, B. C., CLARK, B. R., ASHE, H., HARDY, D. N., JENKINSON, P. Y., CHOU, S.-C., AND SMITH, R. A., 1975, New approach to antifolate treatment of certain cancers as demonstrated in tissue culture, *Proc. Natl. Acad. Sci. U.S.A.*, **72**:4018.

HANDSCHUMACHER, R. E., 1958, Bacterial preparation of orotidine-5'-phosphate and uridine-5'-phosphate, *Nature (London)*, **182**:1090.

HANDSCHUMACHER, R. E., AND PASTERNAK, C. A., 1958, Inhibition of orotidylic acid decarboxylase, a primary site of carcinostasis by 6-azauracil, *Biochim. Biophys. Acta* **30**:451.

HANDSCHUMACHER, R. E., AND WELCH, A. D., 1960, Agents which influence nucleic acid metabolism, in: *The Nucleic Acids*, Vol. III (E. Chargaff and J. N. Davidson, eds.), pp. 453–526, Academic Press, New York.

HANDSCHUMACHER, R. E., CALABRESI, P., WELCH, A. D., BONO, H., FALLON, H., AND FREI, E., III, 1962, Summary of current information on 6-azauridine, *Cancer Chemother. Rep.* **21**:1.

HANKA, L. J., EVANS, J. S., MASON, D. J., AND DIETZ, A., 1966, Microbial production of 5-azacytidine I. Production and biological activity, *Antimicrob. Agents Chemother.* p. 619.

HANZE, A. R., 1967, Nucleic acids IV. The catalytic reduction of pyrimidine nucleosides (human liver deaminase inhibitors), *J. Amer. Chem. Soc.* **89**:6720.

HEIDELBERGER, C., 1965, Fluorinated pyrimidines in: *Progress in Nucleic Acid Research*, Vol. 4 (J. N. Davidson and W. E. Cohen, eds.), p. 1, Academic Press, New York.

HEIDELBERGER, C., 1970, Chemical carcinogenesis, chemotherapy: Cancer's continuing core challenges—G. H. A. Clowes Memorial Lecture, *Cancer Res.* **30**:1549.

HEIDELBERGER, C., 1973, Pyrimidine and pyrimidine nucleoside antimetabolites, in: *Cancer Medicine* (J. F. Holland and E. Frei, III, eds.), pp. 768–791, Lea and Febiger, Philadelphia.

HEIDELBERGER, C., 1975, On the molecular mechanism of antiviral activity of trifluorothymidine, *Ann. N. Y. Acad. Sci.* **255**:317.

HEIDELBERGER, C., LIEBMAN, K. C., HABERS, E., AND BHARGAVA, P. M., 1957, The comparative utilization of uracil-2-C^{14} by liver, intestinal, mucosa and Flexner-Jobling carcinoma in the rat, *Cancer Res.* **17**:399.

HEIDELBERGER, C., KALDON, G., MUKHERJEE, K. L., AND DANNENBERG, P. B., 1960, Studies on fluorinated pyrimidines. XI. *In vitro* studies on tumor resistance, *Cancer Res.* **20**:903.

HEINLE, R. W., AND WELCH, A. D., 1948, Experiments with pteroyl glutamic acid and pteroyl glutamic acid deficiency in human leukemia, *J. Clin. Invest.* **27**:539.

HENDERSON, J. F., AND PATERSON, A. R. P., 1973, *Nucleotide Metabolism*, pp. 173–204, Academic Press, New York.

HITCHINGS, G. H., 1973, Mechanism of action of trimethoprim-sulfa-methoxazole.—I, *J. Infect. Dis.* **128**:5433.

HO, D. H. W., 1973, Distribution of kinase and deaminase in 1-β-D-arabinosylcytosine in tissues of men and mouse, *Cancer Res.* **33**:2816.

HO, D. H. W., 1974, Biochemical studies of a new antitumor agent, O^2,2'-cyclocytidine, *Biochem. Pharmacol.* **23**:1235.

HO, D. H. W., AND FREI, E., III, 1972, Clinical pharmacology of 1-β-D-arabinosylcytosine, *Clin. Pharmacol. Ther.* **12**:944.

HORINISHI, H., AND GREENBERG, D. M., 1972, Purification and properties of thymidylate synthetase from calf thymus, *Biochim. Biophys. Acta* **258**:741.

IVES, D. H., MORSE, P. A., JR., AND POTTER, V. R., 1963, Feedback inhibition of thymidine kinase by thymidine triphosphate, *J. Biol. Chem.* **238**:1467.

JONES, P. A., BENEDICT, W. F., BAKER, M. S., MONDAL, S., RAPP, U., AND HEIDELBERGER, C., 1976, Oncogenic transformation of C3H/10T 1/2 clone 8 mouse embryo cells by halogenated pyrimidine nucleosides, *Cancer Res.* **36**:101.

KALMAN, T. I., AND BARDOS, T. J., 1970, Enzymatic studies relating to the mode of action of 5-mercapto-2'-deoxyuridine, *Mol. Pharmacol.* **6**:621.

KAREV, N. I., 1972, Experience with ftorafur treatment in breast cancer, *Neoplasma* **19**:347.

KARON, M., AND SHIRAKAWA, S., 1969, The locus of action of 1-β-D-arabinofuranosylcytosine in cell cycle, *Cancer Res.* **29**:687.

KARON, M., BENEDICT, W. F., AND RUCKER, N., 1972, Mechanism of 1-β-D-arabinofuranosylcytosine-induced lethality, *Cancer Res.* **32**:2612.

KARON, M., SIEGER, L., LEIMBROCK, S., FINKELSTEIN, J. Z., NESBIT, M. E., AND SWANEY, J. J., 1973, 5-Azacytidine: A new agent for the treatment of acute myelogenous leukemia, *Blood* **42**:359.

KEEFER, R. C., MCNAMARA, D. J., SCHUMM, D. E., BILLMIRE, D. F., AND WEBB, T. E., 1975, Early temporal changes in the uridine kinase isoenzyme profile of the Novikoff hepatoma in response to 5-azacytidine treatment, *Biochem. Pharmacol.* **24**:1287.

KENT, R. J., AND HEIDELBERGER, C., 1972, Fluorinated pyrimidines, XL. The reduction of 5-fluorouridine 5'-diphosphate by ribonucleotide reductase, *Mol. Pharmacol.* **8**:465.

KESSEL, D., 1968, Properties of deoxycytidine kinase partially purified from L1210 cells, *J. Biol. Chem.* **243**:4739.

KLENOW, H., 1962, Further studies on the effect of deoxyadenosine on the accumulation of deoxy-adenosine triphosphate and inhibition of deoxyribonucleic acid synthesis in Ehrlich ascites tumor cells *in vitro*, *Biochim. Biophys. Acta* **61**:885.

KOURI, R. E., KURTZ, S. A., PRICE, P. J., AND BENEDICT, W. F., 1975, 1-β-D-Arabinosylcytosine-induced malignant transformation of hamster and rat cells in culture, *Cancer Res.* **35**:2413.

KOVACS, C. J., HOPKINS, H. A., SIMON, R. M., AND LOONEY, W. B., 1975, Effects of 5-fluorouracil on the cell kinetic and growth parameters of the hepatoma 3924A, *Br. J. Cancer* **32**:42.

KREIS, W., GORDON, C. S., DE JAGER, R., AND KRAKOFF, I. H., 1975, Physiological disposition of 2,2'-anhydro-1-β-D-arabinofuranosylcytosine in humans, *Cancer Res.* **35**:2453.

KUTTER, E., BEUG, A., SLUSS, R., JENSEN, L., AND BRADLEY, D., 1975, The production of undegraded cytosine-containing DNA by bacteriophage T₄ in the absence of dCTPase and endonucleases II and IV, and its effects on T₄-directed protein synthesis, *J. Mol. Biol.* **99**:591.

LABOW, R., AND MALEY, F., 1967, The conversion of deoxyuridine-5'-monophosphate to deoxyuridine-5'-triphosphate in normal and regenerating rat liver, *Biochim. Biophys. Res. Commun.* **29**:136.

LANGEN, P., AND BÄRWOLFF, D., 1975, On the mode of action of 5-vinyl-2'-deoxyuridine, *Biochem. Pharmacol.* **24**:1907.

LEARY, R. P., AND KISLIUK, R. L., 1971, Crystalline thymidylate synthetase from dichloromethotrexate resistant *Lactobacillus casei*, *Prep. Biochem.* **1**:47.

LEE, T., KARON, M., AND MOMPARLER, R. L., 1974, Kinetic studies on phosphorylation of 5-azacytidine with the purified uridine-cytidine kinase from calf thymus, *Cancer Res.* **34**:2482.

LEVITAN, I. B., AND WEBB, T. E., 1969, Effects of 5-azacytidine on polysomes and on the control of tyrosine transaminase activity in rat liver, *Biochim. Biophys. Acta* **182**:491.

LI, L. H., OLIN, E. J., BUSKIRK, H. H., AND REINEKE, L. M., 1970a, Cytotoxicity and mode of action of 5-azacytidine on L1210 leukemia, *Cancer Res.* **30**:2760.

LI, L. H., OLIN, E. J., FRASER, T. J., AND BHUYAN, B. K., 1970b, Phase specificity of 5-azacytidine against mammalian cells in tissue culture, *Cancer Res.* **30**:2770.

LLOYD, H. H., DALMADGE, E. H., AND WILKOFF, L. J., 1972, Kinetics of the reduction in viability of cultured L1210 leukemia cells exposed to 5-azacytidine (NSC-102816), *Cancer Chemother. Rep.* **56:**585.

LORENSON, M. Y., MALEY, G. F., AND MALEY, F., 1967, The purification and properties of thymidylate synthetase from chick embryo extracts, *J. Biol. Chem.* **242:**3332.

MALEY, F., AND MALEY, G. F., 1971, Tetrahydrodeoxyuridylate: A potent inhibitor of deoxycytidylate deaminase, *Arch. Biochem. Biophys.* **144:**723.

MALEY, F., AND MALEY, G. F., 1972, The regulatory influence of allosteric effectors on deoxycytidylate deaminase, in: *Current Topics in Cellular Regulation* (B. L. Horecker and E. R. Stadtman, eds.), pp. 178–228, Academic Press, New York.

MALEY, G. F., AND MALEY, F., 1960, Inhibition of DNA synthesis in chick embryos by deoxyadenosine, *J. Biol. Chem.* **235:**2964.

MANDEL, H. G., 1969, The incorporation of 5-fluorouracil into RNA and its molecular consequences, *Prog. Mol. Subcell. Biol.* **1:**82.

MASKER, W. E., AND HANAWALT, P. C., 1974, Selective inhibition of the semiconservative mode of DNA replication by araCTP, *Biochim. Biophys. Acta* **340:**229.

MATHEWS, C. K., AND COHEN, S. S., 1963, Inhibition of phage-induced thymidylate synthetase by 5-fluorodeoxyuridylate, *J. Biol Chem.* **238:**367.

MCCREDIE, K. B., BODEY, G. P., BURGESS, M. A., GUTTERMAN, J. U., RODRIGUEZ, V., SULLIVAN, M. P., AND FREIREICH, E. J., 1973, Treatment of acute leukemia with 5-azacytidine, *Cancer Chemother. Rep.* **57:**319.

MCHENRY, C. S., AND SANTI, D. V., 1974, A sulfhydryl group is not the covalent catalyst in the thymidylate synthetase reaction, *Biochem. Biophys. Res. Commun.* **57:**204.

MOMPARLER, R. L., 1972, Kinetic and template studies with 1-β-D-arabinofuranosylcytosine 5'-triphosphate and mammalian deoxyribonucleic acid polymerase, *Mol. Pharmacol.* **8:**362.

MOMPARLER, R. L., 1974, A model for the chemotherapy of acute leukemia with 1-β-D-arabinofuranosyl cytosine, *Cancer Res.* **34:**1775.

MOMPARLER, R. L., AND FISHER, G. A., 1968, Mammalian deoxynucleoside kinase. I. Deoxycytidine kinase: Purification, properties and kinetic studies with cytosine arabinoside, *J. Biol. Chem.* **243:**4298.

MOMPARLER, R. L., GOODMAN, J., AND KARON, M., 1975, *In vitro* biochemical and cytotoxicity studies with 1-β-D-arabinosylcytosine and 5-aza-cytidine in combination, *Cancer Res.* **35:**2853.

MOORE, E. C., AND COHEN, S. S., 1967, Effect of arabinonucleotides on ribonucleotide reduction by an enzyme system from rat tumor, *J. Biol. Chem.* **242:**2116.

MORSE, P. A., JR., AND POTTER, V. R., 1965, Pyrimidine metabolism in tissue culture cells derived from rat hepatomas. I. Suspension cell cultures derived from the Novikoff hepatomas, *Cancer Res.* **25:**499.

MULLIGAN, L. T., AND MELLETT, L. B., 1968, Comparative metabolism of cytosine arabinoside and inhibition of deamination by tetrahydrouridine, *Pharmacologist* **10:**167.

MYERS, C. E., YOUNG, R. C., JOHNS, D. G., AND CHABNER, B. A., 1974, Assay of 5-fluorodeoxyuridine 5'-monophosphate pools following 5-fluorouracil, *Cancer Res.* **34:**2682.

NAKAMURA, H., AND SUGINO, Y., 1966, Metabolism of deoxyribonucleotides. III. Purification and some properties of nucleoside diphosphokinase of calf thymus, *J. Biol. Chem.* **241:**4917.

NEIL, G. L., AND HOMAN, E. R., 1973, The effect of dose interval on the survival of L1210 leukemic mice treated with DNA synthesis inhibitors, *Cancer Res.* **33:**895.

NEIL, G. L., MOXLEY, T. E., AND MANAK, R. C., 1970, Enhancement by tetrahydrouridine of 1-β-D-arabinosylcytosine (cytarabine) oral activity in L1210 leukemic mice, *Cancer Res.* **30:**2166.

NESNOW, S., MIYAZAKI, T., KHAWJA, T., MEYER, R. B., JR., AND HEIDELBERGER, C., 1973, Pyrimidine nucleosides related to 5-fluorouracil and thymine, *J. Med. Chem.* **16:**524.

NOVAK, E. K., 1971, Effect of polyene antibiotics on yeasts, *Szeszipar* **19:**4.

OCKEY, C. H., AND ALLEN, T. D., 1975, Distribution of DNA or DNA synthesis in mammalian cells following inhibition with hydroxyurea and 5-fluorodeoxyuridine, *Cancer Res.* **93:**275.

PAČES, V., DOSKOČIL, J., AND ŠORM, F., 1968, Incorporation of 5-azacytidine into nucleic acids of *E. coli*, *Biochim. Biophys. Acta* **161:**352.

PASTERNAK, C. A., AND HANDSCHUMACHER, R. E., 1959, The biochemical activity of 6-azauridine: Interference with pyrimidine metabolism in transplantable mouse tumors, *J. Biol. Chem.* **234:**2992.

PÍSKALA, A., AND ŠORM, F., 1964, Nucleic acid components and their analogues, LI. Synthesis of 1-glycosyl derivatives of 5-azauracil and 5-azacytosine, *Collect. Czech. Chem. Commun.* **29:**2060.

PIZER, L. I., AND COHEN, S. S., 1960, Metabolism of pyrimidine arabinonucleosides and cyclonucleosides in *Escherichia coli*, *J. Biol. Chem.* **235**:2387.

POGOLOTTI, A. L., IVANETLICH, K. M., SOMMER, H., AND SANTI, D. V., 1976, Thymidylate synthetase: Studies on the peptide containing covalently bound 5-fluoro-2'-deoxyuridylate and methylenetetrahydrofolate, *Biochem. Biophys. Res. Commun.* **70**:972.

PRUSOFF, W. H., 1963, A review of some aspects of 5-iododeoxyuridine and azauridine, *Cancer Res.* **23**:1246.

RAŠKA, K., JR., JUROVČIK, M., ŠORMOVA, Z., AND SÖRM, F., 1965, On the metabolism of 5-azacytidine and 5-aza-2'-deoxycytidine in mice, *Collect. Czech. Chem. Commun.* **30**:3006.

REICHARD, P., 1959*a*, The biosynthesis of deoxyribonucleic acid by the chick embryo II. Metabolism of O^2:2'-*cyclo*uridine, *J. Biol. Chem.* **234**:2719.

REICHARD, P., 1959*b*, The enzymic synthesis of pyrimidines, *Adv. Enzymol.* **21**:263.

REICHARD, P., SKÖLD, O., KLEIN, G., RÉVÉSZ, L., AND MAGNUSSON, P.-H., 1962, Studies on resistance against 5-fluorouracil. I. Enzymes of the uracil pathway during development of resistance, *Cancer Res.* **22**:235.

REICHMAN, M., AND PENMAN, S., 1973, The mechanism of inhibition of induction of protein synthesis by 5-azacytidine in HeLa cells, *Biochim. Biophys. Acta* **324**:282.

REICHMAN, M., KARLAN, D., AND PENMAN, S., 1973, Destructive processing of the 45s ribosomal precursor in the presence of 5-aza-cytidine, *Biochim. Biophys. Acta* **299**:173.

REYES, P., 1969, The synthesis of 5-fluorouridine-5'-phosphate by a pyrimidine phosphoribosyl transferase of mammalian origin, I. Some properties of the enzyme from P1534J mouse leukemia cells, *Biochemistry* **8**:2057.

REYES, P., AND HEIDELBERGER, C., 1965, Fluorinated pyrimidines, XXVI. Mammalian thymidylate synthetase; its mechanism of action and inhibition by fluorinated nucleotides, *Mol. Pharmacol.* **1**:14.

ROBBINS, M. J., AND CURRIE, B. L., 1968, The synthesis of 3-deazauridine 4-hydroxy-1-(β-D-ribopentofuranosyl)-2-pyridone, *Chem. Commun.* **2**:1547.

ROSSI, M., MOMPARLER, R. L., NUCCI, R., AND SCARANO, E., 1970, Studies on analogs of isosteric and allosteric ligands of deoxycytidylate aminohydrolase, *Biochemistry* **9**:2539.

RUTMAN, R. J., CANTAROW, A., AND PASCHKIS, K. E., 1954, Studies on 2-acetylaminofluorene carcinogenesis: III. The utilization of uracil-2-C^{14} by preneoplastic rat liver and rat hepatoma, *Cancer Res.* **14**:119.

SANTI, D. V., AND BREWER, C. F., 1973, Model studies of thymidylate synthetase, intramolecular catalysis of 5-hydrogen exchange and 5-hydroxymethylation of 1-substituted uracils, *Biochemistry* **12**:2416.

SANTI, D. V., AND McHENRY, C. S., 1972, 5-Fluoro-2'-deoxyuridylate: Covalent complex with thymidylate synthetase, *Proc. Natl. Acad. Sci. U.S.A.* **69**:1855.

SANTI, D. V., AND SAKAI, T. T., 1971, Thymidylate synthetase model studies of inhibition by 5-trifluoromethyl-2'-deoxyuridylic acid, *Biochemistry* **10**:3598.

SANTI, D. V., McHENRY, C. S., AND SOMMER, H., 1974, Mechanism of interaction of thymidylate synthetase with 5-fluorodeoxyuridylate, *Biochemistry* **13**:471.

SARTORELLI, A. C., 1969. Some approaches to the therapeutic exploitation of metabolic sites of vulnerability of neoplastic cells, *Cancer Res.* **29**:2292.

SARTORELLI, A. C., AGRAWAL, K. C., AND MOORE, E. C., 1971, Mechanism of inhibition of ribonucleoside reductase by α-N-heterocyclic aldehyde thiosemicarbazones, *Biochem. Pharm.* **20**:3119.

SCHINDLER, R., AND WELCH, A. D., 1958, Ribosidation as a means of activating 6-azauracil as an inhibitor of cell reproduction, *Science* **125**:548.

SCHRECKER, A. W., AND URSHEL, M. J., 1968, Metabolism of 1-β-D-arabinofuranosylcytosine in leukemia L1210: Studies with intact cells, *Cancer Res.* **28**:793.

SEIFERTOVÁ, M., VESELÝ, J., AND ŠORM, F., 1968, Effect of 5-azacytidine on developing mouse embryo, *Experientia* **24**:487.

SILAGI, S., 1965, Metabolism of 1-β-D-arabinofuranosyl cytosine in L-cells, *Cancer Res.* **25**:1446.

SILVESTRINI, R., DIMARCO, A., AND DOSDIA, T., 1970, Interference of daunomycin with metabolic events of the cell cycle in synchronized cultures of rat fibroblasts, *Cancer Res.* **30**:966.

SIMONE, J. V., AUR, R. J. A., HUSTO, H. O., AND VERZOSA, M., 1975, Acute lymphocytic leukemia in children, *Cancer* **36**:770.

SINCLAIR, W. K., 1967, Hydroxyurea: Effects on Chinese hamster cells grown in culture, *Cancer Res.* **27**:297.

360

FRANK
MALEY

SKIPPER, H. E., SCHABEL, F. M., AND WILCOX, W. S., 1967, Experimental evaluation of potential anticancer agents. XXI. Scheduling of arabinosylcytosine to take advantage of its S-phase specificity against leukemia cells, *Cancer Chemother. Rep.* **51**:125.

ŠKODA, J., 1963, Mechanism of action and application of azapyrimidines, in: *Progress in Nucleic Acid Research*, Vol. 2 (J. N. Davidson and W. E. Cohen, eds.), pp. 197–219, Academic Press, New York.

SMART, C. R., TOWNSEND, L. B., RUSHO, W. J., EYRE, H. J., QUAGLIANA, J. M., WILSON, M. L., EDWARDS, C. B., AND MANNING, S. J., 1975, Phase I study of ftorafur, an analog of 5-fluorouracil, *Cancer* **36**:103.

SOMMER, H., AND SANTI, D. V., 1974, Purification and amino acid analysis of an active site peptide from thymidylate synthetase containing covalently bound 5-fluoro-2'-deoxyuridylate and methylenetetrahydrofolate, *Biochem. Biophys. Res. Commun.* **57**:689.

ŠORM, F., AND VESELÝ, J., 1964, The activity of a new antimetabolite, 5-azacytidine, against lymphoid leukemia in AK mice, *Neoplasma* **11**:123.

ŠORM, F., PÍSKALA, A., ČIHAK, A., AND VESELÝ, J., 1964, 5-Azacytidine, a new highly effective cancerostatic, *Experientia* **20**:202.

STEINSTROM, M. L., EDELSTEIN, M., AND GRISHAM, J. W., 1974, Effects of ara-CTP on DNA replication and repair in isolated hepatocyte nuclei, *Exp. Cell. Res.* **89**:439.

STEWART, C. D., AND BURKE, P. J., 1971, Cytidine deaminase and development of resistance to arabinosyl cytosine, *Nature (London) New Biol.* **233**:109.

STORM, D. R., AND STROMINGER, J. L., 1974, Binding of bacitracin to cells and protoplasts of *Micrococcus leisodeikticus*, *J. Biol. Chem.* **249**:1823.

STROMINGER, J. L., 1968–1969, Penicillin sensitive enzymatic reactions in bacterial cell wall synthesis, *Harvey Lect.* **64**:179.

SUGINO, Y., TERAOKA, H., AND SHIMONO, H., 1966, Metabolism of deoxyribonucleotides I. Purification and properties of deoxycytidine monophosphokinase in calf thymus, *J. Biol. Chem.* **241**:961.

SUHADOLNIK, R. J., 1970a, Spongosine and arabinosyl nucleosides, in: *Nucleoside Antibiotics*, pp. 123–169, Interscience, New York.

SUHADOLNIK, R. J., 1970b, Azapyrimidine nucleosides, in: *Nucleoside Antibiotics*, pp. 271–297, Interscience, New York.

SWIERKOWSKA, K. M., JASIASKER, J. K., AND STEFFEN, J. A., 1973, 5-Ethyl-2'-deoxyuridine: Evidence for incorporation into DNA and evaluation of biological properties in lymphocyte cultures grown under conditions of amethopterine-imposed thymidine deficiency, *Biochem. Pharmacol.* **22**:85.

TATTERSALL, M. H. N., GANESHAGURU, K., AND HOFFBRAND, A. V., 1974, Mechanisms of resistance to arabinosyl cytosine, *Br. J. Haematol.* **27**:39.

TAYLOR, J. H., HAUT, W. F., AND TUNG, J., 1962, Effects of fluorodeoxyuridine on DNA replication, chromosome breakage and reunion, *Proc. Natl. Acad. Sci. U.S.A.* **48**:190.

VALERIOTE, F. A., BRUCE, W. R., AND MEEKER, B. E., 1966, A model for the action of vinblastine *in vivo*, *Biophys. J.* **6**:145.

VENDETTI, J. M., BARATTA, M. C., GREENBERG, N., ABBOTT, B. T., AND KLINE, I., 1972, Studies on the L1210 antileukemic activity of O-2,2'-cyclocytidine, monoacetate (anhydro-ara-C; NSC-129220)—comparison with cytosine arabinoside (NSC-63878) with respect to treatment schedule dependency, *Cancer Chemother. Rep.* **56**:483.

VESELÝ, J., ČIHAK, A., AND ŠORM, F., 1967, Biochemical mechanisms of drug resistance IV. Development of resistance to 5-azacytidine and simultaneous depression of pyrimidine metabolism in leukemic mice, *Int. J. Cancer* **2**:639.

VONGTAMA, V., DOUGLASS, H. O., MOORE, R. H., HOLYOKE, E. D., AND WEBSTER, J. H., 1975, End results of radiation therapy, alone and combination with 5-fluorouracil in colorectal cancers, *Cancer* **36**:2020.

WALWICK, E. R., ROBERTS, W. K., AND DEKKER, C. A., 1959, Cyclization during the phosphorylation of uridine and cytidine by polyphosphoric acid; a new route to $O^2,2'$-cyclonucleosides, *Proc. Chem. Soc.* p. 84.

WANG, M. C., AND BLOCH, A., 1972, Studies on the mode of action of 3-diazapyrimidines—1. Metabolism of 3-deazauridine and 3-deazacytidine in microbial and tumor cells, *Biochem. Pharmacol.* **21**:1063.

WEBER, G., QUEENER, S. F., AND FERNANDUS, J. A., 1970, Control of gene expression in carbohydrate metabolism and DNA metabolism, in: *Advances in Enzyme Regulation*, Vol. 9 (G. Weber, ed.), pp. 63–95, Pergamon Press, New York.

WEISS, J. W., AND PITOT, H. C., 1975, Effects of 5-azacytidine on nucleolar RNA and the preribosomal particles in Novikoff hepatoma cells, *Biochemistry* **14**:316.

WENTWORTH, D. F., AND WOLFENDEN, R., 1975, On the interaction of 3,4,5,6-tetrahydrouridine with human liver cytidine deaminase, *Biochemistry* **14:**5099.

WILKINSON, D. S., TLSTY, T. D., AND HANAS, R. J., 1975, The inhibition of ribosomal RNA synthesis and maturation in Novikoff hepatoma cells by 5-fluorouridine, *Cancer Res.* **35:**3014.

WILKOFF, L. J., DULMADGE, E. A., AND LLOYD, H., H., 1972, Kinetics of effect of 1-β-D-arabinofuranosylcytosine, its 5'-palmitoyl ester, 1-β-D-arabinofuranosyluracil, and tritiated thymidine on the viability of cultured L1210 cells, *J. Natl. Cancer Inst.* **48:**685.

WOODS, D. D., 1940, The relation of *p*-aminobenzoic acid to the mechanism of the action of sulphanilamide, *Br. J. Exp. Pathol.* **21:**74.

WU, R., AND GEIDUSCHEK, E. P., 1975, The role of replication proteins in the regulation of bacteriophage T$_4$ transcription I. Gene 45 and hydroxymethyl-C-containing DNA, *J. Mol. Biol.* **96:**513.

YATAGANAS, X., STRIFE, A., PEREZ, A., AND CLARKSON, B. D., 1974, Microfluorometric evaluation of cell kill kinetics with 1-β-D-arabinofuranosylcytosine, *Cancer Res.* **34:**2795.

YOUNG, R. S. K., AND FISCHER, G. A., 1968, The action of arabinosylcytosine on synchronously growing populations of mammalian cells, *Biochem. Biophys. Res. Commun.* **32:**23.

13

Folate Antagonists

BRUCE A. CHABNER AND DAVID G. JOHNS

1. Mode of Action of Folate Antagonists: Relationship between Inhibition of Dihydrofolate Reductase and Cytotoxicity

The value of antifolate agents has been clearly established in the therapy of human neoplasms, but the use of these drugs has been complicated by consistent toxicity to normal host tissues. Continuously replicating tissues such as bone marrow, oral and GI epithelium, and reproductive tissue are the most frequent targets for antifolate toxicity. The biochemical mechanism underlying toxicity to these host tissues is thought to be the same as that responsible for toxicity to malignant tissue, i.e., inhibition of dihydrofolate reductase. Significant injury to the liver, brain, and kidneys has also been seen as a consequence of antifolate therapy. These latter toxicities, which are not clearly related to reductase inhibition, will be considered later in this chapter.

The cytotoxicity of methotrexate (MTX), the commonly used antifolate, has been extensively investigated in cell culture and in whole animals, and has been shown to result from the interaction of pharmacological variables that determine the duration and degree of inhibition of DNA synthesis consequent on the depletion of tetrahydrofolate cofactors. The important pharmacological factors are drug concentration and duration of exposure (Goldman, 1975; Pinedo and Chabner, 1976), but intrinsic cell properties such as replication rate (Hryniuk et al., 1969) and levels of dihydrofolate reductase (Bertino, 1963), and the physiological environment of the cell (Pinedo and Chabner, 1976), are also important determinants.

The influence of these factors has been most clearly demonstrated in tissue culture experiments, but these findings have undoubted relevance to the *in vivo* effects of MTX and other antifolates.

BRUCE A. CHABNER AND DAVID G. JOHNS ● Division of Cancer Treatment, National Cancer Institute, National Institutes of Health, Bethesda, Maryland.

364

BRUCE A.
CHABNER
AND
DAVID G.
JOHNS

Central to the present understanding of MTX toxicity is the concept that free intracellular MTX, i.e., MTX in molar excess to the target enzyme, is required for maintaining effective blockade of dihydrofolate reductase (Goldman, 1975). While the binding of MTX to dihydrofolate reductase is essentially stoichiometric under mildly acid conditions (pH 6.0) and in the presence of limited competitive substrate (Bertino *et al.*, 1964), less favorable conditions are found in the intact cell, where physiological pH and higher levels of competitive substrate (dihydro-folate and its polyglutamates) decrease the binding of enzyme and inhibitor. For example, Nixon *et al.* (1973) showed that in the presence of MTX, intracellular folates accumulate as dihydrofolate derivatives, substrates that can compete effectively with the inhibitor for binding to the enzyme. *In vitro* studies of MTX binding to enzyme, in which the formation of enzyme–inhibitor complex has been measured directly (Myers *et al.*, 1975), as well as experiments employing conven-tional enzyme kinetics (Werkheiser, 1961), showed that an excess of free drug is required to inactivate the enzyme completely. This observation assumes great significance in view of indications that dihydrofolate reductase is found in excess in most cells, and only a small fraction of the total enzyme is needed to maintain the intracellular reduced folate pool (Jackson and Harrap, 1973; Sirotnak and Donsbach, 1973). In order to reduce the level of functional dihydrofolate reduc-tase to insignificant concentrations, and thus to terminate DNA synthesis, con-centrations of inhibitor far in excess of enzyme are required.

Explicit evidence for the requirement for free extracellular MTX has come from several sources, but was initially suggested by experiments with the folate-cleaving enzyme carboxypeptidase G_1 (Chabner *et al.*, 1972b). This enzyme, isolated and purified from *Pseudomonas stutzeri*, was able to prevent lethal toxicity of MTX by hydrolysis of residual circulating drug *when given 24 hr after the antifolate*. These findings suggested that toxicity to host tissues was a function of at least two factors: (1) the presence and persistence of free extracellular drug, and (2) the duration of exposure of target tissues to this drug. Similarly, *in vitro* experiments have demonstrated a requirement for free extracellular MTX, and have related this requirement to the need for free intracellular drug. Goldman (1974), using mouse L cells in culture, demonstrated inhibition of incorporation of [³H]deoxyuridine into DNA in the presence of MTX concentrations above 10^{-7} M, with increasing degrees of inhibition as the level of free drug was increased. Removal of free extracellular drug by washing and resuspending cells led to immediate reversal of the inhibition, despite retention of a tightly bound fraction of MTX presumably bound to dihydrofolate reductase. Inhibition of RNA and protein synthesis was also dependent on the presence of free extracellu-lar MTX (Goldman *et al.*, 1975). Sirotnak and Donsbach (1973) showed that drug in excess of the concentration of dihydrofolate reductase was required to inhibit DNA synthesis in GI mucosa and in L1210 cells. The *in vitro* requirement of 10^{-6}M MTX for 50% inhibition of [³H]deoxyuridine incorporation into DNA in L1210 cells was considerably greater than the level of drug required *in vivo* to produce an equivalent effect. An explanation for this difference is not readily apparent, although it has been suggested that the higher proliferative rate of these cells *in vivo* may render them more sensitive to submaximal changes in intracellular tetrahydrofolate levels.

Recognition of the important role of free drug in determining inhibition of DNA synthesis has made it possible to relate pharmacological effects to specific drug concentrations *in vivo*. Initial studies identified the lowest plasma level of drug required for inhibition of DNA synthesis (as determined by [^{3}H]deoxy-uridine incorporation into DNA) in mouse tissues (Chabner and Young, 1973). The lowest plasma concentration of MTX associated with inhibition of DNA synthesis in mouse bone marrow was 10^{-8} M, while inhibition in intestinal epithelium required a slightly lower plasma concentration of MTX (5×10^{-9} M), a finding consistent with the greater cytotoxic effect of the drug for mouse intestinal epithelium. The relative sensitivities of bone marrow and intestinal epithelium were directly compared by Zaharko *et al.* (1974), by means of constant-infusion devices; these workers suggested that differences in sensitivity could be attributed to a difference in the permeability of these tissues to MTX. Chello *et al.* (1975) clearly demonstrated differences in the persistence of free MTX in the more sensitive L1210 cells as compared with intestinal mucosal epithelium following pulse doses of drug, and these differences were ascribed to differences in the affinities of the MTX transport processes of these tissues. This hypothesis is consistent with the results of earlier studies that related the differential sensitivity of a series of murine tumors to their ability to accumulate intracellular MTX during incubation *in vitro* (Kessel *et al.*, 1965).

Thus far, only one study has been performed in man aimed at determining the threshold for inhibition of DNA synthesis by MTX; in 6 patients with ovarian cancer, inhibition of DNA synthesis in bone marrow was associated with minimum drug concentrations in the range of $1-3 \times 10^{-8}$ M (Young and Chabner, 1973).

Delineation of the minimal drug levels required to inhibit DNA synthesis has been useful in interpreting the pharmacokinetic decay patterns of MTX. For example, it has become clear that the slow final phase of drug clearance, having a half-time of 12 hr and associated with plasma levels in the range of $10^{-8}-10^{-7}$ M, may be responsible for significant toxicity to bone marrow and intestinal mucosa (Chabner and Young, 1973). In the presence of renal failure, the half-time for the final phase of drug disappearance may be greatly prolonged (Kristensen *et al.*, 1975), leading to serious toxicity for otherwise nontoxic doses.

The appreciation of minimum toxic drug concentrations, or thresholds, has been helpful in understanding MTX toxicity, but leaves unanswered the question whether drug concentrations above the threshold have increasingly greater cytotoxicity. The relationship between drug level and cytotoxicity to bone marrow has been studied in mice, using constant-infusion devices to set plasma MTX concentration at specific levels (Pinedo *et al.*, 1976*a*). A linear relationship was observed between drug-infusion rates in the range of $1-1000$ μg/kg per min and the plateau concentration of MTX achieved in plasma in the range of $10^{-8}-10^{-5}$ M. It was found that the highest concentrations of drug produced the most rapid depletion of nucleated cells in bone marrow, and that cell loss was a linear function of duration of exposure until a nadir of cell depletion was reached. A

366

BRUCE A.
CHABNER
AND
DAVID G.
JOHNS

common nadir of approximately 30% of original cell count was reached for all levels of drug in the range of 10^{-8}–10^{-5} M, although, as stated above, the nadir was reached most rapidly at highest drug concentrations. The reason for the halt in cell depletion at 30% is not clear from these studies, but may be related to the ancillary inhibitory effects of MTX on RNA and protein synthesis, effects that could prevent cells from further progression into the vulnerable DNA synthetic period of the cell cycle (Bruce *et al.*, 1966).

It appears that the effects of MTX on bone marrow are more complex than reflected in the cell count. During constant-infusion experiments, changes in the myeloid-colony-forming potential of bone marrow have been determined by removing cells from the marrow cavity, washing the pellet free of MTX, and cloning the cells in semisolid methylcellulose media. The decline in the number of myeloid precursor cells parallels the fall in the total number of nucleated cells during the initial 24 hr of drug exposure, but thereafter, the number of myeloid-colony-forming cells either remained constant or increased despite continued drug infusion and despite a continued fall in total nucleated cells, suggesting recruitment of a more primitive stem cell to myeloid-colony-forming potential (Pinedo *et al.*, 1976*b*). A similar enrichment of bone marrow with myeloid-colony-forming cells has been observed after large single doses of MTX (Vogler *et al.*, 1973), and may be responsible for the increased rate of DNA synthesis seen in the recovery phase after large single doses of this drug (Chabner and Young, 1973).

Drug concentration and duration of exposure are the primary determinants of cytotoxicity subject to alteration in the design of clinical schedules; however, the cellular effects of MTX have also been shown to be influenced by multiple factors related to intrinsic cell properties and cell metabolism. The levels of dihydrofolate reductase and the capacity to transport antifolates are both important factors in determining drug effect, and will be considered in detail in the discussion of drug resistance (Section 3). As mentioned previously, the sensitivity of cells to MTX and other cell-cycle-specific agents has also been shown to be greatest during periods of rapid DNA synthesis, with little effect being exerted on nondividing cell populations (Hryniuk *et al.*, 1969). If protein synthesis is inhibited by agents such as L-asparaginase, cells are unable to progress into DNA synthesis, and MTX loses its cytotoxic effect (Capizzi, 1974). This observation has been the basis of a clinical regimen employing MTX, followed by L-asparaginase, the latter terminating the cytotoxic action of the drug (Capizzi, 1975). Since the cytotoxicity of MTX depends on depletion of intracellular reduced folates, it is not surprising that reduced folates such as leucovorin (5-formyltetrahydrofolate) (Goldin *et al.*, 1953, 1955) and 5-methyltetrahydrofolate (Halpern *et al.*, 1975), which bypass the block in reduction of dihydrofolate, are able to protect against the antifolate. Leucovorin protection has been used extensively in the clinical treatment of cancer to terminate the toxic effects of high-dose MTX therapy (see Section 4), and to prevent otherwise lethal toxicity to host organs (Mitchell *et al.*, 1968). It has recently been demonstrated that murine malignant cells in tissue culture lack the capacity to convert 5-methyltetrahydrofolate to the cofactor forms (N^5,N^{10}-methylenetetrahydrofolate, 10-formyltetrahydrofolate, N^5, N^{10}-methenyltetrahydrofolate) required for purine and pyrimidine synthesis. Thus, 5-methyltetrahydrofolate may be the preferred "rescue" agent because of its ability to rescue normal cells without salvage of malignant cells (Halpern *et al.*, 1975).

Nucleoside precursors of DNA are also known to protect cells from antifolate toxicity, by supplying the necessary end products of folate-mediated reactions. Both thymidine and a purine (adenosine, hypoxanthine, or inosine) were necessary to protect mouse bone marrow *in vitro* (Pinedo *et al.*, 1976*a*), a finding consistent with the known inhibitory effects of MTX on purine and pyrimidine synthesis. Experiments *in vivo* have indicated protection of bone marrow of tumor-bearing animals by thymidine alone (Tattersall *et al.*, 1975), but this difference may be due to concomitant elevation of the circulating purine pool as a consequence of tumor lysis. The nucleosides required to reverse MTX toxicity to tumor cells have been studied extensively, with variable results. Tattersall and co-workers examined five leukemic cell lines in detail, and found that two lines required both thymidine and a purine for protection, while thymidine alone provided partial protection of three cell lines (Tattersall *et al.*, 1974). Hryniuk (1972) observed that the early cytotoxic effects of MTX on the L5178Y murine leukemia cell line could be partially prevented by a purine source alone, while complete protection of cells required both thymidine and a purine source. Human CEM leukemia cells in culture require thymidine plus deoxycytidine, the latter being needed to circumvent the thymidine-induced inhibition of dCTP synthesis (Roberts and Warmath, 1975). The foregoing experiments reveal a wide variation in the requirements of malignant cells for nucleoside protection against antifolate toxicity, and the accumulated data furnish no evidence for a constant exploitable difference between normal and malignant cells.

While the influence of exogenous nucleosides on MTX toxicity has been clearly shown, it is not clear what effect endogenous nucleoside pools may have in determining the antitumor action of MTX in clinical or experimental chemotherapy. Recent observations indicate that purine and pyrimidine nucleosides in fetal calf serum may be responsible for the marked MTX resistance of bone marrow cells grown in nondialyzed serum; this resistance can be eliminated by dialysis of serum prior to its use in the culture medium (Pinedo and Chabner, 1976). Grindey and Moran (1975) diminished the cytotoxicity of MTX for L1210 cells by pretreating mice with allopurinol, thus elevating circulating levels of hypoxanthine and xanthine. One would suspect that rapidly growing neoplasms such as Burkitt's lymphoma or oat-cell carcinoma might cause elevated circulating nucleoside levels, particularly in the presence of allopurinol, altering antifolate sensitivity. Further information concerning nucleoside levels in man is needed to establish the possible correlation between nucleoside levels and drug toxicity.

2. Toxicities Unrelated to Inhibition of Dihydrofolate Reductase

While the most significant pharmacological effects of MTX result from inhibition of dihydrofolate reductase, important complications of antifolate

368

BRUCE A.
CHABNER
AND
DAVID G.
JOHNS

chemotherapy that appear to be unrelated to enzyme inhibition have been reported. Renal dysfunction has recently been reported as a consequence of high-dose (>50 mg/kg) infusions (Djerassi *et al.*, 1967; Jaffe and Paed, 1972), and has been associated with delayed drug excretion, ineffective reversal of toxicity by leucovorin, and fatal myelosuppression (Stoller *et al.*, 1975). It has been possible to reproduce the renal toxicity syndrome in monkeys using high-dose drug infusions, and a heavy precipate of MTX-derived material has been identified by light microscopy and autoradiography in the renal tubules of those animals developing renal failure (Fig. 1). This precipitate appears to result from the limited solubility of MTX and possibly 7-hydroxymethotrexate, both weak organic acids, in acid urine. During high-dose infusion, the concentration of MTX in the urine exceeded 2 mM, the limit of MTX solubility at pH 5.7. In less acid solution, MTX solubility rises rapidly. This observation provides the rationale for alkalinization of urine and diuresis during high-dose therapy (Stoller *et al.*, 1975). Jacobs *et al.* (1976) recently reported identification of a metabolite, 7-OH methotrexate, in the urine of both man and monkeys following high-dose infusion. This metabolite, which is even less water-soluble than MTX, represented a significant fraction of drug excreted in later time periods following drug infusion (18–24 and 24–48 hr), and was the major antifolate derivative found in the kidneys of monkeys that developed renal failure. Its role in the renal failure syndrome in

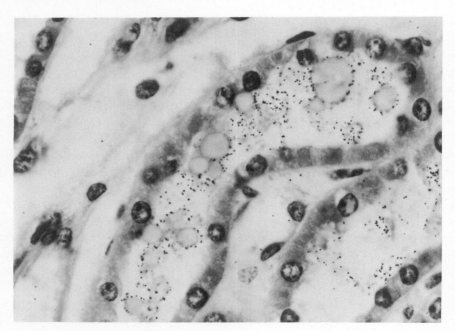

FIGURE 1. Autoradiograph of tissue section 5 μm thick from renal medulla of a rhesus monkey 24 hr after administration of (3'5',9-[^{3}H]) methotrexate (546 μCi), at a dose of 200 mg/kg. ×860. The slide was dipped in Kodak Nuclear Track Emulsion, NTB2 (Eastman Kodak Company, Rochester, New York), exposed for 14 days, developed, and stained with hemotoxylin and eosin. Reproduced by permission of Dr. Samuel A. Jacobs, Department of Medicine, Montefiore Hospital, Pittsburg, Pennsylvania.

man and the enzymatic reaction leading to its production remain unclear at this time. The metabolite is not detectable in human urine after MTX therapy at conventional dose levels.

A second important manifestation of MTX toxicity that may be unrelated to the ability of the drug to inhibit dihydrofolate reductase is a consistent acute elevation of hepatic enzymes during high-dose infusion (Djerassi *et al.*, 1967; Jaffe and Paed, 1972), and the development of cirrhosis in patients receiving continuous low-dose therapy (Dahl *et al.*, 1971). It is not known whether a common mechanism of toxicity underlies both types of hepatic damage, although the rises in SGOT and SGPT (often to 10-fold normal levels) following high-dose infusions have not been associated as yet with the later development of cirrhosis. Whether pathological changes underlie the acute elevations of hepatic enzymes seen in high-dose therapy has not been documented as yet, but there is strong clinical and pathological evidence for chronic hepatotoxicity of MTX in patients with leukemia and psoriasis. The incidence of cirrhosis in psoriatic patients receiving MTX has been estimated to be as high as 14% (Dahl *et al.*, 1971). Predisposition to the development of hepatic fibrosis and cirrhosis has been documented in patients with psoriasis (Berge *et al.*, 1970), and it is possible that the high incidence of cirrhosis in psoriatic patients receiving antifolates represents an interaction of drug toxicity and an already abnormal liver.

The uptake, metabolism, and biliary excretion of MTX in the liver have been studied, primarily in rodents. An active transport mechanism with low affinity for MTX has been found in isolated hepatocytes (Horne *et al.*, 1976). During the initial phases of uptake by the liver in rodents, most of the drug is excreted into the bile and undergoes enterohepatic recirculation (Bischoff *et al.*, 1971). In addition, partial conversion of the drug to a diglutamate metabolite has been documented in the liver in the rat (Baugh *et al.*, 1973) and in man (Jacobs *et al.*, 1975a). The diglutamate metabolite possesses the same ability as the parent compound to inhibit dihydrofolate reductase (Jacobs *et al.*, 1975b) and, in man, is retained in the liver for some months after drug administration (Jacobs *et al.*, 1975a). The enzyme system responsible for MTX diglutamate formation appears to be the same one that forms the folate polyglutamates, although with the folates, longer glutamyl chain-lengths appear to predominate. The metabolic consequences of this long-term retention of MTX diglutamate in liver are unknown, although altered metabolism of folic acid in the liver has been documented in rodents in the presence of MTX, with decreased uptake of [^{3}H]folic acid, and decreased conversion of folate to polyglutamate (Shin *et al.*, 1974). In addition, MTX has been observed to accelerate deposition of lipids in the rat liver (Tuma *et al.*, 1975), due to interference with synthesis of methionine. These changes are reversible by concomitant administration of methionine or choline. The relationship of these metabolic abnormalities to acute or chronic drug toxicity has not been established.

Neurotoxicity related to intrathecal MTX has become an important impediment to the treatment of meningeal leukemia. Acute arachnoiditis in the form of headache, nuchal rigidity, and fever occurs in approximately 30% of patients

370

BRUCE A.
CHABNER
AND
DAVID G.
JOHNS

receiving intrathecal MTX, and usually subsides without specific treatment (Dutt-era *et al.*, 1973). The possible usefulness of intrathecal corticosteroids in preventing this syndrome has been suggested, but remains to be established. More serious complications have been neuropathies, altered consciousness, or seizures, or some combination of these, observed in 10% of patients undergoing treatment for meningeal leukemia, and less frequently, in patients receiving prophylactic intrathecal therapy. These toxicities occasionally progress to a fatal necrotizing encephalopathy (Shapiro *et al.*, 1973), although in most instances, symptoms improve with discontinuation of intrathecal treatment. MTX-induced encephalopathy has been associated with a delay in clearance of MTX from the subarachnoid space, and detection of an elevated level of MTX in the CSF tends to confirm the clinical diagnosis of drug-induced neurotoxicity (Bleyer *et al.*, 1973).

The mechanism of MTX neurotoxicity appears to be unrelated to dihydrofolate reductase inhibition, since the enzyme is not detectable in the CNS (Makulu *et al.*, 1973). A role for folates in the synthesis of neurotransmitters has been suggested by Laduron (1972) and Banerjee and Snyder (1973), although MTX has not been shown to affect these processes directly.

In addition to the significant incidence of neurotoxicity when MTX is administered by the lumbar route, treatment of meningeal leukemia with this drug has other pitfalls, including a high rate of relapse when therapy is discontinued. In an attempt to explain these failures, Shapiro *et al.* (1975) studied the distribution of MTX in the CSF after intraventricular, lumbar, or intravenous administration, and showed that drug given by the lumbar route in small volumes (0.5–5 ml) distributes unreliably into the ventricles. High-dose intravenous administration of 500 mg/M^2 over 24 hr led to therapeutic levels in the spinal fluid approaching 10^{-6} M, while MTX given via an indwelling ventricular shunt provided reproducible therapeutic drug concentrations ($>10^{-6}$ M) for at least a 48-hr period. Bleyer *et al.* (1976) have inserted Ommaya-type ventricular reservoirs into a series of patients with meningeal leukemia, and have used repeated small doses of MTX with the hope of avoiding neurotoxicity while maintaining continuously effective drug levels in the CSF. Preliminary results in 19 patients have indicated fewer neurotoxic symptoms in the patients with Ommaya reservoirs, and equal therapeutic efficacy.

3. Resistance to Folate Antagonists

The sequence of events necessary for MTX to exert its cytocidal action were reviewed in Section 1, and include the following steps: (1) drug uptake by neoplastic cells; (2) tight binding to and inhibition of dihydrofolate reductase; (3) sufficient inhibition of dihydrofolate reductase activity to cause depletion of tetrahydrofolate pools in the target cells; and (4) entry of cells into the S phase during the period of MTX exposure. In light of the multiple obligatory steps involved in cytotoxicity, it is not surprising that resistance of mammalian neo-plasms to MTX may occur by any one of several mechanisms involving alterations in intrinsic cell properties.

Resistance in cells that have no prior history of exposure and adaptation to MTX has been most carefully studied in murine leukemias. Reduced capability to transport MTX and the naturally occurring folates has been documented in the resistant Walker 256 carcinosarcoma in rats (Rosen and Nichol, 1962), and Kessel *et al.* (1965) were able to correlate transport capability with antitumor effect in a series of murine and human tumor cell sources (Kessel *et al.*, 1968). A conflicting view has been offered by Harrap *et al.* (1971), who analyzed multiple biochemical parameters in five murine leukemia cell lines, and correlated sensitivity with the apparent affinity of MTX for dihydrofolate reductase. These authors hypothesized that small decreases in enzyme affinity for MTX would lead to a significant increase in the concentration of free drug required for complete enzyme inhibition. Dihydrofolate reductase with decreased affinity for MTX has been characterized biochemically in studies of a MTX-resistant cell culture line (Albrecht *et al.*, 1972). Hanggi and Littlefield (1975) purified two forms of dihydrofolate reductase in MTX-resistant hamster kidney cells. These forms differed in charge, molecular size, optimum pH, and catalytic activity. It has not been determined whether both enzyme forms are equally sensitive to inhibition by MTX. Bertino and Skeel (1975) have offered preliminary evidence for an altered affinity of enzyme for inhibitor in kinetic studies of enzyme from two patients resistant to MTX, although precise determination of the dissociation constant for the enzyme–inhibitor complex is complicated by the extremely tight binding of MTX to reductase. Direct measurement of enzyme–inhibitor complex forma-tion by competitive binding techniques (Myers *et al.*, 1975) offers considerable promise for allowing more precise determination of the strength of enzyme–inhibitor binding for enzymes from sensitive and resistant cells.

Repeated exposure of sensitive cells, either normal (Bertino *et al.*, 1963) or malignant (Fischer, 1961), to MTX is known to lead to increased levels of the target enzyme dihydrofolate reductase, as a consequence of a decreased rate of enzyme catabolism. Increased enzyme levels have also been documented in anecdotal cases of human leukemia following drug exposure (Hryniuk and Bertino, 1969), and are clearly responsible for resistance in several experimental cell lines (Albrecht *et al.*, 1972; Hanggi and Littlefield, 1975). At present, however, there are no data to indicate the relative importance of increased enzyme, as opposed to other mechanisms of resistance, in patients with neoplastic disease.

The prediction of response to MTX has been investigated by Hryniuk *et al.* (1974), who recently reported that resistance correlated best with the failure of MTX *in vitro* to depress [^{3}H]TdR incorporation into DNA; evidence was pre-sented that this test predicted for response to antineoplastic agents in general, and did not test for susceptibility to a specific biochemical lesion induced by antifo-lates, since depression of [^{3}H]TdR incorporation was not reversible by addition of purines. Earlier work (Hryniuk and Bertino, 1969) had indicated that *de novo*

372

BRUCE A.
CHABNER
AND
DAVID G.
JOHNS

resistance might also be predicted by the failure of MTX to depress thymidylate synthesis (as measured by incorporation of [³H]UdR into DNA) to 1% or less of the pretreatment rate. However, neither the UdR nor the TdR nucleoside incorporation test has been utilized in a prospective clinical trial to determine its usefulness in predicting response.

4. Clinical Applications of Folate Antagonists

As a single agent, MTX has produced responses in a broad spectrum of human neoplasms, and stands with adriamycin and cyclophosphamide as the most useful of the available agents. The highest response rates to antifolates are found in tumors having the most rapid growth rates, such as acute lymphocytic leukemia (Henderson and Samaha, 1969) and choriocarcinoma (Hertz *et al.*, 1961), but activity has also been recognized in slowly replicating solid tumors such as breast and ovarian cancer, head and neck cancer, and epidermoid carcinoma of the lung. In addition, this drug has become the mainstay for prophylaxis and therapy of meningeal leukemia. For a more complete review of clinical aspects of antifolate chemotherapy, the reader is referred to standard texts, such as *Cancer Medicine* (Holland and Frei, 1973).

Schedules of administration have varied widely, e.g., daily dosage in the range of 2–5 mg/M² per day, twice-weekly doses of 25 mg/M², weekly doses of 60 mg/M², and higher single doses in the range of 100–250 mg/M². The clinical tolerance to these doses varies according to the patient's previous exposure to chemotherapy and his bone marrow status. However, an additional factor determining toxicity appears to be the considerable individual variation in MTX pharmacokinetics observed from one patient to the next. Prolongation of the terminal phase of drug disappearance has been observed in patients with diminished renal function, and it has been recommended that the dosage of MTX be reduced in proportion to the reduction in creatinine clearance (Kristensen *et al.*, 1975).

In recent years, single-agent chemotherapy has largely been supplanted by combinations of agents (DeVita and Schein, 1973), or by multimodality regimens employing drugs as well as surgery and irradiation. In this context, drug interactions have assumed increasing importance. For example, it is known that the sequence of administration of drugs may have profound effects on the effectiveness of a regimen; MTX given prior to 5-fluorouracil is less effective than the same combination given in reverse order (Kline *et al.*, 1966), presumably because pretreatment with 5-fluorouracil blocks progression of cells into the MTX-vulnerable DNA synthetic phase. Other agents that halt progression of cells into DNA synthesis, such as arabinosyl cytosine or hydroxyurea, may have similar antagonistic effects on MTX cytotoxicity. Lampkin *et al.*, (1971) demonstrated that MTX can be used to synchronize human myeloblasts *in vivo*, creating an advantageous situation for subsequent treatment with an S-phase-specific agent such as arabinosyl cytosine. Unfortunately, the technical difficulties of determining the

optimum sequence and timing of drug therapy in individual patients have
resulted in the use of simplified treatment schedules paying a minimum of heed to
kinetic or pharmacological considerations.

Although the folate antagonists have been used effectively in the treatment of
many types of cancer, actual cure of established disease has been demonstrated
unequivocally only in the treatment of choriocarcinoma (Hertz *et al.*, 1961), and in
combination therapy of childhood leukemia (Pinkel, 1971). In an effort to
improve the results of antifolate therapy, radical changes have been made in the
dosage and schedule of administration, and treatment has been instituted earlier
in the course of disease. In an attempt to drive high concentrations of drug into
cells resistant to conventional drug schedules, Djerassi *et al.* (1967), Jaffe and Paed
(1972), and others have investigated the safety and efficacy of otherwise lethal
doses of MTX (above 50 mg/kg) given in continuous, short-term (6–24 hr) infusions, followed by leucovorin rescue; consistent responses have been observed in
childhood leukemia (Djerassi *et al.*, 1967), osteogenic sarcoma (Jaffe and Paed,
1972), and bronchogenic carcinoma (Djerassi *et al.*, 1972). Levitt *et al.* (1973) have
employed more prolonged infusions of 250–1000 mg/M^2 for up to 42 hr, followed
by leucovorin rescue, and have observed less toxicity and a slightly improved
response rate in comparison with conventional dose regimens. However, a
syndrome of renal failure, probably resulting from drug precipitation in the renal
tubules, has been seen in some patients receiving 50 mg/kg or more, and has been
associated with fatal myelosuppression (Jaffe and Paed, 1972). This renal toxicity
has been avoided in recent studies by alkalinization of the urine, diuresis, and
monitoring of plasma MTX to determine whether additional leucovorin is
required to protect against high levels of drug (Stoller *et al.*, 1975). The reader is
referred to a comprehensive symposium on the pharmacology of high-dose MTX
administration for a detailed evaluation of the risks, complications, and therapeutic results of this form of therapy (Chabner and Slavik, 1975).

Conventional and high-dose regimens of antifolate therapy have recently been
employed in adjuvant settings, i.e., in patients having surgical resection of all
clinically apparent tumor, but at high risk for development of metastic disease.
Advantages of this type of therapy include (1) the increased effectiveness of
chemotherapy employed against small tumor foci having a high growth fraction,
and (2) treatment at a time when the host is least debilitated by tumor and best able
to tolerate drug-related toxicity. Adjuvant high-dose MTX has decreased the rate
of recurrence of osteogenic sarcoma in preliminary studies (Jaffe *et al.*, 1974), and
in combination with 5-fluorouracil and cyclophosphamide, has markedly
decreased the recurrence rate in women having positive axillary lymph nodes
found at radical mastectomy for breast cancer (Bonadonna *et al.*, 1976). Both
studies will require long-term follow-up to determine whether the delayed early
recurrence rate will be translated into meaningful prolongation of survival, and
cure. Additional risks have to be accepted in the use of extended-duration,
adjuvant therapy, including permanent injury to bone marrow and reproductive tissue, hepatotoxicity, and potential carcinogenesis (Sieber and Adamson,
1975).

374

BRUCE A.
CHABNER
AND
DAVID G.
JOHNS

Two other forms of experimental antifolate chemotherapy have recently been employed in preliminary studies. Capizzi (1975) has investigated a regimen of high-dose MTX followed in 24 hr by L-asparaginase, an enzyme with antileukemic activity that inhibits protein synthesis and prevents MTX toxicity. Beneficial responses including hematological remission were reported in 6 patients with acute lymphocytic leukemia resistant to conventional doses of methotrexate. The study demonstrated conclusive alteration of MTX toxicity, although the therapeutic results may have been largely the result of L-asparaginase effects. In other investigations from the same laboratory, McCullough et al. (1971) have purified a folate-cleaving enzyme, carboxypeptidase G, from *Pseudomonas stutzeri*. This enzyme possesses antitumor activity against the MTX-resistant Walker 256 carcinosarcoma (Chabner *et al.*, 1972*a*). In addition, the enzyme is capable of cleaving circulating MTX (Chabner *et al.*, 1972*b*), and may provide an alternative means of eliminating toxic concentrations of drug in patients who develop renal failure while receiving high-dose MTX. Its utility for therapy or for rescue from MTX toxicity remains to be established.

5. References

ALBRECHT, A. M., BIEDLER, J. L., AND HUTCHISON, D. G., 1972, Two different species of dihydrofolate reductase in mammalian cells differentially resistant to amethopterin and methasquin, *Cancer Res.* **32:**1539.

BANERJEE, S. P., AND SNYDER, S. H., 1973, Methyltetrahydrofolic acid mediates *N*- and *O*-methylation of biogenic amines, *Science* **182:**74.

BAUGH, C. M., KRUMDIECK, C. L., AND NAIR, M. G., 1973, Polyglutamyl metabolites of methotrexate, *Biochem. Biophys. Res. Commun.* **52:**27.

BERGE, G., LUNDQUIST, A., ROSSMAN, H., AND ÅKERMAN, M., 1970, Liver biopsy in psoriasis, *J. Dermatol.* **82:**250.

BERTINO, J. R., 1963, The mechanism of action of the folate antagonists in man, *Cancer Res.* **23:**1286.

BERTINO, J. R., AND SKEEL, R. T., 1975, On natural and acquired resistance to folate antagonists in man, in: *Pharmacological Basis of Cancer Chemotherapy*, pp. 401–468, Williams and Wilkins, Baltimore.

BERTINO, J. R., DONAHUE, D. M., SIMMONS, GABRIO, B. W., SILBER, R., AND HUENNEKENS, F. M., 1963, The "induction" of dihydrofolate reductase activity in leukocytes and erythrocytes of patients treated with amethopterin, *J. Clin. Invest.* **42:**466.

BERTINO, J. R., BOOTH, B. A., CASHMORE, A., BIEBER, A. L., AND SARTORELLI, A. C., 1964, Studies of the inhibition of dihydrofolate reductase by the folate antagonists, *J. Biol. Chem.* **239:**479.

BISCHOFF, K. B., DEDRICK, R. L., ZAHARKO, D. S., AND LONGSTRETH, J. A., 1971, Methotrexate pharmacokinetics, *J. Pharm. Sci.* **60:**1128.

BLEYER, W. A., DRAKE, J. C., AND CHABNER, B. A., 1973, Neurotoxicity and elevated cerebrospinal-fluid methotrexate concentration in meningeal leukemia, *N. Engl. J. Med.* **289:**770.

BLEYER, W. A., POPLACK, D. G., ZIEGLER, J. L., LEVENTHAL, B. G., OMMAYA, A. K., AND CHABNER, B. A., 1976, "Concentration × Time" (C × T) methotrexate (MTX) therapy of meningeal leukemia via a subcutaneous reservoir: A controlled clinical trial, *Proc. Amer. Assoc. Cancer Res.* **17:**253.

BONADONNA, G., BRUSAMOLINO, E., VALAGUSSA, P., ROSSI, A., BRUGNATELLI, L., BRAMBILLA, C., DELENA, M., TANCINI, G., BAJETTA, E., MUSUMECI, R., AND VERONESI, U., 1976, Combination chemotherapy as an adjuvant treatment in operable breast cancer, *N. Engl. J. Med.* **294:**405.

BRUCE, W. R., MEEKER, B. E., AND VALERIOTE, F. A., 1966, Comparison of the sensitivity of normal hematopoietic and transplanted lymphoma colony forming cells to chemotherapeutic agents administered *in vivo*, *J. Natl. Cancer Inst.* **37:**233.

CAPIZZI, R. L., 1974, Schedule-dependent synergism and antagonism between methotrexate and L-asparaginase, *Biochem. Pharmacol.* **23**(Suppl. 2):151.

CAPIZZI, R. L., 1975, Improvement in the therapeutic index of methotrexate (NSC-740) by L-asparaginase (NSC-109229), *Cancer Chemother. Rep. Part 3* **6**:37.

CHABNER, B. A., AND SLAVIK, M. (eds.), 1975, Proceedings of the High-Dose Methotrexate Therapy Meeting, Dec. 19, 1974, *Cancer Chemother. Rep. Part 3* **6**:1.

CHABNER, B. A., AND YOUNG, R. C., 1973, Threshold methotrexate concentration for *in vivo* inhibition of DNA synthesis in normal and tumorous target tissues, *J. Clin. Invest.* **52**:1804.

CHABNER, B. A., CHELLO, P. L., AND BERTINO, J. R., 1972*a*, Antitumor activity of a folate-cleaving enzyme, carboxypeptidase G₁, *Cancer Res.* **32**:2114.

CHABNER, B. A., JOHNS, D. G., AND BERTINO, J. R., 1972*b*, Enzymatic cleavage of methotrexate provides a method for prevention of drug toxicity, *Nature (London)* **239**:395.

CHELLO, P., DONSBACH, R. C., SIROTNAK, F. M., AND HUTCHISON, D. J., 1975, Relevance of membrane transport to therapeutic responsiveness and selective activity with methotrexate in murine tumor models, *Proc. Amer. Assoc. Cancer Res.* **16**:181.

DAHL, M. G. C., GREGORY, M. M., AND SCHEUER, P. J., 1971, Liver damage due to methotrexate in patients with psoriasis, *Br. Med. J.* **1**:625.

DEVITA, V. T., AND SCHEIN, P. S., 1973, The use of drugs in combination for the treatment of cancer, *N. Engl. J. Med.* **288**:998.

DJERASSI, I., FARBER, S., ABIR, E., AND NEIKIRK, W., 1967, Continuous infusion of methotrexate in children with acute leukemia, *Cancer* **20**:233.

DJERASSI, I., ROMINGER, C. J., KIM, J. S., TURCHI, J., SUVRANSKI, U., AND HUGHES, D., 1972, Phase I study of high doses of methotrexate with citrovorum factor in patients with lung cancer, *Cancer* **30**:22.

DUTTERA, M. J., BLEYER, W. A., POMEROY, T. C., LEVENTHAL, C. M., AND LEVENTHAL, B. G., 1973, Irradiation, methotrexate toxicity, and the treatment of meningeal leukemia, *Lancet* **2**:703.

FISCHER, G. A., 1961, Increased levels of folic acid reductase as a mechanism of resistance to amethopterin in leukemic cells, *Biochem. Pharmacol.* **7**:75.

GOLDIN, A., MANTEL, N., GREENHOUSE, S. W., VENDITTI, J. M., AND HUMPHREYS, S. R., 1953, Estimation of the antileukemic potency of the antimetabolite, aminopterin, administered alone and in combination with citrovorum factor or folic acid, *Cancer Res.* **13**:843.

GOLDIN, A., VENDITTI, J. M., HUMPHREYS, S. R., DENNIS, D., AND MANTEL, N., 1955, Studies on the management of mouse leukemia (L1210) with antagonists of folic acid, *Cancer Res.* **15**:742.

GOLDMAN, I. D., 1974, The mechanism of action of methotrexate. I. Interaction with a low-affinity intracellular site required for maximum inhibition of deoxyribonucleic acid synthesis in L-cell mouse fibroblasts, *Mol. Pharmacol.* **10**:257.

GOLDMAN, I. D., 1975, Analysis of the cytotoxic determinants for methotrexate (NSC-740): A role for "free" intracellular drug, *Cancer Chemother. Rep. Part 3* **6**:51.

GOLDMAN, I. D., WHITE, J. C., AND LOFTFIELD, S., 1975, Mechanism of action of methotrexate: III. Free intracellular methotrexate is required for maximal suppression of C¹⁴ formate incorporation into nucleic acids and protein, *Mol. Pharmacol.* **11**:287.

GRINDEY, G. B., AND MORAN, R. G., 1975, Effects of allopurinol on the therapeutic efficacy of methotrexate, *Cancer Res.* **35**:1702.

HALPERN, R. M., HALPERN, B. C., CLARK, B. R., ASHE, H., HARDY, D. N., JENKINSON, P. Y., CHOU, S., AND SMITH, R. A., 1975, New approach to antifolate treatment of certain cancers as demonstrated in tissue culture, *Proc. Natl. Acad. Sci. U.S.A.* **72**:4018.

HANGGI, U. J., AND LITTLEFIELD, J. W., 1975, Isolation and characterization of the multiple forms of dihydrofolate reductase from methotrexate-resistant hamster cells, *J. Biol. Chem.* **249**:1930.

HARRAP, K. R., HILL, B. T., FURNESS, M. E., AND HART, L. I., 1971, Sites of action of amethopterin: Intrinsic and acquired drug resistance, *Ann. N. Y. Acad. Sci.* **186**:312.

HENDERSON, E. S., AND SAMAHA, R. J., 1969, Evidence that drugs in multiple combinations have materially advanced the treatment of human malignancies, *Cancer Res.* **29**:2272.

HERTZ, R., LEWIS, J., JR., AND LIPSETT, M. B., 1961, Five years experience with the chemotherapy of metastatic choriocarcinoma and related trophoblastic tumors in women, *Amer. J. Obstet. Gynecol.* **82**:631.

HOLLAND, J. F., AND FREI, E., III (eds.), 1973, *Cancer Medicine,* Lea and Febiger, Philadelphia.

HORNE, D. W., BRIGGS, W. T., AND WAGNER, C., 1976, A functional, active transport system for methotrexate in freshly isolated hepatocytes, *Biochem. Biophys. Res. Commun.* **68**:70.

HRYNIUK, W. M., 1972, Purineless death as a link between growth rate and cytotoxicity of methotrexate, *Cancer Res.* **32**:1506

376

BRUCE A.
CHABNER
AND
DAVID G.
JOHNS

HRYNIUK, W. M., AND BERTINO, J. R., 1969, Treatment of leukemia with large doses of methotrexate and folinic acid: Clinical–biochemical correlates, *J. Clin. Invest.* **48**:2140.

HRYNIUK, W. H., FISCHER, G. A., AND BERTINO, J. R., 1969, S-Phase cells of rapidly growing and resting populations, *Mol. Pharmacol.* **5**:557.

HRYNIUK, W. H., BISHOP, A., AND FOERSTER, J., 1974, Clinical correlates of *in vitro* effects of methotrexate on acute leukemia blasts, *Cancer Res.* **34**:2823.

JACKSON, R. C., AND HARRAP, K. R., 1973, Studies with a mathematical model of folate metabolism, *Arch. Biochem. Biophys.* **158**:827.

JACOBS, S. A., DERR, C. J., AND JOHNS, D. G., 1975a, Long-term retention of 2,4-diamino-N^{10}-methylpteroylglutamyl-γ-glutamate [MTX(G_1)] by human liver, *Proc. Amer. Assoc. Cancer Res.* **16**:65.

JACOBS, S. A., ADAMSON, R. H., CHABNER, B. A., DERR, C. J., AND JOHNS, D. G., 1975b, Stoichiometric inhibition of mammalian dihydrofolate reductase by the γ-glutamyl metabolite of methotrexate, 4-amino-4-deoxy-N^{10}-methylpteroylglutamyl-γ-glutamate, *Biochem. Biophys. Res. Commun.* **63**:692.

JACOBS, S. A., STOLLER, R. G., CHABNER, B. A., AND JOHNS, D. G., 1976, 7-Hydroxymethotrexate as a urinary metabolite in human subjects and rhesus monkeys receiving high dose methotrexate, *J. Clin. Invest.* **57**:534.

JAFFE, N., AND PAED, D., 1972, Recent advances in the chemotherapy of metastatic osteogenic sarcoma, *Cancer* **30**:1627.

JAFFE, N., FREI, E., III, TRAGGIS, D., AND BISHOP, Y., 1974, Adjuvant methotrexate and citrovorum-factor treatment of osteogenic sarcoma, *N. Engl. J. Med.* **291**:994.

KESSEL, D., HALL, T. C., ROBERTS, D., AND WODINSKY, I., 1965, Uptake as a determinant of methotrexate response in mouse leukemia, *Science* **150**:752.

KESSEL, D., HALL, T. C., AND ROBERTS, D., 1968, Modes of uptake of methotrexate by normal and leukemic human leukocytes *in vitro* and their relation to drug response, *Cancer Res.* **28**:564.

KLINE, I., VENDITTI, J. M., MEAD, J. A. R., TYRER, D. D., AND GOLDIN, A., 1966, The antileukemic effectiveness of 5-fluorouracil and methotrexate in the combination chemotherapy of advanced leukemia, *Cancer Res.* **26**:848.

KRISTENSEN, L. O., WEISMAN, K., AND HUTTERS, L., 1975, Renal function and rate of disappearance of methotrexate from serum, *Eur. J. Clin. Pharmacol.* **8**:439.

LADURON, P., 1972, *N*-Methylation of dopamine to epinine in brain tissue using *N*-methyltetrahydrofolic acid as the methyl donor, *Nature (London) New Biol.* **238**:212.

LAMPKIN, B. C., NAGAO, AND MAUER, A. M., 1971, Synchronization and recruitment in acute leukemia, *J. Clin. Invest.* **50**:2204.

LEVITT, M., MOSHER, M. B., DeCONTI, R. C., FARBER, L. R., SKEEL, R. T., MARSH, J. C., MITCHELL, M. S., PAPAC, R. J., THOMAS, E. D., AND BERTINO, J. R., 1973, Improved therapeutic index of methotrexate with "leucovorin rescue," *Cancer Res.* **33**:1729.

MAKULU, D. R., SMITH, E. F., AND BERTINO, J. R., 1973, Lack of dihydrofolate reductase activity in brain tissue of mammalian species. Possible implications, *J. Neurochem.* **21**:241.

McCULLOUGH, J. M., CHABNER, B. A., AND BERTINO, J. R., 1971, Purification and properties of carboxypeptidase G_1, *J. Biol. Chem.* **246**:7207.

MITCHELL, M. S., WAWRO, N. W., DeCONTI, R. C., KAPLAN, S. R., PAPAC, R., AND BERTINO, J. R., 1968, Effectiveness of high-dose infusions of methotrexate followed by leucovorin in carcinoma of the head and neck, *Cancer Res.* **28**:1088.

MYERS, C. W., LIPPMAN, M. E., ELIOT, H. M., AND CHABNER, B. A., 1975, Competitive protein binding assay for methotrexate, *Proc. Natl. Acad. Sci. U.S.A.* **72**:3683.

NIXON, P. J., SLUTSKY, G., NAHAS, A., AND BERTINO, J. R., 1973, The turnover of folate coenzymes in murine lymphoma cells, *J. Biol. Chem.* **248**:5932.

PINEDO, H. M., AND CHABNER, B. A., 1976, The role of drug concentration, duration of exposure and endogenous metabolites in determining methotrexate cytotoxicity, *Cancer Treatment Rep.*, in press.

PINEDO, H. M., ZAHARKO, D. S., BULL, J. M., YOUNG, R. C., AND CHABNER, B. A., 1976a, Importance of methotrexate plasma concentration (MTX)p and duration of exposure in determining marrow toxicity during continuous infusion, *Proc. Amer. Assoc. Cancer Res.* **17**:104

PINEDO, H. M., CHABNER, B. A., ZAHARKO, D. S., AND BULL, J. M., 1976b, Evidence for early recruitment of granulocytic precursors during high dose methotrexate infusion in mice, *Blood* **48**:301.

PINKEL, D., 1971, Five-year follow-up of "total therapy" of childhood lymphocytic leukemia, *J. Amer. Med. Assoc.* **216**:648.

ROBERTS, D., AND WARMATH, E. V., 1975, Methotrexate inhibition of CCRM-CEM cultures of human lymphoblasts, *Eur. J. Cancer* **11**:771.

ROSEN, F., AND NICHOL, C. A., 1962, Inhibition of the growth of an amethopterin-refractory tumor by dietary restriction of folic acid, *Cancer Res.* **22**:495.

SHAPIRO, W. R., CHERNICK, N. L., AND POSNER, J. B., 1973, Necrotizing encephalopathy following intraventricular instillation of methotrexate, *Arch. Neurol.* **28**:96.

SHAPIRO, W. R., YOUNG, D. F., AND MEHTA, B. M., 1975, Methotrexate distribution in cerebrospinal fluid after intravenous, ventricular and lumbar injections, *N. Engl. J. Med.* **293**:161.

SHIN, Y. S., BUEHRING, K. U., AND STOKSTAD, E. L. R., 1974, The metabolism of methotrexate in *Lactobacillus casei* and rat liver, and the influence of methotrexate on metabolism of folic acid, *J. Biol. Chem.* **249**:5772.

SIEBER, S. M., AND ADAMSON, R. M., 1975, The clastogenic, mutagenic, teratogenic and carcinogenic effects of various antineoplastic agents, in: *Pharmacological Basis of Cancer Chemotherapy*, pp. 401–468, Williams and Wilkins, Baltimore.

SIROTNAK, F. M., AND DONSBACH, R. C., 1973, Differential cell permeability and the basis for selective activity of methotrexate during therapy of the L1210 leukemia, *Cancer Res.* **33**:1290.

STOLLER, R. G., JACOBS, S. A., DRAKE, J. C., LUTZ, R. J., AND CHABNER, B. A., 1975, Pharmacokinetics of high-dose methotrexate, *Cancer Chemother. Rep. Part 3* **6**:19.

TATTERSALL, M. H. N., JACKSON, R. C., JACKSON, S. T. M., AND HARRAP, K. R., 1974, Factors determining cell sensitivity of methotrexate: Studies of folate and deoxyribonucleoside triphosphate pools in five mammalian cell lines, *Eur. J. Cancer* **10**:819.

TATTERSALL, M. H. N., BROWN, B., AND FREI, E., III, 1975, The reversal of methotrexate toxicity with maintenance of antitumor effects, *Nature (London)* **253**:198.

TUMA, D. J., BARAK, A. J., AND SORRELL, M. F., 1975, Interaction of methotrexate with lipotropic factors in rat liver, *Biochem. Pharmacol.* **24**:1327.

VOGLER, W. R., MINGIOLI, E. S., AND GARWOOD, F. A., 1973, The effect of methotrexate on granulocyte stem cells and granulopoiesis, *Cancer Res.* **33**:1628.

WERKHEISER, W. C., 1961, Specific binding of 4-amino analogues by folic acid reductase, *J. Biol. Chem.* **236**:888.

YOUNG, R. C., AND CHABNER, B. A., 1973, An *in vivo* method for monitoring differential effects of chemotherapy on target tissues in animals and man. Correlation with plasma pharmacokinetics, *J. Clin. Invest.* **52**:92A.

ZAHARKO, D. S., DEDRICK, R. L., PEALE, A. L., DRAKE, J. C., AND LUTZ, R. J., 1974, Relative toxicity of methotrexate in several tissues of mice bearing Lewis lung carcinoma, *J. Pharmacol. Exp. Ther.* **189**:585.

14

Plant Alkaloids

WILLIAM A. CREASEY

1. Introduction

The use of plant derivatives for treating human cancer originated in remote antiquity. In the Ebers papyrus, written about 1550 B.C., external application of garlic was recommended for skin disorders that may have included cancer. The same document described the use of the seeds of the autumn crocus, *Colchicum autumnale*, for joint pain, but a role for this plant or the less toxic *C. lingulatum* in treating cancer was not established until the time of Dioscorides in the 1st century A. D. Bittersweet, or woody nightshade, *Solanum dulcamara*, is another plant the use of which as a remedy for cancers, warts, and tumors is very ancient, the plant being listed for this purpose by Galen in the 2nd century A.D. Other plants with long-established folkloric reputations include *Euphorbia esula* and *Croton tiglium* (Kupchan *et al.*, 1976), many members of the lily family (Amaryllidaceae) (Fitzgerald *et al.*, 1958), white bryony, cinquefoil, and asarabaca (Culpeper, 1653). McKenzie (1927) described many other examples, including *Atropa belladonna*, the elder tree (*Sambucus niger*), the mandrake, and surprisingly, the rose. Among its many other reputed uses, ginseng has been employed to treat cancer in Chinese herbal medicine (Leake, 1975). During the 17th and 18th centuries, the doctrine of signatures, which stressed the resemblance between a diseased organ and the plant effective in treating it, was applied widely. This usage brought about the addition of a vast number of new herbal remedies, most of which were, however, of no efficacy whatsoever. As a result, the use of plant preparations became to some extent suspect, and what may be termed a chemical approach to pharmacology finally reached dominance. Nevertheless, as we shall see in this chapter, a

WILLIAM A. CREASEY ● Departments of Internal Medicine and Pharmacology, Yale University School of Medicine, New Haven, Connecticut. Present address: Children's Hospital of Philadelphia and Department of Pharmacology, University of Pennsylvania School of Medicine, Philadelphia, Pennsylvania.

large number of traditional plant remedies have been found to contain active antitumor agents, most often of an alkaloidal nature.

In this chapter, we shall review the pharmacology and touch on the clinical usefulness of a number of classes of alkaloids. There will not be any attempt to compile a comprehensive compendium; rather, examples will be chosen because of their clinical interest or unusual structure, or because they illustrate a variety of mechanisms of action.

2. Metaphase-Arresting Agents: Colchicine, the Vinca Alkaloids, Podophyllotoxin, and Griseofulvin

For the purposes of this discussion, the agents that arrest cell division during metaphase may be grouped together, despite the great disparity in their chemical structures (see Figs. 1–3). This grouping reflects fundamental analogies among these compounds with respect to their biological and biochemical properties. Apart from the vinca alkaloids and compounds related to colchicine, griseofulvin and the derivatives of podophyllotoxin that are not alkaloids belong to this group of drugs. The pharmacology of antimitotic agents in general has been discussed by Dustin (1963), Savel (1966), and Creasey (1975a), and much of the earlier background material will not be considered in detail in this chapter.

2.1. Occurrence

Colchicine occurs in plants of the genus *Colchicum* (Liliaceae), the seeds of the autumn crocus, *C. autumnale*, for example, containing up to 4 g of this alkaloid per kilogram. This drug is the subject of a monograph (Eigsti and Dustin, 1955) that provides a large amount of background material. The chemistry of colchicine derivatives has been reviewed (Wildman and Pursey, 1968). The vinca alkaloids are derived from the Madagascan periwinkle plant, *Vinca rosea* Linn., or more correctly, *Catharanthus roseus* G. Don (Apocynaceae). Leukopenic and antitumor activities were identified during screening of the plant for the hypoglycemic activity traditionally attributed to it. These alkaloids occur in very low concentrations, as little as 3 mg vincristine in 1 kg dry leaves, for example. Various aspects of the botany, chemistry, pharmacology, and clinical use of these agents have been collected in one volume (Taylor and Farnsworth, 1975). The mayapple, *Podophyllum peltatum* Linn. (*Berberidaceae*), contains a resin long used as a remedy for treating warts, as a cathartic, and in more recent times, as a topical agent for condylomata acuminata (Kaplan, 1942). The major active agent in the resin is podophyllotoxin. A number of derivatives have been synthesized and brought to clinical trial. An early review (M. G. Kelly and Hartwell, 1953) may be consulted for background information on podophyllin. Griseofulvin, derived from the molds *Penicillium griseofulvum* Dierckx and *P. janczewskii* Zal., is an antifungal agent effective in certain skin infections; Bent and Moore (1966) summarized much information regarding this drug. Narciclasine, which also causes mitotic arrest, will be discussed later in this chapter. Mescaline has recently been described as a mitotic spindle inhibitor (Harrisson *et al.*, 1976), but will not be discussed further.

2.2. Biological Activity

2.2.1. Mitotic Arrest

Arrest of cell division in metaphase is characteristic of these compounds. It was described first for colchicine in 1934 (Lits, 1934), and since that time, the same type of action has been well documented for the vinca alkaloids (Cardinali *et al.*, 1961; Palmer *et al.*, 1963; George *et al.*, 1965) and griseofulvin (Grisham *et al.*, 1973; Gull and Trinci, 1973). In the case of the podophyllins, mitotic arrest is produced by the parent drug (B. J. Sullivan and Wechsler, 1947) and several derivatives, with the exception of the glycosides VP-16 and VM-26, which have a more pronounced effect on the transition between the late S phase and the prophase (Stähelin, 1970; Misra and Roberts, 1975).

In studies of mitotic arrest, the primary action of antimitotics has been found to occur on the spindle structure. Thus, the process is not to be envisaged as the freezing of mitosis at an intermediate stage, but rather the dissolution of the spindle itself, which prevents progression to anaphase and telophase. Chromosomes may subsequently become dispersed throughout the cytoplasm or associated into unusual groupings.

Mitotic arrest is in general a reversible process for most antimitotic agents. Krishan (1968) detailed the course of recovery for Earle's L cells in culture after exposure to vinblastine. In as little as 4 hr after removal of vinblastine, a large number of the metaphase-blocked and multimicronucleated cells resulting from drug treatment began to divide. However, many aberrations appeared during subsequent divisions of these released cells. The oocytes of the marine annelid *Pectinaria gouldi* (Malawista *et al.*, 1968) and of the starfish *Pisaster ochraceous* (Malawista *et al.*, 1976) represent elegant systems for the study of reversible spindle dissolution. Vinblastine, colcemid, and griseofulvin cause the meiotic spindle to shrink and disappear within a matter of minutes, only to reappear rapidly when the drugs are washed away with sea water. Recovery was not completely reversible when podophyllotoxin and vincristine were the drugs under study. It is interesting to note a similar lack of complete reversibility when HeLa, Chinese hamster fibroblast, and chick spinal ganglion cells were exposed to vincristine (Journey *et al.*, 1968).

Mitotic arrest has commonly been used not only for synchronizing cell cultures, but also for studying cell kinetics. It is evident that care should be taken in interpreting such data if the mitotic arrest should not prove to be completely reversible. Another factor that could enter into such considerations is possible perturbation of the cell cycle by drugs. Thus, while Bruchovsky *et al.* (1965) could find no evidence for any effect of vinblastine on the rate of cell progression into mitosis, varying degrees of reduction in the rates of cells entering prophase have been attributed to colchicine (Mueller *et al.*, 1971), the vinca alkaloids (Cardinali *et al.*, 1968), and podophyllin derivatives (Stähelin, 1970). Chromosome damage is an additional factor, one that has been considered to be minor and secondary in nature (Sentein, 1964). Such a secondary nature certainly fits the observations of Krishan (1968) referred to above. However, chromosomal aberrations induced by vincristine have been described as prominent and similar to those produced by alkylating agents (Gebhart *et al.*, 1969).

The extent of mitotic arrest induced by these agents is subject to alteration by other compounds or experimental conditions. Thus, Marsland (1968) reported that the mitotic arrest produced by colchicine in the eggs of the echinoderm *Lytechinus variegatus* undergoing first cleavage division was enhanced by lowering the temperature or raising the pressure. Adrenalectomy produced a similar potentiation of the antimitotic effect of colcemid on rat hair follicles; adrenal steroids antagonized the effects on the spindle (DeHarven, 1956). Other compounds found to antagonize mitotic-arresting agents are diethylstilbestrol (Cutts, 1968), ATP (Dustin, 1963), and the amino acids tryptophan and glutamic acid (Cutts, 1961). The latter compound acts as a competitive inhibitor of the transport of vinblastine by human leukocytes (Creasey *et al.*, 1971); such an action could form the basis for biological antagonism.

2.2.2. Antitumor Action in Experimental Systems

The antitumor activity of colchicine itself has been demonstrated in Flexner-Jobling carcinoma, Shope rabbit papilloma, carcinoma 63, and various spontaneous tumors (Ludford, 1945). Trimethylcolchicinic acid methyl ether is active against L1210 and, to a lesser extent, P388, whereas L1210 is relatively insensitive to colcemid, which inhibits P388 and, to a much greater extent, adenocarcinoma 755 (Venditti and Abbott, 1967). All four of the major active alkaloids in the periwinkle plant inhibit the growth of P1534 and Freund leukemias. Ridgeway osteogenic sarcoma is sensitive to vinrosidine and vincristine, while Ehrlich ascites carcinoma responds to vinblastine and vinleurosine. Vinblastine and vincristine inhibit the growth of S180 and B82A, the latter tumor also responding to vinrosidine (I. S. Johnson *et al.*, 1963). L1210 is only moderately sensitive to vinblastine and vincristine, two drugs that are potent inhibitors of P388, Walker 256, and the Dunning tumor (Venditti and Abbott, 1967). Vinglycinate is approximately as potent against P1534 leukemia as is vincristine (I. S. Johnson *et al.*, 1966). In cultured mammalian cells, the cell-cycle phases most sensitive were late G_1 and S for vinblastine and S for vincristine (Madoc-Jones and Mauro, 1968). Cross-resistance has been demonstrated between the vinca alkaloids and the anthracyclines adriamycin and daunorubicin in Ehrlich ascites (Danø, 1972). The podophyllin derivative podophyllic acid ethyl hydrazide inhibits the growth of S37 and S180, Walker 256, and, to a lesser extent, Yoshida ascites and L1210 (Stähelin and Cerletti, 1964). Walker 256, L1210, and P1534 leukemia are quite sensitive to VM-26 (Stähelin, 1970). Griseofulvin has not been studied as an antitumor agent, although it does exert striking metaphase arrest and chromosomal disorientation in Walker 256 and a rat lymphosarcoma (Paget and Walpole, 1958).

2.2.3. Antiinflammatory Action

Colchicine derivatives have traditionally been used to treat gouty episodes (Malawista, 1965), but they have only weak antiinflammatory activity in other disorders. Vinblastine (Krakoff, 1965) and griseofulvin (Slonim *et al.*, 1962) can also relieve the pain of gout.

2.2.4. Neuromuscular Actions

Neurological toxicity is a well-documented side effect of colchicine and the vinca alkaloids, although only in the case of vincristine is it the dose-limiting side effect. As described for vincristine by Sandler *et al.* (1969), this toxicity in humans involved asymptomatic depression of the Achilles reflex as its earliest manifestation. Paresthesias of the extremities also developed early. Motor nerve conduction velocity and the Hoffman's reflex were intact at this time. Involvement of the cranial and sensory nerves and slapping gait occurred only in advance cases. These workers postulated a selective effect on the muscle spindle. GI symptoms, notably constipation and even paralytic ileus, as well as muscle weakness, especially of the wrist extensors, are other effects of neurological origin (Casey *et al.*, 1970). In contrast to the work described above, the findings of Bradley *et al.* (1970) and of McLeod and Penny (1969) suggested that reduction of conduction velocities did occur. Among the pathological changes described are axonal degeneration and demyelination produced by direct infusion of colchicine into the region of the sciatic nerve of the mouse (Angevine, 1957), or by treatment of human patients with vinblastine and vincristine (Gottschalk *et al.*, 1968). Other changes noted in rodents receiving single doses of vincristine large enough to cause hindlimb paralysis were lysis of dorsal root ganglion cells and inhibition of Schwann cell proliferation (UY *et al.*, 1967). Effects on nerve cell growth include inhibition by colchicine of axon sprouting in partially denervated muscle (Hoffman, 1952) and retraction of terminal expansion and of the undulating membrane of spinal ganglion cells in culture exposed to vinblastine (Barasa *et al.*, 1970).

There are fast and slow components of axoplasmic transport responsible for movement of storage granules, proteins, and other materials (Keen and Livingston, 1970). Intraocular administration of colchicine to rabbits almost completely inhibited rapid migration of labeled proteins in the optic tract (Karlsson and Sjöstrand, 1969). A similar study in isolated cat sciatic nerves found that vincristine was twice as potent as vinblastine or desacetyl vinblastine amide in inhibiting transport of labeled components (Ochs and Worth, 1975). Both colchicine and vinblastine inhibit the transport of norepinephrine storage granules in adrenergic neurons and of acetylcholine and choline acetyl transferase in cholinergic motor neurons, primarily by affecting the rapidly transportable forms (Dahlström *et al.*, 1975).

Action on the muscle spindle and other myopathies have been described (Tobin and Sandler, 1966; Bradley *et al.*, 1970), and it is evident that muscle cells form a direct target for antimitotic drugs, apart from indirect action through nervous innervation. Degenerative changes in motor end plates, necrosis of muscle fibers, and appearance of spheromembranous bodies were described in rats treated with vincristine (Anderson *et al.*, 1967). Other evidence of damage to muscle produced by vincristine includes reduction in calcium uptake and an altered phospholipid profile of rat skeletal muscle microsomes (Yasin *et al.*, 1973), and an increase in plasma creatine phosphokinase that was correlated with the appearance of muscle cell necrosis (Yasin and Parker, 1975).

2.2.5. Autonomic Actions

Certain of the toxic reactions ascribed to vincristine, such as hypertension (Ueda *et al.*, 1969) or hypotension accompanied by an abnormal Valsalva response (Hancock and Naysmith, 1975), may reflect side effects on the autonomic nervous system. Apart from the interference with the transport of neurotransmitters discussed in Section 2.2.4, which could produce effects such as the delay in release of sympathetic transmitter seen after treatment of rats with colchicine (Lundberg, 1970), there are other sources of autonomic neuropathy. Vinblastine and vincristine both caused a major reduction in the cardiac effects of noradrenergic nerve stimulation and sensitized the myocardium to norepinephrine (Bennett and Gardiner, 1975). In addition, colchicine and vinblastine inhibited the uptake of norepinephrine by adrenergic fibers (Costa and Filogamo, 1970) and of 5-HT and norepinephrine by rat brain synaptosomes (Nomura and Segawa, 1975). Finally, colchicine, vinblastine, griseofulvin, and colcemid inhibited the release of histamine from rat peritoneal mast cells (E. Gillespie *et al.*, 1968).

2.2.6. Morphological Alterations

Padawer (1963) described displacement of the nuclei and anisodiametry of the cytoplasm of mast cells exposed to colchicine, vinblastine, and podophyllotoxin. Subsequently, a wide variety of other changes have been described. Vinblastine induced into normal erythrocytes a rigidity that resembled the hereditary spherocytosis syndrome; colchicine was 10 times less effective than vinblastine (Jacob *et al.*, 1972). Colchicine and vinblastine induce autophagy, a segregation of organelles into membrane-bounded cavities followed by lysis, in Ehrlich ascites and in liver cells (Hirsimäki *et al.*, 1975). Human leukemic lymphoblasts exposed to low levels (0.01–0.1 μg/ml) of vinblastine or vincristine also formed membrane-lined vesicles, which were, however, released from the peripheral cytoplasm. This process closely resembled the formation of platelets from megakaryocytes (Krishan and Frei, 1975), and it is significant that the vinca alkaloids produce a thrombocytosis in rats (Robertson *et al.*, 1970) and humans (Robertson and McCarthy, 1969). Another extremely interesting observation has been the induction of differentiation in T lymphocytes by vinca alkaloids (Sabad, 1975).

2.2.7. Immunologic Effects

The vinca alkaloids inhibited both the formation of antibodies to serum albumin and delayed hypersensitivity in rats (Aisenberg, 1963), although these drugs are not among the more effective immunosuppressive agents. Both colchicine and vincristine inhibit the secretion of IgM antibody (Teplitz *et al.*, 1975), but in contrast to cytochalasins, neither these antimitotics nor colcemid influenced antibody-dependent cytotoxicity measured by lysis of antibody-coated target cells (Gelfand *et al.*, 1975).

2.2.8. *Effects on Secretion and Phagocytosis*

Hyponatremia has been described as a side effect of vincristine therapy; this action was attributed to an inappropriate antidiuretic hormone secretion (R. N. Fine *et al.*, 1966; Slater *et al.*, 1969). Recently, levels of this hormone were shown to increase repetitively after multiple doses of vincristine; the syndrome of inappropriate antidiuretic hormone secretion was prevented by vigorous fluid restriction (Stuart *et al.*, 1975). Other endocrine secretory processes that are affected by antimitotics include thyroid hormone mobilization (Wolff and Bhattacharyya, 1975) and insulin secretion (Lacy *et al.*, 1968), both of which are inhibited, and adrenal steroid release, which is elevated (Chung and Gabourel, 1971). Colchicine and the vinca alkaloids reduce the secretion of plasma lipoproteins (Orci *et al.*, 1973; Stein *et al.*, 1974) and lipoprotein lipase (Chajek *et al.*, 1975) by the liver. The degree of specificity of certain of these effects is suggested by the finding that colchicine inhibited the secretion of catecholamines by perfused rabbit adrenal glands that is evoked by acetylcholine, but not that evoked by potassium (Douglas and Sorimachi, 1972). Antimitotics interfere with lysosomal degranulation and the formation of digestive vacuoles, processes that are vital to phagocytosis (Malawista, 1968).

2.2.9. *Ribosomal Interactions*

Vinblastine brings about the precipitation or formation of aggregates of ribosomes. Such aggregates have been reported after exposure to vinblastine of *Escherichia coli* cells, which lack microtubules (Kingsbury and Voelz, 1969), human leukemic lymphoblasts, and mouse fibroblasts (Krishan and Hsu, 1971). Vinblastine is also able to precipitate ribosomes *in vitro* (Wilson *et al.*, 1970). The aggregation phenomenon may be related to the binding of vinblastine by ribosomes, especially by the lighter subunits. Binding of the alkaloid leads to a reduction in protein synthesis by ribosome preparations (Swerdlow and Creasey, 1975).

2.2.10. *Teratogenesis*

Vinblastine is teratogenic in hamsters (Ferm, 1963) and rats (Cohlan and Kitay, 1965).

2.3. *Structure–Activity Relationships*

2.3.1. *Colchicine*

This agent is a tropolone derivative (Fig. 1) that has been subjected to a number of modifications. Deacetyl-*N*-methylcolchicine (demicolcin; colcemid) and

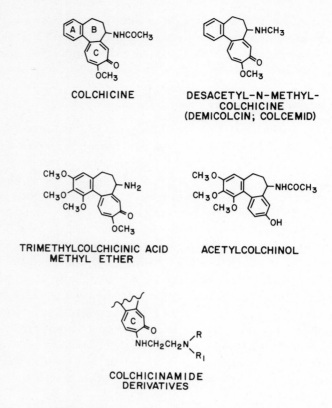

FIGURE 1. Chemical structures of colchicine and colchicine derivatives.

trimethylcolchicinic acid methyl ether are the most commonly used derivatives. Basic colchicinamides, notably the very potent dimethylaminoethylamine and morpholinoethylamine derivatives, have been synthesized (DaRe *et al.*, 1966). The methoxy group of the C ring has been replaced with methylthio and the B ring substituted with *N*-ribosyl side chains to give active compounds (Harmon *et al.*, 1975). Among other colchicinamide derivatives are substituted α-phosphoethanolamines, which are hydrolyzed by a specific prostatic acid phosphatase, introducing the possibility of selectivity for tumors of prostatic origin (Seligman *et al.*, 1975). The major structural requirements for antimitotic activity thus appear to be a methoxy group on ring A and a substituted 7-membered C ring. Modifications of the B ring are not critical (Dustin, 1963).

2.3.2. Vinca Alkaloids

These compounds, which are indole derivatives, possess a dimeric structure consisting of vindoline and catharanthine moieties (Fig. 2). Six of the alkaloids occurring in the periwinkle plant inhibit the growth of tumors (Svoboda and Blake, 1975): vinblastine, vincristine, vinleurosine, vinrosidine, leurosivine, and rovidine. Of these six, the latter two are minor components that have received no adequate study, and only vinblastine and vincristine are of proved clinical value.

Recently, 4- desacetoxyvinblastine has been separated from large amounts of impure vinblastine (Neuss *et al.*, 1975). The sulfate salt is the usual form in which these drugs are available; however, vinleurosine has also been employed as the methiodide. Many semisynthetic derivatives of the vinca alkaloids have been prepared in an effort to overcome the problem of resistance or to modify their spectrum of activity. In general, these modifications have led to reduced activity. This is true of both 6,7-dihydrovinblastine (Noble *et al.*, 1967) and vinglycinate, the 4-*N*,*N*-dimethylaminoacetyl derivative of desacetylvinblastine (Armstrong, 1968), which have only about one-tenth the activity of vinblastine. In the case of manipulations of the 3 and 4 positions of vinblastine to give a series of amides, however, there was evidence of a shift toward an antitumor spectrum more akin to that of vincristine, with a similar molar efficacy, but apparently lower toxicity (Sweeney *et al.*, 1974; Todd *et al.*, 1975).

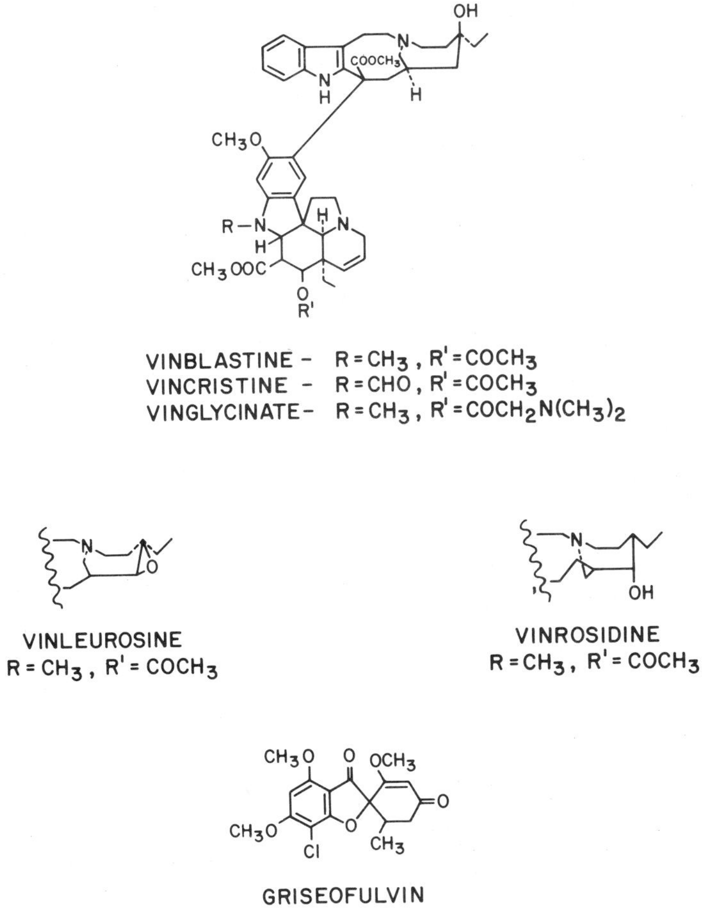

VINBLASTINE – R = CH$_3$, R' = COCH$_3$
VINCRISTINE – R = CHO , R' = COCH$_3$
VINGLYCINATE– R = CH$_3$, R' = COCH$_2$N(CH$_3$)$_2$

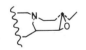

VINLEUROSINE
R = CH$_3$, R' = COCH$_3$

VINROSIDINE
R = CH$_3$, R' = COCH$_3$

GRISEOFULVIN

FIGURE 2. Chemical structures of the vinca alkaloids and griseofulvin.

Certain requirements for activity can be listed:

1. The indole nitrogen of the catharanthine moiety should retain its basic nature; amidation, for example, leads to loss of activity.
2. It has generally been considered that the C-4 position of the vindoline structure should be substituted by acyl or aminoacetyl functions for activity. However, 4-desacetylvinblastine is active, albeit against different tumors from those sensitive to the parent agent.
3. Acetylation of the free hydroxyl functions yields inactive acetates.
4. Reduction with LiAlH$_4$ to carbinols causes total loss of activity, but partial reduction, as by hydrogenation of the C-6,7 double bond, only reduces the activity.

2.3.3. Podophyllotoxin Derivatives

The structural features of these compounds appear in Fig. 3. It is evident that there can be a wide range of substituents on the 1 position without loss of activity. The thenylidene glycoside side chain does appear to modify the biological activity, however, by rendering metaphase arrest a much less prominent feature and accentuating the block in the progress of cells into mitosis (Stähelin, 1970).

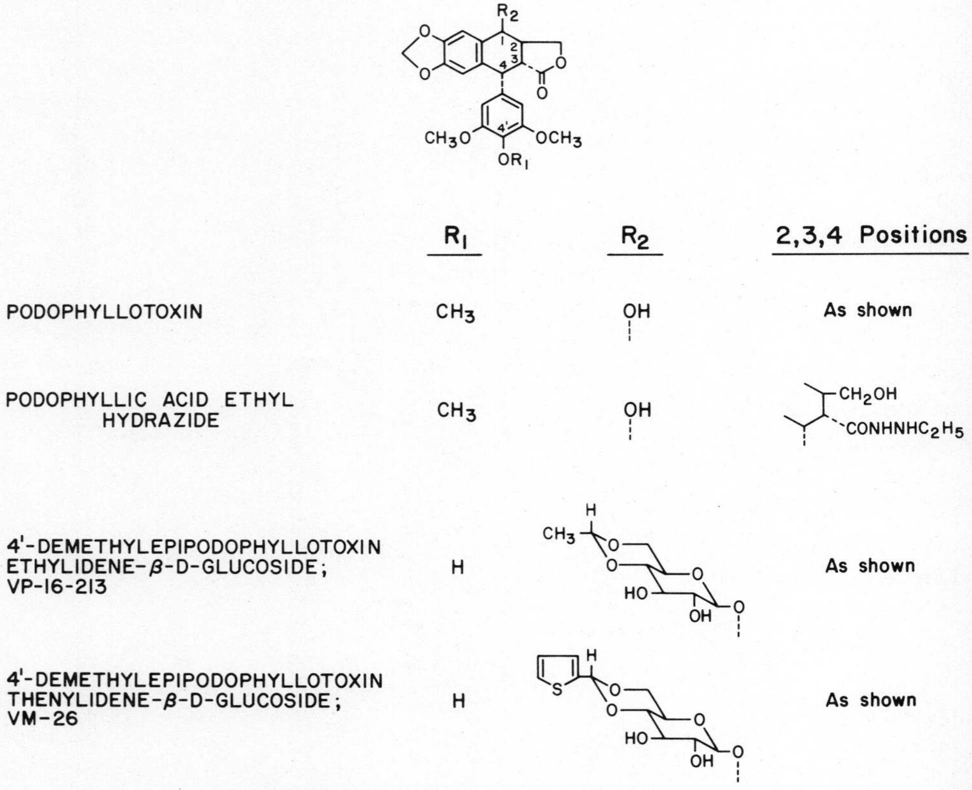

FIGURE 3. Chemical structures of podophyllin derivatives.

2.4.1. Microtubule Interactions

The microtubule system consists of tubules with diameters of about 250 Å, and often many microns in length, that may occur in many regions of the cytoplasm of eukaryote cells. They have not been identified in prokaryote organisms. Although the tubules may occur singly, in general they form assemblies of either loose aggregates near the cell surface or intracellular organelles, or highly structured components of such organelles as the mitotic spindle, cilia, or flagella. Those wishing an in-depth study of the microtuble system and its role in cell function are referred to reviews by Porter (1966), Adelmann *et al.* (1968), Burnside (1975), and Olmsted and Borisy (1973). For our present purposes, it is sufficient to briefly summarize what is known of this system.

The tubules themselves are derived from a number of protofibrils, commonly 13, although 11 and 12 have also been reported. In turn, the fibrils appear to be in equilibrium with the microtubule subunit protein, tubulin, which normally exists as a heterodimer with each chain of molecular weight close to 55,000 (R. E. Fine, 1971). Levels of tubulin appear to be greatest during the late S and G_2 phases of the cell cycle (Klevecz and Forrest, 1975). Recent studies have highlighted the complexity of the assembly process and of the completed microtubules. In addition to the free tubulin of sedimentation coefficient 6S, there are 36S double ring and spiral structures that may serve as nucleation centers for assembly of protofilaments and tubules (Kirschner *et al.*, 1975). In addition, there are high-molecular-weight proteins (Borisy *et al.*, 1975), and in many cases AMP-dependent protein kinases (Soifer *et al.*, 1975), associated with the microtubules. It would appear that hydrophobic interactions are most significant in tubulin polymerization, except at lower temperatures (Engelborghs *et al.*, 1976). Although the whole system of tubulin, free microtubules, and formed microtubule-containing structures may be considered to be in dynamic equilibrium (Fig. 4), certain tubules, notably those of cilia and flagella, are relatively stable and little affected by changes in the pool of precursor subunits, or by treatment with heat, enzymes, or drugs (Behnke and Forer, 1967).

Most of the structures derived from the microtubule system are involved in movement or in maintaining shape or rigidity. For example, the role of micro-tubules in axonal transport may involve the axoplasmic tubules as stationary or moving tracts associated with mitochondria and vesicles (Smith *et al.*, 1975). During mitosis, the decrease in length of the spindle fibers may reflect either loss of subunits from the polar end or microtubules of fixed length sliding over one another (McIntosh *et al.*, 1975). In the latter case, tubule–tubule interactions, or even an actomyosin, could be involved; actin has been detected in the mitotic spindle (Gawadi, 1971). Not all cell movement involves microtubules, however, and it should be stressed that cytokinesis, ameboid motion, cytoplasmic streaming, blood clot retraction, and muscle cell contraction are among the types of motion apparently mediated by the quite separate microfilament (40–70 Å) system, a

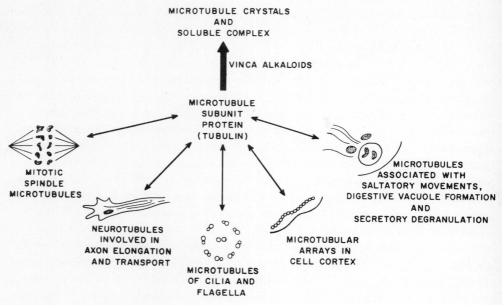

FIGURE 4. Interrelationships of the microtubule system. Microtubules in formed structures are considered to be in equilibrium with the pool of subunit protein, but the kinetics of the equilibria vary widely. The microtubules of cilia and flagella, for example, are relatively stable. Antimitotic agents disturb the equilibrium by forming complexes that deplete the tubulin pool.

system that is uniquely sensitive to the cytochalasins (Wessels *et al.*, 1971; Spooner *et al.*, 1971).

Turning to the antimitotic drugs, it is clear that these drugs exert a profound intervention in the organization and function of the microtubule system (Creasey, 1975*a*,*b*; Wilson, 1975*a*,*b*). This interaction takes the form of binding of the antimitotic drug by tubulin, a process first demonstrated in soluble cytoplasmic preparations (Borisy and Taylor, 1967; Creasey, 1967; Wilson and Friedkin, 1967; Georgatsos *et al.*, 1968). It became apparent very early that the various drugs interacted at different sites. Binding of colchicine was sensitive to urea and increased by the vinca alkaloids, with griseofulvin and *p*-fluorophenylalanine competing for the binding site. In the case of vinblastine, binding was sensitive to sodium chloride, but not to urea, and was stimulated by colchicine, griseofulvin, and *p*-fluorophenylalanine, and inhibited by other vinca alkaloids (Creasey, 1975*b*).

More detailed study has been carried out with purified tubulin preparations. Three types of preparative procedures have been used: isolation by repeated polymerization and dissociation (e.g., Borisy *et al.*, 1975); column chromatography with DEAE cellulose as a major step (e.g., Eipper, 1975); and affinity chromatography (e.g., Morgan and Seeds, 1975). Three classes of binding sites have been demonstrated. There are two sites for GTP, one for colchicine, and two for vinblastine on each molecule of dimer (Bryan, 1972). As reviewed by Wilson (1975*a*), colchicine reacts relatively slowly with its binding site, and the reaction is markedly temperature-dependent, but not affected by changes in pH between 5.5 and 8.5 and in ionic strength from 0.1 to 0.5. Podophyllotoxin competes for the colchicine binding site, but the reaction is less time- and temperature-dependent, and is readily reversible. Bryan (1975) has produced evidence for involvement of a lipid in the tubulin–colchicine binding site. Griseofulvin may not interact in the same way, since polymerization of tubulin is not completely inhibited, as it is by vinblastine, colchicine, and podophyllotoxin. Vinblastine binds more rapidly to its specific sites, for which competition by vincristine and desacetylvinblastine can be demonstrated. In addition, there may be as many as 10–20 low-affinity binding sites per molecule of chick embryo brain tubulin. These sites are involved in precipitation of tubulin and in the formation of microtubule crystals (Wilson, 1975*a*). Such crystals, which are uniquely formed through the action of vinca alkaloids, have been noted in a wide range of cells exposed to these agents, including starfish oocytes (Malawista *et al.*, 1969), human leukocytes and L-strain fibroblasts (Bensch and Malawista, 1969), human blood platelets (White, 1968), rabbit neurons (Kotorii *et al.*, 1971), and even isolated tubulin preparations (Bensch *et al.*, 1969). Crystal formation may be enhanced by colcemid and puromycin (Strahs and Sato, 1973). All such interactions, whether they result in intracellular microtubule crystals or soluble drug–tubulin complex, will deplete the pool of subunit protein. Those structures in rapid equilibrium with the pool will dissociate readily, as does the mitotic spindle. Neurotubules are in a less dynamic state, and thus will dissolve more slowly, while the tubules in cilia and flagella are rather resistant. These interactions with the microtubule system can be invoked to explain most of the biological effects of this class of drugs.

2.4.2. *Effects on Biosynthetic Processes*

While microtubule interaction may underlie many of the biological properties of antimitotics, cytotoxicity is unlikely to depend completely on this essentially reversible phenomenon. In accord with this view is the fact that these agents intervene in many biochemical pathways (Creasey, 1974, 1975*a,b*). It is appropriate to select examples of effects on biochemical pathways, rather than to completely cover the rather extensive literature on the subject.

a. Nucleic Acid Biosynthesis. All the antimitotic agents inhibit the synthesis of nucleic acids. Colchicine inhibits incorporation of purines and pyrimidines into DNA and RNA of mealworm pupas, rat embryos, spleen and regenerating liver, guinea pig intestinal mucosa (Ilan and Quastel, 1966), and Ehrlich ascites carcinoma cells (Creasey and Markiw, 1964). Vinblastine or vincristine or both have been reported to inhibit the synthesis of DNA and RNA in Ehrlich ascites cells (Creasey and Markiw, 1964, 1965), rat spleen and bone marrow (Van Lancker *et al.*, 1966), rat thymus cells (Jones *et al.*, 1966), mouse brain (Agustin and Creasey, 1967), human leukemic leukocytes (Cline, 1968; Creasey, 1968), rat embryos in *in vivo* culture (Krowke *et al.*, 1970), and HEp-2 cells in culture (Wagner and Roizman, 1968). In these studies, the relative sensitivities of DNA and RNA synthesis, as well as of the RNA subfractions, varied considerably. Both vinleurosine (Creasey, 1969) and vinrosidine (Richards *et al.*, 1966) inhibited nucleic acid synthesis in sarcoma 180 and rat thymus cells, respectively. Podophyllic acid ethyl hydrazide inhibited incorporation of precursors into DNA and RNA of mouse mammary tumors and liver *in vivo* (Georgatsos and Karemfyllis, 1968). VM-26 inhibited thymidine incorporation into the DNA of cells in culture (Stähelin, 1970), while VP-16 reduced incorporation of precursors into the DNA and RNA of P815 cells; at low levels of the latter drug (1 μg/ml), enhancement of RNA synthesis occurred (Grieder *et al.*, 1974). Griseofulvin inhibits nucleic acid synthesis in sensitive fungi (El-Nakeeb *et al.*, 1965). The mechanism of these inhibitory actions has not been clarified. However, colchicine does form a complex with DNA that is detectable by optical rotation experiments (Ilan and Quastel, 1966), and vincristine inhibits isolated RNA polymerase preparations (Cline, 1968). In nucleated erythrocytes stimulated with erythropoietin, vinblastine and colcemid prevent the increased activity of cytoplasmic DNA polymerase of high molecular weight (Roodman *et al.*, 1975).

b. Protein Synthesis. Among the reports of inhibition of protein biosynthesis by the vinca alkaloids are those of Warnecke and Seeber (1968) and Creasey and Markiw (1965), who studied Ehrlich ascites cells; Cline (1968), using human leukemic leukocytes; and Krowke *et al.* (1970), who examined rat embryos in *in vivo* culture. The mechanisms involved may include a secondary action through effects on synthesis of RNA, inhibition of amino acid transport (Creasey, 1975*a*), and complex formation with ribosomes (Swerdlow and Creasey, 1975).

c. Lipid Synthesis. The demyelination of nerve fibres mentioned earlier argues for an effect of colchicine and the vinca alkaloids on lipid biosynthesis. Such effects have been demonstrated in the gastrocnemius muscle of rats treated with vincristine (Graff *et al.*, 1967), and in sarcoma 180 ascites cells exposed to vinleurosine (Creasey, 1969) and vincristine (Creasey, 1975*b*). Phospholipid synthesis was the parameter inhibited by these drugs. Total lipid synthesis is also inhibited by vincristine in rat embryos (Krowke *et al.*, 1970).

d. Miscellaneous Effects. Among the changes ascribed to the vinca alkaloids are a fall in rat liver CoA (Mascitelli-Coriandoli and Lanzani, 1963), and inhibition of respiratory processes in L1210 cells (Hunter, 1963), in leukocytes engaged in phagocytosis (Goldfinger *et al.*, 1965), and in a variety of tumor cells (Obrecht and Fusenig, 1966).

2.5. Metabolism and Distribution

Knowledge of the metabolism and distribution of the antimitotic agents, especially in man, is rather incomplete. In the case of colchicine, colorimetric assay disclosed rapid initial urinary excretion in rats, with 50% of the administered dose still in the animals after 16 hr; 10–25% was in the intestine, reflecting biliary excretion (Brues, 1942). Using ^{14}C-labeled colchicine, Back and Walaszek (1953) found a major difference between normal mice, in which around 40% of the body burden was in the spleens, and those bearing sarcoma 180, the spleens of which contained no drug. Levels in the intestine were higher in tumor-bearing mice (38–46% vs. 18–23%), while tumor and liver contents of drug were similar (6–15%). In humans, a mean apparent volume of distribution of 2.1 liters/kg and a plasma half-life of 19.3 min were calculated. Levels of drug within the leukocytes were 3–17 times greater than concentrations in the plasma (Ertel et al., 1969). A radioimmunoassay of colchicine that may be of value for pharmacokinetic studies has been developed (Boudene et al., 1975).

In rats given tritiated vinblastine, about 25% of the administered tritium was in the intestine and its contents 24 hr later, while urinary excretion accounted for a little over 6%. The liver retained 2.9% and the blood 1.6% at this time. Only 2% of the biliary tritium was unchanged vinblastine (Beer and Richards, 1964). Later fractionation of the blood radioactivity in rats showed that 60% was transported in the platelets, 15% in the leukocytes, 10% in the red cells, and 15% in the plasma. All the platelet tritium and 50% of that in the plasma was unchanged drug (Hebden et al., 1970). Platelets may constitute a major storage and transport medium for vinca alkaloids. In dogs, vinblastine showed plasma half-lives of 17–38 min and 3–5 hr. Up to 79% of plasma tritium was protein-bound, and the leukocytes had intracellular drug levels 2–12 times those of the plasma. In 9 days, 12–17% was excreted in the urine, and 30–36% in the feces. The ratio of biliary to plasma tritium varied from 7 to 57, and vinblastine was the major (47–81%) bile component (Creasey et al., 1975). In humans, labeled vinblastine shows a biphasic clearance, with half-lives of about 4 and 190 min. Platelets bound the drug more avidly than leukocytes, and both had higher levels per unit weight of protein than the red cells or plasma, but the latter had the greatest total amount. After 72 hr, 25–41% of the dose had been excreted in the stools, and 19–23% in the urine. Very little unchanged drug was in the stools, but 17–50% of urinary tritium was in the form of vinblastine (Owellen and Hartke, 1975).

Early studies with a KB cell bioassay indicated that after a dose of 1 mg/kg of vincristine to dogs and monkeys, serum levels fell from a range of 0.3–1 mg/ml to 0.02–0.05 mg/ml in 6 hr. In rats, vincristine was not detectable at 3 hr (Dixon et al., 1969), whereas in leukemic children, measurable blood levels were found in 50% after 4 hr (Morasca et al., 1969). Studies with tritiated vincristine in rats showed a biphasic clearance curve, with a secondary plasma half-life of 70 min. Very high tritium levels were found in the intestinal contents due to rapid biliary excretion. The spleen, adrenal, small intestine, and thyroid had unusually high concentrations of radioactivity; although lower, the levels in the heart, lung, kidney, and marrow were significantly above those in the blood (Owellen and Donigian, 1972). Vincristine apparently is translocated by a carrier-mediated transport mechanism in many tumor cells (Bleyer et al., 1975). The existence of such a system could be related to the competitive inhibition of vinblastine uptake by glutamate (Creasey *et al.*, 1971). The vinca alkaloids and colchicine all undergo significant binding (75 and 50%, respectively, at physiological concentrations) by serum proteins, especially the α- and β-globulins (Donigian and Owellen, 1973).

Labeled podophyllotoxin appears to be excreted about equally in the bile (26%) and urine (22%). Metabolism to a nonextractable material, possibly pic-ropodophyllin, is very extensive in mice (Kocsis *et al.*, 1957). The highest concentration of podophyllic acid ethyl hydrazide occurred in the liver and kidney of dogs, rats, mice, and humans. Significant amounts entered bronchocarcinoma and brain tumor tissue (Stähelin and Cerletti, 1964). The human pharmacokinetics of VP-16 fitted a two-compartment open model with a clearance of 13.6 ml/min and metabolism described by a first-order constant of $0.21\ hr^{-1}$ (Allen and Creaven, 1975).

2.6. Clinical Aspects

Many aspects of the clinical use of the vinca alkaloids have been reviewed by I. S. Johnson *et al.* (1963) and DeConti and Creasey (1975). A summary of the most common human toxicities appears in Table 1. It is evident that certain side effects are experienced with approximately the same frequency for both drugs, but vincristine engenders considerably more neurological and lower GI effects, and

TABLE 1
Human Toxicities of the Vinca Alkaloids[a]

Side effect	Approximate incidence (%)	
	Vinblastine	Vincristine
Alopecia	7	8
Constipation	2	16
Cramps	—	3
Depression	2	3
Diarrhea	2	—
Hoarseness	—	13
Ileus	2	—
Jaw pain	—	2
Leukopenia	32	—
Nausea, vomiting	17	—
Paresthesias	8 (includes all neurotoxicity)	>50
Perforated colon	—	2
Phlebitis	2	3
Rectal bleeding and hematuria	1	—
Reduced reflexes	—	31
Stomatitis	3	—
Thrombocytopenia	<1	—
Weakness	—	8

[a] Data derived from DeConti and Creasey (1975).

vinblastine more leukopenia and disturbances of the upper GI tract. The major use of vinblastine is in Hodgkin's disease, but it also may have value in choriocarcinoma. Because of the leukopenia it produces, vinblastine cannot be included in as many combination therapy regimens as vincristine, since most of the other agents in such therapies are also myelosuppressive. Vincristine is of greatest value in Hodgkin's disease, acute lymphoblastic leukemia, lymphosarcomas, reticulumcell sarcoma, Wilms's tumor, Ewing's sarcoma, retinoblastoma, embryonal rhabdomyosarcoma, and in combinations for breast cancer, melanoma, and neuroblastoma (Zubrod, 1974). Of the other vinca alkaloids, vinleurosine sulfate has generally been found to be less effective than vinblastine or vincristine. It produces a shocklike syndrome on rapid intravenous injection, but otherwise its toxicity resembles that of vinblastine (Mathé *et al.*, 1965; Gailani *et al.*, 1966). Vinglycinate may lack cross-resistance to the other vinca alkaloids, but a dose 10 times that of vinblastine is required, making it prohibitively expensive; it generally resembles vinblastine in its spectrum of activity (Armstrong *et al.*, 1967). In general, the future of the vinca alkaloids lies in their effective integration into combination therapy using the general principles discussed by Sartorelli and Creasey (1973): biochemical interactions, avoidance of summation of toxicity, multiple mechanisms for damage to target cells, and cell cycle kinetics.

Although colchicine and its derivatives have been used in the past for treating human cancer (Ludford, 1945), recent interest has centered on trimethylcolchicinic acid methyl ether. Results with malignant melanoma have, however, been disappointing (Stolinsky *et al.*, 1972). A range of tumors, including carcinoma of the breast, Wilms's tumor, reticulum-cell sarcoma, liposarcoma, embryonal cell testicular carcinoma, and oat-cell carcinoma of the lung have shown responses to VP-16. Side effects included nausea and vomiting, stomatitis, diarrhea, leukopenia, alopecia, thrombocytopenia, and pruritis (Falkson and Falkson, 1974; Eagen *et al.*, 1975; Nissen *et al.*, 1975). Further study of these derivatives is warranted.

3. Ellipticine Derivatives

3.1. Occurrence and Chemistry

Ellipticine and 9-methoxyellipticine are uleine alkaloids (pyridocarbazole derivatives) originally isolated from *Ochrosia elliptica* Labill, a small tropical evergreen tree native to Australia, Madagascar, and the Pacific islands; the tree belongs to the tribe Plumiereae of the family Apocynaceae (Goodwin *et al.*, 1959). Alkaloids of this group have subsequently been isolated from other members of the genus *Ochrosia*, as well as the genera *Excavatia* and *Aspidosperma* (Cranwell and Saxton, 1962; Culvenor and Loder, 1966; Svoboda *et al.*, 1968). The chemistry of these alkaloids has been reviewed by Gilbert (1965). The structures of some of the more important derivatives are shown in Fig. 5. Synthetic work with this group of agents has been extensive. Ellipticine itself has been synthesized from formylcarbazole

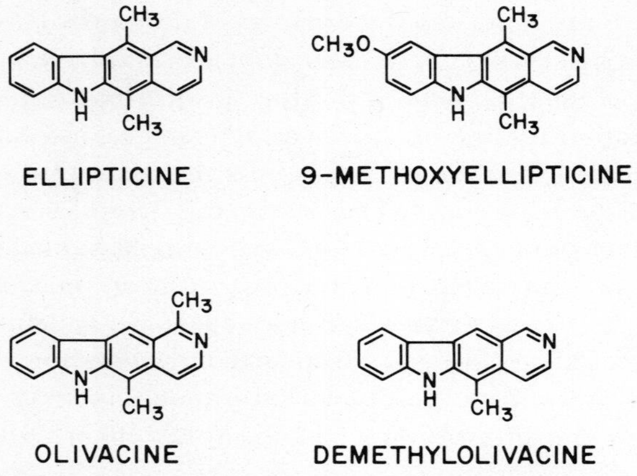

FIGURE 5. Chemical structures of ellipticine and ellipticine derivatives.

precursors (Cranwell and Saxton, 1962; Culvenor and Loder, 1966), from 2,5-
dimethylbenzoic acid via the acetonitrile and a Borsche carbazole ring closure
(Acton *et al.*, 1966), and from indole by condensation with 3-acetyl pyridine,
reduction, and pyrolysis (Woodward *et al.*, 1969). Other derivatives of interest that
have been synthesized include thiaellipticine, in which the carbazole nitrogen is
replaced by sulfur (Fujiwara *et al.*, 1968); 9-methoxyellipticine (Culvenor and
Loder, 1966); olivacine and 1-demethylolivacine (Acton *et al.*, 1966; Mosher *et al.*,
1966); and the dimethoxyellipticines (Guthrie *et al.*, 1975).

3.2. Pharmacological Activity

The alkaloids of this group exert cardiovascular actions. Lower doses of ellipticine
lead to hypotension and bradycardia in dogs and monkeys, followed by slight
persistent hypertension. In isolated heart preparations, high doses of ellipticine
led to prolonged depression of both rate and contractile force. *dl*-Propranolol and
reserpine prevented the cardiac action, suggesting that the alkaloid stimulates
β-receptors (Herman *et al.*, 1971). 9-Hydroxyellipticine shows a cardiotonic action
with increased contractile force at low doses in the dog, but at higher doses,
cardiac output and systolic ejection were reduced (Huu Chanh *et al.*, 1974). In the
latter study, as in one carried out in mice (Paoletti *et al.*, 1974), the Purkinje cells
were affected. Hypotension, bradycardia, and increased carotid blood flow,
coupled with an immediate hemolytic action, maximal at 5 min and declining after
15 min, occurred in monkeys treated with ellipticine. The hemolysis was prevented by preparing the ellipticine in buffer at pH 4 (Herman *et al.*, 1974). Other
toxicities reported have included hypothermia, paraplegia before death and fatty
infiltration of the liver in mice (Paoletti *et al.*, 1974), and increased alkaline
phosphatase and reduced potassium in the blood after 9-hydroxyellipticine (Huu
Chanh *et al.*, 1974). In the latter study, ellipticine, but not its 9-hydroxy derivative,

produced irreversible cardiovascular and respiratory depression when high doses were given to dogs.

Ellipticine and its 9-methoxy derivative were identified in plant extracts through their ability to inhibit the growth of L1210 in mice (Culvenor and Loder, 1966; Venditti and Abbott, 1967; Svoboda *et al.*, 1968; LeMen *et al.*, 1970). In these studies, 9-methoxyellipticine was somewhat more active than the parent alkaloid. The same tumor screen has shown demethylolivacine to be more active than olivacine itself, the increase in life spans being 52–121% and 41%, respectively (Mosher *et al.*, 1966). Extension of such comparative studies to other derivatives disclosed that 9-hydroxyellipticine (LePecq *et al.*, 1973) was more active and less toxic than any other compound studied. In contrast, 9-aminoellipticine was less active than ellipticine (LePecq *et al.*, 1974; Hayat *et al.*, 1974). Ellipticine and 9-methoxyellipticine proved to be almost equally effective in terms of their cytotoxicity for L1210 cells in culture (Li and Cowie, 1974). In a study with L1210 and Chinese hamster (DON) cells in culture, mitosis and early G_1 were the phases of the cell cycle most sensitive to ellipticine. Chromatid breaks, achromatic gaps, and chromatid interchanges were among the aberrations induced in DON cells (Bhuyan *et al.*, 1972).

3.3. Mechanism of Action

Drugs of this group are potent inhibitors of the synthesis of biopolymers. In L1210 cells in culture, DNA, RNA, and protein synthesis were all strongly and irreversibly inhibited by ellipticine, with incorporation of precursors into nucleic acids being most sensitive at lower drug concentrations (0.2–1.0 μg/ml). No inhibition of kinase enzymes or RNA polymerase was evident (Li and Cowie, 1974). Similar findings were made for the action of 9-methoxyellipticine on human embryonic fibroblasts (WI-38) in culture (Garcia-Girault and Macieira-Coelho, 1970). The action on RNA synthesis has been the subject of more intensive experimentation with the finding of a degree of selectivity by ellipticine for inhibition of the synthesis and maturation sequence of 45S nucleolar RNA, the ribosomal RNA precursor (Abelson and Penman, 1975; Snyder *et al.*, 1971). Chain-shortening did not seem to occur, however (Kann and Kohn, 1972). As was stated above, effects on nucleic acid synthesis are not the result of inhibition of enzymes, but rather intervention at the level of the template (Li and Cowie, 1974). The ellipticine ring structure has dimensions similar to those of proflavin, and it binds preferentially to helical DNA with a binding strength greater than that of the acridine. The plane of bound ellipticine is parallel to the plane of the bases. An unwinding angle of about 8° has been calculated, the same as that of proflavin and quinacrine, less than that of actinomycin D (12°), and slightly greater than that of 9-methoxyellipticine (6.8°) (Saucier *et al.*, 1971; Kohn *et al.*, 1975). 9-Hydroxyellipticine, mentioned above for its potent activity against L1210, had a greater apparent DNA binding constant and a larger DNA unwinding angle (12°) than any other derivative examined (LePecq *et al.*, 1974).

WILLIAM
A. CREASEY

3.4. Distribution and Metabolism

The tissue distribution of ellipticine was studied in mice by a spectrophotometric assay sensitive down to 0.5 μg/g. After intraperitoneal injection, the highest drug levels were in the liver, but the agent was also detectable in the brain. Maximal levels of drug in L1210 cells *in vivo* were achieved in 4–6 hr. Metabolism appeared to be minimal (Hardesty and Chaney, 1970). The study was later extended to examine the blood levels, which were generally better with a lactate than with a hydrochloride formulation. Fecal excretion attained 49% in 9 days, whereas there were only traces of drug in the urine (Hardesty *et al.*, 1972). Using ellipticine labeled with ^{14}C, Chadwick *et al.* (1971) followed the distribution and excretion of the alkaloid in dogs and rats. Dogs excreted less than 5% by the urinary route in 24 hr, whereas rats excreted 11% in this time interval. Of this radioactivity, 10% was in the form of ellipticine. Rats excreted up to 70% by the biliary route in a 24-hr period; less than 10% of this was unchanged drug. Dogs also excreted large amounts in the bile, and by 24 hr, the material in dog tissues was mainly metabolites. Levels were detected in the brain, and these might relate to neurological activity.

3.5. Clinical Trials

The lactate formulation of 9-methoxyellipticine was administered to 34 patients (Mathé *et al.*, 1970). There were no responses in the patients with acute lymphoblastic leukemia (10) and Hodgkin's disease (9), but there were 3 complete and 6 partial remissions in the group of 15 patients with acute myeloblastic leukemia. One subject was still in remission after 3 months, and bone marrow improvement in responders occurred over 21–34 days.

4. Camptothecin

4.1. Occurrence and Chemistry

Camptothecin (Fig. 6) is an alkaloid derived from the wood of *Camptotheca acuminata* (Nyssaceae), a tree native to China (Wall *et al.*, 1966). Details of the isolation and structural elucidation of camptothecin and its hydroxy and methoxy derivatives may be found in the review by Shamma and St. Georgiev (1974). Considerable effort has been applied to the partial and complete synthesis of this alkaloid. Total synthesis has been achieved from a variety of starting materials: α-pyrrolidone and *o*-aminobenzaldehyde (Storck and Schultz, 1971); β-aminopropionaldehyde diethyl acetal and dicarbomethoxyacetylene (Volkmann *et al.*, 1971); an indole derivative (Boch *et al.*, 1972); and a pyrroloquinoline (Wani *et al.*, 1972).

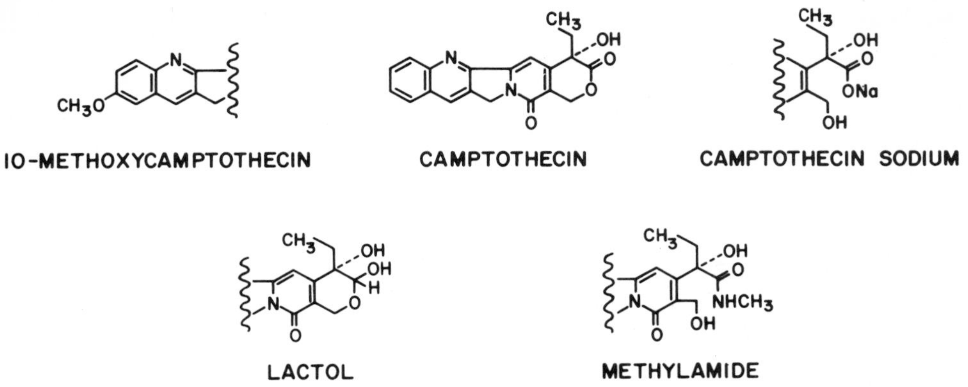

10-METHOXYCAMPTOTHECIN   CAMPTOTHECIN   CAMPTOTHECIN SODIUM

LACTOL   METHYLAMIDE

FIGURE 6. Chemical structures of camptothecin and related drugs.

4.2. Experimental Antitumor Activity

Camptothecin inhibits the growth of a wide range of experimental tumors. The L1210 mouse leukemia was used as the bioassay system during the original isolation of the drug (Wall *et al.*, 1966). Growth of Walker 256 carcinosarcoma is strongly inhibited, although only a moderate increase in survival is attained (DeWys *et al.*, 1968). Subsequently, Gallo *et al.* (1971) established the activity of camptothecin in a large number of tumor systems: L1210, L5178Y, and Novikoff hepatoma *in vitro*; L5178Y, K1964, and P388 (70–90% long-term survivors); plasma-cell tumor YPC-1; mast-cell tumor P815; and a reticulum-cell sarcoma (A-RCS). Studies carried out with DON and L1210 cells indicated that cytotoxicity is greatest during the S phase (Bhuyan *et al.*, 1972; Kessel *et al.*, 1972). Progression of cells from G_2 into mitosis was blocked even at levels of camptothecin as low as 0.01 μg/ml, whereas the S–G_2 transition required about 1000-fold higher concentrations for equivalent blockade (Li *et al.*, 1972). The existence of the G_2/mitosis block had been suggested earlier by Gallo *et al.* (1971).

Antiviral action has been ascribed to camptothecin, an example being the inhibition of fowl plague virus (an influenza virus) replication in BHK21/13 cells (D. C. Kelly *et al.*, 1974).

4.3. Biochemical Actions

The biochemical effects of camptothecin were reviewed recently (Horwitz, 1975). The drug inhibits the biosynthesis of DNA and RNA in HeLa, L5178Y, and L1210 cells (Bosmann, 1970; S. B. Horwitz *et al.*, 1971; Kessel *et al.*, 1972), as well as of vaccinia DNA in HeLa cells (S. B. Horwitz *et al.*, 1972). In our laboratory, we have found that camptothecin inhibits the incorporation of thymidine into the DNA of human peripheral leukemic leukocytes in suspension. Cells from patients with acute myelocytic leukemia were generally the most sensitive to the drug, the

ED_{50} being around 10 $\mu g/ml$ (Creasey, unpublished data). Synthesis of nucleic acids in mitochondria or in *Escherichia coli* cells is not affected by this alkaloid (Bosmann, 1970). While inhibition of protein synthesis has generally been reported as minimal, an interesting exception is the highly selective effect on synthesis of certain influenza virus proteins in infected BHK cells (Minor and Dimmock, 1975). The effects on RNA synthesis lead to a block in the formation of ribosomes (Wu *et al.*, 1971), apparently due to inhibition of the fabrication of heterogeneous nuclear RNA, and a block in the processing of ribosomal precursor RNA. Kessel (1971) did not find the latter block in L1210 cells in culture, but did describe inhibition of the synthesis of ribosomal precursor and heterogeneous nuclear RNA. Certainly, marked reductions in the chain lengths of all nuclear RNA, including precursors of cytoplasmic forms, to give sharp peaks of 24S instead of 45S, and 26S instead of normal heterogeneous nuclear RNA, have been reported (Kann and Kohn, 1972; Abelson and Penman, 1972). When L1210 (Spataro and Kessel, 1972) or HeLa cells, with or without adenovirus type 2 infection (M. S. Horwitz and S. B. Horwitz, 1971; S. B. Horwitz and M. S. Horwitz, 1973), were incubated with camptothecin, and the DNA was then analyzed on alkaline sucrose-density gradients, there was evidence that fragmentation of DNA had occurred. Work by Abelson and Penman (1973), however, in which cells were lysed in neutral sarkosyl, rather than under alkaline conditions, in the presence of camptothecin prior to alkaline density-gradient centrifugation, indicated that the DNA breaks occurred only when DNA was exposed to high pH in the presence of drug, and were thus artifacts. Possibly the alkaloid induces some change that renders the DNA more alkali-labile. It is interesting in this connection that camptothecin induces denatured regions in HeLa-cell DNA that may be visualized by the use of fluorescein-labeled anticytosine antibodies, which react only with single-stranded DNA (Liebeskind *et al.*, 1974). Furthermore, camptothecin induces a transformation of the covalently closed superhelical double-stranded circles of simian virus 40 DNA to relaxed circles containing single-strand breaks. Alkali-labile double-stranded regions were not generated (Rubinstein and Rein, 1974). It is evident that more needs to be known of these interactions.

4.4. Structure–Activity Relationships

Camptothecin, 10-methoxycamptothecin, camptothecin methylamide, and deoxycamptothecin are all of similar activity, while the lactol is less active (S. B. Horwitz, 1975). The functional group of the hydroxylactone E ring must be present to maintain activity, but in a study of a series of compounds having only portions of the camptothecin ring system, it was evident that the D and E rings alone were not sufficient requirements for activity (Bristol *et al.*, 1975).

4.5. Distribution and Metabolism

A fluorometric assay method has been developed for camptothecin that is capable of measuring levels down to 0.005 $\mu g/ml$. Extraction with ethyl acetate and measurement of fluorescence at 434 nm after activation at 370 nm forms the basis of the procedure. Application of the method to dogs treated with camptothecin yielded a value for the plasma half-life of less than 15 min (Hart *et al.*, 1969). On a dosage schedule of 0.5–10 mg/kg by single intravenous injections, a mean initial plasma half-life of 65 min was determined for 12 patients. Of the drug in the plasma, 97.4–98.9% was bound to protein. Urinary recovery averaged 17.4% (3.6–38.9%) in 24 hr. No fluorescent metabolites could be detected (Gottlieb *et al.*, 1970*a,b*).

4.6. Clinical Trials

Camptothecin, in the form of the sodium derivative camptothecin sodium, has been put into both Phase I and Phase II trials in the clinic. In a series of patients reported from the National Institutes of Health (Gottlieb *et al.*, 1970*a,b*), toxicity was tolerable. Dose-related but mild marrow depression occurred in 75% of the cases. Alopecia (33%), vomiting and GI toxicity (33%), and frequently hemorrhagic cystitis (8%), were the other major toxicities. Objective regressions of tumor (>50%) occurred in 5 patients, and some objective responses in 6 others of a total of 18 subjects. The duration of responses was brief, little more than 2 months. In another Phase I trial, a schedule of 20–67 mg/M^2 as weekly doses was compared with 5-day loading courses begun at total doses of 1.5 mg/M^2 each course. Leukopenia was more prolonged after the daily than after weekly treatment; it occurred in 4 of 6 patients receiving a total of 100 mg/M^2. Of 10 evaluable patients, 2 had objective responses after weekly courses, but no clinical benefit was discernible in 8 patients treated with 5-day courses at toxic levels (Muggia *et al.*, 1972). In a Phase II trial of camptothecin for malignant melanoma, no patient of the total of 15 achieved a 50% or greater decrease in tumor mass, although 3 had a lesser, transient response. Toxic effects included myelosuppression (11), nausea and vomiting (9), alopecia (8), diarrhea (3), and hemorrhagic cystitis (1) (Gottlieb and Luce, 1972). Moertel *et al.* (1972), using both single injections every 3 weeks (90–180 mg/M^2) and 5-day courses repeated every 4 weeks at initial total doses of 55–110 mg/M^2, found objective responses in only 2 subjects with large bowel cancer of 61 patients on the study. Thus, in the clinic, camptothecin has not fulfilled the promise suggested by its activity against a wide spectrum of experimental tumors.

5. Benzylisoquinoline and Aporphine Alkaloids

5.1. Occurrence and Chemistry

These alkaloids constitute a heterogeneous group (Fig. 7), since for our purposes we have assembled agents possessing benzylisoquinoline, aporphine, and related ring systems. Two subgroups can be distinguished, the monomeric alkaloids that are composed basically of a single ring system, and the dimeric alkaloids having

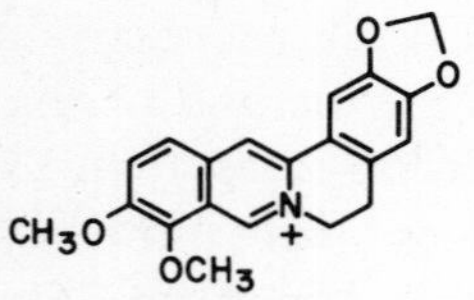

BERBERINE

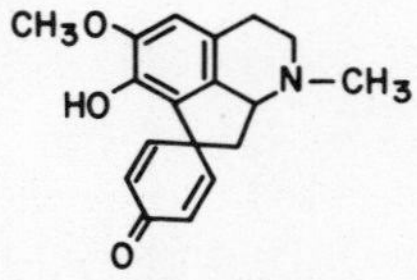

GLAZIOVINE

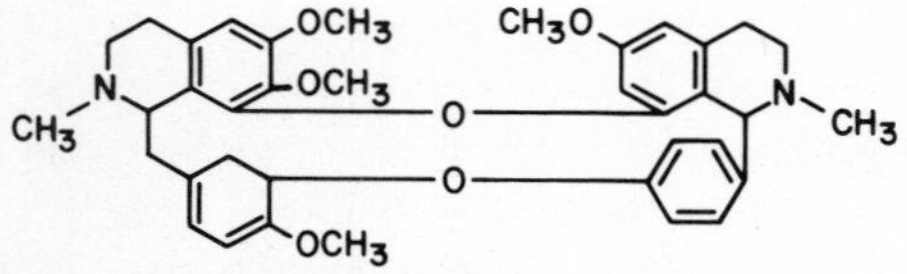

d-TETRANDRINE

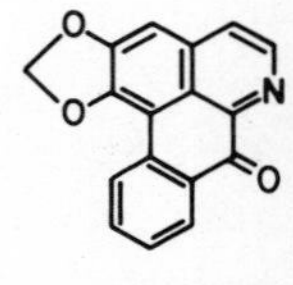

LIRIODENINE

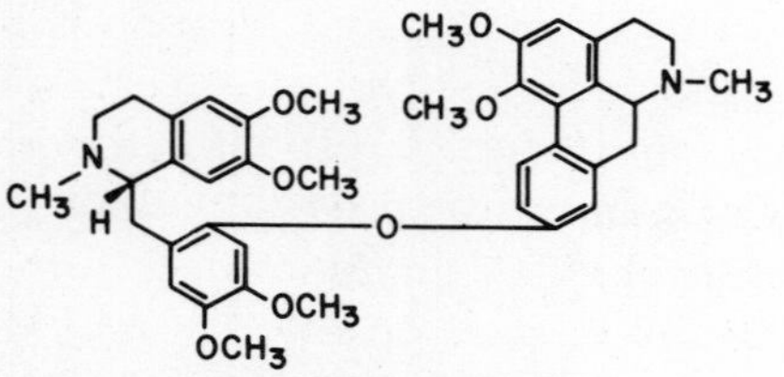

THALICARPINE

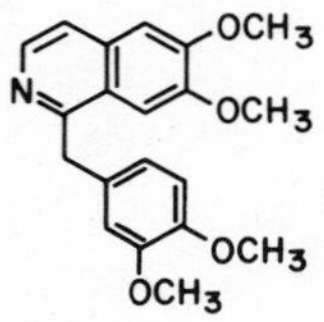

PAPAVERINE

FIGURE 7. Chemical structures of benzylisoquinoline and aporphine alkaloids.

two such systems. Thalicarpine and *d*-tetrandrine are examples of the dimeric alkaloids, while liriodenine, glaziovine, and papaverine belong to the monomeric subgroup. Berberine, which is a benzodioxoloquinolizine derivative, can justifiably be included with the monomeric alkaloids.

The chemistry of the dimeric alkaloids was reviewed by Curcumelli-Rodostamo and Kulka (1967). *d*-Tetrandrine is a major component of the Chinese herbal medicine han-fang chi (Chen and Chen, 1935), which includes several plants of the family Menispermaceae. A number of related alkaloids in addition to *d*-tetrandrine have been isolated from members of this family, notably from *Stephania hernandifolia* Walp. and *Cyclea peltata* Diels (Kupchan *et al.*, 1961). Thalicarpine and related compounds have been isolated from species of the genus *Thalictrum* (Ranunculaceae), especially *T. dasycarpum* and *T. minus elatum* (Kupchan *et al.*, 1967, 1968; Mollov *et al.*, 1968). Papaverine is one of the alkaloids present in the milky exudate of the seed capsules of the opium poppy plant, *Papaver somniferum*; it is a benzylisoquinoline. Liriodenine and glaziovine are aporphine derivatives found in the bark of *Annona glabra* and *A. purpurea*, respectively, which are species of the family Annonaceae (Warthen *et al.*, 1969; Sonnet and Jacobson, 1971). Berberine is isolated from *Hydrastis canadensis* L. (Berberidaceae).

Thalicarpine and *d*-tetrandrine both produce cardiovascular effects, manifested by marked hypotension (Hahn *et al.*, 1966; Gralla *et al.*, 1974). It appears that the drugs exert a direct depressive action on myocardial, vascular, and smooth musculature (Hahn *et al.*, 1966; Herman and Chadwick, 1974), an action that suggests analogies with the monomeric benzylisoquinoline alkaloid papaverine, a well-known smooth muscle relaxant. A similar depressive action, perhaps due to inhibition of depolarization and repolarization of excitable tissue, leading to hypotension, has been ascribed to berberine, a drug that also has anticholinesterase activity (Sabir and Bhide, 1971). *d*-Tetrandrine exhibited antiinflammatory, antipyretic, and analgesic properties in studies carried out with an experimental arthritic state induced by injecting rats with formaldehyde (Berezhinskaya and Nikitina, 1965). Kupchan *et al.* (1961) described *d*-tetrandine as having a *d*-tubocurarinelike effect. Recently, a series of *bis*-benzylisoquinolines were tested for neuromuscular blocking action, and, with the one exception of N,N^1-dimethylberbamine, were found to be much less active than *d*-tubocurarine (Bick and McLeod, 1974).

Antitumor activity of the dimeric alkaloids has been identified by the use of Walker 256 carcinosarcoma (Kupchan, 1966; Hartwell and Abbott, 1969), and by KB cells in monolayer cultures (Mollov *et al.*, 1968). The latter system was also the one used during the isolation and identification of liriodenine (Warthen *et al.*, 1969) and glaziovine (Sonnet and Jacobson, 1971). Berberine showed a level of activity against KB cells exceeding that of thalicarpine (Mollov *et al.*, 1968), but in Ehrlich and lymphoma ascitic tumor cells, this drug was cytostatic only in culture, and was without significant activity *in vivo* (Shvarev and Tsetlin, 1972). Monomeric benzylisoquinolines and aporphines are not generally active tumor inhibitors, whereas many dimeric alkaloids are active cytotoxic agents. Interestingly, there do not seem to be stereospecificity requirements for activity among the latter compounds (Kupchan and Altland, 1973). Papaverine was found to act as a mitotic poison in fertilized eggs of the sea urchin, *Paracentrotus lividus* (Druckrey *et al.*, 1953), and more recently showed significant levels of activity against human neuroblastoma, melanoma, and lymphoblastic cell lines in culture (Helson *et al.*, 1974).

5.3. Mechanism of Action

The dimeric alkaloids thalicarpine and *d*-tetrandrine exhibit a basic similarity in their actions at the molecular level. Thalicarpine inhibited the synthesis of RNA, DNA, and proteins in cultures of L1210 cells (Allen and Creaven, 1973). All species of RNA were depleted, with possibly greater effect on the rapidly labeled heterogeneous nuclear fraction; Abelson and Penman (1975) have claimed that thalicarpine has no RNA specificity. DNA synthesis is the process most sensitive to drug, and the least readily reversible on transfer of the cells to fresh medium.

There was evidence of impaired phosphorylation of nucleosides (Allen and Creaven, 1973). The thalicarpine molecule has the necessary N–O–O triangulation described by Chen (1975) for DNA binding. Whereas there were no spectral shifts on mixing thalicarpine and DNA, equilibrium dialysis measurements indicated that association between these structures did occur (Allen and Creaven, 1974). This type of study has been extended to compare thalicarpine with d-tetrandrine (Creasey, 1976). Both drugs inhibited DNA, RNA, and protein synthesis by S180 ascites cells in suspension, but in intact tumor-bearing mice, significant effects were obtained only on the incorporation of thymidine into DNA. Lipid synthesis and oxidation of glucose were not affected. In this study, both drugs were shown to undergo binding by DNA, RNA, and several synthetic polynucleotides. Thalicarpine showed no affinity for cytosine moieties, while d-tetrandrine associated only poorly with thymine, and not at all with uracil residues in the polynucleotides. Berberine also acts as an inhibitor of the incorporation of nucleosides into DNA and RNA by human leukemic leukocytes and S180 cells. It is bound by DNA, showing affinity for both purine bases, but not for pyrimidines (Creasey, unpublished data).

Papaverine represents a rather special case. It is an inhibitor of cyclic nucleotide phosphodiesterase (Hanna $et\ al.$, 1972), and its action has been ascribed to intracellular accumulation of cAMP (Helson $et\ al.$, 1974), a known modulator of cell growth. However, papaverine appears only to enhance the accumulation of this nucleotide that is induced by agents such as norepinephrine, rather than inducing such an elevation by itself (Schultz $et\ al.$, 1972). Furthermore, papaverine exerts a potent inhibitory effect on respiration in C6 astrocytoma cells (Browning $et\ al.$, 1974), a lesion that could well be relevant to its cytoxicity.

5.4. Distribution and Metabolism

When d-tetrandrine labeled with ^{14}C was given to patients by intravenous infusion over a 60-min period at a dose of 200 mg/M^2, plasma levels of drug fell, with initial and secondary half-lives of 30–120 min and 16–24 hr, respectively. Between 58 and 72% of plasma radioactivity was bound to protein, and the leukocytes were able to concentrate drug to about 6 times the coincident plasma levels. Urinary excretion of the drug accounted at the maximum for about 5% in 24 hr, with more than 80% of the drug unmetabolized. Inhibition of thymidine incorporation into DNA by leukemic leukocytes was evident (DeConti $et\ al.$, 1975). Excretion of papaverine was studied in rats, guinea pigs, rabbits, cats, and dogs after administration of tritium-labeled drug at 5 mg/kg. Except for the rabbit, in which up to 50% of the dose was excreted in the urine in 5 hr, biliary excretion was the principal pathway (80% in rats, 50% in guinea pigs, cats and dogs). Unchanged papaverine was not found, most radioactivity being present in the bile as glucuronides and sulfates. Three monodemethylated metabolites and one didemethylated metabolite were found (Belpaire and Bogaert, 1974).

Both *d*-tetrandrine and thalicarpine have been introduced into clinical trial. *d*-Tetrandrine was given to 32 patients as 1-hr infusions (to obviate cardiovascular effects) on single-dose or 5-day schedules escalating from 50 to 875 mg/M^2. Toxicity included pain and phlebitis at the injection site at dose levels above 200 mg/M^2; hemoglobinemia, hemoglobinuria, and mild anemia above 360 mg/M^2; and nausea, vomiting, tachycardia, and breathlessness above 450 mg/M^2 (DeConti *et al.*, 1975). Thalicarpine was administered to 36 patients as single doses of 200–1900 mg/M^2. At the maximum tolerated dose of 1400 mg/M^2, toxic effects included arm pain, CNS depression, nausea and vomiting, hypo- and hypertension, premature ventricular contractions, and T-wave flattening. The maximum tolerable dose for weekly administration was 1100 mg/M^2 per week × 6 by 2-hr infusions (Creaven *et al.*, 1975).

6. *Ergot Alkaloids*

The ergot alkaloids are produced by the fungus *Claviceps purpurea*, which grows on rye and other cereals. An oxytocic effect has been associated with the fungus for over 2000 years, but it is little more than 6 years since an antitumor action was first ascribed to these alkaloids (Nagasawa and Meites, 1970). Of the naturally occurring agents, ergocornine (Fig. 8) is the most effective inhibitor of the dimethylbenz(α)anthracene-induced rat mammary tumor. The specificity of the drugs for mammary tumors, as well as their ability to inhibit prolactin secretion

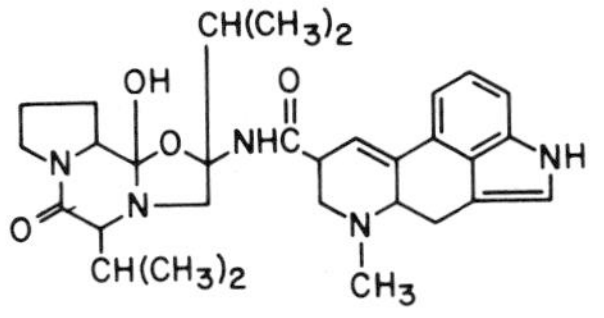

ERGOCORNINE

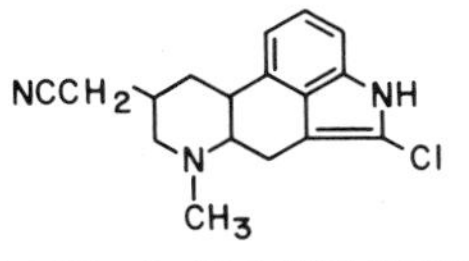

2-CHLORO-6-METHYLERGOLINE
-8β-ACETONITRILE
(LERGOTRILE)

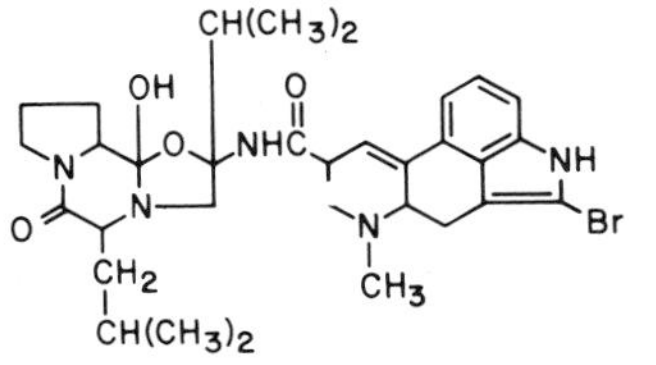

2-BROMO-α-ERGOCRYPTINE

FIGURE 8. Chemical structures of ergot derivatives.

(Lu *et al.*, 1971; Shaar and Clemens, 1972), suggests that this endocrine intervention represents their mechanism of action. This conclusion is supported by the enhanced tumor regression obtained by combination of ergocornine with high doses of estrogen (Quadri *et al.*, 1974), which suppress the release and peripheral action of prolactin. A number of synthetic ergot derivatives (Fig. 8) have been found to possess anticancer activity. They include 2-bromo-α-ergocryptine (Heuson *et al.*, 1970) and several 6-methyl-8-substituted ergolines, notably 2-chloro-6-methylergoline-8β-acetonitrile (lergotrile) (Sweeney *et al.*, 1975). In view of demonstrably increased blood levels of prolactin in many patients with metastatic breast carcinoma (Murray *et al.*, 1972), and a reported 32% incidence of prolactin dependence for this tumor (Salih *et al.*, 1972), lergotrile has undergone a preliminary clinical trial in 16 subjects with advanced breast and prostate cancer; only 1 response was noted (Tallos *et al.*, 1975). Toxic side effects included transient marked hypotension without compensatory tachycardia, and 1 case of transient psychosis. Most subjects experienced initial somnolence and nausea. Despite the low level of activity seen in this initial trial, the possible utility of agents with specificity for prolactin-dependent tumors warrants further study.

7. *Tylophora Alkaloids*

7.1. *Occurrence and Chemical Structure*

The tylophora alkaloids (Fig. 9) are phenanthroindolizidine and phenanthroquinolizidine derivatives isolated from plants of the genus *Tylophora* (Asclepiadacea), notably *T. crebriflora* (Gellert *et al.*, 1962), a plant native to Northern Queensland in Australia. Such alkaloids as tylophorine and tylocrebrine have also been isolated from *Ficus septica* and even from species of the Lauraceae (Govindachari, 1967). A number of pharmacological actions have been ascribed to these

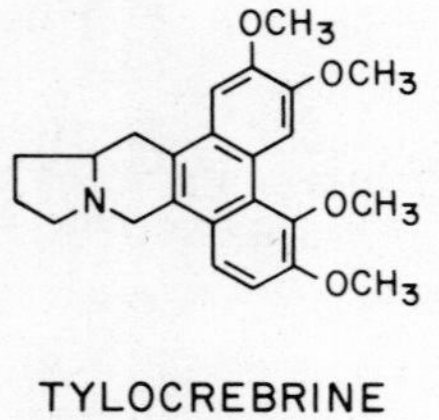

TYLOCREBRINE

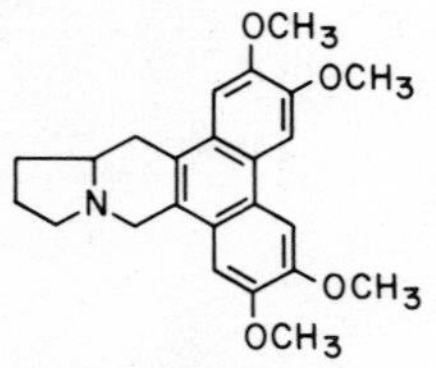

TYLOPHORINE

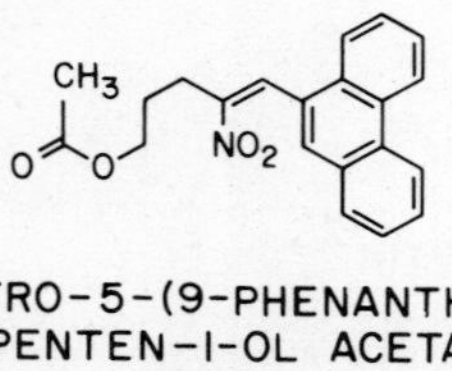

4-NITRO-5-(9-PHENANTHRYL)
-4-PENTEN-I-OL ACETATE

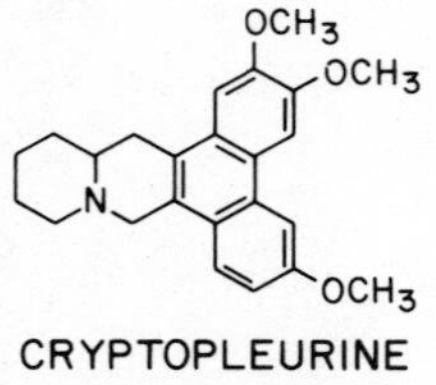

CRYPTOPLEURINE

FIGURE 9. Chemical structures of the tylophora alkaloids.

alkaloids. They are vesicants, are toxic to *Paramecia*, exert a paralyzing action on cardiac muscle and a stimulatory action on the muscles of blood vessels leading to a reduction and then a rise in blood pressure, and, finally, show activity against experimental neoplasms (Govindachari, 1967). The antileukemic effect is presumably associated with the N–O–O triangle structure reviewed by Cheng (1975). Other features are not so critical for activity, however, as indicated by the tumor-inhibitory effects of structures such as 4-nitro-5-(9-phenanthryl)-4-penten-1-ol acetate (Fig. 9) (Zee-Cheng and Cheng, 1969).

7.2. Mechanism of Action

The tylophora alkaloids are inhibitors of protein synthesis in mammalian cells. In Ehrlich ascites carcinoma cells, for example, cryptopleurine was the most effective inhibitor, reducing leucine incorporation by 50% at 2×10^{-8} M. There was no effect on nucleic acid synthesis from uracil, nor on protein synthesis in cell-free systems derived from *Escherichia coli* (Donaldson *et al.*, 1968). In other systems, however, such as HeLa cells and rabbit reticulocytes, as well as isolated polymerase enzymes, inhibition of the biosynthesis of both DNA and RNA occurred, although both processes were less sensitive than the synthesis of protein. The critical step in protein fabrication that is affected by these drugs is the elongation of peptide chains (Huang and Grollman, 1972; Grollman, 1975). The tylophora alkaloids differ from cycloheximide in the irreversibility of their inhibitory action and their lack of effect on chain initiation, but resemble this classic inhibitor of protein synthesis in that sulfhydryl compounds diminish their inhibitory effects (Huang and Grollman, 1972).

8. Miscellaneous Alkaloids

8.1. Acronycine (Acronine)

Acronycine (Fig. 10) is an acridone derivative that occurs, together with the related but inactive alkaloids melicopine and normelicopidine, in the bark of the Australian scrub ash, *Acronychia baueri* Schott (Rutaceae) (Svoboda, 1971; Svoboda *et al.*, 1966). The spectrum of experimental tumors that respond to acronycine is extremely wide, wider indeed than for any other agent. It includes C1498 and B82 leukemias; AKR, L5178Y, S-91, and X-5563 melanomas; Ridgeway osteogenic sarcoma; Shionogi carcinoma 115; and adenocarcinoma 755 (Svoboda *et al.*, 1966; I. S. Johnson *et al.*, 1968). Studies of the mechanism of action of this potent alkaloid show major departures from the pattern of inhibition of nucleic acid biosynthesis believed to characterize most cancer chemotherapy agents. Inhibition of incorporation of external nucleosides into DNA and RNA has been demonstrated, but when incorporation from prelabeled intracellular pools was examined, this inhibition was not evident. The alkaloid did not associate

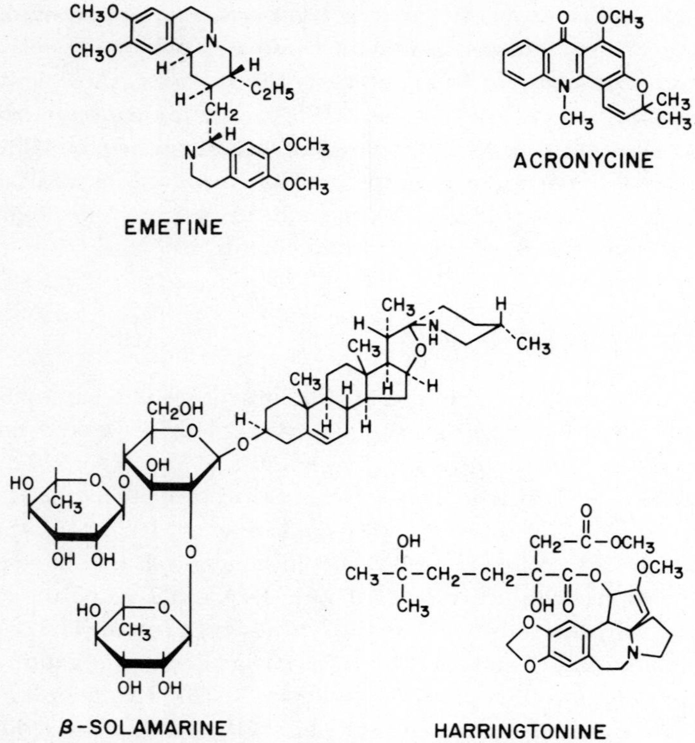

FIGURE 10. Chemical structures of miscellaneous alkaloids.

with DNA or inhibit RNA polymerase systems. Its action appeared to depend on reduction of nucleoside transport through the plasma membrane (Dunn *et al.*, 1973). In a study of the ultrastructure of L5178Y-, cervical carcinoma C-4II-, melanoma HFH-18-, and SV40-induced hamster tumor cells, acronycine caused swelling and destruction of Golgi complexes and mitochondria, binucleation, reduced adhesion to substrata, interference with melanosome dispersion, and cessation of mitotic activity by viable cells at reduced cell density (Tan and Auersperg, 1973). Thus, the drug seems to act by interfering with the structure, function, or turnover of cell-surface components.

When acronycine-O-methyl-^{14}C was administered to various species, hydroxylation appeared to be the major metabolic changes produced in man, dog, rat, and mouse; the chief metabolites were 9- and 11-hydroxyacronycine, with small amounts of dihydroxy derivatives and extensive conjugation. In the guinea pig and the mouse, O-demethylation occurred actively (H. R. Sullivan *et al.*, 1970).

8.2. Emetine

Emetine (Fig. 10) is an ipecac alkaloid derived from the dried root or rhizome of *Cephaëlis ipecacuanha* or *acuminata*, plants that are found in Brazil and Central America. The chemistry of these alkaloids was reviewed by Openshaw (1970). In addition to emetine, cephaëline also occurs in ipecac, and a number of derivatives such as 2-dehydroemetine and tubulosine have been prepared.

Ipecac was used for centuries as a remedy for dysenteries, but it was not until 1912 that its ability to kill *Entamoeba histolytica* was demonstrated *in vitro* (Vedder, 1912). Other pharmacological or toxicological effects of emetine include lowering of blood pressure; myositis, most notably of the myocardium; nausea and vomiting; increased intestinal peristalsis (Klatskin and Friedman, 1948); adrenergic blocking (Ng, 1966); and antiviral action (Grunberg and Prince, 1966; Del Puerto *et al.*, 1968). Druckrey *et al.* (1953) described emetine as a mitotic poison, and subsequently, this drug and its derivatives have shown activity against L1210 *in vivo* (Jondorf *et al.*, 1971), so it is not surprising that many clinical trials have been undertaken, the severe toxicity notwithstanding. Abd-Rabbo (1969) found significant improvement in a patient with Hodgkin's disease, another with chronic myelocytic leukemia, and 2 with bladder cancer of schistosomal origin, out of a total of 25 patients treated with 2,3-dehydroemetine. In a series of 50 patients receiving the same drug, DePierre and Chahinian (1974) obtained 1 complete regression of head and neck cancer, and 5 regressions exceeding 50% in renal, head and neck, cervix, and epidermoid bronchial cancer; lesser improvements were seen in another 8 subjects. Significant improvements after therapy with emetine were also reported in cases of teratoma, thyroid, transitional-cell, and lung cancer (Panettiere and Coltman, 1971). Grollman (1965) reported favorable results using emetine in cases of nonspecific granulomas. On the other hand, Moertel *et al.* (1974) could find no beneficial effects of emetine on GI cancers.

Emetine and related drugs function as inhibitors of protein synthesis, apparently because of conformational analogies to the classic inhibitor cycloheximide (Grollman, 1966, 1967). This effect can be seen in myocardial tissue (Beller, 1968), where it might represent the basis for cardiotoxicity, as well as in HeLa cells, in which inhibition of the synthesis of DNA and of infective viral RNA occurred (Grollman, 1968). Like tylocrebrine, emetine preferentially affects chain elongation (Grollman and Huang, 1973). Gilead and Becker (1971) reported a target-size effect for emetine in HeLa S3 cells, with the synthesis of preribosomal and ribosomal RNS affected at lower drug concentrations than transfer RNA.

Emetine exhibits a pattern of prolonged retention by tissues, especially the kidney, liver, spleen, and lung of both dogs and rodents; urinary excretion was very limited (Gimble *et al.*, 1948; Parmer and Cottrill, 1949). A recent study in mice has indicated, however, that as much as 40% of the dose is excreted in the urine as unchanged drug in 24 hr (Auletta *et al.*, 1974). In rats, 2,3-dehydroemetine is excreted very slowly, 25% at 24 and 34% at 48 hr, with only 1% in the feces. Glucuronides were the major labeled components of the bile, whereas as much as 30–40% of urinary radioactivity was free drug (R. K. Johnson and Jondorf, 1973).

8.3. β-Solamarine

β-Solamarine is the glycoside of a steroidal alkaloid (Fig. 10). It occurs in woody nightshade, *Solanum dulcamara* Linn. (Solanaceae), a plant that has been used medicinally since the time of Galen. This compound showed activity against sarcoma 180 (Kupchan *et al.*, 1965) and Walker 256 carcinosarcoma (Kupchan, 1966).

8.4. Harringtonine

The alkaloid harringtonine (Fig. 10) is derived from the seeds of *Cephalotaxus harringtonia* var. *drupacea* and *harringtonia*. It inhibits the growth of both L1210 and P388 in mice (Powell *et al.*, 1969). The basis of the antitumor action appears to be an effect on protein biosynthesis that is characterized by breakdown of polyribosomes to monosomes (Huang and Grollman, 1972). Subsequent studies have defined the action of this agent more precisely, using HeLa cells and rabbit reticulocyte preparations as the test systems. Some inhibition of the synthesis of DNA, but not of RNA, was observed. On addition of drug to a reticulocyte lysate, there was a delay of 2 min before inhibition of globin synthesis occurred. Binding of poly-U or tRNA to ribosomes, and chain elongation, were unaffected, the major action appearing to be on initiation. As regards structure–activity relationships, neither the side chain alone, nor the alkaloid moiety (cephalotaxine) lacking the side chain, was active. Isoharringtonine, in which the hydroxyl near the end of the side chain is moved to become *cis* with respect to the other hydroxyl, and deoxyharringtonine, which lacks the distal hydroxyl, were active, whereas pseudoharringtonine was not (Huang, 1975). The data of Powell *et al.* (1972) obtained with P388 were similar, but in addition, homoharringtonine with an additional methylene between the two hydroxylated carbons was active, while acetylcephalotaxine was not.

8.5. Pyrrolizidine Alkaloids

The pyrrolizidine alkaloids are widely distributed in nature, presenting major toxicologic problems for livestock. The chemistry and pathogenicity of the group

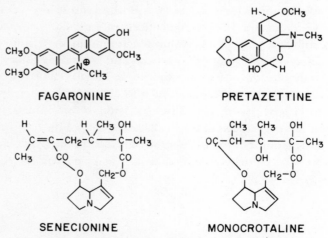

FIGURE 11. Chemical structures of miscellaneous alkaloids.

are the subject of a monograph (Bull *et al.*, 1968). Among the best-known members of this group are monocrotaline and senecionine (Fig. 11), which are found in *Senecio triangularis* Hook (Compositae), a plant that has been used as a folkloric cancer remedy for centuries. The N-oxide of senecionine also occurs naturally, and both this derivative and the parent alkaloid were identified by their activity against Walker 256 (Kupchan and Suffness, 1967). In a survey of 18 alkaloids and their derivatives, Culvenor (1968) established that 10 were active in a five-tumor test screen. Senecionine, lasiocarpine, monocrotaline, heliotrine, and spectabiline were especially active against Walker 256. It appeared that the allylic ester function, which imparts alkylating ability (and hepatotoxicity), was associated with the highest levels of activity.

8.6. Narcissus Alkaloids and Fagaronine

The Amaryllidaceae have been a source of remedies for cancer in virtually every continent since the time of Hippocrates (Fitzgerald *et al.*, 1958). Extracts of the bulbs of the Sacred Lily, *Narcissus tarzetta* L., a medicinal plant grown in the Pacific area, have yielded the alkaloid pretazettine (Fig. 11). This compound appears to be a fairly specific inhibitor of RNA-dependent DNA polymerase, as, for example, the polymerase of avian myeloblastosis virus. The alkaloid combines with the polymerase enzyme rather than affecting the binding of the template to the enzyme, and this is reflected in the noncompetitive kinetics of inhibition. Both antiviral and antitumor activity were demonstrated *in vivo* and *in vitro* (Papas *et al.*, 1973). The alkaloid exhibits significant additive and synergistic antitumor effects against Rauscher leukemia when used in combination with BCNU, cyclophosphamide, actinomycin D, 6-mercaptopurine, and 5-azacytidine (Furusawa *et al.*, 1975).

Another agent, narciclasine, has been isolated from the bulbs of *Narcissus.*. This compound has an amidic nitrogen, and thus is not strictly an alkaloid, although related to many alkaloids found in *Narcissus*. Narciclasine causes metaphase arrest at low levels, but is mitoclastic at higher doses (Ceriotti, 1967); narciprimine, a related compound occurring in the bulbs of many varieties of daffodils that lacks two of the hydroxyl groups, is inactive (Piozzi *et al.*, 1968). Peptide-bond formation is blocked by narciclasine, which binds at the "anisomycin area" of the ribosomal 60S subunit (Carrasco *et al.*, 1975).

Fagaronine is a benzophenanthridine alkaloid (Fig. 11) derived from the roots of *Fagara zanthoxyloides* (Rutaceae) (Tin-wa *et al.*, 1974). This African plant is used as a chewing stick for cleaning teeth, and also appears to have a favorable action on sickling and crenation of erythrocytes (Sofowora and Isaacs, 1971). Fagaronine is a potent antileukemic agent, as reflected by inhibition of the growth of P388 leukemia (Messmer *et al.*, 1972). Like pretazettine, fagaronine appears to be a specific inhibitor of reverse transcriptase, as assayed by its effect on the RNA-directed DNA polymerase of avian myeloblastosis virus, Rauscher leukemia virus, and simian sarcoma virus. Unlike pretazettine, however, fagaronine appears to interact with the A : T template primer (Sethi and Sethi, 1975) to bring about its inhibitory effects. The chemical synthesis of fagaronine has been achieved (J. P. Gillespie *et al.*, 1974).

Although not an alkaloid, the ansa macrolide maytansine deserves mention here, since it belongs to a class of compounds that includes streptovaricins and rifamycins, well-known inhibitors of reverse transcriptase. It is derived from the East African shrubs *Maytenus ovatus* and *M. serrata*, and is the first macrolide to show antitumor activity (Kupchan *et al.*, 1972). Murine tumors L1210, L5178Y, and especially P388, as well as KB cells, are inhibited by this agent. Incorporation of thymidine into DNA is the most sensitive biochemical parameter (Wolpert-Defilippes *et al.*, 1975).

9. Conclusion

In making this survey, many interesting agents have of necessity been omitted in order to maintain the chapter within manageable proportions. The aim throughout has been to illustrate the diversity of the alkaloids and their varied mechanisms of action. In many cases, these mechanisms are but little understood, yet such understanding is essential if these agents are to be integrated effectively into regimens of multidrug and multimodal therapy. It is the author's hope that surveys of the type of this chapter may aid in achieving this goal.

10. References

ABD-RABBO, H., 1969, Chemotherapy of neoplasia (cancer) with dehydroemetine, *J. Trop. Med.* **72:**287.

ABELSON, H. T., AND PENMAN, S., 1972, Selective interruption of high molecular weight RNA synthesis in HeLa cells by camptothecin, *Nature (London) New Biol.* **237:**144.

ABELSON, H. T., AND PENMAN, S., 1973, Induction of alkali labile links in cellular DNA by camptothecin, *Biochem. Biophys. Res. Commun.* **50:**1048.

ABELSON, H. T., AND PENMAN, S., 1975, Selective interruption of RNA metabolism by chemotherapeutic agents, in: *Handbook of Experimental Pharmacology*, Vol. 38, Part II, *Antineoplastic and Immunosuppressive Agents* (A. C. Sartorelli and D. G. Johns, eds.), pp. 571–581, Springer-Verlag, Berlin.

ACTON, E., MOSHER, C. W., FUJIWARA, A. N., CREWS, O. P., DEGRAW, J. I., JR., AND GOODMAN, L., 1966, *Amer. Chem. Soc. Abstr. 152nd Meeting*, New York, p. 30.

ADELMANN, M. R., BORISY, G. G., SHELANSKI, M. L., WEISENBERG, R. C., AND TAYLOR, E. W., 1968, Cytoplasmic filaments and tubules, *Fed. Proc. Fed. Amer. Soc. Exp. Biol.* **27:**1186.

AGUSTIN, B. M., AND CREASEY, W. A., 1967, Effects of vinca alkaloids on the synthesis of RNA in mouse brain, *Nature (London)* **215:**965.

AISENBERG, A. C., 1963, Suppression of immune response by "vincristine" and "vinblastine," *Nature (London)* **200:**484.

ALLEN, L. M., AND CREAVEN, P. J., 1973, Inhibition of macromolecular biosynthesis in cultured L1210 mouse leukemia cells by thalicarpine (NSC 68075), *Cancer Res.* **33:**3112.

ALLEN, L. M., AND CREAVEN, P. J., 1974, Binding of a new antitumor agent, thalicarpine, to DNA, *J. Pharm. Sci.* **63:**474.

ALLEN, L. M., AND CREAVEN, P. J., 1975, Pharmacokinetics of an epipodophyllotoxin derivative (VP-16-213) in man, *Proc. Amer. Assoc. Cancer Res.* **16:**201.

ANDERSON, P. J., SONG, S. K., AND SLOTWINER, P., 1967, The fine structure of spheromembranous degeneration of skeletal muscle induced by vincristine, *J. Neuropathol. Exp. Neurol.* **26**:15.

ANGEVINE, J. B., JR., Nerve destruction by colchicine in mice and golden hamsters, *J. Exp. Zool.* **136**:363.

ARMSTRONG, J. G., 1968, New derivatives of the *Vinca rosea* alkaloids, *Acta Genet. Med. Gemellol.* (*Rome*) **17**:193.

ARMSTRONG, J. G., DYKE, R. W., FOUTS, P. J., HAWTHORNE, J. J. JANSEN, C. J., JR., AND PEABODY, A. M., 1967, Initial clinical experience with vinglycinate sulfate, a molecular modification of vinblastine, *Cancer Res.* **27**:221.

AULETTA, A. E., GERY, A. M., AND MEAD, J. A. R., 1974, Influence of antileukemic (L1210) treatment schedule on disposition of (−)-emetine hydrochloride (NSC 33669) in normal and leukemic mice, *Cancer Res.* **34**:1581.

BACK, A., AND WALASZEK, E. J., 1953, Studies with radioactive colchicine I. The influence of tumors on the tissue distribution of radioactive colchicine in mice, *Cancer Res.* **13**:552.

BARASA, A., MACCOTTA, V., FILOGAMO, G., AND CANAVESE, B., 1970, Azione della vincaleucoblastina (VLB) sui prolungamenti, centrale e periferico, dei neuroni dei gangli spinali coltivati *in vitro*, *Boll. Soc. Ital. Biol. Sper.* **46**:860.

BEER, C. T., AND RICHARDS, J. F., 1964, The metabolism of *Vinca* alkaloids. Part II. The fate of tritiated vinblastine in rats, *Lloydia* **27**:352.

BEHNKE, O., AND FORER, A., 1967, Evidence for four classes of microtubules in individual cells, *J. Cell Sci.* **2**:169.

BELLER, B. M., 1968, Observations of the mechanism of emetine poisoning of myocardial tissue, *Circulation Res.* **22**:501.

BELPAIRE, F. M., AND BOGAERT, M. G., 1974, Species differences in the excretion of papaverine metabolites, *Arch. Intern. Pharmacodyn. Ther.* **208**:362.

BENNETT, T., AND GARDINER, S. M., 1975, The effects of intravenous injections of vinblastine or vincristine on the responses of the rat heart to nerve stimulation and to drugs, *Br. J. Pharmacol.* **53**:444P.

BENSCH, K. G., AND MALAWISTA, S. E., 1969, Microtubule crystals in mammalian cells, *J. Cell Biol.* **40**:95.

BENSCH, K. G., MARANTZ, R., WISNIEWSKI, H., AND SHELANSKI, M., 1969, Induction *in vitro* of microtubular crystals by vinca alkaloids, *Science* **165**:495.

BENT, K. J., AND MOORE, R. H., 1966, The mode of action of griseofulvin, in: *Biochemical Studies of Antimicrobial Drugs* (B. A. Newton and P. E. Reynolds, eds.), pp. 82–110, Cambridge University Press, London.

BEREZHINSKAYA, V. V., AND NIKITINA, S. S., 1965, Antiphlogistic effects of tetrandrine and some aspects of its mechanism of action, *Farmakol. Toksikol.* **28**:77.

BHUYAN, B. K., FRASER, T. J., AND LI, L. H., 1972, Cell cycle phase specificity and biochemical effects of ellipticine on mammalian cells, *Cancer Res.* **32**:2538.

BICK, I. R. C., AND MCLEOD, L. J., 1974, Pharmacological activity of some *bis*-benzylisoquinoline alkaloids, *J. Pharm. Pharmacol.* **26**:988.

BLEYER, W. A., FRISBY, S. A., AND OLIVERIO, V. T., 1975, Uptake of vincristine by murine leukemia cells, *Biochem. Pharmacol.* **24**:633.

BOCH, M., NORTH, T., NELKE, J. M., PIKE, D., RADUNZ, H., AND WINTERFELDT, E., 1972, Die biogenetisch orientierte Total synthese von DL-Camptothecin und 7-Chlorcamptothecin, *Chem. Ber.* **105**:2126.

BORISY, G. G., AND TAYLOR, E. W., 1967, The mechanism of action of colchicine. Binding of colchicine-³H to cellular protein, *J. Cell Biol.* **34**:525.

BORISY, G. G., MARCUM, J. M., OLMSTED, J. B., MURPHY, D. B., AND JOHNSON, K. A., 1975, Purification of tubulin and associated high molecular weight proteins from porcine brain and characterization of microtubule assembly *in vitro*, *Ann. N. Y. Acad. Sci.* **253**:107.

BOSMANN, H. B. 1970, Camptothecin inhibits macromolecular synthesis in mammalian cells but not in isolated mitochondria or *E. coli*, *Biochem. Biophys. Res. Commun.* **41**:1412.

BOUDENE, C., DUPREY, F., AND BOHUON, C., 1975, Radioimmunoassay of colchicine, *Biochem. J.* **151**:413.

BRADLEY, W. G., LASSMAN, L. P., PEARCE, G. W., AND WALTON, J. N., 1970, The neuromyopathy of vincristine in man. Clinical, electrophysiological and pathological studies, *J. Neurol. Sci.* **10**:107.

BRISTOL, J. A., COMINS, D. L., DAVENPORT, KANE, M. J., LYLE, R. E., MALONEY, J. R., AND HORWITZ, S. B., 1975, Analogs of camptothecin, *J. Med. Chem.* **18**:535.

BROWNING, E. T., GROPPI, V. E., JR., AND KON, C., 1974, Papaverine, a potent inhibitor of respiration in C-6 astrocytoma cells, *Mol. Pharmacol.* **10**:175.

BRUCHOVSKY, N., OWEN, A. A., BECKER, A. J., AND TILL, J. E., 1965, Effects of vinblastine on the proliferative capacity of L cells and their progress through the division cycle, *Cancer Res.* **25**:1232.

BRUES, A. M., 1942, The fate of colchicine in the body, *J. Clin. Invest.* **21**:646.

BRYAN, J., 1972, Definition of three classes of binding sites in isolated microtubule crystals, *Biochemistry* **11**:2611.

BRYAN, J., 1975, Preliminary studies on affinity labeling of the tubulin–colchicine binding site, *Ann. N. Y. Acad. Sci.* **253**:247.

BULL, L. B., CULVENOR, C. C. J., AND DICK, A. T., 1968, *The Pyrrolizidinie Alkaloids. Their Chemistry, Pathogenicity and Other Biological Properties*, North-Holland Publishing Company, Amsterdam.

BURNSIDE, B., 1975, The form and arrangement of microtubules: An historical, primarily morphological review, *Ann. N. Y. Acad. Sci.* **253**:14.

CARDINALI, G., CARDINALI, G., AND BLAIR, J., 1961, Stathmokinetic effect of vincaleukoblastine on normal bone marrow and leukemic cells, *Cancer Res.* **21**:1542.

CARDINALI, G., CARDINALI, G., AND CENTURELLI, G., 1968, The *Catharanthus roseus* (*Vinca rosea*) alkaloids: A new class of stathmokinetic agents, *Acta Genet. Med. Gemellol.* (*Rome*) **17**:197.

CARRASCO, L., FRESNO, M., AND VAZQUEZ, D., 1975, Narciclasine: An antitumor alkaloid which blocks peptide bond formation by eukaryotic ribosomes, *FEBS Lett.* **52**:236.

CASEY, E. B., FULLERTON, P. M., AND JELLIFFE, A. W., 1970, Vincristine neurotoxicity: A clinical and electrophysiological study of eighteen patients, *Clin. Sci.* **38**:23P.

CERIOTTI, G., 1967, Narciclasine: An antimitotic substance from *Narcissus* bulbs, *Nature* (*London*) **213**:595.

CHADWICK, M., PLATZ, B. B., AND LISS, R. H., 1971, Physiological disposition of ellipticine in dogs and rats, *Proc. Amer. Assoc. Cancer Res.* **12**:34.

CHAJEK, T., STEIN, O., AND STEIN, Y., 1975, Colchicine-induced inhibition of plasma lipoprotein lipase in the intact rat, *Biochim. Biophys. Acta* **380**:127.

CHEN, K. K., AND CHEN A. L., 1935, The alkaloids of han-fang chi, *J. Biol. Chem.* **109**:681.

CHENG, C. C., 1975, Design of cancer chemotherapeutic agents: Chemical approach, in: *Pharmacological Basis of Cancer Chemotherapy*, pp. 165–196, Williams and Wilkins Co., Baltimore.

CHUNG, L. W. K., AND GABOUREL, J. D., 1971, Adrenal steroid release by vinblastine sulfate and its contribution to vinblastine sulfate effects on rat thymus, *Biochem. Pharmacol.* **20**:1749.

CLINE, M. J., 1968, Effect of vincristine on synthesis of ribonucleic acid and protein in leukaemic leucocytes, *Br. J. Haematol.* **14**:21.

COHLAN, S. Q., AND KITAY, D., 1965, The teratogenic effect of vincaleukoblastine in the pregnant rat, *J. Pediatr.* **66**:541.

COSTA, M., AND FILOGAMO, G., 1970, Effetti della colchicina nella fibre adrenergiche dei plessi nervosi intestinali, *Boll. Soc. Ital. Biol. Sper.* **46**:865.

CRANWELL, P. A., AND SAXTON, J. E., 1962, A synthesis of ellipticine, *J. Chem. Soc.* **1962**:3482.

CREASEY, W. A., 1967, The binding of antimitotic agents by cell-free extracts of tumor cells, *Pharmacologist* **9**:192.

CREASEY, W. A., 1968, Modifications in biochemical pathways produced by the vinca alkaloids, *Cancer Chemother. Rep.* **52**:501.

CREASEY, W. A., 1969, Biochemical effects of the vinca alkaloids—IV. Studies with vinleurosine, *Biochem. Pharmacol.* **18**:227.

CREASEY, W. A., 1974, The vinca alkaloids, *Biochem. Pharmacol.* **23**(Suppl. 2):217.

CREASEY, W. A., 1975*a*, Vinca alkaloids and colchicine, in: *Handbook of Experimental Pharmacology*, Vol. 38, Part II, *Antineoplastic and Immunosuppressive Agents* (A. C. Sartorelli and D. G. Johns, eds.), pp. 670–694, Springer-Verlag, Berlin.

CREASEY, W. A., 1975*b*, Biochemistry of dimeric *Catharanthus* alkaloids in: *The Catharanthus Alkaloids. Botany, Chemistry, Pharmacology and Clinical Use* (W. I. Taylor and N. R. Farnsworth, eds.), pp. 209–236, Marcel Dekker, New York.

CREASEY, W. A., 1976, Biochemical effects of *d*-tetrandrine and thalicarpine, *Biochem. Pharmacol.*, **25**:1887.

CREASEY, W. A., AND MARKIW, M. E., 1964, Biochemical effects of the vinca alkaloids II. A comparison of the effects of colchicine, vinblastine and vincristine on the synthesis of ribonucleic acids in Ehrlich ascites carcinoma cells, *Biochim. Biophys. Acta* **87**:601.

CREASEY, W. A., AND MARKIW, 1965, Biochemical effects of the vinca alkaloids III. The synthesis of ribonucleic acid and the incorporation of amino acids in Ehrlich ascites cells *in vitro*, *Biochim. Biophys. Acta* **103**:635.

CREASEY, W. A., BENSCH, K. G., AND MALAWISTA, S. E., 1971, Colchicine, vinblastine and griseofulvin: Pharmacological studies with human leukocytes, *Biochem. Pharmacol.* **20**:1579.

CREASEY, W. A., SCOTT, A. I., WEI, C. C., KUTCHER, J., SCHWARTZ, A., AND MARSH, J. C., 1975, Pharmacological studies with vinblastine in the dog, *Cancer Res.* **35**:1116.

CREAVEN, P. J., COHEN, M. H., SELAWRY, O. S., TEJADA, F., AND BRODER, L. E., 1975, Phase I study of thalicarpine (NSC-68075), a plant alkaloid of novel structure, *Cancer Chemother. Rep.* **59**:1001.

CULPEPER, N., 1653, *The Complete Herbal*, reprinted for Imperial Chemical Industries by the Kynoch Press, Birmingham, 1953.

CULVENOR, C. C. J., 1968, Tumor-inhibitory activity of pyrrolizidine alkaloids, *J. Pharm. Sci.* **57**:1112.

CULVENOR, C. C. J., AND LODER, J. W., 1966, Ellipticine alkaloids from *Ochrosia* and *Excavatia* species. Isolation and synthesis, *Amer. Chem. Soc. Abstr. 152nd Meeting*, New York, p. 29.

CURCUMELLI-RODOSTAMO, M., AND KULKA, M., 1967, *bis*-Benzylisoquinoline and related alkaloids, in: *The Alkaloids* (R. H. F. Manske, ed.), Vol. 9, pp. 133–174, Academic Press, New York.

CUTTS, J. H., 1961, Changes in mitosis in ascites tumors and normal bone marrow induced by vincaleukoblastine *in vivo*, *Can. Cancer Conf.* **4**:363.

CUTTS, J. H., 1968, Protective action of diethylstilbestrol on the toxicity of vinblastine in rats, *J. Natl. Cancer Inst.* **41**:919.

DAHLSTROM, A., HEIWALL, P. O., HÄGGENDAL, J., AND SAUNDERS, N. R., 1975, Effect of antimitotic drugs on the intraaxonal transport of neurotransmitters in rat adrenergic and cholinergic nerves, *Ann. N. Y. Acad. Sci.* **253**:507.

DANØ, K., 1972, Cross resistance between vinca alkaloids and anthracyclines in Ehrlich ascites tumor *in vivo*, *Cancer Chemother. Rep.* **56**:701.

DaRe, P., MANCINI, V., COLUMBO, G., AND MICCIARELLI, A., 1966, Antimitotic effects of some basic colchicinamides on mammalian cells *in vitro*, *Life Sci.* **5**:211.

DeCONTI, R. C., AND CREASEY, W. A., 1975, Clinical aspects of the dimeric *Catharanthus* alkaloids, in: *The Catharanthus Alkaloids. Botany, Chemistry, Pharmacology and Clinical Use* (W. I. Taylor and N. R. Farnsworth, eds.), pp. 237–278, Marcel Dekker, New York.

DeCONTI, R. C., MUGGIA, F. J., CUMMINGS, F. J., CALABRESI, P., AND CREASEY, W. A., 1975, Clinical and pharmacological studies with d-tetrandrine, *Proc. Amer. Assoc. Cancer Res.* **16**:96.

DeHARVEN, E., 1956, Action de la colchicine et de certaines hormones corticosurréraliennes sur les mitoses des follicules pileux du rat, *Rev. Belge Pathol.* **25**:277.

DEL PUERTO, B. M., TATO, J. C., KOLTAN, A., BURES, O. M., DeCHIERI, P. R., GARCIA, A., ESCARAY, T. I., AND LORENZO, B., 1968, Hepatitis viral en el nino con especial referencia a su tratamiento con emetina, *Prensa Med. Argent.* **55**:818.

DePIERRE, A., AND CHAHINIAN, P., 1974, Dehydroemetin in 50 disseminated carcinomas unresponsive to other drugs, *Proc. Amer. Assoc. Cancer Res.* **15**:11.

DEWYS, W. D., HUMPHREYS, S. R., AND GOLDIN, A., 1968, Studies on therapeutic effectiveness of drugs with tumor weight and survival time indices of Walker 256 carcinoma, *Cancer Chemother. Rep.* **52**:229.

DIXON, G. J., DULMADGE, E. A., MULLIGAN, L. T., AND MELLETT, L. B., 1969, Cell culture bioassay for vicristine sulfate in sera from mice, rats, dogs and monkeys, *Cancer Res.* **29**:1810.

DONALDSON, G. R., ATKINSON, M. R., AND MURRAY, A. W., 1968, Inhibition of protein synthesis in Ehrlich ascites tumor cells by phenanthrene alkaloids tylophorine, tylocrebrine and cryptopleurine, *Biochem. Biophys. Res. Commun.* **31**:104.

DONIGIAN, D. W., AND OWELLEN, R. J., 1973, Interaction of vinblastine, vincristine and colchicine with serum proteins, *Biochem. Pharmacol.* **22**:2113.

DOUGLAS, W. W., AND SORIMACHI, M., 1972, Colchicine inhibits adrenal medullary secretion evoked by acetylcholine without affecting that evoked by potassium, *Br. J. Pharmacol.* **45**:129.

DRUCKREY, H., DANNEBERG, P., AND SCHMÄHL, D., 1953, Mitotic poisons, *Arzeneim. Forsch.* **3**:151.

DUNN, B. P., GOUT, P. W., AND BEER, C. T., 1973, Effects of the antineoplastic alkaloid acronycine on nucleoside uptake and incorporation into nucleic acids by cultured L5178Y cells, *Cancer Res.* **33**:2310.

DUSTIN, P., JR., 1963, New aspects of the pharmacology of antimitotic agents, *Pharmacol. Rev.* **15**:449.

EAGAN, R. T., AHMANN, D. L., HAHN, R. G., AND O'CONNELL, M. J., 1975, Pilot study to determine an intermittent dose schedule for VP16–213, *Proc. Amer. Assoc. Cancer Res.* **16:**55.

EIGSTI, O. J., AND DUSTIN, P., JR., 1955, Colchicine, in: *Agriculture, Medicine, Biology and Chemistry,* Iowa College Press, Ames.

EIPPER, B. A., 1975, Purification of rat brain tubulin, *Ann. N. Y. Acad. Sci.* **253:**239.

EL-NAKEEB, M. A., MCLELLAN, W. L., JR., AND LAMPEN, J. O., 1965, Antibiotic action of griseofulvin on dermatophytes, *J. Bacteriol.* **89:**557.

ENGELBORGHS, Y., HEREMANS, K. A. H., DEMAEYER, L. C. M., AND HOEBEKE, J., 1976, Effect of temperature and pressure on polymerization equilibrium of neuronal microtubules, *Nature (London)* **259:**686.

ERTEL, N., OMOKOKU, B., AND WALLACE, S. L., 1969, Colchicine concentrations in leucocytes, *Arthritis Rheum.* **12:**293.

FALKSON, G., AND FALKSON, H., 1974, Clinical trial of the oral form of 4'-dimethylepipodophyllotoxin-β-D ethylidene glucoside (NSC-141540) VP 16-213, *Proc. Amer. Soc. Clin. Oncol.* **10:**160.

FERM, V. H., 1963, Congenital malformations in hamster embryos after treatment with vinblastine and vincristine, *Science* **141:**426.

FINE, R. E., 1971, Heterogeneity of tubulin, *Nature (London) New Biol.* **233:**283.

FINE, R. N., CLARKE, R. R., AND SHORE, N. A., 1966, Hyponatremia and vincristine therapy. Syndrome possibly resulting from inappropriate antidiuretic hormone secretion, *Amer. J. Dis. Child.* **112:**256.

FITZGERALD, D. B., HARTWELL, J. L., AND LEITER, J., 1958, Tumor-damaging activity in the plant families showing antimalarial activity. Amaryllidaceae, *J. Natl. Cancer Inst.* **20:**763.

FUJIWARA, A. N., ACTON, E. M., AND GOODMAN, L., 1968, Synthesis of thiaellipticine, 5,11-dimethyl-benzothieno[2,3-g]isoquinoline (1), *J. Heterocycl. Chem.* **5:**853.

FURUSAWA, E., SUZUKI, N., FURUSAWA, S., AND LEE, J. Y. B., 1975, Combination chemotherapy of Rauscher leukemia and ascites tumors by *Narcissus* alkaloid with standard drugs and effect on cellular immunity, *Proc. Soc. Exp. Biol. Med.* **149:**771.

GAILANI, S. D., ARMSTRONG, J. G., CARBONE, P. P., TAN, C., AND HOLLAND, J. F., 1966, Clinical trial of vinleurosine sulfate (NSC-90636): A new drug derived from *Vinca rosea* Linn., *Cancer Chemother. Rep.* **50:**95.

GALLO, R. C., WHANG-PENG, J., AND ADAMSON, R. H., 1971, Studies on the antitumor activity, mechanism of action, and cell cycle effects of camptothecin, *J. Natl. Cancer Inst.* **46:**789.

GARCIA-GIRAULT, W., AND MACIEIRA-COELHO, A., 1970, Methoxy-9-ellipticine. II. Analysis *in vitro* of the mechanism of action, *Eur. J. Clin. Biol. Res.* **15:**539.

GAWADI, N., 1971, Actin in the mitotic spindle, *Nature (London)* **234:**410.

GEBHART, W., SCHWANITZ, G., AND HARTWICH, G., 1969, Zytogenetische Wirkung von Vincristin auf menschliche Leukozyten *in vivo* und *in vitro*, *Med. Klin.* **64:**2366.

GELFAND, E. W., MORRIS, S. A., AND RESCH, K., 1975, Antibody-dependent cytotoxicity: Modulation by the cytochalasins and microtubule-disruptive agents, *J. Immunol.* **114:**919.

GELLERT, E., GOVINDACHARI, T. R., LAKSHMIKANTHAM, M. V., RAGADE, I. S., RUDZUTS, R., AND VISWANATHAN, N., 1962, The alkaloids of *Tylophora crebriflora*: Structure and synthesis of tylocrebrine, a new phenanthroindolizidine alkaloid, *J. Chem. Soc.* **1962:**1008.

GEORGATSOS, J. G., AND KAREMFYLLIS, T., 1968, Action of podophyllic acid on malignant tumors—II. Effects of podophyllic acid ethyl hydrazide on the incorporation of precursors into the nucleic acids of mouse mammary tumors and liver *in vivo*, *Biochem. Pharmacol.* **17:**1489.

GEORGATSOS, J. G., KAREMFYLLIS, T., AND SYMEONIDIS, A., 1968, Action of podophyllic acid on malignant tumors—I. Distribution of tritiated podophyllic acid ethyl hydrazide in subcellular fractions of mouse mammary tumors, *Biochem. Pharmacol.* **17:**1485.

GEORGE, P., JOURNEY, L. J., AND GOLDSTEIN, M. N., 1965, Effect of vincristine on the fine structure of HeLa cells during mitosis, *J. Natl. Cancer Inst.* **35:**355.

GILBERT, B., 1965, The alkaloids of *Aspidosperma, Diplorrhyncus, Kopsia, Ochrosia, Pleiocarpa,* and related genera, in: *The Alkaloids* (R. H. F. Manske, ed.), Vol. 8, pp. 335–513, Academic Press, New York.

GILEAD, Z., AND BECKER, Y., 1971, Effect of emetine on ribonucleic acid biosynthesis in HeLa cells, *Eur. J. Biochem.* **23:**143.

GILLESPIE, E., LEVINE, R. J., AND MALAWISTA, S. E., 1968, Histamine release from rat peritoneal mast cells: Inhibition by colchicine and potentiation by deuterium oxide, *J. Pharmacol. Exp. Ther.* **164:**158.

GILLESPIE, J. P., AMOROS, L. G., AND STERMITZ, F. R., 1974, Synthesis of fagaronine. An anticancer benzophenanthridine alkaloid, *J. Org. Chem.* **39:**3239.

GIMBLE, A. I., DAVISON, C., AND SMITH, P. K., 1948, Studies on the toxicity, distribution and excretion of emetine, *J. Pharmacol. Exp. Ther.* **94**:431.

GOLDFINGER, S. E., HOWELL, R. R., AND SEEGMILLER, J. E., 1965, Suppression of metabolic accompaniment of phagocytosis by colchicine, *Arthritis Rheum.* **8**:1112.

GOODWIN, S., SMITH, A. F., AND HORNING, E. C., 1959, Alkaloids of *Ochrosia elliptica* Labill, *J. Amer. Chem. Soc.* **81**:1903.

GOTTLIEB, J. A., AND LUCE, J. K., 1972, Treatment of malignant melanoma with camptothecin (NSC 100880), *Cancer Chemother. Rep.* **56**:103.

GOTTLIEB, J. A., GUARINO, A. M., CALL, J. B., OLIVERIO, V. T., AND BLOCK, J. B., 1970a, Preliminary pharmacologic and clinical evaluation of camptothecin sodium (NSC-100880), *Cancer Chemother. Rep.* **54**:461.

GOTTLIEB, J. A., GUARINO, A. M., OLIVERIO, V. T., AND BLOCK, J. B., 1970b, Preliminary clinical and pharmacological studies with camptothecin sodium (CS), *Proc. Amer. Assoc. Cancer Res.* **11**:31.

GOTTSCHALK, P. G., DYCK, P. J., AND KIELY, J. M., 1968, Vinca alkaloid neuropathy: Nerve biopsy studies in rats and in man, *Neurology* **18**:875.

GOVINDACHARI, T. R., 1967, Tylophora alkaloids, in: *The Alkaloids* (R. H. F. Manske, ed.), Vol. 9, pp. 517–528, Academic Press, New York.

GRAFF, G. L. A., GUENING, C., AND HILDEBRAND, J., 1967., Action du sulfate de vincristine sur le gastrocémien de rat I. Mis en évidence de deux compartments, metaboliquement distincts, pour le phosphate inorganique; effets sur les phosphates organiques acidosolubles et les phospholipides, *C. R. Soc. Biol.* (*Paris*) **161**:2645.

GRALLA, E. J., COLEMAN, G. L., AND JONAS, A. M., 1974, Toxicology studies with *d*-tetrandrine (NSC-77037), a plant alkaloid with vascular and lymphotoxic effects in dogs and monkeys, *Cancer Chemother. Rep. Part 5* **5**:79.

GRIEDER, A., MAURER, R., AND STÄHELIN, H., 1974, Effect of an epipodophyllotoxin derivative (VP 16–213) on macromolecular synthesis and mitosis in mastocytoma cells *in vitro*, *Cancer Res.* **34**:1788.

GRISHAM, L. M., WILSON, L., AND BENSCH, K. G., 1973, Antimitotic action of griseofulvin does not involve disruption of microtubules, *Nature* (*London*) **244**:294.

GROLLMAN, A. P., 1965, Emetine in the treatment of intraabdominal and retroperitoneal non-specific granulomas, *Surg. Gynecol. Obstet.* **120**:792.

GROLLMAN, A. P., 1966, Structural basis for inhibition of protein synthesis by emetine and cycloheximide based on an analogy between ipecac alkaloids and glutarimide antibiotics, *Proc. Natl. Acad. Sci. U.S.A.* **56**:1867.

GROLLMAN, A. P., 1967, Structural basis for the inhibition of protein biosynthesis: Mode of action of tubulosine, *Science* **157**:84.

GROLLMAN, A. P., 1968, Inhibitors of protein biosynthesis. V. Effects of emetine on protein and nucleic acid biosynthesis in HeLa cells, *J. Biol. Chem.* **243**:4089.

GROLLMAN, A. P., 1975, Cytotoxic inhibitors of protein synthesis, in: *Handbook of Experimental Pharmacology*, Vol. 38, Part II, *Antineoplastic and Immunosuppressive Agents* (A. C. Sartorelli and D. G. Johns, eds.), pp. 554–570, Springer-Verlag, Berlin.

GROLLMAN, A. P., AND HUANG, M. T., 1973, Inhibitors of protein synthesis in eukaryotes: Tools in cell research, *Fed. Proc. Fed. Amer. Soc. Exp. Biol.* **32**:1673.

GRUNBERG, E., AND PRINCE, H. N., 1966, Antiviral activity of emetine, 2-dehydroemetine and 2-dehydro-3-noremetine, *Antimicrob. Agents Chemother.* **1966**: 527.

GULL, K., AND TRINCI, A. P. J., 1973, Griseofulvin inhibits fungal mitosis, *Nature* (*London*) **244**:292.

GUTHRIE, R. W., BROSSI, A., MENNONA, F. A., MULLIN, J. G., KIERSTEAD, R. W., AND GRUNDBERG, E., 1975, Ellipticine derivatives, *J. Med. Chem.* **18**:755.

HAHN, R. A., NELSON, J. W., TYE, A., AND BEAL, J. L., 1966, Pharmacological activity of thalicarpine, *J. Pharm. Sci.* **55**:466.

HANCOCK, B. W., AND NAYSMITH, A., 1975, Vincristine-induced autonomic neuropathy, *Br. Med. J.* **3**:207.

HANNA, P. E., O'DEA, AND GOLDBERG, N. D., 1972, Phosphodiesterase inhibition by papaverine and structurally related compounds, *Biochem. Pharmacol.* **21**:2266.

HARDESTY, C. T., AND CHANEY, N. A., 1970, Distribution of the antileukemic agent ellipticine in mouse tissue, *Proc. Amer. Assoc. Cancer. Res.* **11**:34.

HARDESTY, C. T., CHANEY, N. A., AND MEAD, J. A. R., 1972, The effect of route of administration on the distribution of ellipticine in mice, *Cancer Res.* **32**:1884.

HARMON, R. E., SHIAU, G. T., DE, K. K., FICSOR, G., AND FEDESNA, N. E., 1975, Synthesis and evaluation of alkylthiocolchicines and their N-derivatives as antileukemic and antimitotic agents, *Amer. Chem. Soc. Abstr. 169th Meeting*, MEDI 10.

HARRISSON, C. M. H., PAGE, B. M., AND KEIR, H. M., 1976, Mescaline as a mitotic spindle inhibitor, *Nature (London)* **260**:138.

HART, L. G., CALL, J. B., AND OLIVERIO, V. T., 1969, A fluorometric method for determination of camptothecin in plasma and urine, *Cancer Chemother. Rep.* **53**:211.

HARTWELL, J. L., AND ABBOTT, B. J., 1969, Antineoplastic principles in plants: Recent developments in the field, *Adv. Pharmacol. Chemother.* **7**:117.

HAYAT, M., MATHÉ, G., JANOT, M. M., POTIER, P., DAT-XUONG, N., CAVE, A., SEVENET, T., KAN-FAN, C., POISSON, J., MIET, J., LEMEN, J., LEGOFFIC, F., GOUYETTE, A., AHOND, A., DALTON, L. K., AND CONNORS, T. A., 1974, Experimental screening of 3 forms and 19 derivatives or analogs of ellipticine: Oncostatic effect on L1210 leukemia and immunosuppressive effect of 4 of them, *Biomed. Express (Paris)* **21**:101.

HEBDEN, H. F., HADFIELD, J. R., AND BEER, C. T., The binding of vinblastine by platelets in the rat, *Cancer Res.* **330**:1417.

HELSON, L., HELSON, C., LAI, K. B., AND PIH, K., 1974, Papaverine effects on growth and function of tumor cells and lymphocytes, *Proc. Amer. Soc. Clin. Oncol.* **10**:172.

HERMAN, E. H., AND CHADWICK, D. P., 1974, Cardiovascular effects of d-tetrandrine, *Pharmacology* **12**:97.

HERMAN, E., VICK, J., AND BURKA, B., 1971, The cardiovascular actions of ellipticine, *Toxicol. Appl. Pharmacol.* **18**:743.

HERMAN, E. H., LEE, I. P., MHATRE, R. M., AND CHADWICK, D. P., 1974, Prevention of hemolysis induced by ellipticine (NSV-71795) in rhesus monkeys, *Cancer Chemother. Rep. Part 1* **58**:171.

HEUSON, J. C., GAVER, C. W., AND LEGROS, N., 1970 Growth inhibition of rat mammary carcinoma and endocrine changes produced by 2-Br-α-ergocryptine, a suppressor of lactation and nidation, *Eur. J. Cancer* **6**:353.

HIRSIMÄKI, Y., ARSTILA, A. U., AND TRUMP, B. F., 1975, Autophagocytosis: *In vitro* induction by microtubule poisons, *Exp. Cell Res.* **92**:11.

HOFFMAN, H., 1952, Acceleration and retardation of the processes of axon-sprouting in partially denervated muscles, *Aust. J. Exp. Biol. Med. Sci.* **30**:541.

HORWITZ, M. S., AND HORWITZ, S. B., 1971, Intracellular degradation of HeLa and adenovirus type 2 DNA induced by camptothecin, *Biochem. Biophys. Res. Commun.* **45**:723.

HORWITZ, S. B., 1975, Camptothecin, in: *Handbook of Experimental Pharmacology*, Vol. 38, Part II, *Antineoplastic and Immunosuppressive Agents* (A. C. Sartorelli and D. G. Johns, eds.), pp. 649–656, Springer-Verlag, Berlin.

HORWITZ, S. B., AND HORWITZ, M. S., 1973, Effects of camptothecin on the breakage and repair of DNA during the cell cycle, *Cancer Res.* **33**:2834.

HORWITZ, S. B., CHANG, C., AND GROLLMAN, A. P., 1971, Studies on camptothecin: I. Effects on nucleic acid and protein synthesis, *Mol. Pharmacol.* **7**:632.

HORWITZ, S. B., CHANG, C., AND GROLLMAN, 1972, Antiviral action of camptothecin, *Antimicrob. Agents Chemother.* **2**:395.

HUANG, M. T., 1975, Harringtonine, an inhibitor of initiation of protein biosynthesis, *Mol. Pharmacol.* **11**:511.

HUANG, M. T., AND GROLLMAN, A. P., 1972, Mode of action of tylocrebrine: Effects on protein and nucleic acid synthesis, *Mol. Pharmacol.* **8**:538.

HUNTER, J. C., 1963, Effects of vincaleukoblastine sulfate on metabolism of thioguanine-resistant L1210 leukemia cells, *Biochem. Pharmacol.* **12**:283.

HUU CHANH, P., SORBARA, R., DAT-XUONG, N., LEPECQ, J. B., AND PAOLETTI, C., 1974, Actions cardiovasculaires et toxicités de l'hydroxy-9-ellipticine chez le chien, *C. R. Acad. Sci. Ser. D.* **279**:1039.

ILAN, J., AND QUASTEL, J. H., 1966, Effect of colchicine on nucleic acid metabolism during metamorphosis of *Tenebrio molitor* L. and in some mammalian tissues, *Biochem. J.* **100**:448.

JACOB, H., AMSDEN, T., AND WHITE, J., 1972, Membrane microfilaments of erythrocytes: Alteration in intact cells reproduces the hereditary spherocytosis syndrome, *Proc. Natl. Acad. Sci. U.S.A.* **69**:471.

JOHNSON, I. S., ARMSTRONG, J. G., GORMAN, M., AND BURNETT, J. P., JR., 1963, The vinca alkaloids: A new class of oncolytic agents, *Cancer Res.* **23**:1390.

JOHNSON, I. S., HARGROVE, W. W., HARRIS, P. N., WRIGHT, H. F., AND BODER, G. B., 1966, Preclinical studies with vinglycinate, one of a series of chemically derived analogs of vinblastine, *Cancer Res.* **26**:2431.

JOHNSON, I. S., SVOBODA, G. H., POORE, G. A., AND BODER, G. B., 1968, Experimental anti-tumor activity of acronycine, in: *Cancer Chemotherapy* (A. Goldin, ed.), Gann Monograph 2, pp. 177–183, Maruzen Company, Osaka.

JOHNSON, R. K., AND JONDORF, W. R., 1973, Studies on the metabolic fate of (^{14}C)- labeled (±)-2,3-dehydroemetine in the rat, *Xenobiotica* **3**:85.

JONDORF, W. R., ABBOTT, B. J., GREENBERG, N. H., AND MEAD, J. A. R., 1971, Increased life-span of leukemic mice treated with drugs related to (−)-emetine, *Chemotherapy* **16**:109.

JONES, R. G. W., RICHARDS, J. F., AND BEER, C. T., 1966, Biochemical studies with the vinca alkaloids II. Effect of vinblastine on the biosynthesis of nucleic acids and their precursors in rat thymus cells, *Cancer Res.* **26**:882.

JOURNEY, L. J., BURDMAN, J., AND GEORGE, P., 1968, Ultrastructural studies on tissue culture cells treated with vincristine (NSC-67574), *Cancer Chemother. Rep.* **52**:509.

KANN, H. E., JR., AND KOHN, K. W., 1972, Effects of deoxyribonucleic acid-reactive drugs on ribonucleic acid synthesis in leukemia L1210 cells, *Mol. Pharmacol.* **8**:551.

KAPLAN, I. W., 1942, Condylomata acuminata, *New Orleans Med. Surg. J.* **94**:388.

KARLSSON, J. O., AND SJOSTRAND, J., 1969, The effect of colchicine on the axonal transport of protein in the optic nerve and tract of the rabbit, *Brain Res.* **13**:617.

KEEN, P., AND LIVINGSTON, A., 1970, Decline of tissue noradrenalin under the influence of a mitotic inhibitor, *Nature (London)* **227**:967.

KELLY, D. C., AVERY, R. J., AND DIMMOCK, N. J., 1974, Camptothecin: An inhibitor of influenza virus replication, *J. Gen. Virol.* **25**:427.

KELLY, M. G., AND HARTWELL, J. L., 1953, The biological effects and the chemical composition of podophyllin. A review, *J. Natl. Cancer Inst.* **14**:967.

KESSEL, D., 1971, Effects of camptothecin on RNA synthesis in leukemia L1210 cells, *Biochim. Biophys. Acta* **246**:225.

KESSEL, D., BOSMANN, H. B., AND LOHR, K., 1972, Camptothecin effects on DNA synthesis in murine leukemia cells, *Biochim.Biophys. Acta* **269**:210.

KINGSBURY, E. W., AND VOELZ, H.,1969, Induction of helical arrays of ribosomes by vinblastine sulfate in *Escherichia coli, Science* **166**:768.

KIRSCHNER, M. W., SUTER, M., WEINGARTEN, M., AND LITTMAN, D., 1975, The role of rings in the assembly of microtubules *in vitro, Ann. N. Y. Acad. Sci.* **253**:90.

KLATSKIN, G., AND FRIEDMAN, H., 1948, Emetine toxicity in man: Studies on the nature of early toxic manifestations, their relation to dose level, and their significance in determining safe dosage, *Ann. Intern. Med.* **28**:892.

KLEVECZ, R. R., AND FORREST, G. L., 1975, Regulation of tubulin expression through the cell cycle, *Ann. N. Y. Acad. Sci.* **253**:292.

KOCSIS, J. J., WALASZEK, E. J., AND GEILING, E. M., 1957, Disposition of biosynthetically labeled ^{14}C podophyllotoxin in normal and tumor-bearing mice, *Arch Int. Pharmacodyn.* **111**:134.

KOHN, K. W., WARING, M. J., GLAUBIGER, D., AND FRIEDMAN, C. A., 1975, Intercalative binding of ellipticine to DNA, *Cancer Res.* **35**:71.

KOTORII, K., MORI, H., AND YOSHIDA, M., 1971, A peculiar crystalline structure in neurons of rabbits treated with vincristine, *Kurume Med. J.* **18**:57.

KRACKOFF, I. H., 1965, Discussion of conference on gout and purine metabolism, *Arthritis Rheum.* **8**:760.

KRISHAN, A., 1968, Time lapse and ultrastructure studies on the reversal of mitotic arrest induced by vinblastine sulfate in Earle's L. cells, *J. Natl. Cancer Inst.* **41**:581.

KRISHAN, A., AND FREI, E., III, 1975, Morphological basis for the cytolytic effect of vinblastine and vincristine on cultured human leukemic lymphoblasts, *Cancer Res.* **35**:497.

KRISHAN, A., AND HSU, D., 1971, Vinblastine-induced ribosomal complexes. Effect of some metabolic inhibitors on their formation and structure, *J. Cell Biol.* **49**:927.

KROWKE, R., ZIMMERMAN, B., AND MERKER, H. J., 1970, Biochemical and electron microscopic studies of rat embryos in *in vivo* culture, *Naunyn-Schmiedeberg's Arch. Pharmakol.* **266**:382.

KUPCHAN, S. M., 1966, Plants supply promising antitumor agents, *Chem. Eng. News* **44**:64.

KUPCHAN, S. M., AND ATLAND, H. W., 1973, Structural requirements for tumor-inhibitory activity among benzylisoquinoline alkaloids and related synthetic compounds, *J. Med. Chem.* **16**:913.

KUPCHAN, S. M., AND SUFFNESS, M. I., 1967, Tumor inhibitors XXII. Senecionine and senecionine N-oxide, the active principles of *Senecio triangularis*, *J. Pharm. Sci.* **56**:541.

KUPCHAN, S. M., YOKOYAMA, N., AND THYAGARAJAN, B. S., 1961, Menispermaceae alkaloids II. The alkaloids of *Cyclea peltata* Diels, *J. Pharm. Sci.* **50**:164.

KUPCHAN, S. M., BARBOUTIS, S. J., KNOX, J. R., AND LAU CAM, C. A., 1965, Beta-solamarine: Tumor inhibitor isolated from *Solanum dulcamara*, *Science* **150**:1827.

KUPCHAN, S. M., YANG, T. H., VASILIKIOTIS, G. S., BARNES, M. H., AND KING, M. L., 1967, The isolation and structural elucidation of thalidasine, a novel *bis* benzylisoquinoline alkaloid tumor inhibitor from *Thalictrum dasycarpum*, *J. Amer. Chem. Soc.* **89**:3075.

KUPCHAN, S. M., YANG, T. H., KING, M. L., AND BORCHARDT, R. T., 1968, *Thalictrum* alkaloids, VIII. The isolation, structural elucidation, and synthesis of dehydrothalicarpine, *J. Org. Chem.* **33**:1052.

KUPCHAN, S. M., KOMODA, Y., COURT, W. A., THOMAS, G. J., SMITH, R. M., KARIM, A., GILMORE, C. J., HALTIWANGER, R. C., AND BRYAN, R. F., 1972, Maytansine, a novel antileukemic ansa macrolide from *Maytenus ovatus*, *J. Amer. Chem. Soc.* **94**:1354.

KUPCHAN, S. M., UCHIDA, I., BRANFMAN, A. R., DAILEY, R. G., JR., AND FEI, B. Y., 1976, Antileukemic principles isolated from *Euphorbiaceae* plants, *Science* **191**:571.

LACY, P. E., HOWELL, S. L., YOUNG, D. A., AND FINK, C. J., 1968, New hypothesis on insulin secretion, *Nature (London)* **219**:1177.

LEAKE, C. D., 1975, *An Historical Account of Pharmacology to the 20th Century*, Charles C Thomas, Springfield, Illinois.

LEMEN, J., HAYAT, M., MATHÉ, G., GUILLON, J. C., CHENU, E., HUMBLOT, M., AND MASSON, Y., 1970, Methoxy-9-ellipticine lactate. I. Experimental study (oncostatic and immunosuppressive actions; preclinical pharmacology), *Eur. J. Clin. Biol. Res.* **15**:534.

LEPECQ, J. B., GOSSE, C., DAT-XUONG, N., AND PAOLETTI, C., 1973, Un nouveau composé antitumoral: l'Hydroxy-9-ellipticine. Action sur la leucémie L1210 de la souris, *C. R. Acad. Sci. Ser. D* **277**:2289.

LEPECQ, J. B., DAT-XUONG, N., GOSSE, C., AND PAOLETTI, C., 1974, A new antitumoral agent: 9-Hydroxyllipticine. Possibility of a rational design of anticancerous drugs in the series of DNA intercalating drugs, *Proc. Natl. Acad. Sci. U.S.A.* **71**:5078.

LI, L. H., AND COWIE, C. H., 1974, Biochemical effects of ellipticine on leukemia L1210 cells, *Biochim. Biophys. Acta* **353**:375.

LI, L. H., FRASER, T. J., OLIN, E. J., AND BHUYAN, B. K., 1972, Action of camptothecin on mammalian cells in culture, *Cancer Res.* **32**:2643.

LIEBESKIN, D., HORWITZ, S. B., HORWITZ, M. S., AND HSU, K. C., 1974, Immunoreactivity to antinucleoside antibodies in camptothecin treated HeLa cells, *Exp. Cell Res.* **86**:174.

LITS, F., 1934, Contribution a l'étude des réactions cellulaires provoquées par la colchicine, *C. R. Soc. Biol.* **115**:1421.

LU, K. H., KOCH, Y., AND MEITES, J., 1971, Direct inhibition by ergocornine of pituitary prolactin release, *Endocrinology* **89**:229.

LUDFORD, R. J., 1945, Colchicine in the experimental chemotherapy of cancer, *J. Natl. Cancer Inst.* **6**:89.

LUNDBERG, D., 1970, Colchicine-induced delay of the degenerative release of sympathetic transmitter in the conscious rat, *Acta Physiol. Scand.* **80**:430.

MADOC-JONES, J., AND MAURO, F., 1968, Interphase action of vinblastine and vincristine: Differences in their lethal action through the mitotic cycle of cultured mammalian cells, *J. Cell Physiol.* **72**:185.

MALAWISTA, S. E., 1965, The action of colchicine in acute gout, *Arthritis Rheum.* **8**:752.

MALAWISTA, S. E., 1968, Colchicine: A common mechanism for its anti-inflammatory and antimitotic effects, *Arthritis Rheum.* **11**:191.

MALAWISTA, S. E., SATO, H., AND BENSCH, K. G., 1968, Vinblastine and griseofulvin reversibly disrupt the living mitotic spindle, *Science* **160**:770.

MALAWISTA, S. E., SATO, H., CREASEY, W. A., AND BENSCH, K. G., 1969, Vinblastine produces uniaxial birefringent crystals in starfish oocytes, *Fed. Proc. Fed. Amer. Soc. Exp. Biol.* **28**:875.

MALAWISTA, S. E., SATO, H., AND CREASEY, W. A., 1976, Dissociation of the mitotic spindle in oocytes exposed to griseofulvin and vinblastine, *Exp. Cell Res.* **99**:193.

MARSLAND, D., 1968, Cell division-enhancement of the antimitotic effects of colchicine by low temperature and high pressure in the cleaving eggs of *Lytechinus variegatus*, *Exp. Cell Res.* **50**:369.

MASCITELLI-CORIANDOLI, E., AND LANZANI, P., 1963, Effects of *Vinca rosea* Linn. alkaloids on the liver coenzyme A and pantothenic acid, *Arzneim. Forsch.* **13**:1011.

MATHÉ, G., SCHNEIDER, M., BAND, P., AMIEL, J. L., SCHWARZENBERG, L., CATTAN, A., AND SCHLUM-BERGER, J. R., 1965, Leurosine sulfate (NSC-90636) in treatment of Hodgkin's disease, acute lymphoblastic leukemia, and lymphoblastic lymphosarcoma, *Cancer Chemother. Rep.* **49**:47.

MATHÉ, G., HAYAT, M., DEVASSAL, F., SCHWARZENBERG, L., SCHNEIDER, M., SCHLUMBERGER, J. R., JASMIN, C., AND ROSENFELD, C., 1970, Methoxy-9-ellipticine lactate. III. Clinical screening: Its action in acute myeloblastic leukemia, *Eur. J. Clin. Biol. Res.* **15**:541.

MCINTOSH, J. R., CANDE, Z., SNYDER, J., AND VANDERSLICE, K., 1975, Studies on the mechanism of mitosis, *Ann. N. Y. Acad. Sci.* **253**:407.

MCKENZIE, D., 1927, *The Infancy of Medicine*, McMillan, London.

MCLEOD, J. G., AND PENNY, R., 1969, Vincristine neuropathy: An electrophysiological and his-tological study, *J. Neurol. Neurosurg. Psychiatry* **32**:297.

MESSMER, W. M., TIN-WA, M., FONG, H. H. S., BEVELLE, C., FARNWORTH, N. R., ABRAHAM, D. J., AND TROJANEK, J., 1972, Fagaronine, a new tumor inhibitor isolated from *Fagara zanthoxyloides* Lam. (Rutaceae), *J. Pharm. Sci.* **61**:1858.

MINOR, P. D., AND DIMMOCK, N. J., 1975, Inhibition of synthesis of influenza virus proteins: Evidence for two host-cell-dependent events during multiplication, *Virology* **67**:114.

MISRA, N. C., AND ROBERTS, D., 1975, Inhibition by 4'-demethyl-epipodophyllotoxin-9-(4,6-0-2-thenylidene-β-D-glucopyranoside) of human lymphoblast cultures in G_2 phase of the cell cycle, *Cancer Res.* **35**:99.

MOERTEL, C. G., SCHUTT, A. J., REITEMEIER, R. J., AND HAHN, R. G., 1973. Phase II study of camptothecin (NSC-100880) in the treatment of advanced gastrointestinal cancer, *Cancer Chemother. Rep.* **56**:95.

MOERTEL, C. G., SCHUTT, A. J., HAHN, R. G., AND REITEMEIER, 1974, Treatment of advanced gastrointestinal cancer with emetine (NSC-33669), *Cancer Chemother. Rep.* **58**:229.

MOLLOV, N., DUTSCHEWSKA, SILJANOVSKA, K., AND STOJCEV, S., 1968, Cytotoxic effect of alkaloids from *Thalictrum minus elatum* and their derivatives, *C. R. Acad. Bulg. Sci.* **21**:605.

MORASCA, L., RAINISIO, C., AND MASERA, G., 1969, Duration of cytotoxic activity of vincristine in the blood of leukemic children, *Eur. J. Cancer* **5**:79.

MORGAN, J. L., AND SEEDS, N. W., 1975, Properties of tubulin prepared by affinity chromatog-raphy, *Ann. N. Y. Acad. Sci.* **253**:260.

MOSHER, C. W., CREWS, O. P., ACTON, E. M., AND GOODMAN, L., 1966, Preparation and antitumor activity of olivacine and some new analogs, *J. Med. Chem.* **9**:237.

MUELLER, G. A., GAULDEN, M. E., AND DRANE, W., 1971, The effects of varying concentrations of colchicine on the progression of grasshopper neuroblasts into metaphase, *J. Cell Biol.* **48**:253.

MUGIA, F. M., CREAVEN, P. J., HANSEN, H. H., COHEN, M. H., AND SELAWRY, O. S., 1972, Phase I clinical trial of weekly and daily schedules of camptothecin sodium (NSC-100880): Correlation with preclinical studies, *Cancer Chemother. Rep.* **56**:515.

MURRAY, R. M. L., MOZAFFARIAN, G., AND PEARSON, O. H., 1972, Prolactin levels with L-DOPA treatment in metastatic breast carcinoma, in: *Prolactin and Carcinogenesis* (A. Boyns and K. Griffiths, eds.), pp. 158–161, Alpha Omega Alpha Publishing, Cardiff, Wales.

NAGASAWA, H., AND MEITES, J., 1970, Suppression by ergocornine and iproniazid of carcinogen-induced mammary tumors in rats: Effects on serum and pituitary prolactin levels, *Proc. Soc. Exp. Biol. Med.* **135**:469.

NEUSS, N., BARNES, A. J., AND HUCKSTEP, L. L., 1975, Vinca alkaloids XXXV. Desacetoxyvinblastine, a new minor alkaloid from *Vinca rosea* L. (*Catharanthus roseus* G. Don), *Experientia* **31**:18.

NG, N. K. F., 1966, A new pharmacological action of emetine, *Br. Med. J.* **1**:1278.

NISSEN, N. I., HANSEN, H. H., PEDERSEN, H., STROYER, I., DOMBERNOWSKY, P., AND HESSELLUND, M., 1975, Clinical trial of the oral form of a new podophyllotoxin derivative, VP-16-213 (NSC-141540), in patients with advanced neoplastic disease, *Cancer Chemother. Rep.* **59**:1027.

NOBLE, R. L., BEER, C. T., AND MCINTYRE, R. W., 1967, Biological effects of dihydrovinblastine, *Cancer* **20**:885.

NOMURA, Y., AND SEGAWA, T., 1975, Influences of colchicine and vinblastine on the uptake of 5-hydroxytryptamine and norepinephrine by rat brain synaptosomes and small vesicle fractions, *J. Neurochem.* **24**:1257.

OBRECHT, P., AND FUSENIG, N. E., 1966, Die Wirkung von Vincaleukoblastin (Velbe®) auf die Glykolyse von Tumor Zellen, *Eur. J. Cancer* **2**:109.

OCHS, S., AND WORTH, 1975, Comparison of the block of fast axoplasmic transport in mammalian nerve by vincristine, vinblastine and desacetyl vinblastine amide sulfate (DVA), *Proc. Amer. Assoc. Cancer Res.* **16**:70.

OLMSTED, J. B., AND BORISY, G. G., 1973, Microtubules, *Annu. Rev. Biochem.* **42**:507.

OPENSHAW, H. T., 1970, The ipecacuanha alkaloids, in: *Chemistry of the Alkaloids* (S. W. Pelletier, ed.), pp. 85–115, Van Nostrand Reinhold, New York.

ORCI, L., LEMARCHAND, Y., SINGH, A., ASSIMACOPOULOS-JEANNET, F., ROUILLER, C., AND JEANRENAUD, B., 1973, Role of microtubules in lipoprotein secretion by the liver, *Nature (London)* **244**:30.

OWELLEN, R. J., AND DONIGIAN, D. W., 1972, [³H]Vincristine. Preparation and preliminary pharmacology, *J. Med. Chem.* **15**:894.

OWELLEN, R. J., AND HARTKE, C. A., 1975, The pharmacokinetics of 4-acetyl tritium vinblastine in two patients, *Cancer Res.* **35**:975.

PADAWER, J., 1963, Quantitative studies with mast cells, *Ann. N. Y. Acad. Sci.* **103**:87.

PAGET, G. E., AND WALPOLE, A. L., 1958, Some cytological effects of griseofulvin, *Nature (London)* **182**:1320.

PALMER, C. G., WARREN, A. K., AND SIMPSON, P. J., 1963, A comparison of the cytologic effects of leurosine methiodide and vinblastine in tissue culture, *Cancer Chemother. Rep.* **31**:1.

PANETTIERE, F., AND COLTMAN, C. A., 1971, Phase I experience with emetine hydrochloride (NSC 33669) as an antitumor agent, *Cancer* **27**:835.

PAOLETTI, C., CROS, S., SORBARA, R., GOSSE, C., TOLLON, Y., AND MOISAND, C., 1974, Etudes sur la toxicité de la 9-hydroxyellipticine, *C. R. Acad. Sci. Ser. D* **278**:1437.

PAPAS, T. S., SANHAUS, L., AND CIRIGOS, M. A., 1973, Inhibition of DNA polymerase of avian myeloblastosis virus by an alkaloid extract from *Narcissus tazetta* L., *Biochem. Biophys. Res. Commun.* **52**:88.

PARMER, L. G., AND COTTRILL, C. W., 1949, Distribution of emetine in tissues, *J. Lab. Clin. Med.* **34**:818.

PIOZZI, F., FUGANTI, C., MONDELLI, R., AND CERIOTTI, G., 1968, Narciclasine and narciprimine, *Tetrahedron* **24**:1119.

PORTER, K. R., 1966, Cytoplasmic microtubules and their functions, in: *Ciba Found. Symp., Principles of Biomolecular Organization*, pp. 308–356, Little, Brown, Boston.

POWELL, R. G., WEISLEDER, D., SMITH, C. R., JR., AND WOLFF, I. A., 1969, Structure of cephalotaxine and related alkaloids, *Tetrahedron Lett.* **46**:4081.

POWELL, R. G., WEISLEDER, D., AND SMITH, C. R., JR., 1972, Antitumor alkaloids from *Cephalotaxus harringtonia*: Structure and activity, *J. Pharm. Sci.* **61**:1227.

QUADRI, S. K., KLEDZIK, G. S., AND MEITES, J., 1974, Enhanced regression of DMBA-induced mammary cancers in rats by combination of ergocornine with ovariectomy or high doses of estrogen, *Cancer Res.* **34**:499.

RICHARDS, J. F., JONES, R. G. W., AND BEER, C. T., 1966, Biochemical studies with the vinca alkaloids I. Effect on nucleic acid formation by isolated cell suspensions, *Cancer Res.* **26**:876.

ROBERTSON, J. H., AND MCCARTHY, G. M., 1969, Periwinkle alkaloids and the platelet-count, *Lancet* **2**:353.

ROBERTSON, J. H., CROZIER, E. H., AND WOODEND, B. E., 1970, The effect of vincristine on the platelet count in rats, *Br. J. Haematol.* **19**:331.

ROODMAN, G. D., HUTTON, J. J., AND BOLLUM, F. J., 1975, DNA polymerase activities during erythropoiesis. Effects of erythropoietin, vinblastine, colcemid, and daunomycin, *Exp. Cell Res.* **91**:269.

RUBINSTEIN, L., AND REIN, A., 1974, Effect of camptothecin on simian virus 40 DNA, *Nature (London)* **248**:226.

SABAD, A., 1975, Induction of differentiation in thymus-derived lymphocytes by vinca alkaloids, *Proc. Amer. Assoc. Cancer Res.* **16**:153.

SABIR, M., AND BHIDE, N. K., 1971, Study of some pharmacological actions of berberine, *Indian J. Physiol. Pharmacol.* **15**:111.

SALIH, H., H., FLAX, H., BRANDER, W., AND HOBBS, J. R., 1972, Prolactin dependence in human breast cancers, *Lancet* **2**:1103.

SANDLER, S. G., TOBIN, W., AND HENDERSON, E. S., 1969, Vincristine-induced neuropathy. A clinical study of fifty leukemic patients, *Neurology* **19**:367.

SARTORELLI, A. C., AND CREASEY, W. A., 1973, Combination chemotherapy, in: *Cancer Medicine* (J. F. Holland and E. Frei, III, eds.), pp. 707–717, Lea and Febiger, Philadelphia.

SAUCIER, J. M., FESTY, B., AND LEPECQ, J. B., 1971, The change of the torsion of the DNA helix caused by intercalation. II. Measurement of the relative change of torsion induced by various alkylating drugs, *Biochimie* **53**:973.

SAVEL, H., 1966, The metaphase-arresting plant alkaloids and cancer chemotherapy, *Prog. Exp. Tumor Res.* **8**:189.

SCHULTZ, J., HAMPRECHT, B., AND DALY, J. W., 1972, Accumulation of adenosine 3′:5′ cyclic monophosphate in clonal glial cells: Labeling of intracellular adenine nucleotides with radioactive adenine, *Proc. Natl. Acad. Sci. U.S.A.* **69**:1266.

SELIGMAN, A. M., STERNBERGER, N. J., PAUL, B. D., FRIEDMAN, A. E., SHANNON, W. A., JR., WASSERKRUG, H. L., PLAPINGER, R. E., AND LYNM, D., 1975, Design of spindle poisons activated specifically by prostatic acid phosphatase (PAP) and new methods for PAP cytochemistry, *Cancer Chemother. Rep.* **59**:233.

SENTEIN, P., 1964, Action de la vincaleukoblastine sur l'oeuf en segmentation et analyse du mécanisme mitotique, *C. R. Acad. Sci. Paris* **258**:4854.

SETHI, V. S., AND SETHI, M. L., 1975, Inhibition of reverse transcriptase activity of RNA-tumor viruses by fagaronine, *Biochem. Biophys. Res. Commun.* **63**:1070.

SHAAR, C. J., AND CLEMENS, J. A., 1972, Inhibition of lactation and prolactin secretion in rats by ergot alkaloids, *Endocrinology* **90**:285.

SHAMMA, M., AND ST. GEORGIEV, V., 1974, Camptothecin, *J. Pharm. Sci.* **63**:163.

SHVAREV, I. F., AND TSETLIN, A. L., 1972, Antiblastic properties of berberine and its derivatives, *Farmakol. Toksikol.* **35**:73.

SLATER, L. M., WAINER, R. A., AND SERPICK, A. A., 1969, Vincristine neurotoxicity with hyponatremia, *Cancer* **23**:122.

SLONIM, R. R., HOWELL, D. S., AND BROWN, H. E., JR., 1962, Influence of griseofulvin upon acute gouty arthritis, *Arthritis Rheum.* **5**:397.

SMITH, D. S., JÄRLFORS, U., AND CAMERON, B. F., 1975, Morphological evidence for the participation of microtubules in axonal transport, *Ann. N. Y. Acad. Sci.* **253**:472.

SNYDER, A. L., KANN, H. E., JR., AND KOHN, K. W., 1971, Inhibition of the processing of ribosomal precursor RNA by intercalating agents, *J. Mol. Biol.* **58**:555.

SOFOWORA, E. A., AND ISAACS, W. A., 1971, Reversal of sickling and crenation in erythrocytes by the root extract of *Fagara zanthoxyloides*, *Lloydia* **34**:383.

SOIFER, D., LASZLO, A., MACK, K., SCOTTO, J., AND SICONOLFI, L., 1975, The association of a cyclic AMP-dependent protein kinase activity with microtubule protein, *Ann. N. Y. Acad. Sci.* **253**:598.

SONNET, P. E., AND JACOBSON, M., 1971, Tumor inhibitors II: Cytotoxic alkaloids from *Annona purpurea*, *J. Pharm. Sci.* **60**:1254.

SPATARO, A., AND KESSEL, D., 1972, Studies on camptothecin-induced degradation and apparent reaggregation of DNA from L1210 cells, *Biochem. Biophys. Res. Commun.* **48**:643.

SPOONER, B. S., YAMADA, K. M., AND WESSELLS, N. K., 1971, Microfilaments and cell locomotion, *J. Cell Biol.* **49**:595.

STÄHELIN, H., 1970, 4′-Demethyl-epipodophyllotoxin thenylidene glucoside (VM-26), a podophyllum compound with a new mechanism of action, *Eur. J. Cancer* **6**:303.

STÄHELIN, H., AND CERLETTI, A., 1964, Experimentalle Ergebnisse mit den Podophyllum-cytostatica SP-1 und SP-G, *Schweiz. Med. Wochenschr.* **94**:1490.

STEIN, O., SANGER, L., AND STEIN, Y., 1974, Colchicine-induced inhibition of lipoprotein and protein secretion into the serum and lack of interference with secretion of biliary phospholipids and cholesterol by rat liver *in vivo*, *J. Cell Biol.* **62**:90.

STOLINSKY, D. C., JACOBS, E. M., BRAUNWALD, J., AND BATEMAN, J. R., 1972, Further study of trimethyl-colchicinic acid, methyl ether, d-tartrate (TMCA; NSC-36354) in patients with malignant melanoma, *Cancer Chemother. Rep.* **56**:263.

STORCK, G., AND SCHULTZ, A. G., 1971, The total synthesis of dl-camptothecin, *J. Amer. Chem. Soc.* **93**:4074.

STRAHS, K. R., AND SATO, H., 1973, Potentiation of vinblastine crystal formation *in vivo* by puromycin and colcemid, *Exp. Cell Res.* **80**:10.

STUART, M. J., CUASO, C., MILER, M., AND OSKI, F. A., 1975, Syndrome of recurrent increased secretion of antidiuretic hormone following multiple doses of vincristine, *Blood*, **45**:315.

SULLIVAN, B. J., AND WECHSLER, H. I., 1947, The cytological effects of podophyllin, *Science* **105**:433.

SULLIVAN, H. R., BILLINGS, R. E., OCCOLOWITZ, J. L., BOAZ, H. E., MARSHALL, F. J., AND MCMAHON, R. E., 1970, *In vivo* hydroxylation of the alkaloid acronine, an experimental antitumor agent, *J. Med. Chem.* **13**:904.

SVOBODA, G. H., 1971, Recent advances in the search for antitumor agents of plant origin, in: *Pharmacognosy and Phytochemistry* (H. Wagner and L. Hörhammer, eds.), pp. 166–200, Springer-Verlag, Berlin.

SVOBODA, G. H., AND BLAKE, D. A., 1975, The phytochemistry and pharmacology of *Catharanthus roseus* (L.), in: *The Catharanthus Alkaloids. Botany, Chemistry, Pharmacology and Clinical Use* (W. I. Taylor and N. R. Farnsworth, eds.), pp. 45–83, Marcel Dekker, New York.

SVOBODA, G. H., POORE, G. A., SIMPSON, P. J., AND BODER, G. B., 1966, Alkaloids of *Acronychia baueri* Schott I. Isolation of the alkaloids and a study of the antitumor and other biological properties of acronycine, *J. Pharm. Sci.* **55**:758.

SVOBODA, G. H., POORE, G. A., AND MONTFORT, M. L., 1968, Alkaloids of *Ochrosia maculata* Jacq. (*Ochrosia parbonica* Gmel.). Isolation of the alkaloids and study of the antitumor properties of 9-methoxy-ellipticine, *J. Pharm. Sci.* **57**:1720.

SWEENEY, M. J., CULLINAN, G. J., POORE, G. A., AND GERZON, K., 1974, Experimental antitumor activity of vinblastine amides, *Proc. Amer. Assoc. Cancer Res.* **15**:37.

SWEENEY, M. J., POORE, G. A., KORNFELD, E. C., BACH, N. J., OWEN, N. V., AND CLEMENS, J. A., 1975, Activity of 6-methyl-8-substituted ergolines against the 7,12-dimethylbenz[α]anthracene-induced mammary carcinoma, *Cancer Res.* **35**:106.

SWERDLOW, B., AND CREASEY, W. A., 1975, Binding of vinblastine *in vitro* to ribosomes of sarcoma 180 cells, *Biochem. Pharmacol.* **24**:1243.

TALLOS, P., HELLMAN, L., AND KRAKOFF, I. H., 1975, Initial therapeutic trial of 2-chloro-6-methyl-ergoline-8β-acetonitrile methane sulfonate (lergotrile), *Proc. Amer. Assoc. Cancer Res.* **16**:187.

TAN, P., AND AUERSBERG, N., 1973, Effects of the antineoplastic alkaloid acronycine on the ultrastructure and growth patterns of cultured cells, *Cancer Res.* **33**:2320.

TAYLOR, W. I., AND FARNSWORTH, N. R. (eds.), 1975, *The Catharanthus Alkaloids. Botany, Chemistry, Pharmacology and Clinical Use*, Marcel Dekker, New York.

TEPLITZ, R. L., MAZIE, J. C., GERSON, I., AND BARR, K. J., 1975, The effects of microtubular binding agents on secretion of IgM antibody, *Exp. Cell. Res.* **90**:392.

TIN-WA, M., BELL, C. L., BEVELLE, C., FONG, H. H. S., AND FARNSWORTH, N. R., 1974, Potential anticancer agents I: Confirming evidence for the structure of fagaronine, *J. Pharm. Sci.* **63**:1476.

TOBINS, W. E., AND SANDLER, S. G., 1966, Depression of muscle spindle function with vincristine, *Nature (London)* **212**:90.

TODD, G. C., GIBSON, W. R., GRIFFING, W. J., AND MORTON, D. M., 1975, The preclinical study of desacetyl vinblastine amide (DVA), *Proc. Amer. Assoc. Cancer Res.* **16**:70.

UEDA, M., SAWADI, M., KAWAKAMI, M., MINESITA, T., AND TAKEDA, H., 1969, Pressure mechanism of vincristine sulfate, *Jpn. J. Pharmacol.* **19**:324.

UY, Q. L., MOEN, T. H., JOHNS, R. J., AND OWENS, A. H., JR., 1967, Vincristine neurotoxicity in rodents, *Johns Hopkins Med. J.* **121**:349.

VAN LANCKER, J. L., FLANGAS, A. L., AND ALLEN, J., 1966, Metabolic effects of vinblastine. I. The effect of vinblastine on nucleic acid synthesis in spleen and bone marrow, *Lab. Invest.* **15**:1291.

VEDDER, E. B., 1912, An experimental study of the action of ipecacuanha on amoebae, *J. Trop. Med.* **15**:313.

VENDITTI, J. M., AND ABBOTT, B. J., 1967, Studies on oncolytic agents from natural sources. Correlations of activity against animal tumors and clinical effectiveness, *Lloydia* **30**:332.

VOLKMANN, R., DANISHEFSKY, S., EGGLER, J., AND SOLOMON, D. M., 1971, A total synthesis of *dl*-camptothecin, *J. Amer. Chem. Soc.* **93**:5576.

WAGNER, E. K., AND ROIZMAN, B., 1968, Effect of the vinca alkaloids on RNA synthesis in human cells *in vitro*, *Science* **162**:569.

WALL, M. E., WANI, M. C., COOK, C. E., PALMER, K. H., MCPHAIL, A. T., AND SIM, G. A., 1966, Plant antitumor agents. I. The isolation and structure of camptothecin, a novel alkaloidal leukemia and tumor inhibitor from *Camptotheca acuminata*, *J. Amer. Chem. Soc.* **88**:3888.

WANI, M. C., CAMPBELL, H. F., BRINE, G. A., KEPLER, J. A., WALL, M. E., AND LEVINE, S. G., 1972, Plant antitumor agents. IX. The total synthesis of *dl*-camptothecin, *J. Amer. Chem. Soc.* **94**:3631.

WARNECKE, P., AND SEBEBER, S., 1968, Angriffspunkte von Vinca-alkaloiden im Protein- und Nucleinsäure Stoffwechsel, *Z. Krebsforsch.* **71**:361.

WARTHEN, D., GOODEN, E. L., AND JACOBSON, M., 1969, Tumor inhibitors: Liriodenine, a cytotoxic alkaloid from *Annona glabra*, *J. Pharm. Sci.* **58**:637.

WESSELS, N. K., SPOONER, B. S., ASH, J. F., BRADLEY, M. O., LUDUENA, M. A., TAYLOR, E. L., WRENN, J. T., AND YAMADA, K. M., 1971, Microfilaments in cellular and developmental processes, *Science* **171**:135.

WHITE, J. G., 1968, Effects of colchicine and vinca alkaloids on human platelets II. Changes in the dense tubular system and formation of an unusual inclusion in incubated cells, *Amer. J. Pathol.* **53**:447.

WILDMAN, W. C., AND PURSEY, B. A., 1968, Colchicine and related compounds, in: *The Alkaloids* (R. H. F. Manske, ed.), pp. 407–457, Academic Press, New York.

WILSON, L., 1975a, Action of drugs on microtubules, *Life Sci.* **17**:303.

WILSON, L., 1975b, Microtubules as drug receptors: Pharmacological properties of microtubule protein, *Ann. N. Y. Acad. Sci.* **253**:213.

WILSON, L., AND FRIEDKIN, M., 1967, The biochemical events of mitosis II. The *in vivo* and *in vitro* binding of colchicine in grasshopper embryos and its possible relation to inhibition of mitosis, *Biochemistry* **6**:3126.

WILSON, L., BRYAN, J., RUBY, A., AND MAZIA, D., 1970, Precipitation of proteins by vinblastine and calcium ions, *Proc. Natl. Acad. Sci. U.S.A.* **66**:807.

WOLFF, J., AND BHATTACHARYYA, B., 1975, Microtubules and thyroid hormone mobilization, *Ann. N. Y. Acad. Sci.* **253**:763.

WOLPERT-DEFILIPPES, M. K., ADAMSON, R. H., CYSYK, R. L., AND JOHNS, D. G., 1975, Initial studies on the cytotoxic action of maytansine, a novel ansa macrolide, *Biochem. Pharmacol.* **24**:751.

WOODWARD, R. B., IACOBUCCI, G. A., AND HOCHSTEIN, F. A., 1969, The synthesis of ellipticine, *J. Amer. Chem. Soc.* **81**:4434.

WU, R. S., KUMAR, A., AND WARNER, J. R., 1971, Ribosome formation is blocked by camptothecin, a reversible inhibitor of RNA synthesis, *Proc. Natl. Acad. Sci. U.S.A.* **68**:3009.

YASIN, R., AND PARKER, J. A., 1975, Altered plasma creatine phosphokinase activity in vincristine-treated rats, *Biochem. Pharmacol.* **24**:745.

YASIN, R., HUGHES, B. P., AND PARKER, J. A., 1973, The effect of vincristine on the calcium transport and phospholipid composition of rat skeletal muscle microsomes, *Lab. Invest.* **29**:207.

ZEE-CHENG, K. Y., AND CHENG, C. C., 1969, Experimental tumor inhibitors. Antitumor activity of esters of ω-aryl-ψ-nitro-alken-1-ol and related compounds, *J. Med. Chem.* **12**:157.

ZUBROD, C. G., 1974, Agents of choice in neoplastic disease, in: *Handbook of Experimental Pharmacology*, Vol. 38, Part I, *Antineoplastic and Immunosuppressive Agents* (A. C. Sartorelli and D. G. Johns, eds.), pp. 1–11, Springer-Verlag, Berlin.

15

Antibiotics: Nucleic Acids As Targets in Chemotherapy

Irving H. Goldberg, Terry A. Beerman, and Raymond Poon

1. Introduction

Most of the antibiotics that have proved to be of value in the treatment of human cancer affect the function or synthesis, or both, of nucleic acids. Antibiotic inhibitors of protein biosynthesis are considerably less useful because they lack the required selectivity for neoplastic cells (see Goldberg *et al.*, 1975). All the agents discussed in this chapter alter DNA function (replication or transcription or both), but it has not been established in all cases that their cytotoxic or antiproliferative actions are the direct consequences of interference with DNA function. Thus, significant antimitotic (DiMarco *et al.*, 1975) and cell-surface (Murphree *et al.*, 1976) effects may be found at concentrations of a particular agent (e.g., daunomycin or adriamycin) that are too low to alter nucleic acid synthesis significantly. In addition, it is often difficult to distinguish primary from secondary effects on nucleic acids. For instance, agents such as actinomycin or the anthracyclines, adriamycin and daunomycin, bind DNA *in vitro*, but this binding is not associated with DNA-strand breakage, at least under the conditions that have been used; the incubation of these agents with intact cells, however, is associated with DNA-strand scission (Pater and Mak, 1974; Schwartz and Kanter, 1975). Indirect DNA

Irving H. Goldberg, Terry A. Beerman, and Raymond Poon ● Department of Pharmacology, Harvard Medical School, Boston, Massachusetts 02115. Dr. Beerman's present address is Grace Cancer Drug Center, Roswell Park Memorial Institute, Buffalo, New York 14263. Dr. Poon's present address is Division of Hematology, University of California, San Francisco General Hospital, San Francisco, California 94101.

428

IRVING H.
GOLDBERG,
TERRY A.
BEERMAN,
AND RAYMOND
POON

breakage may occur after interference with DNA replication or repair. Accordingly, it is essential to show conclusively that agents that do cut DNA strands *in vitro*, e.g., bleomycin, phleomycin, and neocarzinostatin, do so by the same mechanism *in vivo*. In this regard, it is sobering in any consideration of the primary action or target of a particular agent to recall that since the discovery of streptomycin, some fourteen different "primary" effects have been described for this antibiotic. Relating *in vitro* to *in vivo* effects may also be complicated by significant differences in the concentrations of drug required to produce a given effect, such as inhibition of nucleic acid synthesis. Such differences, of course, might be accounted for by the ability of cells to concentrate or metabolize the antibiotic.

The availability of a series of congeners of an antibiotic is very helpful in determining whether a relationship exists between two or more biological actions, even though the concentrations of drug needed differ significantly, depending on the particular action considered. It then becomes important to determine how extensive a particular effect, e.g., DNA-strand scission, need be before antimitotic or irreversible cell effects are found. In the case of radiation-induced damage to DNA, such considerations have led to the "critical DNA damage" hypothesis (Burki, 1976), and may be important in determining the consequences of antibiotics that interact with or damage DNA in a selective way. Similarly, even though total DNA or RNA synthesis may be minimally affected under conditions leading to a block in cell proliferation, it is possible that the formation of a critical DNA or RNA, comprising only a small fraction of the total, is essential for cell growth.

With the reservations described above in mind, we shall discuss in this chapter a number of antitumor antibiotics that have DNA as a primary target in their mechanism of action. We have not attempted to be all-inclusive; instead, we have selected a relatively small number of agents that illustrate different modes of interfering with DNA function. We have omitted from discussion an important group of agents: the nucleoside antibiotics that act as analogues of nucleic acid precursors. Furthermore, for those antibiotics that we shall consider, we have selected only a small portion of an increasingly vast literature in an effort to focus on unique aspects of their modes of action.

2. Agents That Alter Nucleic Acid Structure and Function

2.1. Intercalators of DNA

The drug intercalation process can be described as the positioning of a planar molecule between the base pairs of DNA, resulting in the unwinding of the double-helical structure. Intercalation is sensitive to factors, such as the ionic environment, that alter the native, double-helical structure of DNA. The intercalation process of drug binding to DNA is often classified as strong binding, and is generally accompanied by a weaker secondary binding of the drug to the negatively charged phosphates of the DNA backbone (ionic bonding).

Interference with the DNA template function through drug intercalation has been demonstrated to cause inhibition of nucleic acid synthesis with DNA-dependent DNA and RNA polymerases (see Gale *et al.*, 1972). Measurements of the binding constant and DNA unwinding angle can be used to determine the degree of intercalation of a drug into DNA *in vitro*. It is possible to show that the extent of *in vivo* inhibition of nucleic acid synthesis and cell growth can be correlated with this level of intercalation, though the actual effectiveness *in vivo* does depend on many cellular properties.

2.1.1. Actinomycin D

Actinomycin D (AMD) (for recent reviews, see Goldberg and Friedman, 1971; Sobell, 1973; Meinhoffer and Atherton, 1973; Hollstein, 1974; Goldberg, 1975*a*) is an extremely toxic peptide-containing antibiotic that forms complexes with DNA *in vivo* and *in vitro*. Complex formation with DNA accounts for the ability of AMD to interfere with nucleic acid synthesis and DNA function, and this effect is responsible for most, if not all, of the biological properties of this antibiotic. AMD selectively blocks the DNA-directed synthesis of RNA in prokaryotic and eukaryotic cells. Almost all cellular RNA fractions are inhibited, although at concentrations of the antibiotic that do not completely prevent RNA formation, certain classes of RNA (in particular ribosomal RNA) are inhibited more than others. One of the species of RNA in animal cells with a formation that is resistant to AMD has a double-stranded structure (Stern and Friedman, 1971) and is synthesized in the nucleoplasm (Stern *et al.*, 1973). The function of this RNA is not yet known. AMD has been shown to act by blocking RNA chain elongation, rather than chain initiation. DNA synthesis by intact cells or by the isolated DNA polymerase is inhibited by AMD, but considerably higher levels of the antibiotic are needed than for comparable inhibition of RNA synthesis.

The definition of the molecular characteristics of the complex formed between AMD and its target, DNA, represents the first elucidation of the structure of a drug–receptor complex at the molecular level. Over the past 15 years, a wealth of information has accumulated on the nature of the complex formed between AMD and DNA (see the reviews cited above for details). The model proposed by Sobell and his co-workers (Sobell, 1973), which is based on the X-ray structure of a crystalline complex of AMD and deoxyguanosine, appears to fit the available data best. In this model, the planar phenoxazone ring system of AMD intercalates between adjacent G-C base pairs of DNA, where the guanine moieties are on opposite DNA strands, and the 2-amino groups of the guanines form a strong hydrogen bond with the carbonyl oxygen atom of the L-threonine residue of the two cyclic pentapeptides of the AMD molecule. The cyclic peptides reside in the minor groove of the DNA—where the RNA polymerase may act—and extend over a distance of about five base pairs. Additional stabilization is provided by hydrophobic interactions between groups on the pentapeptides and the sugar residues. Such hydrophobic interactions, as well as the stacking of guanine and phenoxazone rings, provide stability to the complex, but it is the hydrogen-bonding that plays a key role in the association and explains the requirement for

430

IRVING H.
GOLDBERG,
TERRY A.
BEERMAN,
AND RAYMOND
POON

the 2-amino group of guanine (Goldberg *et al.*, 1962; Cerami *et al.*, 1967) in the binding of AMD to DNA.

This model predicts a preference for the sequence GpC, and this prediction has been supported by studies on the interaction of AMD with a series of deoxydinucleotides (Krugh, 1972). The essential features of this model have also been found to exist in solution, as determined by recent spectral and stopped-flow kinetic studies employing mono-, di-, hexa-, and poly-deoxyribonucleotides (Krugh, 1972; Schara and Müller, 1972; Krugh and Neely, 1973*a,b*; Patel, 1974; Krugh and Chen, 1975; Bittman and Blau, 1975).

As a result of conformational changes within the cyclic pentapeptides induced by the DNA, several forms of the AMD–DNA complex are thought to exist at equilibrium (Müller and Crothers, 1968). In the most stable form of the complex, it is proposed that the peptide rings undergo conformational changes that adapt their structures to interact specifically with the DNA backbone, one ring interacting with each strand in the minor groove of the double helix. The slow reversal of the peptide-ring conformation is considered to account for the slow dissociation of AMD from DNA, and to be the basis for the high order of effectiveness of AMD on the RNA polymerase reaction compared with simpler analogues of the antibiotic that lack the cyclic peptides (Müller and Crothers, 1968). The peptide rings of AMD lie in the minor groove of the DNA, where the path of the advancing RNA polymerase would be blocked, possibly in analogy with the mode of action of the more specific protein repressors. It should be noted, however, that the question as to which groove of the DNA the RNA polymerase functions in is not yet settled; in fact, evidence suggesting that it may not be in the minor groove has been presented (Beabealashvilly *et al.*, 1973). The selective resistance of the DNA polymerase reaction to AMD may be due to the ability of the DNA polymerase system to produce local denaturation of the DNA immediately ahead of the enzyme, which causes the antibiotic to dissociate away much faster (Müller and Crothers, 1968).

AMD has been used widely to study biological phenomena dependent on DNA transcription. The antibiotic has also proved useful in the treatment of certain solid tumors in man. Of special interest is the enhanced effectiveness of AMD as an antitumor drug when administered in sequential combination with radiotherapy. The observed synergistic effect has been related to the interference by AMD with the cellular repair of DNA damage induced by X-rays.

Permeability differences appear to account for the resistance of certain cell lines and transformed cells to AMD (Goldstein *et al.*, 1966; Kessel and Wodinsky, 1968; Simard and Cassingena, 1969; Biedler and Riehm, 1970; Kessel and Bosmann, 1970; Cremisi *et al.*, 1974; Polet, 1975). The degree of resistance to AMD can be correlated with the degree of decreased cellular uptake of the drug. Alteration of the cell membrane by treatment with Tween 80, a potent surfactant, increases both the uptake of the drug and its toxicity (Riehm and Biedler, 1972). Further, it has been found that AMD-resistant murine leukemia cells possess an altered cell-surface glycoprotein fraction (Kessel and Bosmann, 1970). AMD sensitivity has also been related to differences in the rate of efflux of the drug from the cells

(Sawicki and Godman, 1972; Benedetto *et al.*, 1972; Williams and Macpherson, 1973, 1975). Resistant cells have been found to have a higher rate constant for the outward flow of AMD, resulting in a lower concentration of drug at equilibrium. It is of interest that cells that rapidly recover their RNA synthesis after inhibition by high doses of AMD have a low retention for the drug (Benedetto and Djaczenko, 1972). The lower retention has been related to the tendency of the chromatin of these cells to bind AMD in a weaker way (Benedetto *et al.*, 1972). It has been found, however, that the rapid recovery of overall RNA synthesis (and the delayed recovery of cell division) in certain cell lines can be explained only partly by the ability of these cells to eliminate bound AMD (Sawicki and Godman, 1972). It has been postulated that these recoveries may depend to a considerable extent on the stabilities of factors, such as possibly the acidic chromosomal proteins and their RNA messages, to decay during AMD suppression of transcription. How these findings relate to the observation that recovery of RNA synthesis takes place even when AMD is still present in the cell nucleus (Becker and Brenowitz, 1970) remains to be clarified.

2.1.2. Daunomycin and Adriamycin

Daunomycin (DNM), isolated from cultures of *Streptomyces peucetius* (DiMarco *et al.*, 1964), was found to be a potent inhibitor of growth of both normal and tumor cells, inhibiting cell proliferation of rat fibroblasts, HeLa, KB, and Helius-Lettic cells at 0.1 μg/ml (DiMarco *et al.*, 1963). A related anthracycline antibiotic, 14-hydroxydaunomycin, adriamycin (ADR) (Arcamone *et al.*, 1969), also showed strong activity against tumor cells (DiMarco *et al.*, 1969).

DNM binding to duplex DNA *in vitro* was demonstrated by observing that a drug–DNA complex was formed in which the drug's absorption spectrum was suppressed and the sedimentation velocity of the DNA decreased (Calendi *et al.*, 1965). With both DNM and ADR, strong complex formation was found only with native DNA; heat-denatured DNA did not show the expected spectral shift, nor did the DNA sedimentation velocity decrease (Zunino, 1971). Further proof for the drug's preference for duplex DNA was found in studies showing that the replication of T4 phage (containing duplex DNA) was strongly inhibited by DNM, whereas that of Ec9 or S13 (containing single-stranded DNA) phages was not (Calendi *et al.*, 1966).

It was suggested that DNM binds to DNA by intercalation of its chromophore moiety (Kersten *et al.*, 1966), and this model was substantiated by demonstrating that DNM causes changes in the supercoiling of ØX-174 RF (replicative form) DNA in a manner similar to the intercalating drug ethidium bromide (Waring, 1970). Further support for intercalation came from X-ray analysis and model-building of the stereochemical relationships in the DNM–DNA complex. From the model, it was determined that there is a 12° angle of unwinding per drug molecule, and that the amino sugar of DNM resides in the major groove of the DNA, where it can have electrostatic interactions with the negatively charged sugar phosphates (Pigram *et al.*, 1972). More recently, however, it has been found

432

IRVING H.
GOLDBERG,
TERRY A.
BEERMAN,
AND RAYMOND
POON

that the angle of unwinding for ethidium, on which the results with DNM are based, is 26° (Wang, 1974), so that the angle of unwinding for DNM is at least twice that previously proposed. A Scatchard analysis of DNM and ADR binding to DNA revealed two types of binding, classified as strong intercalative binding and weak ionic binding (Zunino *et al.*, 1972). The *N*-acetylated derivative of DNM binds DNA less well, suggesting that the protonated amino group of the sugar residue of DNM provides stabilization to the complex by electrostatic interaction with the negatively charged sugar phosphates of the DNA.

The ability of DNM to inhibit DNA-dependent DNA and RNA polymerases *in vitro* was found to correlate with the ability of DNM to intercalate DNA. Both DNM and ADR have been shown to have about equal inhibition of DNA-dependent DNA and RNA polymerase systems from a variety of mammalian, bacterial, and viral sources (DiMarco *et al.*, 1975). In a study done with *E. coli* DNA polymerase I, DNM inhibition was found to be independent of the A-T content of the template, and even with templates of low A-T content, inhibition at high drug levels was essentially complete (Honikel and Santo, 1972). From this study, it appears that DNM binding to template DNA is not base-pair specific, and that the drug inhibits polymerase function over the entire length of the template DNA. Recent evidence has been presented, however, that DNM binding to DNA may be directly related to the A-T content of the DNA, and that the drug inhibition of DNA synthesis is proportional to the A-T content of the DNA template (DiMarco, 1975).

While intercalative binding by the anthracyclines is essential for their interfering with DNA function, the sensitivity of DNA synthesis to the antibiotics may be determined to a considerable degree by the polymerizing enzyme itself. Differential inhibitory effects of DNM and ADR (as well as other intercalating agents) on nucleotide incorporation by different purified DNA polymerases have been described (Goodman *et al.*, 1974). In an *in vitro* study on the effects of DNM and ADR on three DNA polymerases from T4 bacteriophage mutants (T4D: wild-type levels of polymerase and 3′-exonuclease activities; L56 mutator: lower ratio of 3′-exonuclease to polymerase activity compared with wild type; and L141 antimutator: higher ratio of 3′-exonuclease to polymerase activity compared with wild type), it was found that enzymes with high nuclease-to-polymerase ratios (antimutator enzymes) were the most sensitive to drug inhibition. In fact, low drug levels stimulate the T4D and L56 polymerase systems. In contrast, the exonuclease activities of the three enzymes are equally sensitive to the drug. It was proposed that the stimulation at low drug levels (0.02 mM) might result from intercalation of the DNA template, and that the inhibition at higher drug levels (0.04–0.1 mM) might be due to ionic binding of drug to DNA. Differential effects on the DNA polymerizing or degrading systems in a cell have been postulated as accounting for the selective cytotoxic actions of these agents (Goodman *et al.*, 1974).

In general, ADR is more potent than DNM as an inhibitor of the RNA polymerase from *E. coli* and the DNA polymerase from *Micrococcus lysodeikticus*. For 50% inhibition of DNA or RNA synthesis, somewhat greater levels of DNM are required than of ADR (Zunino *et al.*, 1975*a*). Polymerases from normal rat liver (containing high- and low-molecular-weight P1 and P2 cytoplasmic polymerases and nuclear polymerase) were all significantly inhibited by ADR, and less effectively by DNM (Zunino *et al.*, 1975*b*). ADR inhibited DNA polymerase from mouse sarcoma virus, rat liver, and *Micrococcus leuteus*, while again DNM showed similar but somewhat less activity (Zunino *et al.*, 1975*c*). The mouse sarcoma virus polymerase was more sensitive to inhibition by drug than the polymerases from normal cells, and was the only enzyme to demonstrate competitive inhibition by drug with respect to DNA and to be less inhibited by drug in the presence of Mg^{2+} (Zunino *et al.*, 1974). DNM inhibition of nucleic acid synthesis has been shown to be related to the interaction of drug with the DNA template, and not to be a result of direct drug–polymerase interaction (Mizuno *et al.*, 1975). DNM derivatives with reduced binding to DNA *in vitro* also show reduced capacity to inhibit cell growth and nucleic synthesis *in vivo* (DiMarco *et al.*, 1971).

Inhibition by DNM and ADR of *in vivo* nucleic acid synthesis has been well documented (see the review by DiMarco *et al.*, 1975). In HeLa cells, it was found that DNM inhibited DNA and RNA synthesis equally (Rusconi and DiMarco, 1969). During the cell cycle, DNA synthesis in late S and RNA synthesis in mid G_1 and G_2 were the most sensitive to DNM (Simard, 1967).

DNM and ADR have been found to cause strand scission of cellular DNA when given at therapeutic levels to mice bearing lymphocytic leukemia (Schwartz and Kanter, 1975). In tissue culture studies, it was found that strand scission of cellular DNA occurs at drug levels that do not cause inhibition of cell growth or DNA synthesis.

DNM can inhibit cell growth of synchronized cells at any point during the cell cycle, but the strongest effect with L cells was observed when drug was given during the late S, G_2, or M phase (Mizuno *et al.*, 1975). Treatment of CHO hamster cells with low levels of ADR (0.1 μg/ml) was found to triple the S–G_2 cycle time (Hittelman and Rao, 1975). It was also noted that drug treatment of cells, especially those in the S phase, induced exchanges, gaps, and breaks in the chromosomes. The damage to chromosomes appeared to be related to the S–G_2 cycling delays, since the extent of the delay and the chromosomal damage increased when the drug was given to synchronous cultures during the S phase. S-phase cells were also shown to be more sensitive to ADR than G_2-phase cells in cytoxicity studies (Barranco *et al.*, 1973).

Recently, an analogue of ADR (AD32; *N*-trifluoroacetyladriamycin-14-valerate) has been shown to have greater antitumor activity and less toxicity than ADR or DNM (Israel *et al.*, 1975; Krishan *et al.*, 1976). The activity of this compound is unusual, because the free amino group of ADR that is necessary for complex formation with DNA and biological activity (DiMarco *et al.*, 1971) is converted to an amide in AD32. Another recently discovered anthracycline antibiotic, carminomycin, a desmethyl DNM compound (Brazhnikova *et al.*, 1974; Pettit *et al.*, 1975), has demonstrated potent therapeutic action with low relative cardiotoxicity (Gause *et al.*, 1974).

The therapeutic studies of DNM and ADR are numerous, and a recent publication of *Cancer Chemotherapy Reports* (October 1975) presents some of the latest ones.

434

IRVING H.
GOLDBERG,
TERRY A.
BEERMAN,
AND RAYMOND
POON

2.1.3. Nogalamycin

Nogalamycin, an anthracycline antibiotic isolated from *Streptomyces nogalater* var. *nogalater* (Bhuyan and Dietz, 1965), is an effective inhibitor of KB cell growth (50% inhibition at 0.005 μg/ml) and of RNA and DNA synthesis (Bhuyan and Smith, 1965). Nogalamycin predominantly affects RNA synthesis, and also binds preferentially to DNA containing alternating deoxyadenylic and thymidylic acid (Bhuyan and Smith, 1965; Ward *et al.*, 1965). It has been found that nogalamycin inhibits RNA polymerase and, to a lesser extent, DNA polymerase from KB cells (Reusser and Bhuyan, 1967). Nogalamycin binds to DNA by intercalation (Waring, 1970); in addition, the sugar side chains are presumed to interact with the grooves of the DNA (Das *et al.*, 1974). The inhibitory effects of nogalamycin on nucleic acid synthesis are similar to those found with antinomycin D (see Section 2.1.1), with rRNA synthesis being especially sensitive (Ellem and Rhode, 1970), and chain elongation being primarily affected (Sentenac *et al.*, 1968).

2.1.4. Echinomycin

Another class of intercalating antibiotics are those that possess two intercalating groups and can thus be considered as bifunctional intercalators. An example of such a drug is echinomycin, a quinoxaline antibiotic, which, like single intercalators, is cytotoxic to cells and can inhibit DNA and RNA synthesis both *in vivo* and *in vitro* with DNA-dependent DNA and RNA polymerase systems (see the review by Katagiri *et al.*, 1975).

Echinomycin possesses two quinoxaline-2-carboxylic acid chromophores linked to a cross-bridged cyclic octapeptide dilactone containing both L- and D-amino acids (Dell *et al.*, 1975). The molecule has a pseudosymmetrical structure with a twofold axis of rotational symmetry for the cyclic octapeptide dilactone and its attached quinoxaline ring system. On the basis of these considerations, it was postulated that echinomycin might act as a bifunctional intercalating agent (Waring and Wakelin, 1974). It was known that echinomycin inhibited enzymatic RNA synthesis by binding to native double-helical DNA (not to RNA), and that inhibition was found with DNAs of various base compositions (Ward *et al.*, 1965). In this work, it was shown that as an inhibitor of the RNA polymerase reaction, echinomycin was about 2.5 times more effective than daunomycin and almost 4 times more effective than chromomycin. Evidence in favor of echinomycin binding to DNA by a double intercalation event was provided by the finding that on interaction, the unwinding of the helix was twice that caused by binding of a monofunctional intercalating agent such as ethidium (Waring and Wakelin, 1974). The strongest binding occurs with native duplex DNA, in which there is one binding site for every six base pairs. Intercalation is thought to occur at two symmetrically located binding sites. This model helps to explain the marked potency of echinomycin—which is 4–5 times as effective as actinomycin D—in inhibiting cellular RNA synthesis *in vivo* (Waring and Makoff, 1974).

Bifunctional intercalators, because of their high potency as antimicrobial and antitumor agents and their potential for binding specificity, are promising chemotherapeutic agents. Recently, other double-intercalating agents, the diacridines, have been reported to be good inhibitors of P-388 cells both *in vivo* and *in vitro* (Canellakis *et al.*, 1976).

2.2. Strand Scission of DNA

An interesting class of antitumor drugs are those capable of inducing strand scissions in DNA. The ability to cause fragmentation of cellular DNA may explain the cytotoxicity of these drugs, but there are many aspects of the drug–cell interaction that must be examined before such a conclusion can be placed on a sound footing.

A comparison of drug concentrations and incubation times needed to inhibit cell growth and to cause strand scission of cellular DNA is useful in determining whether a relationship between cytotoxicity and cutting of cellular DNA exists. Even with such evidence, it must be remembered that many of the drugs that cut DNA are relatively high-molecular-weight proteins and glycoproteins, and it is reasonable to question whether they can penetrate to the cellular DNA through both the cell and nuclear membranes. If fragmentation of cellular DNA is the primary mechanism of drug action, then consideration must be given to learning how this effect results in inhibition of cell division and growth.

In many cases, not only can these drugs fragment cellular DNA *in vivo*, but they also cause strand scission of DNA under *in vitro* conditions. Whether the cutting mechanism is identical for *in vivo* and *in vitro* conditions is difficult to prove conclusively, but the existence of both activities does in itself lend support to the idea that fragmentation of the cellular DNA is an important aspect of the drug action. This section will discuss experimental data on a number of these drugs, and will deal with their effects both on isolated and cellular DNA and on the inhibition of cell proliferation.

2.2.1. Bleomycin

The bleomycins are a group of copper-chelating glycopeptides (see Umezawa, 1974, for structures) isolated from *Streptomyces verticillus* and found to have both antitumor and antibacterial activities (Ishizuka *et al.*, 1967). The antibiotic inhibits primarily DNA synthesis in *E. coli*, Ehrlich carcinoma, and HeLa cells (Suzuki *et al.*, 1968). Bleomycin can inhibit DNA and RNA synthesis by isolated DNA-dependent DNA and RNA polymerases from *E. coli* and mouse lymphoma cells (Müller *et al.*, 1975). The DNA polymerase from Rauscher murine leukemia virus is especially sensitive to the antibiotic. *In vivo* DNA synthesis appears to be inhibited selectively. Evidence has been presented that bleomycin preferentially inhibits the DNA polymerase I reaction directed by DNA containing a high A-T content, but stimulates that with DNA containing only G-C (Yamazaki *et al.*, 1973). That DNA is the target of bleomycin action is also supported by the studies of DiCioccio and Sahai Srivastava (1976), in which bleomycin was shown to inhibit DNA polymerases α and β of cells of acute lymphoblastic leukemia origin by interacting with the template DNA.

IRVING H.
GOLDBERG,
TERRY A.
BEERMAN,
AND RAYMOND
POON

On the basis of the observation that bleomycin caused a decrease in the melting temperature of DNA (Nagai *et al.*, 1969), it was found that with both intact cells and isolated DNA, incubation with bleomycin resulted in DNA-strand scissions (Suzuki *et al.*, 1969). More recent studies on the sulfhydryl-stimulated cutting of DNA by bleomycin *in vitro* have revealed that both double-stranded and heat-denatured, single-stranded DNA are cut (Haidle, 1971), indicating that helical structure is not a prerequisite for cutting. Oxidizing agents have also been shown to stimulate bleomycin breakage of DNA (Shirakawa *et al.*, 1971), as does the presence of ribonucleoside triphosphates and Mg^{2+} (Takeshita *et al.*, 1974). RNA does not seem to interact with bleomycin (Asakura *et al.*, 1975), and it appears that its resistance comes from the oxygen at the 2'-C position of ribose, because DNA from phage PBS-1, which contains uracil instead of thymine, is cut by bleomycin (Haidle *et al.*, 1972). Though the detailed mechanism whereby bleomycin cuts DNA is not known, the presence of sulfhydryl agents like 2-mercaptoethanol stimulate the drug activity nearly 20-fold, allowing strand scission of SV40 superhelical DNA at only 0.1 μg drug/ml (Umezawa *et al.*, 1973). The strand scissions have been thought to be nonspecific, and extensive cutting can reduce DNA to acid-soluble material (Haidle, 1971). It should be noted, however, that in these studies, exceedingly high concentrations of drug were used (milligrams per milliliter), and sulfhydryl compound was not present. There is now evidence that in the case of bleomycin-induced strand scissions of the lactose operator DNA, the drug does have a preference for the 3' side of the TpGpT sequence (W. Gilbert, personal communication).

A possible chemical mechanism for the sulfhydryl-requiring bleomycin cutting of DNA is provided by the finding that thymine is released from the DNA, and this release is accompanied by the generation of free aldehyde groups (Müller *et al.*, 1972). It is suggested that the aldehyde formed from the ring-opening of the deoxyribose is a result of hydrolysis of thymine *N*-glycosidic bonds. Phosphodiester bond cleavage is associated with the generation of mainly 5'-phosphoryl-ended DNA fragments (Kuo and Haidle, 1973). The break is claimed not to be repairable by DNA ligase, but since these experiments were done in the presence of the antibiotic, which itself inhibits the ligase at low concentrations (Miyaki *et al.*, 1971), this claim remains to be documented.

When the cutting of DNA by bleomycin was examined in intact mouse L cells at drug levels of 1.0 μg/ml, the DNA isolated on alkaline and neutral sucrose gradients contained 10 single-strand breaks for every double-strand scission (Terasima *et al.*, 1970). This finding is in agreement with the observed preferential formation of single-strand breaks in the *in vitro* assay systems. Partial repair of the cellular DNA could be found 3 min after removing bleomycin and returning the cells to fresh media. In fact, DNA repair in isolated hepatic nuclei (Sartiano *et al.*, 1973) and in *E. coli* dependent on DNA polymerase I has been found to be stimulated by bleomycin (Ross and Moses, 1976). In studies with AH 66 cells (rat ascites hepatoma cells), treatment with 10 μg bleomycin/ml caused the release of DNA from an isolated DNA–membrane complex (Miyaki *et al.*, 1974). Before drug treatment, the complex banded on a CsCl density gradient at a position representing DNA associated with cell membrane ($\rho = 1.55$); after drug treatment, the DNA moved to a heavier density ($\rho = 1.70$) representative of free DNA. Because the concentration of bleomycin needed to obtain free DNA did not produce double-strand breaks in the DNA, it was proposed that bleomycin released the DNA from the membrane by disrupting its point of attachment.

An interesting, but not well understood, observation has been made on the effect of bleomycin on the DNA of nuclei from rat liver. DNA isolated from liver nuclei of rats administered bleomycin was fragmented as expected, but when the liver was perfused prior to isolation of the nuclei, the DNA was not broken (Cox *et al.*, 1974). This result was interpreted as evidence that strand scission of DNA occurs only after cell lysis, and is due to the presence of drug in the blood. The implication is that bleomycin may not actually penetrate the cell, but acts only after the DNA has been released.

In a system in which the extent of bleomycin cutting of cellular DNA varied with the cell line, DNA from sensitive AH 66 cells bound more [^{14}C]bleomycin than did DNA of a resistant subclone (AH 66F), though equal levels of drug were taken up by both cell lines (Miyaki *et al.*, 1975). AH 66F cells contain an enzyme that inactivates bleomycin, and in AH 66 cells, there is 3.5 times less of this enzyme. The level of bleomycin-inactivating enzyme in AH 66F cells, taken together with their low level of free sulfhydryl compounds, has been used to account for the insensitivity of this cell line to bleomycin. The chemotherapeutic effectiveness of bleomycin in the treatment of squamous-cell carcinoma appears to involve a mechanism that parallels the results with AH 66 cells and its resistant subclone (Umezawa, 1974). Using [^{3}H]bleomycin, it was found that drug taken up by the skin and lung were inactivated at slower rates than that in other organs, due to a lower level of bleomycin-inactivating enzyme in these two organs (Umezawa *et al.*, 1972).

Bleomycin treatment of L cells resulted in a prolonged S phase and a retardation of cells through G_2 (Watanabe *et al.*, 1974). Similar interferences with the cell cycle have been found with other agents that damage DNA (Ohara and Terasima, 1972), and these findings support the concept that bleomycin also acts by inducing DNA damage.

2.2.2. Phleomycin

Phleomycin, a copper-containing peptide isolated from *Streptomyces vesticillus* (Maeda *et al.*, 1956), is similar in structure to bleomycin (Takita *et al.*, 1972). The antibiotic inhibits DNA polymerase I *in vitro*, and increases the melting temperature of the DNA (Falaschi and Kornberg, 1964). Studies in which $HgCl_2$ was used as a competitive agent have suggested that phleomycin binds to the carbonyl oxygen at the 2 position of thymidine in DNA (Pietsch and Garrett, 1968). The drug was found to inhibit DNA synthesis in *E. coli* and HeLa S_3 cells, while not affecting RNA synthesis (Tanaka *et al.*, 1963). Phleomycin, like bleomycin, causes single-strand scissions of DNA (adenovirus and phage λ) *in vitro* (Stern *et al.*, 1974). The presence of a reducing agent is required, and cutting is observed at

438

IRVING H.
GOLDBERG,
TERRY A.
BEERMAN,
AND RAYMOND
POON

concentrations near 1 μg antibiotic/ml. Phleomycin also causes fragmentation of cellular DNA in intact *E. coli*, but it has been proposed that this effect is a secondary one that results from the activation of a cellular nuclease by phleomycin (Farrell and Reiter, 1973). In *Bacillus subtilis*, phleomycin nicks the DNA and causes its release from the cell membrane after only 1 min (Reiter *et al.*, 1972). When nuclei isolated from HeLa S_3 cells were treated with phleomycin, there was a breakdown of nuclear DNA and a stimulation of repair synthesis of DNA (R. M. Friedman *et al.*, 1974).

Phleomycin and bleomycin resemble one another in their actions, although there are distinct differences. It is reasonable to expect that both agents damage DNA as a primary event, but that there then ensue other effects, such as nuclease activation, that lead to the extensive degradation of the DNA.

2.2.3. Neocarzinostatin

Neocarzinostatin (NCS), isolated from *Streptomyces carzinostaticus* var. F-14, is a single-chain protein antibiotic of 10,700 mol.wt., the amino acid sequence of which has been determined (Meienhofer *et al.*, 1972). NCS is active against gram-positive bacteria and experimental animal tumors (N. Ishida *et al.*, 1965), and has been used to induce remission in patients with acute leukemia (Hiraki *et al.*, 1974). The protein exists in a tight conformation that is stable to acid and base and possesses two reduction-resistant disulfide bridges. Its biological activity is resistant to most proteolytic enzymes (Samy *et al.*, 1974).

Early studies with *Sarcina lutea* showed that NCS inhibited primarily DNA synthesis, and reduced the cellular DNA to acid-soluble material (Ono *et al.*, 1966). On the other hand, while NCS caused inhibition of DNA synthesis in HeLa cells, cellular DNA was not made acid-soluble (Homma *et al.*, 1970). Recently, however, it has been reported that in HeLa S_3 (Beerman and Goldberg, 1974, 1977; Beerman *et al.*, 1974, 1976) and L1210 (Tatsumi *et al.*, 1974; Sawada *et al.*, 1974) cells grown in culture, NCS concentrations as low as 0.1 μg/ml (10^{-8} M) cause single-strand scissions in the cellular DNA. This effect has also been found in *Bacillus subtilis* (Ohtsuki and Ishida, 1975).

Like the antitumor agents bleomycin and phleomycin, NCS appears to act on cells by inhibiting DNA synthesis, presumably as a result of strand scission of the cellular DNA. The fragmentation of cellular DNA precedes the inhibition of DNA synthesis, and both actions exhibit similar dose–response relationships (Beerman and Goldberg, 1976). That damage to the DNA is responsible for NCS-induced inhibition of DNA synthesis is supported by reconstitution experiments with subcellular components isolated from cells treated with NCS. DNA synthesis of isolated nuclei or cell lysates derived from NCS-treated HeLa S_3 cells is inhibited, but this inhibition can be overcome in cell lysates by adding activated DNA (Beerman and Goldberg, 1977). Further, a cytoplasmic fraction (containing DNA polymerases) from drug-treated cells can stimulate DNA synthesis by nuclei isolated from untreated cells, whereas nuclei from drug-treated cells are not stimulated by the cytoplasmic fraction from untreated cells.

These results indicate that the DNA synthetic apparatus is otherwise intact in treated cells, but that the DNA is no longer an effective template for replication. Additional evidence suggesting that NCS directly damages DNA is the finding that low levels of drug (5×10^{-9} M) stimulate DNA repair in cultured lymphocytes (Tatsumi *et al.*, 1975). Further, an NCS-like antibiotic complex has been shown to induce λ prophage (Heinemann and Howard, 1964; Price *et al.*, 1964), again implicating DNA damage as the mechanism.

NCS causes single-strand scissions in duplex DNA *in vitro* in a reaction strongly dependent on the presence of sulfhydryl compound (Beerman and Goldberg, 1974; Beerman *et al.*, 1977*a*). Strand scissions by NCS were also found with DNAs such as superhelical SV40 or bacteriophage PM2 DNA, duplex linear *E. coli*, and λ bacteriophage DNA, and single-stranded bacteriophage ØX-174 DNA, but not with single- or double-stranded RNA (Beerman *et al.*, 1974). The extent of DNA strand scission depends on the ratio of NCS to DNA, and can be detected at very low levels of drug ($>10^{-8}$ M). Double-strand breaks are found only at high drug concentrations, and are presumably due to the placement of single-strand breaks on opposite DNA chains within a few nucleotides of one another. The breaks bear 5'-phosphoryl termini, and all four deoxymononucleotides are recoverable at the 5'-ends of the cleavage sites, although a higher proportion of dGMP and TMP is consistently found (Poon *et al.*, 1977). The lesions are not reparable with polynucleotide ligase from *E. coli* (Poon *et al.*, 1977) and are not active sites for DNA polymerase I (Kappen and Goldberg, 1976), suggesting that damage exists at the 3' end of the nick. The release of thymine has been detected especially at high levels of NCS (Ishida and Takahashi, 1976; Poon *et al.*, 1977), and the amount of release correlates well with the number of strand scissions (Poon *et al.*, 1977). Data from protection experiments with synthetic and natural DNAs indicate the requirement for thymidylic acid and deoxyadenylic acid in the DNA for cutting (Poon *et al.*, 1977). In DNA–RNA hybrids, riboadenylic acid can substitute for deoxyadenylic acid, whereas ribouridylic acid cannot substitute for thymidylic acid.

Since NCS is a protein isolated from a biological source, it was essential to show that its ability to nick DNA was not due to a contaminating endonuclease, and that this activity went hand-in-hand with the *in vivo* effects under various conditions of purity or denaturation. Thus, similar profiles of heat-inactivation of NCS were found whether activity was measured by the scission of DNA strands *in vitro* or in HeLa cells treated with drug (Beerman *et al.*, 1977*a*). Similarly, by column isoelectric focusing, it was shown that all four activities (inhibition of cell growth and DNA synthesis as well as the strand scission of DNA *in vivo* and *in vitro*) are associated with the same protein band (pH = 3.28) (Beerman *et al.*, 1977*a*). From these data, it was concluded that the cytotoxic activity of NCS and the nicking of DNA strands *in vitro* appear to reside in the same protein.

Even though NCS stimulates DNA repair synthesis, presumably secondary to damaging the DNA (Tatsumi *et al.*, 1975), NCS lowers the template activity of DNA for DNA polymerase I *in vitro* (Kappen and Goldberg, 1977). Accordingly, the damaged 3' end of the break must be excised in the cell before repair synthesis

440

IRVING H.
GOLDBERG,
TERRY A.
BEERMAN,
AND RAYMOND
POON

by DNA polymerase I takes place. There is a correlation between the extent of strand scission and the degree of DNA polymerase I inhibition, maximal inhibition of the polymerase reaction being obtained under conditions promoting maximal strand scission (e.g., pretreatment of DNA but not enzyme with NCS). Experiments in which the amount of drug-treated DNA template was varied at a constant level of DNA polymerase I suggest that the sites associated with NCS-induced breaks are nonfunctional in DNA synthesis, but bind the enzyme. That DNA polymerase I binds to the inactive nick sites was supported by studies using [^{203}Hg]polymerase. These data indicate that the lowering of the template activity of DNA by NCS under conditions of strand scission is due to the generation of a large number of inactive sites that block competitively the binding of DNA polymerase to the active sites on the template. As expected, the inhibition of DNA synthesis can be reversed by increasing the levels of template or polymerase (Kappen and Goldberg, 1977). Since the template activity of NCS-nicked DNA for DNA polymerase I can be markedly increased by treatment with alkaline phosphatase, it appears that a phosphoryl group exists at the 3′ end of the break (Kappen and Goldberg, unpublished data).

NCS irreversibly blocks the growth of CHO Chinese hamster cells at phase G_2 of the cell cycle, as do other agents and treatments (e.g., X-ray) that damage DNA, and the same block is found in synchronized cultures independent of when the drug is added during the cell cycle (Tobey, 1975). Similar results have been found with HeLa S_3 cells (Beerman and Krishan, unpublished data). Also, the drug level needed for detectable cell growth inhibition (0.01 μg/ml, 10^{-9} M) is the same as that needed for detectable strand scission of cellular DNA and inhibition of DNA synthesis (Beerman and Goldberg, to be published).

The data cited are compatible with the concept that the cutting reaction of DNA observed *in vitro* is responsible for the action of NCS in the cell. It will be important to show, however, that the chemical nature of the DNA break produced *in vivo* is the same as that generated *in vitro*. In addition, it is not yet known whether the nucleolytic activity of NCS is a catalytic one; the best available data indicate a requirement for 10 molecules of NCS to produce one break (Beerman and Goldberg, to be published). It is possible, of course, that in the cell an activated species of NCS is generated that does function much more efficiently. Finally, the nature of the interaction of NCS with the cell surface to facilitate presumed uptake of drug remains to be elucidated. In fact, preliminary reports have questioned whether NCS enters the cell at all (Nakamura and Ono, 1974; Lazarus *et al.*, 1976). It is important in this regard to recall that for an increasing number of protein toxins (e.g., diphtheria and cholera toxins, colicins E2 and E3, the plant toxins abrin and ricin; see Kappen and Goldberg, 1977), evidence has been accumulating that contrary to earlier views, they possess inherent—usually enzymatic—activities that can be demonstrated in cell-free systems and can be related to their cytotoxic effects. In most cases, it has been shown that uptake of the toxin or a fragment of it into the cell is required.

2.2.4. Macromomycin

Macromomycin (MCR), a protein antibiotic isolated from *Streptomyces macromomyceticus*, is cytostatic for gram-positive bacteria and has been found to prolong the life of mice bearing L1210 leukemia and sarcoma 180 (Chimura *et al.*, 1968; Yamashita *et al.*, 1976). In studies with HeLa and Yoshida sarcoma cells, MCR at 4 μg/ml inhibited both cell growth and DNA synthesis (Kunimoto *et al.*, 1972). MCR has also been found to increase the life span of mice carrying the fast-growing L1210 or P388 leukemia or the slow-growing B16 melanoma or Lewis lung tumor (Lippman *et al.*, 1975). Interestingly, cell growth resumed when drug-treated cells were exposed to trypsin, indicating that the drug interaction was occurring at a site that exposed it to trypsin, i.e., the cell surface. Presumably the MCR receptor on the cell surface was susceptible to proteolysis by trypsin, since MCR itself is not. Similar results were seen with Ta3Ha and L140 cells, where trypsin released cells blocked at G_2 by MCR (Lippman and Abott, 1973). MCR blocks the growth of HeLa S_3 cells and causes strand scission of cellular DNA and inhibition of DNA synthesis (Beerman *et al.*, to be published). Initial attempts to find an *in vitro* strand scission activity with purified DNAs have not yet been successful, but this may be a matter of finding a proper activator, such as the reducing compound that stimulates cutting with bleomycin, phleomycin, and NCS.

2.3. Covalent Binding

This class of antibiotics interacts with DNA in an irreversible manner. They form covalent adducts with the nucleic acids. One example of such binding is through alkylation of the nucleic acid bases. In the case of antibiotics with a bifunctional alkylating property, cross-linking of the complementary strands of the DNA can occur. If the lesion is not repaired, the immediate consequence is the prevention of the unwinding of the DNA double helix, which would have obvious implications for the process of replication and transcription, thereby upsetting the normal cellular metabolism and causing cytotoxicity.

2.3.1. Mitomycin C

The mitomycins are broad-spectrum antibiotics isolated from *Streptomyces caespitosus* (Hata *et al.*, 1956; Wakaki *et al.*, 1958). Mitomycin C is mutagenic for bacteria (Szybalski, 1958), causes chromosomal translocations in leukocytes (Cohen and Shaw, 1964), and interferes with mitosis in HeLa cells (Djordjevic and Kim, 1968). The drug has therapeutic activity against several solid tumors in man (Moore, 1968).

Mitomycin C possesses several potential active groups, such as the aziridine ring at C-1 and C-2, the carbamate group at C-10, and the dihydroquinone moiety. The antibiotic reacts with purified DNA *in vitro* in the presence of a reducing

442

IRVING H.
GOLDBERG,
TERRY A.
BEERMAN,
AND RAYMOND
POON

agent. The treated DNA, on heat denaturation and quick cooling, renatures rapidly to regain its native hypochromicity and buoyant density (Iyer and Szybalski, 1963, 1964). This result indicates that the drug forms cross-links between the two complementary strands of the DNA molecule. It was also observed that the degree of cross-linking was a function of the G-C content of the DNA molecule. Monofunctional attachment (non-cross-linking) to DNA was observed to be present in a ratio of 10 : 1 to the cross-links (Weissbach and Lisio, 1965). Tomasz *et al.* (1974) recently obtained evidence to propose that the partially reduced semiquinone form of mitomycin (the semiquinone radical) is the reactive intermediate, and that an intercalative mode of interaction precedes the covalent attachment. The aziridine ring is needed for cross-linking activity, but compounds lacking the aziridine ring are potent antibiotics and inhibit cellular DNA synthesis, presumably by intercalative binding to the DNA. The oxygen on position 6 of guanine is possibly the site of covalent attachment in the DNA.

Mitomycin has also been shown to cause cross-links of the DNA *in vivo* (Iyer and Szybalski, 1964). It is proposed that as a result of the cross-linking of the DNA, replication of the chromosome is impaired (Szybalski and Iyer, 1964).

Mitomycin also alkylates RNA, ribosomes, and other cellular macromolecules, but to a lesser extent than DNA (Weissbach and Lisio, 1965).

2.3.2. Anthramycin

Anthramycin, an antibiotic isolated from *Streptomyces refuineus*, has antitumor activities against several experimental tumors in mice. It also has a wide spectrum of antibacterial activity (for reviews, see Horowitz, 1975; Kohn, 1975).

The drug primarily inhibits RNA and DNA synthesis in mammalian cells. It binds to the DNA to inactivate it as a template for nucleic acid synthesis (Kohn *et al.*, 1968; Horowitz and Grollman, 1968). The drug–DNA complex is formed slowly, but is highly stable. The bound antibiotic is not dissociated by sodium lauryl sulfate, dialysis, silver ions, or alkali (Kohn and Spears, 1970). These findings led to the suggestion that the anthramycin–DNA interaction might involve a covalent bond (Kohn and Spears, 1970), although the nature of the bond remains to be identified.

Binding of anthramycin to high-molecular-weight DNA increases the viscosity of the DNA, similar to the effect of intercalating antibiotics. Contrary to the intercalating antibiotics, however, anthramycin does not induce a change in the sedimentation rate of the DNA. Electric dichroism measurements also indicate that the drug is not intercalated between base pairs (Glaubiger *et al.*, 1974).

Anthramycin binds to poly(dG) · poly(dC), but not to poly[d(A-T)] or poly(rG) · poly(rC). It also reacts with heat-denatured DNA, but at a much slower rate. Poly(dG) is much better than poly(dC) in binding the antibiotic. The relationship between drug binding and G-C content of the DNA is not clear, since DNA with high G-C ratio does not complex more readily with the antibiotic than DNA with low G-C content. It is also surprising that the drug does not inhibit RNA

synthesis primed with poly(dG) · poly(dC). The requirement for guanine in the
DNA for binding is further substantiated by the observation that DNA saturated
with anthramycin can no longer bind actinomycin, although other explanations
are possible. It has been found with equilibrium dialysis that at saturating drug
level, one molecule of anthramycin is bound for every eight to nine base pairs of
calf thymus DNA (Kohn *et al.*, 1975; Kohn and Spears, 1970).

2.4. Other Binding

In this category are the antibiotics that have not been assigned to the categories
discussed above either because their known mechanisms of interaction with DNA
are different from the aforementioned types or because not enough is known
about their mechanisms to permit them to be unequivocally classified into these
categories. Their binding to DNA can be demonstrated, and the complex can be
dissociated by certain treatments.

2.4.1. Chromomycin, Mithramycin, and Olivomycin

These related antibiotics were isolated from, respectively, *Streptomyces griseus* in
Japan (Tatsuoka *et al.*, 1958), *Streptomyces plicatus* in the United States (Rao *et al.*,
1962), and *Streptomyces olivoreticulis* in the U.S.S.R. (Gause *et al.*, 1962). Their
biochemical mechanism of action, antitumor effects in animals, and clinical usefulness in man were thoroughly reviewed recently (Gause, 1975*a,b*; Slavik and
Carter, 1975).

These antibiotics appear to have a common mechanism of action. They complex
with DNA and thereby block RNA synthesis. The interaction with DNA is believed
to be mediated by an antibiotic–Mg^{2+} complex (Ward *et al.*, 1965). Complex
formation has also been found to depend on the guanine content and the
presence of native double-helical structure in the DNA. As with actinomycin D,
the 2-amino group of guanine is required for interaction (Cerami *et al.*, 1967).
Heat-denatured calf thymus DNA binds the antibiotic much less effectively
compared with native DNA. The maximum binding with the double-stranded
synthetic poly(dG) · poly(dC) is one molecule of chromomycin per four base pairs,
whereas the single-stranded poly(dC) or poly(dG) is completely inactive in binding chromomycin (Behr *et al.*, 1969). Analogously, these antibiotics do not inhibit
poly[d(A-T)]-directed RNA synthesis at concentrations that completely abolish
the same reaction using calf thymus DNA as template (Ward *et al.*, 1965).

Many properties of the interaction of chromomycin with DNA resemble those
of actinomycin D. However, the bulky sugar substituents at each end of the
chromophores of the chromomycin family of antibiotics make intercalation as the
mode of binding by these antibiotics unlikely. Waring (1971) further showed by
sedimentation analysis that the interaction of these antibiotics with the superhelical ØX174 RF DNA is unlike those patterns usually associated with intercalating
drugs. Recently, it was found that the binding constants of chromomycin
for mouse fibrosarcoma chromatin are 1.5–3 times higher than those

444

IRVING H.
GOLDBERG,
TERRY A.
BEERMAN,
AND RAYMOND
POON

found for mouse liver chromatin (Nayak *et al.*, 1975), possibly reflecting the nature and amount of exposed DNA in the chromatin of normal and neo-plastic tissues.

As a function of its LD_{50}, olivomycin appears to be the most active therapeuti-cally among these antibiotics against lymphosarcoma and transplantable leukosis in mice (Chorin and Rossolimo, 1965; Sedov *et al.*, 1969).

2.4.2. Distamycin A

Distamycin A was isolated from the fermentation products of *Streptomyces distal-licus* (Arcamone *et al.*, 1961). It has marked effects on ascites tumors and certain solid tumors in mice (DiMarco *et al.*, 1962). It is highly inhibitory to the replication of DNA viruses (summarized in Hahn, 1975).

The antibiotic binds DNA, as determined by the shift of the absorption spectrum of the antibiotic (Krey and Hahn, 1970). The complex can be dissociated by various drastic treatments (Zimmer *et al.*, 1971*a,b*). Distamycin A also causes a shift in the melting curve of calf thymus DNA to a higher temperature (Chandra *et al.*, 1970). Viscosity measurements of the complex between drug and superhelical DNA have demonstrated that distamycin does not intercalate between the base pairs in the DNA (Krey *et al.*, 1973). It was also found that the synthetic duplex polymer poly[d(A-T)] causes a greater spectral shift of the antibiotic than poly[d(G-C)] (Krey *et al.*, 1973). The antibiotic also interacts with single-stranded polydeoxyribonucleotides and ØX174 DNA (Krey *et al.*, 1976).

Distamycin has an inhibitory effect on nucleic acid synthesis *in vitro* with purified *E. coli* enzymes at 5×10^{-6} M to 5×10^{-5} M drug (Puschendorf and Grunicke, 1969; Chandra *et al.*, 1970). Using a double-labeling experiment, Puschendorf *et al.* (1974) showed that distamycin inhibits the initiation of T4 DNA-directed RNA synthesis by *E. coli* RNA polymerase, but does not affect RNA chain elongation. They also showed that this defect is the result of the inability of the enzyme to bind to the promoter sites of the drug-treated template. Since distamycin has preference for binding to A-T-rich DNA (Zimmer *et al.*, 1971*b*), and since promoter sites are rich in A-T sequences (LeTalaer and Jeanteur, 1971), it is surmised that the binding of drug to promoter regions alters the conforma-tion of the nucleic acid so as to prevent the formation of the initiation enzyme–DNA complex.

Distamycin does not interact with rRNA by absorption spectrum measurements (Zimmer *et al.*, 1971*a*), but Chandra *et al.* (1971) did find binding of radioactive antibiotic to polyribonucleotides by equilibrium dialysis. The drug (at about 10^{-4} M) also inhibits polymerization of polyuridylic acid-dependent polymeriza-tion of polyphenylalanine (Zimmer and Luck, 1970).

3. Inactivators of Nucleic Acid Polymerizing Enzymes

3.1. DNA and RNA Polymerases

The only antibiotics discovered to date that directly and specifically interact with RNA polymerases are the rifamycins. They specifically inhibit RNA synthesis initiation by binding tightly to the holoenzyme (Wehrli and Staehelin, 1971). They are found to be inhibitory only against prokaryotic RNA polymerases, and are ineffective against eukaryotic enzymes. Nevertheless, several rifamycin derivatives are active against eukaryotic polymerases and will be discussed in Section 3.2 in connection with inhibitors of viral reverse transcriptase. The eukaryotic counterpart to the rifamycins is the mushroom toxin α-amanatin, which specifically binds the RNA polymerase B from eukaryotic cells to prevent chain elongation (Cochet-Meilhac and Chambon, 1974). However, this toxin is too toxic for clinical use.

ANTIBIOTICS:
NUCLEIC ACIDS
AS TARGETS IN
CHEMOTHERAPY

3.1.1. Kanchanomycin

The antibiotic kanchanomycin is of interest, for it combines features of the antibiotics that inactivate the DNA template and those that inactivate the RNA polymerase (Goldberg, 1975b). Kanchanomycin has a broad spectrum of biological activity, being effective as an antimicrobial and an antitumor agent at extremely low concentrations (Liu et al., 1962; Bateman et al., 1965; Fukushima et al., 1973). The structure of kanchanomycin has recently been determined (Gurevich et al., 1972).

Kanchanomycin complexes with polynucleotides in the presence of stoichiometric amounts of divalent cation in a two-step time-dependent reaction (P. A. Friedman et al., 1968a,b). An initial complex forms immediately, and changes with time to a second, more stable complex with different spectral and chemical properties. The antibiotic appears to combine first with Mg^{2+}, and this complex then interacts with DNA or other polynucleotides. Kachanomycin inhibits in vitro RNA and DNA synthesis in two distinctive ways (Joel et al., 1970). While the inhibition of DNA synthesis by kanchanomycin can be overcome by increasing the concentration of DNA (not DNA polymerase), the inhibition of RNA synthesis is overcome by increasing the RNA polymerase concentration. The latter is not reversed by increasing amounts of DNA to which a fixed amount of antibiotic has been previously bound. In a double-reciprocal plot of the kinetics of inhibition, kanchanomycin appears to act as a competitive inhibitor of DNA in DNA synthesis, but as a competitive inhibitor of the RNA polymerase in RNA synthesis. Thus, the inhibition of RNA synthesis by kanchanomycin is not due solely to the binding of the inhibitor to the DNA, but must also involve the inactivation of the RNA polymerase in the complex. It is possible that the enzyme is attracted to sites on the DNA where inhibitor is located, and that excess enzyme can go to sites free of inhibitor. On the other hand, in the case of the DNA polymerase, it is the template function of the DNA that is altered by the antibiotic.

3.2. Tumor Virus Reverse Transcriptase

It has been known for some time that Type C RNA viruses are the causative agents for certain types of tumor in animals (for a review, see Lieber and Todaro, 1975). Recent data have shown that Type-C-virus-related components are also present in certain human cancers (Spiegelman et al., 1973). The reverse transcriptase that is

446

IRVING H.
GOLDBERG,
TERRY A.
BEERMAN,
AND RAYMOND
POON

found in the virions and coded for by the viral gene (Linial and Mason, 1973; Baltimore *et al.*, 1974) is essential for transformation in culture and leukemia development in mice. This potential target for chemotherapy has been the subject of recent reviews (Smith and Gallo, 1974, 1976).

Some derivatives of the antibiotic rifamycin can inhibit the activities of the reverse transcriptase (Gurgo *et al.*, 1971). In an extensive study, Gallo and colleagues screened a number of these derivatives and found good correlation between their effectiveness in the inhibition of reverse transcriptase activity *in vitro* and the inhibition of focus formation and leukemogenesis when the viruses were pretreated with these drugs before infection (Ting *et al.*, 1972; Wu *et al.*, 1973). However, another extensive study (O'Connor *et al.*, 1975) with various rifamycin derivatives failed to show such correlation. With a particular rifamycin derivative (AF/013), other studies have implicated the antitiotic's interaction with cellular enzymes and the plasma membrane (Riva *et al.*, 1972; Scheer, 1975).

It is clear that the rifamycin derivatives are not totally specific for the viral reverse transcriptase, but it is suggested that they have a preference for viral and cellular polymerases (Wu and Gallo, 1974; Thompson *et al.*, 1974). In this regard, the more potent derivatives have been found to bind directly to reverse transcriptase (Wu and Gallo, 1974; Gurgo *et al.*, 1971).

Another class of antibiotics that interact with reverse transcriptase is the streptovaricins, which are structurally similar to the rifamycins (Rhinehart, 1972). The streptovaricins inhibit reverse transcriptase, cellular transformations, and leukemogenesis (Brockman *et al.*, 1971; Carter *et al.*, 1971).

4. Summary and Conclusions

In this discussion, we have focused on the nature of the interaction between antitumor antibiotics and DNA- or nucleic-acid-synthesizing systems. Unfortunately, we do not yet know of antibiotics that have interactions with DNA so specific as to be able to distinguish clearly between sequences in host or tumor DNA. This is not unexpected, since the primary and secondary structures of DNAs have only a limited number of options, and antibiotics, e.g., actinomycin D, usually require for interaction only a very small segment of DNA (as little as one or two base pairs) that is common to varying degrees to all DNAs. Thus, it appears that other factors such as those relating to membrane permeability and drug metabolism may be more important in determining selectivity for tumor over host cells. It should be noted, however, that the accessibility of DNA in chromatin to AMD may be determined to a considerable degree by the state of the proteins associated with it (Ringertz and Bolund, 1969; Pederson and Robbins, 1972). In fact, the physicochemical properties of the chromatin have been postulated as playing a role in the ability of certain cell types to recover RNA synthesis after inhibition by AMD (Benedetto *et al.*, 1972), and might be an important factor in determining the relative sensitivities of different cell types to the drug. This possibility requires further investigation.

The opportunity for drug specificity is considerably greater, however, when the targets are the proteins involved in nucleic acid formation. This is dramatically seen in the case of the antibiotic rifampicin, which is highly specific for the prokaryotic RNA polymerase. The recent report by Springgate and Loeb (1973) that the DNA polymerase of leukemic cells is different, i.e., has mutator properties, from that of nonleukemic cells offers the possibility that agents will be found that interact specifically with the altered enzyme. In the case of the anthracycline antibiotics that intercalate DNA, we have already discussed (Section 2.1.2) evidence that these agents exhibit differential effects on mutant DNA polymerases of bacterial origin. It is of interest that in this case, even though the primary target of the antibiotic is DNA, the ability of the polymerizing or degrading enzymes to function in the presence of the antibiotic will vary with the particular enzyme.

While the search for new antibiotics with higher therapeutic indices continues, efforts to modify chemically available agents to the same end appear promising. It will be of interest to determine whether such modifications have also resulted in changes in the nature of the cellular target. Finally, efforts are being made to modify the physical form in which a cytotoxic antibiotic is delivered to a cancer cell, with the hope that selectivity might be achieved based on unique uptake properties of the cancer and normal cells. Complexes of antibiotic–DNA (Trouet et al., 1972; Ohnuma et al., 1975; Marks and Venditti, 1976) and antibiotic entrapped in lipid bilayers (Gregoriadis, 1973; Rahman et al., 1974) have been used, but the results are too preliminary to determine whether these approaches have any merit, or whether the proposed mechanisms for presumed enhanced selectivity have any basis in fact.

ACKNOWLEDGMENTS

Work done in this laboratory was supported by U.S. Public Health Service Research Grant GM12573 from the National Institute of General Medical Sciences. T. A. Beerman was supported by an Anna Fuller Fund Fellowship, a Sterling Winthrop Fellowship, and an NIH Fellowship. R. Poon was supported by an Anna Fuller Fund Fellowship.

5. References

ARCAMONE, F., BIZIOLI, F., CANEVAZZI, G., AND GREIN, A., 1961, Distamycin and distacin, Chem. Abstr. 55:2012.

ARCAMONE, F., CASSINELLI, G., FANTINI, G., GREIN, A., OREZZI, P., POL, C., AND SPALLA, C., 1969, Adriamycin, 14 hydroxydaunomycin, a new antitumor antibiotic from S. peuncetius var. caesius, Biotechnol. Bioeng. 11:1101.

ASAKURA, H., HORI, M., AND UMEZAWA, H., 1975, Characterization of bleomycin action on DNA, J. Antibiot. 28:537.

BALTIMORE, D., VERMA, I. M., DROST, S., AND MASON, W. S., 1974, Template sensitive DNA polymerase from rous sarcoma virus mutants, Cancer 34:1395.

448

IRVING H.
GOLDBERG,
TERRY A.
BEERMAN,
AND RAYMOND
POON

BARRANCO, S. C., GERNER, E. W., BURK, K. H., AND HUMPHREY, R. M., 1973, Survival and cell kinetics. Effects of adriamycin on mammalian cells, *Cancer Res.* **33**:11.

BATEMAN, J. R., MARSH, A. A., AND STEINFELD, J. L., 1965, Kanchanomycin (NCS-62773): A Phase I study, *Cancer Chemother. Rep.* **44**:25.

BEABEALASHVILLY, R. S., GURSKY, G. V., SAVOTCHKINA, L. P., AND ZASEDATELEV, A. S., 1973, RNA polymerase–DNA complexes. III. Binding of actinomycin D to RNA polymerase–DNA complex, *Biochim. Biophys. Acta* **294**:425.

BECKER, F. F., AND BRENOWITZ, J. B., 1970, The concentration of actinomycin D in hepatocyte nuclei as related to inhibition of ribonucleic acid synthesis, *Biochem. Pharmacol.* **19**:1457.

BEERMAN, T. A., AND GOLDBERG, I. H., 1974, DNA strand scission by the antitumor protein neocarzinostatin, *Biochem. Biophys. Res. Commun.* **59**:1254.

BEERMAN, T. A., AND GOLDBERG, I. H., 1977, The relationship between DNA strand-scission and DNA synthesis inhibition in HeLa cells treated with neocarzinostatin, *Biochim. Biophys. Acta*, in press.

BEERMAN, T. A., GOLDBERG, I. H., AND POON, R., 1974, The interaction of the protein antibiotic neocarzinostatin with DNA, in: *Proceedings of the XIth International Cancer Congress Series No. 353*, Vol. 5, *Surgery, Radiotherapy and Chemotherapy of Cancer*, p. 347, Excerpta Medica, Amsterdam.

BEERMAN, T. A., GOLDBERG, I. H., KAPPEN, L. S., POON, R., AND SUZUKI, H., 1976, Molecular basis of action of cytotoxic antibiotics, in: *Advances in Enzyme Regulation* (G. Weber, ed.), pp. 207–225, Pergamon Press, New York.

BEERMAN, T. A., POON, R., AND GOLDBERG, I. H., 1977, Single-strand nicking of DNA *in vitro* by neocarzinostatin and its possible relationship to the mechanism of drug action, *Biochim. Biophys. Acta*, in press.

BEHR, W., HONIKEL, K., AND HARTMANN, G., 1969, Interaction of the RNA polymerase inhibitor chromomycin with DNA, *Eur. J. Biochem.* **9**:82.

BENEDETTO, A., AND DJACZENKO, W., 1972, 37RC cells rapidly recover their RNA synthesis after inhibition with high doses of actinomycin D, *J. Cell. Biol.* **52**:171.

BENEDETTO, A., DELFINI, C., PULEDDA, S., AND SEBASTIANI, A., 1972, Actinomycin D binding to 37RC and HeLa cell lines, *Biochim. Biophys. Acta* **287**:330.

BHUYAN, B. K., AND DIETZ, A., 1965, Fermentation, taxonomic and biological studies of nogalamycin, *Antimicrob. Agents Chemother.*, p. 836.

BHUYAN, B., AND SMITH, C. G., 1965, Differential interaction of nogalamycin with DNA of varying base composition, *Proc. Natl. Acad. Sci. U.S.A.* **54**:566.

BIEDLER, J. L., AND RIEHM, H., 1970, Cellular resistance to actinomycin D in Chinese hamster cells *in vitro*: Cross-resistance, radioautographic, and cytogeneic studies, *Cancer Res.* **30**:1174.

BITTMAN, R., AND BLAU, L., 1975, Stopped-flow kinetic studies of actinomycin binding to DNAs, *Biochemistry* **14**:2138.

BRAZHNIKOVA, M. G., ZBARSKY, V. B., PONOMARENKO, V. I., AND POTAPOVA, N. P., 1974, Physical and chemical characteristics and structure of carminomycin, a new antitumor antibiotic, *J. Antibiot.* **27**:254.

BROCKMAN, W. W., CARTER, W. A., LI, H. L., REUSSER, F., AND NICHOL, F. R., 1971, Streptovaricins inhibit RNA-dependent DNA polymerase present in an oncogenic RNA virus, *Nature (London)* **230**:249.

BURKI, H. J., 1976, Critical DNA damage and mammalian cell reproduction, *J. Mol. Biol.* **103**:599.

CALENDI, E., DiMARCO, A., REGGIANI, M., SCARPINATO, B. M., AND VALENTINI, L., 1965, On physico-chemical interactions between daunomycin and nucleic acids, *Biochim. Biophys. Acta* **103**:25.

CALENDI, E., DETTORI, R., AND NERI, M. G., 1966, Filamentous sex-specific bacteriophages of *E. coli* K12. IV. Studies on physico-chemical characteristics of bacteriophage Ec9, *Giorn. Microbiol.* **14**:227.

CANCER CHEMOTHERAPY REPORTS, 1975, Fifth new drug seminar on adriamycin, **6**(October):83.

CANELLAKIS, E. S., SHAW, Y. H., HANNERS, W. E., AND SCHWARTZ, R. A., 1976, Diacridines: Bifunctional intercalators I. Chemistry, physical chemistry and growth inhibitory properties, *Biochim. Biophys. Acta* **418**:277.

CARTER, W. A., BROCKMAN, W. W., AND BORDEN, E. C., 1971, Streptovaricins inhibit focus formation by MSV (MLV) complex, *Nature (London) New Biol.* **232**:212.

CERAMI, A., REICH, E., WARD, D. C., AND GOLDBERG, I. H., 1967, The interaction of actinomycin with DNA. Requirement for the 2-amino group of purines, *Proc. Natl. Acad. Sci. U.S.A.* **57**:1036.

CHANDRA, P., ZIMMER, C., AND THRUM, H., 1970, Effect of distamycin A on the structure and template activity of DNA in RNA polymerase system, *FEBS Lett.* **7**:90.

CHANDRA, P., GETZ, A., WACKER, A., VERNI, M. A., CASAZZA, A. M., FIORETTI, A., ARCAMONE, F., AND GHIONE, M., 1971, Some structural requirements for the antibiotic action of distamycin, *FEBS Lett.* **16**:249.

CHIMURA, H., ISHIZUKA, M., HAMADA, M., HORI, S., KIMURA, K., IWANAGA, J., TAKEUCHI, T., AND UMEZAWA, H., 1968, A new antibiotic, macromomycin, exhibiting antitumor and antimicrobial activity, *J. Antibiot.* **21**:44.

CHORIN, V. A., AND ROSSOLIMO, O. K., 1965, An experimental study of the antitumor effect of six antibiotics belonging to the olivomycin group, *Antibiotici* **10**:48.

COCHET-MEILHAC, M., AND CHAMBON, P., 1974, Animal DNA-dependent RNA polymerases. II. Mechanism of the inhibition of RNA polymerase B by amatoxins, *Biochim. Biophys. Acata* **353**:160.

COHEN, M. M., AND SHAW, M. W., 1964, Effects of mitomycin C on human chromosomes, *J. Cell Biol.* **23**:386.

COX, R., DAOUD, A. H., AND IRVING, C. C., 1974, Damage of rat liver deoxyribonucleic acid by bleomycin, *Biochem. Pharmacol.* **23**:3147.

CREMISI, C., SONENSHEIN, G., AND TOURNIER, P., 1974, Studies on the mechanism of actinomycin D resistance of an SV40-transformed hamster cell line, *Exp. Cell Res.* **89**:89.

DAS, G. C., DASGUPTA, S., AND DAS GUPTA, N. N., 1974, Interaction of nogalamycin with DNA, *Biochim. Biophys. Acta* **353**:274.

DELL, A., WILLIAMS, D. H., MORRIS, H. R., SMITH, G. A., FEENEY, J., AND ROBERTS, G. C. K., 1975, Structure revision of the antibiotic echinomycin, *J. Amer. Chem. Soc.* **97**:2497.

DICIOCCIO, R., AND SAHAI SRIVASTAVA. B. I., 1976, Effect of bleomycin on deoxynucleotide-polymerizing enzymes from human cells, *Cancer Res.* **36**:1664.

DIMARCO, A., 1975, Adriamycin (NCS-123127). Mode and mechanism of action, *Cancer Chemother. Rep.* **6**:91.

DIMARCO, A., GAETANI, M., OREZZI, P., SCOTTI, T., AND ARCAMONE, F., 1962, Experimental studies on distamycin A—a new antibiotic with cytotoxic activity, *Cancer Chemother. Rep.* **18**:15.

DIMARCO, A., SOLDATI, M., FIORETTI, A., AND DASDINA, T., 1963, Ricerche sulla attivita della daunomicina su cellule normali e neoplastiche coltivate *in vitro*, *Tumori* **49**:4.

DIMARCO, A., GAETANI, M., DORIGOTTI, L., SOLDATI, M., AND BELLINI, O., 1964, Daunomycin: A new antibiotic with antitumor activity, *Cancer Chemother. Rep.* **38**:31.

DIMARCO, A., GAETANI, M., AND SCARPINATO, B. M., 1969, Adriamycin (NCS-123,127): A new antibiotic with antitumor activity, *Cancer Chemother. Rep.* **53**:33.

DIMARCO, A., ZUNINO, F., SILVESTRINI, R., GAMBARUCCI, C., AND GAMBETTA, R. A., 1971, Interaction of some daunomycin derivatives with DNA and their biological activity, *Biochem. Pharmacol.* **20**:1323.

DIMARCO, A., ARCAMONE, F., AND ZUNINO, F., 1975, Daunomycin (daunorubicin) and adriamycin and structural analogues: Biological activity and mechanism of action, in: *Antibiotics*, Vol. III, pp. 101–128, Springer-Verlag, Berlin.

DJORDJEVIC, B., AND KIM, J. H., 1968, Different lethal effects of mitomycin C and actinomycin D during the division cycle of HeLa cells, *J. Cell Biol.* **38**:477.

ELLEM, K. A. O., AND RHODE, S. L., 1970, Selective inhibition of ribosomal RNA synthesis in HeLa cells by nogalamycin, a dA:dT binding antibiotic, *Biochim. Biophys. Acta* **209**:415.

FALASCHI, F., AND KORNBERG, A., 1964, Phleomycin, an inhibitor of DNA polymerase, *Fed. Proc. Fed. Amer. Soc. Exp. Biol.* **23**:940.

FARRELL, L., AND REITER, H., 1973, Phleomycin-stimulated degradation of deoxyribonucleic acid in *Escherichia coli*, *Antimicrob. Agents Chemother.* **4**:320.

FRIEDMAN, P. A., JOEL, P. B., AND GOLDBERG, I. H., 1969*a*, Interaction of kanchanomycin with nucleic acids. I. Physical properties of the complex, *Biochemistry* **8**:1535.

FRIEDMAN, P. A., LI, T.-K., AND GOLDBERG, I. H., 1969*b*, Interaction of kanchanomycin with nucleic acids. II. Optical rotatory dispersion and circular dichroism, *Biochemistry* **8**:1545.

FRIEDMAN, R. M., STERN, R., AND ROSE, J. A., 1974, Phleomycin stimulation of thymidine triphosphate incorporation by animal cell nuclei, *J. Natl. Cancer Inst.* **52**:693.

FUKUSHIMA, K., ISHIWATA, K., KURODA, S., AND ARAI, T., 1973, Identity of antibiotic P-42-1 elaborated by *Actinomyces tumemacerans* with kanchanomycin and albofungin, *J. Antibiot.* **26**:65.

GALE, E. F., CUNDLIFFE, E., REYNOLDS, P. E., RICHMOND, M. H., AND WARING, M. J., 1972, *The Molecular Basis of Antibiotic Action*, p. 193, John Wiley and Sons, New York.

GAUSE, G. F., 1975*a*, Chromomycin, olivomycin, mithramycin, in: *Handbook of Experimental Pharmacology*, Vol. XXXVIII/2 (A. C. Sartorelli and D. G. Johns, eds.), pp. 615–622, Springer-Verlag, Berlin.

450

IRVING H.
GOLDBERG,
TERRY A.
BEERMAN,
AND RAYMOND
POON

GAUSE, G. F., 1975*b*, Olivomycin, chromomycin and mithramycin, in: *Antibiotics III. Mechanism of Action of Antimicrobial and Antitumor Agents* (J. W. Corcoran and F. E. Hahn, eds.), pp. 197–202, Springer-Verlag, Berlin.

GAUSE, G. F., UKHOLINA, R. S., AND SVESHNIKOVA, M. A., 1962, Olivomycin—a new antibiotic produced by *Actinomyces olivoreticuli, Antibiotiki (Moscow)* 7:34.

GAUSE, G. F., BRAZHNIKOVA, M. G., AND SHORIN, V. A., 1974, A new antitumor antibiotic, carminomycin (NSC-180024), *Cancer Chemother. Rep.* 58:255.

GLAUBIGER, D., KOHN, K. W., AND CHARNEY, E., 1974, The reaction of anthramycin with DNA. III. Properties of the complex, *Biochim. Biophys. Acta* 361:303.

GOLDBERG, I. H., 1975*a*, Actinomycin D, in: *Handbook of Experimental Pharmacology* (A. C. Sartorelli and D. G. Johns, eds.), Vol. XXXVIII/2, pp. 582–592, Springer-Verlag, Berlin.

GOLDBERG, I. H., 1975*b*, Kanchanomycin, in: *Antibiotics III. Mechanism of Action of Antimicrobial and Antitumor Agents* (J. W. Corcoran and F. E. Hahn, eds.), pp. 166–173, Springer-Verlag, New York.

GOLDBERG, I. H., AND FRIEDMAN, P. A., 1971, Antibiotics and nucleic acids, *Annu. Rev. Biochem.* 40:775.

GOLDBERG, I. H., RABINOWITZ, M., AND REICH, E., 1962, Basis of actinomycin action. I. DNA binding and inhibition of RNA-polymerase synthetic reactions by actinomycin, *Proc. Natl. Acad. Sci. U.S.A.* 48:2094.

GOLDBERG, I. H., KAPPEN, L. S., AND SUZUKI, H., 1975, Interaction of carcinostatic antibiotics with macromolecules, in: *Pharmacological Basis of Cancer Chemotherapy*, p. 531, Williams and Wilkins Co., Baltimore.

GOLDSTEIN, M. N., HAMM, K., AND AMROD, E., 1966, Incorporation of tritiated actinomycin into drug-sensitive and drug-resistant HeLa cells, *Science* 151:1555.

GOODMAN, M. F., BESSMAN, M. J., AND BACHUR, N. R., 1974, Adriamycin and daunomycin inhibition of mutant T4 DNA polymerases, *Proc. Natl. Acad. Sci. U.S.A.* 71:1193.

GREGORIADIS, G., 1973, Drug entrapment in liposomes, *FEBS Lett.* 36:292.

GUREVICH, A. I., KARAPETYAN, M. G., KOLOSOV, M. N., OMELCHENKO, V. N., ONOPRIENKO, V. V., PETRENKO, G. I., AND POPRAVKO, 1972, The structure of albofungin, *Tetrahedron Lett.* 18:1751.

GURGO, C., RAY, R. K., THIRY, L., AND GREEN, M., 1971, Inhibitors of the RNA and DNA dependent polymerase activities of RNA tumor viruses, *Nature (London) New Biol.* 229:111.

HAHN, F. E., 1975, Distamycin A and netropsin, in: *Antibiotics III. Mechanism of Action of Antimicrobial and Antitumor Agents* (J. W. Corcoran and F. E. Hahn, eds.), p. 79, Springer-Verlag, New York.

HAIDLE, C. W., 1971, Fragmentation of deoxyribonucleic acid by bleomycin, *Mol. Pharmacol.* 7:645.

HAIDLE, C. W., KUO, M. T., AND WEISS, K. K., 1972, Nucleic acid-specificity of bleomycin, *Biochem. Pharmacol.* 21:3308.

HATA, T., SANO, Y., SUGAWARA, R., MATSUMA, A., KANAMORI, K., SHIMA, T., AND HOSHI, T., 1956, Mitomycin, a new antibiotic from *Streptomyces, J. Antibiotics* 9:141.

HEINEMANN, B., AND HOWARD, A. J., 1964, Induction of lambda-bacteriophage in *Escherichia coli* as a screening test for potential antitumor agents, *Appl. Microbiol.* 12:234.

HIRAKI, K., KAMIMURA, O., TAKAHASHI, I., NAGAO, T., KITAJIMA, K., AND IRINO, S., 1974, Neocarzinostatin: Une approche nouvelle dans la chimiothérapie des leucémies aigues, *Rev. Fr. d'Hemat.* 13:29.

HITTELMAN, W. N., AND RAO, P. N., 1975, The nature of adriamycin-induced cytotoxicity in Chinese hamster cells as revealed by premature chromosome condesation, *Cancer Res.* 35:3027.

HOLLSTEIN, U., 1974, Actinomycin. Chemistry and mechanism of action, *Chem. Rev.* 74:625.

HOMMA, M., KOIDA, T., SAITO-KOIDE, T., KAMO, I., SETO, M., KUMAGAI, K., AND ISHIDA, N., 1970, Specific inhibition of the initiation of DNA synthesis in HeLa cells by neocarzinostatin, *Prog. Antimicrob. Anticancer Chemother. Proc. VI Internat. Congr. Chemother.* 2:410.

HONIKEL, K. O., AND SANTO, R. E., 1972, A model for the *in vitro* inhibition of the DNA polymerase reaction with the base specific antibiotics chromomycin-A$_3$, actinomycin-C$_3$ and daunomycin, *Biochim. Biophys. Acta* 269:354.

HOROWITZ, S. B., 1975, Anthramycin, in: *Handbook of Experimental Pharmocology*, Vol. XXXVIII/2 (A. C. Sartorelli and D. G. Johns, eds.), pp. 642–648, Springer-Verlag, Berlin.

HOROWITZ, S. B., AND GROLLMAN, A. P., 1968, Interactions of small molecules with nucleic acids. I. Mode of action of anthramycin, *Antimicrob. Agents Chemother.* 21.

ISHIDA, N., MIYAZAKI, K., KUMAGAI, K., AND RIKIMARU, M., 1965, Neocarzinostatin, an antitumor antibiotic of high molecular weight, *J. Antibiot.* 18:29.

ISHIDA, R., AND TAKAHASHI, T., 1976, *In vitro* release of thymine from DNA by neocarzinostatin, *Biochim. Biophys. Res. Commun.* 68:256.

ISHIZUKA, M., TAKAYAMA, H., TAKEUCHI, T., AND UMEZAWA, H., 1967, Activity and toxicity of bleomycin, *J. Antibiot.* **20**:15.

ISRAEL, M., MODEST, E. S., AND FREI, E., III, 1975, *N*-Trifluoroacetyladriamycin-14-valerate, an analog with greater experimental antitumor activity and less toxicity than adriamycin, *Cancer Res.* **35**:1365.

IYER, V. N., AND SZYBALASKI, W., 1963, A molecular mechanism of mitomycin action: Linking of complementary DNA strands, *Proc. Natl. Acad. Sci. U.S.A.* **50**:355.

IYER, V. N., AND SZYBALSKI, W., 1964, Mitomycin and porfiromycin: Chemical mechanism of activation and cross-linking of DNA, *Science* **145**:55.

JOEL, P. B., FRIEDMAN, P. A., AND GOLDBERG, I. H., 1970, Interaction of kanchanomycin with nucleic acids. III. Contrasts in the mechanisms of inhibition of ribonucleic acid and deoxyribonucleic acid polymerase reactions, *Biochemistry* **9**:4421.

KAPPEN, L. S., AND GOLDBERG, I. H., 1977, Effect of neocarzinostatin-induced strand-scission on the template activity of DNA for DNA polymerase I, *Biochemistry*, in press.

KATAGIRI, K., YOSHIDA, T., AND SATO, K., 1975, Quinoxaline antibiotics, in: *Antibiotics III. Mechanism of Action of Antimicrobial and Antitumor Agents* (J. W. Corcoran and F. E. Hahn, eds.), pp. 234–251, Springer-Verlag, New York.

KERSTEN. W., KERSTEN, H., AND SZYBALSKI, W., 1966, Physico-chemical properties of complexes between DNA and antibiotics which affect RNA synthesis, *Biochemistry* **5**:236.

KESSEL, D., AND BOSMANN, H. B., 1970, On the characteristics of actinomycin D resistance in L5178Y cells, *Cancer Res.* **30**:2695.

KESSEL, D., AND WODINSKY, I., 1968, Uptake *in vivo* and *in vitro* of actinomycin D by mouse leukemias as factors in survival. *Biochem. Pharmacol.* **17**:161.

KOHN, K. W., 1975, Anthramycin, in: *Antibiotics III. Mechanism of Action of Antimicrobial and Antitumor Agents* (J. W. Corcoran and F. E. Hahn, eds.), pp. 3–11, Springer-Verlag, New York.

KOHN, K. W., AND SPEARS, C. L., 1970, Reaction of anthramycin with DNA, *J. Mol. Biol.* **51**:551.

KOHN, K. W., BONO, V. H., AND KANN, H. E., JR., 1968, Anthramycin, a new type of DNA-inhibiting antibiotic: Reaction with DNA and effect on nucleic acid synthesis in mouse leukemia cells, *Biochim. Biophys. Acta* **155**:121.

KOHN, K. W., GLAUBIGER, D., AND SPEARS, C. L., 1974, The reaction of anthramycin with DNA. II. Studies of kinetics and mechanism, *Biochim. Biophys. Acta* **361**:288.

KREY, A. K., AND HAHN, F. E., 1970, Studies on the complex of distamycin A with calf thymus DNA, *FEBS Lett.* **10**:175.

KREY, A. K., ALLISON, R. G., AND HAHN, F.E., 1973, Interactions of the antibiotic, distamycin A, with native DNA and with synthetic duplex polydeoxyribonucleotides, *FEBS Lett.* **29**:58.

KREY, A. K., OLENICK, J. G., AND HAHN, F. E., 1976, Interactions of the antibiotic distamycin A with monopolymeric single-stranded polydeoxyribonucleotides with ØX174 DNA, *Mol. Pharmacol.* **12**:185.

KRISHAN, A., ISRAEL, M., MODEST, E. J., AND FREI, E., III., 1976, Difference in cellular uptake and cytofluorescence of adriamycin and *N*-trifluoroacetyladriamycin-14-valerate, *Cancer Res.* **36**:2114.

KRUGH, T. R., 1972, Association of actinomycin D and deoxyribonucleotides as a model for binding of the drug to DNA, *Proc. Natl. Acad. Sci. U.S.A.* **69**:1911.

KRUGH, T. R., AND CHEN, Y.-C., 1975, Actinomycin D–deoxynucleotide complexes as models for the actinomycin D–DNA complex. The use of nuclear magnetic resonance to determine the stoichiometry and the geometry of the complexes, *Biochemistry* **14**:4912.

KRUGH, T. R., AND NEELY, J. W., 1973*a*, Actinomycin D–mononucleotide interactions as studied by proton magnetic resonance, *Biochemistry* **12**:1775.

KRUGH, T. R., AND NEELY, J. W., 1973*b*,·Actinomycin D–deoxydinucleotide interactions as a model for binding of the drug to deoxyribonucleic acid. Proton magnetic resonance results, *Biochemistry* **12**:4418.

KUNIMOTO, T., HORI, M., AND UMEZAWA, H., 1972, Macromomycin, an inhibitor of the membrane function of tumor cells, *Cancer Res.* **32**:1251.

KUO, M. T., AND HAIDLE, C. W., 1973, Characterization of chain breakage in DNA induced by bleomycin, *Biochim. Biophys. Acta* **335**:109.

LAZARUS, H., RASO, V., AND SAMY, T. S. A., 1976, Neocarzinostatin—a protein antibiotic with unusual properties, *Proc. Amer. Assoc. Cancer Res.*, 107.

LETALAER, J. Y., AND JEANTEUR, P. H., 1971, Preferential binding of *E. coli* RNA polymerase to A-T rich sequence of bacteriophage lambda DNA, *FEBS Lett.* **12**:253.

452

IRVING H.
GOLDBERG,
TERRY A.
BEERMAN,
AND RAYMOND
POON

LIEBER, M. M., AND TODARO, G. C., 1975, Mammalian type C RNA viruses, in: *Cancer—A Comprehensive Treatise*, Vol. 2, *Viral Carcinogenesis* (F. F. Becker, ed.), p. 91, Plenum Press, New York.

LINIAL, M., AND MASON, W. S., 1973, Characterization of two conditional early mutants of Rous sarcoma virus, *Virology* **53**:258.

LIPPMAN, M. M., AND ABOTT, B. J., 1973, Modification of transplantability and tumor growth following treatment of L1210 leukemia and TA3Ha cells with macromomycin (NSC-170105), *Cancer Chemother. Rep.* **57**:501.

LIPPMAN, M. M., LASTER, W. R., ABOTT, B. J., VENDITTI, J., AND BARATTA, M., 1975, Antitumor activity of macromomycin B (NSC-170105) against murine leukemias, melanoma, and lung carcinoma, *Cancer Res.* **35**:939.

LIU, W.-C., CULLEN, W. P., AND RAO, K. V., 1962, BA-180265: A new cytotoxic antibiotic, *Antimicrob. Agents Chemother.*, p. 767.

MAEDA, K., KOSAKA, H., YAGASHITA, K., AND UMEZAWA, H., 1956, A new antibiotic, phleomycin, *J. Antibiot.* **9**:82.

MARKS, T. A., AND VENDITTI, J. M., 1976, Potentiation of actinomycin D or adriamycin antitumor activity with DNA, *Cancer Res.* **36**:496.

MEIENHOFER, J., AND ATHERTON, E., 1973, Structure–activity relationships in the actinomycins, *Adv. Appl. Microbiol.* **16**:203.

MEIENHOFER, J., MAEDA, H., GLASER, C. B., CZOMBOS, J., AND KUROMIZ, K., 1972, Primary structure of neocarzinostatin, an antitumor antibiotic, *Science* **178**:875.

MIYAKI, M., ONO, T., AND UMEZAWA, H., 1971, Inhibition of ligase reaction by bleomycin, *J. Antibiot.* **24**:587.

MIYAKI, M., KITAYAMA, T., AND ONO, T., 1974, Breakage of DNA–membrane complex by bleomycin, *J. Antibiot.* **27**:647.

MIYAKI, M., ONO, T., HORI, S., AND UMEZAWA, H., 1975, Binding of bleomycin to DNA in bleomycin-sensitive and resistant rat ascites hepatoma cells, *Cancer Res.* **35**:2015.

MIZUNO, N. S., ZAKIS, B., AND DECKER, R. W., 1975, Binding of daunomycin to DNA and the inhibition of RNA and DNA synthesis, *Cancer Res.* **35**:1542.

MOORE, G. E., 1968, Effects of mitomycin C in 346 patients with advanced cancer, *Cancer Chemother. Rep.* **52**:672.

MÜLLER, W., AND CROTHERS, D. M., 1968, Studies on the binding of actinomycin and related compounds, *J. Mol. Biol.* **35**:251.

MÜLLER, W. E. G., YAMAZAKI, Z., BRETER, H. J., AND ZAHN, R. K., 1972, Action of bleomycin on DNA and RNA, *Eur. J. Biochem.* **31**:518.

MÜLLER, W. E. G., TOTSUKA, A., NUSSER, I., ZAHN, R. K., AND UMEZAWA, H., 1975, Bleomycin inhibition of DNA synthesis in isolated enzyme systems and in intact cell systems, *Biochem. Pharmacol* **24**:911.

MURPHREE, S. A., CUNNINGHAM, L. S., HWANG, K. M., AND SARTORELLI, A., 1976, Effects of adriamycin on surface properties of sarcoma 180 ascites cells, *Biochem. Pharmacol.* **25**:1227.

NAGAI, K., YAMAKI, H., SUZUKI, H., TANKA, N., AND UMEZAWA, H., 1969, The combined effects of bleomycin and sulfhydryl compounds on the thermal denaturation of DNA, *Biochim. Biophys. Acta* **179**:165.

NAKAMURA, H., AND ONO, K., 1974, Neocarzinostatin-sepharose in preventing the cell growth of leukemia cells, *Proc. Jpn. Cancer Assoc.*, 33rd Annual Meeting, p. 112.

NAYAK, R., SIRSI, M., AND PODDER, S. K., 1975, Mode of action of antitumor antibiotics. Spectrophotometric studies on the interaction of chromomycin A3 with DNA and chromatin of normal and neoplastic tissue, *Biochim. Biophys. Acta* **38**:195.

O'CONNOR, T. E., SCHIOP-STANSLY, P., SETHI, V. S., HADIDI, A., AND OKANO, P., 1975, Antibiotic control of infection of human or mouse cells with oncorna virus, in: *Pharmacological Basis of Cancer Chemotherapy*, p. 319, Williams and Wilkins, Baltimore.

OHARA, H., AND TERASIMA, T., 1972, Lethal effect of mitomycin-C on cultured mammalian cells, *Gann* **63**:317.

OHNUMA, T., HOLLAND, J. F., AND CHEN, J. H., 1975, Pharmacological and therapeutic efficacy of daunomycin–DNA complex in mice, *Cancer Res.* **35**:1767.

OHTSUKI, K., AND ISHIDA, N., 1975, Mechanism of DNA degradation induced by neocarzinostatin in *Bacillus subtilis*, *J. Antibiot.* **28**:229.

ONO, Y., WATANABE, Y., AND ISHIDA, N., 1966, Mode of action of neocarzinostatin: Inhibition of DNA synthesis and degradation of DNA in *Saccina lutea*, *Biochim. Biophys. Acta* **119**:70.

PATEL, D. J., 1974, Peptide antibiotic–oligonucleotide interactions. Nuclear magnetic resonance investigations of complex formation between actinomycin D and d-ApTpGpCpApT in aqueous solution, *Biochemistry* **13**:2396.

PATER, M. M., AND MAK, S., 1974, Actinomycin D-induced breakage of human KB cell DNA, *Nature (London)* **250**:786.

PEDERSON, T., AND ROBBINS, E., 1972, Chromatin structure and the cell division cycle. Actinomycin binding in synchronized HeLa cells, *J. Cell Biol.* **55**:322.

PETTIT, G. R., EINCH, J. J., HERALD, C. L., ODE, R. H., VONDREDE, R. B., BROWN, P., BRAZHNIKOVA, M. G., AND GAUSE, G. F., 1975, The structure of carminomycin I, *J. Amer. Chem. Soc.* **97**:7387.

PIETSCH, P., AND GARRETT, H., 1968, Primary site of reaction in the *in vitro* complex of phleomycin and DNA, *Nature (London)* **219**:488.

PIGRAM, W. J., FULLER, W., AND HAMILTON, L. D., 1972, Stereochemistry of intercalation: Interaction of daunomycin with DNA, *Nature (London) New Biol.* **235**:17.

POLET, H., 1975, Role of the cell membrane in the uptake of ^{3}H-actinomycin D by mammalian cells *in vitro, J. Pharmacol. Exo. Ther.* **192**:270.

POON, R., BEERMAN, T. A., AND GOLDBERG, I. H., 1977, Characterization of the DNA strand-breakage *in vitro* by the antitumor protein neocarzinostatin, *Biochemistry*, in press.

PRICE, K. E., BUCK, R. E., AND LEIN, J., 1964, System for detecting inducers of lysogenic *Escherichia coli* W1709 (λ) and its applicability as a screen for antineoplastic antibiotics, *Appl. Microbiol.* **12**:428.

PUSCHENDORF, B., AND GRUNICKE, H., 1969, Effect of distamycin A on the template activity of DNA in a DNA polymerase system, *FEBS Lett.* **4**:355.

PUSCHENDORF, B., BECKER, H., BOHLANDT, D., AND GRUNICKE, H., 1974, Effects of distamycin A on T4 DNA-directed RNA synthesis, *Eur. J. Biochem.* **49**:531.

RAHMAN, Y.-E., CERNY, E. A., TOLLAKSEN, S. L., WRIGHT, B. J., NANCE, S. L., AND THOMSON, J. F., 1974, Liposome-encapsulated actinomycin D: Potential in cancer chemotherapy, *Proc. Soc. Exp. Biol. Med.* **146**:1173.

RAO, K. V., CULLEN, W. P., AND SOGIN, B. A., 1962, A new antibiotic with antitumor properties, *Antibiot. Chemother.* **12**:182.

REITER, H., MILEWSKIY, M., AND KELLEY, P., 1972, Mode of action of phleomycin on *Bacillus subtilis, J. Bacteriol.* **111**:586.

REUSSER, F., AND BHUYAN, B. K., 1967, Comparative studies with three antibiotics binding to deoxyribonucleic acid, *J. Bacteriol.* **94**:576.

RIEHM, H., AND BIEDLER, J. L., 1972, Potentiation of drug effect by Tween 80 in Chinese hamster cells resistant to actinomycin D and daunomycin, *Cancer Res.* **32**:1195.

RINEHART, K. L., JR., 1972, Antibiotics with ANSA rings, *Acc. Chem. Res.* **5**:57.

RINGERTZ, N. R., AND BOLUND, L., 1969, Actinomycin binding capacity of deoxyribonucleoprotein, *Biochim. Biophys. Acta* **174**:147.

RIVA, S., FIETTA, A., AND SILVESTRI, L. G., 1972, Mechanism of action of a rifamycin derivative (AF/013) which is active on the nucleic acid polymerases insensitive to rifampicin, *Biochem. Biophys. Res. Commun.* **49**:1263.

ROSS, S. L., AND MOSES, R. E., 1976, Effect of bleomycin on deoxyribonucleic acid synthesis in toluene-treated *Escherichia coli* cells, *Antimicrob. Agents Chemother.* **9**:239.

RUSCONI, A., AND DIMARCO, A., 1969, Inhibition of nucleic acid synthesis by daunomycin and its relationship to the uptake of the drug in HeLa cells, *Cancer Res.* **29**:1509.

SAMY, T. S. A., ATREYI, M., MAEDA, H., AND MEIENHOFER, J., 1974, Selective tryptophan oxidation in the antitumor protein neocarzinostatin and effects on conformation and biological activity, *Biochemistry* **15**:1007.

SARTIANO, G. P., WINKELSTEIN, A., LYNCH, W., AND BOGGS, S. S., 1973, Effects of bleomycin on PHA-stimulated lymphocytes and isolated hepatic nuclei, *J. Antibiot.* **26**:437.

SAWADA, H., TATSUMI, K., SASADA, M., SHIRAKAWA, S., NOKAMURA, T., AND WAKISAKA, G., 1974, Effect of neocarzinostatin on DNA synthesis in L1210 cells, *Cancer Res.* **34**:3341.

SAWICKI, S. G., AND GODMAN, G. C., 1972, On the recovery of transcription after inhibition by actinomycin D, *J. Cell Biol.* **55**:299.

SCHARA, R., AND MÜLLER, W., 1972, Über die Wechselwirkung des Actinomycin C₃ mit Mono-, Di- und Oligonucleotiden, *Eur. J. Biochem.* **29**:210.

SCHEER, U., 1975, The rifamycin derivative AF/013 is cytolytic, *Mol. Pharmacol.* **11**:883.

SCHWARTZ, H. S., AND KANTER, P. M., 1975, Cell interactions: Determinants of selective toxicity of adriamycin (NSC-123127) and daunorubicin (NSC-82151), *Cancer Chemother. Rep.* **6**:107.

454

IRVING H.
GOLDBERG,
TERRY A.
BEERMAN,
AND RAYMOND
POON

SEDOV, K. A., SOROKINA, I. B., BERLIN, Y. A., AND KOLOSOV, M. N., 1969, Olivomycin and related antibiotics. XXIII. Effect of olivomycins, chromomycins and mithramycins on leucosis LA of mice, *Antibiotiki* **14:**721.

SENTENAC, A., SIMON, E. J., AND FROMAGEOT, P., 1968, Initiation of chains by RNA polymerase and the effects of inhibitors studied by a direct filtration technique, *Biochim. Biophys. Acta* **161:**299.

SHIRAKAWA, I., AZEGAMI, M., ISHII, S., AND UMEZAWA, H., 1971, Reaction of bleomycin with DNA. Strand scission of DNA in the absence of sulfhydryl or peroxide compounds, *J. Antibiot.* **24:**761.

SIMARD, R., 1967, The binding of actinomycin D-³H to heterochromatin as studied by quantitative high resolution radioautography, *J. Cell. Biol.* **35:**716.

SIMARD, R., AND CASSINGENA, R., 1969, Actinomycin resistance in cultured hamster cells. Cancer cells, *Cancer Res.* **29:**1590.

SLAVIK, N., AND CARTER, S. K., 1975, Chromomycin A₃, mithramycin, and olivomycin: Antitumor antibiotics of related structure, in: *Advances in Pharmacology and Chemotherapy*, Vol. 12 (S. Garattin, A. Goldin, F. Hawkins, and I. J. Kopin, eds.), p. 1, Academic Press, New York.

SMITH, R. G., AND GALLO, R. G., 1974, Agents which inhibit reverse transcriptase, *Life Sci.* **15:**1711.

SMITH, R. G., AND GALLO, R. C., 1976, Prospects for biologic and pharmacologic inhibition of RNA tumor viruses, *Biochem. Pharmacol.* **25:**491.

SOBELL, H. M., 1973, The stereochemistry of actinomycin binding to DNA and its implications in molecular biology, *Prog. Nucleic Acid Res.* **13:**153.

SPIEGELMAN, S., AXEL, R., BAXT, W., GULATI, S., HEHLMAN, R., KUFE, D., AND SCHLOM, J., 1973, The relevance of RNA tumor viruses to human cancers, in: *Sixth Miles International Symposium on Molecular Biology* (R. F. Beers, ed.), p. 282, Johns Hopkins University Press, Baltimore.

SPRINGGATE, C. F., AND LOEB, L. A., 1973, Mutagenic DNA polymerase in human leukemic cells, *Proc. Natl. Acad. Sci. U.S.A.* **70:**245.

STERN, R., AND FRIEDMAN, R. M., 1971, Ribonucleic acid synthesis in animal cells in the presence of actinomycin, *Biochemistry* **10:**3635.

STERN, R., TWANMOH, A., AND COOPER, H. L., 1973, Site of actinomycin-resistant RNA synthesis in animal cells, *Exp. Cell Res.* **78:**136.

STERN, R., ROSE, J. A., AND FRIEDMAN, R. M., 1974, Phleomycin-induced cleavage of deoxyribonucleic acid, *Biochemistry* **13:**307.

SUZUKI, H., NAGAI, K., YAMAKI, H., TANAKA, N., AND UMEZAWA, H., 1968, Mechanism of action of bleomycin. Studies with the growing culture of bacterial and tumor cells, *J. Antibiot.* **21:**379.

SUZUKI, H., NAGAI, K., YAMAKI, H., TANAKA, N., AND UMEZAWA, H., 1969, On the mechanism of action of bleomycin: Scission of DNA strands *in vitro* and *in vivo*, *J. Antibiot.* **232:**446.

SZYBALSKI, W., 1958, Special microbiological systems. II. Observation on chemical mutagenesis in microorganisms, *Ann. N. Y. Acad. Sci.* **76:**475.

SZYBALSKI, W., AND IYER, V. N., 1964, Cross-linking of DNA by enzymatically or chemically activated mitomycins and porfiromycin, *Fed. Proc. Fed. Amer. Soc. Exp. Biol.* **23:**946.

TAKESHITA, M., HORWITZ, S. B., AND GROLLMAN, A. P., 1974, Bleomycin, an inhibitor of vaccinia virus replication, *Virology* **60:**455.

TAKITA, T., MURAOKA, Y., YOSHIOKA, T., FUJI, A., MAEDA, H., AND UMEZAWA, H., 1972, The chemistry of bleomycin. IX. The structures of bleomycin and phleomycin, *J. Antibiot.* **25:**755.

TANAKA, N., YAMAGUCHI, Y., AND UMEZAWA, H., 1963, Mechanism of action of phleomycin. I. Selective inhibition of DNA synthesis in *E. coli* and in HeLa cells, *J. Antibiot.* **16:**86.

TATSUMI, K., NAKAMURA, T., AND WAKISAKA, G., 1974, Damage of mammalian cell DNA *in vivo* and *in vitro* induced by neocarzinostatin, *Gann* **65:**459.

TATSUMI, K., SAKANE, T., SAWADA, M., SHIRAKAWA, S., NAKAMURA, T., AND WAKISAKA, G., 1975, Unscheduled DNA synthesis in human lymphocytes treated with neocarzinostatin, *Gann* **66:**441.

TATSUOKA, S., NAKAZAWA, K., MIYAKE, A., KAZIWARA, K., AARAMAKI, Y., SHIBATA, M., TANAKE, K., HAMADA, Y., HITOMI, H., MIYAMOTO, M., MIZUNO, K., WATANABE, J., ISHIDATA, M., YOKOTANI, H., AND ISHIKAWA, I., 1958, Isolation, anticancer activity and pharmacology of a new antibiotic, chromomycin, *Gann* **49:**23.

TERASIMA, T., YASUKAWA, M., AND UMEZAWA, H., 1970, Breaks and rejoining of DNA in cultured mammalian cells treated with bleomycin, *Gann* **61:**513.

THOMPSON, F. M., TISCHLER, A. S., ADAMS, J., AND CALVIN, M., 1974, Inhibition of three nucleotide polymerases by rifamycin derivatives, *Proc. Natl. Acad. Sci. U.S.A.* **71:**107.

TING, R. C., YANG, S. S., AND GALLO, R. C., 1972, Reverse transcriptase. RNA tumor virus transformation and derivatives of rifamycin SV, *Nature (London) New Biol.* **236:**163.

TOBEY, R. A., 1975, Different drugs arrest cells at a number of distinctive stages in G2, *Nature (London)* **245**:245.

TOMASZ, M., MERCADO, C. M., OLSON, J., AND CHATTERJIE, N., 1974, The mode of interaction of mitomycin C with DNA and other polynucleotides *in vitro*, *Biochemistry* **31**:4878.

TROUET, A., DEPREZ-DECAMPENEERE, D., AND DEDUVE, C., 1972, Chemotherapy through lysosomes with DNA–daunomycin complex, *Nature (London) New Biol.* **239**:110.

UMEZAWA, H., 1974, Chemistry and mechanism of action of bleomycin, *Fed. Proc. Fed. Amer. Soc. Exp. Biol.* **33**:2296.

UMEZAWA, H., TAKEUCHI, T., HORI, S., SAWA, T., ISHIZUKA, M., ICHIKAWA, T., AND KOMAI, T., 1972, Studies on the mechanism of antitumor effect of bleomycin on squamous cell carcinoma, *J. Antibiot.* **25**:409.

UMEZAWA, H., ASAKURA, H., ODA, K., HORI, S., AND HORI, M., 1973, The effect of bleomycin on SV40 DNA: Characteristics of bleomycin action which produces a single scission in a superhelical form of SV40 DNA, *J. Antibiot.* **26**:521.

WAKAKI, S., MARUMO, H., TOMIOKA, K., SHIMIZU, G., KATO, E., KAMADA, H., KUDO, S., AND FUJIMOTO, Y., 1958, Isolation of new fractions of antitumor mitomycins, *Antibiot. Chemother.* **8**:228.

WANG, J., 1974, Interactions between twisted DNAs and enzymes: The effects of superhelical turns, *J. Mol. Biol.* **87**:797.

WARD, D. C., REICH, E., AND GOLDBERG, I. H., 1965, Base specificity in the interaction of polynucleotides with antibiotic drug, *Science* **149**:1259.

WARING, M., 1970, Variation of the supercoils in closed circular DNA by binding of antibiotics and drugs: Evidence for molecular models involving intercalation, *J. Mol. Biol.* **54**:247.

WARING, M., 1971, Binding of drugs to supercoiled circular DNA: Evidence for and against intercalation, *Prog. Mol. Subcell. Biol.* **2**:216.

WARING, M., AND MAKOFF, A., 1974, Breakdown of pulse-labeled ribonucleic acid and polysomes in *Bacillus megaterium*: Action of streptolydigin, echinomycin and triostins, *Mol. Pharmacol.* **10**:214.

WARING, M. J., AND WAKELIN, L. P. G., 1974, Echinomycin: A bifunctional intercalating antibiotic, *Nature (London)* **252**:653.

WATANABE, M., TAKABE, Y., KATSUMATA, T., AND TERASIMA, T., 1974, Effects of bleomycin on progression through the cell cycle of mouse L-cells, *Cancer Res.* **34**:878.

WEHRLI, W., AND STAEHELIN, M., 1971, Action of the rifamycins, *Bacteriol. Rev.* **35**:290.

WEISSBACH, A., AND LISIO, A., 1965, Alkylation of nucleic acids by mitomycin C and porifiromycin, *Biochemistry* **4**:196.

WILLIAMS, J. G., AND MACPHERSON, I. A., 1973, The differential effect of actinomycin D in normal and virus-transformed cells, *J. Cell. Biol.* **57**:148.

WILLIAMS, J. G., AND MACPHERSON, I. A., 1975, The uptake of actinomycin D by normal and virus transformed BHK21 hamster cells, *Exp. Cell Res.* **91**:237.

WU, A. M., AND GALLO, R. C., 1974, Interaction between murine type-C virus RNA-directed DNA polymerases and rifamycin derivatives, *Biochim. Biophys. Acta* **340**:419.

WU, A. M., TING, R. C., AND GALLO, R. C., 1973, RNA-directed DNA polymerases and virus-induced leukemia in mice, *Proc. Natl. Acad. Sci. U.S.A.* **70**:1298.

YAMASHITA, T., NAOI, N., WATANABE, K., TAKEUCHI, T., AND UMEZAWA, H., 1976, Further purification and characterization of macromycin, *J. Antibiot.* **29**:415.

YAMAZAKI, K. Z., MÜLLER, W. E. G., AND ZAHN, R. K., 1973, Action of bleomycin on programmed synthesis. Influence on enzymatic DNA, RNA and protein synthesis, *Biochim. Biophys. Acta* **308**:412.

ZIMMER, C., AND LUCK, G., 1970, Optical rotatory dispersion properties of nucleic acid complexes with the oligopeptide antibiotics distamycin A and netropsin, *FEBS Lett.* **10**:339.

ZIMMER, C., REINERT, K. E., LUCK, G., WAHNERT, U., LOKER, G., AND THRUM, H., 1971*a*, Interaction of the oligopeptide antibiotics netropsin and distamycin A with nucleic acids, *J. Mol. Biol.* **58**:329.

ZIMMER, C., PUSCHENDORF, B., GRUNICKE, H., CHANDRA, P., AND VEANER, H., 1971*b*, Influence of netropsin and distamycin A on the secondary structure and template activity of DNA, *Eur. J. Biochem.* **21**:269.

ZUNINO, F., 1971, Studies on the mode of interaction of daunomycin and its derivatives with DNA, *FEBS Lett.* **18**:249.

ZUNINO, F., GAMBETTA, R. A., DIMARCO, A., AND ZACCARA, A., 1972, Interaction of daunomycin and its derivatives with DNA, *Biochim. Biophys. Acta* **277**:489.

ZUNINO, F., DIMARCO, A., ZACCARA, A., AND LUONI, G., 1974, The inhibition of RNA polymerase by daunomycin, *Chem.–Biol. Interact.* **9**:25.

456

IRVING H.
GOLDBERG,
TERRY A.
BEERMAN,
AND RAYMOND
POON

Zunino, F., Gambetta, R. A., and DiMarco, A., 1975*a*, The inhibition *in vitro* of DNA polymerase and RNA polymerases by daunomycin and adriamycin, *Biochem. Pharmacol.* **24**:309.

Zunino, F., Gambetta, R., Colombo, A., Luoni, G., and Zaccara, A., 1975*b*, DNA polymerase of rat liver. Partial characterizations and effect of various inhibitors, *Eur. J. Biochem.* **60**:495.

Zunino, F., Gambetta, R., DiMarco, A., Zaccara, A., and Luoni, G., 1975*c*, A comparison of the effects of daunomycin and adriamycin on various DNA polymerases, *Cancer Res.* **35**:754.

16

Enzyme Therapy

JACK R. UREN AND ROBERT E. HANDSCHUMACHER

1. General Considerations of Enzymes as Therapeutic Agents

1.1. Comparisons with Other Chemotherapeutic Agents

Most chemotherapeutic agents function either by depriving cells of an adequate quantity of metabolic precursors, e.g., purine, pyrimidine, and folate antagonists, or by modifying the structures of existing cellular components, e.g., alkylating and intercalating agents. Enzymes have been used in experimental therapeutic trials following these same mechanistic principles. Asparaginase, glutaminase, arginase, methioninase, β-tyrosinease, phenylalanine ammonia lyase, xanthine oxidase, and a folic-acid-degrading enzyme (carboxypeptidase G) have been used to deprive cells of metabolic precursors, while DNase, RNase, neuraminidase, proteolytic enzymes, abrin, ricin, and diphtheria toxin have been used to modify existing cellular components. Enzymes differ from other chemotherapeutic agents, however, in that their macromolecular nature probably restricts their cellular permeability and consequently their accessibility to substrates. This very macromolecular nature enables enzymes to demonstrate a high degree of substrate specificity that can be very useful in restricting their cytotoxicity toward specific tissues, e.g., asparaginase therapy of asparagine-dependent leukemia cells.

1.2. Optimal Characteristics of Enzymes for Enzyme Therapy

Certain thermodynamic and kinetic criteria must be satisfied if an enzyme is to be used to deplete a particular substrate *in vivo*: (1) the substrate–product equilibrium must be sufficiently toward product formation to deplete substrate; (2) the

JACK R. UREN ● Sidney Farber Cancer Institute, Harvard University, Boston, Massachusetts. ROBERT E. HANDSCHUMACHER ● Department of Pharmacology, Yale University School of Medicine, New Haven, Connecticut.

enzyme–substrate affinity ($1/K_m$) must be in a proper relationship to the substrate concentration in the environment; (3) the substrate decomposition rate (V_{max}) must be adequate to achieve and maintain the depleted state in the face of repletion by donor tissues; (4) the enzyme's stability and activity characteristics with respect to pH and temperature must be compatible with the physiological conditions; (5) cosubstrates or activators must be present in an adequate concentration in the environment; (6) the substrate specificity must be sufficiently restrictive to avoid destruction of essential metabolites in the host; and (7) the products of enzyme catalysis must be neither toxic nor readily converted back to the original substrate.

1.3. Biological Limitations of Enzyme Therapy

Even if an enzyme with suitable kinetic and thermodynamic properties is isolated, many biological properties of the host will determine its therapeutic effectiveness. The greatest difficulty is substrate accessibility. Proteins that exceed 60,000 mol.wt. are greatly retarded in their vascular permeability (Goldstein *et al.*, 1974). Many enzymes exceed this molecular weight, and would be largely confined to the intravascular space. Furthermore, the extracellular concentration of substrate in many cases will be either nonexistent or greatly reduced, as compared with the intracellular concentration, since many nutrients or intermediates in metabolism are actively transported and concentrated within cells. Low substrate concentrations require the use of enzymes with low K_m and high V_{max} values. In some cases, the substrate accessibility is even further reduced by the binding of the nutrient to a carrier protein, e.g., fatty acids bound to serum albumin. In addition, the limited vascular permeability of injected enzymes allows sanctuaries for neoplastic cells to exist in the extravascular space within organs that demonstrate a large capacity for substrate synthesis.

In nonimmunized animals, very little is known about the mechanisms of plasma clearance of foreign proteins (Pearsall and Weiser, 1970). Although factors such as isoelectric point (Rutter and Wade, 1971), state of aggregation (Thorbecke *et al.*, 1960), and sialic acid content (Morell *et al.*, 1971) have been shown to influence the rate of plasma clearance of specific proteins, it is not possible to draw any general conclusions. In mice, the lactic-dehydrogenase-elevating virus causes a marked increase in the plasma half-life of exogenous and endogenous proteins (Riley, 1968). Since this virus is generally associated with transplantable mouse tumors, the half-life of enzymes being evaluated for antitumor activity in this species may be extended as much as 10-fold, as in the case of asparaginase (Riley *et al.*, 1970). There are no comparable examples documented for other species.

Not unexpectedly, immunologic reactions after repeated injection of enzymes prepared from other species are a major limitation to systemic treatment. In the case of asparaginase therapy, hypersensitivity reactions ranging from mild allergic reactions to severe anaphylactic shock occur in approximately 25% of patients (Hrushesky, personal communication). This problem can be minimized by short courses of enzyme therapy for remission induction, rather than maintenance therapy. It should also be noted that enzymes would rarely be given as single agents, and proper combinations with immunosuppressive chemotherapeutic agents might reduce the incidence of allergic reactions. In addition to the hazard of severe allergic reactions, the development of antibodies against a therapeutic enzyme can cause a greatly accelerated clearance of the enzyme from the plasma.

With enzyme therapy, as with all other forms of chemotherapy, biological resistance must be anticipated. In the treatment of tumors with requirements for a "nonessential" amino acid, the frequency of nutritionally independent mutants in a population of cancer cells is likely to be similar to the frequency of drug-resistant cells in that population (1 in 10^6–10^8 cells). Since at least 10^8 neoplastic cells are present at the time of diagnosis or relapse, some resistant cells will almost certainly exist. This fact underscores the need for a combination of enzyme therapy and chemotherapy or radiotherapy. Particularly important is the selection of combinations in which each component shows different host toxicities.

The expanding technology for immobilization of enzymes offers many possibilities to enhance the role of enzyme therapy. Such procedures not only afford high concentrations of enzyme, but also frequently increase dramatically the stability of the enzyme to denaturation with minimal changes in kinetic properties. One can envision extracorporeal enzyme reactors consisting of enzyme-lined tubes through which blood would be bypassed and the concentration of substrate for that enzyme in the plasma reduced to desired levels, based on the activity of the matrix-bound enzyme and the duration of exposure. Engasser and Horvath (1976) have defined theoretical and practical considerations that limit this technique, since classic solution enzyme kinetics may not apply. However, if substrate replenishment to the plasma is sufficiently slow and the biological sensitivity of the tumor to the depleted substrate is great, this system could have several advantages. It could permit utilization of enzymes that normally are cleared too rapidly to be useful, and possibly minimize or eliminate the development of immune reactions against the enzyme. This would be particularly true if substrate access to the enzyme is through a semipermeable membrane that could prevent passage of lymphocytes, macrophages, or even other macromolecules (e.g., antibodies, proteases). As indicated in Section 1.2, the kinetics of synthesis, as well as the metabolism of a target substrate in donor tissues and the distributional factors governing its access to the tumor cell, must all be considered as potentially limiting the effectiveness of matrix-bound enzymes.

Finally, substrate depletion *in vivo* must create an environment around the tumor cells that will not only reduce the rate of growth, but, more important, also actually cause cell death. As with chemotherapeutic agents, definition of the biochemical action leading to substrate depletion or an effect on a particular path in intermediary metabolism or macromolecule synthesis may be a far distance from the actual reason for lethality.

A summary of important enzymatic and biological considerations for optimal enzyme therapy is presented in Table 1.

TABLE 1
Desirable Properties of an Enzyme for Therapy

Enzymatic	Biological
Equilibrium favoring product formation	Vascular permeability
High substrate affinity ($1/K_m$)	Low rate of substrate synthesis by host
Rapid rate of substrate decomposition (V_{max})	Minimal serum protein binding of substrate
Suitable stability	Low immunogenicity
Adequate cofactor and cosubstrate concentrations	Long plasma half-life
Restrictive substrate specificity	Infrequent resistant cell types
Low product toxicity	

2. Nonessential Amino Acid Depletion

2.1. Asparagine Depletion

Although enzyme therapy has been suggested in the past by many authors, and limited studies have been undertaken, the appearance of this chapter is almost solely predicted on the effectiveness of L-asparaginase from *Escherichia coli* or *Erwinia carotovora* as a treatment for acute lymphoblastic leukemia. This section will not attempt an exhaustive review of the literature covering this development, which exceeds 750 reports. Several comprehensive reviews that document progress up to the time of their publication have been prepared (Grundmann and Oettgen, 1970; Bernard *et al.*, 1970). Primarily nonclinical aspects of the field were covered in reviews by Cooney and Handschumacher (1970), Wriston and Yellin (1973), and Cooney and Rosenbluth (1975). Clinical experience with asparaginase therapy and associated biochemical, immunologic, and toxicologic ramifications were reviewed by Adamson and Fabro (1968), Land *et al.* (1972), Capizzi *et al.* (1970), and Holcenberg and Roberts (1977). The most complete compilation of the clinical effects of this enzyme in more than 8000 patients was made by Hrushesky (personal communication) at the Division of Cancer Treatment of the National Cancer Institute. In this chapter, specific principles of enzyme therapy as exemplified by L-asparaginase will be discussed as prototypic guides.

Asparaginase therapy did not originate as a logical exploitation of the specific nutritional requirement of certain neoplastic cells for L-asparagine. Kidd (1953) observed that guinea pig serum was capable of causing regression of the Gardner lymphoma in mice. Initially, complement activity or other immunologic factors were suspected to be responsible, but Broome (1963*a, b*) demonstrated that fractionation of the serum for antitumor activity resulted in a parallel purification of L-asparaginase activity. At about the same time, Newman and McCoy (1956) and Haley *et al.* (1961) showed that a select group of experimental tumors in cell culture had an apparently unique nutritional requirement for the amino acid L-asparagine when compared with the majority of cell lines. Practical development of these leads was limited until Mashburn and Wriston (1964) purified L-asparaginase from *E. coli* and demonstrated essentially equivalent antitumor activity. The next eight years of research and clinical trials in large measure defined the current status of this radical departure from previous modes of therapy. Referring to the characteristics described earlier as essential for a therapeutically useful enzyme, it will become apparent that the bacterial asparaginase preparations are at present the only enzymes discussed in this chapter that have an established role in human therapy.

2.1.1. Enzyme Properties

A wide variety of bacterial sources have been surveyed for asparaginase preparations with antitumor activity. At present, the two clinically important enzymes are prepared from the human commensal *E. coli* and the vegetation-decomposing species *Erwinia carotovora*. The *E. coli* enzyme has a tetrameric structure with identical subunits of about 32,000 mol.wt. (Laboureur *et al.*, 1971). The primary structure of the monomer was reported by Maita *et al.* (1974) for *E. coli* A-1-3, confirming portions of the sequence established for *E. coli* B by Gumprecht and Wriston (1973). The degree of dissociation of tetramer under physiological conditions is very minor, and concentrated solutions of the enzyme tend to form higher aggregates of the tetrameric structure (P. P. K. Ho and Millikin, 1970). There are four active sites on the tetrameric form of the enzyme, as determined by covalent binding of the asparagine analogue 5-diazo-4-oxo-L-norvaline (Jackson and Handschumacher, 1970), but enzyme activity is lost in urea solutions, a condition that causes dissociation of the tetramer (Shifrin *et al.*, 1971). The enzyme varies in its isoelectric point (pI 4.6–5.5), depending on the strain or organism and mode of purification (reviewed by Wriston and Yellin, 1973). It does not contain detectable carbohydrate residues or phosphate groups. L-Asparagine is the preferred natural substrate (K_m 1×10^{-5} M), and the specific activity is 300–400 units (μmol/min)/mg in homogeneous preparations. Substrate activity is also observed with a variety of naturally occurring amino acids, including L-glutamine (3%), D-asparagine (2%), and L-β-cyanoalanine (3%), as well as with the acid analogues aspartate hydroxamate (15%), 5-diazo-4-oxo-L-norvaline (2%), and diamino succinamide (50%). The enzyme prepared from *Erwinia carotovora* is also tetrameric, but has a higher isoelectric point and specific activity. It possesses relatively greater glutaminase activity, and has been chemically modified to delay biological clearance (Rutter and Wade, 1971). Minor substrate activity for *E. coli* or *Erwinia carotovora* enzyme has been reported using a very wide variety of amino acid derivatives (reviewed by Cooney and Rosenbluth, 1975), as well as some macromolecular derivatives of asparagine (Howard and Carpenter, 1972). There is no conclusive evidence, however, that these minor activities play a significant role in the biological effects of L-asparaginase therapy. However, the glutaminase activity, an intrinsic catalytic function of homogeneous preparations of the enzyme, may be responsible for certain of the biological effects, particularly the toxic effects, of various bacterial asparaginase preparations. Selective reduction of the glutaminase activity has been attempted by chemical modification, but with limited success (Liu and Handschumacher, 1972).

Since diffusion of the tetrameric enzyme through capillary walls into intercellular spaces is very limited, numerous attempts have been made to modify the enzyme by chemical means to produce active subunits that would not reassemble into tetramers (Shifrin and Grochowski, 1972; Hare and Handschumacher, 1973). In no case was there more than a 10% retention of activity in preparations that may have had a greater degree of subunit dissociation.

Matrix-bound asparaginase has been employed by several groups in an effort to reduce plasma and hence tissue concentrations of asparagine without direct access of immunocompetent cells or possibly proteolytic enzymes to the asparaginase. The solid supports have included plastics, glass, gels, semipermeable capsules, and collagen (reviewed by Cooney and Rosenbluth, 1975). The technology for implantation or extracorporeal circulation is available, but in general is cumbersome for the necessarily long periods of asparagine depletion required. Some of the conditions to be met if this technique is to be useful should be considered. Studies in patients undergoing renal dialysis showed that removal of one-third of the asparagine from plasma in each pass through an artificial kidney at an arteriovenous bypass rate of 300 ml/min failed to alter plasma levels of asparagine in 8 patients (Cooney *et al.*, 1970). Even if complete removal were to be achieved on each pass, it seems unlikely that sufficient blood could be directed through the machine over prolonged periods to effect reductions in plasma concentrations of asparagine sufficient to arrest cell growth or cause lysis, since in experimental leukemias, about 1/50 of the normal plasma concentration of asparagine sustains 50% of the normal growth rate.

Repletion of plasma pools of asparagine from tissue stores and *de novo* synthesis in many normal tissues is very rapid, and thus the rate of hydrolysis of plasma asparagine must be extremely rapid. If as little as 10 units of free asparaginase is released into the circulation, however, plasma concentrations of asparagine will remain undetectable for many hours. In several of the *in vivo* experiments with matrix-bound enzyme, plasma concentrations of asparagine remained depressed for up to 24 hr after removal of the device. In light of a $T_{1/2}$ (repletion rate) of about 20 min for the plasma pool of asparagine in normal individuals, these prolonged depressions almost certainly are the result of dissociation of small amounts of enzyme from the matrix into the vascular system. In at least one report, this dissociation has been documented by enzymatic and immunologic methods (Cooney and Rosenbluth, 1975).

2.1.2. Biochemical Effects of Asparaginase in Vitro and in Vivo

The selectivity of asparaginase therapy in animals reflects the inability of many experimental lymphoid tumors to synthesize asparagine (Broome, 1963*b*; Patterson and Orr, 1969). Biochemical studies with cells from experimental (Prager and Bachynsky, 1968) and human neoplasms (Haskell and Canellos, 1969) indicate that the majority of these cells also have undetectable synthetase activity prior to therapy. Although it might be hoped that this activity would serve as a means of predicting the sensitivity of experimental and human disease, these workers have shown that in some cases, neoplastic cells are apparently capable of derepressing asparagine synthetase and thus escaping from the lethal effect of depleted levels of circulating asparagine. Asparagine synthetase activity is low in most normal tissues, but in response to the nutritional stress created by an asparagine-free diet or asparaginase treatment, the activity increases (Patterson and Orr, 1969). This adaptive increase in enzyme activity is presumably the reason Becker and Broome (1967) observed inhibition of the initial but not subsequent waves of mitosis in regenerating rat livers. Asparagine synthetase is very sensitive to product inhibition by asparagine (Horowitz and Meister, 1972); hence, whole-cell measurements of enzymatic capability must recognize the inhibitory effect of intracellular pools of asparagine (Chou and Handschumacher, 1972). Asparagine is also concentrated within cells from extracellular spaces by an active transport reaction. Each of the preceding factors conditions the response to systemic asparaginase. As important, however, is the consequence of asparagine depletion within the cell. As might be expected, the synthesis of protein is most sensitive to asparagine depletion. What was not predictable and remains an enigma is the rapidity with which asparaginase treatment results in lysis of sensitive lymphoblasts in culture (Summers and Handschumacher, 1971), as well as the dissolution of large tumor masses in animals (Kidd, 1953; Old *et al.*, 1967) and humans (Capizzi *et al.*, 1970). It was attractive to consider these results to be a consequence of direct attack by asparaginase on cell membranes, but in cell culture systems, equivalent rates of lysis can be observed by culturing sensitive cell lines in medium devoid of asparagine (Summers and Handschumacher, 1973).

Some consideration must be given to the degree of asparagine depletion that must be achieved to effect cell kill. To sustain half-maximal growth rates, some experimental leukemias require approximately 1×10^{-6} M asparagine (Haley *et al.*, 1961). Since normal plasma levels in humans are about 4×10^{-5} M, even a 97% reduction in the plasma pool would reduce the rate of growth by only half if human cells in the blood have similar requirements. Of even greater importance is removal of asparagine from intercellular spaces in the tissues. In these areas, leukemic cells may continue proliferation using asparagine released from adjacent normal cells, the synthetase of which would have been activated by the systemic depletion of preformed asparagine. These sanctuaries for growth are of great importance with asparaginase, since the tetramer enzyme with a molecular weight of about 135,000 is largely confined to the vascular spaces, and is present in lymph and interstitial spaces at low levels (P. H. W. Ho *et al.*, 1970). Virtually no enzyme enters the CSF.

Preliminary studies have shown that killing of murine leukemic cells that have infiltrated various organs is not uniform. In fact, very minimal cell death was observed in the liver, an organ known to have very high concentrations of asparagine. Furthermore, the liver has been demonstrated to be a chemostat probably responsible for the maintenance of plasma levels of asparagine (Woods and Handschumacher, 1973). It can either hydrolyze excess asparagine with an intrinsic asparaginase activity or increase asparagine synthetase to permit controlled release of the amino acid into the blood. If asparagine synthesis is blocked by inhibitors, the controlled release continues until hepatic pools of the amino acid are depleted.

Since sensitivity to asparaginase is known to require a loss or gross depletion of asparagine synthetase, it is not surprising that under the selective pressures of asparaginase therapy *in vivo* or in cell culture, mutant sublines can be selected for biological resistance. Repeated exposure to increasing levels of asparaginase has selected for some highly resistant lines. It is of interest that these and some of the naturally resistant tumor cell types have levels of asparagine synthetase that exceed by severalfold that found in most normal tissues (Horowitz *et al.*, 1968). During the course of tumor therapy, however, sensitive cells must develop only minimal levels of synthetase to achieve resistance. It has been shown with murine cell lines that these initially selected mutants exhibit a repressible form of the synthetase (Uren *et al.*, 1974).

The dependence of sensitive cells on the uptake and utilization of exogenous asparagine, as well as the potential for inhibition of asparagine synthesis, has made synthesis of asparagine analogues an attractive approach. With respect to utilization of exogenous asparagine, however, the sensitivity of tumor cell lines to asparaginase does not correlate with their ability to transport and use exogenous asparagine. In planning the development of inhibitors of asparagine synthetase as an adjunct to therapy with asparaginase, levels of synthetase activity in different normal tissues must be considered. Cooney and Rosenbluth (1975) showed that of all tissues surveyed, the greatest activity was observed in extracts of the pancreas and parathyroid glands. Horowitz *et al.* (1968) had shown earlier that rat testes and brain had modestly high levels of this enzyme. It is uncertain whether high intrinsic activity is indicative of great need or an excess capability for asparagine synthesis. The hypoinsulinemia observed in some patients would favor the view that high synthetase activity can be equated with a greater requirement.

Many compounds have been tested as inhibitors of asparagine synthetase (reviewed by Cooney and Rosenbluth, 1975). Recently, homoserine adenylate (P. K. Chang, 1976), an analogue of the proposed transition state in the reaction, has been shown to be a very active inhibitor. The use of such compounds in combination with enzyme therapy to deplete the natural substrate must take into account the possible effects of the analogues on asparaginase. Nevertheless, selective toxicity for the tumor might be observed if inhibition of asparagine synthetase in normal tissues can be titered so that their ability to feed adjacent or distal tumor cells can be eliminated, and yet allow them to retain enough synthesis to sustain their own synthesis of protein. Since asparagine is not known to subserve any function other than peptide assembly, and in some cases provides a point of attachment for the oligosaccharide chains of glutoproteins, asparagine analogues are unlikely to damage other metabolic functions in the cell.

2.1.3. Toxic Reactions

Most of the toxicity seen in animals or humans after intensive therapy with asparaginase (Whitecar *et al.*, 1970) can be directly attributed to inhibition of the synthesis of excreted proteins. These toxic reactions have included hypoglycemia consequent to suppressed insulin synthesis (Ohnuma *et al.*, 1969; Haskell *et al.*, 1969), defective clotting because of reduced levels of prothrombin and other clotting factors (Haskell *et al.*, 1969; Bettigole *et al.*, 1970), hypoalbuminemia (Capizzi *et al.*, 1970), and a severe hypocalcemia in rabbits as a consequence of reduced function of the parathyroid glands (Cooney and Rosenbluth, 1975). It is difficult to assign responsibility for these effects solely to asparagine depletion. In general, they are seen only at dosage levels that have been shown to deplete glutamine as well as asparagine (Miller *et al.*, 1969). As indicated earlier, the availability of an asparaginase preparation that did not have intrinsic glutaminase activity could resolve this question, and possibly increase the selectivity and effectiveness of asparaginase therapy. Enzyme prepared from guinea pig serum does not hydrolyze glutamine, but isolation from this source is not practical. A recent report suggests that asparaginase isolated from *Vibrio succinogenes* has antitumor activity and very low glutaminase activity (Distasio and Niederman, 1976). This source bears further development, since the enzyme does not cross-react immunologically with the enzyme from *E. coli*. The subsequent discussion of amidase enzymes with much greater activity on glutamine will put some of these observations in perspective.

In planning for use in combination therapy protocols, it would be useful to define the cycle specificity of asparaginase therapy. Bosmann (1972) reported that there is inhibition of protein and glycoprotein synthesis through the cell cycle, but that primary inhibition occurs during the S phase. Saunders (1972) indicated that lysis of both proliferating and nonproliferating cells occurred with asparaginase, and that passage of cells from the G_1 into the S phase was blocked.

2.1.4. Immunologic Reactions

The most common reason for terminating therapy with asparaginase is the development of allergic reactions. Although as many as 25% of all patients given intravenous therapy develop some hypersensitivity reactions, only about 9% of these have been sufficiently severe to have been classified as anaphylactic (Hrushesky, personal communication). This represents a remarkably low incidence of reaction to the injection of a bacterial protein, over a 10–20 day period and repeated at monthly intervals. Undoubtedly, this low incidence is conditioned by the fact that asparaginase can be shown to be a mild immunosuppressive agent in animals (Schwartz, 1969) and man (Ohno and Hersh, 1970). *In vitro* studies with lymphocytes indicate that blastogenic transformation requires adequate levels of asparagine (Astaldi *et al.*, 1969); the possible relationships of this inhibition of normal blastogenesis and the effects of asparaginase as an antileukemic agent are discussed by Astaldi (1972). It is not clear whether lymphocyte transformation is affected by enzyme depletion of glutamine (Hersh, 1971; Baechtel *et al.*, 1976). Transient lymphatic involution has been observed as a consequence of asparaginase therapy. It appears, however, that lymphoid cells are capable of adapting to prior asparaginase therapy by derepressing asparagine synthetase. The humoral immune response appears to follow that for other antigens, with early appearance of IgM and IgG and a secondary response of predominantly IgG antibodies (Peterson *et al.*, 1971). It has also been shown that the enzyme–antibody complex retains considerable activity, and that the enzyme is stabilized in this form to various denaturing conditions (Zyk, 1973). Formation of the complex *in vivo* results in greatly accelerated rates of clearance, a finding that is frequently but not always associated with anaphylactic reactions in patients (Peterson *et al.*, 1971). In mice, immune clearance is associated with a rapid return of asparagine levels in the plasma and loss of antitumor effects (Vadlamudi *et al.*, 1970; Goldberg *et al.*, 1973).

There is evidence to suggest that regression and curves of experimental lymphomas depend on an immune response to the tumor challenge (Ryan and Curtis, 1973). Survival is reduced in T-cell-depleted animals, and response to therapy is optimal, if therapy is delayed for several days after tumor implantation. This latter increase in response is due in part to the establishment of the LDH virus normally passaged along with most murine tumors, which delays clearance of asparaginase activity from $T_{1/2}$ of 3 hr to about 18 hr. However, immunosuppression by antilymphocyte serum or radiation prevented expression of the antitumor effect.

The lack of cross-reactivity to asparaginase from *Erwinia carotovora* in patients sensitized to the *E. coli* preparation has extended useful enzyme therapy in patients with lymphoblastic leukemia (Ohnuma *et al.*, 1972). Enzyme from this alternative source has a similar antitumor spectrum in experimental animals. Its intrinsic immunosuppressive effect is 10 times greater than the *E. coli* enzyme in the lymphocyte blastogenic assay, possibly because of its greater glutaminase activity (Han and Ohnuma, 1972). Both enzymes were approximately equally potent in suppressing antibody response in mice to sheep erythrocytes, and neither influenced cell-mediated responses in guinea pigs (Ashworth and MacLennan, 1974). Others have indicated that *E. coli* enzyme can exert a significant immunosuppressive effect in the renal graft rejection model in rats, an action potentiated by combination therapy with cytoxan (Levin and Merrill, 1972). In some circumstances, treatment with asparaginase before the time of tumor implantation can enhance metastatic spread of experimental tumors, presumably because of a temporary suppression of the host immune response (Deodhar, 1973).

2.1.5. Clinical Results

The clinical evaluation of *E. coli* asparaginase as an antitumor agent now includes approximately 8000 patients. A recent review of all clinical data by Hrushesky (personal communication) affords a comprehensive tabulation and evaluation of efficacy and toxicity in man. With the use of asparaginase as a single agent, the primary indication for asparaginase therapy is as induction therapy in acute lymphoblastic leukemia. Complete remission rates of about 40% have been noted in end-stage disease of children. With the use of asparaginase in combination with other drugs, remission rates of about 60% were seen in advanced cases in both children and adults. In combination with vincristine and prednisone, asparaginase produced a 95% complete remission rate in previously untreated acute lymphoblastic leukemia. There is also evidence that it prolongs the duration of remission (Ortega *et al.*, 1975).

Minimal activity has been noted in poorly differentiated non-Hodgkins lymphomas of children. When asparaginase is used in combination with other drugs, 15% of patients with acute myelogenous leukemia achieved complete remission; when used as a single drug, however, it is much less effective.

The recommended dosage schedule is 6000 IU/M^2 thrice weekly for 3 or 4 weeks, or 1000 IU/kg for 10 days after vincristine and prednisone. Preliminary studies by one group suggest that the incidence of severe allergic reactions may be greatly reduced by intramuscular rather than intravenous administration (Newton *et al.*, 1973). Because of the hazard of anaphylactic reactions (9% of all patients), it is generally not recommended for maintenance therapy, and second courses must be used with caution. Unlike many drugs, schedule dependency is not evident, except that intermittent therapy (weekly) predisposes to allergic reactions (Nesbitt *et al.*, 1970). Other dose-limiting toxicities include pancreatitis, particularly in adults and diabetics, CNS toxicity that may relate to high serum levels of ammonia, and hepatotoxicity manifest as altered liver function tests and hypoalbuminemia.

Although current usage is limited to induction therapy of ALL immediately after vincristine and prednisone, other combination studies are in progress that may change the scope of therapeutic action of asparaginase. Capizzi *et al.* (1971) and Capizzi (1975) demonstrated that asparaginase could almost completely nullify the toxic effects of large doses of methotrexate in cell culture and experimental animals if it was given at an appropriate interval before the antifolate. Capizzi and co-workers extended these studies to man, and showed that patients previously refractory to methotrexate have been able to tolerate very much larger doses of methotrexate (400 mg/M^2 every 9 to 10 days) if asparaginase is given 24 hr later (Capizzi *et al.*, 1974). Remissions have been observed in 8 of 10 acute lymphoblastic leukemias previously refractory to methotrexate. Similar reductions in the toxicity of other appropriately scheduled cytotoxic agents have been observed, which suggests that asparaginase might find use in combination therapy of solid tumors even if it is not active alone.

2.2. Glutamine Depletion

Glutamine is synthesized by the amidation of glutamic acid by the enzyme glutamine synthetase. Unlike the case with asparagine synthetase, diminished levels of glutamine synthetase in malignant cells compared with their normal cell counterparts have not been observed. However, therapeutic trials with the glutamine analogues 6-diazo-5-oxo-L-norleucine and azaserine have shown significant antitumor effects in mice and some improvement in humans (Ellison *et al.*,

1954). These observations and the requirements of malignant cells for glutamine in culture have made glutamine a logical candidate for depletion therapy.

Glutaminases with antitumor activity have been isolated from *Acinetobacter glutaminasificans*, *Pseudomonas aureofaciens* (Schmid and Roberts, 1974), *Pseudomonas aeruginosa* (Oki *et al.*, 1973), *Pseudomonas* 7a (Roberts, 1976), and *Achromobacter* (Spiers and Wade, 1976). These enzymes are not strictly glutaminases, since they show high levels of asparaginase activity as well (reviewed by Holcenberg *et al.*, 1973). The treatment of mice with the *Acinetobacter* enzyme will reduce both asparagine and glutamine concentrations in tissues. It was proposed that the therapeutic effect may depend on the combined depletion of both these amino acids (Holcenberg *et al.*, 1975*b*). The glutaminase–asparaginase enzymes have antitumor activity against the asparaginase-resistant Ehrlich carcinoma, Taper liver tumor, and Meth A sarcoma. Greater toxicity has been found with the glutaminase–asparaginase enzymes than with *E. coli* asparaginase, including leukopenia, thrombocytopenia, and reduced splenic weight (Schmid and Roberts, 1974). Recently, a glutaminase–asparaginase was isolated from *Pseudomonas* 7a (Roberts, 1976) that has a long plasma half-life in mice (13 hr), and is effective against solid tumors in mice (Roberts and Schmid, 1976). The *Achromobacter* asparaginase–glutaminase of Spiers and Wade (1976) has a very short half-life in man ($T_{1/2} = 80$ min), but can reduce plasma glutamine (and asparagine) concentrations to undetectable levels when given as a continuous infusion for 28 days. Objective improvement was seen in 7 patients with acute lymphoblastic and myeloid leukemia, 4 of whom were resistant to asparaginase (Spiers and Wade, 1976). All 7 patients had objective but transient improvement in their disease state, but nausea and vomiting, marrow toxicity, and metabolic acidosis were seen. Further clinical studies are needed to assess the potential role of this enzyme in solid tumors as well as the leukemias.

2.3. Arginine Depletion

Arginine is a nonessential amino acid that is normally derived from the urea cycle, but in some cancer cells, the rate of synthesis of this amino acid may not be adequate. Ohnuma *et al.* (1971) showed that a 50–60% reduction in the incorporation of [³H]uridine into RNA and DNA by cells from patients with acute myelocytic leukemia occurred when the cells were incubated in media containing no arginine. Uridine uptake in cells from patients with acute lymphocytic leukemia was only minimally (6–24%) affected by the arginine deprivation. In cell culture, both the L5178Y and L1210 mouse lymphosarcoma lose viability when incubated in media that contain less than 8×10^{-6} M arginine (Storr and Burton, 1974). Furthermore, the addition of purified arginase to the culture media reduces the viability of L5178Y and L1210 cells (Storr and Burton, 1974), and inhibits the growth rate of Jensen sarcoma (Wolf and Ransberger, 1972). Recently, it has been shown that arginine is required for the replication of Marek's disease herpes virus in Japanese quail embryo fibrolasts (Mikami *et al.*, 1974), and the replication of Shope fibroma virus in rabbit kidney cells (Newcomb and Minocha, 1973).

Reports on the *in vivo* antitumor effects of purified arginase have been less definitive. Positive therapeutic responses have been observed with adenocarcinoma in mice (Neukomm *et al.*, 1949; Vrat, 1951) and Walker carcinoma in rats (Wolf and Ransberger, 1972). Other workers have not observed antitumor effects (Storr and Burton, 1974; Cooney and Rosenbluth, 1975; Greenberg and Sassenrath, 1953). The plasma concentration of arginine was reduced 86% at 3 hr, and returned to normal within 8 hr, after 200 IU arginase was given to mice bearing lymphosarcoma 6C3HED. No decrease in the concentration of arginine in the tumor or liver was observed. The half-life of the injected enzyme was about 8 hr in these experiments (Greenberg and Sassenrath, 1953). A probable reason for these poor therapeutic responses is the low substrate affinity ($K_m = 1.8 \times 10^{-2}$ M at pH 7.0) of the injected liver arginases (Roholt and Greenberg, 1956). A reinvestigation of the *in vivo* effects of arginine depletion created by an arginine decarboxylase isolated from *E. coli* (W. H. Wu and Morris, 1973) would be of interest. This purified enzyme has a K_m of 3×10^{-5} M, and might be much more effective in depleting circulating levels of this amino acid.

2.4. Tyrosine Depletion

Tyrosine is formed by hydroxylation of phenylalanine by the enzyme phenylalanine hydroxylase. Dietary restrictions of phenylalanine and tyrosine have been shown to inhibit the growth of pigmented S91 melanomas in mice, but a nonpigmented S37 sarcoma was not affected by the diet (Demopoulos, 1966*a*). In humans, positive clinical responses in advanced malignant melanomas to a reduction in dietary intake of phenylalanine and tyrosine have been reported (Demopoulos, 1966*b*). A possible explanation for these results is that the extensive utilization of tyrosine for melanin synthesis imposes an enhanced tyrosine dietary requirement on the pigmented melanoma cells. Consequently, these cells are preferentially inhibited by dietary restrictions of phenylalanine and tyrosine. Melanoma cells are not the only tumors that may respond to this form of therapy. Lorincz *et al.* (1969) reported that the growth rates of hepatomas are reduced in animals on a diet low in phenylalanine and tyrosine, and Ohnuma *et al.* (1971) reported that cells derived from patients with acute lymphocytic leukemia and acute myelocytic leukemia have a greatly reduced ability to incorporate [^{3}H]uridine into macromolecules when cultured in media deprived of tyrosine.

A recent report describes the effects of tyrosine phenol lyase on the growth of B-16 melanoma (Meadows *et al.*, 1976). This enzyme degrades tyrosine to phenol, pyruvate, and ammonia with a K_m value of 0.28 mM. The enzyme had a plasma half-life of 6–7 hr, and significantly inhibited the growth of B-16 melanoma in mice. Plasma concentrations of tyrosine dropped to about 50% of control values

7 hr after the injection of 160 IU/kg, and returned to normal within 26 hr. Presumably, a larger dose of this enzyme or an enzyme with a lower K_m would enhance the depletion of tyrosine, and may enhance therapeutic effectiveness.

2.5. Cystine Depletion

Cysteine is a nonessential amino acid derived from methionine and serine. The cystine nutritional requirements of human leukemic cells in long-term culture were reported by Foley *et al.* (1969). They observed that a number of human leukemic cell lines had an absolute requirement for cystine, regardless of the ploidy of the chromosomal complement and the cell population density. The cysteine precursor cystathionine could not substitute for cystine in the media. Using short-term culture techniques, Ohnuma *et al.* (1971) confirmed the cystine requirement for cells derived from patients with acute lymphocytic and myelocytic leukemia. Lymphoid cell lines derived from normal individuals or patients with infectious mononucleosis retained the ability to grow on cystathionine in the absence of cysteine (Lazarus *et al.*, 1974; Livingston *et al.*, 1976). The mechanism of this difference was related to the higher activity of cystathionase (the last enzyme in cystine biosynthesis) in normal cells as compared with the malignant cell lines. Livingston *et al.* (1976) demonstrated that the cystathionase activity in thymocytes decreased as thymic tumors were induced by Maloney type C virus.

An attempt to exploit this nutritional difference was reported by Uren and Lazarus (1975). From *Enterobacter cloacae*, they isolated cysteine desulfhydrase, which degrades cystine to pyruvate, H_2S, and ammonia. The enzyme demonstrated a K_m of 0.4 mM and a specific activity of 420 IU/mg. Rat liver cystathionase was also shown to degrade cysteine with a K_m of 0.1 mM and a specific activity of 0.28 IU/mg. Both enzymes inhibited the growth of murine L1210 and human CEM leukemic cells in culture, but the cysteine desulfhydrase required the presence of a reducing agent to reduce cystine to cysteine. The desulfhydrase was rapidly cleared from mice with a half-life of 12 min, and the cystathionase had a half-life of 2 hr. No *in vivo* antileukemic evaluation of these two enzymes has been reported to date.

2.6. Serine Depletion

In mammals, serine is formed from 3-phosphohydroxypyruvic acid, or from glycine and 5,10-methylene tetrahydrofolic acid. Regan *et al.* (1969) reported that in serine-deficient media, cells from human chronic granulocytic leukemia and normal human bone marrow greatly inhibited incorporation of precursors into macromolecules, whereas normal diploid fibroblasts did not. No attempts at serine depletion by inhibiting synthesis or enzymatic degradation have been reported. A reasonable candidate for this may be serine dehydrase from *Clostridium acidiurici*. Sagers and Carter (1971) reported that this enzyme is highly specific for serine, with a K_m value of 7.8 mM and specific activity of 2140 IU/mg.

3. Essential Amino Acid Depletion

3.1. Introduction

Restrictions of certain essential amino acids in the diet of tumor-bearing animals have been shown to inhibit tumor growth. The growth of sarcoma 180 in mice was consistently and significantly less when the animals were fed synthetic diets deficient in each of the following amino acids: valine, leucine, isoleucine, threonine, phenylalanine, histidine, or methionine (Skipper and Thomson, 1958). In rats bearing the Walker tumor, the rate of tumor growth was considerably reduced when the animals were force-fed diets deficient in methionine, isoleucine, or valine, and, to a lesser extent, phenylalanine, histidine, or tryptophan (Sugimura *et al.*, 1959). Theuer (1971) fed mice bearing the BW10232 adenocarcinomas a series of diets with a graded depletion of the essential amino acids. He observed that reduced dietary levels of tryptophan, threonine, leucine, or methionine inhibited tumor growth, but caused weight loss in the host as well; however, reduced dietary levels of phenylalanine, valine, or isoleucine inhibited tumor weight without affecting host weight. Taken together, it appears that isoleucine and valine dietary restriction consistently showed substantial antitumor effects. A preliminary report on the antitumor activity of a leucine dehydrogenase from *Bacillus sphaericus* (Oki *et al.*, 1973) has not been confirmed (Roberts *et al.*, 1974).

3.2. Phenylalanine Depletion

The effects of the dietary restrictions of phenylalanine and tyrosine cited support the proposal that enzymic phenylalanine destruction might inhibit tumor growth. Abell *et al.* (1972) demonstrated that phenylalanine ammonialyase (K_m 0.25 mM) will deaminate phenylalanine to produce cinnamic acid and to a lesser extent tyrosine to form coumaric acid. The enzyme inhibited the growth of human leukemic and murine L5178Y lymphoblasts. The products of the reaction, cinnamic and coumaric acids, were without effect in this system. *In vivo*, the enzyme at a dosage of 100 IU/kg depleted phenylalanine to 3% of control values in 7 hr, and maintained it at 12% of control levels for 2 days (Abell *et al.*, 1973). Mice bearing the L5178Y lymphoblastic leukemia showed a mean increase in survival, discounting the "cured" mice, of only 17% over controls after receiving 100 IU/kg every 8 hr for 5 days; however, 43% "cures" were reported. Although a recent report was unable to confirm activity with this enzyme (Roberts *et al.*, 1976), further exploration of phenylalanine and tyrosine depletion seems warranted.

3.3. Methionine Depletion

Reports of the effects of dietary depletion of methionine on the Walker carcinosarcoma in rats were discussed in Section 3.1. More recently, Halpern *et al.*

(1974) presented evidence that homocystine can substitute for methionine to support the growth of normal fibroblasts. For three malignant cell lines, however, homocystine could not substitute for methionine. These observations suggest that normal tissues may be rescued from the effects of methionine deprivation by homocystine, but malignant cells may not be.

Kreis and Hession (1973a, b) described an enzyme from *Clostridium sporogenes* that will degrade methionine to methanethiol, ammonia, and α-ketobutyric acid. Unfortunately, the enzyme degrades homocysteine and cysteine more rapidly than methionine, and shows a very high K_m (80–90 mM) for methionine. The enzyme was shown to inhibit the growth of P815 and L1210 in tissue culture. At 1 hr after an intravenous injection into mice of 250 IU of the enzyme/kg, the plasma concentration of methionine was reduced to 8% of control value, but returned to normal within 24 hr; the enzyme had a plasma half-life of 4 hr. After 6 consecutive days of 1100 IU/kg per day, the Walker carcinosarcoma 256 showed a 45–48% reduction in tumor diameter when compared with nontreated controls. Diets deprived of methionine caused a 23–37% reduction in tumor diameter during a comparable period of time, but also caused much greater weight loss of the host. An enzyme that shows a greater substrate specificity with better kinetic properties should improve the therapeutic responses observed with this type of therapy.

3.4. Other Essential Amino Acid Depletions

Some enzymes that have not been previously examined for antineoplastic activity and have reasonable kinetic properties toward the degradation of certain essential amino acids are presented in Table 2. Therapeutic trials in experimental animals with these enzymes may be worthwhile.

TABLE 2

Kinetic Properties of Amino Acid Degrading Enzymes

Enzyme	Source	K_m (mM)	Specific activity (IU/mg)	pH optimum	Comments
Threonine deaminase (biosynthetic) Burns (1971)	*Salmonella typhimurium*	1.6	450	9–10	Degrades serine at $\frac{1}{3}$ rate. Inhibited by isoleucine ($K_I = 5 \times 10^{-5}$ M).
Threonine deaminase (degradative) Shizuta and Tokushige (1971)	*Escherichia coli*	11	900	7.5–9.0	Degrades serine ($K_m = 5$ mM). Needs 10 mM AMP.
Trypotophanase Morino and Snell (1970)	*Escherichia coli* B	0.3	26.5	8.0	Also degrades cysteine and serine.
Histidine decarboxylase Recsei and Snell (1970)	*Lactobacillus* 30a	0.36	80	4.0–6.5	Above pH 6.5, the K_m increases greatly.

Vitamins, functioning in a catalytic role as coenzymes, are pivotal in many areas of tumor metabolism. The differential sensitivity of some tumors to either vitamin deficiency or vitamin antagonists points logically to the development of enzymes that could induce a vitamin-depleted state. This approach is particularly attractive, since the amount of substrate to be removed is much smaller than with amino acids. Furthermore, vitamins in general cannot be synthesized, and thus one does not face the problem of rapid replenishment of tissue stores.

A prototype enzyme has been the carboxypeptidase G_1 isolated from *Pseudomonas stutzeri*, which hydrolyzes glutamatic acid from reduced and non-reduced folic acid derivatives (McCullough *et al.*, 1971). This enzyme has been shown to inhibit the growth of several leukemias in culture, but was not particularly active *in vivo*. This may be related in part to the high serum levels of folates in mice compared with dogs and humans. Although the enzyme has a reasonably low K_m (10^{-5}), it must act on substrate concentrations in a region of 10^{-8} M. In addition, the tissue stores of folate derivatives are extensive, and preliminary courses of treatment in mice led to minimal depletion. The Walker 256 carcinosarcoma growth as a solid tumor is sensitive to dietary depletion of folates, but resistant to methotrexate; as might be hoped, carboxypeptidase G_1 also caused a 43–99% increase in survival time (Chabner *et al.*, 1972a). This difference may reflect the fact that methotrexate exerts the majority of its effects on thymidylate synthetase because of the coupling of that reaction to dihydrofolate reductase. Carboxypeptidase G_1, however, depletes all forms of folate coenzymes, and thus has an effect on purine and amino acid biosynthesis, as well as other folate-catalyzed reactions.

Preliminary clinical studies have indicated that the enzyme is rapidly cleared ($T_{1/2} = 6$–10 hr), but that it is capable of causing a reduction of circulating folates (Bertino *et al.*, 1974). Further studies await the preparation of larger quantities of this enzyme and the possible development of matrix-bound forms that could extend its effectiveness. An alternative use for the enzyme derives from the fact that methotrexate is also a substrate ($K_m = 4 \times 10^{-6}$ M). It has been possible to "rescue" experimental animals (Chabner *et al.*, 1972b) and man (Bertino *et al.*, 1974) from toxic doses of this folate antagonist by subsequent treatment with carboxypeptidase G_1. The immunosuppressive activity of this enzyme compared with asparaginase is not known at this time, but allergic reactions have been observed (Bertino *et al.*, 1974).

Another candidate for enzyme depletion is riboflavin (for a thorough review, see Rivlin, 1973). As early as 1943, the effect of riboflavin deficiency on tumor growth was noted. Many investigators have extended these observations, and some evidence exists for an effect of riboflavin deficiency on the rate of tumor growth in man (Lane *et al.*, 1964; Lane and Smith, 1971). Riboflavin analogues have also been shown to inhibit tumor growth, and can be used to create an apparently deficient state. It is of interest that the Novikoff hepatoma, which is sensitive to riboflavin deficiency *in vivo*, does not show any change in the concentration of FAD compared with tumors from normal animals at a time when the liver stores of FAD are seriously depleted (Rivlin *et al.*, 1973). It would seem that even more complete depletion might be created by use of a riboflavin-degrading enzyme, an approach that has not been reported.

Most of the other vitamins could be considered potential candidates for enzyme depletion studies. It might be appropriate to pay particular attention to enzymes that degrade pyridoxine, since vitamin B_6 analogues have been shown to exert antitumor effects, and B_6 deficiency inhibits tumor growth (Mihich and Nichol, 1965; Tryfiates and Morris, 1974). Similarly, nicotinamide could be considered an appropriate target, since antitumor activity has been reported for the analogue 6-amino-nicotinamide (Shapiro *et al.*, 1957; McColl *et al.*, 1957; Herter *et al.*, 1961). One report suggests that pantothenic acid deficiency inhibits tumor growth (Morris, 1947). There do not seem to be any suggestive leads to link fat-soluble vitamin deficiency to tumor inhibition.

5. Immunologic Enhancement

5.1. Neuraminidase

Aside from asparaginase, the most widely investigated enzyme therapy in malignant disease has employed neuraminidase. This enzyme, isolated from *Vibrio cholerae* or *Clostridium perfringens*, will cleave the glycoside linkages between sialic acid residues and mucopolysaccharides on the surfaces of cells. Injection of tumor cells treated with this enzyme may elicit an enhanced immune response, which will either retard the growth of established tumors of the same cell line or prevent successful takes by injection of untreated tumor cells (Simmons *et al.*, 1971; Sethi and Brandis, 1973). Several points of evidence support a specific immunologic basis for these effects: (1) heat-inactivated enzyme is without an effect; (2) the enzyme is without effect in an immunosuppressed animal; and (3) the tumor inhibitory activity is specific to the type of tumor, and other tumors bearing a shared mammary tumor virus antigen did not regress (Simmons and Rios, 1973*a*; Simmons *et al.*, 1971). Experiments have shown that the extent of treatment is important. L1210 cells treated *in vitro* with 250 U *V. cholerae* neuraminidase/ml evoked a less vigorous immune response than cells treated with 50 U/ml (Sethi and Brandis, 1973). Recently, Sedlacek *et al.* (1975) reported that injection with a mitomycin- and neuraminidase-treated cell suspension derived from a spontaneous mammary tumor would cause the remaining tumors in that dog to regress if 2×10^7 tumor cells were given; if 10^8 cells were given, tumor growth was accelerated. Direct injection of neuraminidase into spontaneous mammary adenocarcinoma in mice will retard tumor growth, but the best effects were observed with combination therapy including the nonspecific immunostimulant Bacillus Calmette-Guerin (BCG) (Simmons and Rios, 1973*b*). Varied results have been reported in the treatment of melanoma in humans with combination therapies that include neuraminidase treatment. Patients whose disease was confined to the skin, subcutaneous tissues, and lymph nodes seemed to benefit most, whereas patients whose disease had progressed to the visceral, skeletal, or central nervous system showed no benefit (Shingleton *et al.*, 1975; Seigler *et al.*, 1974). A preliminary report indicates that in patients with AML in whom a remission was induced by chemotherapy, the duration of remission was at least 4-fold longer in patients receiving chemotherapy plus intradermal neuraminidase-treated allogenic leukemic cells than in patients receiving chemotherapy alone (Bekesi *et al.*, 1976).

5.2. Proteolytic Enzymes

The intratumor injection of a proteolytic enzyme mixture termed "Wobe-Mugos" into spontaneous mammary adenomas in rats has been reported to cause tumor regression in 70% of the animals at a dose of 50 mg per injection. This therapy is reported to show a selective action on the tumor, with healthy tissues being "respected" by the enzymes (Weigelt, 1974; Wolf and Ransberger, 1972). The daily infusion of Protease 1 from *Aspergillus oryzae* (brinase) into patients with acute leukemia produced autocytotoxic antibodies and remission in 3 of 5 patients. The mechanisms of these effects are thought to include: (1) a direct cytolytic activity of the enzyme on the leukemic cells; (2) a reduction in antiplasmin, so that plasmin can act unopposed as a cytotoxic agent; and (3) the release or exposure of tumor antigens that enhance antibody formation (Thornes *et al.*, 1972). It must be recognized that in all these examples, a foreign protein is being injected, and at least a portion of any response observed may result from nonspecific stimulation of the immune response by such antigenic material.

5.3. Amino Acid Depletion

Sections 2 and 3 described the antitumor effects of diets deficient in certain amino acids. Jose and Good (1973) presented evidence that the dietary effects may not relate solely to the nutritional requirements of the tumor. Diets reduced in the amino acids phenylalanine and tyrosine, valine, threonine, methionine and cystine, isoleucine, and tryptophan reduced the production of hemagglutinating and "blocking" antibody responses with no loss in cytotoxic cell-mediated immunity. Limitations of arginine, histidine, and lysine in the diets depressed the humoral immune responses only slightly. Dietary restriction of leucine appeared to depress cytotoxic cell-mediated immunity, with little effect on serum blocking activity. Depletion of the nonessential amino acid asparagine by asparaginase therapy has been shown to suppress both cell-mediated and humoral immunity (Hersh, 1973). Since the balance between the humoral antibody response and cell-mediated cytotoxicity may affect the rate of tumor growth (see Hersh, Volume 6), these factors should be considered in the interpretation of amino acid depletions created by specific enzyme therapy.

JACK R.
UREN AND
ROBERT E.
HANDSCHUMACHER

6. Enzymes That Function Intracellularly

6.1. Xanthine Oxidase

Xanthine oxidase, an enzyme not detected in most malignant tissues, catalyzes the oxidation of both hypoxanthine and xanthine, the products of purine catabolism, to uric acid. A hypothesis concerning the basic properties of cancer cells formulated by Potter (1958) proposed that malignant tissues have deletions in the catabolic enzymes, which in turn stimulate the cell's synthetic ability. It was suggested that an injection of the catabolic enzyme xanthine oxidase may reestablish a balance between the synthetic and catabolic processes within the cell, and return cell growth rates to those of normal tissues. Haddow *et al.* (1958) injected purified bovine xanthine oxidase into mice bearing a spontaneous mammary tumor. The rate of tumor growth was decreased and the enzyme activity in the livers and tumors increased 2.5-fold. These results, which are discussed in greater detail by Bergel (1961), have not been extended.

6.2. Nucleases

Ribonuclease (RNase) has been reported to retard the growth of a spontaneous mammary carcinoma in mice (Bergel, 1961). However, the enzyme has been shown to be ineffective against the Ehrlich ascites carcinoma (Lamirande, 1961) and the tumors in the standard screen of the National Cancer Institute (Cooney and Rosenbluth, 1975). Sartorelli (1964) also reported the lack of an antitumor effect of RNase toward the sarcoma 180 tumor, but observed synergistic responses with a combination of RNase and actinomycin D therapy. A possible interpretation of these results was that actinomycin D inhibited the repair of RNA cleaved by the nuclease. Blumberg (1974) suggested that actinomycin D, RNase, or a combination of both, might exert this therapeutic effect by preventing synthesis of the RNA component of tumor angiogenesis factor. Recently, Bartholeyns and Baudhuin (1976) showed that inactivated RNase retains its tumor growth inhibitory activity *in vitro*. They suggest that this activity may result from an increased lability of lysosomes in the cells.

Deoxyribonuclease (DNase) has been shown to increase the survival of Ehrlich ascites carcinoma in mice from 34 to 67% (Lamirande, 1961). Data reported from the Drug Evaluation Branch of the National Cancer Institute showed that DNase is without demonstrable antineoplastic activity in their panel of experimental tumors (Cooney and Rosenbluth, 1975). A protein that may have nuclease activity and does show antineoplastic activity toward solid tumors and acute leukemia in man is neocarzinostatin (Beerman and Goldberg, 1974; Goldberg *et al.*, Chapter 15, Section 2.2.3). A catalytic, as opposed to stoichiometric, role in scission of the DNA strands by neocarzinostatin has yet to be established. These results suggest that other nucleases such as restriction endonucleases (Boyer, 1974) might be examined for antineoplastic activity.

Two plant proteins—abrin, isolated from *Abrus precatorius,* and ricin, from *Ricinus communis*—increase the survival of mice bearing the Ehrlich ascites tumor (Lin *et al.,* 1970). Olsnes *et al.* (1974) showed that these proteins each consist of two subunits, one of which binds to the cell surface, while the other enters the cell and inhibits protein synthesis. The mechanism by which the subunit inhibits protein synthesis is not completely elucidated, but it must be a catalytic action, since one toxin molecule can inactivate thousands of ribosomes in a cell-free system. A bacterial toxin isolated from *Corynebacterium diphtheriae* will increase the survival of mice bearing the Ehrlich ascites tumor or inhibit the rate of growth of the tumor as a solid form (Buzzi and Maistrello, 1973). The diphtheria toxin had been shown to inhibit protein synthesis by catalyzing a reaction between NAD and Elongation Factor II to form an inactive adenosine diphosphoribosyl derivative of Elongation Factor II (Gill *et al.,* 1973). Exotoxin A, which has a mechanism of action similar to diphtheria toxin, as well as cholera toxin and *E. coli* enterotoxin, which has two subunits (Kolata, 1975), might be candidates as antineoplastic agents.

7. The Future of Enzyme Therapy

7.1. Selection of Enzymes

This review of enzymes under consideration and being used to treat malignant disease suggests that when a qualitative or quantitative nutritional requirement of cancer cells is established, the kinetic properties of a depleting enzyme may be a limiting factor in the therapeutic response. This is particularly true for the enzymes arginase and methioninase, and is probably true for β-tyrosine phenol lyase, cystathionase, and carboxypeptidase G_1. At present, enzymes are obtained either by screening various microorganisms and plant and animal species for an enzyme with the desired kinetic properties or by selecting a microorganism capable of growth on the substrate of interest as a sole source for carbon or nitrogen or both (enrichment culture techniques; see Hayashi, 1955). While these procedures almost always produce an organism that has a desired enzyme, the kinetic properties of that enzyme are not always suitable. Attempts have been made to direct evolution of certain enzymes to improve their kinetic properties, as well as to define the process of evolution (Rigby *et al.,* 1974; Hegeman and Rosenberg, 1970). Organisms with more efficient enzymes than their parental strains have been selected (Betz *et al.,* 1974; T. T. Wu *et al.,* 1968), but more commonly, superproduction of the wild-type enzyme occurs. Future progress in understanding the mechanisms of evolution may lead to generalized procedures for the selection of more efficient enzymes.

Another future solution to these problems may be chemical synthesis or modification of enzymes. Chemical modification procedures have been used to alter enzyme specificity. The carboxyl group responsible for the binding of arginine and lysine residues to trypsin has been chemically modified; the modified enzyme lost activity toward basic substrates, but would still react with nonspecific titrants such as diisopropylfluorophosphate (DFP) (Feinstein *et al.*, 1969). Asparaginase has been modified by nitration with a greater loss of glutaminase activity than of asparaginase activity (Liu and Handschumacher, 1972). Hemoglobin S has been reacted with cyanate, and the carbamylated protein has a greater oxygen affinity than the native structure (Manning *et al.*, 1974). As more knowledge is gained about enzyme structure and function, it may be possible to alter enzyme specificities in more meaningful ways. We may even predict that the chemical synthesis of enzymes or active fragments with the desired specificity and activity will occur.

7.2. Overcoming the Biological Limitations

7.2.1. Substrate Accessibility

As indicated in Section 1, the macromolecular nature of enzymes restricts their vascular permeability, and consequently their substrate accessibility. Attempts have been made to create smaller enzymes by either subunit dissociation or the production of active fragments by limited proteolysis. To date, the preparation of active subunits of asparaginase by chemical modification procedures has been unsuccessful (Hare and Handschumacher, 1973; Shifrin and Grochowski, 1972). Aspartate transcarbamylase, on the other hand, has been dissociated by treatment with mercurials from an enzyme of 310,000 daltons to 96,000 daltons with retention of catalytic activity, but with loss of regulatory feedback inhibition activity (Gerhart and Schachman, 1965). The production of active fragments by limited proteolysis in general greatly reduces catalytic activity, e.g., staphylococcal nuclease (Sachs *et al.*, 1974). Perhaps cross-linkage followed by limited proteolysis may stabilize active site conformations and catalytic activity.

The observation that the plant and bacterial toxins have cell-binding capability as well as enzyme-mediated cytotoxicity suggests that enzyme penetration into cells may be aided by attachment to lectins or tumor-specific antibodies. The ability of antibodies to enhance the cytotoxicity of various anticancer agents including enzymes has been reported (Rubens, 1974), but much development work remains to establish the validity of this approach to human disease.

7.2.2. Drug Resistance and Host Sanctuaries

Depletion of nonessential amino acids with enzymes has had only limited success, partially because malignant cells become resistant by the expression of increased biosynthetic capacity for the depleted amino acid, and organs that have a large capacity for the biosynthesis of the depleted amino acid may act as sanctuaries for malignant cells. Attempts have been made to improve the effectiveness of enzyme therapy by combining the amino-acid-destroying enzyme with compounds that interfere with the amino acid biosynthesis. Uren and Handschumacher (1974) combined asparagine analogues and asparaginase therapy, with only limited success. The glutamine analogue 5-chloro-4-oxo-norvaline (CONV) has been combined with high doses of asparaginase, possibly taking advantage of the minor but significant glutaminase activity of the enzyme, to achieve synergistic responses in experimental animals (Burchenal *et al.*, 1970). The synergism between ribonuclease and actinomycin D was discussed in Section 6.2.

7.2.3. Clearance and Antigenicity of Foreign Proteins

Rapid rates of plasma clearance and the antigenicities of foreign proteins have continually plagued the enzyme therapist. Fortunately, some progress has been made in overcoming these difficulties. Chemical modification procedures have been used to alter both the rates of plasma clearance and the antigenicity. Both the *Erwinia* asparaginase and the *Acinetobacter* glutaminase–asparaginase have been chemically modified to decrease the isoelectric point and increase the plasma half-life (Rutter and Wade, 1971; Holcenberg *et al.*, 1975*a*). The increasing understanding of the role of carbohydrate groups in regulating the plasma half-lives of glycoproteins (Morell *et al.*, 1971; Rogers and Kornfeld, 1971) has led Holcenberg *et al.* (1975*b*) to glycosylate glutaminase–asparaginase. These procedures have increased the plasma half-life of the enzyme 4–15 fold. Glycosylation of the *E. coli* asparaginase increased the clearance rate severalfold (Marsh *et al.*, 1976). Further studies may produce generalized procedures to increase plasma half-lives of foreign proteins. Another approach may be the attachment of the foreign enzyme to a long-lived host component, such as a red blood cell, to determine whether it will act as a carrier to prolong the half-life of the foreign enzyme (Chen and Richardson, 1974). These procedures may also increase the antigenicity of the protein.

Chemical modification may also decrease antigenicity. Minor decreases in asparaginase antigenicity have been reported by acetylation (Makino *et al.*, 1975) and maleylation and amidination (Hare and Handschumacher, 1973). Extensive changes in antigenicity of trypsin have been reported by attachment of polyalanyl side chains (Arnon and Neurath, 1970), and of immunoglobulin G by attachment of polyhomocysteinyl side chains (Kendall, 1972). These more extensive modifications should be investigated with enzymes of therapeutic interest. Possibly, classes of antigenically distinct, chemically modified enzymes can be generated to treat patients who show immunogenic reactions to the parent enzyme, in the same way that *Erwinia* asparaginase is now used to treat patients who react to *E. coli* asparaginase. Rather than masking antigenetic determinants, it may also be possible to characterize and isolate the antigenic amino acid sequences and inject these sequences into the patients to develop immunologic tolerance to these determinants.

Another solution to these problems may be the introduction of a physical barrier between the therapeutic enzyme and the immune recognition and clearance mechanisms of the host. T. M. S. Chang (1971) and Chong and Chang (1974) entrapped asparaginase in semipermeable nylon microcapsules and injected these microcapsules into mice. The microcapsules prolonged the ability of asparaginase to deplete asparagine from the blood, and were more effective at increasing the survival of mice implanted with lymphosarcoma. The pore size in the microcapsules is too small to allow antibodies or proteases to interact with the entrapped enzyme. The ability to entrap enzymes would also permit development of therapy with multienzyme complexes, in which the product of the first enzyme may be the substrate for the next. This approach could be used to shift unfavorable equilibria to completion or to detoxify unwanted products. Similarly, one enzyme may be used to generate cofactors or cosubstrates for another. If encapsulation procedures can be expanded to generate long-lived circulating microcapsules, the real value of "artificial cells" may be realized. The modification of erythrocytes with entrapment of foreign proteins by a hemolysis technique was reported by Ihler *et al.* (1973), and may offer an immunologically neutral means of introducing enzymes. These procedures have been shown not to alter the transport capability or, in preliminary trials, the life span of the modified erythrocytes (Ihler *et al.*, 1975). It should be recognized that the success of this approach requires that the target substrate and its products have an adequate permeation rate or be transported across the erythrocyte membrane.

7.3. Conclusion

In conclusion, enzyme therapy has moved from a theoretical concept to a recognized mode of treatment in at least one case, asparaginase. The continuing search for qualitative or quantitative differences in the nutritional requirements of cancer cells or their susceptibility to catalytic alteration will undoubtedly uncover other targets for modification by enzymes. The high degree of specificity of enzymes, as well as rapidly expanding competence in macromolecular chemistry, assures that such biochemical leads can be developed for therapeutic evaluation.

ACKNOWLEDGMENTS

Work in these laboratories was supported by USPHS Grants CA10101 and CA10748, by American Cancer Society Grant PDT-47P, and by NCI Grants CA06516 and CA18917.

8. References

ABELL, C. W., STITH, W. J., AND HODGKINS, D. S., 1972, The effects of phenylalanine ammonia-lyase on leukemic lymphocytes *in vitro*, *Cancer Res.* **32:**285.
ABELL, C. W., HODGKINS, D. S., AND STITH, W. J., 1973, An *in vivo* evaluation of the chemotherapeutic potency of phenylalanine ammonia-lyase, *Cancer Res.* **33:**2529.
ADAMSON, R. H., AND FABRO, S. 1968, Antitumor activity and other biologic properties of L-asparaginase (NSC-109229)—a review, *Cancer Chemother. Rep.* **52**(6):617.

ARNON, R., AND NEURATH, H., 1970, Immunochemical studies on bovine trypsin and trypsinogen derivatives, *Immunochemistry* **7**:241.

ASHWORTH, L. A. E., AND MACLENNAN, A. P., 1974, Comparison of the L-asparaginases from *Escherichia coli* and *carotovora* as immunosuppressants, *Cancer Res.* **34**:1353.

ASTALDI, G., 1972, Is L-asparaginase an antiblastic agent? *Haematologia* **6**:433.

ASTALDI, G., BURGIO, G. R., KRC, J., GENOVA, R., AND ASTALDI, A. A., JR., 1969, L-Asparaginase and blastogensis, *Lancet* **1**:423.

BAECHTEL, F. S., GREGG, D. E., AND PRAGER, M. D., 1976, The influence of glutamine, its decomposition products, and glutaminase on the transformation of human and mouse lymphocytes, *Biochim. Biophys. Acta* **421**:33.

BARTHOLEYNS, J., AND BAUDHUIN, P., 1976, Inhibition of tumor cell proliferation by dimerized ribonuclease, *Proc. Natl. Acad. Sci. U.S.A.* **73**:573.

BECKER, F. F., AND BROOME, J. D., 1967, L-Asparaginase: Inhibition of early mitosis in regenerating rat liver, *Science* **156**:1602.

BEERMAN, T. A., AND GOLDBERG, I. H., 1974, DNA strand scission by the antitumor protein neocarzinostatin, *Biochem. Biophys. Res. Commun.* **59**:1254.

BEKESI, J. G., HOLLAND, J. F., CUTTNER, J., SILVER, R., COLEMAN, M., JAROWSKI, C., AND VINCEGUERRA, V., 1976, Immunotherapy in acute myelocytic leukemia (AML) with neuraminidase (N'ASE) treated allogenic myeloblasts with or without MER, *Proc. Amer. Assoc. Cancer Res.* **35**:184.

BERGEL, F., 1961, *Chemistry of Enzymes in Cancer*, pp. 65–70, Charles C Thomas, Springfield, Illinois.

BERNARD, J., BOIRON, M., JACQUILLAT, C., WEIL, M., AND LEVY D. (eds.), 1970, *La L-Asparaginase*, Editions du Centre National de la Recherche Scientifique, Paris.

BERTINO, J. R., SKEEL, R., MAKULU, D., MCINTOSH, S., UHOCH, J., AND CHABNER, B., 1974, Initial clinical studies with carboxypeptidase G₁ (CPG₁): A folate depleting enzyme, *Clin. Res.* **22**:483a.

BETTIGOLE, R. E., HIMELSTEIN, E. S., OETTGEN, H. F., AND CLIFFORD, G. O., 1970, Hypofibrinogenemia due to L-asparaginase: Studies of fibrinogen survival using autologous ^{131}I-fibrinogen, *Blood* **35**:195.

BETZ, J. L., BROWN, P. R., SMYTH, M. J., AND CLARKE, P. H., 1974, Evolution in action, *Nature (London)* **247**:261.

BLUMBERG, N., 1974, Tumor angiogenesis factor: Speculations on an approach to cancer chemotherapy, *Yale J. Biol. Med.* **47**:71.

BOSMANN, H. B., 1972, Antineoplastic drug activity in the mitotic cycle—effects of six agents on macromolecular synthesis in synchronous mammalian leukemic cells, *Biochem. Pharmacol.* **21**:1977.

BOYER, H. W., 1974, Restriction and modification of DNA: Enzymes and substrates, *Fed. Proc. Fed. Amer. Soc. Exp. Biol.* **33**:1125.

BROOME, J. D., 1963a, Evidence that the L-asparaginase of guinea pig serum is responsible for its antilymphoma effects. I. Properties of the L-asparaginase of guinea pig serum in relation to those of the antilymphoma substance, *J. Exp. Med.* **118**:99.

BROOME, J. D., 1963b, Evidence that the L-asparaginase of guinea pig serum is responsible for its antilymphoma effects. II. Lymphoma 6C3HED cells cultured in a medium devoid of L-asparagine lose their susceptibility to the effects of guinea pig serum *in vivo*, *J. Exp. Med.* **118**:121.

BURCHENAL, J. H., CLARKSON, B. D., DOWLING, M. D., GEE, T., HAGHBIN, M., AND TAN, C. T. C., 1970, Experimental and clinical studies of L-asparaginase in combination therapy, in: *La L-Asparaginase* (J. Bernard, M. Boiron, C. Jacquillat, M. Weil, and D. Levy, eds.), pp. 243–248, Editions de Centre National de la Recherche Scientifique, Paris.

BURNS, R. O., 1971, L-Threonine deaminase—biosynthetic (*Salmonel la typhimurium*), in: *Methods in Enzymology* (H. Tabor and C. W. Tabor, eds.), Vol. 17B, pp. 555–560, Academic Press, New York.

BUZZI, S., AND MAISTRELLO, I., 1973, Inhibition of growth of Ehrlich tumors in Swiss mice by diphtheria toxin, *Cancer Res.* **33**:2349.

CAPIZZI, R. L., 1975, Improvement in the therapeutic index of L-asparaginase by methotrexate, *Cancer Chemother. Rep.* **6**(3):37.

CAPIZZI, R. L., BERTINO, J. R., AND HANDSCHUMACHER, R. E., 1970, L-Asparaginase, *Annu. Rev. Med.* **21**:433.

CAPIZZI, R. L., SUMMERS, W. P., AND BERTINO, J. R., 1971, L-Asparaginase induced alteration of methotrexate activity in mouse leukemia L5178Y, *Ann. N. Y. Acad. Sci.* **186**:302.

CAPIZZI, R., CASTRO, O., ASPNES, G., BOBROW, S., BERTINO, J., FINCH, S., AND PEARSON, H., 1974, Treatment of acute lymphocytic leukemia (ALL) with intermittent high dose methotrexate (MTX) and asparaginase, *Proc. Amer. Assoc. Cancer Res.* **15**:182.

CHABNER, B. A., CHELLO, P. L., AND BERTINO, J. R., 1972a, Antitumor activity of a folate-cleaving enzyme, carboxypeptidase G1, *Cancer Res.* **32**:2114.

CHABNER, B. A., JOHNS, D. G., AND BERTINO, J. R., 1972b, Enzymic cleavage of methotrexate provides a method for prevention of drug toxicity, *Nature (London)* **239:**395.

CHANG, P. K., 1976, *O*-L-Homoserine-5'-adenylate (USAMP). Esterification of 5'-adenylic acid with the gamma-hydroxyl group of L-homoserine, in: *Synthetic Procedures in Nucleic Acid Chemistry,* Vol. III (L. Townsend, ed.), John Wiley and Sons, New York.

CHANG, T. M. S., 1971, The *in vivo* effects of semipermeable microcapsules containing L-asparaginase on 6C3HED lymphosarcoma, *Nature (London)* **229:**117.

CHEN, L. F., AND RICHARDSON, T., 1974, Enzyme derivatives containing reactive groups. Immobilization of alpha-amylase on human erythrocytes, *Pharmacol. Res. Commun.* **6:**273.

CHONG, E. O. S., AND CHANG, T. M. S., 1974, *In vivo* effects of intraperitoneally injected L-asparaginase solution and L-asparaginase immobilized within semipermeable nylon microcapsules with emphasis on blood L-asparaginase, "body" L-asparaginase, and plasma L-asparagine levels, *Enzyme* **18:**218.

CHOU, T. C., AND HANDSCHUMACHER, R. E., 1972, Production of L-asparagine by tumor cells and the effect of asparagine analogs, *Biochem. Pharmacol.* **21:**39.

COONEY, D. A., AND HANDSCHUMACHER, R. E., 1970, L-Asparaginase and L-asparagine metabolism, *Annu. Rev. Pharmacol.* **10:**421.

COONEY, D. A., AND ROSENBLUTH, R. J., 1975, Enzymes as therapeutic agents, *Adv. Pharmacol. Chemother.* **12:**185.

COONEY, D. A., CAPIZZI, R. L., AND HANDSCHUMACHER, R. E., 1970, Evaluation of L-asparagine metabolism in animals and man, *Cancer Res.* **30:**929.

DEMOPOULOS, H. B., 1966a, Effects of low phenylalanine–tyrosine diets on S91 mouse melanomas, *J. Natl. Cancer Inst.* **37:**185.

DEMOPOULOS, H. B., 1966b, Effects of reducing the phenylalanine–tyrosine intake of patients with advanced malignant melanoma, *Cancer* **19:**657.

DEODHAR, S. D., 1973, Enhancement of metastases by L-asparaginase in allogeneic and isogeneic mouse tumor systems, *Adv. Exp. Med. Biol.* **29:**519.

DISTASIO, J. A., AND NIEDERMAN, R. A., 1976, Purification and characterization of L-asparaginase with antilymphoma activity from *Vibrio succinogenes, J. Biol. Chem.* **251:**6929.

ELLISON, R. R., KARNOFSKY, D. A., STERNBERG, S. S., MURPHY, M. L., AND BURCHENAL, J. H., 1954, Clinical trials of *O*-diazoacetyl-L-serine (azaserine) in neoplastic disease, *Cancer* **7:**801.

ENGASSER, J.-M., AND HORVATH, C., 1976, Diffusion and kinetics with immobilized enzymes, in: *Applied Biochemistry and Bioengineering,* Vol. I (L. B. Wingard, Jr., E. Katzir-Katchalski, and L. Goldstein, eds.), pp. 127–220, Academic Press, New York.

FEINSTEIN, G., BODLAENDER, P., AND SHAW, E., 1969, The modification of essential carboxylic acid side chains of trypsin, *Biochemistry* **8:**4949.

FOLEY, G. E., BARELL, E. F., ADAMS, R. A., AND LAZARUS, H., 1969, Nutritional requirements of human leukemic cells. Cystine requirements of diploid cell lines and their heteroploid variants, *Exp. Cell Res.* **57:**129.

GERHART, J. C., AND SCHACHMAN, H. K., 1965, Distinct subunits for the regulation and catalytic activity of aspartate transcarbamylase, *Biochemistry* **4:**1054.

GILL, D. M., PAPPENHEIMER, A. M., AND UCHIDA, T., 1973, Diphtheria toxin, protein synthesis, and the cell, *Fed. Proc. Fed. Amer. Soc. Exp. Biol.* **32:**1508.

GOLDBERG, A. I., COONEY, D. A., GLYNN, J. P., HOMAN, E. R., GASTON, M. R., AND MILMAN, H. A., 1973, The effects of immunization to L-asparaginase on antitumor and enzymatic activity, *Cancer Res.* **33:**256.

GOLDSTEIN, A., ARONOW, L., AND KALMAN, S., 1974, *Principles of Drug Action: The Basis of Pharmacology,* p. 166, John Wiley and Sons, New York.

GREENBERG, D. M., AND SASSENRATH, E. N., 1953, Lack of effect of high potency arginase on tumor growth, *Cancer Res.* **13:**709.

GRUNDMANN, E., AND OETTGEN, H. F. (eds.), 1970, *Experimental and Clinical Effects of L-Asparaginase,* Springer-Verlag, New York—Heidelberg—Berlin.

GUMPRECHT, J. G., AND WRISTON, J. C., 1973, Purification and partial sequencing of cyanogen bromide peptides from L-asparaginase of *Escherichia coli, Biochemistry* **12:**4869.

HADDOW, A., LAMIRANDE, G. P., BERGEL, F., BRAY, R. C., AND GILBERT, D. A., 1958, Antitumor and biochemical effects of purified bovine xanthine oxidase in C3H and C mice, *Nature (London)* **182:**1144.

HALEY, E. E., FISCHER, G. A., AND WELCH, A. D., 1961, The requirement for L-asparagine of mouse leukemia cells L5178Y in culture, *Cancer Res.* **21:**532.

HALPERN, B. C., CLARK, B. R., HARDY, D. N., HALPERN, R. M., AND SMITH, R. A., 1974, The effect of replacement of methionine by homocystine on survival of malignant and normal adult mammalian cells in culture, *Proc. Natl. Acad. Sci. U.S.A.* **71**:1133.

HAN, T., AND OHNUMA, T., 1972, L-Asparaginase: *In vitro* inhibition of blastogenesis by enzyme from *Erwinia catotovora*, *Nature (London) New Biol.* **239**:50.

HARE, L. E., AND HANDSCHUMACHER, R. E., 1973, Physical and biological properties of acetamidino-, β-dimethylaminopropionamidino-, and maleyl-L-asparaginase, *Mol. Pharmacol.* **9**:534.

HASKELL, C. M., AND CANELLOS, G. P., 1969, L-Asparaginase resistance in human leukemia—asparagine synthetase, *Biochem. Pharmacol.* **18**:2578.

HASKELL, C. M., CANELLOS, G. P., LEVENTHAL, B. G., CARBONE, P. P., BLOCK, J. B., SERPICK, A. A., AND SELAWRY, O. S., 1969, L-Asparaginase: Effects in patients with neoplastic disease, *N. Engl. J. Med.* **281**:1028.

HAYASHI, O., 1955, Special techniques for bacterial enzymes. Enrichment culture and adaptive enzymes, in: *Methods in Enzymology* (S. P. Colowick and N. O. Kaplan, eds.), Vol. 1, pp. 126–137, Academic Press, New York.

HEGEMAN, G. D., AND ROSENBERG, S. L., 1970, The evolution of bacterial enzyme systems, *Annu. Rev. Microbiol.* **24**:429.

HERSH, E. M., 1971, L-Glutaminase: Suppression of lymphocyte blastogenic responses *in vitro*, *Science* **172**:736.

HERSH, E. M., 1973, Immunosuppressive enzymes, *Transplant. Proc.* **5**:1211.

HERTER, F. P., WEISSMAN, S. G., THOMPSON, H. G., HYMAN, G., AND MARTIN, D. S., 1961, Clinical experience with 6-amino nicotinamide, *Cancer Res.* **21**:31.

HO, P. H. W., THETFORD, B., CARTER, C. J. K., AND FREI, E., 1970, Clinical pharmacologic studies of L-asparaginase, *Clin. Pharmacol. Ther.* **11**:408.

HO, P. P. K., AND MILLIKIN, E. B., 1970, Multiple forms of L-asparaginase, *Biochim. Biophys. Acta* **206**:196.

HOLCENBERG, J. S., AND ROBERTS, J., 1977, Enzymes as drugs, *Annu. Rev. Pharmacol.* **17**.

HOLCENBERG, J. S., ROBERTS, J., AND DOLOWY, W. C., 1973, Glutaminases as antineoplastic agents, in: *The Enzymes of Glutamine Metabolism* (S. Prusiner and G. Stadtman, eds.), pp. 277–292, Academic Press, New York and London.

HOLCENBERG, J. S., SCHIMER, G., TELLER, D. C., AND ROBERTS, J., 1975a, Biologic and physical properties of succinylated and glycosylated *Acinetobacter* glutaminase–asparaginase, *J. Biol. Chem.* **250**:4165.

HOLCENBERG, J. S., TANG, E., AND DOLOWY, W. C., 1975b, Effect of *Acinetobacter* glutaminase–asparaginase treatment on free amino acids in mouse tissues, *Cancer Res.* **35**:1320.

HOROWITZ, B., AND MEISTER, A., 1972, Glutamine-dependent asparagine synthetase from leukemia cells, *J. Biol. Chem.* **247**:6708.

HOROWITZ, B., MADRAS, B. K., MEISTER, A., OLD, L. S., BOYCE, E. A., AND STOCKERT, E., 1968, Asparagine synthetase activity of mouse leukemias, *Science* **160**:533.

HOWARD, J. B., AND CARPENTER, F. H., 1972, L-Asparaginase from *Erwinia carotovora*. Substrate specificity and enzymatic properties, *J. Biol. Chem.* **247**:1020.

IHLER, G. M., GLEW, R. H., AND SCHNURE, F. W., 1973, Enzyme loading of erythrocytes, *Proc. Natl. Acad. Sci. U.S.A.* **70**:2663.

IHLER, G. M., LANTZY, A., PURPURA, J., AND GLEW, R. H., 1975, Enzymatic degradation of uric acid by urease-loaded human erythrocytes, *J. Clin. Invest.* **56**:595.

JACKSON, R. C., AND HANDSCHUMACHER, R. E., 1970, *Escherichia coli* L-asparaginase. Catalytic activity and subunit nature, *Biochemistry* **9**:3585.

JOSE, D. G., AND GOOD, R. A., 1973, Quantitative effects of nutritional essential amino acid deficiency upon immune responses to tumors in mice, *J. Exp. Med.* **137**:1.

KENDALL, P. A., 1972, Antibody labelling for electron microscopy: Immunochemical properties of immunoglobulin G heavily labeled with methylmercury after thiolation by homocysteine thiolactone, *Biochim. Biophys. Acta* **257**:101.

KIDD, J. D., 1953, Regression of transplanted lymphomas induced *in vivo* by means of normal guinea pig serum, *J. Exp. Med.* **98**:565.

KOLATA, G. B., 1975, Intracellular bacterial toxins: Origins and effects, *Science* **190**:969.

KREIS, W., AND HESSION, C., 1973a, Isolation and purification of L-methionine-α-deamino-γ-mercaptomethane-lyase (L-methionase) from *Clostridium sporogenes*, *Cancer Res.* **33**:1862.

KREIS, W., AND HESSION, C., 1973b, Biological effects of enzymatic deprivation of L-methionine in cell culture and an experimental tumor, *Cancer Res.* **33**:1866.

LABOUREUR, P., LANGLOIS, C., LABROUSSE, M., BOUDON, M., EMERAUD, J., SAMAIN, J. F., AGERON, M., AND DUMESNIL, Y., 1971, L-Asparaginases *d'Escherichia coli*. II. Pluralite et origine des formes moleculaires. Relations avec l'activite biologique, *Biochimie* **53**:1157.

LAMIRANDE, G. D., 1961, Action of deoxyribonuclease and ribonuclease on the growth of Ehrlich ascites carcinoma in mice, *Nature (London)* **192**:52.

LAND, V. J., SUTOW, W. W., FERNBACH, D. J., LANE, D. M., AND WILLIAMS, T. E., 1972, Toxicity of L-asparaginase in children with advanced leukemia, *Cancer* **30**:339.

LANE, M., AND SMITH, F. E., 1971, Induced riboflavin deficiency in treatment of patients with lymphomas and polycythemia vera, *Proc. Amer. Assoc. Cancer Res.* **12**:85.

LANE, M., ALFREY, C. P., MENGEL, C. E., DOHERTY, M. A., AND DOHERTY, J., 1964, The rapid induction of human riboflavin deficiency with galactoflavin, *J. Clin. Invest.* **43**:357.

LAZARUS, H., BARELL, E. F., OPPENHEIM, S., AND KRISHAN, A., 1974, Divergent properties of two human lymphocytic cell lines isolated from a single specimen of peripheral blood, *In Vitro* **9**:303.

LEVIN, B., AND MERRILL, J. P., 1972, Immunosuppressive effects of cyclophosphamide and L-asparaginase in the inbred rat renal transplant model, *Transplantation* **13**:160.

LIN, J. Y., TSERNG, K. Y., CHEN, C. L., LIN, L. T., AND TUNG, T. C., 1970, Abrin and ricin: New antitumor substances, *Nature (London)* **227**:292.

LIU, Y. P., AND HANDSCHUMACHER, R. E., 1972, Nitroasparaginase: Subunit cross-linkage and altered substrate specificity, *J. Biol. Chem.* **247**:66.

LIVINGSTON, D. M., FERGUSON, C., GALLOGLY, R., AND LAZARUS, H., 1976, Accumulation of cystine auxotrophic thymocytes accompanying Type C viral leukemogenesis in the mouse, *Cell* **7**:41.

LORINCZ, A. B., KUTTNER, R. E., AND BRANDT, M. B., 1969, Tumor response to phenylalanine–tyrosine limited diets, *J. Amer. Diet. Assoc.* **54**:198.

MAITA, T., MOROKUMA, K., AND MATSUDA, G., 1974, Amino acid sequence of L-asparaginase from *Escherichia coli*, *J. Biochem.* **76**:1351.

MAKINO, H., SATOH, H., KUROIWA, Y., YANAZAKI, S., TAMAURA, Y., AND INADA, Y., 1975, Immunochemical properties of asparaginase modified by chemical substitutions, *Immunochemistry* **12**:183.

MANNING, J. M., CERAMI, A., GILLETTE, P. N., DEFURIA, F. G., AND MILLER, D. R., 1974, Biochemical and physiological properties of carbamylated hemoglobin S, *Adv. Enzymol.* **40**:1.

MARSH, J. W., DENIS, I., AND WRISTON, J. C., 1976, Effect of glycosylation on clearance of E. coli asparaginase in mice, *Fed. Proc.* **35**:1371.

MASHBURN, L. T., AND WRISTON, J. C., 1964, Tumor inhibitory effect of L-asparaginase from *Escherichia coli*, *Arch. Biochem. Biophys.* **105**:450.

McCOLL, J. D., RICE, W. B., AND ADAMKIEWICZ, V. W., 1957, Inhibition of Walker carcinoma 256 by 6-amino nicotinamide, *Can. J. Biochem.* **35**:795.

McCULLOUGH, J. L., CHABNER, B. A., AND BERTINO, J. R., 1971, Purification and properties of carboxypeptidase G₁, *J. Biol. Chem.* **246**:7207.

MEADOWS, G. G., DiGIOVANNI, J., MINOR, J., AND ELMER, G. W., 1976, Some biological properties and an *in vivo* evaluation of tyrosine phenol-lyase on growth of B-16 melanoma, *Cancer Res.* **36**:167.

MIHICH, E., AND NICHOL, A. A., 1965, Antitumor effects of methylglyoxal-*bis*-(*N*⁴-methylthiosemicarbazone) and their potentiation in pyridoxine-deficient animals, *Cancer Res.* **25**:794.

MIKAMI, T., OHUMA, M., AND HAYASHI, T. T. A., 1974, Requirement of arginine for the replication of Marek's disease herpes virus, *J. Gen. Virol.* **22**:115.

MILLER, H. K., SALSER, J. S., AND BALIS, M. E., 1969, Amino acid levels following L-asparagine amidohydrolase (EC.3.5.1.1) therapy, *Cancer Res.* **29**:183.

MORELL, A. G., GREGORIADIS, G., SCHEINBERG, I. H. HICKMAN, J., AND ASHWELL, G., 1971. The role of sialic acid in determining the survival of glycoproteins in the circulation, *J. Biol. Chem.* **246**:1461.

MORINO, Y., AND SNELL, E. E., 1970, Tryptophanase (*Escherichia coli B*), in: *Methods in Enzymology* (H. Tabor and C. W. Tabor, eds.), Vol. 17A, pp. 439–446, Academic Press, New York.

MORRIS, H. P., 1947, Effects on the genesis and growth of tumors associated with vitamin intake, *Ann. N. Y. Acad. Sci.* **49**:119.

NESBITT, M., CHARD, R., EVANS, A., KARON, M., AND HAMMOND, D., 1970, Intermittent L-asparaginase therapy for acute childhood leukemia, *Proceedings of the 10th International Cancer Congress*, p. 447.

NEUKOMM, S., THOMPSON, C. B., AND BIOSSONNAZ, M., 1949, Action de l'arginase pure sur la croissance du cancer greffe de la souris, *Experientia* **5**:239.

NEWMAN, R. E., AND MCCOY, T. A., 1956, Dual requirement of Walker carcinosarcoma 256 *in vitro* for asparagine and glutamine, *Science* **124:**124.

NEWCOMB, E., AND MINOCHA, H. C., 1973, Amino acid requirement for fibroma virus replication in rabbit kidney cells, *Amer. J. Vet. Res.* **34:**261.

NEWTON, W. A., ERTEL, I. J., NESBIT, M., THATCHER, L. G., KARON, M., AND HAMMOND, G. B., 1973, Effective dose of L-asparaginase in acute leukemia, *Proc. Amer. Assoc. Cancer Res.* **14:**78.

OHNO, R., AND HERSH, E. M., 1970, Immunosuppressive effects of L-asparaginase, *Cancer Res.* **30:**1605.

OHNUMA, T., HOLLAND, J. F., NAGEL, G., AND ST. ARNEAULT, G., 1969, Effects of L-asparaginase in acute myelocytic leukemia, *J. Amer. Med. Assoc.* **210:**1919.

OHNUMA, T., WALIGUNDA, J., AND HOLLAND, J. F., 1971, Amino acid requirements *in vitro* of human leukemic cells, *Cancer Res.* **31:**1640.

OHNUMA, T., HOLLAND, J. F., AND MEYER, P., 1972, *Erwinia carotovora* asparaginase in patients with prior anaphylaxis to asparaginase from *E. coli*, *Cancer* **30:**376.

OKI, T., SHIRAI, M., OHSHIMA, M., YAMAMOTO, T., AND SODA, K., 1973, Antitumor activities of bacterial leucine dehydrogenase and glutaminase A, *FEBS Lett.* **33:**286.

OLD, L. J., BOYSE, E. A., CAMPBELL, H. A., BRODEY, R. S., FIDLER, J., AND TELLER, J. D., 1967, Treatment of lymphosarcoma in the dog with L-asparaginase, *Cancer* **20:**1066.

OLSNES, S., REFSNES, K., AND PIJL, A., 1974, Mechanism of action of the toxic lectins abrin and ricin, *Nature (London)* **249:**627.

ORTEGA, J., NESBIT, M., DONALDSON, M., WEINER, J., HITTLE, R., AND KARON M., 1975, L-Asparaginase, vincristine and prednisone for induction of first remission in acute lymphocytic leukemia (ALL), *Proc. Amer. Assoc. Cancer Res.* **16:**140.

PATTERSON, M. K., JR., AND ORR, G. R., 1969, Regeneration, tumor, dietary and L-asparaginase effects on asparagine biosynthesis in rat liver, *Cancer Res.* **29:**1179.

PEARSALL, N. N., AND WEISER, R. S., 1970, *The Macrophage*, p. 65, Lea and Febiger, Philadelphia.

PETERSON, R. G., HANDSCHUMACHER, R. E., AND MITCHELL, M. S., 1971, Immunological responses to L-asparaginase, *J. Clin. Invest.* **50:**1080.

POTTER, V. R., 1958, The biochemical approach to the cancer problem, *Fed. Proc. Fed. Amer. Soc. Exp. Biol.* **17:**691.

PRAGER, M. D., AND BACHYNSKY, N., 1968, Asparagine synthetase in normal and malignant tissues: Correlation with tumor sensitivity to asparaginase, *Arch. Biochem. Biophys.* **127:**645.

RECSEI, P. A., AND SNELL, E. E., 1970, Histidine decarboxylase of *Lactobacillus* 30a. VI. Mechanism of action and kinetic properties, *Biochemistry* **9:**1492.

REGAN, J. D., VODOPICK, H., TAKEDA, S., LEE, W. H., AND FAULCON, F. M., 1969, Serine requirement in leukemic and normal blood cells, *Science* **163:**1452.

RIGBY, P. W. J., BURLEIGH, B. D., AND HARTLEY, B. S., 1974, Gene duplication in experimental enzyme evolution, *Nature (London)* **251:**200.

RILEY, V., 1968, Role of the LDH-elevating virus in leukemia therapy by asparaginase, *Nature (London)* **220:**1245.

RILEY, V., CAMPBELL, H. A., AND STOCK, C. C., 1970, Asparaginase clearance: Influence of the LDH-elevating virus, *Proc. Soc. Exp. Biol. Med.* **133:**3.

RIVLIN, R. S., 1973, Riboflavin and cancer: A review, *Cancer Res.* **33:**1977.

RIVLIN, R. S., HORNIBROOK, R., AND OSNOS, M., 1973, Effects of riboflavin deficiency upon concentrations of riboflavin mononucleotide and flavin adenine dinucleotide in Novikoff hepatoma in rats, *Cancer Res.* **33:**3019.

ROBERTS, J., 1976, Purification and properties of highly potent antitumor glutaminase–asparaginase from *Pseudomonas* 7a, *J. Biol. Chem.* **251:**2119.

ROBERTS, J., AND SCHMID, F. A., 1976, Biological and antineoplastic properties of a novel *Pseudomonas* glutaminase–asparaginase with high therapeutic efficacy, *Proc. Amer. Assoc. Cancer Res.* **17:**26.

ROBERTS, J., SCHMID, F. A., AND TAKAI, K., 1974, The *in vivo* effects of leucine dehydrogenase from *Bacillus sphaericus*, *FEBS Letters* **43:**56.

ROBERTS, J., SCHMID, F. A., AND TAKAI, K., 1976, *In vivo* effects of phenylalanine ammonia lyase, *Cancer Treatment Rep.* **60:**261.

ROGERS, J. C., AND KORNFELD, S., 1971, Hepatic uptake of proteins coupled to feteuin glycopeptide, *Biochem. Biophys. Res. Commun.* **45:**622.

ROHOLT, O. A., AND GREENBERG, D. M., 1956, Liver arginase. IV. Effects of pH on kinetics of manganese-activated enzyme, *Arch. Biochem. Biophys.* **62:**454.

RUBENS, R. D., 1974, Antibodies as carriers of anticancer agents, *Lancet* **1974:**498.

RUTTER, D. A., AND WADE, H. E., 1971, The influence of the iso-electric point of L-asparaginase upon its persistence in the blood, *Br. J. Exp. Pathol.* **52:**610.

RYAN, W. L., AND CURTIS, G. L., 1973, Immunity and asparaginase suppression of tumor growth, *J. Natl. Cancer Inst.* **51:**147.

SACHS, D. H., SCHECHTER, A. N., EASTLAKE, A., AND ANFINSEN, C. B., 1974, Immunological distinction between the possible origins of enzymatic activity in a polypeptide fragment of staphylococcal nuclease, *Nature (London)* **251:**242.

SAGERS, R. D., AND CARTER, J. E., 1971, L-Serine dehydratase (*Clostridium acidiurici*), in: *Methods in Enzymology* (H. Tabor and C. W. Tabor, eds.), Vol. 17B, pp. 351–356, Academic Press, New York.

SARTORELLI, A. C., 1964, Combination chemotherapy with actinomycin D and ribonuclease: An example of complementary inhibition, *Nature (London)* **203:**877.

SAUNDERS, E. F., 1972, The effect of L-asparaginase on the nucleic acid metabolism and cell cycle of human leukemia cells, *Blood* **39:**575.

SCHMID, F. A., AND ROBERTS, J., 1974, Antineoplastic and toxic effects of *Acinetobacter* and *Pseudomonas* glutaminase–asparaginase, *Cancer Chemother. Rep.* **58:**829.

SCHWARTZ, R. S., 1969, L-Asparaginase acts as an immunosuppressant in mice, *Nature (London)* **224:**275.

SEDLACEK, H. H., MEESMANN, H., AND SEILER, F. R., 1975, Regression of spontaneous mammary tumors in dogs after injection of neuraminidase-treated tumor cells, *Int. J. Cancer* **15:**409.

SEIGLER, H. F., SHINGLETON, W. W., AND PICKRELL, K. L., 1974, Intralesional BCG, intravenous immuno lymphocytes, and immunization with neuraminidase-treated tumor cells to manage melanoma, *Plast. Reconstr. Surg.* **55:**294.

SETHI, K. K., AND BRANDIS, H., 1973, Neuraminidase induced loss in the transplantability of murine leukemia L1210, induction of immunoprotection and the transfer of induced immunity to normal DBA/2 mice by serum and peritoneal cells, *Br. J. Cancer* **27:**106.

SHAPIRO, D. M., DIETRICH, L. S., AND SHILS, M. E., 1957, Quantitative biochemical differences between tumor and host as a basis for cancer chemotherapy, V. Niacin and nicotinamide, *Cancer Res.* **17:**600.

SHIFRIN, S., AND GROCHOWSKI, B. J., 1972, L-Asparaginase from *Escherichia coli* B. Succinylation and subunit interaction, *J. Biol. Chem.* **247:**1048.

SHIFRIN, S., LUBORSKY, S. W., AND GROCHOWSKI, B. J., 1971, L-Asparaginase from *Escherichia coli* B. Physiocochemical studies of the dissociation process, *J. Biol. Chem.* **246:**7708.

SHINGLETON, W. W., SEIGLER, H. F., STOCKS, L. H., AND DOWNS, R. W., 1975, Management of recurrent melanoma of the extremity, *Cancer* **35:**574.

SHIZUTA, Y., AND TOKUSHIGE, M., 1971, Threonine deaminase—degradative (*Escherichia coli*), in: *Methods in Enzymology* (H. Tabor and C. W. Tabor, eds.), Vol. 17B, pp. 575–580, Academic Press, New York.

SIMMONS, R. L., AND RIOS, A., 1973a, Differential effect of neuraminidase on the immunogenicity of viral associated and private antigens of mammary carcinomas, *J. Immunol.* **111:**1820.

SIMMONS, R. L., AND RIOS, A., 1973b, Neuraminase treated cells and their role in cancer immunotherapy, in: *Birth Defects: Original Article Series* (D. Bergsma, ed.), Vol. 9, pp. 223–228, Williams and Wilkins, Baltimore.

SIMMONS, R. L., RIOS, A., LANDGREN, G., RAY, P. K., MCKHANN, C. F., AND HAYWOOD, G. R., 1971, Immunospecific regression of methylcholanthrene fibrosarcoma with the use of neuraminidase, *Surgery* **70:**38.

SKIPPER, H. E., AND THOMSON, J. R., 1958, A preliminary study of the influence of amino acid deficiencies on experimental cancer chemotherapy, in: *Ciba Found. Symp.: Amino Acids and Peptides with Antimetabolic Activity* (G. E. W. Wolstonholme and C. M. O'Connor, eds.), pp. 38–61, Little, Brown and Co., Boston.

SPIERS, A. S. D., AND WADE, H. E., 1976, Bacterial glutaminase in treatment of acute leukaemia, *Br. Med. J.* **1:**1317.

STORR, J. M., AND BURTON, A. F., 1974, The effects of arginine deficiency on lymphoma cells, *Br. J. Cancer* **30:**50.

SUGIMURA, T., BIRNBAUM, S. M., WINITX, M., AND GREENSTEIN, J. P., 1959, Quantitative nutritional studies with water-soluble, chemically defined diets. VIII. The forced feeding of diets each lacking in one essential amino acid, *Arch. Biochem. Biophys.* **81:**448.

SUMMERS, W. P., AND HANDSCHUMACHER, R. E., 1971, L5178Y asparagine-dependent cells and independent clonal sublines: Toxicity of 5-diazo-4-oxo-L-norvaline, *Biochem. Pharmacol.* **20:**2213.

SUMMERS, W. P., AND HANDSCHUMACHER, R. E., 1973, The rate of mutation of L5178Y asparagine-independence and its biological consequences, *Cancer Res.* **33**:1775.

THEUER, R. C., 1971, Effect of essential amino acid restriction on the growth of female C57BL mice and their implanted BW10232 adenocarcinomas, *J. Nutr.* **101**:223.

THORBECKE, G. J., MAURER, P. H., AND BENACERAFF, B., 1960, The affinity of the reticulo-endothelial system for various modified serum proteins, *Br. J. Exp. Pathol.* **41**:190.

THORNES, R. D., DEASY, P. F., CARROLL, R., REEN, D. C., AND MACDONELL, J. D., 1972, The use of the proteolytic enzyme brinase to produce autocytoxicity in patients with acute leukemia and its possible role in immunotherapy, *Cancer Res.* **32**:280.

TRYFIATES, G. P., AND MORRIS, H. P., 1974, Effect of pyridoxine deficiency on tyrosine transaminase activity and growth of four Morris hepatomas, *J. Natl. Cancer Inst.* **52**:1259.

UREN, J. R., AND HANDSCHUMACHER, R. E., 1974, Evaluation of asparagine analogs as cancer chemotherapeutic agents, *Proc. Amer. Assoc. Cancer Res.* **15**:124.

UREN, J. R., AND LAZARUS, H., 1975, Enzymatic approaches to cyst(e)ine depletion therapy, *Proc. Amer. Assoc. Cancer Res.* **16**:144.

UREN, J. R., SUMMERS, W. P., AND HANDSCHUMACHER, R. E., 1974, Enzymatic and nutritional evidence for two-stage expression of the asparagine synthetase locus in L5178Y murine leukemia mutants, *Cancer Res.* **34**:2940.

VADLAMUDI, S., PADARATHSINGH, M., WARAVDEKAR, V. S., AND GOLDIN, A., 1970, Factors influencing the therapeutic activity of L-asparaginase (NSC 109229) in leukemic (L5178Y) mice, *Cancer Res.* **30**:1467.

VRAT, V. A., 1951, Inhibitory effects of arginase on mammary adenocarcinoma transplants in strain A mice, *Permanente Found. (Oakland, Calif.) Med. Bull.* **9**:49.

WEIGELT, O., 1974, Die Wirkung intratumoral applizierter proteolytischer Enzyme auf spontane Mamma-adenome bei weiblichen Sprague-Dawley Ratten, *Arzneim. Forsch.* **24**:549.

WHITECAR, J. P., BODEY, G. P., HARRIS, J. E., AND FREIREICH, E. J., 1970, L-Asparaginase, *N. Engl. J. Med.* **282**:732.

WOLF, M., AND RANSBERGER, K., 1972, *Enzyme Therapy*, Vantage Press, New York.

WOODS, J. S., AND HANDSCHUMACHER, R. E., 1973, Hepatic regulation of plasma L-asparagine, *Amer. J. Physiol.* **224**:740.

WRISTON, J. C., AND YELLIN, T. O., 1973, L-Asparaginase: A review, *Adv. Enzymol.* **39**:185.

WU, T. T., LIN, E. C. C., AND TANAKA, S., 1968, Mutants of *Aerobacter aerogenes* capable of utilizing xylitol as a novel carbon source, *J. Bacteriol.* **96**:447.

WU, W. H., AND MORRIS, D. R., 1973, Biosynthetic arginine decarboxylase from *Escherichia coli*: Purification and properties, *J. Biol. Chem.* **248**:1687.

ZYK, N., 1973, Modification of L-asparaginase EC-2 by homologous antibodies, *Biochim. Biophys. Acta* **302**:420.

17

Hydrazines and Triazenes

Willi Kreis

1. Introduction

Hydrazines, but not triazines, have been identified in a small number of biological substances. Those used in cancer chemotherapy are synthetic products, are relatively unstable, and provide biologically active groups on their decomposition and metabolism. The basic moieties of hydrazine, $H_2N–NH_2$, and triazene, $NH_2–N=NH$, are substituted with aromatic and aliphatic groups on both ends of their nitrogen bridges; these substituents probably also provide a limited stability to the respective molecules. While a large number of derivatives in both groups have been synthesized and evaluated for biological activity, the representatives reported in this chapter are few, and are the most interesting ones from both the therapeutic and the theoretical points of view.

2. Hydrazines

2.1. Introduction: History, Chemistry, and General Remarks

Hydrazine and hydrazine derivatives have yet to be found and clearly identified as intermediary or end products in the metabolism of mammalian cells. So far, there is no evidence that hydrazine, as often postulated, is an intermediary product in nitrogen fixation by leguminous plants of microorganisms (Lehninger, 1970). Naturally occurring hydrazines and hydrazine derivatives have been isolated and identified, however, in tobacco and tobacco smoke (Liu and Hoffmann, 1973) and in several mushrooms (for a survey, see Toth, 1975). Synthetic hydrazines are used in rocket fuels, laboratory reagents (*The Merck Index*, 1968), and ripening agents (Gowing and Leeper, 1955). The prominent place of synthetic hydrazine

Willi Kreis ● Memorial Sloan–Kettering Cancer Center, New York, New York 10021.

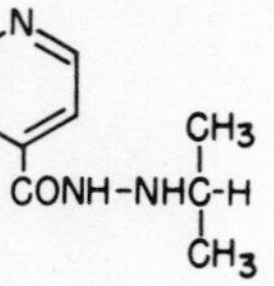

FIGURE 1. Iproniazide (Marsilid).

derivatives in human biology is undoubtedly in the field of monoamine oxidase inhibitors. Studies pertaining to this highly important group of drugs were initiated when a tuberculostatic hydrazine derivative, iproniazide (Marsilid) (Fig. 1), proved to be too toxic in the routine treatment of tuberculosis, as excessive psychic stimulation was encountered.

Monoamine oxidases destroy three important stimulators of the CNS, serotonin, epinephrine, and norepinephrine, and thus assure the regulation of a highly complex physiological balance. Initiated by these findings, a large number of amine oxidase inhibitors, mostly hydrazine derivatives, have been synthesized in many laboratories. At present, the most useful pharmacological action of these agents consists in the elevation of the mood of depressed patients.

2.2. 1-Methyl-2-p-(isopropylcarbamoyl)benzylhydrazine Hydrochloride (MBH)

For reviews on MBH (procarbazine, Matulane, Natulan, NSC 77213), see Jelliffe and Marks (1965), Stock (1967), Sartorelli and Creasey (1969), Carter (1970), Oliverio (1973), Reed (1975), and Livingston and Carter (1970b).

2.2.1. Development

In the search for monoamine oxidase inhibitors, chemists and biologists at Hoffman-La Roche synthesized and tested a large number of hydrazines and hydrazides (Zeller et al., 1963). A by-product of these efforts was a group of substituted hydrazines with the general formula

$$R-CH_2-NH-NH-CH_3$$

that exhibited antineoplastic activity (Bollag and Grunberg, 1963). Of particular interest were compounds in which R represented substituted benzyl groups. The two compounds shown in Fig. 2 proved to be of special potency and interest. Of the two, MBH proved to be less toxic, and was further investigated and developed. Significantly, MBH proved to be active against a number of solid murine tumors, especially Walker carcinosarcoma 256 of the rat and sarcoma 180 of the mouse

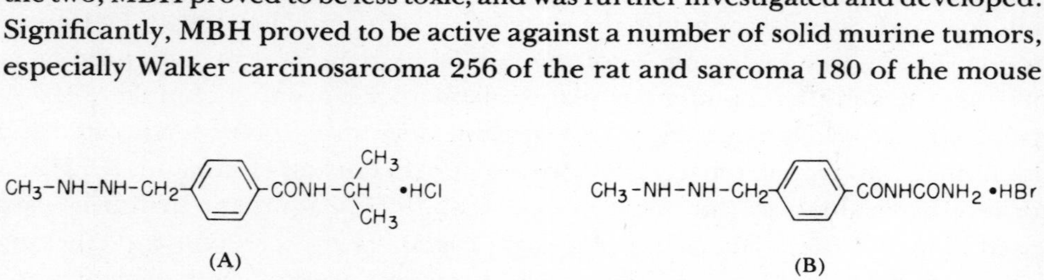

(A)   (B)

FIGURE 2. (A) 1-Methyl-2-p-(isopropylcarbamoyl)benzylhydrazine hydrochloride (Natulan, Matulane, procarbazine, MBH, NSC 77213); (B) 1-methyl-2-p-allophanoylbenzylhydrazine hydrobromide.

(Bollag and Grunberg, 1963; Grunberg, 1970). Also, MBH was active against mouse neoplasm L1210, but only in its solid form, by all routes of administration (intraperitoneal, subcutaneous, and oral), whereas the ascites form of L1210 did not respond to intraperitoneal treatment with MBH. Both the solid and the ascites form of Ehrlich carcinoma, however, responded to intraperitoneal treatment with MBH (Bollag and Grunberg, 1963); at a higher dosage, the ascites form responded significantly better than the solid form. Apparently, differences in uptake and metabolism are responsible for sensitivity and specificity. The most sensitive tumor proved to be the Walker carcinosarcoma 256 of rats: as little as 10 mg/kg resulted in 100% tumor inhibition (Bollag and Grunberg, 1963). Other experimental tumors responding to MBH were sarcoma 180; mammary adenocarcinoma E0771 of mice; the ascites (Kreis, 1970a, b) and solid forms of P815 in mice and Dunning leukemia in Fischer rats (Oliverio et al., 1964); a spontaneous mammary tumor in C3H mice (Gelzer and Loustalot, 1967); uterine epithelioma (Guérin) T-8, Murphy-Sturm lymphosarcoma, Flexner Jobling carcinoma, and human epidermoid carcinoma No. 3 of the rat (Bollag and Grunberg, 1963; Grunberg, 1970); and the human adenocarcinoma No. 1 growing in the hamster cheek pouch in the series of Grunberg (1970), but not in the study of Goldenberg and Witte (1967). In dogs, an intracerebrally implanted gliosarcoma responded to MBH by prolongation of the life span (Merker et al., 1975). A remarkable advantage of MBH is that intraperitoneal and oral administration (Bollag and Grunberg, 1963) and intraperitoneal, oral, and subcutaneous administration (Grunberg, 1970) showed comparable results in the experiments in which the different routes of administration had been compared.

Resistance to MBH was first obtained by Bollag and Grunberg (1963) in Ehrlich ascites carcinoma; it developed after 7–9 passages in mice treated with MBH. A Walker 256 carcinosarcoma in rats, made resistant to cyclophosphamide, still responded well to MBH (W. Bollag, personal communication). A large number of clinical investigations indicate no cross-resistance of MBH with any of the conventional antitumor drugs, including alkylating agents (d'Alessandri et al., 1963; Brunner and Young, 1965; Samuels et al., 1967; Boehnel and Stacher, 1966; Kenis, 1968). Resistance to MBH in Ehrlich ascites cells (Gutterman et al., 1969) developed rapidly when the cells were exposed during the phase of DNA synthesis, and slowly when the DNA synthesis was depressed. In resistant cells, two new metacentric chromosomes appeared during each cell mitosis.

2.2.2. Metabolism

The metabolism of MBH has been studied extensively, both in vitro and in vivo. Figure 3 presents a summary of verified and hypothetical metabolic pathways. Identified metabolic end products of MBH in mice, rats, dogs, and humans and some in vitro systems are carbon dioxide (Dost and Reed, 1967; Dewald et al., 1969; Baggiolini et al., 1965; Schwartz et al., 1967; Kreis, 1970b), methane (Dost and Reed, 1967; Schwartz et al., 1967), formaldehyde (Wittkop et al., 1969; Schwartz, 1966), methylamine (Schwartz, 1966), N-isopropylterephthalamic acid

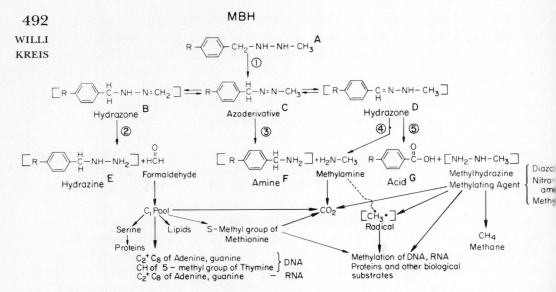

FIGURE 3. Current concepts of the metabolism of MBH as compiled from the literature. The compounds in brackets are as yet unidentified. See the text for a discussion.

(Raaflaub and Schwartz, 1965; Oliverio, 1970), and methylated purines and pyrimidines (Brookes, 1965; Kreis, 1970*a*, *b*; Kreis and Yen, 1965). As diagrammed in Fig. 3, the first step in the metabolism is the oxidation of MBH (A) to its azo derivative (C), which does not necessarily depend on the microsomal hydroxylase (Baggiolini *et al.*, 1969; Gale *et al.*, 1967). Whereas the azo derivative (C) of MBH has been identified *in vivo* (Raaflaub and Schwartz, 1965), the two likely isomerization products, hydrazone (B) and hydrazone (D), are, at this time, hypothetical reaction products. Hydrazone (B) is probably the reaction product involved in oxidative release of C_1-units, and as such, contributing to the C_1 or formate pool. Oxidative splitting of the $-N{=}CH_2$ double bond would lead primarily to formaldehyde, which has been isolated and identified in small amounts in the expiration air of rats after administration of MBH labeled with ^{14}C in the *N*-methyl group (Schwartz, 1966). The C_1-pool is responsible for the *in vivo* labeling of proteins, lipids, DNA, and RNA (C_2 and C_8 of adenine and guanine; CH of the 5-methyl group of thymine), and probably, but to a small extent only, for one C and one H atom of the 5-methyl group of methionine (Kreis, 1970*a*). That methylamine, *in vivo*, is more efficiently oxidized to CO_2 than is MBH (Schwartz, 1966) leaves pathways 2 and 3, at best, subjects for speculation. Furthermore, that neither hydrazine (E) nor amine (F) has been found *in vivo* or *in vitro*, but only acid (G) of pathway 4 (Fig. 3), suggests caution in the proposed pathways.

Azoderivative (C) is the most likely precursor of methylamine. The latter is rapidly excreted in rat urine in substantial amounts after injection of MBH into rats (Schwartz, 1966). The splitting of a N–N bond *in vivo* is not new, but had been reported as early as 1937 in the metabolism of Prontosil (Fuller, 1937). In findings of the investigation by Schwartz (1966), methylamine is also the major urinary metabolite of methylhydrazine, and is excreted unchanged in urine up to about 30% after injection of methylamine to rats; however, the bulk of the injected methylamine is rapidly oxidized to CO_2 (Schwartz, 1966). At present, there is no evidence that methylamine in rats produces more than just traces of methane (Schwartz, 1966), although no special analysis was performed for the detection of methane other than the trapping of the expired air at $-80°C$; therefore, with this reservation in mind, it is unlikely that methylamine is of importance in the methylation of DNA, RNA, and protein. Thus, while the fate of methylamine is reasonably well established in rats, its pathway of production from MBH is still open to discussion.

The strong increase (300%) of urinary methylamine excretion after administration of certain monoamine oxidase inhibitors containing the hydrazine moiety, as observed by Davis and DeRopp (1961), is probably not responsible for the labeled methylamine excretion after MBH injection, since that effect was due to a stimulation of the regular methylamine production, and the monoamine oxidase inhibitors used (pheniprazine and iproniazid) were not methylhydrazine derivatives. Since sarcosine and creatine are the most likely precursors of methylamine in the rat (Davis and DeRopp, 1961), however, a flow of N-methyl-derived radioactivity of MBH through this pathway could be excluded completely only with the help of MBH double-labeled in the methyl group, whereas Schwartz (1966) used only 1-methyl-^{14}C-labeled material. Comparing the rate of methane and CO_2 formation from monomethylhydrazine and MBH, Dost and Reed (1967) and Dost *et al.* (1966) came to the conclusion that monomethylhydrazine might be an intermediary derivative in the metabolism of MBH (Fig. 3, pathway 5). Although methylhydrazine has not yet been isolated as a reaction product of MBH metabolism, pyridoxalmethylhydrazone has been isolated from mice injected with MBH and pyridoxal (Chabner *et al.*, 1969). Dewald *et al.* (1969) concluded, from experiments with intact rats and perfused rat liver, that the main pathway for CO_2 production from MBH involved the primary N–C bond cleavage, rather than the intermediary formation of methylhydrazine. Supportive of this argument is the fact that monomethylhydrazine is devoid of carcinogenic activity, whereas MBH is a strong carcinogen (Kelly *et al.*, 1969; Adamson, 1970). Hydrazone (D) is more likely to be of significance for methylation of macromolecules, and possibly for part or even total release of the other MBH-derived metabolites.

N-Isopropylterephthalamic acid (G), a split and oxidation product of hydrazone (D), has been identified in significant amounts in blood and urine of humans (Raaflaub and Schwartz, 1965), and in various animal species (Oliverio *et al.*, 1964), and has also been derived from MBH in perfused rat liver (Baggiolini *et al.*, 1969). During the cleavage of the C=N double bond, several products are probably being formed that so far have not been identified. Theoretically, methylhydrazine, methyldiazene, diazomethane, and monomethylnitrosamine are intermediary products, which could possibly produce the alkylating radicals, methylamine and CO_2. The last two intermediary products were suggested as active methylating agents by Magee and Farber (1962). Methyldiazene produces large amounts of methane by chemical decomposition (Tsuji and Kosower, 1971). At this point, it is important to mention that the N-methyl group is apparently crucial for the activity of MBH: if it was absent, or if it was replaced by an ethyl group, inactive compounds resulted (Schwartz *et al.*, 1968). Oxidation products of MBH, however, such as N-isopropyl-α-[methylazo]-p-toluamide and N-isopropyl-α-[methylazoxy]-p-toluamide, still show activity, but usually of a lower grade and with a lower therapeutic index than MBH (Bollag *et al.*, 1964). Enzymatic aspects of the metabolism of MBH were published by Reed (1970), Baggiolini *et al.* (1969), and Dewald *et al.* (1969).

Obviously, special importance had to be attributed to the N-methyl group of MBH. Evidence for transmethylation of that N-methyl group onto DNA and RNA was first given by Brookes (1965): after 18-hr exposure of HeLa cells in tissue culture to ^{3}H-labeled MBH, both DNA and RNA were significantly labeled. However, most of the labeling was located in guanine and adenine, and no significant labeling was found in the form of 7-methylguanine. However, in 7-day-old Landschutz ascites tumors grown *in vivo* in Swiss mice and exposed 17 hr to 250 mg [^{3}H]MBH/kg, significant activity was found to be present in the form of 7-methylguanine. Brookes (1965) indicated that each ascites cell would contain approximately 1.2 million alkylated guanine moieties, and yet, from a comparison with the alkylation by other monofunctional alkylating agents, concluded that the relatively low level of alkylation would not be expected to be lethal, although it might well lead to mutation. 7-Methylguanine was found in RNA to about the same extent as in DNA. No evidence was given for the intact transfer of the MBH-methyl group onto the DNA or RNA.

Another indication of transmethylation of the N-methyl group was also obtained in experiments with P815-neoplasm-bearing mice: in the urine of mice treated with N-methyl-labeled [^{14}C]MBH, 7-methylguanine, 1-methyladenine, and 1-methylhypoxanthine were compared with guanine, adenine, and hypoxanthine. The radioactivity ratios clearly indicated transfer of the intact N-methyl group, as well as the feeding of the C_1-pool by oxidative demethylation of the N-methyl group (Kreis *et al.*, 1966). When intermolecularly double-labeled N-methyl[^{14}C^{3}H$_3$]MBH (^{3}H:^{14}C ratio about 3:1) was administered to P815-ascites-bearing mice and the purine and pyrimidine bases derived from cytoplasmic RNA were evaluated for ^{3}H:^{14}C ratios, it became clear that guanine and adenine received their ^{14}C and ^{3}H labeling through the C_1-pool (ratios of ^{3}H:^{14}C close to 2:1 and 1:1, respectively), whereas 5-methylcytosine, 1-methylguanine, 7-methylguanine, and 1-methyladenine obviously had had to receive the bulk of their labeling by intact transfer of the N-methyl group, since the ^{3}H:^{14}C ratios were in the neighborhood of 3:1 and higher (Kreis, 1970a).

Thus, while the pathways for the production of the reacting CH$_3$-radicals are still open to speculation, the fact of methylation of DNA and RNA is well established. The purpose of Fig. 3 is to indicate the complexity of the metabolic pathways, as compiled from many studies, rather than to indicate firmly established channels of metabolism of MBH. It must also be pointed out that different tissues and different species might well handle the compound differently, a fact contributing to specificity, toxicity, or lack of one or both.

2.2.3. *Mechanism of Action*

The question pertaining to cycle specificity has not received sufficient attention, and cannot be answered from the information published. The reported suppression of the mitosis by prolongation of the interphase (S or G_2 phase) (Rutishauser and Bollag, 1967) does not provide a definite answer.

The original study on the reaction mechanism of MBH by Berneis *et al.* (1963) was based primarily on the chemical nature of MBH (Zeller *et al.*, 1963), and on the observation by Rutishauser and Bollag (1963) of chromatid breaks* and reunions in Ehrlich ascites cells. Under the influence of MBH or MBH-derived material, viscosity determinations of DNA *in vitro* revealed an exponential drop of the specific viscosity over several days when the system was kept in the presence of molecular oxygen. Replacement of oxygen by nitrogen or the addition of peroxidase or catalase reduced the breakdown of DNA almost completely. Hydrogen peroxide is a by-product of autooxidation of MBH at 37°C. These findings supported the hypothesis of hydrogen-peroxide-induced degradation of DNA reported by Butler and Smith (1950). Berneis *et al.* (1963) concluded that the slow release of hydrogen peroxide, providing OH radicals, was the principal cause for DNA degradation by MBH. A synergistic effect on *in vitro* double breaks of DNA was observed by combining MBH treatment with ionizing radiation (Berneis *et al.*, 1966). It was suggested that unstable peroxide products were responsible for this effect. While these *in vitro* experiments have a striking effect on DNA, the authors did not claim that a similar effect would take place *in vivo*. Indeed, it is unlikely that sufficient amounts of hydrogen peroxide could accumulate in tissues for such a reaction to take place. Efforts to identify the breakdown of DNA *in vivo* with this drug's activity have failed (Sartorelli and Tsunamura, 1966; Koblet and Diggelmann, 1968; Gale *et al.*, 1967; Kreis, unpublished results).

A closer look at the hydrogen peroxide hypothesis (Kreis, 1970*b*) reveals the following facts: For a 5-fold increase of the survival time of Ehrlich-ascites-bearing mice, 6 intraperitoneal injections of 180 and 360 mg hydrogen peroxide/kg were necessary (Krementz and Youngblood, 1962). The dosage of MBH necessary to produce 180 mg hydrogen peroxide/kg in connection with the oxidation of MBH would be roughly 2700 mg/kg; according to Bollag and Grunberg (1963), this dosage is well beyond the lethal dose. Also, 300 mg MBH/kg injected into Ehrlich-ascites-bearing mice for 7 days produced an increase of survival time of 310%. This dosage of 300 mg MBH/kg could provide only about 20 mg H_2O_2, which is far below the 180 mg/kg necessary for the significantly increased survival time reported by Krementz and Youngblood (1962). Gale *et al.* (1967) reported that an MBH solution, stored for 10 days and containing 400% more hydrogen peroxide than a solution stored for 4 days only, produced similar inhibition of DNA synthesis in Ehrlich ascites tumor cells *in vitro*. They concluded that H_2O_2 was not the inhibitory component of MBH. It is likely that catalases and peroxidases, which are abundantly available in many mammalian tissues, would rapidly destroy hydrogen peroxide, and thus prevent

---

* Chromosomal aberrations under the influence of MBH were also observed in humans (Vormittag, 1974).

its accumulation in the target cells. Thus, while H_2O_2 production may be a contributing factor in the reaction mechanism of MBH, it certainly is not the major one. Several investigators have reported *in vitro* and *in vivo* inhibition of DNA synthesis (Sartorelli and Tsunamura, 1966; Trepel *et al.*, 1967; Weitzel *et al.*, 1967*a*; Gale *et al.*, 1967), RNA synthesis (Sartorelli and Tsunamura, 1966; Weitzel *et al.*, 1967*a*, *b*; Kreis, 1970*a*; Gale *et al.*, 1967), and protein synthesis (Sartorelli and Tsunamura, 1966; Weitzel *et al.*, 1967*b*; Koblet and Diggelmann, 1968) under the influence of MBH.

The proposed reduction of intracellular purine bases and nucleosides due to the action of isopropylcarbonamid (Weitzel *et al.*, 1967*b*) is unlikely to be of importance, since their phosphorylated DNA and RNA precursors are provided sufficiently and by other pathways in the *de novo* synthesis. The trapping of amino acids by condensation with isopropyl-4-formylbenzamide by the Schiff reaction (Weitzel *et al.*, 1967*b*) remains highly speculative as long as such condensation products have not been identified. A reasonable explanation for DNA and RNA inhibition would be a possible carbamyl phosphate blockage and subsequent decomposition of the activated carbonate by MBH or its metabolites, similar to the reported effect of hydrazine (McKinley *et al.*, 1967). No such studies have been reported so far for MBH.

Inhibition of polysome breakdown and binding of MBH to microsomes and polysomes as evidenced in *in vitro* studies by Koblet and Diggelmann (1968) need further investigation and confirmation. Obviously, there is a discrepancy in the reported findings in these studies with purified DNA and the *in vivo* experiments. Compatible with the *in vivo* inhibition of DNA, RNA, and protein synthesis is the observed *in vivo* methylation of DNA and RNA (Brookes, 1965; Kreis, 1970*a*, *b*) and the inhibition of the synthesis and normal methylation of transfer RNA (Kreis, 1970*b*; Kreis *et al.*, 1968). As demonstrated by Fig. 4, there is a distinct discrepancy in the pattern of *in vivo* labeling in cytoplasmic RNA, when the methionine-derived methylation is compared with the methylation by MBH. It is likely, therefore, that the aberrant methylation pattern observed in cytoplasmic RNA (Kreis, 1970*a*, *b*) after administration of MBH leads to a malfunction of RNA and, consequently, to impaired protein DNA and RNA synthesis. Alterations of the function of tRNA as a result of deficiency of methylation have been reported by Revel and Littauer (1966). The reported reversal of the chemotherapeutic action of MBH by simultaneous or previous administration of large amounts of L-methionine (Kreis, 1970*b*) and the partial reversal of the teratogenic action of MBH by methionine (Chaube and Murphy, 1969) suggest a possible interference of MBH with the normal methylation of RNA and DNA. While these studies do not exclude other possible interferences in the normal biochemistry of cells treated with MBH, they give, by cause and effect, a reasonable explanation for the *in vivo* action of MBH.

2.2.4. Physiological Disposition

Initial pharmacological disposition studies performed by Schwartz *et al.* (1967) with three differently labeled species of MBH revealed substantial differences of

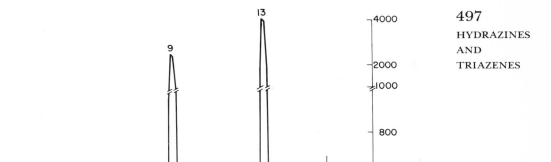
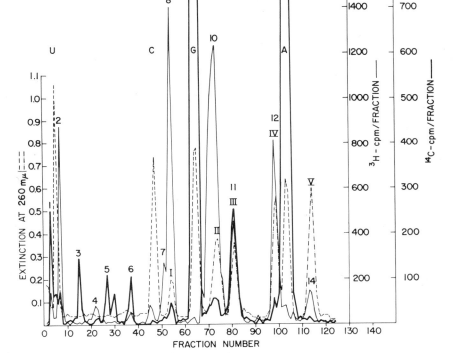

FIGURE 4. Base analysis of a $HClO_4$ hydrosylate of 12 mg dried cytoplasmic RNA, extracted 4 hr after a single intraperitoneal injection of a mixture of 2.24 mg L-methionine[C^3H_3] (specific activity, 106.5 mCi/mmole) per kilogram and 200 mg MBH[^{14}C] (6.04 mCi/mmole) per kilogram. After the hydrolysis of the RNA, 0.2 mg of the following cold methylated bases was added (identified in chart by the Roman numerals at the tops of the respective absorbance peaks at 260 nm): 5-methylcytosine (I), 1-methylguanine + N^2-methylguanine (common peak II), 7-methylguanine (III), 1-methyladenine (IV), and 6-methyladenine (V) (— · — · —). (– – –) The normally occurring bases uracil (U), cytosine (C), guanine (G), and adenine (A), and absorption between the peaks. Light solid lines: ^3H counts derived from the ^3H atoms of the methyl group of methionine; heavy solid lines: ^{14}C counts derived from the ^{14}C atoms of the N-methyl group of MBH. From Kreis (1970a).

distribution of radioactivity for the three compounds. At 30 min after administration of MBH (^{14}C-labeled in the N-methyl group) in rats bearing Walker carcinosarcoma 256, the highest values of radioactivity were found in the kidneys, small intestines, and liver; intermediary values in the heart, muscle, testes, bone marrow, spleen, and lungs; and the lowest values in plasma and tumor. At 60 min after injection, a similar pattern of distribution was revealed, but generally at a slightly lower level. Of the radioactivity of the ^{14}C-methyl-labeled MBH, 30% appeared in the form of CO_2 within about 8 hr, with a peak at 30–60 min after the injection. Formaldehyde was accounted for in the expiration air to about 0.1%. The bulk of the radioactivity derived from MBH, ^{14}C-labeled in the carbamide group, appeared in the urine of rats (intraperitoneal administration) and dogs (intravenous administration) to about 67–70% within the first 24 hr, while only small amounts were found in the feces. According to Oliverio (1970), N-isopropyl terephthalamic acid and its glucuronide were identified in mouse urine. In rats, CO_2 (30%) and unchanged MBH plus methylamine (together, about 35% of the radioactivity administered) were identified (Schwartz, 1966); N-isopropyl terephthalamic acid was not mentioned in this study.

In humans, MBH disappears rapidly from the bloodstream, with a half-life of about 7 min. Concomitant with the decrease of MBH, an increase of the azo derivative was observed, the derivative being subsequently further metabolized to N-isopropyl terephthalamic acid (Raaflaub and Schwartz, 1965). The latter was identified in plasma, and was excreted through the kidneys. This urinary metabolite accounted for about 40% of the MBH administered. The unchanged MBH was not detected in human urine (Raaflaub and Schwartz, 1965). After injecting radioactive MBH, ^{14}C-labeled in the carbamide group, in humans, Schwartz *et al.* (1967) found about 70% and 4–9% of the radioactivity in urine and feces, respectively; after the injection of N-methyl-labeled MBH, they found 20% of radioactivity in the form of CO_2. Obviously, about 30% of the urinary radioactivity remains unidentified. Of special interest is the rapid equilibration of the drug or metabolites in the plasma and CSF in both dogs and humans. In patients, peak CSF values were obtained $1–1\frac{1}{2}$ hr after intravenous or oral administration of the drug. No information was given as to qualitative analysis of the material observed in the spinal fluid (Oliverio, 1970).

2.2.5. Toxicity

The LD_{50} values for acute toxicity of MBH in animals are presented in Table 1. In man, doses of 1500 mg/M^2 or higher must be used with extreme caution (Chabner *et al.*, 1973).

The most consistent chronic toxicity in all species studied was impairment of hematopoiesis, as presented in Table 2. Further toxicities observed are presented in Table 3.

2.2.6. Other Biological Effects

MBH is also a powerful carcinogen! In (BALB/c × DBA/2)F_1 mice, MBH and azo compound (C) and hydrazone (D) (see Fig. 3) induced multiple pulmonary tumors with high incidence. N-Isopropylterephthalamic acid [acid (G)] exhibited considerably less carcinogenicity, and no such effect was found with methylhydrazine, N-isopropyl-*p*-formylbenzamine, or benzylhydrazine. MBH

TABLE 1

LD$_{50}$ Values for Acute Toxicity of MBH[a]

Species	Administration mode	LD$_{50}$ (mg/kg)
Mouse	Single, intravenous	300
Mouse	Single, oral	700
Rat	Single, intravenous	350
Rat	Single, oral	1400

[a] From Miller (1970).

TABLE 2

Hematopoietic Toxicity of Chronic MBH in Various Species[a]

Species	Dosage for toxicity	Leukopoiesis	Thrombopoiesis	Erythropoiesis
Rat	≥ 20 mg/kg · day for 4–6 weeks	Lymphopenia	Less impairment than of lymphopoiesis	No effect
Dog	≥ 20 mg/kg · day for 4–6 weeks	Granulopenia	Less impairment than of granulopoiesis	Hemolytic anemia with Heinz bodies[b]
Humans	5 mg/kg · day for 3–5 weeks	Leukopenia	Thrombopenia	Anemia (moderate)

[a] From Miller (1970).

[b] With extensive hemosiderin deposits in the spleen, liver, kidney, and bone marrow. This is a hydrazine effect!

TABLE 3

Other Toxicities of MBH in Various Species

Species	Toxicity	References
Rat	Atrophy of testes, alopecia Increase in ketone bodies and slight hypocalcemia	Miller (1970)
Dog	Atrophy of testes, alopecia	Miller (1970), Oliverio (1970)
Humans[a,b]	Gastrointestinal *Frequent*: nausea, vomiting *Rare*: stomatitis, diarrhea Central nervous system *Rare*: pain, myalgia, arthralgia, lethargy and drowsiness, hyperexcitability, euphoria, ataxia, nystagmus Dermatological Occasional dermatitis	d'Alessandri *et al.* (1963), Brunner and Young (1965), Sears (1971), Samuels (1971), Livingston and Carter (1970b)

[a] Some of the neurotoxic effects may be due to a pyridoxine depletion induced by inhibition of pyridoxal phosphokinase by hydrazone formation (Oliverio, 1970). In some instances, intravenous administration of vitamin B$_6$ is helpful.

[b] MBH is a monoamine oxidase inhibitor.

and azo compound (C) also induced leukemia and cystadenoma of the kidney (Kelly *et al.*, 1969). Such neoplasms were induced in mice at doses of 200–400 mg/kg i.p. or 250 mg/kg p.o. weekly for 8 weeks. In Osborn–Mendel rats (Adamson, 1970), MBH induced, at doses of 50–250 mg/kg i.p. (4 weeks) followed by p.o. for a further 3 weeks (once weekly), mammary tumors (adenocarcinomas) in both sexes (more frequently in females than in males); other neoplasms were situated in the kidneys, lungs, jejunum, blood, muscle, and skin. In a total of 27 rhesus, cynomolgus, and African green monkeys, only 2 gave evidence of carcinogenic action of MBH (Adamson, 1970). Deckers *et al.*, (1974) reported the induction by MBH of mammary, uterine, and ear duct tumors in female rats (R strain).

Teratogenic effects produced by MBH in rats were reported by Chaube and Murphy (1969). Increased doses (12 mg/kg on day 12 to 250 mg/kg on day 17) of MBH on days 5, 6, 9–12, 14, and 17 of gestation (but not on day 7 or 8) caused tail, appendicular, and brain defects, facial clefts, and cleft palate and shortened jaws. The pattern of defects depended on the day of administration of the drug. The estimated maternal LD_{100} was 550 mg/kg. L-Methionine could reverse this MBH effect only partially. Both the carcinogenic and the teratogenic effects of MBH suggest an interference with the nucleic acid metabolism.

Early in the development of MBH, the effect of the drug on immunologic reactions was studied. Suppression of the immunologic system by MBH, as evaluated by the immune response against tumor heterografts, was first reported by Bollag (1963). Only pretreatment with MBH (before implantation of the graft) resulted in delayed rejection of the heterograft; treatment after implantation had no effect on the growth of the tumor. When primary skin homograft reactions were evaluated, it became evident that methylhydrazine derivatives, MBH among them, produced significant prolongation of the survival of the graft in mice (Floersheim, 1963). Increased survival time of second-set skin homografts (50–70%) in inbred mice with strong histocompatibility differences [C57BL ← (CBA × C57BL)F_1], strong antigenic differences, and *H-2* locus disparity (C57BL ← CBA) was noticed under the influence of MBH and 1-methyl-2-*p*-allophanoylbenzylhydrazine hydrobromide. No such graft survival was found with cyclophosphamide and azathioprine. A small, retarded rejection due to the two hydrazine derivatives was also observed in the combinations C3H ← C⁻ and CBA ← A (Floersheim, 1966).

The immunosuppressive effect of MBH has been used, with some success, in systemic lupus erythematosus (Deicher, 1972), macroglobulinemia Waldenstroem (Mitron and Schubert, 1973), and chronic polyarthritis (Thumb *et al.*, 1972; Fellinger, 1973). The successful transplantation of bone marrow under immunosuppression by a combination of cyclophosphamide, procarbazine, and antithymocyte globin was reported by Kersey *et al.* (1975).

2.2.7. Clinical Use

The first clinical investigations by Martz *et al.* (1963) and d'Alessandri *et al.* (1963) revealed the therapeutic effect of MBH in malignant lymphomas. A large number of subsequent papers (Brunner and Young, 1965; Kenis *et al.*, 1966; Mathé *et al.*, 1963; Brulé *et al.*, 1965; Falkson *et al.*, 1965; Hope-Stone, 1965; Todd, 1965; Dawson, 1965; Jelliffe *et al.*, 1965; Backhouse and Sicher, 1966; Spies and Snyman, 1966; DeVita, 1966; Young, 1970; Sears, 1971; Samuels, 1971) dealt with the administration of MBH as a single agent.

In a survey of the results of treatment with MBH alone, Livingston and Carter (1970*b*) found a 69% objective response rate in over 300 cases of lymphomas, especially in Hodgkin's disease, in which 37% attained the status of complete response. As to the response rate in recticulum-cell sarcoma and lymphosarcoma, these authors concluded that MBH is probably inferior to vincristine or cytoxan, but not to nitrogen mustard or vinblastine. In the same survey, the authors reported a response rate varying from 6 to 39% for bronchogenic carcinoma; the best effect was seen in "oat-cell" carcinomas, the least effect in squamous-cell bronchogenic cancer. Some activity was also reported against malignant melanoma. MBH has been inadequately tried in acute leukemia, although the survey cites 2 responders besides the reported "objective regression" in adult leukemia (Martz *et al.*, 1963). The same survey cites antitumor activity of MBH for embryonal-cell carcinoma of the testes, ovarian carcinoma, bladder cancer, and neuroblastoma. Other applications of MBH included polycythemia vera (Fischer and Martin, 1972), carcinomas of the lung and melanomas (Alberto, 1974; Oberfield, 1975), and reticulum-cell sarcoma, mycosis fungoides, and malignant mesothelioma (Falkson *et al.*, 1965). Marked improvement in 9 patients with Dupuytren's disease was reported by Aron (1968). MBH is usually administered at a dose of 50–200 mg/M² per day p.o. until either toxicity or maximum response appears.

Single-drug treatment with MBH has now been replaced, almost exclusively, by a combination of drugs. Normally, drugs of different reaction mechanism and possibly not overlapping toxicity, but with demonstrated individual activity in the disease to be treated, make up successsful combinations.

MBH has been used in several multiple-drug treatment programs (DeVita *et al.*, 1970; Brunner *et al.*, 1973; Raich *et al*, 1975; Gutin *et al.*, 1975). MOPP is probably the most successful and most widely known combination in which MBH is a component (DeVita *et al.*, 1970). With this combination, consisting of nitrogen mustard, vincristine (oncovin), procarbazine (MBH), and prednisone, administered to lymphoma patients in six 2-week cycles with 2-week rest periods between cycles, a complete suppression of Hodgkin's disease can be achieved in 70–80% of previously untreated patients (De Vita *et al.*, 1970; Bull *et al.*, 1970; Rosenberg and Kaplan, 1970; Carter, 1973; Fine, 1974; Frei, 1974; Goldsmith and Carter, 1974). Other combinations, subsequently developed and used for different malignomas, include a combination of 1,3-*bis*(2-chloroethyl)-1-nitrosurea (BCNU), vincristine, prednisone, and procarbazine for Stages III and IV Hodgkin's disease (Brunner *et al.*, 1973); cyclophosphamide, vincristine, prednisone, and procarbazine (COPP) for lymphomas (Raich *et al.*, 1975); MBH, vincristine, and BCNU for malignant brain tumors (Gutin *et al.*, 1975); and vincristine, procarbazine, melphalan, and prednisone for myelomas (Jacobs and Dubovsky, 1975).

Complications of such intensive chemotherapy (or radiotherapy or both) may be the appearance of second malignancies (Canellos *et al.*, 1975), teratogenic effects (Garret, 1974; Menutti *et al.*, 1975) in fetuses exposed to such treatment during gestation, chromosomal abnormalities (Vormittag, 1974), and severe damage to germinal epithelium (Arseneau *et al.*, 1974).

2.3. Hydrazine Sulfate and Miscellaneous Hydrazine Derivatives

With the intention of interrupting a "metabolic circuit, composed of glycolysis in cancer tissue and gluconeogenesis in normal liver tissue," Gold (1970, 1971, 1973) evaluated the response of four experimental tumors to hydrazine sulfate (NSC 150014). Gold reported growth inhibition of Walker 256 (Gold, 1971) and other solid experimental tumors such as B16 melanoma, Murphy Sturm lymphosarcoma, and L1210 solid leukemia (Gold, 1973). The rationale was to block phosphoenolpyruvate carboxykinase (PEPCK), an enzyme essential to the synthesis of glucose-6-phosphate from lactate. Tarnowski and Stock (personal communication), however, could not find growth inhibition by hydrazine sulfate in four mouse tumors (sarcoma 180, Meth A sarcoma, B16 melanoma, and Ridgeway osteogenic sarcoma), and only moderate results were found in Walker 256 carcinosarcoma.

In subsequent clinical trials reported by Gold (1974), of 10 patients with a variety of advanced cancer, such as breast, ovarian, prostatic, colonic, bronchogenic, and lymphomatous tumors, 6 patients exhibited subjective improvement (return of appetite, cessation of weight loss and weight gain, decrease of pain) or objective improvement (reduction of tumor size, total obliteration of tumor, disappearance of effusion) or both, with minimal side effects (minor gastritis, torpor, weakness).

Contrary to Gold's report (1974), Ochoa *et al.* (1975), in a study in which 29 patients with disseminated, nonresectable neoplasms received adequate therapy with hydrazine sulfate, observed no significant subjective or objective responses. Toxicity (neurological impairment, especially, and GI toxicity) was significant. These authors concluded that further clinical utilization was not warranted at present.

2.3.1. 1-Acetyl-2-picolinoylhydrazine

1-Acetyl-2-picolinoylhydrazine (NSC 68626), at a dosage of 100 mg/kg, produced 80–100% inhibition of Walker carcinosarcoma 256 in rats (Laszlo *et al.*, 1969). In clinical evaluations, this compound has been disappointing (Olson *et al.*, 1969; Laszlo *et al.*, 1969; Wilson *et al.*, 1970; Sutow *et al.*, 1975).

2.3.2. Other Hydrazine Derivatives

Other hydrazines under investigation for antitumor activity were dithiocarbamoylhydrazine (Shay *et al.*, 1964), hydrazino acids (Pollack *et al.*, 1964; Wilson *et*

al., 1970), 2-isonicotinoylhydrazino-5-nitrosotropine *N*-oxide (Arakawa, 1964),
*bis*oxime sulfonates and *bis*quaternary hydrazones (Remers *et al.*, 1967), orotic
acid hydrazine (Golovinskii *et al.*, 1970), derivatives of 2-hydrazino-5-
nitropyridine (Prescott and Caldes, 1970), and acylhydrazines (Rutner *et al.*,
1974).

3. Triazenes

3.1. Introduction

Triazenes have experienced long-standing use in the synthesis of azo dyes, in the
rubber industry, and in the production of high-octane gasoline. Tumor-
inhibitory activity of a triazene, a phenyl derivative, was first reported by Clarke *et
al.* (1955). Subsequently, imidazole triazenes with potential anticancer activity
[5(or 4)-substituted triazeno imidazole-4(or 5)-carboxamides] were synthesized by
Shealy *et al.* (1962*a*, *b*). Thus, two main lines of triazenes have been pursued for
antitumor therapy: (1) phenyltriazenes, and (2) imidazole triazenes.

For reviews on imidazole triazenes, see Shealy (1970), Oliverio (1973), Loo
(1975), and Livingston and Carter (1970*c*).

3.2. Phenyltriazenes

The growth-inhibitory activity of 3,3-dimethyl-1-phenyltriazene (PDT) (Fig. 5) in
subcutaneous mouse sarcoma 180, as reported by Clarke *et al.* (1955), was
attributed to the formation of a diazonium ion. This compound proved to be the
most promising of a large series of compounds tested, mostly triazene derivatives.
Subsequently, PDT and two related triazene derivatives (3,3-dimethyl-1-*p*-
nitrophenyltriazene and 3,3-dimethyl-1-*p*-tolyltriazene) exhibited carcinostatic
activity in mouse leukemia 82, whereas no activity was found in the L1210 test
neoplasm (Burchenal *et al.*, 1956). A decrease of the oncogenic potential of L1210
leukemia due to repeated treatment of 10–15 transplant generations with PDT
and 1-phenyl-3-monomethyltriazene (PMT) was later reported by Schmid and
Hutchison (1973). These same authors (Schmid and Hutchison, 1974) also
reported a moderate increase of survival time in L1210 mouse leukemia due to the
treatment with PMT and PDT. PMT also produced papillomas in two strains of
mice.

3.3. Imidazole Triazenes

3.3.1. History, Chemistry, and General Remarks

In 1923, Windaus and Langenbeck (1923) described the synthesis of 5-
aminoimidazole-4-carboxamide (AIC) (Fig. 6), which they used for the synthetic

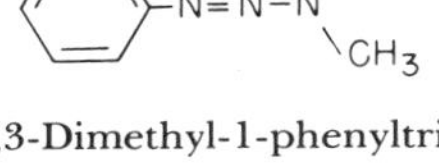

FIGURE 5. 3,3-Dimethyl-1-phenyltriazene (PDT).

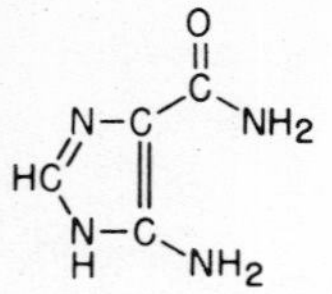

FIGURE 6. 5-Aminoimidazole-4-carboxamide (AIC).

preparation of purines. In the *de novo* biosynthesis of purines (Fig. 7), the starting material is α-5-phosphoribosyl-1-pyrophosphate (PRPP), on which, in many subsequent steps, the purine ring is built up at position 1 of the ribose moiety. One of the intermediary products is 5-aminoimidazole-4-carboxamide ribonucleotide, which, after introduction (from N^{10}-formyltetrahydrofolate) of a formate group and ring closure, is converted to inosinic acid. For reviews of details, see Greenberg and Jaenicke (1957) and Buchanan (1960). With the expectation that imidazole-4-carboxamide derivatives might be of interest in cancer chemotherapy, Shealy and co-workers (Shealy *et al.* 1961, 1962*a*; Shealy, 1970) synthesized a number of such compounds. The prototype of triazene compounds, 5-(3,3-dimethyl-1-triazeno)imidazole-4-carboxamide (DIC, NSC 45388) (Fig. 8), revealed tumor inhibition in mouse leukemia L1210, sarcoma 180, and adenocarcinoma 755 (solid forms) (Shealy *et al.*, 1962*b*), and was selected for clinical evaluation. DIC and its derivatives also inhibited Walker carcinosarcoma of rats (Shealy *et al.*, 1968), and a human malignant melanoma established in nude mice by serial transplantation (Povlsen and Jacobsen, 1975). DIC is more stable in aqueous and alcoholic solutions than its demethylation product, 5-(3-monomethyl-1-triazeno)imidazole-4-carboxamide (MIC), which releases AIC during decomposition (Shealy and Krauth, 1966*a*). Screening of large numbers of triazene derivatives in L1210 murine leukemia revealed that these compounds, with at least one methyl group (of the two alkyl groups), are the most effective ones (Shealy and Krauth, 1966*a*). Hano *et al.* (1965, 1968), studying a series of mono- and dialkyltriazenoimidazolcarboxamides in Ehrlich carcinoma, found DIC and the dipropyltriazene derivative to be the most active ones, whereas AIC stimulated significantly the growth of the solid form of Ehrlich carcinoma (Hano *et al.*, 1965). The hazards of structure–activity evaluations and speculations are evidenced by the fact that 5-[3,3-*bis*(2-chloroethyl)-1-triazeno]imidazole-4-carboxamide (BIC, NSC 82196) was the most potent derivative in L1210 mouse leukemia, both in the

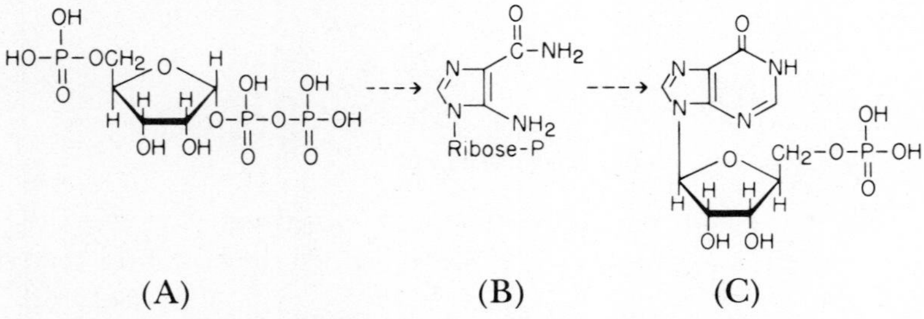

(A)   (B)   (C)

FIGURE 7. (A) α-5-Phosphoribosyl-1-pyrophosphate (PRPP); (B) 5-aminoimidazole-4-carboxamide ribonucleotide; (C) inosinic acid.

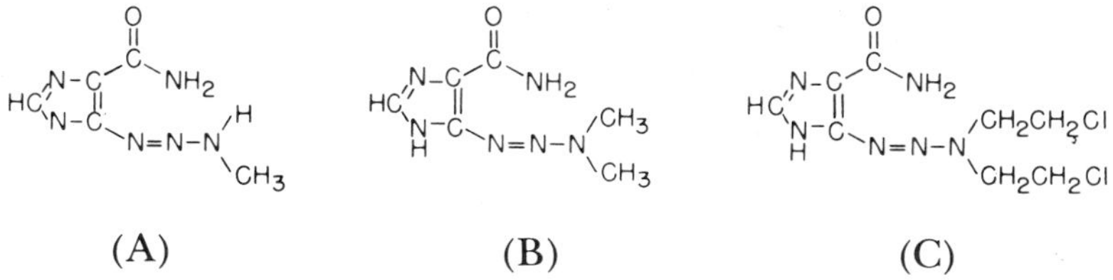

FIGURE 8. (A) 5-(3-Monomethyl-1-triazeno)imidazole-4-carboxamide (MIC, NSC 407347); (B) 5-(3,3-dimethyl-1-triazeno)imidazole-4-carboxamide (DIC, NSC 45388); (C) 5-[3,3-*bis*(2-chloroethyl)-1-triazeno]imidazole-4-carboxamide (BIC, NSC 82196).

initial form (Shealy and Krauth, 1966*b*) and in the advanced form (Hoffmann *et al.*, 1968). It is possible that the structural relationship of part of the BIC molecule to nitrogen mustard (mechlorethamine) (Livingston and Carter, 1970*a*) (Fig. 9) is responsible for this phenomenon. Supporting this explanation might be the findings of Kline *et al.* (1971), in which a line resistant to DIC was still sensitive to BIC. Not fitting this explanation is the fact that an L1210 line resistant to BIC exhibited cross-resistance to DIC and nitrosoureas, while it was still sensitive to melphalan and cyclophosphamide (Tyrer *et al.*, 1969). An L1210 line resistant to 6-mercaptopurine revealed marginal cross-resistance to BIC, but no resistance to DIC (Wodinsky *et al.*, 1968). DIC produced similar results in L1210 when administered intraperitoneally, subcutaneously, or orally (Goldin and Venditti, 1970).

3.3.2. Metabolism

Skibba *et al.* (1970*a*), studying the metabolism of DIC in rats, found oxidative *N*-demethylation of DIC *in vitro* by rat liver microsomes, as well as *in vivo*, after intraperitoneal injection of ^{14}C-methyl-labeled DIC (Fig. 10, step 1). The resulting MIC spontaneously decomposes to AIC (step 3) and a methylating agent. This pathway has been described as taking place in man (Householder and Loo, 1969*a*, *b*; Skibba *et al.*, 1970*a*, *c*) and rats (Skibba *et al.*, 1970*a*), and also *in vitro* in human and animal tumor tissues (Mizuno and Humphrey, 1972). Subsequently, trans-methylation of the methyl group of MIC onto the 7 position of guanine of rat liver DNA and RNA takes place. There is good evidence that the methyl group is transferred intact, since adenine and guanine of the same DNA and RNA preparations exhibited only trace amounts of radioactivity (Skibba *et al.*, 1970*a*).

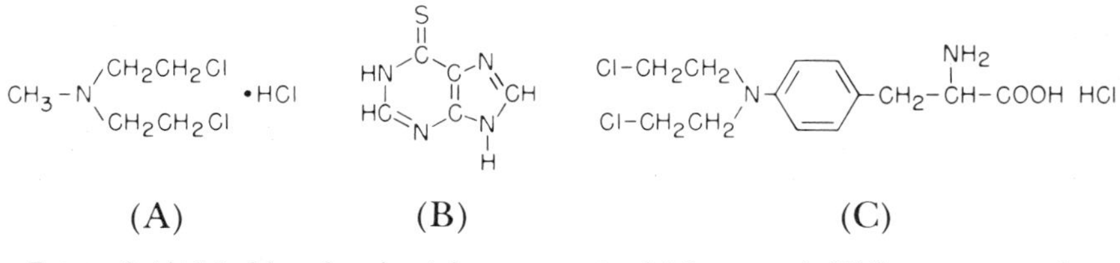

FIGURE 9. (A) Mechlorethamine (nitrogen mustard, Mustargen); (B) 6-mercaptopurine; (C) melphalan (phenylalanine mustard, Alkeran, L-PAM, L-sarcolysin).

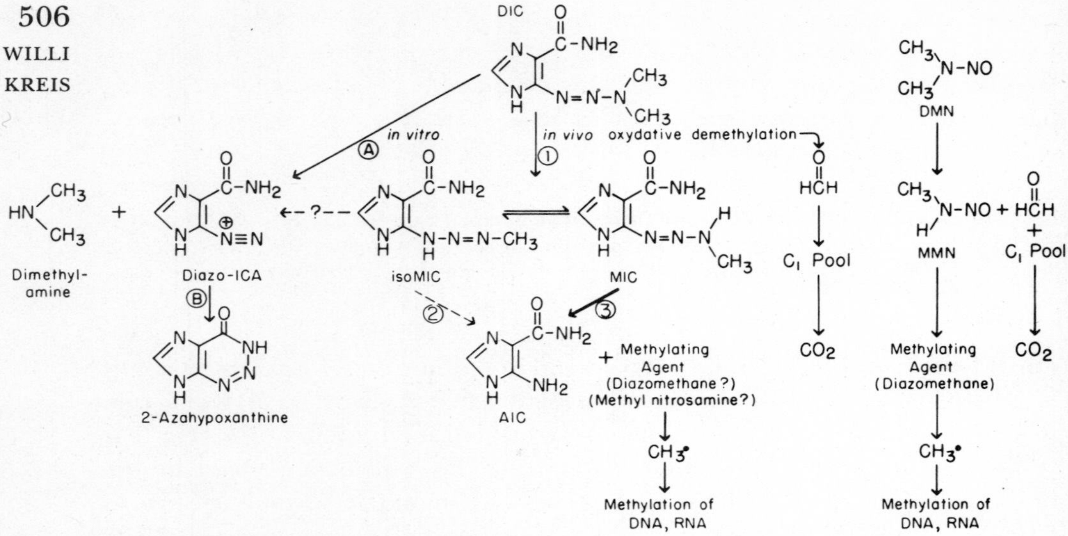

FIGURE 10. Current concepts of the metabolism of DIC and DMN as compiled from the literature.

Of the injected radioactivity of DIC, 4% was recovered within 6 hr in the form of CO_2 in the expiration air; pretreatment of the rats with prochlorperazine or phenobarbital increased this amount to 8.1 and 10.5%, respectively. Of the radioactivity in the rat experiments, 45% is unaccounted for. In the *in vitro* experiment with rat liver, not only AIC but also formaldehyde was identified. In 1 patient, after oral administration of the labeled DIC, 21.4% of the radioactivity was recovered within 6 hr in the form of $^{14}CO_2$, and 26% in urine within the same time. This urinary value is comparable to two other reported studies (Loo *et al.*, 1968; Skibba *et al.*, 1969). *In vitro* (but not *in vivo*), at low pH, and under the influence of UV light, DIC decomposes to diazoimidazole carboxamide (Diazo-ICA) plus dimethylamine (Fig. 10, pathway A). Diazo-ICA is then converted, under ring closure, to 2-azahypoxanthine (Beal *et al.*, 1975). The latter compound has also been identified in the urine of dogs, after administration of BIC (Vogel *et al.*, 1970). At present, there is no indication that DIC might be converted, through MIC or iso-MIC or both, to Diazo-ICA. The method used by these authors would not allow the evaluation of a possible expiration of $^{14}CH_4$.

Skibba *et al.* (1970a) compared the metabolism of DIC with that of dimethylnitrosamine (DMN) (Magee and Barnes, 1967), and proposed the sequence of reactions indicated in Fig. 10. For DIC, formaldehyde, carbon dioxide, and AIC have been properly identified; for DMN, formaldehyde and CO_2 were identified. Diazomethane, or any other methylating agent so far, lacks clear-cut identification for both compounds, although it is a likely reaction product in both instances.

3.3.3. Reaction Mechanism

For the phenyltriazenes, such as PMT and PDT, there is good evidence from studies by Preussman *et al.* (1969a) and Krüger *et al.* (1971) that PDT is enzymatically deaminated to PMT, with simultaneous release of formaldehyde. PMT then

acts like an alkylating agent, providing the methyl group of 7-methylguanine of
RNA and DNA (Krüger *et al.*, 1971) of liver in rats treated *in vivo* with PDT.
According to Dimroth (1903), phenylmethyltriazene reacts like a stabilized
diazomethane. The methylation of nucleic acids by DIC was reported by Skibba *et*
al. (1970*b*) and Skibba and Bryan (1971). In view of the identification of aniline in
in vitro reactions with PDT and of methemoglobinemia *in vivo* in acute
toxicity experiments with several triazenes (a consequence of aniline toxicity)
(Preussmann *et al.*, 1969*a*), the reaction mechanism by alkylation as proposed for
PDT, and by inference for DIC, is at present the most likely one.

5-Diazoimidazole-4-carboxamide (NSC 22420), which is devoid of the *N*-
alkylating moiety of DIC and BIC, still exhibits carcinostatic activity in animal
tumor systems (Shealy *et al.*, 1961). Therefore, for triazenoimidazoles, besides the
mechanism by alkylation, an interference with purine synthesis and metabolism is
likely (Newell and Tucker, 1968; Hoshi *et al.*, 1968; Loo *et al.*, 1967). A substantial
inhibition by DIC of DNA, RNA, and protein synthesis in *Bacillus subtilis* was
attributed by Saunders and Schultz (1972) to 4-diazoimido-5-carboxamide, which
is a photodecomposition product of DIC, and is itself highly inhibitory. These
authors also reported that DIC (in contrast to 5-fluorouracil) is lethal to both
proliferating and nonproliferating cells, implying that DIC is not a cycle-specific
agent. Wilkoff *et al.* (1968), in experiments with L1210 cells in tissue cultures, came
to the same conclusion.

As mentioned already for MBH, it is also possible that different tissues will
metabolize these triazenes in different ways, and thus react differently to the
emerging reaction products. This differing metabolism will, in turn, also contribute to the sensitivity and specificity of this group of compounds.

3.3.4. *Physiological Disposition*

DIC, injected intravenously 20 mg/kg (400 mg/M²) into dogs, exhibited a plasma
half-life of about 36 min; in man, the half-life after intravenous injection (133–
270 mg/M²) was 35 min (Loo *et al.*, 1968). In both species, the volume of distribution exceeded total body water content. In man, after oral administration (30–
260 mg/M²), the half-life of the drug was 111 min. Urinary excretion in dogs, after
intravenous injection, was completed within 6 hr and amounted to only 17%, as
compared with 43% in humans within the same time. In man, this 43% was
unchanged DIC. Trace amounts of at least one unidentified metabolite of DIC
were detected in the urine of both dogs and humans. After oral administration to
patients, an average of 19% of the dose was excreted in the urine, indicating
incomplete resorption of DIC from the GI tract. DIC enters the CSF to a low
degree: at equilibrium in constant infusion of DIC into dogs, CSF levels of only
14% of the plasma levels were reached (Loo *et al.*, 1968). Later, Skibba *et al.*
(1970*c*) and Householder and Loo (1969*b*) reported urinary AIC excretion
following intravenous or oral administration of DIC to patients: 20% of the
intravenously administered DIC was excreted as AIC in the urine within 24 hr;
after oral administration, the corresponding value was 16.5%. AIC in the urine
after DIC administration was also reported by Braunshtein and Vilenkina (1958),

McGeer *et al.* (1961), and Coward and Smith (1965), and AIC in human and animal tumor tissue by Mizuno and Humphrey (1972). Radioactive $[^{14}C]CO_2$, after administration of $[^{14}C]$methyl-labeled DIC, was detected by Skibba *et al.* (1970*a*) in rats at amounts of 4% within 6 hr after intraperitoneal injection, and in one patient up to 21.4% within 6 hr after oral administration of DIC. A significant increase in urinary excretion of radioactivity was found when 2-^{14}C-labeled DIC, instead of $[^{14}C]$dimethyl-DIC (92% vs. 47–73% of injected radioactivity), was used in mice (Household and Loo, 1969*a*); this difference most likely results from the expiration of CO_2, although other volatile substances, such as formaldehyde and methane, also must be taken into consideration.

Uptake of both BIC and DIC into L1210 cells *in vitro* was found to be nonsaturable and temperature-sensitive; lines resistant to DIC and BIC exhibited no impairment for drug accumulation (Kessel, 1971).

BIC, ^{14}C-labeled in the 2 position of the imidazole ring and administered intraperitoneally and orally to mice, produced a transient accumulation of radioactivity in the liver and kidneys (the pathways of excretion) (Vogel *et al.*, 1970). Excretion, after intraperitoneal administration, occurred predominantly through the urine. The GI absorption after oral administration (as evaluated by comparing the urinary excretion of radioactivity after intraperitoneal and oral administration of the ^{14}C-labeled drug) was 60–70%. In dogs, the plasma half-life was 2 hr after intravenous administration, and urinary excretion amounted to about 64% of the administered dosage (Vogel *et al.*, 1970). With a colorimetric assay, however, the average plasma half-life in dogs was evaluated to be only 3 min (Loo, 1975). This discrepancy is best explained by a rapid chemical conversion. The drug was not excreted unchanged, but was identified predominantly (60%) in the form of an ionic transformation product. Besides a small amount of radioactive 2-azahypoxanthine, the remaining urinary excretion product was not identified. GI absorption was "poor and erratic." After both intravenous and oral administration, permeation into the CSF was negligible (Vogel *et al.*, 1970).

For reasons of instability and light-sensitivity, the only physiological distribution studies in man were performed with orally administered BIC labeled in the *N*-ethyl side chains with ^{14}C. In the plasma, CSF, and pleural fluid, levels of radioactivity were extremely low (Vogel *et al.*, 1971*b*). From radioactivity recovered in urine and feces, these investigators concluded a probable erratic absorption of the drug from the GI tract, a predominant excretion of radioactivity in urine, and there the main excretion product to be an ionic transformation product of the original drug. Interestingly, in one patient, about 10% of the radioactive material was recovered in the form of expired CO_2.

3.3.5. Toxicity

DIC, the most important triazene derivative in clinical cancer chemotherapy, caused nausea and vomiting. Myelosuppression and leukopenia, followed by thrombocytopenia, were the dose-limiting toxic symptoms. It was recommended that the dose be kept within 200–500 mg/M^2 for a 5-day schedule, repeated with intervening 3-week intervals (Luce *et al.*, 1970). "Flu"-like syndromes with high temperatures and hepatotoxicity were also observed. At high dosages of DIC, diarrhea was observed in some patients (C. Young, personal communication). With BIC, nausea, vomiting, and myelosuppression were the most prominent toxic symptoms reported (Vogel *et al.*, 1971*b*).

3.3.6. Other Biological Effects

DIC has a strong *in vitro* inhibitory activity against gram-positive and gram-negative bacteria, fungi, mycobacteria, algae, and yeasts (Shealy *et al.*, 1967; Pittillo and Hunt, 1967*a*; Hunt and Pittillo, 1967), as well as toward some lines of *Escherichia coli* and *Streptococcus faecalis* resistant to a variety of antibiotics (Pittillo and Hunt, 1967*b*), and *in vivo* activity against *Staphylococcus aureus* in mice (Pittillo and Hunt, 1967*a*). BIC demonstrated only minimal antimicrobial activity (Pittillo and Hunt, 1967*c*). BIC also suppressed experimental allergic encephalomyelitis probably due to a delayed hypersensitivity reaction (Vogel *et al.*, 1969).

PDT (Preussmann *et al.*, 1969*b*) and PMT (Preussman and von Hodenberg, 1970), as well as DIC (Skibba *et al.*, 1970*d*; Beal *et al.*, 1975), are strong carcinogens. DIC induced thymic lymphosarcomas and mammary adenocarcinomas in rats. PDT also acts as a "direct" mutagen in at least three different test systems (Vogel *et al.*, 1973).

3.3.7. Clinical Use

While the phenyltriazenes have not yet had any clinical trials, DIC and BIC have been evaluated in many human malignancies. DIC as a single agent first proved to be active in malignant melanoma (Loo *et al.*, 1967; MacDonald *et al.*, 1967; Skibba *et al.*, 1969; Luce *et al.*, 1970; Gottlieb and Serpick, 1971; Vogel *et al.*, 1971*a*; Cowan and Bergsagel, 1971; Burke *et al.*, 1971; Ahmann *et al.*, 1972). Subsequently, objective antitumor responses were also obtained in lymphosarcoma, fibrosarcoma, squamous-cell carcinoma of the lung, Hodgkin's disease, and oat-cell carcinoma of the lung (Luce *et al.*, 1970); lung cancer (Kingra *et al.*, 1971); Hodgkin's disease, lymphosarcoma, and mycosis fungoides (Frei *et al.*, 1972); and neuroblastoma and rhabdomyosarcoma (Finklestein *et al.*, 1975). When DIC is given intravenously as a single agent, the usual dosage is now 250 mg/M^2 per day for 5 days, repeated at intervals of 3 weeks.

When DIC was used in combination with vincristine in malignant melanoma, no improvement was observed over the use of DIC alone (Ahmann *et al.*, 1975). DIC in combination with adriamycin produced objective responses in cancer of the kidney, liver, and lungs, testicular tumors, lymphosarcomas, rhabdomyosarcomas, hepatomas, and mesotheliomas (Gottlieb *et al.*, 1972), and the combination of DIC with vincristine and cyclophosphamide improved the response rate of widespread metastatic neuroblastoma of children (Finkelstein *et al.*, 1974). A combination of 5-fluorouracil (5-FU), DIC, vincristine, and 1,3-*bis*(2-chloroethyl)-1-nitrosurea (BCNU) produced objective responses in breast cancer, colon carcinoma, rectal carcinoma, cholangiocellular carcinoma, adenocarcinoma of unknown origin, ovarian carcinoma, and myeloblastosis (Van Eden *et al.*, 1972).

BIC as a single agent has been less successful than DIC: in Phase I (Lane and Talley, 1972) and Phase II (Ahmann *et al.*, 1973; Moertel *et al.*, 1972) studies, only patients with malignant melanoma (Falkson *et al.*, 1972) showed partial response. Response was also reported in lymphoma, but not in patients with childhood leukemia (Vogel *et al.*, 1971*b*). Levine *et al.*, (1975) reported a definite response in a variety of brain tumors.

4. Conclusions and Perspectives

Hydrazines and triazenes, related by structure and probably also by mechanism of action, have established themselves as useful agents in cancer chemotherapy. The pathways of their discovery and development as carcinostatic agents are significantly different: while the first hydrazines came into action in a screening program for amine oxidase inhibition, imidazole triazenes were designed and produced to interfere specifically with the *de novo* synthesis of purines. Their biological relationship is most obvious in the mechanism of action, since both groups of compounds (including the phenoltriazenes) are proven alkylating (predominantly methylating) agents, although probably not in the classic sense: their methylation of purines (and also partly pyrimidines) of DNA and RNA so far is the only well-substantiated evidence for interference with vital functions of the affected cells.

Significant differences in their chemotherapeutic action (sensitivity and specificity) are an expression of different functional capabilities of individual cells or tissues, and are ultimately due to differences in their structure and enzymatic makeup.

Side effects of hydrazines and triazenes, such as the reported immunosuppression and inhibition of the monoaminooxidase, carcinogenesis, and teratogenesis, must always be taken seriously; it is likely that the last two are related to the mechanism of action of these drugs.

The prospects and future for these drugs probably lie in their use in combinations with other agents of different reaction mechanisms. While such studies in patients are ongoing in many hospitals, it must be pointed out that our understanding of the action of each of these individually is still very limited.

Only extensive studies of both malignant and normal cells at the molecular level will allow us to ultimately understand and optimize the management of cancer by chemotherapy. Sensitivity and specificity are terms we have to learn to comprehend, and subsequently learn to manipulate.

ACKNOWLEDGMENTS

The author is indebted to Dr. Charles W. Young and Dr. Edward Miller for critical review, and to Mrs. Patricia Higgins for help in the preparation of this manuscript. This work was supported in part by Grant CA-08748 from the National Cancer Institute and Grant T45 from the American Cancer Society.

5. References

ADAMSON, R. H., 1970, Carcinogenicity studies with procarbazine, in: *Proceedings of the Chemotherapy Conference on Procarbazine (Matulane: NSC-77213): Development and Application* (S. K. Carter, ed.), pp. 29–33, U.S. Government Printing Office, Washington, D.C.

AHMANN, D. L., HAHN, R. G., AND BIESEL, H. F., 1972, Clinical evaluation of 5-(3,3-dimethyl-1-triazeno)imidazole-4-carboxamide (NSC 45388), melphalan (NSC 8806), and hydroxyurea (NSC 32065) in the treatment of disseminated malignant melanoma, *Cancer Chemother. Rep.* **56**:369.

AHMANN, D. L., BISEL, H. F., AND HAHN, R. G., 1973, Difficulties designing clinical trials as exemplified by a phase 2 drug evaluation of 5[3,3-*bis*(2-chloroethyl(-1-triazenol]imidazole-4-carboxamide and 1-(2-chloroethyl)-3-cyclohexyl-1-nitrosourea in patients with disseminated breast cancer, *Cancer Res.* **33**:1707.

AHMANN, D. L., HAHN, R. G., BISEL, H. F., EAGAN, R. T., AND EDMONSON, J. H., 1975, Comparative study of methyl-CCNU (NSC 95441) with cyclophosphamide (NSC 26271) and 5-(3,3-dimethyl-1-triazeno)imidazole-4-carboxamide (NSC 45388) with vincristine (NSC 67574) in patients with disseminated melanoma, *Cancer Chemother. Rep. Part 1* **59**:451.

ALBERTO, P., 1974, Facteurs pronostiques dans la chimiothérapie des cancer bronchiques, *Schweiz. Med. Wochenschr.* **104**:268.

ARAKAWA, M., 1964, Antitumor action of 7-numbered ring compounds. IV. Pharmacology of 2-isonicotinoylhydrazino-5-nitrosotropone *N*-oxide (RCH 1003), *Folia Pharmacol. Jpn.* **60**:471.

ARON, E., 1968, Le traitement médical de la maladie de Dupuytren par un agent cytostatique (methyl-hydrazine), *Presse Med.* **76**:1956.

ARSENEAU, J. C., CANELLOS, G. P., DEVITA, V. T., AND SHERIUS, R. J., 1974, Recently recognized complications of cancer chemotherapy, *Ann. N. Y. Acad. Sci.* **230**:481.

BACKHOUSE, T. W., AND SICHER, K., 1966, Initial experiences with methylhydrazine, a new cytotoxic agent, *Clin. Radiol.* **17**:132.

BAGGIOLINI, M., BICKEL, M. H., AND MESSIHA, F. S., 1965, Demethylation *in vivo* of Natulan, a tumor-inhibiting methylhydrazine derivative, *Experientia* **21**:334.

BAGGIOLINI, M., DEWALD, B., AND AEBI, H., 1969, Oxidation of *p*-(*N*′-methylhydrazinomethyl)-*N*-isopropylbenzamide (procarbazine) to the methylazo derivative and oxidative cleavage of the N²–C bond in the isolated perfused rat liver, *Biochem. Pharmacol.* **18**:2187.

BEAL, D. D., SKIBBA, J. L., CROFT, W. A., COHEN, S. M., AND BRYAN, G. T., 1975, Carcinogenicity of the antineoplastic agent, 5-(3,3-dimethyl-1-triazeno)-imidazole-4-carboxamide, and its metabolites in rats, *J. Natl. Cancer Inst.* **54**:951.

BERNEIS, K., KOFLER, M., BOLLAG, W., KAISER, A., AND LANGEMANN, A., 1963, The degradation of deoxyribonucleic acid by new tumour inhibiting compounds: The intermediate formation of hydrogen peroxide, *Experientia* **19**:132.

BERNEIS, K., BOLLAG, W., KOFLER, M., AND LUTHY, H., 1966, The enhancement of the after effect of ionizing radiation by a cytotoxic methylhydrazine derivative, *Eur. J. Cancer* **2**:43.

BOEHNEL, J., AND STACHER, A., 1966, Über die Wirkung eines Zytostatikums aus der Methylhydrazinereihe bei malignen Haemoblastosen, *Wien Med. Wochenschr.* **116**:468.

BOLLAG, W., 1963, Suppression of the immunological reaction by methylhydrazines, a new class of antitumour agents, *Experientia* **19**:304.

BOLLAG, W., AND GRUNBERG, E., 1963, Tumour inhibitory effects of a new class of cytotoxic agents: Methylhydrazine derivatives, *Experientia* **19**:130.

BOLLAG, W., KAISER, A., LANGEMANN, A., AND ZELLER, P., 1964, Methylazo and methylazoxy compounds; new types of antitumour agents, *Experientia* **20**:503.

BRAUNSHTEIN, A. E., AND VILENKINA, G. I. A., 1958, Chromatographic determination of 4(5)-aminoimidazole-5(4)carboxamide and its presence in human and animal urine, *Biokhimiya* **23**:887.

BROOKES, P., 1965, Studies of the mode of action of Ibenzmethyzin, in: *Natulan (Ibenzmethyzin)* (A. M. Jelliffe and J. Marks, eds.), pp. 9–12, John Wright and Sons, Bristol.

BRULÉ, G., SCHLUMBERGER, J. R., AND GRISCELLI, C., 1965, *N*-Isopropyl-α-2-methylhydrazino-*p*-toluamide hydrochloride (NSC 77213) in treatment of solid tumors, *Cancer Chemother. Rep.* **44**:31.

BRUNNER, K. W., AND YOUNG, C. W., 1965, A methylhydrazine derivative in Hodgkin's disease and other malignant neoplasms. Therapeutic and toxic effects studied in 51 patients, *Ann. Intern. Med.* **63**:69.

BRUNNER, K. W., MAURICE, P., AND SONNTAG, R. W., 1973, CCNU [1,(2-chloroethyl)-3-cyclohexyl-1-nitrosourea] und BCNU [1,3,-bis(2-chloroethyl)1-nitrosourea] sowie BCNU-kombinationen beim Lymphogranuloma Hodgkin Stadium III and IV, in: *Leukämie und Maligne Lymphome, Pathophysiologie, Klinik, Chemo- und Immunotherapie* (A. Stacher, ed.), pp. 401–413, Urban and Schwarzenberg, Munich.

BUCHANAN, J. M., 1960, Biosynthesis of purine nucleotides, in: *The Nucleic Acids*, Vol. 3 (E. Chargaff and J. N. Davidson, eds.), pp. 303–322, Academic Press, New York.

BULL, J. M., DE KIEWIET, J. W. C., ROSENBERG, S. A., AND KAPLAN, H. S., 1970, Cyclic chemotherapy (MOPP) combined with extended field radiotherapy for Hodgkin's disease, *Clin. Res.* **18:**189.

BURCHENAL, J. H., DAGG, M. K., BEYER, M., AND STOCK, C. C., 1956, Chemotherapy of leukemia. VII. Effect of substituted triazenes on transplanted mouse leukemia (22273), *Proc. Soc. Exp. Biol. Med.* **91:**398.

BURKE, P. J., McCARTHY, W. H., AND MILTON, G. W., 1971, Imidazole carboxamide therapy in advanced malignant melanoma, *Cancer* **27:**744.

BUTLER, J. A. V., AND SMITH, K. A., 1950, Degradation of deoxyribonucleic acid by free radicals, *Nature (London)* **165:**847.

CANELLOS, G. P., ARSENEAU, J. C., DEVITA, V. T., WHANG-PENG, J., AND JOHNSON, R. E. C., 1975, Second malignancies complicating Hodgkin's disease in remission, *Lancet* **1:**947.

CARTER, S. K. (ed.), 1970, *Procarbazine (Matulane: NSC 77213): Development and Application,* Bethesda: Cancer Therapy Evaluation Branch, National Cancer Institute, U.S. Government Printing Office (1971 0-440-316), Washington, D.C.

CARTER, S. K., 1973, Useful agents in lymphomas and solid tumors, *Consultant* **13:**45.

CHABNER, B. A., DEVITA, V. T., CONSIDINE, N., AND OLIVERIO, V. T., 1969, Plasma pyridoxal phosphate depletion by the carcinostatic procarbazine, *Proc. Soc. Exp. Biol. Med.* **132:**1119.

CHABNER, B. A., SPONZO, R., HUBBARD, S., CANELLOS, G. P., YOUNG, R. C., SCHEIN, P. S., AND DEVITA, V. T., 1973, High-dose intermittent intravenous infusion of procarbazine (NSC 77213), *Cancer Chemother. Rep. Part 1* **57:**361.

CHAUBE, S., AND MURPHY, M. L., 1969, Fetal malformations produced in rats by N-isopropyl-alpha-(2-methylhydrazino)-p-toluamide hydrochloride (procarbazine), *Teratology* **2:**23.

CLARKE, D. A., BARCLAY, R. K., STOCK, C. C., AND RONDESTVEDT, C. S., JR., 1955, Triazenes as inhibitors of mouse sarcoma 180, *Proc. Soc. Exp. Biol. Med.* **90:**484.

COWAN, D. H., AND BERGSAGEL, D. E., 1971, Intermittent treatment of metastatic malignant melanoma with high-dose 5-(3,3-dimethyl-1-triazeno)imidazole-4-carboxamide (NSC 45388), *Cancer Chemother. Rep.* **55:**175.

COWARD, R. F., AND SMITH, P., 1965, Determination of urinary 4-aminoimidazole-5-carboxamide, *Clin. Chim. Acta* **12:**206.

D'ALESSANDRI, A., KEEL, H. J., BOLLAG, W., AND MARTZ, G., 1963, Erste klinische Erfahrung mit einem neuen Zytostatikum, *Schweiz. Med. Wochenschr.* **93:**1018.

DAVIS, J. E., AND DEROPP, R. S., 1961, Metabolic origin of urinary methylamine in the rat, *Nature (London)* **190:**636.

DAWSON, W. B., 1965, Ibenzmethyzin in the management of late Hodgkin's disease, in: *Natulan (Ibenzmethyzin)* (A. M. Jelliffe and J. Marks, eds.), pp. 31–34, John Wright and Sons, Bristol.

DECKERS, C., DECKERS-PASSAU, L., MAISIN, J., GAUTHIER, J. M., AND MACE, F., 1974, Carcinogenicity of procarbazine, *Z. Krebsforsch.* **81:**79.

DEICHER, H., 1972, Empfehlungen zur immunsuppresiven Therapie beim lupus erythematodes visceralis, *Monatsschr. Kinderheilkd.* **120:**249.

DEVITA, V., 1966, Preliminary clinical studies with Ibenzmethyzin, *Clin. Pharmacol. Ther.* **7:**542.

DEVITA, V. T., JR., SERPICK, A. A., AND CARBONE, P. P., 1970, Combination chemotherapy in the treatment of advanced Hodgkin's disease, *Ann. Intern. Med.* **73:**881.

DEWALD, B., BAGGIOLINI, M., AND AEBI, H., 1969, N-Demethylation of p-(N'-methylhydrazinomethyl)-N-isopropyl benzamide (procarbazine), a cytostatically active methyl-hydrazine derivative, in the intact rat and in the isolated perfused rat liver, *Biochem. Pharmacol.* **18:**2179.

DIMROTH, O., 1903, Synthesen mit Diazobenzolimid, *Ber. Dtsch. Chem. Ges.* **36:**909.

DOST, F. N., AND REED, D. J., 1967, Methane formation *in vivo* from N-isopropyl-α-(2-methylhydrazino)-p-toluamide hydrochloride, a tumor-inhibiting methylhydrazine derivative, *Biochem. Pharmacol.* **16:**1741.

DOST, F. N., REED, D. J., AND WANG, C. H., 1966, The metabolic fate of monomethylhydrazine and unsymmetrical dimethylhydrazine, *Biochem. Pharmacol.* **15:**1325.

FALKSON, G., DE VILLIERS, P. C., AND FALKSON, H. C., 1965, N-Isopropyl-α-(2-methylhydrazino)-p-toluamide hydrochloride (NSC 77213) for treatment of cancer patients, *Cancer Chemother. Rep.* **46**:7.

FALKSON, G., VAN DER MERWE, A. M., AND FALKSON, H. C., 1972, Clinical experience with 5-[3,3-*bis*(2-chloroethyl)-1-triazeno]imidazole-4-carboxamide (NSC 82196) in the treatment of metastatic malignant melanoma, *Cancer Chemother. Rep.* **56**:671.

FELLINGER, K., 1973, Neuere Behandlungsmethoden in der Rheumatologie, *Wien. Med. Wochenschr.* **123**:609.

FINE, M. H., 1974, Treatment of Hodgkin's disease, standard treatment (review), *Ariz. Med.* **31**:364.

FINKLESTEIN, J. Z., LEIKIN, S., EVANS, A., KLEMPERER, M., BERNSTEIN, I., HITTLE, R., AND HAMMOND, G. D., 1974, Combination chemotherapy for metastatic neuroblastoma, *Proc. Amer. Assoc. Cancer Res. Amer. Soc. Clin. Oncol.* **15**:44.

FINKELSTEIN, J. Z., ALBO, V., ERTEL, I., AND HAMMOND, D., 1975, 5-(3,3-Dimethyl-1-triazeno)imidazole-4-carboxamide (NSC 45388) in the treatment of solid tumors in children, *Cancer Chemother. Rep.* **59**:351.

FISCHER, M., AND MARTIN, H., 1972, Zur Diagnostik and Therapie der Polycythaemia vera, *Dtsch. Aerztebl.* **69**:418.

FLOERSHEIM, G. L., 1963, Verlängerte Überlebenszeit von Hauthomotransplantaten durch ein Methylhydrazinderivat, *Experientia* **19**:546.

FLOERSHEIM, G. L., 1966, Effect of methylhydrazine derivatives on the survival of second-set skin homografts, *Nature (London)* **211**:638.

FREI, E., III, 1974, Combination chemotherapy, *Proc. R. Soc. Med.* **67**:425.

FREI, E., III, LUCE, J. K., TALLEY, R. W., VAITKEVICIUS, V. K., AND WILSON, H. E., 1972, 5-(3,3-Dimethyl-1-triazeno)imidazole-4-carboxamide (NSC 45388) in the treatment of lymphoma, *Cancer Chemother. Rep.* **56**:667.

FULLER, A. T., 1937, Is p-aminobenzenesulfonamide the active agent in Prontosil therapy?, *Lancet* **1**:194.

GALE, G. R., SIMPSON, J. G., AND SMITH, A. B., 1967, Studies of the mode of action of N-isopropyl-α-(2-methylhydrazino)-p-toluamide, *Cancer Res.* **27**:1186.

GARRETT, M. J., 1974, Teratogenic effects of combination chemotherapy, *Ann. Intern. Med.* **80**:667.

GELZER, J., AND LOUSTALOT, P., 1967, Biological and chemotherapeutic studies on primary mammary tumor in C3H and C3HO mice, *Int. J. Cancer* **2**:179.

GOLD, J., 1970, Inhibition of Walker 256 intramuscular carcinoma by administration of L-tryptophan, *Oncology* **24**:291.

GOLD, J., 1971, Inhibition of Walker 256 intramuscular carcinoma in rats by administration of hydrazine sulfate, *Oncology* **25**:66.

GOLD, J., 1973, Inhibition by hydrazine sulfate and various hydrazides of *in vivo* growth of Walker 256 intramuscular carcinoma, B-16 melanoma, Murphy Sturm lymphosarcoma and L-1210 solid leukemia, *Oncology* **27**:69.

GOLD, J., 1974, Use of hydrazine sulfate in advanced cancer patients: Preliminary results, *Proc. Amer. Assoc. Cancer Res. Amer. Soc. Clin. Oncol.* **15**:83.

GOLDENBERG, D. M., AND WITTE, S., 1967, The activity of Ibenzmethyzin hydrochloride against the human transplantable tumours, human epithelioma No. 3 and human adenoma No. 1, *Experientia* **23**:234.

GOLDIN, G., AND VENDITTI, J. M., 1970, *In vivo* testing of antitumor agents, in: *Progress in Anticancer Chemotherapy, Proceedings of the 6th International Congress of Chemotherapy*, Vol. II, pp. 864–877, University Park Press, Baltimore.

GOLDSMITH, M. A., AND CARTER, S. K., 1974, Combination chemotherapy of advanced Hodgkin's disease, a review, *Cancer* **33**:1.

GOLOVINSKII, E., EMANUILOV, E., AND MARKOV, G. G., 1970, The effect of orotic acid hydrazide on the growth of neurospora crassa and on the development of Ehrlich ascitic tumor, *Vopr. Med. Khim.* **16**:293.

GOTTLIEB, J. A., AND SERPICK, A. A., 1971, Clinical evaluation of 5(3,3-dimethyl-1-triazeno)imidazole-4-carboxamide in malignant melanoma and other neoplasms: Comparison of twice-weekly and daily administration schedules, *Oncology* **25**:225.

GOTTLIEB, J. A., BAKER, L. H., QUAGLIANA, J. M., LUCE, J. K., WHITECAR, J. P., SINKOVICS, J. G., RIVKIN, S. E., BROWNLEE, R., AND FREI, E., III, 1972, Chemotherapy of sarcomas with a combination of adriamycin and dimethyl triazeno imidazole carboxamide, *Cancer* **30**:1632.

GOWING, D. P., AND LEEPER, R. W., 1955, Induction of flowering in pineapple by beta-hydroxyethylhydrazine, *Science* **122**:1267.

GREENBERG, G. R., AND JAENICKE, L., 1957, On the activation of the one-carbon unit for the biosynthesis of purine nucleotides, in *Ciba Found. Symp.: Chemistry and Biology of Purines* (G. E. W. Wolstenholme and C. M. O'Connor, eds.), pp. 204–232, J. & A. Churchill, London.

GRUNBERG, E., 1970, Experimental tumor inhibitory activity of procarbazine, in: *Proceedings of the Chemotherapy Conference of Procarbazine (Matulane: NSC 77213): Development and Application* (S. K. Carter, ed.), pp. 9–18, U.S. Government Printing Office, Washington, D.C.

GUTIN, P. H., WILSON, C. B., KUMAR, A. R. V., BOLDREY, E. B., LEVIN, V., POWELL, M., AND ENOT, K. J., 1975, Phase II study of procarbazine, CCNU, and vincristine combination chemotherapy in the treatment of malignant brain tumors, *Cancer* **35:**1398.

GUTTERMAN, J., HUANG, A. T., AND HOCHSTEIN, P., 1969, Studies on the mode of action of *N*-isopropyl-alpha-(2-methylhydrazino)-*p*-toluamide, *Proc. Soc. Exp. Biol. Med.* **130:**797.

HANO, K., AKASHI, A., YAMAMOTO, I., NARUMI, S., HORII, Z., AND NINOMIYA, I., 1965, Antitumor activity of 4(or 5)-aminoimidazole-5(or 4)-carboxamide derivatives, *Gann* **56:**417.

HANO, K., AKASHI, A., YAMAMOTO, I., NARUMI, S., AND IWATA, H., 1968, Further investigation of the carcinostatic activity of 4(or5)-aminoimidazole-5(or 4)-carboxamide derivatives: Structure–activity relationship, *Gann* **59:**207.

HOFFMAN, G., KLINE, I., GANG, M., TYRER, D. D., VENDITTI, J. M., AND GOLDIN, A., 1968, Influence of treatment schedules and route of administration on the chemotherapy of murine leukemia L1210 with 5(or 4)-[3,3-*bis*(2-chloroethyl)-1-triazeno]imidazole-4 (or 5)-carboxamide (NSC 82196), *Cancer Chemother. Rep.* **52:**715.

HOPE-STONE, H., 1965, Ibenzmethyzin in the treatment of reticulosis, in: *Natulan (Ibenzmethyzin)* (A. M. Jelliffe and J. Marks, eds.), pp. 15–19, John Wright and Sons, Bristol.

HOSHI, A., KUMAGAI, K., AND KURETANI, K., 1968, Studies on antitumor agents. I. Antitumor activity of 5(4)-amino-4(5)-imidazole carboxamide analogs, *Chem. Pharm. Bull.* **16:**2080.

HOUSEHOLDER, G. E., AND LOO, T. L., 1969*a*, Elevated urinary excretion of 4-aminoimidazole-5-carboxamide in patients after intravenous injection of 4-(3,3-dimethyl-1-triazeno)imidazole-5-carboxamide, *Life Sci.* **8:**533.

HOUSEHOLDER, G. E., AND LOO, T. L., 1969*b*, Physiologic disposition of 4-(dimethyltriazeno)imidazole-5-carboxamide, *Pharmacologist* **11:**280.

HUNT, D. E., AND PITTILLO, R. F., 1967, Methyl 5(or 4)-(3,3-dimethyl-1-triazeno)imidazole-4(or 5)-carboxylate (NSC 87982): Mouse tissue concentrations as determined by microbiological assay, *Proc. Soc. Exp. Biol. Med.* **125:**919.

JACOBS, P., AND DUBOVSKY, D., 1975, Letter: Treatment of myeloma, *Br. Med. J.* **1:**625.

JELLIFFE, A. M., AND MARKS, J. (eds.), 1965, *Natulan (Ibenzmethyzin)*, John Wright and Sons, Bristol.

JELLIFFE, A. M., BLECHEN, N. M., AND FENNER, M. L., 1965, Ibenzmethyzin in the treatment of solid tumours, in: *Natulan (Ibenzmethyzin)* (A. M. Jelliffe and J. Marks, eds.), pp. 53–55, John Wright and Sons, Bristol.

KELLY, M. G., O'GARA, R. W., YANCEY, S. T., GADEKAR, K., BOTKIN, C., AND OLIVERIO, V. T., 1969, Comparative carcinogenicity of *N*-isopropyl-*α*-(2-methylhydrazino)-*p*-toluamide HCl (procarbazine hydrochloride), its degradation products, other hydrazines and isonicotinic acid hydrazide, *J. Natl. Cancer Inst.* **42:**337.

KENIS, Y., 1968, Le traitement de la maladie de Hodgkin generalisée par la procarbazine (Natulan), *Bruxelles-Med.*, **48:**447–456.

KENIS, Y., DE SMEDT, J., AND TAGNON, H. J., 1966, Action du Natulan dans 94 cas de tumeurs solides, *Eur. J. Cancer* **2:**51.

KERSEY, J., ROLOFF, J., KOKENESS, S., JOHNSON, F. L., NESBITT, M., AND KRIVIT, W., 1975, Retransplantation of human bone marrow. Two immunosuppressive drug regimens, *Transplantation* **19:**475.

KESSEL, D., 1971, Transport and accumulation of triazenoimidazoles by L1210 cells, *Cancer Res.* **31:**135.

KINGRA, G. S., COMIS, R., OLSON, K. B., AND HORTON, J., 1971, 5-(3,3-Dimethyl-1-triazeno)imidazole-4-carboxamide (NSC 45388) in the treatment of malignant tumors other than melanoma, *Cancer Chemother. Rep.* **55:**281.

KLINE, I., WOODMAN, R. J., GANG, M., AND VENDITTI, J. M., 1971, Effectiveness of antileukemic agents in mice inoculated with leukemia L1210 variants resistant to 5-(3,3-dimethyl-1-triazeno)imidazole-4-carboxamide (NSC 45388) or 5-[3,3-*bis*(2-chloroethyl)-1-triazeno]imidazole-4-carboxamide (NSC 82196), *Cancer Chemother. Rep.* **55:**9.

KOBLET, H., AND DIGGELMANN, H., 1968, Action of Ibenzmethyzin [*N*-isopropyl-*α*-(2-methylhydrazine)-*p*-toluamide-hydrochloride, Natulan®, IMTH] on protein synthesis in the rat liver, *Eur. J. Cancer* **4:**45.

KREIS, W., 1970a, Metabolism of an antineoplastic methylhydrazine derivative in a P815 mouse neoplasm, *Cancer Res.* **30**:82.

KREIS, W., 1970b, Mechanism of action of procarbazine, in: *Proceedings of the Chemotherapy Conference on Procarbazine (Matulane: NSC 77213): Development and Application* (S. K. Carter, ed.), pp. 35–44, U.S. Government Printing Office, Washington, D.C.

KREIS, W., AND YEN, W., 1965, An antineoplastic C^{14}-labeled methylhydrazine derivative in P815 mouse leukemia. A metabolic study, *Experientia* **21**:284.

KREIS, W., PIEPHO, S. B., AND BERNHARD, H. V., 1966, Studies on the metabolic fate of the ^{14}C-labeled methyl group of a methylhydrazine derivative in P815 mouse leukemia, *Experientia* **22**:431.

KREIS, W., BURCHENAL, J. H., AND HUTCHISON, D. J., 1968, Influence of a methylhydrazine derivative on the *in vivo* transmethylation of the 5-methyl group of methionine onto purine and pyrimidine bases of RNA, *Proc. Amer. Assoc. Cancer Res.* **9**:38.

KREMENTZ, E. T., AND YOUNGBLOOD, J. W., 1962, The effect of peroxides on experimental tumors in mice, *Proc. Amer. Assoc. Cancer Res.* **4**:335.

KRÜGER, F. W., PREUSSMANN, R., AND NIEPELT, N., 1971, Mechanism of carcinogenesis with 1-aryl-3,3-dialkyl-triazenes. III. *In vivo* methylation of RNA and DNA with 1-phenyl-3,3-[^{14}C]-dimethyltriazene, *Biochem. Pharmacol.* **20**:529.

LANE, M., AND TALLEY, R. W., 1972, A phase I study of 5-(3,3-*bis*(2-chloroethyl)-1-triazeno)-imidazole-4-carboxamide (TIC mustard), *Proc. Amer. Assoc. Cancer Res.* **13**:125.

LASZLO, J., DURANT, J., AND LOEB, V., 1969, Clinical pharmacologic study of 1-acetyl-2-picolinoyl hydrazine (NSC 68626), *Cancer Chemother. Rep.* **53**:131.

LEHNINGER, A. L., 1970, *Biochemistry: The Molecular Basis of Cell Structure and Function,* Worth Publishers, New York.

LEVINE, V. A., CRAFTS, D., WILSON, C. B., KABRA, P., HAUSCH, C., BOLDREY, E., ENOT, J., AND NEELY, M., 1975, Imidazole carboxamides: Relationship of lipophilicity to activity against intracerebral murine glioma 26 and preliminary phase II clinical trial of 5-[3,3-*bis*(2-chloroethyl)-1-triazeno]-imidazole-4-carboxamide (NSC 82196) in primary and secondary brain tumors, *Cancer Chemother. Rep. Part 1* **59**:327.

LIU, Y. Y., AND HOFFMANN, D., 1973, Quantitative chemical studies on tobacco smoke. Quantitative analysis of hydrazine in tobacco and cigarette smoke, *Anal. Chem.* **46**:885–889.

LIVINGSTON, R. B., AND CARTER, S. K. (eds.), 1970a, *Single Agents in Cancer Chemotherapy,* pp. 3–24, IFI/Plenum Press, New York—Washington—London.

LIVINGSTON, R. B., AND CARTER, S. K. (eds.), 1970b, Procarbazine, in: *Single Agents in Cancer Chemotherapy,* pp. 318–336, IFI/Plenum Press, New York—Washington—London.

LIVINGSTON, R. B., AND CARTER, S. K. (eds.), 1970c, Dimethyl triazeno imidazole carboxamide, in: *Single Agents in Cancer Chemotherapy,* pp. 373–374, IFI/Plenum Press, New York—Washington—London.

LOO, T. L., 1975, Triazenoimidazole derivatives, in: *Antineoplastic and Immunosuppressive Agents, Part II* (A. C. Sartorelli and D. G. Johns, eds.), pp. 544–553, Springer-Verlag, New York—Heidelberg—Berlin.

LOO, T. L., STRASSWENDER, E. A., JARDINE, J. H., AND FREI, E., III, 1967, Clinical pharmacological studies on 5-(dimethyltriazeno)-imidazole-4-carboxamide (NSC 45388), *Proc. Amer. Assoc. Cancer Res.* **8**:42.

LOO, T. L., LUCE, J. K., JARDINE J. H., AND FREI, E., III, 1968, Pharmacologic studies of the antitumor agent 5-(dimethyltriazeno)imidazole-4-carboxamide, *Cancer Res.* **28**:2448.

LUCE, J. K., THURMAN, W. G., ISAACS, B. L., AND TALLEY, R. W., 1970, Clinical trials with the antitumor agent 5(3,3-dimethyl-1-triazeno)imidazole-4-carboxamide (NSC 45388), *Cancer Chemother. Rep.* **54**:119.

MACDONALD, C., WOLLNER, N., GHAVIMI, F., AND ZWEIG, J., 1967, Phase I study of imidazole, carboxamide dimethyltriazeno (ICD), *Proc. Amer. Assoc. Cancer Res.* **8**:43.

MAGEE, P. N., AND BARNES, J. M., 1967, Carcinogenic nitroso compounds, *Adv. Cancer Res.* **10**:164.

MAGEE, P. N., AND FARBER, E., 1962, Toxic liver injury and carcinogenesis. Methylation of rat-liver nucleic acids by dimethylnitrosamine *in vivo*, *Biochem. J.* **83**:114.

MARTZ, G., D'ALLESSANDRI, A., AND KEEL, H. J., 1963, Preliminary clinical results with a new antitumor agent RO-4-6467, *Cancer Chemother. Rep.* **33**:5.

MATHÉ, G., SCHWEISGUTH, O., SCHNEIDER, M., AMIEL, J. L., BERUMEN, L., BRULÉ, G., CATTAN, A., AND SCHWARZENBERG, L. B., 1963, Methyl-hydrazine in treatment of Hodgkin's disease and various forms of haematosarcoma and leukaemia, *Lancet* **2**:1077.

MCGEER, P. L., MCGEER, E. G., AND GRIFFIN, M. C., 1961, Excretion of 4-amino-5-imidazolecarboxamide in human urine, *Can J. Biochem. Physiol.* **39**:591.

McKINLEY, S., ANDERSON, C. D., AND JONES, M. E., 1967, Studies on the action of hydrazine, hydroxylamine and other amines in the carbamyl phosphate synthetase reaction, *J. Biol. Chem.* **242**:3381.

MENUTTI, M. T., SHEPARD, T. H., AND MELLMAN, W. J., 1975, Fetal renal malformation following treatment of Hodgkin's disease during pregnancy, *Obstet. Gynecol.* **46**:194.

THE MERCK INDEX, 1968, 8th Ed., Merck & Co., Rahway, New Jersey.

MERKER, P. C., WODINSKY, I., MAZRIMAS, M., AND WALKER, M. D., 1975, Chemotherapy of a dog-brain tumor transplanted intracerebrally (I.C.) in neonatal beagles, *Proc. Amer. Assoc. Cancer Res.* **16**:184.

MILLER, E., 1970, Development of procarbazine, in: *Proceedings of the Chemotherapy Conference on Procarbazine (Matulane: NSC 77213): Development and Application* (S. K. Carter, ed.), pp. 3–7, U.S. Government Printing Office, Washington, D.C.

MITRON, P. S., AND SCHUBERT, J. C. F., 1973, Zur Therapie der Macroglobulinämie Waldenstroem mit Procarbazin, in: *Leukämie und maligne Lymphome. Pathophysiologie, Klinik, Chemo- and Immunotherapie* (A. Stacher, ed.), pp. 319–325, Urban and Schwarzenberg, Munich.

MIZUNO, N. S., AND HUMPHREY, E. W., 1972, Metabolism of 5-(3,3-dimethyl-1-triazeno)-imidazole-4-carboxamide (NSC 45388) in human and animal tumor tissue, *Cancer Chemother. Rep. Part 1* **56**:465.

MOERTEL, C. G., SCHUTT, A. J., REITEMEIER, R. J., AND HAHN, R. G., 1972, Phase II study of 5[3,3-*bis*(2-chloroethyl)-1-triazeno]imidazole-4-carboxamide (NSC 82196) in advanced gastrointestinal cancer, *Cancer Chemother. Rep.* **56**:267.

NEWELL, P. C., AND TUCKER, R. G., 1968, Biosynthesis of the pyrimidine moiety of thiamine. A new route of pyrimidine biosynthesis involving purine intermediates, *Biochem. J.* **106**:279.

OBERFIELD, R. A., 1975, Recent trends in chemotherapy of solid tumors, *Med. Clin. North Amer.* **59**:399.

OCHOA, M., JR., WITTES, R. E., AND KRAKOFF, I. H., 1975, Trial of hydrazine sulfate (NSC 150014) in patients with cancer, *Cancer Chemother. Rep. Part 1* **59**:1151.

OLIVERIO, V. T., 1970, Pharmacologic disposition of procarbazine, in: *Proceedings of the Chemotherapy Conference on Procarbazine (Matulane: NSC 77213): Development and Application* ((S. K. Carter, ed.), pp. 19–28, U.S. Government Printing Office, Washington, D.C.

OLIVERIO, V. T., 1973, Derivatives of triazenes and hydrazines, in: *Cancer Medicine* (J. F. Holland and E. Frei, III, eds.), pp. 806–817, Lea and Febiger, Philadelphia.

OLIVERIO, V. T., DENHAM, C., DeVITA, V. T., AND KELLY, M. G., 1964, Some pharmacologic properties of a new antitumor agent, *N*-isopropyl-*α*-(2-methylhydrazino)-*p*-toluamide hydrochloride (NSC 77213), *Cancer Chemother. Rep.* **42**:1.

OLSON, K. B., HORTON, J., PRATT, K. L., PALADINE, W. J., JR., CUNNINGHAM, T., SULLIVAN, J., HOSLEY, H., AND TREBLE, D. H., 1969, 1-Acetyl-*p*-picolinoylhydrazine (NSC 68626) in the treatment of advanced cancer, *Cancer Chemother. Rep.* **53**:291.

PITTILLO, R. F., AND HUNT, D. E., 1967*a*, Broad-spectrum antimicrobial activity of a new triazenoimidazole, *Appl. Microbiol.* **15**:531.

PITTILLO, R. F., AND HUNT, D. E., 1967*b*, Inhibition of nucleic acid and protein sythesis in *Escherichia coli* by a new triazenoimidazole (32503), *Proc. Soc. Exp. Biol. Med.* **126**:555.

PITTILLO, R. F., AND HUNT, D. E., 1967*c*, 5(or 4)-[3,3-*Bis*(2-chloroethyl)-1-triazeno]imidazole-4(or 5)-carboxamide (NSC 82196): Microbiologic evaluation and assay, *Cancer Chemother. Rep.* **51**:213.

POLLACK, G., YELLIN, H., AND CARMI, A., 1964, Hydrazino acids, II. Alkyl-, aralkyl-hydrazinoacids, *J. Med. Chem.* **7**:220.

POVLSEN, C. O., AND JACOBSEN, G. K., 1975, Chemotherapy of a human malignant melanoma transplanted in the nude mouse, *Cancer Res.* **35**:2790.

PRESCOTT, B., AND CALDES, G., 1970, Potential antitumor agents. Derivatives of 2-hydrazino-5-nitropyridine, *J. Pharm. Sci.* **59**:101.

PREUSSMANN, R., AND VON HODENBERG, A., 1970, Mechanism of carcinogenesis with 1-aryl-3,3-dialkyltriazenes. II. *In vivo* alkylation of guanosine RNA and DNA with arylmonoalkyltriazenes to form 7-alkylguanine, *Biochem. Pharmacol.* **19**:1505.

PREUSSMANN, R., VON HODENBERG, A., AND HENGY, H., 1969*a*, Mechanism of carcinogenesis with 1-aryl-3,3-dialkyltriazenes. Enzymatic dealkylation by rat liver microsomal fraction *in vitro*, *Biochem. Pharmacol.* **18**:1.

PREUSSMANN, R., DRUCKREY, H., IVANKOVIC, S., AND VON HODENBERG, A., 1969*b*, Chemical structure and carcinogenicity of aliphatic hydrazo, azo and azoxy compounds and of triazenes, potential *in vivo* alkylating agents, *Ann. N. Y. Acad. Sci.* **163**:697.

RAAFLAUB, J., AND SCHWARTZ, D. E., 1965, Über den Metabolismus eines cytostatisch wirksamen Methylhydrazin-Derivatives (Natulan), *Experientia* **21**:44.

RAICH, P. C., KORST, D. R., AND DESSEL, B. H., 1975, Randomized study of lymphoma therapy, *Proc. Amer. Assoc. Cancer Res.* **16**:182.

REED, D., 1970, Metabolism and mechanism of action of procarbazine, in: *Proceedings of the Chemotherapy Conference on Procarbazine (Matulane: NSC 77213): Development and Application* (S. K. Carter, ed.), pp. 45–56, U.S. Government Printing Office, Washington, D.C.

REED, D. J., 1975, Procarbazine, in: *Antineoplastic and Immunosuppressive Agents, Part II* (A. C. Sartorelli and D. G. Johns, eds.), pp. 747–765, Springer-Verlag, New York—Heidelberg—Berlin.

REMERS, W. A., GIBS, G. J., AND WEISS, M. J., 1967, *Bis*oxime sulfonates and *bis*quaternary hydrazones, *J. Med. Chem.* **10**:274.

REVEL, M., AND LITTAUER, U. Z., 1966, The coding properties of methyl-deficient phenylalanine transfer RNA from *Escherichia coli*, *J. Mol. Biol.* **15**:389.

ROSENBERG, S. A., AND KAPLAN, H. S., 1970, Hodgkin's disease and other malignant lymphomas, *Calif. Med.* **113**:23.

RUTISHAUSER, A., AND BOLLAG, W., 1963, Cytological investigations with a new class of cytotoxic agents: Methylhydrazine derivatives, *Experientia* **19**:131.

RUTISHAUSER, A., AND BOLLAG, W., 1967, Untersuchungen über den Wirkungsmechanismus von Procarbazine (Natulan), *Experientia* **23**:222.

RUTNER, H., LEWIN, N., WOODBURY, E. C., MCBRIDE, T. J., AND RAO, K. V., 1974, Anti-tumor activity of some acylhydrazines, *Cancer Chemother. Rep.* **58**:803.

SAMUELS, M. L., 1971, Procarbazine as a single agent in the treatment of solid tumors, in: *Proceedings of the Chemotherapy Conference on Procarbazine (Matulane: NSC 77213): Development and Application* (S. K. Carter, ed.), pp. 67–76, U.S. Government Printing Office, Washington, D.C.

SAMUELS, M. L., LEARY, W. V., ALEXANIAN, R., HOWE, C. D., AND FREI, E., III, 1967, Clinical trials with *N*-isopropyl-α-(2-methylhydrazino)-*p*-toluamide hydrochloride in malignant lymphoma and other disseminated neoplasia, *Cancer* **20**:1187.

SARTORELLI, A. C., AND CREASEY, W. A., 1969, Cancer chemotherapy, *Annu. Rev. Pharmacol.* **9**:51.

SARTORELLI, A. C., AND TSUNAMURA, S., 1966, Studies on the biochemical mode of action of a cytotoxic methylhydrazine derivative, *N*-isopropyl-α-(-2-methylhydrazino)-*p*-toluamide, *Mol. Pharmacol.* **2**:275.

SAUNDERS, P. P., AND SCHULTZ, G. A., 1972, Role of 4-diazoimidazole-5-carboxamide in the action of the antitumor agent 5(4)-(3,3-dimethyl-1-triazeno)imidazole-4-(5)carboxamide in *Bacillus subtilis*, *Biochem. Pharmacol.* **21**:2065.

SCHMID, F. A., AND HUTCHISON, D. J., 1973, Decrease in oncogenic potential of L1210 leukemia by triazenes, *Cancer Res.* **33**:2161.

SCHMID, F. A., AND HUTCHISON, D. J., 1974, Chemotherapeutic, carcinogenic and cell-regulatory effects of triazenes, *Cancer Res.* **34**:1671.

SCHWARTZ, D. E., 1966, Comparative metabolic studies with Natulan, methylhydrazine and methylamine in rats, *Experientia* **22**:212.

SCHWARTZ, D. E., BOLLAG, W., AND OBRECHT, P., 1967, Distribution and excretion studies of procarbazine in animals and man, *Arzneim.-Forsch.* **17**:1389.

SCHWARTZ, D. E., BRUBACHER, G. B., AND VECCHI, M., 1968, Metabolic formation of methane from *N*-methyl-substituted hydrazine compounds and carcinostatic activity, in: *Radioactive Isotopes in Pharmacology* (P. G. Waser and B. Glasson, eds.), pp. 351–355, John Wiley and Sons, New York.

SEARS, M. E., 1971, Clinical trials with procarbazine, in: *Proceedings of the Chemotherapy Conference on Procarbazine (Matulane: NSC 77213): Development and Application* (S. K. Carter, ed.), pp. 63–65, U.S. Government Printing Office, Washington, D.C.

SHAY, H., GRUENSTEIN, M., AND SHIENKIN, M. B., 1964, Inhibition of mammary cancer in rats by a dithiocarbamoylhydrazine (ICI-33828), *Cancer Res.* **24**:998.

SHEALY, Y. F., 1970, Synthesis and biological activity of 5-aminoimidazoles and 5-triazenoimidazoles, *J. Pharm. Sci.* **59**:1533.

SHEALY, Y. F., AND KRAUTH, C. A., 1966a, Imidazoles. II. 5(or 4)-(Monosubstituted triazeno)imidazole-4(or 5)carboxamides, *J. Med. Chem.* **9**:34.

SHEALY, Y. F., AND KRAUTH, C. A., 1966b, Complete inhibition of mouse leukemia L1210 by 5(or 4)[3,3-*bis*(2-chloroethyl)-1-triazeno]imidazole-4(or 5)-carboxamide (NSC 82196), *Nature (London)* **210**:208.

SHEALY, Y. F., STRUCK, R. F., HOLUM, L. B., AND MONTGOMERY, J. A., 1961, Synthesis of potential anticancer agents. XXIX. 5-Diazoimidazole-4-carboxamide and 5-diazo-v-triazole-4-carboxamide, *J. Org. Chem.* **26**:2396.

SHEALY, Y. F., KRAUTH, C. A., AND MONTGOMERY, J. A., 1962a, Imidazoles. I. Coupling reactions of 5-diazoimidazole-4-carboxamide, *J. Org. Chem.* **27**:2150.

SHEALY, Y. F., MONTGOMERY, J. A., AND LASTER, W. R., JR., 1962b, Antitumor activity of triazenoimidazoles, *Biochem. Pharmacol.* **11**:674.

SHEALY, Y. F., KRAUTH, C. A., PITTILLO, R. F., AND HUNT, D. E., 1967, A new antifungal and antibacterial agent, methyl 5(or 4)-(3,3-dimethyl-1-triazeno)imidazole-4(or 5)-carboxylate, *J. Pharm. Sci.* **56**:147.

SHEALY, Y. F., KRAUTH, C. A., CLAYTON, S. J., SHORTNACY, A. T., AND LASTER, W. R., JR., 1968, Imidazoles. V. 5(or 4)-(3-Alkyl-3-methyl-1-triazeno)imidazole-4(or 5)-carboxamides, *J. Pharm. Sci.* **57**:1562.

SKIBBA, J. L., AND BRYAN, G. T., 1971, Methylation of nucleic acids and urinary excretion of ^{14}C-labeled 7-methylguanine by rats and man after administration of 4(5)-(3,3-dimethyl-1-triazeno)imidazole-5-(4)-carboxamide, *Toxicol. Appl. Pharmacol.* **18**:707.

SKIBBA, J. L., RAMIREZ, G., BEAL, D. D., AND BRYAN, G. T., 1969, Preliminary clinical trial and the physiologic disposition of 4(5)-(3,3-dimethyl-1-triazeno)imidazole-5(4)-carboxamide in man, *Cancer Res.* **29**:1944.

SKIBBA, J. L., BEAL, D. D., RAMIREZ, G., AND BRYAN, G. T., 1970a, N-Demethylation of the antineoplastic agent 4(5)-(3,3-dimethyl-1-triazeno–imidazole-5-(4)carboxamide by rats and man, *Cancer Res.* **30**:147.

SKIBBA, J. L., JOHNSON, R. O., AND BRYAN, G. T., 1970b, Carcinogenicity and possible mode of action of 4(5)-(3,3-dimethyl-1-triazeno)imidazole-5(4)-carboxamide (NSC 45388, DIC), *Proc. Amer. Assoc. Cancer Res.* **11**:73.

SKIBBA, J. L., RAMIREZ, G., BEAL, D. D., AND BRYAN, G. T., 1970c, Metabolism of 4(5)-(3,3-dimethyl-1-triazeno)imidazole-5(4)-carboxamide to 4(5)-aminoimidazole-5(4)-carboxamide in man, *Biochem. Pharmacol.* **19**:2043.

SKIBBA, J. L., ERTURK, E., AND BRYAN, G. T., 1970d, Induction of thymic lymphosarcoma and mammary adenocarcinomas in rats by oral administration of the antitumor agent 4(5)-(3,3-dimethyl-1-triazeno)imidazole-5(4)-carboxamide, *Cancer* **26**:1000.

SPIES, S. K., AND SNYMAN, H. W., 1966, Procarbazine (Natulan) in the treatment of Hodgkin's disease and other lymphomas, *S. Afr. Med. J.* **40**:1061.

STOCK, J. A., 1967, Other antitumor agents, *Exp. Chemother.* **5**:333.

SUTOW, W. W., KOMP, D., VIETTI, T. J., AND PINKERTON, D., 1975, Clinical trials with 1-acetyl-2-picolinoylhydrazine (NSC 68626) in children, *Cancer Chemother. Rep. Part 1* **59**:341.

THUMB, N., KOLARZ, G., WEIDINGER, P., AND HORAK, W., 1972, Spätergebnisse der immunsuppressiven Therapie bei chronischer Polyarthritis, *Z. Rheumaforsch. (Suppl. 2)* **31**:387.

TODD, I. D. H., 1965, Further experience with Ibenzmethyzin, in: *Natulan (Ibenzmethyzin)* (A. M. Jelliffe and J. Marks, eds.), pp. 20–25, John Wright and Sons, Bristol.

TOTH, B., 1975, Synthetic and naturally occurring hydrazines as possible cancer causative agents, *Cancer Res.* **35**:3693.

TREPEL, F., STOCKHUSEN, G., RASTETTER, J., AND BEGEMANN, H., 1967, Zytostatikawirkungen auf die Nukleinsäure und Proteinsynthese von benignen und malignen Lymphomen, *Chemotherapia* **12**:182.

TSUJI, T., AND KOSOWER, E. M., 1971, Diazenes. VI. Alkyl diazenes, *J. Amer. Chem. Soc.* **93**:1992.

TYRER, D. D., KLINE, I., GANG, M., GOLDIN, A., AND VENDITTI, J. M., 1969, Effectiveness of antileukemic agents in mice inoculated with a leukemia L1210 variant resistant to 5-[3,3-bis(2-chloroethyl)-1-triazeno]imidazole-4-carboxamide (NSC 82196), *Cancer Chemother. Rep. Part 1* **53**:229.

VAN EDEN, E. B., FALKSON, G., VAN DYK, J. J., VAN DER MERWE, A. M., AND FALKSON, H. C., 1972, 5-Fluorouracil (5-FU; NSC 19893), 5-(3,3-dimethyl-1-triazeno)imidazole-4-carboxamide (NSC 45388), vincristine (NSC 67574), and 1,3-bis(2-chloroethyl)-1-nitrosourea (BCNU; NSC 409962) given concomitantly in the treatment of solid tumors in man, *Cancer Chemother. Rep. Part 1* **56**:107.

VOGEL, C. L., DEVITA, V. T., LISAK, R. P., AND KIES, M. W., 1969, Suppression of experimental allergic encephalomyelitis by NSC 82196, a new imidazole carboxamide derivative, *Cancer Res.* **29**:2249.

VOGEL, C. L., DENHAM, C., WAALKES, T. P., AND DEVITA, V. T., 1970, The physiological disposition of the carcinostatic imidazole-4(or 5)-carboxamide-5(or 4)-[3,3-bis(2-chloroethyl)-1-triazeno] (NSC 82196) (imidazole mustard) in mice and dogs, *Cancer Res.* **30**:1651.

VOGEL, C. L., COMIS, R., ZIEGLER, J. L., AND KIRYABWIRE, J. W. M., 1971a, Clinical trials of 5-(3,3-dimethyl-1-triazeno)imidazole-4-carboxamide (NSC 45388) given intravenously in the treatment of malignant melanoma in Uganda, *Cancer Chemother. Rep.* **55**:143.

VOGEL, C. L., DEVITA, V. T., DENHAM, C., FOLEY, H. T., FIELD, R. B., AND CARBONE, P. P., 1971b, Preliminary clinical trials and clinical pharmacologic studies with 5-[3,3-bis(2-chloroethyl)-1-triazeno]imidazole-4-carboxamide (NSC 82196) given orally, Cancer Chemother. Rep. 55:159.

VOGEL, E., FAHRIG, R., AND OBE, G., 1973, Triazenes, a new group of indirect mutagens. Comparative investigations of the genetic effects of different aryldialkyltriazenes using Saccharomyces cerevisiae, the host mediated assay, Drosophila melanogaster, and human chromosomes in vitro, Mutat. Res. 21:123.

VORMITTAG, W., 1974, Zytostatische immunodepressive Therapie, chromosomale Aberationen und karzinogene Wirkung, Wien. Klin. Wochenschr. 86:69.

WEITZEL, G., SCHNEIDER, F., FRETZDORFF, A. M., DURST, J., AND HIRSCHMANN, W. D., 1967a, Untersuchungen zum cytostatischen Wirkungsmechanismus der Methylhydrazine II, Hoppe-Seyler's Z. Physiol. Chem. 348:433.

WEITZEL, G., SCHNEIDER, F., HIRSCHMANN, W. D., DURST, J., THAUER, R., OCHS, H., AND KUMMER, D., 1967b, Untersuchungen zum cytostatischen Wirkungsmechanismus der Methylhydrazine III, Hoppe-Seyler's Z. Physiol. Chem. 348:443.

WILKOFF, L. J., DULMADGE, E. A., AND DIXON, G. J., 1968, Kinetics of the effect of 5(or 4)-(3,3-dimethyl-1-triazeno)-imidazole-4(or 5)-carboxamide (NSC 45388) and 5(or 4)-[3,3-bis(2-chloroethyl)-1-triazeno]-imidazole-4(or 5)-carboxamide (NSC 82196) on the reproductive integrity of cultured leukemia L1210 cells, Cancer Chemother. Rep. 52:725.

WILSON, K. S., RICCI, J. A., AND GROBMYER, A. J., III, 1970, Treatment of carcinoma of the lung with 1-acetyl-2-picolinoylhydrazine (NSC 68626), Cancer Chemother. Rep. 54:243.

WINDHAUS, A., AND LANGENBECK, W., 1923, Über die 4(5)-Nitro-imidazole-5(4)carbon Säure, Ber. Dtsch. Chem. Ges. 56B:683.

WITTKOP, J. A., PROUGH, R. A., AND REED, D. J., 1969, Oxidative demethylation of N-methylhydrazines by rat liver microsomes, Arch. Biochem. Biophys. 134:308.

WODINSKY, I., SWINIARSKI, J., AND KENSLER, C. J., 1968, Spleen colony studies of leukemia L1210. IV. Sensitivities of L1210 and L1210/6-MP to triazenoimidazole carboxamides—a preliminary report, Cancer Chemother. Rep. 52:393.

YOUNG, C., 1970, Single-agent therapy with procarbazine, in: Proceedings of the Chemotherapy Conference on Procarbazine (Matulane: NSC 77213): Development and Application (S. K. Carter, ed.), pp. 51–62, U.S. Government Printing Office, Washington, D. C.

ZELLER, P., GUTMANN, H., HEGEDUS, B., KAISER, A., LANGEMANN, A., AND MULLER, M., 1963, Methylhydrazine derivatives, a new class of cytotoxic agents, Experientia 19:129.

18

Antitumor Effects of Interferon

Ion Gresser

1. Introduction*

Interferon was first described in 1957 by Isaacs and Lindenmann (1957) and characterized as "an antiviral substance produced by the cells of many vertebrates in response to virus infection. It appears to be of protein or polypeptide nature, it is antigenically distinct from virus, and it acts by conferring on cells resistance to the multiplication of a number of different viruses" (Isaacs, 1963). Although this description still has some validity today, there is considerable evidence indicating that interferon is not a selective antiviral substance, but that it can also affect both cell division and cell function.

Shortly after its discovery, interferon was shown to inhibit the multiplication of oncogenic viruses both in cell culture and in experimental animals. In investigations of the mechanism of the inhibitory effect of interferon on several virus-induced murine leukemias, it was found that interferon preparations also inhibited the growth of murine transplantable tumors of both viral and nonviral origin. Although the mechanism of this effect was not entirely clear, it was shown that interferon could inhibit the multiplication of tumor cells and exert important effects on the immune system. Partly on the basis of these observations, selected patients with malignancies, especially osteosarcoma, were treated with interferon, and the preliminary results of these clinical trials are most encouraging.

* Abbreviations in this chapter: *Viruses*: (MSV) murine sarcoma virus; (NDV) Newcastle disease virus; (RLV) Rauscher leukemia virus; (RSV) Rous sarcoma virus; (WNV) West Nile virus. *Other terms*: (ALS) antilymphocytic serum; (CAM) chorioallantoic membrane; (C-IF) crude interferon preparation; (COAM) chlorite-oxidized oxyamylose; (EA) Ehrlich ascites; (ERC) erythropoietin-responsive cells; (P-IF) purified (leukocyte) interferon preparation.

Ion Gresser • Institut de Recherches Scientifiques sur le Cancer, Villejuif, France.

521

The purpose of this chapter is to summarize the experimental results pertaining to the antitumor effects of interferon, and to discuss possible mechanisms of action. Several points should be borne in mind. First, since interferon has not been completely purified, it is possible that some antitumor effects observed with crude interferon preparations are due to a factor (or factors) other than interferon. Although the evidence seems very convincing that many of the different biological effects of interferon (other than antiviral effects) observed in cell culture experiments are due to interferon itself, it is somewhat more difficult to provide comparable evidence in *in vivo* experiments, which require considerably greater amounts of interferon. Second, viral and nonviral inducers of interferon have also been shown to exert antitumor effects. Since these inducers exert multiple effects on cells, it is difficult to determine the extent to which results obtained are due to the production of interferon. Nevertheless, for the sake of completeness, the antitumor effects of interferon inducers have also been included in this review.

For the most part, this chapter will be concerned only with data from *in vivo* experimentation. Work concerning the effect of interferon on the multiplication of oncogenic viruses in cell culture, on the multiplication of tumor or normal cells in culture, or on other biological effects of interferon *in vitro* will not be considered in detail, but will be mentioned only when directly pertinent to the antitumor effects of interferon.

First, I will review in some detail the experimental results on the antitumor effects of exogenous interferon and interferon inducers in animals infected with oncogenic viruses or inoculated with transplantable tumor cells or chemical carcinogens. Recent work on the effect of exogenous interferon on the normal animal will be included. I will then discuss the possible mechanisms of the antitumor effects of interferon, and then review some of the preliminary results of interferon treatment of patients with neoplastic disease.

2. Effect of Exogenous Interferon and Interferon Inducers on the Development of Tumors in Animals Infected with Oncogenic Viruses

2.1. Exogenous Interferon

2.1.1. Virus-Induced Neoplasms

It was demonstrated in 1960 (Atanasiu and Chany, 1960) that pretreatment of hamsters with crude interferon preparations prior to inoculation of polyoma virus delayed the appearance of tumors, decreased the number of tumor-bearing animals, and increased animal survival. Likewise, inoculation of interferon onto the chorioallantoic membrane of the chick embryo inhibited the formation of Rous sarcoma virus (RSV) pocks (Strandström *et al.*, 1962), and injection of both crude and semipurified interferon inhibited tumor development in chicks when administered prior to infection with RSV (Lampson *et al.*, 1963). Treatment was ineffective when initiated as early as 6 hr after viral inoculation (Lampson *et al.*,

1963). In contrast to the results to be described on the effect of exogenous interferon on the evolution of the murine leukemias or on transplantable tumors, interferon treatment initiated "after the first appearance of pin-point size (RSV) tumors was of no consequence in terms of size of resulting tumor" (Lampson *et al.*, 1963). Likewise, pretreatment of rabbits with "facteur inhibiteur" (similar if not identical to interferon) also inhibited the development of Shope-virus-induced fibromas, but had no effect on the growth of established tumors (Kishida *et al.*, 1965).

The Friend and Rauscher murine leukemias are examples of subacute infectious processes, and viral multiplication occurs throughout the course of the disease. Daily intraperitoneal or subcutaneous administration of potent crude or semipurified mouse brain or serum–spleen interferon inhibited the development of the characteristic splenomegaly induced by Friend virus in Swiss and DBA/2 mice (Gresser *et al.*, 1966, 1967a,c–e). Interferon was ineffective when administered for only 3 days, even though treatment preceded viral inoculation (Gresser *et al.*, 1967a). In contrast, initiation of interferon treatment 48 hr or even 1 week *after* inoculation of virus (at a time when splenomegaly had already developed) proved effective, provided the treatment was continued throughout the 1-month test period (Gresser *et al.*, 1967a,c–e). Likewise, the continued administration of interferon delayed the evolution of various manifestations of Rauscher disease in Balb/c mice, i.e., hepatosplenomegaly, leukocytosis, and anemia, and also prolonged the mean survival time of virus-infected mice (Gresser *et al.*, 1968a). Histological examination of mice inoculated with Friend and Rauscher viruses confirmed the clinical evaluation and revealed a marked decrease in the extent of tumor involvement in the spleen, liver, and bone marrow of interferon-treated mice compared with control mice (Gresser *et al.*, 1967c,e, 1968a). Less infectious virus was present in the spleens of interferon-treated mice than in the spleens of control mice, as determined by biological assay and electron microscopy (Gresser *et al.*, 1967e, 1968a).

Little work has been done by other investigators on the effect of exogenous interferon on mice infected with leukemia viruses, probably because of the necessity of obtaining large amounts of potent interferon to permit repeated administration. In the experiments of Vandeputte *et al.* (1967), interferon did not protect mice inoculated with Rauscher virus, and Wheelock (1967a) found that pretreatment of mice with interferon did not protect them against Friend virus infection. In the former experiments, the titer of interferon may have been too low, and in the later experiments, treatment may not have been continued long enough. In a subsequent study, Wheelock and Larke (1968) found that the daily intraperitoneal inoculation of interferon for "10 days commencing 31 days after Friend virus infection prolonged survival by an average of 9 days." Continuation of interferon treatment beyond this period, however, did not further increase the survival time. Evidence was presented that leukemic mice were "not completely refractory to the leukemia inhibiting effects of interferon," since inoculation of statolon induced the production of interferon "with subsequent further prolongation of life" (Wheelock and Larke, 1968).

Glasgow and Friedman (1969) reported that only one or two inoculations of interferon given either subcutaneously with Rauscher leukemia virus (RLV), or 24 and 48 hr thereafter, was sufficient to delay the appearance of leukemia. The choice of suckling mice of a randomly bred strain (CD-1) that develop resistance to RLV with age may have been responsible for the marked sensitivity to the protective effects of interferon. Tóth *et al.*, (1971) found that daily intraperitoneal injection of small amounts of interferon (900 U) increased slightly but significantly the survival of 2-month-old Balb/c mice inoculated with RLV.

There have been conflicting results concerning the effects of interferon on mice inoculated with the murine sarcoma viruses. On one hand, Chany and Robbe-Maridor (1969) and Weinstein *et al.* (1971) found that interferon did not affect tumorigenesis in newborn or weanling Balb/c mice inoculated with the Moloney strain of murine sarcoma virus (MSV), whereas De Clercq and De Somer (1971) and Berman (1970) did observe inhibition of tumor development in newborn and weanling mice. Rhim and Huebner (1971) observed a very slight effect, but only small amounts of interferon were injected.

Graft vs. host disease in mice results in the activation of latent type C leukemia viruses that are presumed to cause the subsequent development of malignant lymphomas in some of these mice (Hirsch *et al.*, 1970a; Armstrong *et al.*, 1972). Hirsch *et al.* (1973a) found that daily interferon treatment of F_1 (Balb/c and A/J) mice after inoculation of Balb/c spleen cells reduced the incidence of virus activation (as determined by the XC cell assay), modified the histological appearance of the GVH reaction, and completely prevented (18-month observation period) the development of lymphomas in these mice, in contrast to an incidence of lymphoma in 7/14 GVH mice not treated with interferon (Hirsch *et al.*, 1976). It is of interest to note that activation of C type viruses also occurs after skin homografts (Hirsch *et al.*, 1973b), but, in contrast to the preceding system, interferon treatment of these mice did not inhibit viral activation, even though the multiplication of the C type viruses obtained after skin homograft could be inhibited by interferon in *in vitro* assays (Hirsch *et al.*, 1976). The reasons for this difference in the two systems are not clear.

Herpes saimiri virus induces a malignant lymphoma in several nonhuman primates (Laufs and Fleckenstein, 1973; Laufs and Meléndez, 1973), and multiplication of the virus is inhibited in interferon-treated owl monkey kidney cells (Laufs *et al.*, 1974). In determining the effect of interferon on the development of lymphoma, Laufs *et al.* (1974) injected 2CT marmoset monkeys with human leucocyte interferon (100,000 U) intraperitoneally 6 hr prior to infection and 20,000 U every second day thereafter. Although tumor development was not inhibited, and all 4 monkeys (2 interferon-treated and 2 control) died of malignant lymphoma, the survival time of the interferon-treated monkeys was longer than that of untreated monkeys (i.e., 37 and 50 days, compared with 28 and 30 days). When interferon was administered *after* infection of CJ marmosets, no therapeutic effect was observed.

Rabin *et al.* (1976) reported a "temporary remission" of leukemia in herpes-virus-inoculated owl monkeys treated with 200,000–400,000 U human leukocyte interferon.

2.1.2. Spontaneous Neoplasms

The lymphoid leukemia of AKR mice is an excellent experimental model for determining the effect of chemotherapeutic agents on a spontaneously appearing neoplastic disease that bears certain similarities to human lymphoma. The Gross virus, which is thought to be the etiologic agent, is transmitted vertically. In the experiments of Gresser *et al.* (1968*b*, 1969*a*), newborn AKR mice were inoculated with concentrated preparations of mouse brain interferon or control "normal" brain extract, or were kept without treatment. In an initial experiment, interferon treatment continued daily for the first 3 months of life diminished the incidence of lymphoid leukemia in *male* mice and increased the survival time (Gresser *et al.*, 1968*b*, 1969*a*). No difference was detected between treated and untreated female mice. (Perhaps the failure of interferon treatment of female mice was related to the greater natural susceptibility of female mice to the leukemic process.) In a second experiment, however, daily interferon treatment was continued from birth for 1 year (Gresser *et al.*, 1969*a*). The survival time of both male and female mice was considerably prolonged: The mean days of death for two groups of control male mice were 260 and 282 days, and 385 days for interferon-treated mice. The mean days of death for control female mice were 229 and 233 days, and 312 days for interferon-treated mice. Furthermore, the incidence of leukemia was reduced from 95% in control mice to 63% in interferon-treated mice (Gresser *et al.*, 1969*a*). Interferon treatment was also shown to increase the survival time of male and female AKR mice "superinfected" at birth with an extract of leukemic tissue (Gresser *et al.*, 1969*a*). Graff *et al.* (1970) demonstrated that treatment of AKR mice 6–8 months old with potent interferon preparations also resulted in a delay in the appearance of leukemia. In a recent study, Bekesi *et al.* (1976) found that interferon treatment of preleukemic AKR mice was associated with a marked reduction of virus titer (in mouse tails, using the XC focus assay; Rowe *et al.*, 1970) and a significant delay in the appearance of primary lymphoma. It was of interest that the reduction of virus titer in interferon-treated mice was not transient, and even 85 days after cessation of treatment, virus titers remained low.

All these experiments were undertaken in preleukemic mice. It is, however, a severe test of the value of an antitumor drug to determine its therapeutic efficacy after diagnosis of lymphoma in AKR mice, since at this time there are approximately 10^9 leukemic cells (Skipper *et al.*, 1969), and death occurs on the average 13–18 days later (Rudali and Jullien, 1966; Schabel *et al.*, 1969; Skipper *et al.*, 1972; Strauss *et al.*, 1973; Bekesi and Holland, 1973). It is perhaps not surprising, therefore, that most drugs useful in the treatment of human malignancy delayed AKR mouse death by only a few days after diagnosis (Skipper *et al.*, 1969, 1972; Bekesi and Holland, 1973; Frei *et al.*, 1974). Frei *et al.* (1974) found that only 4 of

27 compounds useful in cancer chemotherapy increased mean survival time 100% or more after diagnosis of lymphoma in AKR mice. Graff *et al.* (1970) reported that daily inoculation of more than 10^5 U interferon/day into mice with "advanced leukemia" caused reduction of nodes and spleen within 24–36 hr. Reduction varied from animal to animal, ranging from 40 to 75%, "with a prolongation of life to 4.7 times that of control animals" (Graff *et al.*, 1970). Kassel and co-workers (Kassel, 1970; Kassel *et al.*, 1972) referred to interferon as "carcinolytic," since no effect was observed on "normal, noninfected animals" (Graff *et al.*, 1970). The development of techniques for the production of large quantities of partially purified mouse interferon of high titer (Tovey *et al.*, 1974) enabled Gresser and his co-workers (1976) to determine the effect of considerably more potent interferon preparations (i.e., 6.4×10^6 mouse interferon reference U/dose) than had previously been used on the survival of AKR mice after diagnosis of the lymphoma. Daily inoculation of these interferon preparations beginning *after* clinical diagnosis of lymphoma increased average survival by approximately 100%. Interferon treatment appeared to delay the evolution of the lymphoma, but in contradistinction to the results of Graff *et al.* (1970), regression of tumor was not observed. The therapeutic effects observed with interferon in AKR mice compared very favorably with reported results obtained using standard anticancer chemotherapeutic substances in this system.

Came and Moore (1971, 1972) showed that the evolution of another spontaneously appearing virus-associated tumor, the mouse mammary carcinoma, can also be delayed by repeated inoculation of interferon. The authors noted that despite the inhibitory effect of interferon on tumor development, no decrease was observed in the amount of mammary tumor antigen in the milk of interferon-treated mice. (As the authors point out, however, the immune diffusion test used is not highly sensitive.)

2.2. Interferon Inducers

2.2.1. Viral Inducers

a. Activity on Oncogenic RNA Viruses. Not all examples of viral interference are mediated by interferon. In many of the experiments to be mentioned, it is difficult to know whether interferon is the factor responsible for the inhibition of tumor development induced by oncogenic viruses.

In some experiments, it is likely that interferon played some role. For example, Shirodkar (1965) described the "blocking effect" of West Nile virus (WNV) on the subsequent development of RSV-induced tumors. The transient nature of the protective effect and the finding that WNV could be inoculated in the contralateral wing (in relation to RSV inoculation) suggested that interferon was probably responsible for this inhibitory effect. Antirabies vaccine and fixed rabies virus were also shown to inhibit the development of RSV tumors in chicks (Kravchenko *et al.*, 1967). Although the authors state that this inhibition was due to "the activity of viral particles and not to interferon," it is possible that the "viral particles" induced the synthesis of endogenous interferon. Stim (1970) observed the inhibitory effect of Cocal arbovirus on Friend leukemia, and suggested that interferon might be responsible.

In other experiments, it seems unlikely that viral interference was mediated by interferon. Jungeblut and Kodza (1962) showed that injection of guinea pigs with a wild strain of LCM virus significantly increased the life span of guinea pigs inoculated with cell-free leukemic material (leukemia L2C). Inoculation of both newborn and adult mice with LCM virus 1–2 days prior to inoculation of RLV was associated with a marked prolongation of the incubation period and a delayed mortality (Barski and Youn, 1964; Youn and Barski, 1966). In some instances, the protection was complete. The findings that (1) prior infection with potent interferonogenic viruses such as WNV or vaccinia virus did not confer protection and (2) persistence of LCM virus infection itself was related to the degree of protection (interferon has not been detected in the serum of mice with chronic LCM virus infection) suggested that in the experimental model, interferon may not have been responsible for the therapeutic effects.

Repeated inoculation of newborn AKR mice with irradiated cell-free extracts of AKR leukemic spleens (Gross virus) was found to decrease the subsequent incidence of leukemia (Latarjet, 1964). Likewise, infection of newborn AKR mice with nonleukemogenic C-type murine viruses (from cell culture) 4–5 hr before challenge with highly leukemogenic passage A Gross virus delayed the appearance of leukemia and prolonged mouse survival (Barski and Youn, 1971). It is unlikely that either of these results can be attributed to the production of interferon. (Neither the spleen extracts used by Latarjet nor the nonleukemogenic viruses utilized in the experiments of Barski and Youn were interferonogenic when inoculated intravenously into mice; Gresser, unpublished observations.)

Oker-Blom and Strandström (1965a,b) found that Coxsackie virus inhibited tumor formation induced by RSV on the chorioallantoic membrane (CAM) of embryonated eggs. Intravenous or intramuscular injections of Coxsackie A10 virus into chickens (Coxsackie virus does not multiply in chickens) prior to inoculations of cell suspensions or cell-free filtrates of RSV tumors were also shown to retard the development of tumors (Oker-Blom and Strandström, 1956a). Since Oker-Blom and his colleagues showed that UV-inactivated influenza virus strain PR 8 and exogenous interferon also interfered with the effects of RSV on the CAM (Strandström et al., 1962), it seemed possible that interferon may also have been responsible for the earlier results utilizing Coxsackie virus. Coxsackie virus, however, did not induce detectable levels of interferon in chick cells (Oker-Blom and Leinikki, 1965) or in chickens (Oker-Blom and Gresser, unpublished observations), so that this appears to be an example of viral interference not mediated by interferon.

Wheelock (1966, 1967b) investigated the effect of Sendaï virus on the development of Friend leukemia of mice. Since inoculation of Sendaï virus 3 or even 6 weeks prior to inoculation of Friend virus still inhibited subsequent splenomegaly (the effect of interferon has been shown to be of short duration, i.e., days), and since other potent interferonogenic viruses proved ineffective, Wheelock (1966, 1967b) interpreted his results as being due to a direct virus interference, rather than to interferon. In a subsequent study, however, Wheelock and Larke (1968) presented some evidence that the beneficial effects following inoculation of Sendaï virus in Friend-virus-infected mice were related at least in part to the production of interferon.

A reciprocal interference between mammary tumor virus and the Moloney leukemia virus in mice was reported by Squartini *et al.* (1967). As in the preceding studies, it is virtually impossible to determine whether low (and probably non-detectable) amounts of interferon were of importance.

b. Activity on Oncogenic DNA Viruses. Preinfection of adult hamsters with herpes virus was associated with an almost complete inhibition of polyoma-virus-induced hemangiomas (Barski, 1963).

2.2.2. Nonviral Inducers

Statolon, synthetic polynucleotides, and pyran copolymer have been the most widely used nonviral interferon inducers, and they will be considered in that order.

a. Activity on Oncogenic RNA Viruses. Statolon is a fermentation product of the mold *Penicillium stoloniferum* (the active interferon-inducing factor is a double-stranded RNA virus; Kleinschmidt *et al.*, 1968; Banks *et al.*, 1968). Regelson and Foltyn (1966) and Wheelock (1967a) demonstrated that one injection (intra-peritoneal) of statolon either before or after inoculation of Friend virus inhibited the development of splenomegaly and increased mouse survival. An inhibitory effect was noted even when statolon was injected 30 days after inoculation of Friend virus (Wheelock and Larke, 1968). Some statolon-treated mice failed to develop leukemia, and proved resistant to rechallenge with Friend virus (Wheelock, 1967a; Wheelock *et al.*, 1969). Evidence was presented that Friend virus remained latent in these apparently clinically normal mice, and Wheelock *et al.* (1971) postulated that the enhanced activity of immunologic mechanisms in statolon-treated mice suppressed the disease. (Statolon was less effective in mice pretreated with antilymphocytic sera; Wheelock, 1971.) Wheelock and his co-workers have suggested that statolon induces interferon initially, which probably somewhat inhibits Friend virus multiplication and results in clearance of viremia (Toy *et al.*, 1973). This endogenous interferon (detectable for 4 days after statolon inoculation) is probably not responsible for the conversion of the lethal Friend disease into a latent infection (30–90% of virus-infected mice; Wheelock *et al.*, 1969; Wheelock and Caroline, 1970). For example, Newcastle disease virus (NDV) or the complex of polyriboinosinic–polyribocytidylic acids (poly-I.C) (Field *et al.*, 1967) does not induce remissions, even though they induce more interferon than statolon (Toy *et al.*, 1973). Thus, statolon probably exerts an anti-Friend-disease effect independently of its capacity to induce interferon. Wheelock and his co-workers found that statolon-treated Friend-virus-injected mice produced more neutralizing, cell-binding cytotoxic antibody to Friend virus than did unprotected mice developing leukemia (Wheelock *et al.*, 1971, 1972). The appearance of leukemia in aging statolon-protected mice appeared to be related to a decline in levels of antibody to the virus. Since Friend virus infection is associated with a depression of the humoral antibody response (Ceglowski and Friedman, 1968), it was of interest that statolon counteracted the immunodepressant effect of Friend virus and restored the capacity to produce normal levels of antibody (to sheep red blood cells) (Weislow *et al.*, 1973). Likewise, M. H. Levy and Wheelock (1975) found that statolon also restored macrophage function depressed by Friend virus infection. Thus, in summary, the anti-Friend-disease effect of statolon appears to be more one of stimulation and restoration of diminished host defenses (humoral, probably cell-mediated and macrophage), rather than an antiviral effect mediated by interferon (Weislow and Wheelock, 1975*a*; Wheelock *et al.*, 1974). In this regard, it was of interest that the efficacy of statolon in Friend disease was increased when chlorite-oxidized oxyamylose (COAM) (an interferon inducer and immunoadjuvant) was also injected (Weislow and Wheelock, 1975*b*).

Statolon has also been shown to provide significant protection against the development of sarcomas in newborn Swiss mice injected with Friend pseudotype sarcoma virus (Rhim and Huebner, 1969).

Perhaps the most widely investigated of the synthetic nucleic acid interferon inducers has been poly-I.C. Youn *et al.* (1968) reported the inhibition of Rauscher disease in mice treated with poly-I.C. The response to poly-I.C has proved variable, however, and other workers have found that poly-I.C is not strikingly beneficial in altering the events in experimental Friend leukemia, the effects being strongly influenced by the time of initiating treatment, the amount of drug given, and the number and frequency of doses administered (Larson *et al.*, 1969*b*; Sarma *et al.*, 1971). Slamon (1973) showed that poly-I.C protected neonatal rats infected with murine erythroblastosis virus from developing the erythroblastosis response, but did not affect the development of neoplasia.

Poly-I.C administered before or even several days after inoculation of MSV markedly inhibited the development of tumors (Sarma *et al.*, 1969, 1971; Pearson *et al.*, 1969; Baron *et al.*, 1970; De Clercq and Merigan, 1971; Kende and Glynn, 1971). "Repeated injections initiated even after the establishment of small tumor nodules were also effective" (Sarma *et al.*, 1969). The degree of protection provided by poly-I.C in mice inoculated with MSV was similar to that observed in mice treated with statolon (Rhim and Huebner, 1969). Weinstein *et al.* (1971), however, found that the efficacy of poly-I.C was determined by the dose of MSV inoculated. Marked differences in the response to the antitumor effects of poly-I.C were observed in different strains of mice. Although poly-I.C induced as much interferon in NZB mice as in other strains, the NZB mice were not protected. De Clercq and De Somer (1971) found that tumor growth in NMRI mice infected neonatally with MSV was inhibited by repeated doses of poly-I.C.

They inferred that the antitumor effects observed were entirely due to the production of interferon. Poly-I.C was effective in inducing regression of established MSV-induced tumors even when inoculated 40–60 days after viral inoculation (De Clercq and Stewart, 1974). Nemes *et al.* (1969) observed a minimal protective effect in poly-I.C-treated chicks inoculated with RSV.

Synthetic polyanions such as pyran copolymer (maleic acid–divinyl ether copolymer) also induce interferon, and several have proved inhibitory in Friend and Rauscher disease of mice (Regelson and Foltyn, 1966; Regelson, 1967; Chirigos *et al.*, 1969; Schuller *et al.*, 1975; Morahan *et al.*, 1976). It was suggested that pyran injected intraperitoneally activated peritoneal macrophages, and thus enhanced elimination of Friend virus when the virus was inoculated intraperitoneally (Schuller *et al.*, 1975). Pyran exerted no protective effect when inoculated intraperitoneally if Friend virus was injected intravenously (Schuller *et al.*, 1975). In contrast to the findings of Wheelock on the effect of statolon in mice pretreated with antilymphocytic serum, Hirsch *et al.* (1970*b*, 1972, 1973*c*) found that pyran copolymer did protect immunodepressed mice inoculated with Rauscher virus against early erythroblastosis and late lymphomas, and decreased the incidence of leukemia in immunodepressed AKR mice. (As in the experiments referred to in Section 2.1.2 with exogenous interferon in AKR mice, pyran was more effective in male than in female AKR mice.) Hirsch *et al.* (1973*c*) suggested that the antitumor effects of pyran copolymer were secondary to macrophage activation and enhanced phagocytosis.

COAM, an interferon inducer (Claes *et al.*, 1970), also inhibited tumor growth in NMRI mice infected neonatally with MSV (De Clercq and De Somer, 1972). With the exception of the experiments with poly-I.C referred to above (De Clercq and Stewart, 1974), none of these interferon inducers has been reported to induce regression of established MSV tumors.

Tilorone hydrochloride, an oral interferon inducer in mice, has also been shown to inhibit splenomegaly in Friend-virus-infected mice (Barker *et al.*, 1971*a,b*; Rheins *et al.*, 1971; Rana *et al.*, 1975).

Barker *et al.* (1971*b*) investigated the effect of sequential administration of nonviral inducers, poly-I.C, statolon, tilorone hydrochloride, and Sendaï virus on the evolution of Friend disease, and observed an increase in mean mouse survival time and an inhibition of spleno-hepatomegaly.

b. Activity on Oncogenic DNA Viruses. Compared with the more popular RNA oncogenic virus animal systems, the DNA oncogenic viruses have received less attention. Larson *et al.* (1969*a*) investigated the effect of poly-I.C, the double-stranded replicative form of MV 9 coliphage, pyran copolymer, and endotoxin on adenovirus 12 oncogenesis in newborn hamsters. Some reduction of internal but not of subcutaneous tumors was noted when poly-I.C was injected before, but not after, virus inoculation. Since the homopolymers poly-I and poly-C were also protective (homopolymers induce little or no interferon), and since poly-I.C was more active in female hamsters than in males, the authors suggested that the effects may have been mediated through immune mechanisms, rather than through the production of interferon. [The same group found that "single or multiple doses of poly-I.C given i.p. before or after subcutaneous inoculation of SV40 virus in newborn hamsters had little or no effect on the percentage of animals developing subcutaneous tumors later in life" (Larson *et al.*, 1970).]

Initiation of poly-I.C treatment before or 7–21 days after inoculation of polyoma virus inhibited the development of tumors in rats (Vandeputte *et al.*, 1970). The authors suggested that although production of interferon may have accounted for the inhibitory effects observed when poly-I.C was inoculated prior to virus challenge, it seemed most likely that immunologic mechanisms were responsible when poly-I.C was injected after virus inoculation.

Hirsch *et al.* (1972) showed that pyran copolymer also inhibited the development of polyoma-induced tumors in immunodepressed mice.

2.2.3. Spontaneous Neoplasms

Neither poly-I.C nor statolon was reported to be effective in delaying the manifestations of the spontaneously appearing lymphoid leukemia in AKR mice (Meier *et al.*, 1970*a,b*).

Weekly inoculation of poly-I.C proved as effective as exogenous interferon in delaying mammary tumors in RIII mice (Came and Moore, 1971). Neonatal injection of polycarboxylate was associated with a slight degree of inhibition of mammary tumors (Billiau *et al.*, 1971), as was treatment of newborn mice with poly-A.U (a poor interferon inducer) (Lacour *et al.*, 1972, 1975).

2.2.4. Enhancement of Viral Oncogenesis with Interferon Inducers

Several investigators have noted that at times, interferon inducers enhance rather than inhibit viral oncogenesis. This enhancement has usually been observed when viruses or nonviral interferon inducers were inoculated *prior to* infection with the test oncogenic virus. Thus, injection of Guaroa virus (W. Turner *et al.*, 1968), NDV (Steeves *et al.*, 1969), or Sindbis virus (Rheins *et al.*, 1971) enhanced Friend disease in mice.

Gresser (unpublished observations) noted that one intraperitoneal injection of statolon afforded protection to mice with Friend disease in accord with the observations of Wheelock (1967*a*), but that repeated intraperitoneal injections appeared to enhance splenomegaly. Larson and his co-workers (Larson *et al.*, 1969*b*; Hilleman, 1970*a,b*) found that the response of Friend-virus-inoculated mice to poly-I.C depended on drug dosage and the time of administration. Thus, enhancement rather than inhibition was observed under some experimental conditions. Likewise, a purified double-stranded RNA from a *Penicillium* culture enhanced Friend disease when inoculated before infection (and inhibited the disease when inoculated 5 days after viral infection) (Pilch and Planterose, 1971). The studies of De Clercq and Merigan (1971) emphasized the age of mice used, since poly-I.C inhibited tumor formation when mice 4–6 days old were inoculated with MSV, but enhanced tumor formation in 20-day-old mice inoculated with MSV. Similar results, i.e., enhancement of MSV oncogenesis in weanling mice, were obtained by Gazdar and co-workers (Gazdar *et al.*, 1972; Gazdar and Ikawa, 1972) after inoculation of several different interferon inducers, poly-I.C, NDV, pyran copolymer, and tilorone hydrochloride. Schuller, Morahan, and their co-workers (Schuller *et al.*, 1975; Morahan *et al.*, 1976) found that Friend disease could be either inhibited or enhanced by pyran copolymer, depending on the route of injection of the drug.

To date, there is one report of enhancement of viral oncogenesis after administration of exogenous interferon. Gazdar *et al.* (1972) found that mouse serum interferon inoculated locally 1 day prior to injection of MSV accelerated the appearance of tumors. (Some accelerating effect was also observed when the control preparation was injected.) Interferon administered systemically did not exhibit this enhancing effect.

Since interferon has been shown to inhibit DNA synthesis in stimulated lymphocytes *in vitro* (Lindahl-Magnusson *et al.*, 1972), inhibit lymphocyte sensitization and multiplication *in vivo* (Cerottini *et al.*, 1973; De Maeyer-Guignard *et al.*, 1975), inhibit antibody formation *in vitro* and *in vivo* (Gisler *et al.*, 1974; Johnson *et al.*, 1975; Braun and Levy, 1972; Brodeur and Merigan, 1974; Chester *et al.*, 1973) and delayed hypersensitivity *in vivo* (De Maeyer *et al.*, 1975), it is perhaps not surprising that large amounts of interferon injected *prior to* inoculation of an antigenic oncogenic virus might enhance subsequent tumor growth by depressing lymphocyte sensitization and multiplication. Likewise, it seems likely that inoculation of a good inducer of endogenous interferon prior to injection of an oncogenic virus (or transplantable tumor) might also be accompanied by an enhancement of tumor growth (provided the development of the tumor is influenced by the host's immunologic response).

3. Effect of Exogenous Interferon and Interferon Inducers on the Growth of Transplantable Tumors in Animals

3.1. Exogenous Interferon

In experiments on the effect of exogenous interferon on mice infected with the Friend and Rauscher viruses, less infectious virus was recovered from the spleens of interferon-treated mice than from the spleens of control mice, and fewer foci of tumor cells were observed in the spleens of treated mice than in the spleens of untreated mice (Gresser *et al.*, 1967*d,e*, 1968*a*). It seemed logical, therefore, to assume that these findings were causally related; i.e., repeated administration of interferon had inhibited viral multiplication, and consequently, the evolution of the leukemic process had been retarded. It was theoretically possible, however, that interferon preparations might also have inhibited multiplication of the tumor cells themselves or have stimulated, in some undefined manner, the host's mechanisms of defense and enhanced tumor-cell rejection (Gresser *et al.*, 1967*d,e*).

To explore this possibility, Gresser and his co-workers determined the effect of exogenous interferon on mice inoculated with various types of allogeneic and syngeneic tumor cells, of viral and nonviral origin. Their results may be summarized as follows: the repeated daily intraperitoneal administration of mouse interferon preparations inhibited the growth of several transplantable ascitic tumors (Ehrlich, RC19, EL4, and L1210), and markedly increased the survival of tumor-inoculated mice of different strains (Balb/c, DBA/2, C57B1/6) (Gresser *et al.*, 1969*b,c*, 1970*a*; Gresser and Bourali, 1969, 1970*a*). For example, after inoculation of 2000–3000 RC19 tumor cells (equivalent to approximately 500 LD_{50}), only 3.7% of Balb/c mice survived more than 22 days, whereas 98% of interferon-treated mice survived beyond this period (Gresser *et al.*, 1969*c*). The mean survival of Balb/c mice inoculated with 10^4 Ehrlich ascites (EA) cells (equivalent to 10^3–10^4 LD_{50}) was 18 days, and no mouse survived beyond day 22. In contrast, 90% of interferon-treated mice survived more than 6 months without any evidence of tumor, and were considered cured (Gresser and Bourali, 1970*a*). Optimal antitumor effects in these experiments were noted when contact between interferon and tumor cells was maximal (i.e., interferon and tumor cells inoculated intraperitoneally), although interferon also proved effective when inoculated at a site distant from that of tumor implantation. Interferon treatment limited to the period preceding inoculation of tumor cells was ineffective; treatment was effective only when continued *after* tumor inoculation. Interferon treatment was less effective in mice bearing solid tumor nodules than in mice inoculated with ascitic cells (Gresser *et al.*, 1969*b,c*, 1970*a*; Gresser and Bourali, 1970*a*).

The efficacy of interferon treatment in increasing mouse survival was directly related to the inhibition of tumor growth, and was inversely proportional to the number of cells inoculated, as illustrated in Table 1. In following the kinetics of

TABLE 1

Relationship Between Efficacy of Interferon Preparations in Increasing Survival of Balb/c Mice and Number of Ehrlich Ascites Cells Inoculated[a]

Number of cells inoculated per mouse	Treatment[b]	Number of mice surviving		Mean harmonic survival (days)	P	Confidence interval (0.95)
		>30 days/ Total number of mice[c]	>60 days/			
10^6	None	0/11		11		10–13
	Interferon	7/11	2/11	29	<0.0001	21–46
10^5	None	1/11	0/11	16		14–19
	Interferon	10/11	4/11	59	<0.0001	36–154
10^4	None	1/11	0/11	18		16–22
	Interferon	11/11	9/11	231	<0.0001	91–∞
10^3	None	0/11		19		17–21
	Interferon	11/11	8/11	133	0.0001	103–189

[a] Reprinted through the courtesy of the *Journal of the National Cancer Institute* from Gresser and Bourali (1970*a*).
[b] Interferon preparations intraperitoneally (40,000 U) were initiated 24 hr after inoculation of tumor cells and continued daily for a month thereafter.
[c] Equal number of male and female Balb/c mice.

Ehrlich ascites cell multiplication in the peritoneal cavity of mice treated with interferon, it was apparent that the inhibitory effect occurred in the days immediately following initiation of interferon treatment (Gresser and Bourali, 1970a). Toward the 6th day after inoculation of EA or RC19 tumor cells, phagocytosis of tumor cells by macrophages was observed in interferon-treated mice, but not in control mice (Gresser et al., 1970a; Gresser and Bourali, 1970a). Surviving interferon-treated tumor-inoculated mice showed an enhanced specific resistance to reinoculation of tumor cells (Gresser et al., 1970a; Gresser and Bourali, 1970a).

The Lewis lung carcinoma has been considered a useful model for the evaluation of potential antitumor chemotherapeutic drugs (Zubrod, 1972). When implanted subcutaneously, this tumor rapidly metastasizes to the lung. Very few standard antitumor drugs, however, are effective in inhibiting growth of this tumor (Zubrod, 1972; Mayo, 1972). Table 2 illustrates the inhibitory effect of interferon treatment on the growth of the primary subcutaneous tumor and on the development of pulmonary metastases (Gresser and Bourali, 1972). A therapeutic effect was observed even when interferon treatment was initiated 6 days after implantation of the tumor, at a time when subcutaneous nodules were already palpable (Gresser and Bourali, 1972).

TABLE 2

Inhibition of the Primary 3LL Tumor and Pulmonary Metastases by Interferon Preparations[a]

Expt. No.	Treatment	Number of mice	Primary tumor		Pulmonary metastases	
			Geometric mean weight (g)	Confidence interval (0.95)	Geometric mean number	Confidence interval (0.95)
1	None	17	6.5 NS[b]	(5.8–7.4)	17.9 NS[b]	(12.4–25.7)
	Control brain	16	5.8	(4.9–6.9)	29.9	(22.4–41.9)
	Interferon	19	3.6 P < 0.001	(3.2–4.0)	4.2 P < 0.001	(2.6–6.9)
2	None	19	4.7	(3.9–5.6)	30	(23.1–39.2)
	Interferon (day + 1 to day 20)	20	2.6 P < 0.001	(2.1–3.1)	7.7 P < 0.001	(4.9–12.2)
	Interferon (day + 6 to day 20)	20	2.9 NS[b]	(2.3–3.6)	6.1 NS[b]	(4.0–9.2)

[a] Reprinted through the courtesy of *Nature (London) New Biology* from Gresser and Bourali-Maury (1972).
[b] Not significant.

Very little work other than that just cited has been done to date on the effect of exogenous interferon on transplantable tumors. Coraggio *et al.* (1965) demonstrated the inhibitory effect of cell culture interferon on a polyoma-induced transplantable sarcoma of mice. They suggested that the integration of viral genome in the cellular DNA was important for the proliferation of the tumor, and that the antitumor action of interferon was mediated by its antiviral activity. Ferris *et al.* (1971) reported inhibition of two tumors, Ehrlich carcinoma and a carcinogen-induced lymphatic leukemia, implanted subcutaneously, by intraperitoneal injections of interferon.

Rossi and his co-workers found that the multiplication of transplantable Friend leukemia cells in the spleens of irradiated mice was inhibited by daily treatment of recipient mice with exogenous brain or cell culture interferon or interferon inducers (Rossi *et al.*, 1975). Since proliferation of Friend leukemia cells in this system was independent of the multiplication of Friend virus, the authors suggested that the antitumor effects of interferon were not mediated by antiviral effect, but rather by a direct inhibitory effect on the proliferation of the injected cells.

Pudov (1971) determined the effect of intravenous inoculation of human leukocyte interferon on the transplantable Brown–Pearce carcinoma in rabbits (human leukocyte interferon exerts a marked antiviral effect on rabbit cells *in vitro*) (Desmyter *et al.*, 1968). Metastases were observed in 6 of 14 interferon-treated rabbits, and in 12 of 14 control rabbits.

Takeyama *et al.* (1975) observed no increase in survival time in interferon-treated mice inoculated with several transplantable tumors (inoculum of 10^5–10^6 tumor cells). When the interferon was concentrated 7-fold (to a titer of 3.3×10^5 IU) and the number of cells inoculated was reduced, a slight but significant increase in survival was noted (23% for mice inoculated with L1210 cells, and 43% for mice inoculated with EA cells).

Chirigos and Pearson (1973) determined the effect of interferon treatment on the recurrence of a transplantable murine leukemia after initial treatment of the mouse with BCNU, which had reduced the tumor mass. BCNU alone, administered on the 7th day at a time when systemic disease was present, increased mean survival 130%, and resulted in a cure in 25% of mice. Exogenous interferon alone (50,000 U) did not increase survival. When interferon treatment followed Carmustine (BCNU) treatment, however, a synergistic effect was observed, with a marked increase in mean survival and an overall cure rate of 72%. These results are important in underlining the potential usefulness of combining interferon with antitumor chemotherapeutic drugs.

3.2. Interferon Inducers

3.2.1. Viral Inducers

The phenomenon of viral oncolysis was a subject of intense research 20 and more years ago. Regression or delay of tumor growth was observed in laboratory animals inoculated with viruses, and it was supposed that the viruses multiplied within the tumor cells (or in some instances induced a "toxic effect" in the absence of viral multiplication), causing destruction of the tumor. In retrospect, however, it seems likely that several different biological phenomena were grouped together as examples of "viral oncolysis." In several experiments, mice and rats were inoculated with large amounts of infectious or noninfectious arboviruses and myxoviruses under conditions that are now known to be optimal for the production of interferon (i.e., intravenous inoculation with high-titered viral preparations). We will cite some of these examples here, referring the reader to a previous review (Gresser, 1972) for a more detailed discussion of viral oncolysis and appropriate references.

Intravenous inoculation of vaccinia virus in mice with established transplantable leukemia or sarcoma was associated with a prolongation of survival (Turner *et al.*, 1948; Turner and Mulliken, 1950). Similar results (i.e., increased survival time and overall survival) were obtained in rats injected with either active or UV-irradiated inactive vaccinia virus 11 days after inoculation of leukemia cells. The therapeutic effect was directly related to the dose of virus inoculated (Zakay-Roness and Bernkopf, 1964). (This finding is consistent with the interpretation that production of interferon was responsible.)

Inoculation of several arboviruses (i.e., WNV, Ilheus, and Russian spring–summer encephalitis viruses) afforded a slight protection to mice injected intraperitoneally with 10^5–10^6 AK4 leukemic cells (Southam and Epstein, 1953). Inoculation of Guaroa virus proved inhibitory for Ehrlich and sarcoma 180 ascites tumors and increased mouse survival by a few days, but no effect was observed on subcutaneous solid tumors (Krulwich *et al.*, 1962). [Inhibition of tumor growth has not always been observed after inoculation of viruses or nonviral interferon inducers. Pierce *et al.* (1959) reported that sublethal doses of Egypt 101 virus "shortened the life-span of animals bearing leukemia L4946 and accelerated the leukemic leukocytosis" (see the discussion in Section 2.2.4).]

Nadel and Haas (1956) observed increased survival of guinea pigs bearing the transplantable leukemia L2B/N by inoculation of LCM from 2 days before to 7 days after transplantation of the leukemia. It was of interest that sequential injection of other viruses (which might also have induced interferon) did not add significantly to the protective effects of LCM virus. Inoculation of LCM virus did not protect mice bearing L1210 tumors. (In retrospect, it would be of interest to know whether LCM induces interferon in guinea pigs and to what titer.)

Molomut and Padnos (1965) reported that inoculation of mice with M-P virus (related if not identical to lymphocytic choriomeningitis virus) resulted in an inhibition of the development of several different transplantable tumors, as well as the spontaneously appearing lymphoid leukemia of AKR mice and the mammary carcinoma of C3H mice. (Tumor inhibition in mice by M-P-virus-induced interferon was reported by the same group.)

Southam and Epstein (1953) found that inoculation of NDV conferred a "slight antileukemic effect" on mice bearing the transplantable AK4 leukemia.

a significant protection on mice inoculated with RC19 tumor cells (Gresser *et al.*,
1969*b*,*c*; Gresser and Bourali, 1969) and EA cells (unpublished observations).
Rhim and Huebner (1971) reported that NDV and poly-I.C increased survival of
mice inoculated with EA cells.

3.2.2. Nonviral Interferon Inducers

Zeleznick and Bhuyan (1969) reported that repeated injections of poly-I.C
increased the survival of mice with L1210 ascites. Since poly-I.C was not cytotoxic
or cytostatic for L1210 cells *in vitro*, they inferred that poly-I.C induced a host
factor that was cytostatic. "It is logical to assume that the active material is
interferon" (Zeleznick and Bhuyan, 1969). H. B. Levy *et al.* (1969, 1970, 1971)
reported that repeated inoculation of poly-I.C inhibited the growth of several
transplantable tumors (of viral and nonviral origin) of mice. In the case of the
reticulum-cell sarcoma and the adenovirus-12-induced tumor, "initiation of
treatment after the tumor was grown to moderate size caused a regression of the
tumor" (Levy *et al.*, 1969). It is of particular interest in terms of the mode of action
of poly-I.C that tumor regression appeared to be due to "massive necrosis and
sloughing" (H. B. Levy *et al.*, 1969). This finding suggests the possibility that
poly-I.C (like endotoxin) may act on blood vessels, and thus affect the blood supply
of the tumor. The most resistant group of tumors tested were leukemias, and the
most sensitive tumors were the reticulum-cell sarcomas, implanted either subcutaneously or peritoneally. Adamson *et al.* (1969) found that poly-I.C was most
effective against the mouse reticulum-cell sarcoma and the Walker 256 rat
carcinosarcoma.

Bart and Kopf (1969) reported inhibition by poly-I.C of the growth of a murine
malignant melanoma of nonviral origin. When the tumor cell inoculum was
reduced, poly-I.C inhibited the growth of both lightly melanized and heavily
melanized tumors, and increased mouse survival (2 of 19 treated mice were
considered cured) (Bart *et al.*, 1971). In their recent work, Bart *et al.* (1975) appear
to favor the interpretation that interferon was responsible for the antitumor
effects because (1) there appeared to be a relationship between levels of endogenous serum interferon and antimelanoma effects (Bart *et al.*, 1973), and (2) poly-I.C
was effective in inhibiting growth of B16 melanoma in thymectomized
immunosuppressed mice—so that presumably it was not acting through any
immunoadjuvant effect.

This last point emphasizes the difficulty in understanding the mechanism of the
antitumor activity of poly-I.C. Since most workers (with exceptions; see Webb *et
al.*, 1972) have found that at antitumor doses, poly-I.C is not cytotoxic *in vitro*, it
has been suggested that it acts by enhancing cellular and humoral immune
mechanisms (Turner *et al.*, 1970; Kreider, 1970; Svec *et al.*, 1972). Several
investigators, however, agree with the findings of Bart *et al.* (1975), and do not
ascribe the poly-I.C-induced antitumor activity to immunoenhancement (Kende
and Glynn, 1971; Fisher *et al.*, 1972; Potmesil and Goldfeder, 1972; Kreider and

Benjamin, 1972), since poly-I.C inhibited antitumor effects in immunodepressed animals.

Ball and McCarter (1971) found that poly-I.C was most effective in inhibiting the growth of a transplantable tumor when tumor cells and poly-I.C were both inoculated intraperitoneally (100% survival at 1 year). When poly-I.C and tumor were injected by different routes, however, there was only a slight protective effect, or even an enhancing effect on tumor growth. Meier *et al.* (1970*b*) reported the ineffectiveness of poly-I.C on transplantable tumors in mice induced by methylcholanthrene. (Examination of their published data, however, suggests some increased survival in some of the poly-I.C-treated tumor-inoculated mice.) Other investigators have also noted that poly-I.C was not always effective in laboratory animals with transplantable tumors. "Single or multiple doses of varying amounts of poly-I.C administered i.p. before and/or after subcutaneous inoculation of virus free SV40 tumor cells had little or no effect on the rate of tumor appearance in hamsters" (Larson *et al.*, 1970). [It is of interest that poly-I.C induces little interferon in hamsters (Larson *et al.*, 1970).] Rhim and Huebner (1971) found that poly-I.C exhibited only a weak antitumor effect in hamsters inoculated with RLV-induced transplantable tumors.

Another interferon inducer, tilorone hydrochloride, was found to inhibit three rodent tumors, but was ineffective against three other transplantable tumors (including L1210) (Adamson, 1971*a*; Adamson and Ting, 1971). When inoculated intraperitoneally, it proved more effective than either rifampicin or poly-I.C in mice bearing the Walker 256 carcinosarcoma (Adamson, 1971*b*). Tilorone proved ineffective in inhibiting the Lewis lung carcinoma and the B-16 melanoma in mice, and when it was inoculated prior to injection of tumor cells, tilorone even accelerated the development of tumors (Morahan *et al.*, 1974).

Regelson (1968) has reviewed the extensive bibliography on the antitumor activity of different polyanions. As stated above, pyran copolymer induces the production of interferon (Regelson, 1967), and when administered prior to inoculation of sarcoma 180 tumor cells, it inhibited subsequent tumor growth (Regelson, 1968). Pyran proved effective in inhibiting both the Lewis lung carcinoma and the B-16 melanoma, even when treatment was begun 6–7 days after tumor implantation (Morahan *et al.*, 1974). Snodgrass *et al.* (1975) attributed the inhibition of the growth of the primary Lewis lung carcinoma and of pulmonary metastases by pyran to an infiltration of the tumor by cells of the histiocyte–macrophage series that were cytotoxic for the tumor (Snodgrass *et al.*, 1975; Kaplan *et al.*, 1974, 1976; Morahan and Kaplan, 1976). Herling (1975) found that pyran injected intravenously 24 hr prior to intravenous injection of B-16 melanoma cells decreased the number of liver metastases, but exerted no effect when injected 3 days after tumor-cell inoculation. As in the experiments by Morahan's group, Herling suggested that activation of liver macrophages by pyran was responsible for the antitumor effects.

At present, it seems unlikely that interferon plays much of a role, if any, in the antitumor effects of pyran copolymer.

4.1. Exogenous Interferon

4.1.1. Chemically Induced Neoplasms

Salerno *et al.* (1972) reported that repeated administration of exogenous interferon (2500 U/dose) beginning on the 5th day of life inhibited the subsequent development of subcutaneous fibrosarcomas and lung adenomas induced by 3-methylcholanthrene in CF-1 mice. Thus, none of 26 interferon-treated mice developed either lung adenomas or subcutaneous tumors, in contrast to 8 of 18 mice with adenomas and 11 of 18 mice with subcutaneous tumors in the control group. Kishida *et al.* (1971) observed a slight delay in the appearance of tumors in 20 methylcholanthrene-injected mice treated with interferon, but all mice eventually developed tumors.

4.1.2. Radiation-Induced Leukemia

Ionizing radiation induces the development of lymphosarcomas in C57B1 mice, and the viruses (Rad LV) extracted from such tumors induce morphologically identical neoplasms in susceptible mice. Repeated administration of interferon for 9 weeks resulted in a significant delay in the development of tumors in mice inoculated with Rad LV and a decrease in the final incidence of tumors (Lieberman *et al.*, 1971). Continued administration of interferon did not alter the evolution of lymphoma induced in mice by irradiation with 168 rads (in agreement with unpublished experimental results of De Maeyer *et al.*). When a submaximal dose of X rays (i.e., 130 rads) was utilized, a slight but significant reduction in the incidence of lymphoma was observed in interferon-treated mice (Lieberman *et al.*, 1971).

4.2. Nonviral Interferon Inducers

4.2.1. Chemically Induced Neoplasms

There are several reports that administration of poly-I.C also inhibited the development of tumors induced by chemical carcinogens. Gelboin and Levy (1970) observed an inhibition of skin tumors induced by 9,10-dimethylbenzanthracene either alone or followed by weekly application of croton oil. Kreibich *et al.* (1970) also investigated the effect of poly-I.C on chemical carcinogenesis induced by DMBA or methylcholanthrene. The ultimate response depended on several experimental conditions, such as time of treatment relative to induction or promotion of carcinogenesis. Elgjo and Degré (1973) found that repeated administration of poly-I.C (maintained during the whole experimental period) inhibited two-stage skin carcinogenesis in mice induced by 3-methylcholanthrene. Since poly-I.C was ineffective when started 4 weeks after tumor initiation, the authors concluded that poly-I.C affected "processes occurring during promotion." Ball and McCarter (1971), however, found that poly-I.C significantly enhanced the incidence of thymic lymphomas induced by DMBA, whereas it reduced the incidence of thymic lymphomas induced by neonatal irradiation. Glaz (1972) found that statolon (at different doses and regimens) was ineffective in inhibiting metholcholanthrene-induced tumors in two strains of mice.

5. Effect of Exogenous Interferon and Interferon Inducers on Normal Animals

5.1. Exogenous Interferon

Most drugs that exert significant antitumor activity have also proved toxic for the host, and the margin of safety between antitumor activity and toxicity has often been narrow. Although many experiments on the *in vivo* antiviral activity of interferon have been undertaken, little is known concerning its effect on normal animals. This question is clearly of importance in the evaluation of the clinical usefulness of interferon. Gresser *et al.* (1967a) found that repeated injections (intraperitoneal) of concentrated mouse brain or mouse serum–spleen interferon preparations induced ascites in mice. It is probable that the large amounts of noninterferon protein in these preparations were responsible for this effect, since ascites was not observed when preparations with greater specific activities were injected.

A series of experiments undertaken by Gresser and co-workers suggested that interferon was in fact not toxic for mice at concentrations that demonstrated a clear-cut antitumor effect. Thus, AKR mice were inoculated with concentrated brain interferon daily from birth for 3 months in one experiment, and for 1 year in a second experiment. These mice developed normally, and the monthly weights for interferon-treated mice were comparable to those of untreated mice or mice treated with normal brain extract (Gresser *et al.*, 1969a).

In another experiment, AKR and C3H mice were inoculated subcutaneously daily from birth for 28 days with concentrated mouse brain interferon preparations, concentrated normal brain extract, or saline. Interferon-treated mice grew and developed as well as control mice, and no macroscopic or microscopic abnormalities were observed when these mice were sacrificed on day 28 (Gresser and Bourali, 1970b). Likewise, no evidence of toxicity was observed in adult Swiss mice inoculated daily with brain interferon preparations (Gresser *et al.*, 1967e). Graff *et al.* (1970) inoculated mice with more than 100,000 U interferon, and stated that it was without "any apparent effect on normal, non-infected animals."

Since interferon had been shown to inhibit the multiplication of both tumor and "normal" mouse cells in cell culture, the question remained whether more potent preparations of interferon than had been previously used could also inhibit cell division in the normal animal. Cerottini *et al.* (1973) transferred splenic lymphocytes from donor C57B1/6 mice to irradiated DBA/2 mice and found that administration of potent interferon preparations, poly-I.C, or NDV to the DBA/2 mice inhibited the multiplication of donor lymphocytes. To determine whether interferon acted by inhibiting the multiplication of transferred allogeneic lymphocytes or by stimulating a residual immune response in the irradiated host, syngeneic bone marrow cells were transferred to irradiated mice. As in the experiments with allogeneic lymphocytes, interferon treatment of the irradiated mice resulted in an inhibition of the multiplication of transferred syngeneic cells (Cerottini *et al.*, 1973).

Likewise, potent preparations of exogenous interferon were shown to inhibit the regeneration of liver in mice after partial hepatectomy (Frayssinet *et al.*, 1973). The total amount of RNA and DNA in the liver increased in untreated hepatectomized mice, but not in interferon-treated hepatectomized mice, and autoradiographic analysis indicated that fewer liver cells were labeled in interferon-treated mice than in control mice.

The availability of potent partially purified mouse interferon preparations (Tovey *et al.*, 1974) enabled Gresser and his co-workers (Gresser *et al.*, 1975a) to reexamine the effect of exogenous interferon on the development and growth of newborn mice. The titer and the specific activity of the interferon preparations used in these experiments were approximately 100-fold greater than those used in their earlier experiments. Newborn Swiss or C3H mice injected daily subcutaneously with mouse cell culture interferon preparations (titer 1 : 800,000) seemed to develop and grow normally for the first 6–7 days of life (Gresser *et al.*, 1975a). In

TABLE 3

Lethality of Mouse Interferon Preparations for Newborn Swiss or C3H Mice[a]

Expt. No.	Mouse strain	Type of mouse interferon	Injected with:				
			Mouse interferon	Control preparation	Inactivated mouse interferon	Human interferon	Uninoculated
1	Swiss	C-243[b]	21/21[c] (13 ± 1)[d]	0/23	NT[e]	NT	0/27
2	Swiss	C-243[b]	23/23 (11 ± 1)	0/11	NT	NT	0/22
3	Swiss	C-243[b]	22/22 (13 ± 2)	NT	NT	NT	0/21
4	Swiss	C-243[b]	26/26 (9 ± 1)	0/18	NT	0/23[f]	0/53
5	Swiss	C-243[b]	15/15 (10 ± 1)	NT	0/15[g]	NT	0/19
6	C3H	C-243[b]	15/15 (9 ± 1)	0/30	0/15[h]	NT	0/18
7	Swiss	L[i]	6/7 (14 ± 1)	NT	NT	NT	0/18
		TOTALS:	128/129	0/82	0/30	0/23	0/178

[a] Reprinted through the courtesy of *Nature* (*London*) from Gresser *et al.* (1975a).
[b] A different mouse C-243 cell interferon preparation titering 1 : 800,000 was used in each of Experiments 1–6.
[c] Number of mice dead/total number of mice injected. Based on survival at 1 month. Newborn mice dying in the first 2 days of life are not included.
[d] Mean day of death ± S.D.
[e] Not tested.
[f] The titer of the human leucocyte interferon was 1 : 2,000,000 [MRC reference interferon (69/19) U], as assayed on human diploid fibroblasts.
[g] Inactivated by heating at 60°C for 1 hr. Residual titer: 1 : 100,000.
[h] Inactivated by treatment with 0.02 M sodium periodate at pH 4 for 3 hr at 4°C. Residual titer: 1 : 600.
[i] The titer of the Sendaï-virus-induced L-cell interferon was 1 : 240,000.

the ensuing few days, an increasing difference in weight was observed between interferon-treated mice and their control littermates. Interferon-treated mice died between days 8 and 14 (Table 3). Diffuse hepatic cell degeneration appeared to be the immediate cause of death. The only other histological abnormalities were some diminution of the cortical region of the thymus in some mice, and poorly differentiated germinal follicles in the spleen. These results constituted the first report of untoward effects associated with interferon treatment of the normal animal. Evidence was presented that interferon itself was the responsible factor. Further work will be necessary to determine whether lower doses of interferon may cause adverse effects that will develop later in life. These findings would seem relevant to the treatment of patients with interferon—especially newborn infants and possibly pregnant women. It should be emphasized, nevertheless, that adult patients have been treated for extended periods of time ($1\frac{1}{2}$ years) with potent preparations of human leukocyte interferon without apparent untoward effects (see Section 7).

5.2. Interferon Inducers

There is considerable evidence that inoculation of viral and nonviral interferon inducers is often associated with considerable toxicity. The *in vivo* toxicity of viral and nonviral interferon inducers was reviewed in some detail previously (Gresser, 1972), and will not be discussed further, since there is no clear-cut evidence to date that the toxicity of interferon inducers is due to interferon itself. It is worth mentioning, however, that the experimental conditions utilized in most experiments designed to elicit "toxicity" are those usually considered optimal for the induction of interferon, i.e., high-titered virus preparations inoculated intravenously or intraperitoneally, or amounts of inducer that elicit interferon production. In fact, it has been suggested that poly-I.C may act in the intact animal as a stimulator of interferon precisely because of its toxic effects (Absher and Stinebring, 1969; De Clercq and Merigan, 1970; Leonard *et al.*, 1969). K. H. Huang and Landay (1969) found that injection of mice with NDV enhanced the lethality of endotoxin in mice, and concluded that the enhanced lethality was mediated by interferon. Likewise, inoculation of NDV increased the incidence and rate of deaths in mice infected with several gram-positive and gram-negative bacteria (Hugh *et al.*, 1971). These authors suggested that interferon might be responsible for the enhanced toxicity.

Actinomycin D has been shown to increase markedly the sensitivity of mice to the toxic effects of minute quantities of endotoxin (Pieroni *et al.*, 1970) and poly-I.C (Pieroni *et al.*, 1971). Were endogenous interferon responsible for the toxicity resulting from injection of poly-I.C or endotoxin, one might expect that actinomycin D would also render mice sensitive to exogenous interferon. In a series of experiments (Chedid and Gresser, unpublished observations), concentrated mouse brain interferon was administered to actinomycin-D-treated mice. No toxicity was observed.

We will consider here only the mechanisms of the antitumor effects of exogenous interferon. In many instances, the antitumor effects of several interferon inducers are probably not mediated by interferon, and interferon production appears to be incidental to their activity.

6.1. Virus-Induced Neoplasms

When interferon was administered to hamsters prior to inoculation of polyoma virus, a delay in the appearance of tumors, a decrease in the number of tumor-bearing animals, and an increased animal survival were observed (Atanasiu and Chany, 1960). Since the oncogenicity of polyoma virus in hamsters is proportional to the viral inoculum (a complete cycle of viral multiplication is not observed), it is likely that interferon inhibited viral replication and an early virus-dependent event that leads to cellular transformation. Likewise, administration of interferon to chicks and rabbits *prior to* inoculation of RSV (Strandström *et al.*, 1962; Lampson *et al.*, 1963) and Shope fibroma virus (Kishida *et al.*, 1965) probably inhibited the development of tumors by inhibiting viral multiplication.

In contrast to these studies, it was found that in mice inoculated with the Friend and Rauscher leukemia viruses, it was necessary to continue the administration of interferon after viral infection to obtain an effect. Treatment confined to the period immediately preceding and following viral inoculation proved totally ineffective, whereas repeated inoculation of interferon *after* viral inoculation inhibited the evolution of the various manifestations of these leukemias and increased the mean survival time (Gresser *et al.*, 1967a,c–e, 1968a; Wheelock and Larke, 1968). Since the Friend and Rauscher leukemias are examples of subacute infectious processes, and viral multiplication occurs throughout the course of the disease, the most likely explanation of the effects observed was that continued repression of viral multiplication by interferon was responsible for the inhibitory effect on the evolution of these leukemias. This interpretation implies that successive cycles of viral multiplication in various organs are in some manner causally related to the progressive increase in the number of "tumor" cells in Friend and Rauscher disease.

The recent work of Smadja-Joffe, Jasmin, and their co-workers supports this interpretation. They suggest that Friend disease is a disease of dysregulation of erythropoiesis, rather than a neoplastic disease (Smadja-Joffe *et al.*, 1973, 1975, 1976; Fredrickson *et al.*, 1975; Jasmin *et al.*, 1976). Friend virus, which multiplies in host tissues, acts on erythropoietin-responsive cells (ERCs) and stimulates them to differentiate into short-lived proerythroblast cells, most of which die rapidly. This cell loss is compensated for by an increase in the stem cell compartment and a continuous supply of target cells (ERCs) resulting from physiological feedback mechanisms. These ERCs are in turn infected by Friend virus. Thus, the process is a continuum dependent on the supply of two essential elements—virus and target cells. According to the work of these authors, Friend "leukemic" cells are characterized by a limited capacity of proliferation and a short life span, and these cells are neither malignant nor clonogenic (Smadja-Joffe *et al.*, 1975, 1976). [The appearance of transplantable Friend cells with malignant characteristics would be an infrequent secondary event, and not representative of Friend disease, according to the model proposed by Smadja-Joffe and Jasmin (Smadja-Joffe *et al.*, 1975, 1976; Jasmin *et al.*, 1976).]

Interferon might act, therefore, at several steps in Friend disease: (1) By inhibiting viral multiplication. [Less infectious virus was present in the spleens of interferon-treated mice than in the spleens of control mice, as determined by biological assay and electron microscopy (Gresser *et al.*, 1967d,e, 1968a).] (2) By inhibiting the multiplication of precursor stem cells and thus reducing the number of ERCs, which are the target cells for Friend virus (Fredrickson *et al.*, 1975). [Injection of myleran, which reduces the number of precursor stem cells and ERCs, markedly reduces the capacity of Friend virus to induce splenomegaly (Fredrickson *et al.*, 1975).] In this regard, Rossi *et al.* (1975) (as mentioned in Section 3.1) found that interferon treatment of mice was associated with an inhibition of the multiplication of transplantable Friend cells.

There are other possible sites of interferon action in Friend disease that may be mentioned:

1. Interferon might promote erythroid differentiation. In the experiments of Gresser *et al.* (1967c,d), not only was the extent of Friend cell involvement less marked in interferon-treated mice than that in control leukemic mice, but also there appeared to be numerous foci of erythroid maturation from proerythroblasts to normoblastic elements. This cellular maturation was seldom observed in untreated leukemic mice.

2. Interferon might counteract the deleterious effects that accompany infection of mice with oncogenic viruses [see the discussion of the effect of statolon on Friend leukemia in Section 2.2.2a]. Tóth *et al.* (1971) suggested that the anti-Rauscher-disease effect was mediated by an enhanced immunologic response in interferon-treated mice.

In summary, however, we favor the following interpretation: interferon may act, on one hand, by inhibiting multiplication of the virus, which is essential for maintaining the disease; on the other hand, it may decrease the supply of target cells for the Friend virus by inhibiting the multiplication of primitive stem cells and ERCs. We should emphasize that this interpretation is in accord with the model of the pathogenesis of Friend disease proposed by Smadja-Joffe and Jasmin (Smadja-Joffe *et al.*, 1973, 1975, 1976; Fredrickson *et al.*, 1975; Jasmin *et al.*, 1976). If, however, Friend disease is in fact a neoplastic disease and the Friend cells are malignant proliferating cells, then interferon might act by inhibiting tumor cell multiplication, as will be discussed in the ensuing paragraphs.

Smadja-Joffe and Jasmin have suggested (Smadja-Joffe *et al.*, 1976; Jasmin *et al.*, 1976) that Friend leukemia is a useful model for understanding the physiopathology of human chronic lymphoid leukemia. Perhaps human interferon would prove a useful adjunct in the treatment of these diseases.

6.2. Transplantable Tumors

Whereas interferon may well act in virus-induced neoplasms principally or in part because of its antiviral activity, it seems to us unlikely that this action can explain its antitumor effect in animals inoculated with transplantable tumors. In these experimental systems, the tumors observed are due to the progressive multiplication of the tumor cells inoculated, and not to a progressive transformation of host cells by viruses that may be present in many of these transplantable tumors.

We may divide the possible mechanism(s) of the antitumor activity of interferon into two categories:

1. A direct effect of interferon on the tumor cells themselves—either inhibiting their multiplication or modifying their tumorigenicity.
2. An action on the host and an enhancement of the host's capacity to reject the tumor.

6.2.1. Inhibition by Exogenous Interferon of Tumor-Cell Multiplication

In experiments on the effect of interferon on the growth of ascitic tumors, it was found that optimal therapeutic results were obtained when intimate contact between interferon and tumor cells was maximal, e.g., when both interferon and tumor cells were inoculated intraperitoneally (Gresser *et al.*, 1969*b*, 1970*a*; Gresser and Bourali, 1970*a*). The effect of interferon was seen early after inoculation of tumor cells. Thus, when mice were injected with Ehrlich tumor cells and treated with interferon and then sacrificed in the ensuing days, fewer tumor cells were recovered from their peritoneal cavities than from the peritoneal cavities of control mice (Gresser and Bourali, 1970*a*). These observations suggested that interferon might be inhibiting the multiplication of tumor cells in the peritoneal cavity, and led Gresser and his co-workers to investigate the effect of interferon on cell division *in vitro*. Their work and that of other investigators has shown that under appropriate experimental conditions, one can demonstrate inhibition by interferon of the multiplication of both murine and human tumor and normal cells in culture (Paucker *et al.*, 1962; Fontaine-Brouty-Boyé *et al.*, 1969; Gresser *et al.*, 1970*b*, 1973; Lindahl-Magnusson *et al.*, 1971; Kishida *et al.*, 1971; S. H. S. Lee *et al.*, 1972; O'Shaughnessy *et al.*, 1972; Knight, 1973; Hilfenhaus and Karges, 1974; Gaffney *et al.*, 1973; McNeill and Fleming, 1971; McNeill and Gresser, 1973; Adams *et al.*, 1975). Some of the evidence indicating that interferon itself is the responsible factor may be summarized as follows:

1. Crude and purified preparations of mouse interferon, regardless of the tissue of orgin and the interferon inducer employed (viral or nonviral), inhibited the multiplication of murine cells (Fontaine-Brouty-Boyé *et al.*, 1969; Gresser *et al.*, 1970*b*), whereas heterologous interferon (prepared with similar inducers) inactivated mouse interferon, and mock interferon preparations were ineffective.
2. Comparison of the antiviral activity of different highly purified interferon preparations and their inhibitory activity on cell multiplication (using a

sensitive assay based on 50% inhibition of colony formation in agarose; Gresser *et al.*, 1971*a*) showed a parallelism in their activities (Gresser *et al.*, 1973). The kinetics of production of both activities and the kinetics of loss of activity after heating were also parallel (Gresser *et al.*, 1973).

3. When human leukocyte interferon was boiled in the presence of SDS and urea under nonreducing or reducing conditions and subjected to electrophoresis in SDS polyacrylamide gels, there was a direct quantitative correlation between the antiviral activity of a given fraction and its inhibitory activity on cell multiplication (Stewart *et al.*, 1976).

4. Cultivation of L1210 cells in the presence of interferon resulted in the selection of a subline of L1210 cells resistant to both the antiviral activity of interferon and the inhibitory activity on cell division (Gresser *et al.*, 1970*b,c*, 1974*a*).

Inhibition of cell multiplication by interferon was not associated with an increased cell death (Fontaine-Brouty-Boyé *et al.*, 1969; Gresser *et al.*, 1970*c*). There is no evidence that interferon is cytotoxic, but it does delay the rate of cell multiplication. The results of a photomicrocinematographic analysis of the effect of interferon on mouse mammary tumor cells indicate that there is a progressive prolongation of the cell-generation time (Collyn d'Hooghe *et al.*, unpublished observations). Tovey *et al.* (1975) cultivated mouse L1210 cells under steady-state conditions of a chemostat, and also observed inhibition of cell division after addition of interferon.

The experimental results from cell culture studies indicate, therefore, that interferon can inhibit tumor-cell multiplication, and under certain experimental conditions, interferon probably inhibits tumor-cell multiplication in the animal. Nevertheless, there are certain difficulties in extrapolating from the cell culture experiments to conditions in the animal. For example, to observe inhibition of tumor-cell multiplication *in vitro*, it was found necessary to keep interferon in the nutrient medium for several hours (Gresser *et al.*, 1970*c*). Is the interferon one injects into mice sufficient to inhibit tumor-cell multiplication? In view of the rapid disappearance of interferon from the circulation (Gresser *et al.*, 1967*b*), is there sufficient contact between interferon and tumor cells? Or is there some system of amplification of interferon effect in the animal that is not observed in *in vitro* systems?

6.2.2. Effect of Exogenous Interferon on the Tumorigenicity and on the Surfaces of Tumor Cells

Gresser *et al.* (1971*b*) found that cultivation of murine L1210 cells in the presence of mouse interferon for 24 hr was associated with a reduction of more than 100-fold in the tumorigenicity of these cells for mice. Likewise, these interferon-treated cells showed a comparable decrease in their capacity to form colonies in semisolid agar. Kishida *et al.* (1971) also observed that interferon treatment of tumor cells *in vitro* resulted in a decreased tumorigenicity. (These results suggested the possibility that interferon treatment might be accompanied by a change in the surfaces of these tumor cells that rendered them incapable of

multiplying in the animal or of forming colonies in agarose.) Lindahl *et al.* (1973)
showed that treatment with mouse interferon preparations does in fact result in
changes in the cell surface, as exemplified by an enhanced capacity to absorb an
alloantiserum. [Enhancement of the expression of surface H-2 antigens was also
observed on interferon-treated thymocytes and splenic lymphocytes (Lindahl *et
al.*, 1974), and on these cells taken from interferon-treated mice (Lindahl *et al.*,
1976).] Likewise, interferon-treated L1210 cells showed an enhanced capacity to
bind radioactive concanavalin A (Huet *et al.*, 1974). Thus, one may postulate that
interferon may act directly on the tumor cells *in vivo* by altering the cell surface in
some manner and thereby modifying cell behavior (possibly also rendering tumor
cells more easily eliminated by host cells). [In Section 3.1, we referred to the
experiments in which phagocytosis of Ehrlich tumor cells by peritoneal macrophages was observed in interferon-treated mice, but not in control mice
(Gresser and Bourali, 1970*a*).]

6.2.3. Effect of Exogenous Interferon on the Host's Mechanisms

To determine whether interferon might also act by enhancing in some manner
the capacity of the host to reject transplanted tumors, Gresser *et al.* (1972) injected
mice with leukemia L1210 cells derived from interferon-sensitive or interferon-
resistant cell lines (Gresser *et al.*, 1970*c*, 1974*a*). The finding that interferon
treatment increased the survival of mice inoculated with interferon-resistant
L1210 cells suggested that the antitumor effect in these mice did not result from a
direct inhibitory effect on tumor-cell multiplication (since the cells were resistant
to this effect), but that inhibition of tumor growth was mediated in some manner
by the host. In mice inoculated with interferon-sensitive L1210 cells, both
mechanisms may have been operative (i.e., a direct inhibitory effect on cell
multiplication and a host-mediated effect), since a greater protective effect of
interferon was observed in mice inoculated with interferon-sensitive L1210 cells
than in mice inoculated with the interferon-resistant L1210 cells (Gresser *et al.*,
1972).

How is this host antitumor effect mediated?

a. Immune System. Apart from its effect on cell division (referred to above),
interferon can also modify the function of differentiated cells. Table 4 lists, for
heuristic reasons, some of the effects of interferon on cells in culture. For example,
interferon may inhibit or enhance the production of specific proteins (Stewart *et
al.*, 1971; Friedman, 1966; Nebert and Friedman, 1973); it enhances the phagocytic capacity of macrophages (K. Y. Huang *et al.*, 1971; Imanishi *et al.*, 1975); it
exerts important effects on lymphocytes and on the immune response. *In vitro*,
interferon can inhibit DNA synthesis in lymphocytes stimulated by PHA or by
allogeneic lymphocytes (Lindahl-Magnusson *et al.*, 1972; Blomgren *et al.*, 1974;
Gericke *et al.*, 1973); when added early, it inhibits antibody formation *in vitro*
(Gisler *et al.*, 1974; Johnson *et al.*, 1975); when added late, after sensitization has

TABLE 4

Effects of Interferon on Cells[a]

A. Inhibition of replication of
   intracellular parasites
   a. Virus
   b. Chlamydiae
   c. Rickettsiae
   d. Bacteria
   e. Protozoa

B. Inhibition of cell function
   a. Cell division
   b. Production of interferon
   c. Generation of antibody-forming cells

C. Enhancement of cell function
   a. Production of specific proteins, such as
      interferon "priming" and aryl hydrocar-
      bon hydroxylase
   b. Phagocytosis by macrophages
   c. Cytotoxicity by sensitized lymphocytes
   d. Generation of antibody-forming cells
   e. Expression of H-2 antigens
   f. Susceptibility of cells to toxicity of
      double-stranded nucleic acids and vac-
      cinia virus

[a] Reprinted from P. Lindahl, 1974, Doctoral thesis, Karolinska Institutet, Stockholm.

occurred, it can increase the number of plaque-forming cells (Gisler *et al.*, 1974). Likewise, it can enhance the cytotoxicity of sensitized lymphocytes for target cells (Lindahl *et al.*, 1972). In the mouse, interferon administration can inhibit the multiplication of lymphocytes transferred to irradiated recipients (Cerottini *et al.*, 1973), inhibit a primary antibody response (Braun and Levy, 1972; Chester *et al.*, 1973; Brodeur and Merigan, 1974), delay the rejection of allogeneic skin grafts (De Maeyer *et al.*, 1973; Mobraaten *et al.*, 1973; Hirsch *et al.*, 1974), and inhibit delayed hypersensitivity reactions (De Maeyer *et al.*, 1975).

Thus, one might suggest that the antitumor effect of interferon might be mediated in part by lymphocytes and macrophages, which are considered important in host rejection of allografts or transplantable tumors. Chernyakhovskaya, Svet-Moldavsky, and co-workers (Svet-Moldavsky and Chernyakhovskaya, 1967; Chernyakhovskaya *et al.*, 1970; Slavina *et al.*, 1974; Svet-Moldavsky *et al.*, 1974) suggested that interferon rendered normal lymphocytes cytotoxic for tumor cells, and proposed this mechanism to explain the antitumor effects of interferon. Lindahl and her co-workers, however, were unable to demonstrate this effect of interferon on normal lymphocytes, and reported that only the cytotoxicity of previously sensitized lymphocytes could be enhanced by interferon (Lindahl *et al.*, 1972).

Gresser and Bourali-Maury undertook experiments on the efficacy of interferon treatment in tumor-inoculated mice pretreated either with antilymphocytic sera (ALS) or X-irradiation to depress lymphocytes or with silica to depress macrophages. Interferon proved as effective in ALS-pretreated tumor-inoculated mice as in mice not receiving ALS. Pretreatment of mice with silica diminished somewhat, but did not abolish, the antitumor effect (Gresser and Bourali-Maury, 1973). Thus, there was no evidence to suggest that the interferon-associated host antitumor component was mediated by lymphocytes or macrophages. In this regard, it is of interest that the antitumor effect of the interferon inducer poly-I.C (which is known to enhance the immune response; Turner *et al.*, 1970) may also not be mediated by lymphocytes (Potmesil and Goldfeder, 1972; Fisher *et al.*,

1972; Kreider and Benjamin, 1972). Thus, immunosuppression of mice with X-ray or ALS did not eliminate the antitumor effect of poly-I.C. Likewise, pyran copolymer protected immunosuppressed mice against tumor development induced by polyoma and RSV (Hirsch *et al.*, 1972). Thus, it is not sufficient to infer that because a substance has an immunoadjuvant effect the antitumor activity is dependent on enhancement of the host's immunologic reactivity. [The work of Wheelock and his co-workers (see Section 2.2.2) suggests, however, that the antitumor activity of statolon is based on its immunoenhancing activity.]

One other point appears relevant to a discussion of a possible interferon-induced host-mediated antitumor effect: Several nonviral interferon inducers (BCG, endotoxin, pyran copolymer) all exert an antitumor effect when injected days or weeks prior to inoculation of tumor cells, and are relatively ineffective when injected after tumor inoculation. In contrast, interferon was effective only when administered repeatedly *after* tumor inoculation, and was ineffective when treatment was limited to the period preceding tumor grafting (Gresser and Bourali, 1970*a*).

b. Other Host-Mediated Mechanisms. It is becoming clear that tumor cells secrete a variety of soluble factors that affect the host. Patients with cancer often exhibit diminished cell-mediated immune responsiveness. Although it is possible that such deficiency may precede the development of cancer (failure of "immune surveillance" has been considered an important factor in the emergence of cancer), it seems equally possible that in some instances, the tumor itself may be the cause of the depressed immune response, by the liberation of immunosuppressive substances. Thus, in experimental animals, it has been shown that transfer of cell-free tumor ascitic fluid to normal mice results in an inhibition of the antibody response to sheep erythrocytes (Grohsman and Nowotny, 1972; Hrsak and Morotti, 1973; Yamazaki *et al.*, 1973), abrogation of lymphocyte "trapping" (Frost and Lance, 1973), and enhancement of the growth of a transplantable tumor (Mocarelli *et al.*, 1973). That the lymphocytes of tumor-bearing animals are probably potentially reactive, but are only temporarily depressed by an inhibitor, is suggested by the findings that bone marrow, thymus, and spleen cells from these mice exhibit immunologic competence when transferred to syngeneic irradiated recipients (Mocarelli *et al.*, 1973). Gresser *et al.* (1975*b*) showed that cell-free Ehrlich ascitic fluid from tumor-bearing mice and the nutrient medium from Ehrlich cells maintained *in vitro* contained a factor or factors that when transferred to normal mice delayed rejection of skin allografts and enhanced the growth of a syngeneic transplantable tumor. Both types of preparations inhibited DNA synthesis in lymphocytes stimulated by PHA, suggesting that Ehrlich tumor cells released a factor which impaired the normal lymphocytic response to allo and tumor antigens.

In addition to immunosuppressive factors, tumors secrete factors that appear to stimulate proliferation of both tumor and normal cells (Baserga and Kisieleski, 1961; Rev-Kury *et al.*, 1966; Lyon, 1970; Chouroulinkov *et al.*, 1971; Morgan and Cameron, 1973; Suddith *et al.*, 1975), increase the blood supply of tumors

(Folkman *et al.*, 1971), inhibit phagocytosis by macrophages (Fauve *et al.*, 1974), and stimulate osteoclasts (Mundy *et al.*, 1974). I suggest the generic name *oncotrophins* for the ensemble of factors secreted by tumors. These factors facilitate the growth of the tumor, either by inhibiting the host's capacity to reject the tumor, by stimulating tumor-cell division by increasing blood supply of the tumor, or by some other mechanism(s). Perhaps interferon might counteract some of the deleterious effects of these tumor-secreted substances. We may cite two examples to illustrate this point:

1. In mice inoculated with EA cells, many of the peritoneal macrophages were observed in mitosis, and others appeared poorly differentiated. Phagocytosis of tumor cells by macrophages was not observed (Gresser and Bourali, 1970*a*). [Chouroulinkov *et al.* (1971) subsequently found that EA cells liberated a factor or factors capable of stimulating mitosis of macrophages *in vitro*.] In interferon-treated mice, however, macrophages did not divide, they were well differentiated, and they phagocytosed tumor cells (Gresser and Bourali, 1970*a*).
2. Kassel *et al.* (1973) suggested that the antitumor effect of interferon was mediated through restoration of a deficient complement level in AKR leukemic mice. According to these investigators, C5 is the antileukemic complement component in normal serum.

c. Pure Speculation. It is becoming clear that the histocompatibility complex is in reality a functional unit comprising several genes that are important in the defense of the organism not only against foreign agents (i.e., viruses, parasites), but also in the recognition and maintenance of "self." As mentioned briefly above (Section 6.2.2), it was found that thymocytes and splenic lymphocytes from interferon-treated mice exhibit an enhanced expression of surface H-2 antigens (Lindahl *et al.*, 1976). Recent experiments suggest that interferon also enhances the expression of H-2 antigens on normal nonlymphoid cells (Gresser and Vignaux, unpublished results). It seems to us entirely conceivable that there are cellular antitumor mechanisms within tissues that are not at all mediated by lymphocytes and macrophages—that all cells have an inherent capacity to distinguish "like from unlike," and that this system of recognition serves to prevent implantation of tumor cells (metastases) and to localize metastatic foci when they do occur. Although there are no other data on the effect of interferon on the expression of surface antigens other than on H-2 and on θ (which was not affected; Lindahl *et al.*, 1974), it may be that by enhancing the expression of certain surface antigens, interferon enhances the inherent capacity of cells in an organ such as the spleen or liver to recognize and reject tumor cells that probably have distinguishable "new" surface antigens.

6.3. Spontaneous Neoplasms

In the example cited in Section 2.1.2, interferon increased the survival (approximately 100%) in AKR mice *after* diagnosis of the lymphoma (Gresser *et al.*, 1976). Very few chemotherapeutic compounds, when used singly, prolong survival of

AKR mice by more than a few days after diagnosis of lymphoma (Skipper *et al.*, 1969, 1972; Frei *et al.*, 1974). The increased survival times of mice receiving potent interferon preparations indicated that interferon is a good anti-AKR-leukemic drug (Frei *et al.*, 1974). What is the mechanism of the antitumor effect of interferon treatment initiated so late in the course of this neoplastic disease?

Since the majority of AKR lymphoma cells multiply exponentially and have a short generation time (Metcalf and Wiadrowski, 1966), it is likely that a considerable tumor-cell loss accompanies this marked cellular proliferation. Thus, any decrease or delay in tumor cell proliferation and/or increase in tumor-cell death should be of some therapeutic benefit. Since the evidence indicates that interferon is not cytocidal, it seems likely that the therapeutic effects of interferon in AKR mice may be related to a direct inhibitory effect of interferon on the multiplication of the lymphoma cells themselves. Perhaps even a slight delay in the rate of tumor cell multiplication shifts the balance in favor of cell loss over cell proliferation. (As stated above, interferon may also inhibit tumor growth indirectly by acting on the host.) The role of the Gross virus at this terminal stage of the disease is unknown, but it seems less likely that the therapeutic effects of interferon at this stage are related to antiviral activity.

6.4. Summary

In summary, we believe that the effect of interferon in animals infected with some oncogenic viruses can be attributed to inhibition of viral replication or inhibition of the early events following viral infection. In those experimental systems in which continued administration of interferon proved effective *after* inoculation of oncogenic viruses, the effect may be due in part to an antiviral effect, and in part to a direct action of interferon on the multiplication of precursor cells or tumor cells themselves. In animals bearing autochthonous tumors or grafted with transplantable tumors, the effects appear to be due in part to a direct inhibition of the multiplication of the tumor cells, and in part to an effect on the host, the nature of which remains to be defined. We must learn more of the interaction of interferon with host cells and understand how so many apparently different effects are triggered by this "polypractic substance" (Gresser, 1975) before we can clarify the mechanism by which interferon can confer protection on animals infested with viruses, protozoa, or tumor cells.

7. Use of Exogenous Interferon and Interferon Inducers in the Treatment of Patients with Neoplastic Disease

7.1. Exogenous Interferon

7.1.1. Source of Interferon

The major obstacle in undertaking clinical trials with exogenous interferon has stemmed from the difficulty of providing large amounts of potent semipurified interferon and the cost involved (Hilleman, 1969, 1970a; Finter, 1970; Gresser, 1971). Suspensions of human leukocytes have provided a good and convenient source of human interferon (Gresser, 1961; Falcoff et al., 1966; Strander and Cantell, 1966, 1967; Cantell et al., 1968; Strander, 1971). For the routine large-scale production of interferon, however, it will probably prove necessary to use cells in culture—either normal diploid human embryonic fibroblasts (Havell and Vilcek, 1972) or a cell line such as a lymphoblastoid cell line (Strander et al., 1975; Tovey et al., 1974). The former has the advantage of being a "normal" cell, but the quantity of interferon obtained may well be limited for industrial-scale production, since these cells are cultivated in monolayer culture. Lymphoblastoid cells, however, can be cultivated in suspension cultures, and have been shown to produce reasonable quantities of interferon when the necessary technical conditions have been defined (Strander et al., 1975; Tovey et al., 1974; Sano et al., 1974). [At present, the best interferon-producing lymphoblastoid cell is one derived from a patient (Namalwa) with Burkitt's disease. About 10,000 U interferon are obtained from 10^7 cells infected with NDV or Sendaï viruses (Strander et al., 1975; Tovey et al., unpublished observations). It seems likely, however, that with further screening, a higher interferon-producing cell will be found.] These lymphoblastoid cells could be cultivated in fermenter tanks of 3000 liters, as currently used for the cultivation of BHK cells for the production of foot and mouth disease vaccines. Thus, the amount of interferon obtained would be limited only by the size and number of the tanks available. The disadvantage of this system stems from the use of a tumor-cell line for the production of interferon destined for use in patients. This objection may be less valid if the interferon were used in patients with malignancies or to treat life-threatening viral diseases (e.g., severe viral hepatitis, viral encephalitis, rabies, Lassa fever) for which there is no effective treatment. Increasing progress in the production of interferon, however, should render this objection more hypothetical than real, and it seems likely to us that purified human lymphoblastoid interferon might eventually be used in the treatment of common viral diseases (e.g., herpes keratitis).

For the present, the apparent species-specificity of interferon necessitates the use of human cells. Since a number of exceptions to the rule of species-specificity have been discovered in recent years (Desmyter et al., 1968; Levy-Koenig et al., 1970; Gresser et al., 1974b), it may be that future investigations will reveal a nonprimate source of interferon active on human cells. It should be emphasized that should interferon prove to be of clinical value, new methodology for its large-scale production and semipurification will certainly follow. One has only to recall that initially the cost and difficulties in the production of penicillin also seemed awesome.

7.1.2. Results of Exogenous Interferon Therapy

Despite the encouraging results from animal experiments, interferon therapy has not yet received a fair evaluation in man. The majority of workers in universities or in industry have until quite recently remained skeptical as to the usefulness of exogenous interferon. Falcoff *et al.* (1966) administered human leukocyte interferon of relatively low titer (1.5×10^3 U/ml) to 18 patients with acute leukemia for prolonged periods of time. The treatment was reported as being well tolerated, and the general impression as to the therapeutic results was favorable. "The average survival appeared increased, although no final conclusion can be drawn at present" (Falcoff *et al.*, 1966). That any interferon has become available at all for clinical trials has been in large part due to the persistent and patient efforts of Cantell and his associates in Helsinki during the past 10 years, and their generous collaboration with investigators in Sweden, Great Britain, and the United States. The production of human leukocyte interferon has been expanded in Finland during recent years, and 5.0×10^{10} units were prepared in 1974 (Cantell, 1975).

Strander and his colleagues at the Karolinska Institute in Stockholm have administered human leukocyte interferon (Strander and Cantell, 1966, 1967; Cantell *et al.*, 1968; Strander, 1971; Cantell, 1970), prepared by Cantell, to patients with a variety of malignancies. Repeated injections of the earlier crude interferon preparations (C-IF) ($1–3 \times 10^6$ U i.m. 3 times weekly) was well tolerated, although some minor reactions (i.e., fever) were observed shortly after initiation of treatment (Strander *et al.*, 1973a,b; Cantell, 1975; Strander and Cantell, 1974). A more purified leukocyte interferon preparation (P-IF) has recently been developed (Cantell, 1975), and unpleasant side effects are usually not encountered (Strander *et al.*, 1976a). No serious toxic effects have been noted. In some instances, the individual dose of interferon injected has been 2×10^7 U (Cantell, 1975). Although interferon is rapidly cleared from the circulation in man and animals (Subrahmanyan and Mims, 1966; Baron *et al.*, 1966; Ho and Postic, 1967a; Gresser *et al.*, 1967b; Pyhälä and Cantell, 1974), intramuscular injection of 2×10^5 U C-IF or P-IF/kg body weight maintained a level of 10^2 U/ml plasma for about 12 hr (Cantell *et al.*, 1974). A plateau of interferon in the CSF of monkeys ($\frac{1}{30}$ the plasma level) was also obtained after intramuscular injection (Habif *et al.*, 1975). It is not known whether therapeutic effects are related to maintenance of blood levels of interferon. In fact, the results of some studies of Gresser *et al.* (1969d) on the effect of exogenous interferon on encephalomyocarditis viral infection in mice suggested that a high concentration of interferon, if only for a short time, might be more important than sustained levels of interferon at a low concentration. On the other hand, it may be that maintenance of a blood level is important in the treatment of patients with malignancy.

Since 1972, Strander and his co-workers have directed most of their efforts to the treatment of patients with osteosarcoma. They chose this malignancy for the following reasons: (1) The prognosis of this disease was poor. Until the recent introduction of adriamycin (Cortes *et al.*, 1972) and high doses of methotrexate with citrovorum rescue (Djerassi *et al.*, 1970, 1972; Jaffe *et al.*, 1974; Frei *et al.*, 1975), therapy consisted of primary amputation, or preoperative irradiation followed usually 6 months later by amputation (Lee and MacKenzie, 1964). Pulmonary metastases occurred in approximately 50% of patients by 6 months, and only 20% of patients were alive 2 years after diagnosis. (2) Since statistics of survival did not appear to differ significantly from one country to another, they could treat a few patients intensively with interferon and compare their results with historical control groups (Swedish, American, or English all being essentially the same) (Frei *et al.*, 1975). (3) There was some indication at the time the studies were undertaken that a virus might be important in the genesis of osteosarcoma in man (Cohen *et al.*, 1972; Finkel *et al.*, 1975). (4) Interferon had been shown to inhibit the multiplication of tumor cells *in vitro* (Gresser *et al.*, 1970*b*,*c*). In the course of the clinical trials, it was found that human leukocyte interferon also inhibited *in vitro* the multiplication of cells of some cell lines derived from osteosarcomatous tissue (Strander and Cantell, 1974).

Patients with osteosarcoma of the long bones without detectable metastases on admission to the Karolinska Hospital were selected for treatment with leukocyte interferon (Strander *et al.*, 1976*a*). Local resection of the primary tumor, rather than amputation of a limb, was done whenever possible (Strander *et al.*, 1976*a*). Patients received $2-3 \times 10^6$ U C-IF or P-IF (when available) 3 times a week for $1\frac{1}{2}$ years. Although the number of treated patients is still small, the preliminary results are most encouraging. As can be seen in Table 5, there appears to be a significant delay in the appearance of pulmonary metastases and an increased survival in patients receiving leukocyte interferon compared with historical control patients.

Although Strander and his co-workers believe that some failures of interferon therapy may have been due to a large tumor burden (Strander *et al.*, 1976*a*) (this is in agreement with studies in mice), they did undertake interferon treatment in a

TABLE 5

Patients with Osteosarcoma Treated with Human Leukocyte Interferon at the Radiumhemmet, Karolinska Hospital[a,b]

Observation period (years)	Historical control (Karolinska Hospital)		Interferon-treated	
	Pulmonary metastases[c]	Deaths	Pulmonary metastases[c]	Deaths
$\frac{1}{2}$	15/33	6/33	1/12	0/12
	(45%)	(18%)	(9%)	(0%)
1	28/33	15/33	3/11	1/11[d]
	(84%)	(45%)	(27%)	(9%)
$1\frac{1}{2}$	29/33	23/33	4/10	2/10
	(87%)	(69%)	(40%)	(20%)
2	29/33	27/33	4/7	1/7
	(87%)	(81%)	(57%)	(14%)
$2\frac{1}{2}$	29/33	28/33	3/5	1/5
	(87%)	(84%)	(60%)	(20%)
3	29/33	28/33	3/4	1/4
	(87%)	(84%)	(75%)	(25%)

[a] Results of Dr. Hans Strander and co-workers as of January 1976.
[b] The diagnosis of osteosarcoma of the long bones in these patients was established by histological examination of a tumor biopsy, and the diagnosis was confirmed by independent examination of the histological sections by several pathologists.
[c] Based on X ray.
[d] This patient died in an accident.

patient with advanced Hodgkin's disease (lymphocyte predominance, Stage IV B) (Blomgren *et al.*, 1976). The patient received 5×10^6 U P-IF i.m. daily. After 2–3 weeks of treatment, "B symptoms disappeared, diseased nodes and pulmonary infiltrations decreased in size and laboratory values normalized." After $1\frac{1}{2}$ months of treatment, "the rate of improvement slowed down, and a stationary phase of about 4 months was followed by clinical progression of the disease" despite continued interferon treatment (Blomgren *et al.*, 1976). Strander and his co-workers also recently observed partial remission in a patient with multiple myeloma. A decrease was noted in the number of myeloma cells and γ-globulin produced, with a return toward normal hemoglobin levels (Strander *et al.*, unpublished observations).

7.1.3. *Effect of Exogenous Interferon Therapy on Viral Infections in Patients with Malignancy*

It is of considerable interest that Strander and his colleagues observed a decreased incidence of viral infections among patients treated with leukocyte interferon, since patients with malignancy and those treated with many chemotherapeutic drugs are very susceptible to common viral infections, which can often prove lethal. "It is remarkable that no virus disease has ever developed during the interferon treatment in any of the patients at the Karolinska Sjukhuset—33 patients in all—although some of them have received interferon for almost 2 years. The patients all have malignant diseases which are known to predispose to infections. Five adults with herpes zoster [3 disseminated and 2 localized] re-covered quickly upon administration of interferon . . . the clinical and laboratory observations collected previously and in this report suggest that viral infections can be controlled in leukaemic children by intramuscular injections of human leukocyte interferon" (Ahström *et al.*, 1974).

Similarly, in an epidemiologic study, Strander and his co-workers compared the incidence of acute (presumably viral) infections in 8 patients with osteosarcoma treated with interferon with the incidence among their family members. Their results suggested that the former group was less severely ill than their nontreated, otherwise healthy family contacts (Strander *et al.*, 1976b).

Merigan and his associates investigated the effect of human leukocyte inter-feron on varicella–zoster infections in a randomized double-blind series involving over 85 patients with malignancy (Jordan *et al.*, 1974; Merigan *et al.*, 1976). A total of 17 patients with varicella were treated shortly after onset of rash. Interferon treatment exerted only a slight effect on skin lesions and visceral involvement. Patients with herpes zoster had a 5-fold lesser frequency of visceral complications compared with placebo-treated subjects.

Emödi *et al.* (1975) reported that interferon treatment of patients with herpes zoster (6 of 37 patients had a malignancy) resulted in a decrease in pain and a rapid clearing of skin lesions. These findings are also in accord with the observations of Strander's group, who reported rapid recovery in several patients with localized zoster (Strander and Cantell, 1974).

The use of viruses for the treatment of neoplasia presents a number of disadvantages and has met with little success (Southam, 1960; Southam and Moore, 1952). Wheelock and Dingle (1964) reported an unexpectedly prolonged course in a patient with acute myelogenous leukemia inoculated with different myxoviruses and two arboviruses (chosen for their interferon-inducing capacity). Although the patient eventually succumbed, transient clinical improvement occurred after each injection (with the exception of Sindbis virus).

In view of the recent findings that different bacteria and bacterial products induce the production of interferon, it might be interesting for historical reasons to know whether Coley's "toxines" induce interferon. In 1894, Coley (1894) stated:

> The curative action of erysipelas upon malignant tumors is an established fact. This action is much more powerful in sarcoma than carcinoma. This action is chiefly due to the soluble toxines of the erysipelas streptococcus, which may be isolated and used with safety and accuracy. This action is greatly increased by the addition of the toxines of bacillus prodigiosus.

Although the use of Coley's toxines was eventually abandoned, the use of bacteria or bacterial products in the treatment of neoplasia has recently reemerged in the form of BCG (Mathé, 1971). It seems unlikely to us, however, that the antitumor effects of BCG and bacterial products are mediated by interferon. BCG can protect experimental animals even when inoculated weeks or months *prior to* tumor challenge (at a time when any effect of interferon would probably have waned) (Old *et al.*, 1963). The mechanism by which BCG exerts antitumor effects is of considerable practical and theoretical importance, since it also induces strong antiviral (Old *et al.*, 1963) and antiprotozoal effects (Clarke *et al.*, 1976) in experimental animals.

Polyanions have also been utilized in chemotherapy, but in many instances; toxicity (Regelson, 1968) has precluded their usefulness. For example, pyran copolymer was used in Phase 1 studies in 67 patients with advanced cancer, and toxic effects included thrombocytopenia, pyrexia, and hypotension (Regelson, 1973). Attempts are being made to develop nontoxic pyran copolymers that exert antitumor activity and are devoid of toxicity (Morahan *et al.*, 1974; Breslow *et al.*, 1973). It seems unlikely, however, that the antitumor effects of pyran copolymers are related to their interferon-inducing capacity (for references, see Regelson *et al.*, 1973).

Despite the initial hopes of using poly-I.C as an antitumor agent in patients (Mathé *et al.*, 1970; DeVita *et al.*, 1970; Young, 1971), the results have proved discouraging (DeVita *et al.*, 1970; H. B. Levy *et al.*, 1975). Nordlund *et al.* (1970) found that a nuclease in human serum hydrolyzed poly-I.C, perhaps accounting for the low levels of interferon induced in man by this synthetic nucleotide (Levy *et al.*, 1975). Levy and his co-workers prepared a complex of poly-I.C with poly-L-lysine and carboxymethyl cellulose, which has proved to be 5–10 times more resistant to hydrolysis by primate serum than uncomplexed poly-I.C (Levy *et al.*,

1975). This compound does induce interferon in subhuman primates (Levy *et al.*, 1975) and man (Levy *et al.*, unpublished observations), and its efficacy as an antitumor drug will soon be evaluated in patients (Robinson *et al.*, 1976).

7.3. Possibilities for Combined Exogenous–Endogenous Interferon Therapy

Although the relative advantages and disadvantages of exogenous vs. endogenous interferon therapy have been amply discussed, there are very few experiments comparing the relative efficacy of each (Gresser *et al.*, 1969*d*; Gresser and Bourali, 1969; Rhim and Huebner, 1971). Perhaps there will be a place for combined therapy, and at least one study in animals has suggested the usefulness of combined exogenous and endogenous therapy (Gresser *et al.*, 1969*d*).

The efficacy of many antitumor chemotherapeutic substances is enhanced when they are used in combination therapy, rather than alone. It would seem worthwhile to determine the value of combining some form of interferon therapy with standard antitumor drugs (see Section 3.1 and Chirigos and Pearson, 1973), provided of course the latter do not block interferon action (St. Geme *et al.*, 1969).

8. Speculations on the Usefulness of Exogenous Interferon in the Treatment of Patients with Malignancy

8.1. As an Antitumor Drug

As we have shown in this chapter, a considerable body of experimental data indicates that interferon does exert antitumor effects in experimental animals. It seems clear that when sufficient interferon is administered, it is effective in delaying the evolution of a neoplastic disease. In virtually all instances, however, complete regression of a well-established tumor mass has not been observed, and the animal is not cured by the interferon preparations currently available. There is no evidence to indicate that interferon is selective in inhibiting tumor growth, but it can slow tumor growth at interferon doses that do not appear injurious to the host. On the basis of the results of animal studies to date, therefore, it seems unlikely to us that interferon will prove to be a "miracle" drug for the treatment of cancer. It should be emphasized, however, that no toxicity has been encountered in adult mice inoculated with as much as 10^6 U interferon daily, and it is possible that more pronounced antitumor effects will be obtained by increasing this dose by a factor of 10 or 100. Furthermore, predictions of the therapeutic value of a drug based on animal systems can be hazardous. Most of the experimental systems used are ones in which a grafted tumor or an autochthonous tumor grows rapidly and death follows quickly and inexorably. In patients, the odds are not so overwhelmingly in favor of the cancer. Therapy is designed toward reduction of tumor mass, since elimination of every tumor cell is virtually impossible. Thus, an equilibrium appears to exist in patients between host defenses and tumor growth—an equilibrium that is less evident in animal systems, in which only a few tumor cells can prove lethal. If we are correct in suggesting that interferon can exert effects on normal cell division and host-cell function, interferon may prove to be of greater value in the treatment of patients with malignancy than the results of animal experimentation suggest.

The clinical studies of Strander, Cantell, and their co-workers in the treatment of patients with osteosarcoma support this optimistic view. The results of animal experimentation might not have led one to predict such success in the treatment of a solid metastasizing tumor, and yet their preliminary results are clearly significant (see Table 5). They have observed regression of tumor in a patient with Hodgkin's disease (Strander *et al.*, 1976*b*) and in a patient with multiple myeloma (Strander *et al.*, unpublished observations). It is thus impossible to predict which malignancies may prove amenable to interferon treatment. It will be necessary to try (beginning perhaps with those tumors for which current therapy is of little or no avail) to determine the efficacy of interferon alone or in combination with antitumor drugs.

8.2. As an Antiviral Drug

Although this chapter has been concerned entirely with the antitumor effects of interferon and its biological effects other than antiviral effects, interferon is still the most effective broad-spectrum antiviral substance known. Interferon inhibits the replication of both RNA- and DNA-containing viruses in cell culture, and it protects experimental animals against viruses inducing either a localized or systemic infection. Despite the prediction of numerous investigators over the years that exogenous interferon would not be of any therapeutic value in treating virus-infected animals (Hilleman, 1963, 1965, 1968, 1969; Wagner, 1965; Merigan, 1967; Lampson *et al.*, 1967; Lockart, 1967; Ho and Postic, 1967*b*), the results clearly demonstrate that it *is* effective, even when small doses of interferon are administered (Gresser, 1971).

It seems to us very likely that interferon will prove to be of considerable value in preventing and treating the often severe viral infections that occur in patients with malignancy, and in patients treated with cytotoxic–immunosuppressive drugs. Again, the preliminary studies of Strander, Cantell, and their associates referred to in Section 7.1.3 indicate the potential usefulness of interferon as an antiviral drug in these patients.

8.3. Other Uses

In the discussion of the mechanism of the antitumor effects of interferon, we have touched on a number of the effects of interferon on cell division and cell function. It is evident that interferon can exert different effects on the immune system. The possibility exists that interferon might be useful in inhibiting or enhancing the immunologic reactivity of patients.

Lastly, it seems only fitting to emphasize how little we know of the mode of action of interferon or other physiological substances similar to interferon, and that interferon may have uses still not dreamed of in our philosophy.

ACKNOWLEDGMENTS

I gratefully acknowledge the excellent assistance of Mrs. F. Zambetti in the preparation of this manuscript for publication.

I am deeply grateful for the many kindnesses shown to me over the years by Drs. John F. Enders, Lewis Thomas, and the late Sidney Farber. I dedicate this chapter to them and to the late Dr. Francisco Duran-Reynals.

9. References

ABSHER, M., AND STINEBRING, W. R., 1969, Endotoxin-like properties of poly I. poly C, an interferon stimulator, *Nature (London)* **223**:715.

ADAMS, A., STRANDER, H., AND CANTELL, K., 1975, Sensitivity of the Epstein–Barr virus transformed human lymphoid cell lines to interferon, *J. Gen. Virol.* **28**:207.

ADAMSON, R. H., 1971a, Antitumor activity of tilorone hydrochloride against some rodent tumors: Preliminary report, *J. Natl. Cancer Inst.* **46**:431.

ADAMSON, R. H., 1971b, Antitumour activity of two antiviral drugs—rifampicin and tilorone, *Lancet* **1**:398.

ADAMSON, R. H., AND TING, R. C., 1971, The antitumor activity of the interferon inducer tilorone hydrochloride, *Bacteriol. Proc.*, p. 196.

ADAMSON, R. H., FABRO, S., HOMAN, E. R., O'GARA, R. W., AND ZENDZIAN, R. P., 1969, Pharmacology of polyriboinosinic:polyribocytidylic acid, a new antiviral and antitumor agent, in: *Antimicrobiol Agents and Chemotherapy*, p. 148, *American Society of Microbiology*, 1970, Bethesda, Maryland.

AHSTRÖM, L., DOHLWITZ, A., STRANDER, H., CARLSTRÖM, G., AND CANTELL, K., 1974, Interferon in acute leukaemia in children, *Lancet* **1**:166.

ARMSTRONG, M. Y. K., BLACK, F. L., AND RICHARDS, F. F., 1972, Tumour induction by cell-free extracts derived from mice with graft-versus-host disease, *Nature (London) New Biol.* **235**:153.

ATANASIU, P., AND CHANY, C., 1960, Action d'un interféron provenant de cellules malignes sur l'infection expérimentale du hamster nouveau-né par le virus du polyome, *C. R. Acad. Sci. Paris* **251**:1687.

BALL, J. K., AND MCCARTER, J. A., 1971, Effect of polyinosinic–polycytidylic acid on induction of primary or transplanted tumors by chemical carcinogen or irradiation, *J. Natl. Cancer Inst.* **46**:1009.

BANKS, G. T., BUCK, K. W., CHAIN, E. B., HIMMELWEIT, F., MARKS, J. E., TYLER, J. M., HOLLINGS, M., LAST, F. T., AND STONE, O. M., 1968, Viruses in fungi and interferon stimulation, *Nature (London)* **218**:542.

BARKER, A. D., RHEIMS, M. S., AND WILSON, H. E., 1971a, Tilorone hydrochloride: Its effect on Friend virus leukemia in mice, *Bacteriol. Proc.*, p. 188.

BARKER, A. D., RHEINS, M. S., AND WILSON, H. E., 1971b, Amelioration of Friend virus leukemia by sequential administration of viral and nonviral interferon inducers, *Proc. Soc. Exp. Biol. Med.* **137**:981.

BARON, S., BUCKLER, C. E., MCCLOSKEY, R. V., AND KIRSCHSTEIN, R. L., 1966, Role of interferon during viremia, I. Production of circulating interferon, *J. Immunol.* **96**:12.

BARON, S., DUBUY, H., BUCKLER, C. E., JOHNSON, M. L., PARK, J., BILLIAU, A., SARMA, P., AND HUEBNER, R. J., 1970, Induction of interferon and viral resistance in animals by polynucleotides, *Ann. N. Y. Acad. Sci.* **173:**568.

BARSKI, G., 1963, Interférence entre les virus d'herpès et de polyome chez le hamster adulte *in vivo, C. R. Acad. Sci. Paris* **256:**5459.

BARSKI, G., AND YOUN, J. K., 1964, Interférence entre la chorioméningite lymphocytaire et la leucémie de souris de Rauscher, *C. R. Acad. Sci. Paris* **259:**4191.

BARSKI, G., AND YOUN, J. K., 1971, Protection of mice against Gross leukemia by interfering action of nonleukemogenic C-type murine viruses inoculated into newborns, *J. Natl. Cancer Inst.* **47:**575.

BART, R. S., AND KOPF, A. W., 1969, Inhibition of the growth of murine malignant melanoma with synthetic double-stranded ribonucleic acid, *Nature (London)* **224:**372.

BART, R. S., KOPF, A. W., AND SILAGI, S., 1971, Inhibition of the growth of murine malignant melanoma by polyinosinic–polycytidylic acid, *J. Invest. Dermatol.* **56:**33.

BART, R. S., KOPF, A. W., VILCEK, J. T., AND LAM, S., 1973, Role of interferon in the anti-melanoma effects of poly (I).poly (C) and Newcastle disease virus, *Nature (London) New Biol.* **245:**229.

BART, R. S., LAM, S., COOPER, J. S., AND KOPF, A. W., 1975, Retention of anti-melanoma effect of polyinosinic–polycytidylic acid in neonatally thymectomized, irradiated, leukopenic mice, *J. Invest. Dermatol.* **65:**285.

BASERGA, R., AND KISIELESKI, W. E., 1961, Cell proliferation in tumor-bearing mice, *Arch. Pathol.* **72:**142.

BEKESI, J. G., AND HOLLAND, J. F., 1973, Combined chemotherapy and immunotherapy of transplantable and spontaneous murine leukemia in DBA/2 and AKR mice, in: *Investigation and Stimulation of Immunity in Cancer Patients* (G. Mathé and R. Weiner, eds), Vol. 1, Editions du Centre National la Recherche Scientifique, Paris, and Springer-Verlag, Heidelberg.

BEKESI, J. G., ROBOZ, J. P., ZIMMERMAN, E., AND HOLLAND, J. F., 1976, Treatment of spontaneous leukemia in AKR mice with chemotherapy, immunotherapy, or interferon, *Cancer Res.* **36:**631.

BERMAN, L. D., 1970, Inhibition of oncogenicity of murine sarcoma virus (Harvey) in mice by interferon, *Nature (London)* **227:**1349.

BILLIAU, A., LEYTEN, R., VANDEPUTTE, M., AND DE SOMER, P., 1971, Inhibition of development of mammary tumors in C3H mice by neonatal administration of polycarboxylate, *Life Sci.* **10:**643.

BLOMGREN, H., STRANDER, H., AND CANTELL, K., 1974, Effect of human leukocyte interferon on the response of lymphocytes to mitogenic stimuli *in vitro, Scand. J. Immunol.* **3:**697.

BLOMGREN, H., CANTELL, K., JOHANSSON, B., LAGERGREN, C., RINGBORG, U., AND STRANDER, H., 1976, Interferon therapy in Hodgkin's disease—a case report, *Acta Med. Scand.* **199:**527.

BRAUN, W., AND LEVY, H. B., 1972, Interferon preparations as modifiers of immune responses, *Proc. Soc. Exp. Biol. Med.* **141:**769.

BRESLOW, D. S., EDWARDS, E. I., AND NEWBERG, N. R., 1973, Divinyl ether–maleic anhydride (pyran) copolymer: The effect of molecular weight on biological activity, *Nature (London) New Biol.* **246:**160.

BRODEUR, B. R., AND MERIGAN, T. C., 1974, Suppressive effect of interferon on the humoral immune response to sheep red blood cells in mice, *J. Immunol.* **113:**1319.

CAME, P. E., AND MOORE, D. H., 1971, Inhibition of spontaneous mammary carcinoma of mice by treatment with interferon and poly I:C, *Proc. Soc. Exp. Biol. Med.* **137:**304.

CAME, P. E., AND MOORE, D. H., 1972, Effect of exogenous interferon treatment on mouse mammary tumors, *J. Natl. Cancer Inst.* **48:**1151.

CANTELL, K., 1970, Preparation of human leukocyte interferon, in: *Symposia Series on Immunobiological Standardization*, Vol. 14, No. 6, Karger, Basel and New York.

CANTELL, K., 1975, Towards clinical use of interferon, *Proc. Gen. Assembly Jpn. Med. Soc.*, Kyoto, **18:**614.

CANTELL, K., STRANDER, H., HADHAZY, G., AND NEVANLINNA, H. R., 1968, How much interferon can be prepared in human leukocyte suspensions?, in: *The Interferons* (G. Rita, ed.), p. 223, Academic Press, New York and London.

CANTELL, K., PYHÄLÄ, L., AND STRANDER, H., 1974, Circulating human interferon after intramuscular injection into animals and man, *J. Gen. Virol.* **22:**453.

CEGLOWSKI, W. S., AND FRIEDMAN, H., 1968, Immunosuppression by leukemia viruses. I. Effect of Friend disease virus on cellular and humoral hemolysin responses of mice to a primary immunization with sheep erythrocytes, *J. Immunol.* **101:**594.

CEROTTINI, J. C., BRUNNER, K. T., LINDAHL, P., AND GRESSER, I., 1973, Inhibitory effect of interferon preparations and inducers on the multiplication of transplanted allogeneic spleen cells and syngeneic bone marrow cells, *Nature (London) New Biol.* **242:**152.

CHANY, C., AND ROBBE-MARIDOR, F., 1969, Enhancing effect of the murine sarcoma virus (MSV) on the replication of the mouse hepatitis virus (MHV) *in vitro*, *Proc. Soc. Exp. Biol. Med.* **131**:30.

CHERNYAKHOVSKAYA, I. Y., SLAVINA, E. G., SVET-MOLDAVSKY, G. J., 1970, Antitumor effect of lymphoid cells activated by interferon, *Nature (London)* **228**:71.

CHESTER, T. J., PAUCKER, K., AND MERIGAN, T. C., 1973, Suppression of mouse antibody producing spleen cells by various interferon preparations, *Nature (London)* **246**:92.

CHIRIGOS, M. A., AND PEARSON, J. W., 1973, Cure of murine leukemia with drug and interferon treatment, *J. Natl. Cancer Inst.* **51**:1367.

CHIRIGOS, M. A., TURNER, W., PEARSON, J., AND GRIFFIN, W., 1969, Effective antiviral therapy of two murine leukemias with an interferon-inducing synthetic carboxylate copolymer, *Int. J. Cancer* **4**:267.

CHOUROULINKOV, I., GUILLON, J. C., LASNE, C., AND GENTIL, A., 1971, Images de division observées sur des marcrophages de la cavité péritonéale de souris en culture *in vitro*, *C. R. Acad. Sci. Paris* **272**:2013.

CLAES, P., BILLIAU, A., DE CLERCQ, E., DESMYTER, J., SCHONNE, E., VANDERHAEGHE, H., AND DE SOMER, P., 1970, Polyacetal carboxylic acids: A new group of antiviral polyanions, *J. Virol.* **5**:313.

CLARK, I. A., ALLISON, A. C., AND COX, F. E., 1976, Protection of mice against *Babesia* and *Plasmodium* with B.C.G., *Nature (London)* **259**:309.

COHEN, A. M., KETCHAM, A. S., AND MORTON, D. L., 1972, Cellular immunity to a common human sarcoma antigen and its specific inhibition by sera from patients with growing sarcomas, *Surgery* **72**:560.

COLEY, W. B., 1894, Treatment of inoperable malignant tumors with the toxines of erysipelas and the *Bacillus prodigiosus*, *Trans. Amer. Surg. Assoc.* **12**:183.

CORAGGIO, F., COTO, V., FANTONI, V., GALEOTA, C. A., AND LAVEGAS, E., 1965, Azione di un interferon, proveniente de culture *in vitro* di cellule embrionali di topo infettate col virus del polioma, su un tumore trapiantabile nel topo (ceppo C 57), *Boll. Ist. Sieroter. Milan.* **44**:64.

CORTES, E. P., HOLLAND, J. F., WANG, J. J., AND SINKS, L. F., 1972, Doxorubicin in disseminated osteosarcoma, *J. Amer. Med. Assoc.* **221**:1132.

DE CLERCQ, E., AND DE SOMER, P., 1971, Role of interferon in the protective effect of the double-stranded polyribonucleotide against murine tumors induced by Moloney sarcoma virus, *J. Natl. Cancer Inst.* **47**:1345.

DE CLERCQ, E., AND DE SOMER, P., 1972, Effect of chlorite-oxidized oxyamylose on Moloney sarcoma virus-induced tumor formation in mice, *Eur. J. Cancer* **8**:535.

DE CLERCQ, E., AND MERIGAN, T. C., 1970, Induction of interferon by nonviral agents, *Arch. Intern. Med.* **126**:94.

DE CLERCQ, E., AND MERIGAN, T. C., 1971, Moloney sarcoma virus-induced tumors in mice: Inhibition or stimulation by (poly-I).(poly-C), *Proc. Soc. Exp. Biol. Med.* **137**:590.

DE CLERCQ, E., AND STEWART, W. E., II, 1974, Regression of autochthonous Moloney sarcoma virus-induced tumors in mice treated with polyriboinosinic–polyribocytidylic acid, *J. Natl. Cancer Inst.* **52**:591.

DE MAEYER, E., MOBRAATEN, L., AND DE MAEYER-GUIGNARD, J., 1973, Prolongation par l'interféron de la survie des greffes de peau chez la souris, *C. R. Acad. Sci. Paris* **277**:2101.

DE MAEYER, E., DE MAEYER-GUIGNARD, J., AND VANDEPUTTE, M., 1975, Inhibition by interferon of delayed-type hypersensitivity in the mouse, *Proc. Natl. Acad. Sci. U.S.A.* **72**:1753.

DE MAEYER-GUIGNARD, J., CACHARD, A., AND DE MAEYER, E., 1975, Delayed-type hypersensitivity to sheep red blood cells: Inhibition of sensitization by interferon, *Science* **190**:574.

DESMYTER, J., RAWLS, W. E., AND MELNICK, J. L., 1968, A human interferon that crosses the species line, *Proc. Natl. Acad.Sci. U.S.A.* **59**:69.

DEVITA, V., CANELLOS, G., CARBONE, P., BARON, S., LEVY, H., AND GRALNICK, H., 1970, Clinical trials with the interferon (InF) inducer polyinosinic–cytidilic acid (PIC), *Amer. Assoc.Cancer Res.* **11**:21.

DJERASSI, I., ROMINGER, C. J., KIM, J., TURCHI, J., AND MEYER, E., 1970, Methotrexate-citrovorum in patients with lung cancer, *Proc. Amer. Soc. Cancer Res.* **11**:21.

DJERASSI, I., ROMINGER, C. J., KIM, J. S., TURCHI, J., SUVANSRI, U., AND HUGHES, D., 1972, Phase I study of high doses of methotrexate with citrovorum factor in patients with lung cancer, *Cancer* **30**:22.

ELGJO, K., AND DEGRÉ, M., 1973, Polyinosinic–polycytidylic acid in two-stage skin carcinogenesis. Effect on epidermal growth parameters and interferon induction in treated mice, *J. Natl. Cancer Inst.* **51**:171.

EMÖDI, G., RUFLI, T., JUST, M., AND HERNANDEZ, R., 1975, Human interferon therapy for herpes zoster in adults, *Scand. J. Infect. Dis.* **7**:1.

FALCOFF, E., FALCOFF, R., FOURNIER, F., AND CHANY, C., 1966, Production en masse, purification partielle et caracterisation d'un interféron destiné à des essais thérapeutiques humains, *Ann. Inst. Pasteur* **11**:562.

FAUVE, R. M., HEVIN, B., JACOB, H., GAILLARD, J. A., AND JACOB, F., 1974, Antiinflammatory effects of murine malignant cells, *Proc. Natl. Acad. Sci. U.S.A.* **71**:4052.

FERRIS, P., PADNOS, M., AND MOLOMUT, N., 1971, Tumor inhibition in mice by M-P virus-induced interferon, *Fed. Proc. Fed. Amer. Soc. Exp. Biol.* **30**:241.

FIELD, A. K., TYTELL, A. A., LAMPSON, G. P., AND HILLEMAN, M. R., 1967, Inducers of interferon and host resistance. II. Multistranded synthetic polynucleotide complexes, *Proc. Natl. Acad. Sci. U.S.A.* **58**:1004.

FINKEL, M. P., REILLY, C. A., JR., AND BISKIS, B. O., 1975, Viral etiology of bone cancer, *Front. Radiat. Ther. Oncol.* **10**:28.

FINTER, N. B., 1970, Exogenous interferon in animals and its clinical implications, *Arch. Intern. Med.* **126**:147.

FISHER, J. C., COOPERBAND, S. R., AND MANNICK, J. A., 1972, The effect of polyinosinic–polycytidylic acid on the immune response of mice to antigenically distinct tumors, *Cancer Res.* **32**:889.

FOLKMAN, J., MERLER, E., ABERNATHY, C., AND WILLIAMS, G., 1971, Isolation of a tumor factor responsible for angiogenesis, *J. Exp. Med.* **133**:275.

FONTAINE-BROUTY-BOYÉ, D., GRESSER, I., MACIEIRA-COELHO, A., ROSENFELD, C., AND THOMAS, M. T., 1969, Cancérologie—Inhibition *in vitro* de la multiplication des cellules leucémiques murines L1210 par des préparations d'interféron, *C. R. Acad. Sci. Paris* **269**:406.

FRAYSSINET, C., GRESSER, I., TOVEY, M., AND LINDAHL, P., 1973, Inhibitory effect of potent interferon preparations on the regeneration of mouse liver after partial hepatectomy, *Nature (London)* **245**:146.

FREDRICKSON, T., TAMBOURIN, P., WENDLIN, F., JASMIN, C., AND SMAJDA, F., 1975, Target cell of the polycythemia-inducing Friend virus: Studies with myleran, *J. Natl. Cancer Inst.* **55**:443.

FREI, E., III, SCHABEL, F. M., AND GOLDIN, A., 1974, Comparative chemotherapy of AKR lymphoma and human hematological neoplasia, *Cancer Res.* **34**:184.

FREI, E., III, JAFFE, N., TATTERSALL, M. H. N., PITMAN, S., AND PARKER, L., 1975, New approaches to cancer chemotherapy with methotrexate, *N. Engl. J. Med.* **292**:846.

FRIEDMAN, R. M., 1966, Effect of interferon treatment on interferon production, *J. Immunol.* **96**:872.

FROST, P., AND LANCE, E. M., 1973, Abrogation of lymphocyte trapping by ascitic tumours, *Nature (London)* **246**:101.

GAFFNEY, E. V., PICCIANO, P. T., AND GRANT, C. A., 1973, Inhibition of growth and transformation of human cells by interferon, *J. Natl. Cancer Inst.* **50**:871.

GAZDAR, A. F., AND IKAWA, Y., 1972, Synthetic RNA and DNA polynucleotides: *In vivo* and *in vitro* enhancement of oncogenesis by a murine sarcoma virus, *Proc. Soc. Exp. Biol. Med.* **140**:1166.

GAZDAR, A. F., STEINBERG, A. D., SPAHN, G. F., AND BARON, S., 1972, Interferon inducers: Enhancement of viral oncogenesis in mice and rats, *Proc. Soc. Exp. Biol. Med.* **139**:1132.

GELBOIN, H. V., AND LEVY, H. B., 1970, Polyinosinic–polycytidylic acid inhibits chemically induced tumorigenesis in mouse skin, *Science* **167**:205.

GERICKE, D., KORNHUBER, B. C. G., AND CHANDRA, P., 1973, Immunosuppressive activity of a heat-stable factor associated with interferon, *Naturwissenschaften* **10**:482.

GISLER, R. H., LINDAHL, P., AND GRESSER, I., 1974, Effects of interferon on antibody synthesis *in vitro*, *J. Immunol.* **113**:438.

GLASGOW, L. A., AND FRIEDMAN, S. B., 1969, Interferon and host resistance to Rauscher virus-induced leukemia, *J. Virol.* **3**:99.

GLAZ, E. T., 1972, Study on the effect of statolon on methylcholanthrene oncogenesis in mice, *Tumori* **58**:185.

GRÄFF, S., KASSEL, R., AND KASTNER, O., 1970, Interferon, *Trans. N. Y. Acad. Sci.* **32**:545.

GRESSER, I., 1961, Production of interferon by suspensions of human leukocytes, *Proc. Soc. Exp. Biol. Med.* **108**:799.

GRESSER, I., 1971, Clinical use of exogenous interferon, in: *Viruses Affecting Man and Animals* (M. Saunders and M. Schaeffer, eds), p. 416, W. H. Green, St. Louis, Missouri.

GRESSER, I., 1972, Anti-tumor effects of interferon, in: *Advances in Cancer Research*, Vol. XVI (G. Klein and S. Weinhouse, eds), p. 97, Academic Press, New York.

GRESSER, I., 1975, Interferon therapy: Obvious and not so obvious applications, *Acta Med. Scand.* **197**:49.

GRESSER, I., AND BOURALI, C., 1969, Exogenous interferon and inducers of interferon in the treatment of Balb/c mice inoculated with RC19 tumor cells, *Nature (London)* **223**:844.

GRESSER, I., AND BOURALI, C., 1970a, Antitumor effects of interferon preparations in mice, *J. Natl. Cancer Inst.* **45**:365.

GRESSER, I., AND BOURALI, C., 1970b, Development of newborn mice during prolonged treatment with interferon, *Eur. J. Cancer* **6**:553.

GRESSER, I., AND BOURALI, C., 1972, Inhibition by interferon preparations of a solid malignant tumour and pulmonary metastases in mice, *Nature (London) New Biol.* **236**:78.

GRESSER, I., AND BOURALI-MAURY, C., 1973, The antitumor effect of interferon in lymphocyte and macrophage-depressed mice, *Proc. Soc. Exp. Biol. Med.* **144**:896.

GRESSER, I., COPPEY, J., FALCOFF, E., AND FONTAINE, D., 1966, Action inhibitrice de l'interféron brut sur le développment de la leucémie de Friend chez la souris, *C. R. Acad. Sci. Paris* **263**:586.

GRESSER, I., COPPEY, J., FALCOFF, E., AND FONTAINE, D., 1967a, Interferon and murine leukemia. I. Inhibitory effect of interferon preparations on development of Friend leukemia in mice, *Proc. Soc. Exp. Biol. Med.* **124**:84.

GRESSER, I., FONTAINE, D., COPPEY, J., FALCOFF, R., AND FALCOFF, E., 1967b, Interferon and murine leukemia. II. Factors related to the inhibitory effect of interferon preparations on development of Friend leukemia in mice, *Proc. Soc. Exp. Biol. Med.* **124**:91.

GRESSER, I., COPPEY, J., FONTAINE-BROUTY-BOYÉ, D., FALCOFF, R. AND FALCOFF, E., 1967c, Interferon and murine leukaemia. III. Efficacy of interferon preparations administered after inoculation of Friend virus, *Nature (London)* **215**:174.

GRESSER, I., COPPEY, J., FONTAINE-BROUTY-BOYÉ, D., FALCOFF, E., FALCOFF, R., ZAJDELA, F., BOURALI, C., AND THOMAS, M. T., 1967d, The effect of interferon preparations on Friend leukaemia in mice, in: *Ciba Found. Symp. Interferon* (G. E. W. Wolstenholme and M. O'Conner, eds.), p. 240.

GRESSER, I., FALCOFF, R., FONTAINE-BROUTY-BOYÉ, D., ZAJDELA, F., COPPEY, J., AND FALCOFF, E., 1967e, Interferon and murine leukemia. IV. Further studies on the efficacy of interferon preparations administered after inoculation of Friend virus, *Proc. Soc. Exp. Biol. Med.* **126**:791.

GRESSER, I., BERMAN, L., DE THÉ, G., BROUTY-BOYÉ, D., COPPEY, J., AND FALCOFF, E., 1968a, Interferon and murine leukemia. V. Effect of interferon preparations on the evolution of Rauscher disease in mice, *J. Natl. Cancer Inst.* **41**:505.

GRESSER, I., COPPEY, J., AND BOURALI, C., 1968b, Action inhibitrice de l'interféron brut sur la leucémie lymphoïde des souris AKR, *C. R. Acad. Sci. Paris* **267**:1900.

GRESSER, I., COPPEY, J., AND BOURALI, C., 1969a, Interferon and murine leukemia. VI. Effect of interferon preparations on the lymphoid leukemia of AKR mice, *J. Natl. Cancer Inst.* **43**:1083.

GRESSER, I., BOURALI, C., LÉVY, J. P., FONTAINE-BROUTY-BOYÉ, D., AND THOMAS, M. T., 1969b, Cancérologie—Prolongation de la survie des souris inoculées avec des cellules tumorales et traitées avec des préparations d'interféron, *C. R. Acad. Sci. Paris* **268**:994.

GRESSER, I., BOURALI, C., LEVY, J. P., FONTAINE-BROUTY-BOYÉ, D., AND THOMAS, M. T., 1969c, Increased survival in mice inoculated with tumor cells and treated with interferon preparations, *Proc. Natl. Acad. Sci. U.S.A.* **63**:51.

GRESSER, I., FONTAINE-BROUTY-BOYÉ, D., BOURALI, C., AND THOMAS, M. T., 1969d, A comparison of the efficacy of endogenous, exogenous and combined endogenous–exogenous interferon in the treatment of mice infected with encephalomyocarditis virus, *Proc. Soc. Exp. Biol. Med.* **130**:236.

GRESSER, I., BOURALI, C., CHOUROULINKOV, I., FONTAINE-BROUTY-BOYÉ, D., AND THOMAS, M. T., 1970a, Treatment of neoplasia in mice with interferon preparations, *Ann. N. Y. Acad. Sci.* **173**:694.

GRESSER, I., BROUTY-BOYÉ, D., THOMAS, M. T., AND MACIEIRA-COELHO, A., 1970b, Interferon and cell division. I. Inhibition of the multiplication of mouse leukemia L1210 cells *in vitro* by interferon preparations, *Proc. Natl. Acad. Sci. U.S.A.* **66**:1052.

GRESSER, I., BROUTY-BOYÉ, D., THOMAS, M. T., AND MACIEIRA-COELHO, A., 1970c, Interferon and cell division. II. Influence of various experimental conditions on the inhibition of L1210 cell multiplication *in vitro* by interferon preparations, *J. Natl. Cancer Inst.* **45**:1145.

GRESSER, I., THOMAS, M. T., BROUTY-BOYÉ, D., AND MACIEIRA-COELHO, A., 1971a, Interferon and cell division. V. Titration of the anticellular action of interferon preparations, *Proc. Soc. Exp. Biol. Med.* **137**:1258.

GRESSER, I., THOMAS, M. T., AND BROUTY-BOYÉ, D., 1971b, Effect of interferon treatment of L1210 cells *in vitro* on tumor and colony formation, *Nature (London)* **231**:20.

GRESSER, I., MAURY, C., AND BROUTY-BOYÉ, D., 1972, On the mechanism of the antitumor effect of interferon in mice, *Nature (London)* **239**:167.

GRESSER, I., BANDU, M. T., TOVEY, M., BODO, G., PAUCKER, K., AND STEWART, W., II, 1973, Interferon and cell division. VII. Inhibitory effect of highly purified interferon preparations on the multiplication of leukemia L1210 cells, *Proc. Soc. Exp. Biol. Med.* **142:**7.

GRESSER, I., BANDU, M. T., AND BROUTY-BOYÉ, D., 1974a, Interferon and cell division. IX. Interferon-resistant L1210 cells: Characteristics and origin, *J. Natl. Cancer Inst.* **52:**553.

GRESSER, I., BANDU, M. T., BROUTY-BOYÉ, D., AND TOVEY, M., 1974b, Pronounced antiviral activity of human interferon on bovine and porcine cells, *Nature (London)* **251:**543.

GRESSER, I., TOVEY, M. G., MAURY, C., AND CHOUROULONKOV, I., 1975a, Lethality of interferon preparations for new-born mice, *Nature (London)* **258:**76.

GRESSER, I., VIGNAUX, F., MAURY, C., AND LINDAHL, P., 1975b, Factor(s) from Ehrlich ascites cell responsible for delayed rejection of skin allografts in mice and its assay on lymphocytes *in vitro, Proc. Soc. Exp. Biol. Med.* **149:**83.

GRESSER, I., MAURY, C., AND TOVEY, M., 1976, Interferon and murine leukemia. VII. Therapeutic effect of interferon preparations after diagnosis of lymphoma in AKR mice, *Int. J. Cancer* **17:**647.

GROHSMAN, J., AND NOWOTNY, A., 1972, The immune recognition of TA3 tumors, its facilitation by endotoxin and abrogation by ascites fluid, *J. Immunol.* **109:**1090.

HABIF, D. V., LIPTON, R., AND CANTELL, K., 1975, Interferon crosses the blood–cerebrospinal fluid barrier in monkeys, *Proc. Soc. Exp. Biol. Med.* **149:**287.

HAVELL, E. A., AND VILCEK, J., 1972, Production of high-titered interferon in cultures of human diploid cells, *Antimicrob. Agents Chemother.* **2:**476.

HERLING, I. M., 1975, Decrease in experimental liver metastasis in mice after treatment with pyran copolymer, *J. Med.* **6:**33.

HILFENHAUS, J., AND KARGES, H. E., 1974, Growth inhibition of human lymphoblastoid cells by interferon preparations, obtained from human leukocytes, *Z. Naturforsch.* **29c:**618.

HILLEMAN, M. R., 1963, Interferon in prospect and perspective, *J. Cell. Comp. Physiol.* **62:**337.

HILLEMAN, M. R., 1965, Immunologic, chemotherapeutic and interferon approaches to control of viral disease, *Amer. J. Med.* **38:**751.

HILLEMAN, M. R., 1968, Approaches to prevention of leukemia in man, in: *Perspectives in Leukemia,* p. 272, Grune and Stratton, New York.

HILLEMAN, M. R., 1969, Toward control of viral infections of man, *Science* **164:**506.

HILLEMAN, M. R., 1970a, Prospects for the use of double-stranded ribonucleic acid (poly I:C) inducers in man, *J. Infect. Dis.* **121:**196.

HILLEMAN, M. R., 1970b, Double-stranded RNAs (poly I:C) in the prevention of viral infections, *Arch. Intern. Med.* **126:**109.

HIRSCH, M. S., BLACK, P. H., TRACY, G. S., LEIBOWITZ, S., AND SCHWARTZ, R. S., 1970a, Leukemia virus activation in chronic allogeneic disease, *Proc. Natl. Acad. Sci. U.S.A.* **67:**1914.

HIRSCH, M. S., BLACK, P. H., WOOD, M. L., AND MONACO, A. P., 1970b, Immunosuppression, interferon inducers, and leukemia in mice, *Proc. Soc. Exp. Biol. Med.* **134:**309.

HIRSCH, M. S., BLACK, P. H., WOOD, M. L., AND MONACO, A. P., 1972, Effects pf pyran copolymer on oncogenic virus infections in immunosuppressed hosts, *J. Immunol.* **108:**1312.

HIRSCH, M. S., ELLIS, D. A., PROFFITT, M. R., BLACK, P. H., AND CHIRIGOS, M. A., 1973a, Effects of interferon on leukaemia virus activation in graft versus host disease, *Nature (London)New Biol.* **244:**102.

HIRSCH, M. S., ELLIS, D. A., BLACK, P. H., MONACO, A. P., AND WOOD, M. L., 1973b, Leukemia virus activation during homograft rejection, *Science* **180:**500.

HIRSCH, M. S., BLACK, P. H., WOOD, M. L., AND MONACO, A. P., 1973c, Effects of pyran copolymer on leukemogenesis in immunosuppressed AKR mice, *J. Immunol.* **111:**91.

HIRSCH, M. S., ELLIS, D. A., BLACK, P. H., MONACO, A. P., AND WOOD, M. L., 1974, Immunosuppressive effects of an interferon preparation *in vivo, Transplantation* **17:**234.

HIRSCH, M. S., BLACK, P. H., AND PROFFITT, M. R., 1976, Interferon effects on immunologically activated murine leukemia viruses, *Monogr. Natl. Cancer Inst.*, in press.

HO, M., AND POSTIC, B., 1967a, Renal excretion of interferon, *Nature (London)* **214:**1230.

HO, M., AND POSTIC, B., 1967b, Prospects for applying interferon to man, in: *Vaccines Against Viral and Rickettsial Diseases of Man, Int. Conf. Pan Amer. Health Organ. Sci. Publ.* **147:**632.

HRSAK, I., AND MAROTTI, T., 1973, Immunosuppression mediated by Ehrlich ascites fluid, *Eur. J. Cancer* **9:**717.

HUANG, K. H., AND LANDAY, M. E., 1969, Enhancement of the lethal effects of endotoxins by interferon inducers, *J. Bacteriol.* **100:**1110.

HUANG, K. Y., DONAHOE, R. M., GORDON, F. B., AND DRESSLER, H. R., 1971, Enhancement of phagocytosis by interferon-containing preparations, *Infect. Immun.* **4:**581.

HUET, C., GRESSER, I., BANDU, M. T., AND LINDAHL, P., 1974, Increased binding of concanavalin A to interferon-treated murine leukemia L1210 cells, *Proc. Soc. Exp. Biol. Med.* **147:**52.

HUGH, R., HUANG, K. Y., AND ELLIOTT, T. B., 1971, Enhancement of bacterial infections in mice by Newcastle disease virus, *Infect. Immun.* **3:**488.

IMANISHI, J., YOKOTA, Y., KISHIDA, T., MUKAINAKA, T., AND MATSUO, A., 1975, Phagocytosis-enhancing effect of human leukocyte interferon preparation of human peripheral monocytes *in vitro*, *Acta Virol.* **19:**52.

ISAACS, A., 1963, Interferon, in: *Advances in Virus Research*, Vol. X, p. 1, Academic Press, New York.

ISAACS, A., AND LINDEMANN, J., 1957, Virus interference, I. The interferon, *Proc. R. Soc. London Ser. B.* **147:**258.

JAFFE, N., FREI, E., III, TRAGGIS, D., AND BISHOP, Y., 1974, Adjuvant methotrexate and citrovorum-factor treatment of osteogenic sarcoma, *N. Engl. J. Med.* **291:**994.

JASMIN, C., SMADJA-JOFFE, F., KLEIN, B., AND KERDILES-LEBOUSSE, C., 1976, Physiopathology of human and virus-induced murine leukemias, *Cancer Res.* **36:**603.

JOHNSON, H. M., SMITH, B. G., AND BARON, S., 1975, Inhibition of the primary *in vitro* antibody response by interferon preparations, *J. Immunol.* **114:**403.

JORDAN, G. W., FRIED, R. P., AND MERIGAN, T. C., 1974, Administration of human leukocyte interferon in Herpes zoster. I. Safety, circulating antiviral activity, and host responses to infection, *J. Infect. Dis.* **130:**56.

JUNGLEBUT, C. W., AND KODZA, H., 1962, Interference between lymphocytic choriomeningitis virus and the leukemia-transmitting agent of leukemia L2C in guinea pigs, *Arch. Ges. Virusforsch.* **12:**552.

KAPLAN, A. M., MORAHAN, P. S., AND REGELSON, W., 1974, Induction of macrophage-mediated tumor-cell cytotoxicity by pyran copolymer, *J. Natl. Cancer Inst.* **52:**1919.

KAPLAN, A. M., WALKER, P. L., AND MORAHAN, P. S., 1976, Tumor cell cytotoxicity versus cytotasis of pyran activated macrophages, *Monogr. Natl. Cancer Inst.*, in press.

KASSEL, R. L., 1970, Carcinolytic effects of interferon, *Clin. Obstet. Gynecol.* **13:**910.

KASSEL, R. L., PASCAL, R. R., AND VAS, A., 1972, Interferon-mediated oncolysis in spontaneous murine leukemia, *J. Natl. Cancer Inst.* **48:**1155.

KASSEL, R. L., OLD, L. J., CARSWELL, E. A., FIORE, N. C., AND HARDY, W. D., JR., 1973, Serum-mediated leukemia cell destruction in AKR mice, *J. Exp. Med.* **138:**925.

KENDE, M., AND GLYNN, J. P., 1971, Modifications of the response of autochthonous Moloney sarcoma virus-induced tumors to poly-I.C. by DEAE-dx, *Chemotherapy* **16:**281.

KISHIDA, T., KATO, S., AND NAGANO, Y., 1965, Effet du facteur inhibiteur du virus sur le fibrome de Shope, *C. R. Soc. Biol.* **159:**782.

KISHIDA, T., TODA, S., TOÏDA, A., AND HATTORI, T., 1971, Effet de l'interféron sur la cellule maligne de la souris, *C. R. Soc. Biol.* **169:**1498.

KLEINSCHMIDT, W. J., ELLIS, L. F., VAN FRANK, R. M., AND MURPHY, E. B., 1968, Interferon stimulation by a double-stranded RNA of a mycophage in statolon preparations, *Nature (London)* **220:**167.

KNIGHT, E., 1973, Interferon: Effect on the saturation density to which mouse cells will grow *in vitro*, *J. Cell. Biol.* **56:**846.

KRAVCHENKO, A. T., VORONIN, E. S., AND KOSMIADI, G. A., 1967, Effects of anti-rabies vaccine and fixed rabies virus on the development of tumours caused by Rous sarcoma, *Acta Virol.* **11:**145.

KREIBICH, G., SÜSS, R., KINZEL, V., AND HECKER, E., 1970, On the biochemical mechanism of tumorigenesis in mouse skin. III. Decrease in tumor yields by poly I/C administered during initiation of skin by an intragastric dose of 7,12 dimethylbenz[α]anthracene, *Z. Krebsforsch.* **74:**383.

KREIDER, J. W., 1970, Prevention of polyinosinic–polycytidylic acid inhibition of tumor growth by immunosuppression, *Fed. Proc. Fed. Amer. Soc. Exp. Biol.* **29:**621 (abstract).

KREIDER, J. W., AND BENJAMIN, S. A., 1972, Tumor immunity and the mechanism of polyinosinic–polycytidylic acid inhibition of tumor growth, *J. Natl. Cancer Inst.* **49:**1303.

KRULWICH, T. A., JACOBS, C. F., WEISMAN, J. H., AND SOUTHAM, C. M., 1962, Studies of six new viruses in tumor-bearing mice, *Cancer Res.* **22:**322.

LACOUR, F., SPIRA, A., LACOUR, J., AND PRADE, M., 1972, Polyadenylic–polyuridylic acid, an adjunct to surgery in the treatment of spontaneous mammary tumors in C3H/He mice and transplantable melanoma in the hamster, *Cancer Res.* **32:**648.

LACOUR, F., DELAGE, G., AND CHIANALE, C., 1975, Reduced incidence of spontaneous mammary tumors in C3H/He mice after treatment with polyadenylate–polyuridylate, *Science* **187**:256.

LAMPSON, G. P., TYTELL, A. A., NEMES, M. M., AND HILLEMAN, M. R., 1963, Purification and characterization of chick embryo interferon, *Proc. Soc. Exp. Biol. Med.* **112**:468.

LAMPSON, G. P., TYTELL, A. A., FIELD, A. K., NEMES, M. M., AND HILLEMAN, M. R., 1967, Inducers of interferon and host resistance. I. Double-stranded RNA from extracts of *Penicillium funicolosum*, *Proc. Natl. Acad. Sci. U.S.A.* **58**:782.

LARSON, V. M., CLARK, W. R., AND HILLEMAN, M. R., 1969a, Influence of synthetic (poly-I.C.) and viral double-stranded ribonucleic acids on adenovirus 12 oncogenesis in hamsters, *Proc. Soc. Exp. Biol. Med.* **131**:1002.

LARSON, V. M., CLARK, W. R., DAGLE, G. E., AND HILLEMAN, M. R., 1969b, Influence of synthetic double-stranded ribonucleic acid, poly-I.C. on Friend leukemia in mice, *Proc. Soc. Exp. Biol. Med.* **132**:602.

LARSON, V. M., PANTELEAKIS, P. N., AND HILLEMAN, M. R., 1970, Influence of synthetic double-stranded ribonucleic acid (poly-I.C.) on SV40 viral oncogenesis and transplant tumor in hamsters, *Proc. Soc. Exp. Biol. Med.* **133**:14.

LATARJET, R., 1964, Action inhibitrice d'extraits leucémiques isologues irradiés sur la leucémogénèse spontanée de la souris AKR, *Ann. Inst. Pasteur* **106**:1.

LAUFS, R., AND FLECKENSTEIN, B., 1973, Susceptibility to herpes virus saimiri and antibody development in Old and New World monkeys, *Med. Microbiol. Immunol.* **158**:227.

LAUFS, R., AND MELÉNDEZ, L. V., 1973, Oncogenicity of herpes virus ateles in monkeys, *J. Natl. Cancer Inst.* **51**:599.

LAUFS, R., STEINKE, H., JACOBS, C., HILFENHAUS, J., AND KARGES, H., 1974, Influence of interferon on the replication of onconogenic herpes virus in tissue cultures and in nonhuman primates, *Med. Microbiol. Immunol.* **160**:285.

LEE, E. S., AND MACKENZIE, D. H., 1964, Osteosarcoma—a study of the value of preoperative megavoltage radiotherapy, *Br. J. Surg.* **51**:252.

LEE, S. H. S., O'SHAUGHNESSY, M. V., AND ROZEE, K. R., 1972, Interferon induced growth depression in diploid and heteroploid human cells, *Proc. Soc. Exp. Biol. Med.* **139**:1438.

LEONARD, B. J., ECCLESTON, E., AND JONES, D., 1969, Toxicity of interferon inducers of the double-stranded RNA type, *Nature (London)* **224**:1023.

LEVY, H. B., LAW, L. W., AND RABSON, A. S., 1969, Inhibition of tumor growth by polyinosinic–polycytidylic acid, *Proc. Natl. Acad. Sci. U.S.A.* **62**:357.

LEVY, H. B., ASOFSKY, R., RILEY, F., GARAPIN, A., CANTOR, H., AND ADAMSON, R., 1970, The mechanism of the antitumor action of Poly I:Poly C, *Ann. N. Y. Acad. Sci.* **173**:640.

LEVY, H. B., ADAMSON, R., CARBONE, P., DEVITA, V., GAZDAR, A., RHIM, J., WEINSTEIN, A., AND RILEY, F., 1971, Studies on the antitumor action of poly I.Poly C, in: *Biological Effects of Polynucleotides* (R. F. Beers, Jr., and W. Braun, eds.), p. 55, Springer-Verlag, New York—Heidelberg—Berlin.

LEVY, H. B., BAER, G., BARON, S., BUCKLER, C. E., GIBBS, C. J., IADAROLA, M. J., LONDON, W. T., AND RICE, J., 1975, A modified polyriboinosinic–polyribocytidylic acid complex that induces interferon in primates, *J. Infect. Dis.* **132**:434.

LEVY, M. H., AND WHEELOCK, E. F., 1975, Impaired macrophage function in Friend virus leukemia: Restoration by statolon, *J. Immunol.* **114**:962.

LEVY-KOENIG, R. E., GOLGHER, R. R., AND PAUCKER, K., 1970, Immunology of interferons. II. Heterospecific activities of human interferons and their neutralization by antibody, *J. Immunol.* **104**:791.

LIEBERMAN, M., MERIGAN, T. C., AND KAPLAN, H. S., 1971, Inhibition of radiogenic lymphoma development in mice by interferon, *Proc. Soc. Exp. Biol. Med.* **138**:575.

LINDAHL, P., LEARY, P., AND GRESSER, I., 1972, Enhancement by interferon of the specific cytotoxicity of sensitized lymphocytes, *Proc. Natl. Acad. Sci. U.S.A.* **69**:721.

LINDAHL, P., LEARY, P., AND GRESSER, I., 1973, Enhancement by interferon of the expression of surface antigens on murine leukemia L1210 cells, *Proc. Natl. Acad. Sci. U.S.A.* **70**:2785.

LINDAHL, P., LEARY, P., AND GRESSER. I., 1974, Enhancement of the expression of histocompatibility antigens of mouse lymphoid cells by interferon *in vitro*, *Eur. J. Immunol.* **4**:779.

LINDAHL, P., GRESSER, I., LEARY, P., AND TOVEY, M., 1976, Interferon treatment of mice: Enhanced expression of histocompatibility antigens on lymphoid cells, *Proc. Natl. Acad. Sci. U.S.A.* **73**:1284.

LINDAHL-MAGNUSSON, P., LEARY, P., AND GRESSER, I., 1971, Interferon and cell division, VI. Inhibitory effect of interferon on the multiplication of mouse embryo and mouse kidney cells in primary cultures, *Proc. Soc. Exp. Biol. Med.* **138**:1044.

LINDAHL-MAGNUSSON, P., LEARY, P., AND GRESSER, I., 1972, Interferon inhibits DNA synthesis induced in mouse lymphocyte suspensions by phytohaemagglutinin or by allogeneic cells, *Nature (London) New Biol.* **273:**120.

LOCKART, R. Z., JR., 1967, Recent progress in research on interferons, *Prog. Med. Virol.* **9:**451.

LYON, G. M., JR., 1970, Growth stimulation of tissue culture cells derived from patients with neuroblastoma, *Cancer Res.* **30:**2521.

MATHÉ, G., 1971, Active immunotherapy, *Adv. Cancer Res.* **14:**1.

MATHÉ, G., AMIEL, J. L., SCHWARZENBERG, L., SCHNEIDER, M., HAYAT, M., DE VASSAL, F., JASMIN, C., ROSENFELD, C., SAKOUHI, M., AND CHOAY, J., 1970, Remission induction with poly IC in patients with acute lymphoblastic leukaemia (preliminary results), *Eur. J. Clin. Biol. Res.* **15:**671.

MAYO, J. G., 1972, Biologic characterization of the subcutaneously implanted Lewis lung tumor, *Cancer Chemother. Rep.* **3:**325.

MCNEILL, T. A., AND FLEMING, W. A., 1971, The relationship between serum interferon and an inhibitor of mouse haemopoietic colonies *in vitro*, *Immunology* **21:**761.

MCNEILL, T. A., AND GRESSER, I., 1973, Inhibition of haemopoietic colony growth by interferon preparations from different sources, *Nature (London) New Biol.* **244:**173.

MEIER, H., MYERS, D. D., AND HUEBNER, R. J., 1970a, Statolon-therapy of spontaneous viral-caused mouse tumors, *Naturwissenchaften* **57:**6.

MEIER, H., MYERS, D. D., AND HUEBNER, R. J., 1970b, Differential effect of a synthetic polyribonucleotide complex on spontaneous and transplanted leukemia in mice, *Life Sci.* **9:**653.

MERIGAN, T. C., 1967, Interferon's promise in clinical medicine, *Amer. J. Med.* **43:**817.

MERIGAN, T. C., RAND, K. H., ADBALLAH, P. S., JORDAN, G. W., FELDMAN, S., AND FRIED, R. P., 1976, Administration of human leukocyte interferon in varicella–zoster infections. II. Preliminary controlled trials to establish effective dosage in patients with malignancy, *J. Infect. Dis.*, in press.

METCALF, D., AND WIADROWSKI, M., 1966, Autoradiographic analysis of lymphocyte proliferation in the thymus and in the thymic lymphoma tissue, *Cancer Res.* **26:**483.

MOBRAATEN, L. E., DE MAEYER, E., AND DE MAEYER-GUIGNARD, J., 1973, Prolongation of allograft survival in mice by inducers of interferon, *Transplantation* **16:**415.

MOCARELLI, P., VILLA, M. L., GAROTTA, G., PORTA, C., BIGI, G., AND CLERICI, E., 1973, Reversibility of the immunodepression due to Ehrlich ascites carcinoma, *J. Immunol.* **111:**973.

MOLOMUT, N., AND PADNOS, M., 1965, Inhibition of transplantable and spontaneous murine tumours by the M-P virus, *Nature (London)* **208:**948.

MORAHAN, P. S., AND KAPLAN, A. M., 1976, Macrophage activation and antitumor activity of biologic and synthetic agents, *Int. J. Cancer* **17:**82.

MORAHAN, P. S., MUNSON, J. A., BAIRD, L. G., KAPLAN, A. M., AND REGELSON, W., 1974, Antitumor action of pyran copolymer and tilorone against Lewis lung carcinoma and B-16 melanoma, *Cancer Res.* **34:**506.

MORAHAN, P. S., SCHULLER, G. B., SNODGRASS, M. J., AND KAPLAN, A. M., 1976, Paradoxical effects of immunopotentiators on tumors and tumor viruses, *J. Infect. Dis.* **133S:**A249.

MORGAN, W. W., AND CAMERON, I. L., 1973, Effect of fast-growing transplantable hepatoma on cell proliferation in host tissue of the mouse, *Cancer Res.* **33:**441.

MUNDY, G. R., RAISZ, L. G., COOPER, R. A., SCHECHTER, G. P., AND SALMON, S. E., 1974, Evidence for the secretion of an osteoclast stimulating factor in myeloma, *N. Engl. J. Med.* **291:**1041.

NADEL, E. M., AND HAAS, V. H., 1956, Effect of the virus of lymphocytic choriomeningitis on the course of leukemia in guinea pigs and mice, *J. Natl. Cancer Inst.* **17:**221.

NEBERT, D. W., AND FRIEDMAN, R. M., 1973, Stimulation of aryl hydrocarbon hydroxylase induction in cell cultures by interferon, *J. Virol.* **11:**193.

NEMES, M. M., TYTELL, A. A., LAMPSON, G. P., FIELD, A. K., AND HILLEMAN, M. R., 1969, Inducers of interferon and host resistance. VI. Antiviral efficacy of poly-I.C. in animal models, *Proc. Soc. Exp. Biol. Med.* **132:**776.

NORDLUND, J. J., WOLFF, S. M., AND LEVY, H. B., 1970, Inhibition of biologic activity of poly I:poly C by human plasma, *Proc. Soc. Exp. Biol. Med.* **133:**439.

OKER-BŁOM, N., AND LEINIKKI, P., 1965, Effect of Coxsackie virus of group A and B on Rous sarcoma virus, *Arch. Ges. Virusforsch.* **17:**448.

OKER-BLOM, N., AND STRANDSTRÖM, H., 1956a, Effect of Coxsackie virus on the growth of the Rous sarcoma in embryonated chicken eggs, *Ann. Med. Exp. Fenn.* **34:**293.

OKER-BLOM, N., AND STRANDSTRÖM, H., 1956b, Effect of Coxsackie virus on the growth of the Rous sarcoma in chickens, *Ann. Med. Exp. Fenn.* **34:**301.

OLD, L. J., BENACERRAF, B., AND STOCKERT, E., 1963, Increased resistance to Mengo virus following infection with bacillus Calmette-Guérin, *Colloq. Int. C.N.R.S.*, No. 115, p. 319.

O'SHAUGHNESSY, M. V., LEE, S. H. S., AND ROZEE, K. R., 1972, Interferon inhibition of DNA synthesis and cell division, *Can. J. Microbiol.* **18:**145.

PAUCKER, K., CANTELL, K., AND HENLE, W., 1962, Quantitative studies on viral interference in suspended L cells. III. Effect of interfering viruses and interferon on the growth rate of cells, *Virology* **17:**324.

PEARSON, J. W., TURNER, W., EBERT, P. S., AND CHIRIGOS, M. A., 1969, Effectiveness of therapy with a multistranded synthetic polynucleotide complex against a murine sarcoma virus, *Appl. Microbiol.* **18:**474.

PIERCE, M., CARTER, R. E., AND RIGOR, E., 1959, Studies on the relationship of viral infections to leukemia in mice, *Cancer* **12:**222.

PIERONI, R. E., BRODERICK, E. J., BUNDEALLY, A., AND LEVINE, L., 1970, A simple method for the quantitation of submicrogram amounts of bacterial endotoxin, *Proc. Soc. Exp. Biol. Med.* **133:**790.

PIERONI, R. E., BUNDEALLY, A. E., AND LEVINE, L., 1971, The effect of actinomycin D on the lethality of poly I:C, *J. Immunol.* **106:**1128.

PILCH, D. J. F., AND PLANTEROSE, D. N., 1971, Effects on Friend disease of double-stranded RNA of fungal origin, *J. Gen. Virol.* **10:**155.

POTMESIL, M., AND GOLDFEDER, A., 1972, Inhibitory effect of polyinosinic:polycytidylic acid on the growth of transplantable mouse mammary carcinoma, *Proc. Soc. Exp. Biol. Med.* **139:**1392.

PUDOV, V. I., 1971, The influence of interferon on metastasization of Brown–Pearce carcinoma, *Bull. Exp. Biol. Med. (USSR)* **8:**91.

PYHÄLÄ, L., AND CANTELL, K., 1974, Clearance of human interferon in rabbits induced to make rabbit interferon, *Proc. Soc. Exp. Biol. Med.* **146:**394.

RABIN, H., ADAMSON, R. H., NEUBAUER, R. H., CICMANEC, J. L., AND WALLEN, W. C., 1976, Pilot studies with human interferon in herpes virus saimiri induced lymphoma in owl monkeys, *Cancer Res.* **36:**715.

RANA, M. W., PINKERTON, H., AND RANKIN, A., 1975, Effect of rifamycin and tilorone derivatives on Friend virus leukemia in mice, *Proc. Soc. Exp. Biol. Med.* **150:**32.

REGELSON, W., 1967, Prevention and treatment of Friend leukemia virus (FLV) infection by interferon-inducing synthetic polyanions, in: *The Reticuloendothelial System and Atherosclerosis* (N. R. DiLuzio and R. Paoletti, eds.), p. 315, Plenum Press, New York.

REGELSON, W., 1968, The antitumor activity of polyanions, in: *Advances in Chemotherapy* (A. Goldin, F. Hawking, and R. J. Schnitzer, eds.), Vol. 3, p. 303, Academic Press, New York.

REGELSON, W., 1973, Host modulation of resistance to infection and neoplasia, *Annu. Rep. Med. Chem.* **8:**160.

REGELSON, W., AND FOLTYN, O., 1966, Prevention and treatment of Friend leukemia virus (FLV) infection by polyanions and phytohemagglutinin, *Proc. Amer. Assoc. Cancer Res.* **7:**58.

REGELSON, W., MORAHAN, P., KAPLAN, A. M., BAIRD, L. G., AND MUNSON, J. A., 1973, Synthetic polyanions: Molecular weight, macrophage activation, and immunologic response, *Excerpta Med. Int. Congr.* Ser. No. 325, p. 97.

REV-KURY, L. H., KURY, G., AND FIREDELL, G. H., 1966, Thymidine uptake in livers of tumor-bearing hamsters, *Arch. Pathol.* **82:**77.

RHEINS, M. S., BARKER, A. D., AND WILSON, H. E., 1971, The amelioration of Friend virus leukemia by the sequential administration of a series of viral and nonviral interferon inducers, *Bacteriol. Proc.*, p. 188.

RHIM, J. S., AND HUEBNER, R. J., 1969, Inhibitory effect of statolon on virus-induced sarcoma of mice, *Antimicrob. Agents Chemother.*, p. 177.

RHIM, J. S., AND HUEBNER, R. J., 1971, Comparison of the antitumor effect of interferon and interferon inducers, *Proc. Soc. Exp. Biol. Med.* **136:**524.

ROBINSON, R. A., DEVITA, V. T., LEVY, H. B., BARON, S., HUBBARD, S. P., AND LEVINE, A. S., 1976, A Phase I–II trial of multiple-dose polyriboinosinic–polyribocytidylic acid (poly I–poly C) in patients with leukemia or solid tumors, in preparation.

ROSSI, G. B., MARCHEGIANI, M., MATARESE, G. P., AND GRESSER, I., 1975, Inhibitory effect of interferon on multiplication of Friend leukemia cells *in vivo*, *J. Natl. Cancer Inst.* **54:**993.

ROWE, W. P., PUGH, W. E., AND HARTLEY, J. W., 1970, Plaque assay techniques for murine leukemia viruses, *Virology* **42:**1136.

RUDALI, G., AND JULLIEN, P., 1966, Notes originales sur l'utilisation des leucémies spontanées des souris pour les recherches chimiothérapeutiques, *Rev. Fr. Etud. Clin. Biol.* **11:**183.

SALERNO, R. A., WHITMIRE, C. E., GARCIA. I. M., AND HUEBNER, R. J., 1972, Chemical carcinogenesis in mice inhibited by interferon, *Nature (London) New Biol.* **239**:31.

SANO, E., MATSUI, Y., AND KOBAYASHI, S., 1974, Production of mouse interferon with high titers in a large-scale suspension culture system, *Jpn. J. Microbiol.* **18**:165.

SARMA, P. S., SHIU, G., NEUBAUER, R. H., BARON, S., AND HUEBNER, R. J., 1969, Virus-induced sarcoma of mice: Inhibition by a synthetic polyribonucleotide complex, *Proc. Natl. Acad. Sci. U.S.A.* **62**:1046.

SARMA, P. S., NEUBAUER, R. H., AND RABSTEIN, L., 1971, Murine sarcoma and leukemia viral infection of mice. Effect of long-term treatment with poly-I.C., *Proc. Soc. Exp. Biol. Med.* **137**:469.

SCHABEL, F. M., JR., SKIPPER, H. E., TRADER, M. W., LASTER, W. R., JR., AND SIMPSON-HERREN, L., 1969, Spontaneous AK leukemia (lymphoma) as a model system, *Cancer Chemother. Rep.* **53**:329.

SCHULLER, G. B., MORAHAN, P. S., AND SNODGRASS, M., 1975, Inhibition and enhancement of Friend leukemia virus by pyran copolymer, *Cancer Res.* **35**:1915.

SHIRODKAR, M. V., 1965, The blocking effect of West Nile virus on production of sarcoma by Rous virus in chickens, *J. Immunol.* **95**:1121.

SKIPPER, H. E., SCHABEL, F. M., JR., TRADER, M. W., AND LASTER, W. R., JR., 1969, Response to therapy of spontaneous, first passage, and long passage lines of AK leukemia, *Cancer Chemother. Rep.* **53**:345.

SKIPPER, H. E., SCHABEL, F. M., JR., TRADER, M. W., LASTER, W. R., JR., SIMPSON-HERREN, L., AND LLOYD, H. H., 1972, Basic and therapeutic trial results obtained in the spontaneous AK leukemia (lymphoma) model—end of 1971, *Cancer Chemother. Rep.* **56**:273.

SLAMON, D. J., 1973, Protective effect of the double-stranded polyribonucleotide, polyinosinic–polycytidylic acid, against rat erythroblastosis induced by murine erythroblastosis virus, *J. Natl. Cancer Inst.* **51**:851.

SLAVINA, E. G., LENEVA, N. V., AND SVET-MOLDAVSKY, G. J., 1974, Sensitivity of target cells to the cytotoxic effects of lymphocytes induced by interferon, *Folia Biol. (Prague)* **20**:231.

SMADJA-JOFFE, F., JASMIN, C., MALAISE, E. P., AND BOURNOUTIAN, C., 1973, Study of the cellular proliferation kinetics of Friend leukemia, *Int. J. Cancer* **11**:300.

SMADJA-JOFFE, F., JASMIN, C., KERDILES, C., AND KLEIN, B., 1975, Friend leukemia: A model for the physiopathology of human chronic leukemia, *Eur. J. Cancer* **11**:831.

SMADJA-JOFFE, F., KLEIN, B., KERDILES, C., FEINENDEGEN, L., AND JASMIN, C., 1976, Study of cell death in Friend leukemia, *Cell Tissue Kinet.* **9**:131.

SNODGRASS, M. J., MORAHAN, P. S., AND KAPLAN, A. M., 1975, Histopathology of the host response to Lewis lung carcinoma: Modulation by pyran, *J. Natl. Cancer Inst.* **55**:455.

SOUTHAM, C. M., 1960, Present status of oncolytic virus studies, *Trans. N. Y. Acad. Sci.* **83**:551.

SOUTHAM, C. M., AND EPSTEIN, J. D., 1953, The effect of Russian encephalitis and other viruses on mouse leukemia, *Cancer Res.* **13**:581.

SOUTHAM, C. M., AND MOORE, A. E., 1952, Clinical studies of viruses as antineoplastic agents with particular reference to Egypt 101 virus, *Cancer* **5**:1025.

SQUARTINI, F., OLIVI, M., BOLIS, G. B., RIBACCHI, R., AND GIRALDO, G., 1967, Reciprocal interference between mouse mammary tumour virus and leukaemia virus, *Nature (London)* **214**:730.

STEEVES, R. A., MIRAND, E. A., THOMSON, S., AND AVILA, L., 1969, Enhancement of spleen focus formation and virus replication in Friend virus-infected mice, *Cancer Res.* **29**:1111.

STEWART, W. E., II, GOSSER, L. B., AND LOCKART, R. Z., JR., 1971, Priming: A nonantiviral function of interferon, *J. Virol.* **7**:792.

STEWART, W. E., II, GRESSER, I., TOVEY, M. G., BANDU, M-T., AND LE GOFF, S., 1976, Identification of the cell multiplication inhibitory factors in interferon preparations as interferons, *Nature* **262**:300.

ST. GEME, G. W., JR., HORRIGAN, D. S., AND TOYAMA, P. S., 1969, The effect of 6-mercaptopurine on the synthesis and action of interferon, *Proc. Soc. Exp. Biol. Med.* **130**:852.

STIM, T. B., 1970, Interference of Cocal virus with Friend leukemia virus-induced splenomegaly in DBA/2J mice, *Proc. Soc. Exp. Biol. Med.* **134**:413.

STRANDER, H., 1971, Production of interferon by suspended human leukocytes, Thesis monograph, Karolinska Institutet, Stockholm, Sweden.

STRANDER, H., AND CANTELL, K., 1966, Production of interferon by human leukocytes *in vitro*, *Ann. Med. Exp. Fenn.* **44**:265.

STRANDER, H., AND CANTELL, K., 1967, Further studies on the production of interferon by human leukocytes *in vitro*, *Ann. Med. Exp. Fen.* **45**:20.

STRANDER, H., AND CANTELL, K., 1974, Studies on antiviral and antitumor effects of human leukocyte interferon *in vitro* and *in vivo*, *Proceedings of a Tissue Culture Association Workshop, Tissue Culture Association Monograph No. 3*, Rockville, Maryland, p. 49.

STRANDER, H., CANTELL, K., CARLSTRÖM, G., AND JACOBSSON, P. A., 1973a, Clinical and laboratory investigations on man: Systemic administration of potent interferon to man, *J. Natl. Cancer Inst.* **51**:733.

STRANDER, H., JACOBSSON, P. A., CARLSTRÖM, G., AND CANTELL, K., 1973b, Administration of potent interferon to patients with malignant diseases, *Cancer Cytol.* **13**:18.

STRANDER, H., MOGENSEN, K. E., AND CANTELL, K., 1975, Production of human lymphoblastoid interferon, *J. Clin. Microbiol.* **1**:116.

STRANDER, H., CANTELL, K., INGIMARSSON, S., JAKOBSSON, P. A., NILSONNE, U., AND SÖDERBERG, G., 1976a, Interferon treatment of osteogenic sarcoma—a clinical trial, *J. Natl. Cancer Inst.*, in press.

STRANDER, H., CANTELL, K., CARLSTRÖM, G., INGIMARSSON, S., JAKOBSSON, P. A., AND NILSONNE, U., 1976b, Acute infections in interferon-treated osteosarcoma patients—preliminary report of a comparative study, *J. Infect. Dis.*, in press.

STRANDSTRÖM, H., SANDELIN, K., AND OKER-BLOM, N., 1962, Inhibitory effect of Coxsackie virus, influenza virus, and interferon on Rous sarcoma virus, *Virology* **16**:384.

STRAUSS, M. J., CHOI, S. C., AND GOLDIN, A., 1973, Increased life-span in AKR leukemia mice treated with prophylactic chemotherapy, *Cancer Res.* **33**:1724.

SUBRAHMANYAN, T. P., AND MIMS, C. A., 1966, Fate of intravenously administered interferon and the distribution of interferon during virus infections in mice, *Br. J. Exp. Pathol.* **47**:168.

SUDDITH, R. L., KELLY, P. J., HUTCHISON, H. T., MURRAY, E. A., AND HABER, B., 1975, *In vitro* demonstration of an endothelial proliferative factor produced by neural cell lines, *Science* **190**:682.

SVEC, J., NOVOTNA, L., AND THURZO, V., 1972, Toward control of tumour and virus growth by helical RNA. I. Effect of poly I:C on tumour transplantation resistance in animals bearing tumours of viral and non-viral origin, *Neoplasma* **19**:447.

SVET-MOLDAVSKY, G. J., AND CHERNYAKHOVSKAYA, I. JU., 1967, Interferon and the interaction of allogeneic normal and immune lymphocytes with L-cells, *Nature (London)* **215**:1299.

SVET-MOLDAVSKY, G. J., NEMIROVSKAYA, B. M., OSIPOVA, T. V., SLAVINA, E. G., ZINZAR, S. N., KARMONOVA, N. V., AND MOROZOVA, L. F., 1974, Interferonogenicity of antigens and "early" cytotoxicity of lymphocytes, *Folia Biol. (Prague)* **20**:225.

TAKEYAMA, H., NISHIWAKI, H., YAMADA, K., ITO, Y., AND NAGATA, I., 1975, Experimental studies on antitumor effects of interferon, personal communication in *Interferon Scientific Memoranda*, Memo I-A 164/1.

TÓTH, F. D., VACZI, L., AND BERENCSI, C., 1971, Effect of interferon treatment on the tumour-specific antibody response of Balb/c mice infected with Rauscher virus, *Acta Microbiol. Acad. Sci. Hung.* **18**:109.

TOVEY, M. G., BEGON-LOURS, J., AND GRESSER, I., 1974, A method for the large-scale production of potent interferon preparations, *Proc. Soc. Exp. Biol. Med.* **146**:809.

TOVEY, M. G., BROUTY-BOYÉ, D., AND GRESSER, I., 1975, Early effect of interferon on mouse leukemia cells cultivated in a chemostat, *Proc. Natl. Acad. Sci. U.S.A.* **72**:2265.

TOY, S. T., WEISLOW, O. S., AND WHEELOCK, E. F., 1973, Suppression of established Friend virus leukemia by statolon. VII. Relative roles of interferon and the immune response in development of FV-dormant infections, *Proc. Soc. Exp. Biol. Med.* **143**:726.

TURNER, J. C., AND MULLIKEN, B., 1950, Effects of intravenous vaccinia in mice with sarcoma 180 or leukemia 9417, *Cancer* **3**:354.

TURNER, J. C., MULLIKEN, B., AND KRITZLER, R. A., 1948, Influence of vaccine virus on a transmissible leukemia of mice, *Proc. Soc. Exp. Biol. Med.* **69**:304.

TURNER, W., CHIRIGOS, M. A., AND SCOTT, D., 1968, Enhancement of Friend and Rauscher leukemia virus replication in mice by Guaroa virus, *Cancer Res.* **28**:1064.

TURNER, W., CHAN, S. P., AND CHIRIGOS, M. A., 1970, Stimulation of humoral and cellular antibody formation in mice by poly I:C, *Proc. Soc. Exp. Biol. Med.* **133**:334.

VANDEPUTTE, M., DE LAFONTEYNE, J., BILLIAU, A., AND DE SOMER, P., 1967, Influence and production of interferon in Rauscher virus infected mice, *Arch. Ges. Virusforsch.* **20**:235.

VANDEPUTTE, M., DATTA, S. K., BILLIAU, A., AND DE SOMER, P., 1970, Inhibition of polyoma-virus oncogenesis in rats by polyriboinosinic–ribocytidylic acid, *Eur. J. Cancer* **6**:323.

WAGNER, R. R., 1965, Interferon: A review and analysis of recent observations, *Amer. J. Med.* **38**:726.

WEBB, D., BRAUN, W., AND PLESCIA, O. J., 1972, Antitumor effects of polynucleotides and theophylline, *Cancer Res.* **32**:1814.

WEINSTEIN, A. J., GAZDAR, A. F., SIMS, H. L., AND LEVY, H. B., 1971, Lack of correlation between interferon induction and antitumour effect of poly I–poly C, *Nature (London) New Biol.* **231**:53.

WEISLOW, O. S., AND WHEELOCK, E. F., 1975a, Depression of humoral immunity to sheep erythrocytes *in vitro* by Friend virus leukemic spleen cells: Induction of resistance by statolon, *J. Immunol.* **114:**211.

WEISLOW, O. S., AND WHEELOCK, E. F., 1975b, Suppression of established Friend virus leukemia by statolon: Potentiation of statolon's leukemosuppressive activity by chlorite-oxidized oxyamylose, *Infect. Immun.* **11:**129.

WEISLOW, O. S., FRIEDMAN, H., AND WHEELOCK, E. F., 1973, Suppression of established Friend virus leukemia by statolon. V. Reversal of virus-induced immunodepression to sheep erythrocytes, *Proc. Soc. Exp. Biol. Med.* **142:**401.

WHEELOCK, E. F., 1966, The effects of nontumor viruses on virus-induced leukemia in mice: Reciprocal interference between Sendaï virus and Friend leukemia virus in DBA/2 mice, *Proc. Natl. Acad. Sci. U.S.A.* **55:**774.

WHEELOCK, E. F., 1967a, Effect of statolon on Friend virus leukemia in mice, *Proc. Soc. Exp. Biol. Med.* **124:**855.

WHEELOCK, E. F., 1967b, Inhibitory effects of Sendaï virus on Friend virus leukemia in mice, *J. Natl. Cancer Inst.* **38:**771.

WHEELOCK, E. F., 1971, Mechanism of suppression of established Friend virus leukemia by statolon, *Bacteriol. Proc.*, p. 241.

WHEELOCK, E. F., AND CAROLINE, N. L., 1970, Suppression and emergence of established Friend virus leukemia: Clinical remission after statolon treatment, *Ann. N. Y. Acad. Sci.* **173:**582.

WHEELOCK, E. F., AND DINGLE, J. H., 1964, Observations on the repeated administration of viruses to a patient with acute leukemia. A preliminary report, *N. Engl. J. Med.* **271:**645.

WHEELOCK, E. F., AND LARKE, R. P., 1968, Efficacy of interferon in the treatment of mice with established Friend virus leukemia, *Proc. Soc. Exp. Biol. Med.* **127:**230.

WHEELOCK, E. F., CAROLINE, N. L., AND MOORE, R. D., 1969, Suppression of established Friend virus leukemia by statolon, *J. Virol.* **4:**1.

WHEELOCK, E. F., CAROLINE, N. L., AND MOORE, R. D., 1971, Suppression of established Friend virus leukemia by statolon. III. Development of FV-leukemogenic and FV-immunogenic activities in bloods, spleens, and lymph nodes, *J. Natl. Cancer Inst.* **46:**797.

WHEELOCK, E. F., TOY, S. T., CAROLINE, N. L., SIBAL, L. R., FINK, M. A., BEVERLY, P. C., AND ALLISON, A. C., 1972, Suppression of established Friend virus leukemia by statolon. IV. Role of humoral antibody in the development of a dormant infection, *J. Natl. Cancer Inst.* **48:**665.

WHEELOCK, E. F., TOY, S. T., WEISLOW, O. S., AND LEVY, M. H., 1974, Restored immune and nonimmune functions in Friend virus leukemic mice treated with statolon, *Prog. Exp. Tumor Res.* **19:**369.

YAMAZAKI, H., NITTA, K., AND UMEZAWA, H., 1973, Immunosuppression induced with cell-free fluid of Ehrlich carcinoma ascites and its fractions, *Gann* **64:**83.

YOUN, J. K., AND BARSKI, G., 1966, Interference between lymphocytic choriomeningitis and Rauscher leukemia in mice, *J. Natl. Cancer Inst.* **37:**381.

YOUN, J. K., BARSKI, G., AND HUPPERT, J., 1968, Inhibition de leucémigenèse virale chez la souris par traitement avec polynucléotides synthétiques, *C. R. Acad. Sci. Paris* **267:**816.

YOUNG, C. W., 1971, Interferon induction in cancer with some observations on the clinical effects of poly I:C, *Med. Clin. North Amer.* **55:**721.

ZAKAY-RONESS, Z., AND BERNKOPF, H., 1964, Effect of active and ultraviolet-irradiated inactive vaccinia virus on the development of Shay leukemia in rats, *Cancer Res.* **24:**373.

ZELEZNICK, L. D., AND BHUYAN, B. K., 1969, Treatment of leukemic (L1210) mice with double-stranded polyribonucleotides, *Proc. Soc. Exp. Biol. Med.* **130:**126.

ZUBROD, C. G., 1972, Chemical control of cancer, *Proc. Natl. Acad. Sci. U.S.A.* **69:**1042.

19

The Physiology of Endocrine Therapy

KELLY H. CLIFTON

> *I say now merely that all glands with an external secretion have at the same time, like the testicles, an internal secretion. The kidneys, the salivary glands, the pancreas are not merely organs of elimination. They are like the thyroid, the spleen, etc., organs giving to the blood important principles, either in a direct manner, or by resorption after their external secretion.*
> —*Charles-Edouard Brown-Sequard, 1891 letter quoted by Olmsted*
> *(1946), p. 216*

1. Endocrine Feedback and Homeostasis

1.1. The Beginnings of Endocrine Therapy

The near truth of Messr. Brown-Sequard's credo has only recently become recognized with the rapidly expanding knowledge of the prostaglandins and related compounds. Brown-Sequard was notable on several levels (Olmsted, 1946). He was the last in the line of great French experimentalists who dominated physiology during the 19th century. At the age of 62, he ascended to the Chair of Medicine at the University of Paris vacated by the death of his contemporary and rival, Claude Bernard. He had an intuitive conviction that the nervous and endocrine systems were intimately associated. And he, probably more than any other, was responsible for the burgeoning interest in the physiological effects of

KELLY H. CLIFTON ● Radiobiology Laboratories, Departments of Human Oncology and Radiology, University of Wisconsin Medical School, Madison, Wisconsin 53706.

organ extracts that ultimately led to the identification of hormones. Indeed, 30 years before Banting and Best, he attempted to reverse the symptoms of diabetes with pancreatic extracts.

In his later years, Messr. Brown-Sequard was preoccupied with the rejuvenating action of injections of testicular extracts. Because of his enthusiastic reports of their beneficial effects on his own person, the therapeutic efficacy of such extracts was tested against all manner of disease. A decade before Beatson (1896) performed his first oophorectomy in the treatment of breast cancer, Brown-Sequard had received reports of four breast cancer patients who were said to have benefited from his testis preparations. Indeed, among the recordings he made of his own physiological state before and after daily testis extract injection, there is detailed a marked increase in the distance he could propel a jet of urine, suggesting that he may have inadvertently instituted the first hormonal therapy for prostatic enlargement.

Although Brown-Sequard's contemporaries demonstrated the reversal of thyroparathyroidectomy-induced tetanus by injection of glandular extracts and the correction of experimental diabetes by pancreatic grafts, the practical application of endocrine therapy to clinical cancer was possible only after another half century of hormone isolation and experimentation. No matter that he was often overenthusiastic or downright wrong; without Brown-Sequard's intuition and flair, it might have been a good deal longer.

In this selective and speculative chapter, a model illustrating neuroendocrine feedback regulation, perhaps similar to that envisioned by Brown-Sequard, is discussed, exploitable sites for therapeutic intervention are reviewed, and the actions of a new group of chemical messengers—the prostaglandins—as yet unexploited in cancer therapy, are briefly described. The author can claim neither originality nor comprehensiveness for the literature review, but accepts responsibility for any errors in fact or conclusion.

1.2. Hormonal Feedback Regulation

1.2.1. Feedback Systems

The concept of feedback regulation of the several hypothalamic–hypophyseal–end-organ axes is essential to an appreciation of rational endocrine therapy (Clifton and Sridharan, 1975; Furth, 1975). It is often helpful to consider a mathematical model to illustrate how a biological system might operate, and occasionally to test the limits of one's concepts of its operation. In so doing, the temptation to confuse the model with reality must be avoided. It is a truth that a model can only be consistent or inconsistent with the data. In the former case, the model is *not proved* adequate. In the latter case, it is unequivocally proved *inadequate.*

With these reservations in mind, a simple computer simulation of a hypothalamic–pituitary–end-organ axis is described below. This program was designed to maintain the circulating levels of an end-organ hormone, T, within normal range, and to bring the levels back to normal when there has been an excursion from normal. In it, R (the hypothalamic hypophysiotropin) was assumed to be released into the hypophyseal portal system and to stimulate the production and release of S (the anterior pituitary hormone). S was assumed to be released into the general circulation, by which it reached the end-organ gland and stimulated the synthesis and release of T. Maintenance of each hormone within normal limits (arbitrarily set at near 1.0) was assumed due to one long-loop and two short-loop feedback mechanisms.

The long-loop feedback system was designed with the assumption that there is a site within the CNS, probably within the hypothalamus, that monitors the blood levels of T. If the level of T rises above 1.0, the amount of R released into the portal system is reduced, the secretion of S by the pituitary is thereby decreased, and stimulation of the T-secreting end-organ is lessened. If T falls below 1.0, R secretion increases, S increases, and the end-organ is stimulated to secrete more T. This is the principal system operating during nonstressful situations.

The first of the short-loop systems (short-loop I) involves the inhibition of hypophyseal S secretion directly by circulating T levels above a critical point. It is assumed that high levels of the end-organ hormone T act directly on the S-secreting cells of the anterior pituitary. This feedback loop is designed to function under unusual circumstances in which the blood titer of T somehow— perhaps by dietary accident or other intake from an exogenous source—reaches a dangerously high level.

The second short-loop feedback system (short-loop II) involves direct inhibition of hypothalamic R release by elevated S titers. This inhibition ultimately serves to prevent large "overshoots" and continued major oscillation around normal in the titers of S, and as a consequence of T, during correction of major deviations of T from normal.

Figures 1 and 2 show computer simulation of how such a system might work to correct two extreme deviations in T titers. In Fig. 1, it was assumed that T had abruptly fallen to 20% of the normal level, an unlikely but illustrative circumstance. The low T titer is detected by the hypothalamus (long-loop feedback),

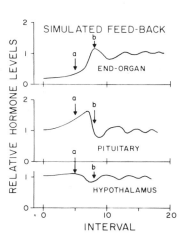

FIGURE 1. Results of computer simulation of hypothalamic–hypophyseal–end-organ axis feedback correction of a situation in which the end-organ hormone T had fallen to 20% of the normal level. The simulation program incorporates one long-loop and two short-loop feedback systems (see the text).

and an immediate modest rise in release of R into the hypophyseal portal system results. This in turn causes an increase in S release by the pituitary. By the time interval indicated by *a*, the end-organ has begun to respond with increased secretion of T. It is of importance to note that at interval *a*, the titers of R have peaked and thereafter decrease toward the norm. This occurs by short-loop feedback II—the direct suppression of R release by elevated S titers. Because the return of R to normal requires time, however, S continues to increase after R has peaked.

At point *b*, T has reached and, indeed, modestly exceeds normal, and R has passed a minimum below norm brought about by the high levels of S. As a result of the low R titers, S is now rapidly decreasing. Thereafter, the levels of all three hormones oscillate about normal, primarily as a result of the long-loop feedback effect of T on R.

In Fig. 2, initial T levels are assumed to be 5 times normal—an equally unlikely event. Under the influence of short-loop I, T directly suppresses S production by the pituitary, and by long-loop, T suppresses R release. As a result, T titers begin to fall. By the time interval *a*, when T has returned about halfway to normal, the pituitary secretion of S has reached its minimum, and hypothalamic release of R has passed its minimum. Time interval *b* marks the transition point from the control of T levels by short-loop I to control by long-loop feedback, and soon thereafter, the levels of all three hormones oscillate within narrow limits around normal. During this normal oscillation, at time interval *c*, it can be seen that the oscillations in R precede the oscillations in S, which in turn precede those in T.

Does this simple model bear any resemblance to reality? In quantitative aspects, no, but qualitatively, yes. It describes in a general fashion the control of thyroid

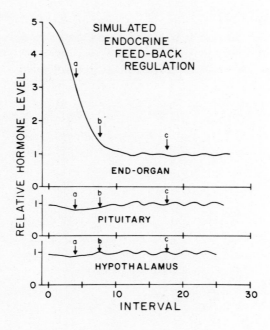

FIGURE 2. Results of computer simulation of feedback correction of a situation in which end-organ hormone T had increased to 5 times normal levels. Same program as in Fig. 1 (see the text).

hormone secretion. The hypothalamus contains thyroid hormone accumulation sites, and thyroid hormone suppresses hypothalamic release of thyrotropin-releasing hormone (TRH); i.e., there is a long-loop feedback. Elevated thyrotropic hormone (TtH) levels also suppress TRH release directly—as short-loop feedback II. And evidence from thyrotropic tumor induction studies indicates direct suppression of hypophyseal TtH release by elevated thyroid hormone levels—as in short-loop I (cf. Furth, 1975; Clifton and Sridharan, 1975). The other hypothalamic–hypophyseal–end-organ axes are also controlled by interlocking short- and long-loop feedback systems.

Why present a model based on the hypothalamic–hypophyseal–thyroid feedback mechanism when it might be said that steroid hormones are more relevant to cancer therapy? Well, thyroid neoplasia is a not insignificant problem, particularly among those exposed to ionizing radiation during infancy or childhood (*BEIR Report*, 1972; Beebe and Kato, 1975). TRH was one of the first of the hypophysiotropins to be recognized (Greer *et al.*, 1960; cf. Furth *et al.*, 1973). And finally, the broad outline of feedback regulation of thyroid hormone is one of the best understood of the axes. The control of glucocorticoid secretion is similar in many respects, acting through adrenocorticotropin-releasing hormone (ARH) and adrenocorticotropin (AtH). Testicular androgens in high titers inhibit luteinizing-hormone-releasing hormone (LRH) and gonadotropin release, and hypophyseal gonadotropin titers markedly increase in castrated animals (cf. Turner and Bagnara, 1971). CNS regulation is superimposed on this long-loop system, and through it, responses to environmental factors are possible. For example, day length controls most seasonal breeding cycles via this pathway.

The hypothalamic–hypophyseal–ovarian axis is perhaps the most complex of these systems, involving differentiation of two new glands—the follicular wall and the corpus luteum—during each female cycle (cf. Turner and Bagnara, 1971). The differentiation of these in cyclic sequence depends in turn on the capacity for cyclic activity within the hypothalamic–pituitary system. That the cyclic capacity of the female lies within the hypothalamus is illustrated by the fact that follicular development, ovulation, and corpus luteum formation resume when male anterior pituitary tissue is grafted in immediate vascular contact with the hypothalamus in histocompatible hypophysectomized females (Nikitovitch-Winer and Everett, 1958*a*, *b*). Ovulation of the ripe Graafian follicle and corpus luteum formation depend on a rapid rise in gonadotropin titers, during which luteinizing hormone (LH) may reach 50 times, and follicle-stimulating hormone (FSH) 5 times, proestrous titers in the rat (Meites *et al.*, 1972). The rapid rise is followed by an equally rapid fall. In species such as cats and rabbits in which ovulation of the mature follicle is induced by copulation, the gonadotropin surge is the result of a surge in LRH, which is brought about by nervous stimulation of the hypothalamus as a reflex response to copulatory stimulation of the uterine cervix. Estrogen is concentrated in specific regions within the hypothalamus (Keefer and Stumpf, 1975), and in spontaneously ovulating species, such as mice, dogs, and man, the preovulatory LRH and gonadotropin surges are brought about by a surge of estrogen from the ripened follicle (Nett *et al.*, 1975; cf. Turner and Bagnara, 1971). This paradoxical action of estrogen on LRH and gonadotropin release is acute and is in contrast to the inhibition of LRH and gonadotropin synthesis and secretion that results from continuously elevated estrogen levels, and to the hypersection of gonadotropins that follows ovariectomy (cf. Turner and Bagnara, 1971). The latter may be suppressed by exogenous estrogen *or* progesterone. The relative quantities of these hormones required for suppression of gonadotropin secretion suggest, however, that estrogens are the prime ovarian hormones in the control of the normal ovulatory cycle (Byrnes and Meyer, 1951; cf. Turner and Bagnara, 1971).

Mammotropin (MtH, prolactin) and somatotropin (StH, growth hormone) differ from the other anterior pituitary hormones in that their synthesis and release are controlled by hypothalamic hypophysiotropins, mammotropin-inhibiting hormone (MIH) and SIH (somatostatin), which inhibit rather than stimulate MtH and StH production and release, respectively (Talwalker *et al.*, 1963; Meites and Nicholl, 1966; Brazeau *et al.*, 1973; Friesen, 1973; Kraicer and Hymer, 1974; Arimura *et al.*, 1975). MIH is, in turn, inhibited by the neural stimulation of suckling, which leads to peaks of serum MtH during nursing, and by elevated estrogen levels. Indeed, the preovulatory surge of estrogen is followed by a surge in MtH as well as FSH and LH (Meites *et al.*, 1972). In contrast to the inhibitory effects of prolonged elevation of estrogen on secretion of LH, continuous high estrogen titers stimulate continuous MtH release, and in laboratory rats and mice, multiplication of the mammotropes, the MtH-secreting cells (Clifton and Meyer, 1956; cf. Furth and Clifton, 1966). Estrogens accumulate in the anterior pituitary (Gardner and Eisenfeld, 1975), and the action of estrogens on MtH secretion is not restricted to inhibition of MIH release, but also includes a direct stimulatory action on MtH secretion and mammotrope division (Clifton and Furth, 1961).

It is not yet clear whether there is a separate hypothalamic releasing hormone for either MtH or StH. Administration of TRH causes MtH release *in vivo* and *in vitro* (Bowers *et al.*, 1971; Meites, 1973; Mueller *et al.*, 1973; Rivier and Vale, 1974; Smith and Convey, 1975). When rats were exposed to low temperatures, however, TtH was increased but MtH decreased, and the opposite occurred at elevated temperatures (Mueller *et al.*, 1974). Thus, the role of TRH in MtH secretion under normal conditions remains obscure.

Some lessons for the endocrine therapist are clear, however. There are a number of points within neuroendocrine feedback systems that are subject, currently or potentially, to interruption or modulation, with profound effects on tumor metabolism and growth. Conversely, because of the interlocking nature of the feedback regulation loops, there is the possibility of internal compensation for the changes brought about by therapeutic intervention. And finally, for the same reasons, there is the possibility that intervention at one point can have unexpected, perhaps untoward, effects at other sites within the system. Further discussion of aspects of neuroendocrine mechanisms can be found in the reviews of Meites (1970), Guillemin (1971), Blackwell and Guillemin (1973), Furth *et al.* (1973), Furth (1975), and Clifton and Sridharan (1975).

The specificity of action of a given hormone resides in the specificity of the hormone receptor system on or within the target cell. The consequences of hormone action on a given target cell may vary as a result of previous or concurrent exposure to other hormones, or among target cells as a result of embryonic differentiation.

It is generally agreed that the principal thyroid hormones—thyroxin and triiodothyronine—bring about their effects, both on metabolic activity at the peripheral tissue level and within the hypothalamus and anterior pituitary, after entry into the cytoplasm of the target cells. There, the primary site of action appears to be on the oxidative enzyme system of the mitochondria. Since many cells convert thyroxin to triiodothyronine (Sterling *et al.*, 1973), and the conversion rate is directly related to tissue metabolic rate, it has been suggested that the conversion is necessary for full hormone action.

Of the hormone receptor systems, those of the steroid hormones have been the most thoroughly studied. And of these, estrogen receptors have received the most attention because of their obvious relevance to two of man's greatest problems—one, overpopulation, a species-threatening problem, and the other, cancer, a problem affecting altogether too many individuals. Estrogens enter the cellular cytosol in a temperature-independent fashion, and are there bound by an 8S receptor protein (McGuire and Julian, 1971; Jensen *et al.*, 1972). This binding occurs with an extraordinarily high affinity (dissociation constant of 0.1 to 10 nM), about 10,000 times greater than that of most enzyme–substrate complexes (Baulieu, 1975). A temperature-dependent transport of the estrogen–receptor complex into the nucleus is accompanied by an allosteric transition to 5S configuration, which activates the "executive site" of the hormone–receptor complex. The latter then brings about its effects by interaction with an intranuclear "acceptor," presumably a nucleohistone–chromatin structure. Gene activation ensues. Weak estrogens have lesser binding affinities than strong estrogens. Dissociation of the hormone–receptor complex with subsequent hormone catabolism can occur at any stage in the process (Baulieu, 1975).

The progesterone receptor is one of the uterine proteins that are synthesized in response to the action of the estrogen–receptor complex. The detectable quantities of the latter are increased by estrogen administration, which probably accounts for the well-known estrogen "priming" of progesterone action (cf. Turner and Bagnara, 1971). Progesterone itself appears to accelerate the decay of its own receptor protein (Baulieu, 1975), illustrating what might be termed an "ultrashort" intracellular hormonal feedback system.

Current information indicates that a sequence similar to that of estrogen reception and action obtains with corticoids and androgens as well. Testosterone is first metabolized to 5α-dihydrotestosterone in the target tissue; the latter binds with the cytosol receptor protein to form a 3.5S complex, and is then transported to the nucleus (Wilson, 1972; Voigt *et al.*, 1975). The dihydrotestosterone receptor has been described in the epididymis, prostate, seminal vesicles, preputial gland, testes, and kidneys (Voigt *et al.*, 1975).

Receptors for the small-molecular-weight catecholamines, the larger peptidic hypophysiotropins, and the even larger peptide hormones such as those of the anterior pituitary are all located on the plasma membrane. The action of all is believed to be mediated at least in part by inhibition or stimulation of synthesis of cyclic nucleotides such as adenosine-3',5'-monophosphate (cAMP) (Robison *et al.*, 1968). For example, MtH has been found to bind to the plasma membranes of mouse, rat, and rabbit mammary cells, and to some tumor cells, and placental lactogen and growth hormone compete for the binding sites at a lower affinity (Turkington, 1972; Birkinshaw and Falconer, 1972; Turkington *et al.*, 1973; Friesen *et al.*, 1973; Kelly *et al.*, 1974). The binding affinity of MtH to receptor protein on rat mammary tissue and carcinoma cells is high ($K_d = 2$–7×10^{-9} M), and the receptor is destroyed by proteolytic enzymes (Costlow *et al.*, 1975). Binding is followed by activation of a cAMP-dependent protein kinase. The nature and quantity of the proteins synthesized as a result of this action are dependent on the spectrum of other hormones to which the mammary cell is exposed at the time and has been exposed to (cf. Clifton and Sridharan, 1975).

Further discussion of hormone–target cell interactions can be found in the reviews of Robison *et al.* (1968), Mueller (1971), Jensen *et al.* (1972), O'Malley and Means (1972), Wilson (1972), Bresciani *et al.* (1973), Pitot and Yatvin (1973), Cuatrecasas (1974), King and Mainwaring (1974), Clifton and Sridharan (1975), and Baulieu (1975).

2. Exploitation of Endocrine Feedback Systems

2.1. Therapy-Sensitive Sites in Feedback Systems: Introduction

The efficacy of endocrine therapy for cancer depends on the fact that many species of cancer cells retain responsiveness to normal regulatory mechanisms; in fact, abnormalities in such regulatory mechanisms can play a role in the oncogenic process (cf. Furth, 1975; Clifton and Sridharan, 1975). The very complexity of endocrine regulatory systems renders them susceptible to therapeutic manipulation at many levels, from the receptor site on or within the target cancer cell to the release of controlling hormone secretion at sites remote from the target cell. Currently or potentially employable procedures for therapeutic manipulation of the endocrine system are summarized in Table 1, and examples are discussed in the following sections.

Because the efficacy of endocrine therapy depends on retention of responsiveness to hormones by the target cancer cells, because this retention varies among tumors of the same type, and because some endocrine therapies involve surgical or other ablative procedures, it is enormously important that methods be developed for selection of patients for whom hormonal therapy is appropriate. One approach in advanced breast cancer has been to test for the presence of estrogen receptors in biopsy or surgical tumor samples. Jensen *et al.* (1972) reported a clinical series in which 77% of those human breast tumors with

TABLE 1
Current and Potential Therapeutic Exploitation of the Endocrine System

I. Reduce hormone levels by:
    A. Surgical or radiotherapeutic ablation of:
        1. The gland that secretes a cancer-stimulating hormone
        2. Another gland that controls secretion of the cancer-stimulating hormone
    B. Clinical suppression of hormone secretion by:
        1. A drug that interferes with hormone synthesis or release
        2. A drug that acts elsewhere in the feedback system to suppress secretion of the hormone
II. Reduce effectiveness of the hormone on the cancer cell by:
    A. A competitor for the hormone receptor site
    B. A substance that alters the target-cell response to the stimulating hormone
III. Potentially, utilize hormones to:
    A. Sensitize target cells to cytotoxic agents
    B. Carry cytotoxic or sensitizing agents to target cells

detectable estrogen receptors responded to endocrine therapy, whereas only 4% of those without receptors responded. Other reports, however, have not been as encouraging (Bresciani *et al.*, 1973). The latter may be related in part to the fact that the usual receptor assay measures only the first of a complex sequence of steps. For example, carcinogen-induced rat mammary carcinomas retain marked but variable hormone responsiveness (Huggins *et al.*, 1959; Kim *et al.*, 1960; Kim and Depowski , 1975). Most of those that are unaffected by gonadectomy contain no estrogen receptor in their cytosol (McGuire and Julian, 1971; Jensen *et al.*, 1972). When uterine cytosol receptor–estrogen complex was mixed with chromatin from one such tumor, however, the estrogen–receptor complex bound to the latter as in the nuclei of responsive cells (McGuire *et al.*, 1972). In other tumors, estrogen receptor protein is present, and appears similar to that of hormone-responsive tumor lines, but the tumors do not regress after ovariectomy (Boylan and Wittliff, 1975). Thus, the presence of estrogen receptors within a mammary neoplasm bears no absolute relationship to hormone responsiveness, and further prognostic aids are required.

Horwitz *et al.* (1975) screened human tumors that contained estrogen receptors, and found that 55–60% of these tumors also contained progesterone receptor proteins. In a small series, only those mammary cancers with both receptors responded to endocrine ablation.

Much experimental evidence indicates that estrogen action on mammary tissue is in large part mediated via stimulation of MtH secretion (cf. Furth, 1973), and specific plasma membrane MtH receptors have been found on hormone-responsive rat and mouse mammary carcinoma cells (Kelly *et al.*, 1974; Turkington, 1974; Costlow *et al.*, 1975). Such receptors were markedly reduced in nonresponsive tumor lines. Study of the clinical responsiveness and progesterone and MtH receptors as well as estrogen receptors is called for.

Recently, Voigt *et al.* (1975) found that a hormone-independent subline of rat prostate carcinoma was deficient both in the capacity to convert testosterone to 5α-dihydrotestosterone and in androgen acceptor protein, as compared with the androgen-responsive tumor from which it was derived.

Alternative prognostic screening procedures based on measurement of a hormone-mediated response have been suggested, and some have the advantage that positive results demonstrate that an entire series of biochemical steps remain under hormonal influence. Hobbs *et al.* (1973) suggested that the persistence of both histologic integrity and dehydrogenase activity in biopsy samples cultured in the presence or absence of hormones might be employed as an indication of hormone responsiveness. C. Lee *et al.* (1975) described a synergism between estradiol and prolactin on the incorporation *in vitro* of [^{3}H]leucine into protein in dimethylbenzanthracene-induced mammary carcinoma tissue from regressing tumors in rats that had been ovariectomized, and Arbogast and De Sombre (1975) found stimulation of RNA synthesis by estradiol in homogenates of similarly regressing tumors. Furthermore, the effect could be demonstrated only if the cytosol fraction contained estrogen receptor protein, and only if the nuclei were from hormone-dependent regressing tumors. These techniques might form the basis for screening procedures.

Dao and Libby (1972) and Dao (1973) investigated the correlation between the ability of breast cancer tissue from postmenopausal women to sulfurylate estradiol and dehydroepiandrosterone (DHEA) and the subsequent response to adrenalectomy. Among those cases in which the ratio of DHEA:estradiol sulfation was equal to or greater than 1.0, 73% responded. Only 15% of those with ratios of less than 1.0 responded. And none of the 30 cases in which no sulfokinase activity was found received benefit from the surgery. Rose and Liskowski (1976) found that all but the near-terminal cases of those breast cancer patients with elevated corticosteroid sulfate excretion also had demonstrable estrogen receptors in their tumors. They suggest that corticosteroid sulfate excretion, particularly when coupled with positive receptor assay, may be an improved indicator of hormone responsiveness.

Continuing efforts in this area can be expected to aid greatly in the design of individualized therapeutic regimens.

2.2. Reduction in Hormone Levels

2.2.1. Ablative Procedures

The association between the male secondary sexual characteristics and the testes was obvious to mankind millenia before Brown-Sequard and the advent of scientific endocrinology, as witness the eunuchs of Chinese and Persian harems and the angel-voiced *castrati* of the medieval Roman Church. It remained for Beatson (1896) to establish the relationship between the ovaries and breast neoplasia, however, and ablation of the gonads is still an important therapeutic procedure for the most common neoplasms of Western females (breast cancer; cf. Seidman, 1969) and males (prostatic cancer; cf. Castro, 1974). The physiological basis for a positive response to these procedures is different in the two situations.

The effectiveness of orchiectomy for prostatic cancer is generally agreed to be due to the removal of the primary source of testosterone, the most active of the androgens. The experimental literature documents the atrophy of the male accessory sex glands—prostate, seminal vesicles, and preputial—after castration, and their hypertrophy on administration of exogenous androgen (cf. Turner and Bagnara, 1971). The stimulatory effect of androgens on neoplastic prostate growth thus represents the persistence of responsiveness to a hormone that under normal circumstances serves a beneficial regulatory function in maintenance of prostate size and function.

Radiological "castration" is not employed therapeutically for prostatic cancer because the androgen-secreting Leydig cells are relatively radioresistant, and the necessary radiation dose is therefore excessive. Because androgen secretion is not dependent on gametogenesis, radiation doses sufficient to cause temporary or permanent sterility may have little effect on androgen production (cf. Rubin and Casarett, 1968).

The efficacy of oophorectomy in 25% of premenopausal women with breast cancer (Lewison, 1961) depends on more complicated endocrine interrelationships. As noted above, estrogens both inhibit hypothalamic MIH release and directly stimulate hypophyseal release of MtH, as well as acting directly at the mammary cell level to moderate MtH action. Estrogen secretion by the ovary depends on follicular maturation, which includes the concurrent differentiation of a primary oocyte and its associated granulosa–theca cell complex. The absence of oogonial stem cells, and the limited number, incapacity for repopulation, and high radiosensitivity of the partially differentiated primary oocytes, renders the induction of sterility by low radiation doses (400 rads or less; cf. Rubin and Casarett, 1968) a viable alternative to surgical oophorectomy to markedly reduce cyclic estrogen secretion. Either surgical oophorectomy or radiotherapeutic sterilization also removes the source or suppresses production of progesterone.

The efficacy of therapeutic adrenalectomy, usually performed concurrently or soon after oophorectomy in premenopausal patients, or without oophorectomy after menopause, is probably due to removal of a secondary source of estrogens or perhaps estrogen precursors that are converted to estrogen elsewhere in the body (Adams and Wong, 1972; Dao, 1973; Griffiths et al., 1972). Thus, both oophorectomy and adrenalectomy depend for effectiveness in the main on removal of the sources of a hormone that in turn stimulates secretion of a second cancer-stimulating hormone, as well as acting directly on the cancer cells. Of the ablative procedures, hypophysectomy—the most extreme—goes to the heart of the matter, removing the source of TtH, AtH, and StH, as well as MtH and the gonadotropins. The interrelationship between steroid hormones and the hypophysis is illustrated by the fact that 90% of those patients who had previously responded to gonadectomy or adrenogonadectomy later responded to hypophysectomy. Of those who had not responded to steroid-secreting-gland removal, only 10% benefited from hyphophysectomy (Miller, 1970).

2.2.2. *Suppression of Hormone Secretion*

The earliest and most commonly used suppressants of hormone production are themselves hormones or hormonally active substances. For example, the administration of thyroid hormone after partial or complete thyroidectomy for thyroid cancer or goiter serves the dual function of maintaining the metabolic rate and, importantly, suppressing TRH release and TtH secretion. In the absence of exogenous thyroid hormone, thyroidectomy would result in release of TRH, and any remaining normal or neoplastic thyroid cells would be subjected to proliferative stimulation by elevated TtH levels (Sinha and Meites, 1965; cf. Turner and Bagnara, 1971).

Similarly, estrogens are widely used in the treatment of prostatic cancer (Castro, 1974). Their effects may be dual—a direct suppressive action on the prostatic cells and an indirect suppressive action—inhibition of hypothalamic LRH release, which secondarily suppresses hypophyseal LH release, and tertiarily reduces testicular production of prostate-stimulating androgens. The direct suppressive action on the prostate cells may be related to a cross-reaction with receptor protein, which normally binds androgen. For example, two cytosol receptor species were found in experimental androgen-dependent mammary carcinoma cells of a tumor strain that regressed on estrogen administration. One receptor bound estrogen with high affinity, but did not bind androgen. The other bound testosterone with high affinity, but bound estrogen also, albeit at a lower affinity (Baulieu, 1975). Estrogen apparently competes for the androgen receptor, and thereby blocks or reduces androgen action and prevents growth of this tumor line.

The hypothalamic hypophysiotropins are small peptide hormones (cf. Clifton and Sridharan, 1975). As they and their analogues become available in synthetic form, they may have great promise in direct regulation of hypophyseal function. For example, a synthetic MIH would be of great interest in experimental and clinical breast cancer work.

Some nonhormonal drugs show promise as endocrine active agents. The release of MIH is controlled, at least in part, by catacholamines. L-Dopa and the monoamine oxidase inhibitors iproniazid, pargyline, and related compounds increase MIH release and suppress serum MtH titers (Meites, 1972*a,b*). Ergot drugs, such as 2-bromo-α-ergotamine, both stimulate MIH release and directly inhibit MtH secretion (Meites, 1972*a*). Methotrexate and phenestrin suppressed the preovulatory MtH surge in rats and increased serum estrogens (Kuo *et al.*, 1975). In addition, Kuo *et al.* investigated the effects of estradiol mustard, testosterone mustard, 5-fluorouracil, vinblastine, vincristine, nitrogen mustard, and 1,3-*bis*(2-chloroethyl)-1-nitrosourea (BCNU) on serum estrogens, progesterone, MtH, and LH, and on changes in endocrine glands and end-organs. All but testosterone mustard increased either or both serum estradiol and estrone, and had varying effects on progesterone and LH. These agents, and probably other chemotherapeutic drugs, thus produce changes in the endocrine system that may be *either* synergistic *or* antagonistic to the intended effect of therapy (Kuo *et al.*, 1975).

It is to be hoped that endocrine-mediated pharmacological therapy will one day render more drastic ablative procedures obsolete.

2.3. Reduction in Hormone Effectiveness

2.3.1. Competitive Agents

This avenue is just beginning to be exploited. Once again, the greatest interest has centered on the development of "antiestrogens." Chemically, the antiestrogens currently available can be classified as "impeded estrogens" (derived from 17β-estradiol or diethylstilbestrol), or are derived from polycyclic phenols (derivatives of diphenylethylene, chlortriansene, dihydronaphthalene, diphenylindene, or nitrostyryl compounds) (Fig. 3). All except MER-25 have been shown to have some estrogenic properties (cf. Lunan and Klopper, 1975), and indeed, naturally occurring estriol has antiuterotropic effects when tested in conjunction with estradiol (cf. MacMahon et al., 1973). Furthermore, the estrogenic:antiestrogenic ratio may vary with the organ and the species studied. To be effective, the concentration of antiestrogen must approach or exceed 20 times that of natural estrogens present, and some give rise to toxic side effects in humans (Lunan and Klopper, 1975).

The "impeded" estrogens such as dimethylstilbestrol and ent-17β-estradiol compete for the estrogen binding sites on the cytosol estrogen receptor protein in the cancer cells and elsewhere in the endocrine system (Korenman, 1972). The nonsteroidal compounds such as chlomiphene and tamoxifen may act by binding to a different site on the receptor molecule in such a fashion that they alter the estrogen affinity of the receptor site. Several antiestrogens have received application in nonneoplastic gynecological disorders (Lunan and Klopper, 1975).

The nitrostyryl compound C1628, which has little uterotropic activity, was found by DeSombre and Arbogast (1974) to cause regression of a majority of

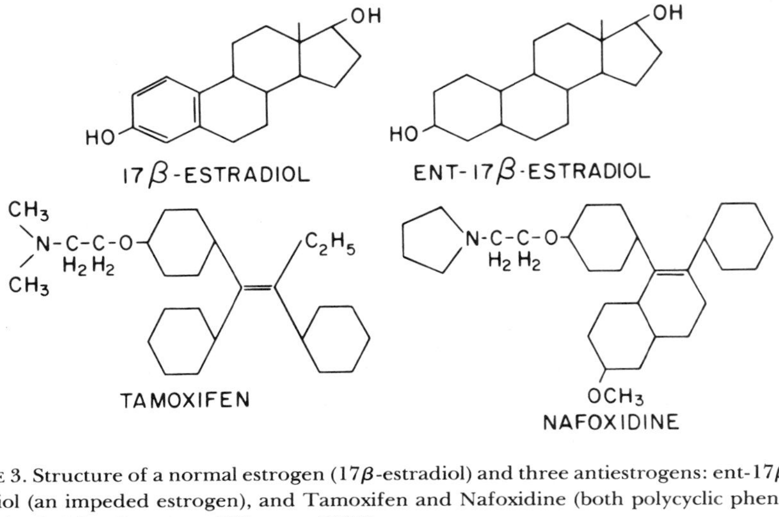

FIGURE 3. Structure of a normal estrogen (17β-estradiol) and three antiestrogens: ent-17β-estradiol (an impeded estrogen), and Tamoxifen and Nafoxidine (both polycyclic phenol derivatives). After Lunan and Klopper (1975).

dimethylbenzanthracene-induced mammary carcinomas in Sprague-Dawley rats. Of these carcinomas, 24% disappeared, and an additional 37% decreased in size by more than half. The latter regrew, despite continuing therapy, as did 27% of those that disappeared. Rapidly growing tumors that appeared soon after carcinogen treatment were the most responsive to therapy.

Results of early clinical trials in advanced breast cancer patients with nafoxidine and tamoxifen, both polycyclic phenol derivatives, are promising, and experimental evidence suggests that combined treatment regimes may be very useful. For example, regression of carcinogen-induced rat mammary carcinomas was enhanced by a combination of ovariectomy or high estrogen dosage with the MtH inhibitor ergocornine (Quadri *et al.*, 1974).

Specific antisera to the plasma membrane MtH-receptor site have been produced by Shiu and Friesen (1976), and were shown to block MtH action on normal rabbit mammary cells. A related possibility is the development of protein hormone competitors. As hormone and binding site structures become better known and understood, receptor-competing antihormonal peptides that could play an important therapeutic role in endocrine-related neoplasia may well be developed.

2.3.2. Alteration of Target Cancer Cell Responsiveness

The effectiveness of high-dose estrogen therapy for breast cancer is probably due to a modification of the target cancer cell response to MtH. High-dose estrogen therapy reduces growth of experimental mammary carcinomas in rats, even though the estrogen causes a concurrent increase in blood titers of MtH. If MtH levels are further increased in such animals by injection or by pituitary grafts, experimental mammary cancer growth is resumed (Nagasawa and Yanai, 1971; Meites *et al.*, 1971). The suppressive effect of high-dose estrogen therapy is thus dependent on a *relative* excess of estrogen over MtH. In a recent short communication, Meites *et al.* (1976) reported that high estrogen levels cause a reduction in MtH receptors on the plasma membranes of hormone-responsive mammary carcinoma cells.

A transplantable rat mammary carcinoma has been observed in the author's laboratory that grows well in the presence of elevated MtH in combination with glucocorticoid deficiency, and poorly or not at all in animals with high MtH levels and intact adrenals. Both MtH and glucocorticoids are requisite to differentiation for milk secretion (Clifton and Furth, 1960), and glucocorticoid deficiency potentiates mammary carcinoma induction by irradiation followed by high MtH levels (Clifton *et al.*, 1975). It seems likely that in the presence of elevated MtH and glucocorticoids, the cells of this experimental tumor differentiate at least partially for milk secretion. As a result, the cancer cell machinery is diverted from proliferation toward a terminal differentiation.

A neuroblastoma cell line can be caused to "differentiate" in culture by addition of cAMP or an inhibitor of cAMP phosphodiesterase. Loss of tumor-forming capacity accompanies this differentiation, and there is an increase in the response to acetylcholine, dopamine, guanosine triphosphate, and prostaglandin E_1 (Prasad *et al.*, 1975). Thus, some nonhormonal—albeit, in this case, hormone-metabolism-linked—compounds may cause shifts in "differentiation" that alter tumor cell responses to hormones.

2.4. Potential Hormone Utilization

2.4.1. Sensitization to Other Agents

The cytotoxicity of ionizing radiation and many chemotherapeutic and radiosensitizing drugs is dependent on the phase of the cell cycle at the time of exposure. For example, actinomycin D interferes with nuclear synthesis of messenger RNA, and thus inhibits production of protein enzymes, whereas the precursor molecule 5-fluorouracil (5-FU) and its product, 5-fluoro-2'-deoxyuridine (FUdR, a thymidine analogue), act by blocking the enzyme thymidylate synthetase, thus suppressing DNA synthesis. The radiosensitizing thymidine analogue 5-iodo-2'-deoxyuridine (IUdR) does not bind to the synthetase enzyme, but like thymidine is built into DNA (cf. Vermund and Gollin, 1968). Thus, the specificity of such agents is cell-cycle-, not neoplasia-, dependent, as witness the high turnover rate in normal tissues—bone marrow, intestinal epithelium—that are most sensitive to their effects. It is now generally recognized that although tumors are characterized by high proliferative rates, most contain significant numbers of slowly dividing or nondividing cells that might serve as a therapy-resistant reservoir and be responsible for local recurrence (cf. Fabrikant, 1972).

The dose limitation of both chemo- and radiotherapy is normal tissue tolerance to these powerful agents. Many procedures, e.g., radiation dose fraction regimes or local drug infusion, are employed to increase the therapeutic ratio—the ratio of damage to the neoplastic tissue as compared with that to the normal tissues. In those situations in which a significant fraction of neoplastic cells are not dividing rapidly and the neoplastic cells retain responsiveness to hormonal stimulation, the therapeutic ratio might well be increased by transient stimulation with exogenous hormone during radio- or chemotherapy, e.g., by MtH or estrogen treatment in breast cancer, or androgen administration in prostatic carcinoma. Although attractive, the possible risks in stimulating the proliferative rate of a neoplasm would make mandatory that clinical application be preceded by extensive and convincing experimental results.

2.4.2. Hormones As Carriers

To utilize hormone specificity to deliver cytotoxic or radiosensitizing agents directly to the target tumor cells is an appealing possibility. For example, boron is characterized by a high neutron cross section. On interaction with a neutron, an atom of boron disintegrates, yielding an atom of lithium and an accelerated α-particle according to the reaction $^{10}B(n, \alpha)^7Li$. The α-particle, a doubly charged helium nucleus, yields all its energy by dense ionization within about 9 μm of its site of origin. Such particles are highly damaging to any cells they traverse, and the damage is highly localized.

Attempts to utilize ^{10}B for "neutron capture therapy" have met with limited experimental success (Zahl *et al.*, 1940; Soloway, 1964). This therapy is based on the premise that if ^{10}B can be administered in a form that will concentrate in the neoplastic tissue to a greater extent than in surrounding normal tissues, when accelerated neutrons are administered, the very localized release of α-particle energy will result primarily in damage to the neoplastic cells. A major difficulty has been to achieve a sufficient beneficial ratio in boron concentration.

Certain boron-containing compounds can be coupled to proteins with minimal alteration in specificity or reactivity (Mallinger *et al.*, 1972). Carter and associates have suggested (cf. Mallinger *et al.*, 1972) that if these could be coupled to tumor-specific antibodies, a high localized concentration of boron might thereby be achieved. Alternatively, if they could be coupled to protein hormones or to antibodies to hormone binding sites—as, for example, to MtH or anti-MtH receptor (cf. Shiu and Friesen, 1976)—without destruction of specificity, a highly beneficial ratio of boron concentration in breast cancer: normal tissue might be achieved, with a corresponding increase in therapeutic ratio on exposure to neutrons.

As more is learned of target-cell metabolism of hormones, other potentially cytotoxic agents might be coupled to them that would be reactive after concentrating on or entering into target cells either while still bound or after hydrolytic or other intracellular release.

3. Potential Cancer Therapeutic Agents—The Prostaglandins and Related Compounds

3.1. Source and Structure

Since Brown-Sequard, it has been the suspicion of most endocrine physiologists that those organs classically included in the "endocrine system"—the hypophysis, thyroid, parathyroid, adrenal cortex and medulla, pancreatic islets, and gonads— were the sources of but the most obvious chemical messengers. On the face of it, the control and integration of growth, renewal, and function requires information transfer—and hence chemical messengers—within and among tissues on a much wider scale than could be explained by the products of these glands. This conclusion was further strengthened by the recognition of the GI hormones, the renin–hypertensinogen complex, and the hemopoiesis-controlling factors. And the emergence of a series of small messenger molecules of ubiquitous distribution, postulated intracellular as well as intercellular function, and minimally exploited, perhaps great, therapeutic potential has added to the list.

The prostaglandins (PGs)—so named for the site from which they were first extracted (von Euler, 1935)—are 20-carbon, unsaturated carboxylic acids contain-

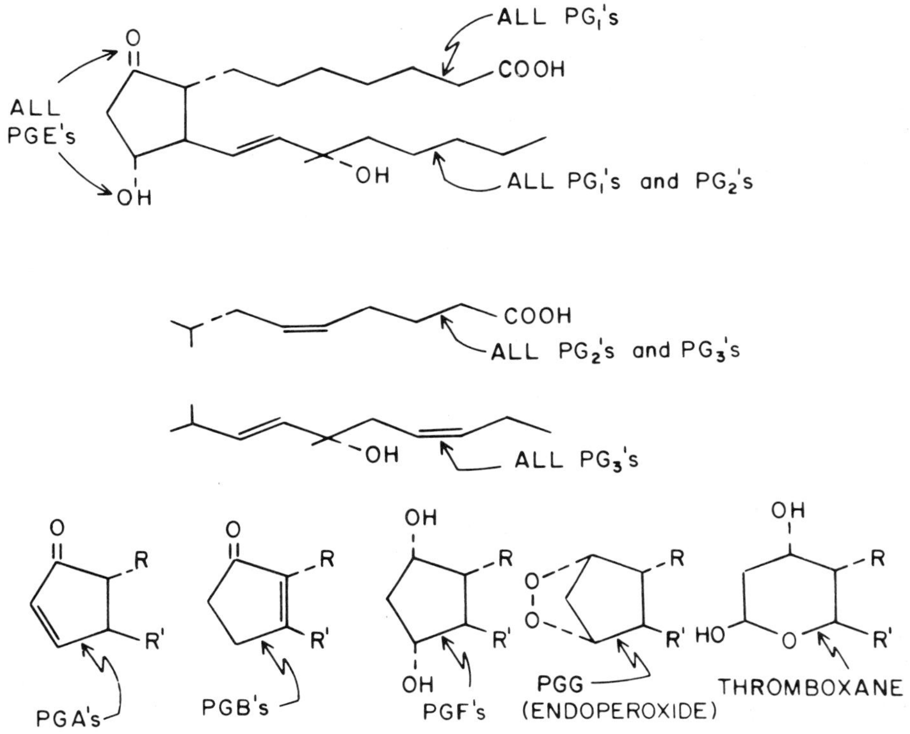

FIGURE 4. Structure of prostaglandins and related compounds. After Katz and Katz (1974) and Kolata (1975).

ing a 5-carbon ring (Fig. 4; cf. Bergstrom, 1967; Katz and Katz, 1974; Weeks, 1974; Russell *et al.*, 1975). Their immediate precursors are *bis*-homo-γ-linolenic and archidonic acids of the cellular phospholipid pool, which are in turn derived from dietary linoleic and linolenic acids. The synthetase system, which catalyzes conversion of the precursors into PGE and F *in vitro*, resides in the subcellular microsomal fraction (Hinman and Weeks, 1972). PGA and PGB are derived from PGE and F by further enzymatic action (Pike, 1972). The PG synthetase system has been found in most tissues, and there is apparently no storage of PGs in active form. The richest known mammalian PG source is human seminal fluid, but PGs are not restricted to vertebrates, having been found in high concentration in gorgonian coelenterates (Pike, 1972).

Although PGs are produced during many biological processes, the addition of exogenous PGs does not in all cases set off the process; indeed, added PGs may inhibit it. This dilemma may be solved by further study of the effects of two closely related and recently recognized classes of compounds—PG endoperoxides and thromboxanes (Fig. 4), the latter so called because of their initial isolation from thrombocytes. It now appears that the active PG-related agent in thrombocyte aggregation is thromboxane A_2, for which PG endoperoxide is a precursor. PG endoperoxides are very, and thromboxane A_2 enormously, labile in neutral aqueous solution (cf. Kolata, 1975). Although the PGs themselves may ultimately prove to be precursors or modulators of thromboxane action or production, they have been studied in their own right, and possess significant and important biological effects.

3.2. Prostaglandin Pharmacology

Prostaglandins have been most intensively studied in relationship to their roles in vascular physiology and reproduction. The vascular and reproductive effects appear to be largely mediated by actions on smooth or cardiac muscle. Vascular actions include pressor effects in many species (DuCharme and Weeks, 1967), cardiac rate control (Vergroesen *et al.*, 1967), control of renal blood distribution, and a possible role in essential hypertension (J. B. Lee, 1967; McGiff *et al.*, 1974). Effects on reproduction include stimulation of myometrial contractility and a consequent role in premature labor (Bygdeman *et al.*, 1967), sperm transport (Labhsetwar, 1974), initiation of parturition, and involution of the corpus luteum (Kirton *et al.*, 1972). PG effects on myometrial contractility involve modulation of intracellular calcium release and restorage in the sarcoplasmic reticulum. Released intracellular calcium triggers contraction of the actomycin filaments (Carsten, 1972).

PGs interact with other pressor hormones. PGE_1 inhibits vasopressin-induced cAMP formation in renal collecting tubules (Orloff and Grantham, 1967) and epinephrine-induced cAMP formation in the toad bladder (Steinberg and Vaughan, 1967). In general, it may be said that PGEs are the major class released as the result of nervous stimulation, and that they usually inhibit adrenergic transmission at a postjunctional level. In some cases, this effect results from inhibition of transmitter release at the nerve terminus. PGFs, in contrast, facilitate responses to sympathetic nerve stimulation, may increase the response of effector organs to norepinephrine, and facilitate catecholamine release by the adrenal medulla. PGF_2 and E_1 are believed to compete for the same receptor sites on vascular smooth muscle (Brody and Kadowitz, 1974).

Recent data suggest that PGs play a role in the function of the hypothalamic–hypophyseal system. PGF_2 appears in cerebral venous blood of anestrous sheep in a regular circhoral rhythm. When estradiol is infused to induce LH release, the magnitude of F_2 pulses is at first suppressed, but returns and even exceeds normal concurrently with the estrogen-induced preovulatory LH surge. Roberts and McCracken (1975) suggest that the estrogen effect is mediated through modulation of PG release by the brain. Ovulation has been induced in pentobarbital-blocked rats by administration of PGE_2 (Labhsetwar, 1974), and in rats in late pregnancy, acute PGE_1 administration induced release of TtH and MtH, and at the highest doses, LH (D'Angelo *et al.*, 1975). In adult male rat pituitary glands *in vitro*, in contrast, PGE_1, E_2, F_1, or F_2 administration was found to potentiate hypothalamic-extract-induced TtH release, but at the doses employed, did not consistently alter LH, FSH, or MtH release. All significantly increased StH release, however, and there was a parallel increase in hypophyseal cAMP concentration.

Administration of indomethacin, a PG synthetase inhibitor, suppressed StH and TtH release, but potentiated hypothalamic-hormone-induced gonadotropin release (Sundberg *et al.*, 1975).

3.3. Prostaglandins and Tumors

PGs are released by a number of clinical and experimental tumors, and their effects on both tumor-associated syndromes and on tumor growth are under expanding investigation. PGE_2 and F_2 are increased in the sera of medullary thyroid cancer patients, appear in media of cultured medullary cancer cells, and may be responsible for the diarrhea commonly seen in such cases. The severity of vasomotor complaints in patients with Kaposi's sarcoma increases in direct relationship to the E_2 and F_2 serum titers. Tissue PGs are elevated in ganglioneuromas, neuroblastomas, pheochromocytomas, and pancreatic alpha cell tumors. All these are also characterized by secretion of amine peptides (cf. Jaffe, 1974). Experimental evidence suggests that PG production may be related to tumor growth rate and characteristics. Tan *et al.* (1974) found that PGE_2 is the major PG product of both normal rat mammary gland and carcinogen-induced mammary tumors. The neoplasms were richest both in the capacity to synthesize PG and in PG concentration. In addition, cells from the mouse fibrosarcoma strain HSDM release PGE_2 and cause bone resorption *in vitro*. *In vivo*, this tumor causes elevated serum E_2 and calcium. Treatment of HSDM-grafted mice with the PG synthetase inhibitor indomethacin decreased both serum calcium and E_2, and slowed both tumor growth and bone resorption (Tashjian *et al.*, 1974). Indomethacin also reduced the number of bone metastases from grafted Walker carcinosarcoma in rats (cf. Jaffe, 1974). Experimental tumor strain $BP8/P_1$ and sarcoma 180, as well as Maloney sarcoma virus-induced tumors in mice, release PGs. In tumors of the latter type, indomethacin reduced PG production and final tumor size, but had no effect on cAMP.

Paradoxically, in four cultured cell lines—HeLa, HEp2, L, and HT-29—cell division appears to be inversely related to PG production and concentration. Decreased proliferation results from addition of PGE_1 or stimulation of endogenous PG synthesis by addition of dibutyryl cAMP. Addition of indomethacin increases proliferation.

Evidence of differentiation can be induced in a cultured neuroblastoma cell line by addition of cAMP to the medium, or by adding an inhibitor (R020-1724) of cAMP phosphodiesterase. This "differentiation" is accompanied by an increase in RNA, protein, cell size, and the enzymes tyrosine hydroxylase, choline acetyltransferase, and acetylcholinesterase, and by a loss in tumorigenicity. Acetylcholine, dopamine, and guanosine triphosphate (GTP) all increase adenylate cyclase more in the "differentiated" than in the undifferentiated neuroblastoma cell line, and PGE_1 potentiates the GTP effect (Prasad *et al.*, 1975).

Recent preliminary evidence indicates that the response of the vasculature of the V2 rabbit carcinoma to norepinephrine and to PGE_2 differs from that of surrounding normal tissues (Rankin and Phernetton, 1976). If this is a common phenomenon, it might be utilized to increase the therapeutic ratio of drugs or radiation or both.

This brief selective overview was designed primarily to call attention to a group of natural molecules with diverse, often paradoxical, effects. It is presented with the conviction that the PGs and related endoperoxides and thromboxanes will one day find important clinical application in cancer therapy.

4. Closing Remarks

As hormone excess or deficiency may accelerate or even cause neoplasia by perversion of a normal target cell response—i.e., as an abnormal hormonal environment may precipitate neoplasia in a normal cell population (cf. Furth, 1975; Clifton and Sridharan, 1975)—just so the efficacy of endocrine therapy is dependent on at least partial retention of hormone responsiveness by neoplastic cells. Considering the relatively small changes in proliferative rate and cell life span and function required to produce excess cell masses—tumors—in metazoans, it would be surprising if neoplastic tissues did not often retain vestigial responsiveness to normal regulatory mechanisms. After all, cancer biochemists have been preoccupied for decades with the search for chemical characteristics unique to cancer cells with but limited success. Indeed, cancer cells have more features in common with normal cells than features in which they differ. The specificity of endocrine therapy is unique among anticancer modalities, and is in marked contrast to those therapies that depend only or primarily on rapid proliferation of their target cells. As more is learned of hormone receptor sites, hormone interactions, and more subtle intercellular messenger molecules, this specificity and effectiveness will be increased.

The use of hormones in combined therapy has yet to be fully exploited. In such use, the tendency to consider hormones as just another class of cytotoxic agents comparable to the bacterial antimetabolites should be avoided. That cytotoxicity that some hormones may possess for some specific cells is most probably the result of induction of partial or complete terminal differentiation—not the result of interference with an essential metabolic process.

Finally, in the use of endocrine manipulation in therapy—whether by surgery or irradiation or hormone or drug administration—it should be recognized that the response of a target cell to a given hormone may depend on past or concurrent exposure to other hormones. It should also be recognized that alterations in the elegant feedback regulatory system can lead to sometimes unpredicted and untoward effects at other sites.

ACKNOWLEDGMENTS

Work in this laboratory is supported by American Cancer Society Grant PDT-46Q, National Cancer Institute Grant CA-13881, and Cancer Center Grant

CA-14520, National Cancer Institute. The author acknowledges with gratitude the aid of Ms. Linda Frentzel.

5. References

ADAMS, J. B., AND WONG, M., 1972, Paraendocrine behavior of human breast cancer, in: *Estrogen Target Tissues and Neoplasia* (T. L. Dao, ed.), pp. 125–150, University of Chicago Press, Chicago.

ARBOGAST, L. Y., AND DE SOMBRE, E. R., 1975, Estrogen-dependent *in vitro* stimulation of RNA synthesis in hormone-dependent mammary tumors in the rat, *J. Natl. Cancer Inst.* **54:**483–485.

ARIMURA, A., SATO, H., COY, D. H., AND SCHALLY, A. V., 1975, Radioimmunoassay for GH-release inhibiting hormone, *Proc. Soc. Exp. Biol. Med.* **148:**784–789.

BAULIEU, E., 1975, Steroid receptors and hormone receptivity, *J. Amer. Med. Assoc.* **234:**404–409.

BEATSON, G. T., 1896, On treatment of inoperable cases of carcinoma of the mamma: Suggestions for a new method of treatment, with illustrative cases, *Lancet* **2:**104.

BEEBE, G. W., AND KATO, H., 1975, Cancers other than leukemia, *J. Radiat. Res. (Japan) Suppl.,* pp. 97–107.

BEIR REPORT, 1972, *The Effects on Population of Exposure to Low Levels of Ionizing Radiation* (Report of the Advisory Committee on the Biological Effects of Ionizing Radiations), National Academy of Sciences—National Research Council, Washington, D.C.

BERGSTROM, S., 1967, Isolation, structure and action of the prostaglandins, in: *Prostaglandins: Nobel Symposium 2* (S. Bergstrom and B. Samuelsson, eds.), pp. 21–30, Interscience Publishers, New York.

BIRKINSHAW, M., AND FALCONER, I. R., 1972, The localization of prolactin labelled with radioactive iodine in rabbit mammary tissue, *J. Endocrinol.* **55:**323.

BLACKWELL, R. E., AND GUILLEMIN, R., 1973, Hypothalamic control of adenohypophysial secretions, *Annu. Rev. Physiol.* **35:**357.

BOWERS, C. Y., FRIESEN, H. G., HWANG, P., GUYDA, H. J., AND FOLKERS, K., 1971, Prolactin and thyrotropin release in man by synthetic pyriglutamyl-histidyl-prolinamide, *Biochem. Biophys. Res. Commun.* **45:**1033.

BOYLAN, E. S., AND WITTLIFF, J. L., 1975, Specific estrogen binding in rat mammary tumors induced by 7,12-dimethyl(α)benzanthracene, *Cancer Res.* **35:**506–511.

BRAZEAU, P., VALE, W., BURGESS, R., LING, N., BUTCHER, M., RIVIER, J., AND GUILLEMIN, R., 1973, Hypothalamic polypeptide that inhibits the secretion of immunoreactive pituitary growth hormone, *Science* **179:**77–79.

BRESCIANI, F., NOLA, E., SICO, V., AND PUCA, G. A., 1973, Early stages in estrogen control of gene expression and its derangement in cancer, *Fed. Proc. Fed. Amer. Soc. Exp. Biol.* **32:**2126–2132.

BRODY, M. J., AND KADOWITZ, P. J., 1974, Prostaglandins as modulators of the autonomic nervous system, *Fed. Proc. Fed. Amer. Soc. Exp. Biol.* **33:**48–60.

BYGDEMAN, M., KWAN, S., AND WIQVIST, N., 1967, The effect of prostaglandin E_1 on human pregnant myometrium *in vivo,* in: *Prostaglandins: Nobel Symposium 2* (S. Bergstrom and B. Samuelsson, eds.), pp. 93–96, Interscience Publishers, New York.

BYRNES, W. W., AND MEYER, R. K., 1951, The inhibition of gonadotrophic hormone secretion by physiological doses of estrogen, *Endocrinology* **48:**133–136.

CARSTEN, M. E., 1972, Prostaglandin's part in regulating uterine contraction by transport of calcium, in: *The Prostaglandins: Clinical Applications in Human Reproduction* (E. M. Southern, ed.), pp. 59–66, Futura Publishing Co., Mt. Kisco, New York.

CASTRO, J. E., 1974, *The Treatment of Prostatic Hypertrophy and Neoplasia,* University Park Press, Balitmore.

CLIFTON, K. H., AND FURTH, J., 1960, Ducto-alveolar growth in mammary glands of adrenogonadectomized male rats bearing mammotropic pituitary tumors, *Endocrinology* **66:**803.

CLIFTON, K. H., AND FURTH, J., 1961, Changes in hormone sensitivity of pituitary mammotropes during progression from normal to autonomous, *Cancer Res.* **21:**913.

CLIFTON, K. H., AND MEYER, R. K., 1956, Mechanism of anterior pituitary tumor induction by estrogen, *Anat. Rec.* **125:**65.

CLIFTON, K. H., AND SRIDHARAN, B. N., 1975, Endocrine factors and tumor growth, in: *Cancer: A Comprensive Treatise,* Vol. 3 (F. F. Becker, ed.), pp. 249–285, Plenum Press, New York.

CLIFTON, K. H., SRIDHARAN, B. N., AND DOUPLE, E. B., 1975, Mammary carcinogenesis-enhancing effect of adrenalectomy in irradiated rats with pituitary tumor MtT-F4, *J. Natl. Cancer Inst.* **55:**485–487.

COSTLOW, M. E., BUSCHOW, R. A., RICHERT, N. J., AND McGUIRE, W. L., 1975, Prolactin and estrogen binding in transplantable hormone-dependent and autonomous rat mammary carcinoma, *Cancer Res.* **35:**970–974.

CUATRECASAS, P., 1974, Membrane receptors, *Annu. Rev. Biochem.* **43:**169.

D'ANGELO, S. A., WALL, N. R., AND BOWERS, C. Y., 1975, Prostaglandin administration to pregnant rats: Effects on pituitary–target gland systems of mother, fetus and neonate, *Proc. Soc. Exp. Biol. Med.* **148:**227–235.

DAO, T. L., 1973, Advances in breast cancer research, in: *Perspectives in Cancer Research and Treatment* (G. P. Murphy, ed.), pp. 31–49, A. R. Liss, New York.

DAO, T. L., AND LIBBY, P. R., 1972, Steroid sulfate formation in human breast tumors and hormone dependency, in: *Estrogen Target Tissues and Neoplasia* (T. L. Dao, ed.), pp. 181–200, University of Chicago Press, Chicago.

DeSOMBRE, E. R., AND ARBOGAST, L. Y., 1974, Effect of antiestrogen C1628 on the growth of rat mammary tumors, *Cancer Res.* **34:**1971–1976.

DuCHARME, D. W., AND WEEKS, J. R., 1967, Cardiovascular pharmacology of prostaglandin $F_{2\alpha}$, a unique pressor agent, in: *Prostaglandins: Nobel Symposium 2* (S. Bergstrom and B. Samuelsson, eds.), pp. 173–181, Interscience Publishers, New York.

FABRIKANT, J. I., 1972, *Radiobiology*, Year Book Medical Publishers, Chicago.

FRIESEN, H. G., 1973, Prolactin, its control and clinical significance, *Clinc. Sci.* **44**(2):2p.

FRIESEN, H., TOLIS, G., SHIU, R., AND HUANG, P., 1973, Studies on human prolactin: Chemistry, radioreceptor assay and clinical significance, in: *Human Prolactin: Proceedings of the International Symposium on Human Prolactin* (J. L. Pasteels and C. Robyn, eds.), pp. 11–23, American Elsevier, New York.

FURTH, J., 1973, The role of prolactin in mammary carcinogenesis, in: *Human Prolactin: Proceedings of the International Symposium on Human Prolactin* (J. L. Pasteels and C. Robyn, eds.), pp. 233–248, American Elsevier, New York.

FURTH, J., 1975, Hormones as etiological agents in neoplasia, in: *Cancer: A Comprehensive Treatise*, Vol. 1 (F. F. Becker, ed.), pp. 75–120, Plenum Press, New York.

FURTH, J. AND CLIFTON, K. H., 1966, Experimental pituitary tumors, in: *The Pituitary Gland*, Vol. 2 (G. W. Harris and B. T. Donovan, eds.), pp. 460–498, Butterworths, London.

FURTH, J., UEDA, G., AND CLIFTON, K. H., 1973, The pathophysiology of pituitaries and their tumors: Methodological advances, in: *Methods in Cancer Research*, Vol. 10 (H. Busch, ed.), pp. 201–277, Academic Press, New York.

GARDNER, W. U., AND EISENFELD, A. J., 1975, Accumulation of ^{3}H-estradiol in the vaginas and pituitary glands of mice of inbred strains, *Proc. Soc. Exp. Biol. Med.* **148:**909–912.

GREER, M. A., YAMADA, T., AND IINO, S., 1960, The participation of the nervous system in the control of thyroid function, *Ann. N. Y. Acad. Sci.* **86:**667–675.

GRIFFITHS, K., JONES, D., CAMERON, E. H. D., GLEAVE, E. N., AND FORREST, A. P. M., 1972, Transformation of steroids by mammary cancer tissue, in: *Estrogen Target Tissues and Neoplasia* (T. L. Dao, ed.), pp. 151–162, University of Chicago Press, Chicago.

GUILLEMIN, R., 1971, Hypothalamic control of the secretion of adenohypophysial hormones, *Adv. Metab. Disord.* **5c:**1.

HINMAN, J. W., AND WEEKS, J. R., 1972, The prostaglandins: Biology and biochemistry, in: *The Prostaglandins: Clinical Applications in Human Reproduction* (E. M. Southern, ed.), pp. 31–36, Futura Publishing Co., New York.

HOBBS, J. R., SALIH, H., FLAX, H., AND BRANDER, W., 1973, Prolactin dependence among human breast cancers, in: *Human Prolactin* (J. L. Pasteels and C. Robyns, eds.), pp. 249–258, Excerpta Medica, Amsterdam, and American Elsevier, New York.

HORWITZ, K. B., McGUIRE, W. L., PEARSON, O. H., AND SEGALOFF, A., 1975, Predicting response to endocrine therapy in human breast cancer: A hypothesis, *Science* **189:**726, 727.

HUGGINS, C., BRIZIARELLI, G., AND SUTTON, H., 1959, Rapid induction of mammary carcinoma in the rat and the influence of hormones on the tumors, *J. Exp. Med.* **109:**25.

JAFFE, B. M., 1974, Prostaglandins and cancer: An update, *Prostaglandins* **6:**453–461.

JENSEN, E. V., BLOCK, G. E., SMITH, S., KYSER, K., AND DE SOMBRE, E. R., 1972, Estrogen receptors and hormone dependency, in: *Estrogen Target Tissues and Neoplasia* (T. L. Dao, ed.), pp. 23–57, University of Chicago Press, Chicago.

KATZ, R. L., AND KATZ, G. J., 1974, Prostaglandins—basic and clinical considerations, *Anesthesiology* **40**:471–493.

KEEFER, D. A., AND STUMPF, W. E., 1975, Atlas of estrogen-concentrating cells in the central nervous system of the squirrel monkey, *J. Comp. Neurol.* **160**:419–441.

KELLY, P. A., BRADLEY, C., SHIU, R. P. C., MEITES, J., AND FRIESEN, H. G., 1974, Prolactin binding to rat mammary tumor tissue, *Proc. Soc. Exp. Biol. Med.* **146**:816–819.

KIM, U., AND DEPOWSKI, M. J., 1975, Progression from hormone dependence to autonomy in mammary tumors as an *in vivo* manifestation of sequential clonal selection, *Cancer Res.* **35**:2068–2077.

KIM, U., FURTH, J., AND CLIFTON, K. H., 1960, Relation of mammary tumors to mammotropes. III. Hormone responsiveness of transplanted mammary tumors, *Proc. Soc. Exp. Biol. Med.* **103**:646.

KING, R. J. B., AND MAINWARING, W. I. P., 1974, *Steroid–Cell Interactions*, Butterworths, London.

KIRTON, K. T., GUTKNECHT, G. D., BERGSTROM, K. K., WYNGARDEN, L. J., AND FORBES, A. D., 1972, in: *The Prostaglandins: Clinical Applications in Human Reproduction* (E. M. Southern, ed.), pp. 37–46, Futura Publishing Co., Mt. Kisco, New York.

KOLATA, G. B., 1975, Research news: Thromboxanes, the power behind the prostaglandins? *Science* **190**:770.

KORENMAN, S. G., 1972, Human breast cancer as a steroid hormone target, in: *Estrogen Target Tissues and Neoplasia* (T. L. Dao, ed.), pp. 59–67, University of Chicago Press, Chicago.

KRAICER, J., AND HYMER, W. C., 1974, Purified somatotrophs from rat adenohypophysis: Response to secretagogues, *Endocrinology* **94**:1525–1530.

KUO, E. Y. H., ESBER, H. J., TAYLOR, D. J., AND BOGDEN, A. E., 1975, Effects of cancer chemotherapeutic agents on endocrine organs and serum levels of estrogens, progesterone, prolactin, and luteinizing hormone, *Cancer Res.* **35**:1975–1980.

LABHSETWAR, A. P., 1974, Prostaglandins and the reproductive cycle, *Fed. Proc. Fed. Amer. Soc. Exp. Biol.* **33**:61–77.

LEE, C., OYASU, R., AND CHEN, C., 1975, *In vitro* interaction of estrogen and prolactin on hormone-dependent rat mammary tumors, *Proc. Soc. Exp. Biol. Med.* **148**:224–226.

LEE, J. B., 1967, Chemical and physiological properties of renal prostaglandins: The antihypertensive effects of medullin in essential human hypertension, in: *Prostaglandins: Nobel Symposium 2* (S. Bergstrom and B. Samuelsson, eds.), pp. 197–210, Interscience Publishers, New York.

LEWISON, E. F., 1961, Prophylactic versus therapeutic castration in the total treatment of breast cancer, in: *Proceedings of the Fourth National Cancer Conference*, pp. 263–265, Lippincott, Philadelphia.

LUNAN, C. B., AND KLOPPER, A., 1975, Antiestrogens: A review, *Clin. Endocrinol.* **4**:551–572.

MACMAHON, B., COLE, P., AND BROWN, J., 1973, Etiology of human breast cancer: A review, *J. Natl. Cancer Inst.* **50**:21.

MALLINGER, A. G., JOZWIAK, E. L., AND CARTER, J. C., 1972, Preparation of boron-containing bovine γ-globulin as a model compound for a new approach to slow neutron therapy of tumors, *Cancer Res.* **32**:1947–1950.

MCGIFF, J. C., CROWSHAW, K., AND ITSHOVITZ, H. D., 1974, Prostaglandins and renal function, *Fed. Proc. Fed. Amer. Soc. Exp. Biol.* **33**:39–47.

MCGUIRE, W. L., AND JULIAN, J. A., 1971, Comparison of macromolecular binding of estradiol in hormone-dependent and hormone-independent rat mammary carcinoma, *Cancer Res.* **31**:1440.

MCGUIRE, W. L., HUFF, K., JENNINGS, A., AND CHAMNESS, G. C., 1972, Mammary carcinoma: A specific biochemical defect in autonomous tumors, *Science* **175**:335.

MEITES, J., 1970, *Hypophysiotropic Hormones of the Hypothalamus: Assay and Chemistry*, Williams and Wilkins, Baltimore.

MEITES, J., 1972a, Relation of prolactin and estrogen to mammary tumorigenesis in the rat, *J. Natl. Cancer Inst.* **48**:1217.

MEITES, J., 1972b, The relation of estrogen and prolactin to mammary tumorigenesis in the rat, in: *Estrogen Target Tissues and Neoplasia* (T. L. Dao, ed.), pp. 275–286, University of Chicago Press, Chicago.

MEITES, J., 1973, Control of prolactin secretion in animals, in: *Human Prolactin: Proceedings of the International Symposium on Human Prolactin* (J. L. Pasteels and C. Robyn, eds.), pp. 104–118, American Elsevier, New York.

MEITES, J., AND NICOLL, C. S., 1966, Adenohypophysis; prolactin, *Annu. Rev. Physiol.* **28**:57.

MEITES, J., CASSELL, E., AND CLARK, J., 1971, Estrogen inhibition of mammary tumor growth in rats; counteraction by prolactin, *Proc. Soc. Exp. Biol. Med.* **137**:1225.

MEITES, J., LU, K. H., WUTTKE, W., WELSCH, C. W., NAGASAWA, H., AND QUADRI, S. K., 1972, Recent studies on functions and control of prolactin secretion in rats, *Recent Prog. Horm. Res.* **28**:171.

MEITES, J., KLEDZIK, G., BRADLEY, C., MARSHALL, S., AND CAMPBELL, G., 1976, Role of prolactin receptors in inhibition of mammary tumor growth by large doses of estrogen, *Proceedings of the 10th Meeting on Mammary Cancer in Experimental Animals and Man*, Kobe, Japan, March 29–31, p. 93, (abstract).

MILLER, T. R., 1970, Hypophysectomy, in: *Breast Cancer: Early and Late* (The University of Texas, M. D. Anderson Hospital and Tumor Institute at Houston), pp. 377–380, Year Book Medical Publishers, Chicago.

MUELLER, G. P., 1971, Estrogen action: A study of the influence of steroid hormones on genetic expression, *Biochem. Soc. Symp.* **32**:1–29.

MUELLER, G. P., CHEN, H. J., AND MEITES, J., 1973, *In vivo* stimulation of prolactin release in the rat by synthetic TRH, *Proc. Soc. Exp. Biol. Med.* **144**:613–615.

MUELLER, G. P., CHEN, H. T., DIBBIT, J. A., CHEN, H. J., AND MEITES, J., 1974, Effects of warm and cold temperatures on release of TSH, GH, and prolactin in rats, *Proc. Soc. Exp. Biol. Med.* **147**:698–700.

NAGASAWA, H., AND YANAI, R., 1971, Reduction by pituitary isograft of inhibitory effect of large dose of estrogen on incidence of mammary tumors induced by carcinogen in ovariectomized rats, *Int. J. Cancer* **8**:463.

NETT, T. M., AKBAR, A. M., PHEMISTER, R. D., HOLST, P. A., REICHERT, L. E., AND NISWENDER, G. D., 1975, Levels of luteinizing hormone, estradiol and progesterone in serum during the estrous cycle and pregnancy in the beagle bitch, *Proc. Soc. Exp. Biol. Med.* **148**:134–139.

NIKITOVICH-WINER, M., AND EVERETT, J. W., 1958a, Comparative study of luteotropin secretion by hypophysial autotransplants in the rat: Effects of site and stages of the estrous cycle, *Endocrinology* **62**:522.

NIKITOVICH-WINER, M., AND EVERETT, J. W., 1958b, Functional restitution of pituitary grafts re-transplanted from kidney to median eminence, *Endocrinology* **63**:916.

OLMSTED, J. M. D., 1946, *Charles-Edouard Brown-Sequard: A Nineteenth Century Neurologist and Endocrinologist*, The Johns Hopkins Press, Baltimore.

O'MALLEY, B. W., AND MEANS, A., 1972, Molecular biology and estrogen regulation of target growth and differentiation, in: *Estrogen Target Tissues and Neoplasia* (T. L. Dao, ed.), pp. 3–22, University of Chicago Press, Chicago.

ORLOFF, J., AND GRANTHAM, J., 1967, The effect of prostaglandin (PGE_1) on the permeability response of rabbit collecting tubules to vasopressin, in: *Prostaglandins: Nobel Symposium 2* (S. Bergstrom and B. Samuelsson, eds.), pp. 143–146, Interscience Publishers, New York.

PIKE, J. E., 1972, Prostaglandin chemistry, in: *The Prostaglandins: Clinical Applications in Human Reproduction* (E. M. Southern, ed.), pp. 23–36, Futura Publishing Co., Mt. Kisco, New York.

PITOT, H. C., AND YATVIN, M. B., 1973, Interrelationships of mammalian hormones and enzyme levels *in vivo*, *Physiol. Rev.* **53**:228.

PRASAD, K. N., GILMER, K. N., SAHU, S. K., AND BECKER, G., 1975, Effect of neurotransmitters, guanosine triphosphate, and divalent ions on the regulation of adenylate cyclase activity in malignant and adenosine cyclic 3'5'-monophosphate-induced "differentiated" neuroblastoma cells, *Cancer Res.* **35**:77–81.

QUADRI, S. K., KLEDZIK, G. S., AND MEITES, J., 1974, Enhanced regression of DMBA-induced mammary cancers in rats by combination of ergocornine with ovariectomy or high doses of estrogen, *Cancer Res.* **34**:499–501.

RANKIN, J. H. G., AND PHERNETTON, T., 1976, Effect of prostaglandin E_2 on blood flow to the V2 carcinoma, *Fed. Proc. Fed. Amer. Soc. Exp. Biol.* **35**:297 (abstract).

RIVIER, C., AND VALE, W., 1974, *In vivo* stimulation of prolactin secretion in the rat by thyrotropin releasing factor, related peptides and hypothalamic extracts, *Endocrinology* **95**:978–983.

ROBERTS, J. S., AND McCRACKEN, J. A., 1975, Prostaglandin F_2 production by the brain during estrogen-induced secretion of luteinizing hormone, *Science* **190**:894–896.

ROBISON, G. A., BUTCHER, R. W., AND SUTHERLAND, E. W., 1968, Cyclic AMP, *Annu. Rev. Biochem.* **37**:199.

ROSE, D. P., AND LISKOWSKI, L., 1976, Corticosteroid sulfate excretion and estrogen receptors in breast cancer, *Clin. Chim. Acta* **67**:183–188.

RUBIN, P., AND CASARETT, G. W., 1968, *Clinical Radiation Pathology*, Vol. 1, W. B. Saunders Company, Philadelphia.

RUSSELL, P. T., EBERLE, A. J., AND CHENG, H. C., 1975, The prostaglandins in clinical medicine. A developing role for the clinical chemist, *Clin. Chem.* **21**:653–666.

SEIDMAN, H., 1969, *Cancer of the Breast: Statistical and Epidemiological Data*, American Cancer Society, New York.

SHIU, R. P. C., AND FRIESEN, H. G., 1976, Blockade of prolactin action by an antiserum to its receptors, *Science* **192**:259–261.

SINHA, D., AND MEITES, J., 1965, Effects of thyroidectomy and thyroxine on hypothalamic concentration of "thyrotropin releasing factor" and pituitary content of thyrotropin in rats, *Neuroendocrinology* **1**:4.

SMITH, V. G., AND CONVEY, E. M., 1975, TRH-stimulation of prolactin release from bovine pituitary cells, *Proc. Soc. Exp. Biol. Med.* **149**:70–74.

SOLOWAY, A. H., 1964, Boron compounds in cancer therapy, in: *Progress in Boron Chemistry* (H. Steinberg and A. L. McCloskey, eds.), pp. 203–234, MacMillan Co., New York.

STEINBERG, D., AND VAUGHAN, M., 1967, *In vitro* and *in vivo* effects of prostaglandins on free fatty acid metabolism, in: *Prostaglandins: Nobel Symposium 2* (S. Bergstrom and B. Samuelsson, eds.), pp. 109–121, Interscience Publishers, New York.

STERLING, K., BRENNER, M. A., AND SALDANHA, V. F., 1973, Conversion of thyroxine to triiodothyronine by cultured human cells, *Science* **179**:1000.

SUNDBERG, D. K., FAWCETT, C. P., ILLNER, P., AND MCCANN, S. M., 1975, The effect of various prostaglandins and a prostaglandin synthetase inhibitor on rat anterior pituitary cyclic AMP levels and hormone release *in vitro*, *Proc. Soc. Exp. Biol. Med.* **148**:54–59.

TALWALKER, P. K., RATNER, A., AND MEITES, J., 1963, *In vitro* inhibition of pituitary prolactin synthesis and release by hypothalamic extract, *Amer. J. Physiol.* **205**:213.

TAN, W. C., PRIVETT, O. S., AND GOLDYNE, M. E., 1974, Studies of prostaglandins in rat mammary tumors induced by 7,12-dibenz[α]anthracene, *Cancer Res.* **34**:3229.

TASHJIAN, A. H., VOELKEL, E. F., GOLDHABER, P., AND LEVINE, L., 1974, Prostaglandins, calcium metabolism and cancer, *Fed. Proc. Fed. Amer. Soc. Exp. Biol.* **33**:81–86.

TURKINGTON, R. W., 1972, Molecular aspects of prolactin, in: *Lactogenic Hormones* (G. E. W. Wolstenholme and J. Knight, eds.), pp. 111–127, Churchill Livingstone, Edinburgh.

TURKINGTON, R., 1974, Prolactin receptors in mammary carcinoma cells, *Cancer Res.* **34**:758–763.

TURKINGTON, R. W., FRANTZ, W. L., AND MAJUMDER, G. P., 1973, Effector–receptor relations in the action of prolactin, in: *Human Prolactin: Proceedings of the International Symposium on Human Prolactin* (J. L. Pasteels and C. Robyn, eds.), pp. 24–34, American Elsevier, New York.

TURNER, C. D., AND BAGNARA, J. T., 1971, *General Endocrinology*, W. B. Saunders Co., Philadelphia.

VERGROESEN, A. J., DEBOER, J., AND GOTTENBOS, J. J., 1967, Effects of prostaglandins on perfused isolated rat hearts, in: *Prostaglandins: Nobel Symposium 2* (S. Bergstrom and B. Samuelsson, eds.), pp. 211–218, Interscience Publishers, New York.

VERMUND, H., AND GOLLIN, F. F., 1968, Mechanisms of action of radiotherapy and chemotherapeutic adjuvants: A review, *Cancer* **21**:58–76.

VOIGT, W., FELDMAN, M., AND DUNNING, W. F., 1975, 5α-Dihydrotestosterone-binding proteins and androgen sensitivity in prostatic cancers of Copenhagen rats, *Cancer Res.* **35**:1840–1846.

VON EULER, U. S., 1935, Über die specifische blutdruckenskende Substanz des menschlichen Prostata- und Samensblasenskretes, *Klin. Wochenschr.* **14**:1182, 1183.

WEEKS, J. R., 1974, Prostaglandins: Introduction, *Fed. Proc. Fed. Amer. Soc. Exp. Biol.* **33**:37, 38.

WILSON, J. D., 1972, Recent studies in the mechanism of action of testosterone, *N. Engl. J. Med.* **287**:1284–1291.

ZAHL, P. A., COOPER, F. S., AND DUNNING, J. R., 1940, Some *in vivo* effects of localized nuclear disintegration products on a transplantable mouse sarcoma, *Proc. Natl. Acad. Sci. U.S.A.* **26**:589–598.

20

New Anticancer Drug Design: Past and Future Strategies

MARTIN A. APPLE

1. Synopsis of Cancer Treatment Research

1.1. Three Degrees of Cancer Advancement: Advanced, Previsible, and First Cell

The current strategies we have used for the conquest of the advanced cancer, i.e., one big enough to see, have involved less planned strategy and more the historical accretion of procedures such as surgery (Veronesi, 1973), radiation therapy (Kligerman, 1974), drug therapy (Salmon and Apple, 1976; Sartorelli and Johns, 1974; Carter and Slavik, 1974; Cline and Haskell, 1975), immunotherapy (Fefer, 1974; von Leyden and Blumenthal, 1902), and others (Hahn, 1975). In the innovative clinical thinking, we see attempts to integrate these modalities of therapy (Bloedorn *et al.*, 1961; Cohen *et al.*, 1971; Mathé *et al.*, 1970) and to enhance the effectiveness within each modality—e.g., to develop and utilize radiosensitizers that will make radiation therapy selective for cancer (Dewey and Humphrey, 1965; Erikson and Szybalski, 1963) or radiation protectors that will protect normal cells but not cancer from radiation, or, alternatively, to enhance the effectiveness of chemotherapy by the use of drug combinations (Goldin *et al.*, 1968, 1974; Nathanson *et al.*, 1969; E. Henderson and Samaha, 1969).

In the past, there has been discussion of the specific "search-and-destroy" tool, the so-called "magic-bullet cure" for cancer, but we have yet to develop any information or strategy that would allow us to create such an effective tool with facility. Perhaps chemo- and immunotherapy (Mathé *et al.*, 1969) still offer the greatest future hope of high specificity.

MARTIN A. APPLE ● University of California Medical School, San Francisco, California 94143.

Within the realm of the previsible cancers, which are now usually undiagnosable, we need to improve our detection of the microfocus of cancer by developing improved methods of detecting released markers from the cancer cell, or by creating new "homing pigeons" that zero in on the tumor cells we seek and emit amplified messages (Edwards and Hayes, 1970). A second approach, once we detect cancer as a microfocus, is to block the microcolony-specific events, such as neoangiogenesis (Folkman and Cotnan, 1976), because such blockades have great potential to prevent tumor growth and progression. Third, within this realm of preclinical cancer, we need to devise microcolony-specific kill methods, perhaps by enhancing those things we know about the specificity of susceptibility, such as the limitations of our immunosuppression techniques for coping with large cancers, but not necessarily tiny ones (Folkman and Cotnan, 1976), or the use of cycle-specific drugs (Schabel, 1975b).

In the third realm or area of attack on cancer, we need to prevent the first cancer cell from forming. Our current approach to doing so has been to identify human carcinogens and to evaluate their significance *in vitro* or in animal model studies (Upton, 1968; Gelhorn, 1958; Druckrey *et al.*, 1967). More important, our epidemiologic methods suggest a human carcinogen only if it increases some infrequent cancer. If, however, a factor increased lung, breast, or GI cancer by 10,000 cases per year, this factor might be undetectable by our current methods because the increase would be invisible against the background of 100,000 new patients with cancer at that site annually.

Perhaps we need to alter the human response to human carcinogens. Certainly our own experience of three or four decades in discovering and verifying that viruses cause animal cancers (Wolfe *et al.*, 1971; Bittner and Little, 1937; Andervont and Bryan, 1944; Rous, 1911; Rowe *et al.*, 1971; Rickard *et al.*, 1969; Scolnick and Parks, 1973; Opler, 1967; Kelloff *et al.*, 1970; Rapp and Duff, 1972), or that cigarette smoking is related to the cause of many of our lung cancers (Hammond and Horn, 1958; Haenszel *et al.*, 1962), has not led us to effective removal of these carcinogens from the environment. Perhaps, then, we need to look also at the more practical alternative approach; i.e., assuming we will be exposed, how might we prevent the exposure from becoming cancer? If, for example, certain enzyme systems are required to form epoxides from aromatic hydrocarbon in cigarette smoking (Nebert and Gelboin, 1968), might we intervene and interfere with the capacity of these enzymes to function in the cases in which they create proximate carcinogens from the chemicals of cigarette smoking?

In order to prevent cancer, we need to discover people at specific risk for cancer *as individuals*. We can specify the medical or family histories of women that would predispose them to having a 25% chance of developing breast cancer (Wynder, 1959; Anderson, 1971), but we do so only with the understanding that we will predict incorrectly 3 out of 4 times, for specific individuals. How can we specifically identify that 1 woman in 12 who will develop breast cancer (MacMahon *et al.*, 1970) and distinguish her from the 90% of women who will not? How can we identify that specific individual who smokes cigarettes who will develop lung cancer as opposed to those many individuals in the same exposure groups who will not?

Finally, we need to develop methods that prevent carcinogens from acting in the exposed high-risk individual. We need to learn how to alter gene expression to reverse a transformation process once begun, perhaps by use of new drugs and other forms of molecular intervention within a cell that is becoming a cancer.

1.2. Current Treatment Modalities

Since many of the methodologies that we will need to solve cancer as a clinical problem have not yet been developed, we must look at the problem of cancer therapy in its most promising form, which is the utilization of drug or chemotherapy for the treatment once it is evident as the advanced (i.e., detectable) state.

The basic biological processes in the pathophysiology of cancer include the development of the initial or primary tumor and the subsequent invasion and subsequent metastases of the tumor, which finally lead to death (Strauli, 1970).

Let us examine the various modes of cancer therapy that have been used. Surgery, historically first, has been the primary choice of therapeutic approach, and can produce a significant number of cured cases (Halsted, 1907). Obviously, the limitation of surgery is the excision of a visible tumor. The same goes, with perhaps slightly less limitation, for the historically second and often appended approach to therapeutics for cancer, the use of ionizing radiation therapy. That is, to verify the effect quantitatively, we must have the target in sight in order to aim the ionizing radiation at the tumor, although we can radiate fields that are likely to contain minitumors and decrease or delay the incidence of visible recurrence in those sites (Fletcher, 1970).

Among the three major therapeutic regimens currently demonstrably effective (Holland and Frei, 1974), however, chemotherapy offers the hope of an ultimate cure because of the ability of drugs to seek out tumor cells that are not visible or those in sites we had not predicted and destroy them.

In order to understand how we can best approach the design of new anticancer drugs that may ultimately cure cancer, we must examine the current status of drugs and the many factors previously discussed at length. For example:

1. How do cancer cells differ from their normal counterparts?
2. What are the mechanisms by which anticancer drugs act, and what strategies have been used to discover them?
3. What is the potential of the quantitative structure-activity relationships analysis, or QSAR strategy, and how does it compare with the drug-receptor analysis strategy?

Last, let us examine the discovery of new drugs and some strategies that might improve this current approach to discovery.

2. The Biochemical Differences of Cancer Cells

Much of the effort of oncologic research of this century has been spent seeking *the* major biochemical difference between cancer cells and their normal counterparts.

The assumption that there is a single difference and that it would be discoverable from searching the biochemical information available up to now has led to a cataloging of all the biochemical events so far discovered in normal and counterpart cancer cells.

It is possible to divide all the biochemical discoveries into: (1) discoveries about energy-utilizing reactions, such as those catalyzed by ligases, or, in some instances, similar reactions catalyzed by transferase enzymes in cells; (2) those reactions that break down the molecules built up by energy-using reactions, e.g., those catalyzed by the oxidoreductases, hydrolases, and lyases enzyme classes; and (3) the non-energy-utilizing, non-rate-limiting, and incidental metabolic reaction categories (Weber, 1966a,b).

While previous major strategies attempting to uncover the cancer-unique "biochemical" (usually metabolic) differences and clarify them have not proved totally successful, each has led to an improved understanding. One such strategy, the use of "minimal deviation" tumors, was an attempt to eliminate all the background noise in future study caused by using advanced, maximally deviated cancers and comparing them with their normal, often nongrowing counterparts (Morris, 1965; Pitot, 1966). Another approach was the molecular correlation concept, which collated a wealth of data and studies to further extrapolate and clarify and summarize much available information (Weber and Lea, 1966; Weber, 1966a,b).

A clear summary model we may use to explain the basic biochemical differences of cancer cells as they have so far been elucidated that arises from these two concepts is shown by the tripartite metabolic epitome in Fig. 1. The upward-pointing arrow at left in each diagram indicates the rate at which all the cell ligase and transferase reactions (category 1) are occurring. The downward-pointing arrow at right indicates the rate at which the oxidoreductase, hydrolase, and lyase reactions (category 2) are generally occurring. The horizontal arrow at the bottom indicates the rate at which the incidental, non-rate-limiting, non-energy-yielding reactions (category 3) are occurring in cells. If we now look at the question of how the cancer cells differ from their normal counterparts, and we consider the relative thicknesses of the arrows as representing the proportional rates of occurrence of these reaction categories, we see in the category of amino acid metabolism that the arrow at left, indicating ligase and transferase reactions, is tremendously enhanced in cancer cells as compared with the normal counterparts. The arrow at right, representing the breakdown into energy-yielding

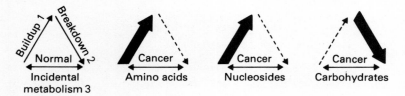

FIGURE 1. Summary models of metabolic changes with increasing malignancy (see the text).

reactions, is very much diminished in the metabolism of most amino acids in most cancer cells, and perhaps decreased directly as a function of the degree of malignancy. The reactions that do not fit clearly in either of the two prior categories do not seem as yet to be cataloged as showing any significant increase that is consistently found, and therefore cannot be represented by either as a consistent trait (Weber, 1966a,b,; Weinhouse, 1960).

The metabolism of nucleosides by cancer cells is similarly enhanced in their flow into ligase and transferase reactions (category 1) in direct proportion to their degree of malignancy, and extraordinarily decreased in their flow into oxidoreductase, hydrolase, and, perhaps, lyase reactions (category 2). Those metabolic pathway reactions that are considered to be different from those in these two categories are not consistently demonstrable as being shifted in either direction in cancer cells or as a degree of malignancy (Elford et al., 1970; Weber, 1966a,b; Morris, 1965).

In contrast, the metabolism of carbohydrates is quite frequently diminished in the ligase–transferase reaction category (1), e.g., the rate of storage of glycogen, whereas the oxidoreductase–hydrolase-lyase reaction category (2), e.g., glycolysis (Warburg, 1956), is often enormously enhanced in cancer cells, and at one time was thought to be the primary lesion that led to the formation of the cancer cell. Those metabolic reactions that are non-rate-limiting in general in the metabolism of carbohydrates do not seem to fluctuate consistently up or down either as a function of increasing malignancy or as an absolute difference between the normal cell and its cancer counterpart (Weber and Cantero, 1957; Busch and Starbuck, 1964; Morris, 1965).

The picture that emerges from this model is that cancer cells are distinguished by having shifted their catabolism of amino acids and nucleotides into anabolic pathways building up polyamino acids and polynucleotides—e.g., enzymes, DNA, and RNA—and by having utilized the breakdown of carbohydrate energy for the creation of these immense polymerized molecules. If this is indeed the state of our knowledge, in essence we have defined the main nonunique metabolic shifts of every continuously growing cell as it differs from its normal resting counterpart, and have not really adequately studied or distinguished the growing cancer cell from the growing normal cell. It appears that this major summary of reactions represents the same kind of changes that occur in normal cells stimulated to rapid division, e.g., tissue regenerations, embryo growth, and healing (Potter, 1969; Potter et al., 1972).

One interesting finding, that of reverse transcription (Temin and Baltimore, 1972; Apple, 1973), has led us to a study of those biochemical mechanisms of information transfer that have been found more cancer-specific in terms of cell metabolism than other biochemical/metabolic processes. Recent observations, however, suggest that reverse transcription is again a process that is (1) possibly not unique to cancer (Temin and Mizutani, 1974; Sarin and Gallo, 1974) or to oncorna viruses and (2) not the *sine qua non* for the origin, explanation, or definition of all cancer cells. What is perhaps most biochemically unique about cancer cells has been the least exploited in terms of development of drugs, i.e., a basic difference in gene expression: the failure to cease some gene expression and failure to stop cell division. It is this failure to stop cell division apparently regulated by membranes and genetic expression of the nuclear DNA that seems to suggest that the basic biochemical events just described are not uniquely able to describe a cancer cell. The failure of the cell to stop division, not necessarily that it has accelerated its rate of division, seems to be the hallmark property of cancer, and the failure of the genes to shut down in the intermitotic time represents the area of major interest in probably finally defining cancer cells.

3. The Major Mechanisms by Which All Anticancer Drugs with Known Mechanisms of Action Appear to Work

There appear to be four classes of mechanisms by which all the effective current cancer drugs seem to act. One class of mechanism appears to be that of the enzyme allosteric pseudoregulator. A second is that of the active site competitor of an enzyme. This class has two subcategories: one in which the drug stops all product formation, and another in which the drug is incorporated into a malfunctioning product. A third class precludes the proper formation of the enzyme–substrate complex by acting on substrates. The fourth class follows the binding of drug to protein receptors of highly specific, possibly nonenzymic, function. We can thus look on the majority of reactions by which anticancer drugs work as interfering with enzyme catalyses. It is especially convenient to divide this interference with these mechanisms as a way of representing a synopsis of previous information (Sartorelli and Johns, 1974, 1975; Salmon and Apple, 1976), and put emphasis on new conceptual approaches to drug action and interaction.

3.1. Action at Enzyme Regulatory Centers

This mechanism consists in interference with the regulatory property by which the enzyme rate is modulated. If an enzyme reaction occurring at some key branch pathway in metabolism is decreased in rate by 99.99%, i.e., if a reaction that is normally occurring at 10^6 molecules/sec turnover is decreased to a rate of 1000 or 100 molecules/sec turnover, the cell experiences, for all practical purposes, an annihilation of that enzyme function. Enzyme regulation is a well-documented event.

Among the major mechanisms by which enzyme rates are modulated are the infrequent cases of stimulation of the enzyme rates through various direct activity mechanisms (Apple and Greenberg, 1972; Massey, 1953), induction of new enzyme synthesis (Knox, 1966; Monod and Cohn, 1952; Monod, 1960), repression of existing enzyme synthesis (Ames and Garry, 1959; Umbarger, 1969), and one that acts through a fine-tuning mechanism of rate modulation directly on the enzyme, now generally termed *allosteric regulation* (Feigelson, 1968; Caskey *et al.*, 1964; Monod *et al.*, 1965; Gerhart and Pardee, 1964; Gerhart and Schachman,

605

NEW
ANTICANCER
DRUG
DESIGN:
PAST AND
FUTURE
STRATEGIES

1965), even though it has not been documented to be so in every instance. Frequently, allosteric regulation of enzyme activity occurs by the feedback of an end product in a metabolic pathway in order to prevent its own synthesis, in a thermostatlike control mechanism.

In one well-documented case, that of aspartate carbamyl transferase, the enzyme complex contains a mixture of polypeptides, some portion of which act as catalytic subunits, and others of which act as regulatory subunits without catalytic powers themselves, but with the ability to modulate the rate of the catalytic subunit (Gerhart and Schachman, 1965; Changeaux *et al.*, 1968). 6-Mercaptopurine (6-MP) *in vivo* is metabolized to form a ribotide, and is then eventually either oxidized to a 6-thiouric acid or methylated to 6-methylmercaptopurine-ribotide. Thus, there are three main metabolites of 6-MP: its ribotide, its methylated ribotide form (MMPRP), and its oxidation product, thiourate (TU) (Allan *et al.*, 1966; Caldwell, 1969; Lukens and Herrington, 1957). In the early synthetic pathway of purine metabolism, ribose-5-phosphate is converted through a series of steps to aminoimidazolecarboxamide ribotide (AICR) (R. W. Miller *et al.*, 1959; Lukens and Buchanan, 1959), which is subsequently metabolized through a series of steps to form inosinic acid (hypoxanthine ribotide), which itself is aminated to adenylic acid (Hartman and Buchanan, 1959; Flaks *et al.*, 1957). Adenylic acid is subsequently converted through a series of steps to ATP and biochemicals such as DNA, RNA, NADH, and CoA (Kit, 1970; Hartman, 1970). Obviously, any cessation in the supply of adenylic acid would cause a cessation in the production of almost every major metabolite required for growth and energy coupling within the cell. It is not surprising, then, to find that the level of adenylic acid in cells would be regulated through a supply mechanism such as the synthesis of inosinic acid. When the adenylate supply is completely depleted, e.g., because of the rapid need for the synthesis of ATP, DNA, RNA, and other biochemicals during the period of rapid cell growth, then the cell is called upon to produce much more. On the other hand, if all these growth processes were to cease, for example, during the G_0 phase or G_1 phase of cell division, the quiescent cell would conserve energy, and cease the unnecessary production of adenylic acid or inosinic acid. The conversion of inosinic acid to adenylic acid is a tightly coupled process, and it appears that 6-MP ribotide (MPRP) interferes with the conversion process of inosinic acid to adenylic acid (Atkinson *et al.*, 1964). Recent research work has suggested, however, that the most important mechanism by which 6-MP acts is through the formation of metabolite MMPRP. MMPRP seems to act as a false feedback inhibitor of the conversion of ribose-5-phosphate to AICR, a glutamine-requiring step (Bennett *et al.*, 1965; LePage and Jones, 1961; McCollister *et al.*, 1964).

Normally, in a cell, either inosinic acid or adenylic acid acts as the feedback regulator of the enzymic synthesis of AICR, and therefore would serve as the cell's thermostatic regulator (J. Henderson and Khoo, 1965) (see Fig. 2). When the supply of inosinic acid or adenylic acid is at a peak, it directs the shutdown of synthesis of AICR; when both are completely depleted, then the probability decreases that the purine nucleotides can continue to occupy the enzyme regulatory site by which they shut off AICR synthesis, and the enzyme then functions

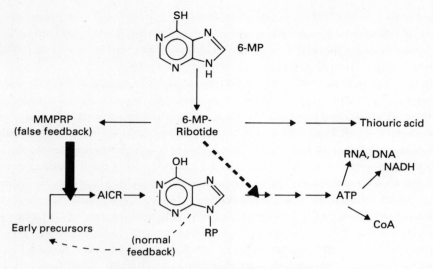

FIGURE 2. Inhibition of enzyme regulation.

maximally to provide adenylate. Instead, when 6-MP is introduced into a cell, the MMPRP metabolite acts as a false feedback regulator, tightly binding the AICR-synthesizing enzyme and shutting down AICR synthesis, but the cell now becomes depleted of crucially needed adenylic acid. This distinctive class of mechanism by which a clinical drug works is represented by very few examples other than 6-MP. Its success suggests that this class of activities is a prototype for the creation and development of a variety of additional new anticancer drugs.

3.2. Action at Enzyme Catalytic Centers

A second group of the four mechanisms by which all the anticancer drugs work is the group that works at enzyme active centers. We will divide this group of drugs that act competitively into two subcategories. The first comprises those drugs with a time of occupancy of the active center of the enzyme that is very brief and can be reversed by the addition of the normal metabolite. Additionally, instead of blocking catalytic product formation, the drug may occupy the enzyme and be incorporated into a key dysfunctional product. The second subcategory comprises those metabolite-structure-analogue drugs that bind the enzyme center and fail to rapidly release or be readily replaced by the presence of normal metabolites (tight-binding drugs) and can eventually be reversed in their activities, the pseudoirreversible inhibitors.

In the first subcategory, the readily reversed active center competitor, we will look at two examples with somewhat different mechanisms. The first example is the drug cytosine arabinoside, Ara-C. Ara-C is converted metabolically in cells into a corresponding ribotide triphosphate, Ara-CTP (Furth and Cohen, 1968). Ara-CTP has on its outside physical surface the same properties as cytidine deoxynucleotide (dCTP); however, when Ara-CTP occupies the active enzyme center of DNA polymerase, it appears that the function of DNA synthesis on the template cannot proceed. It can be reversed by dCTP, allowing reversal of inhibition; then the synthesis can proceed.

The second example of drugs that occupy active enzyme centers is that of 6-thiogaunine, which, as the ribotide 6TdGTP, occupies the enzyme active center of DNA polymerase and is incorporated into a product DNA (LePage, 1960, 1963) that is dysfunctional. That is, even though the drug acts as an enzyme center competitive inhibitor of normal DNA synthesis, some of it can be incorporated into DNA, producing an additional mechanism of damage to the cell.

In the second subcategory of the group of drugs that act as active center competitor inhibitors, the pseudoirreversibly bound, we have two examples, 5-fluorouracil (5-FU) and amethopterin or methotrexate (MTX). The 5-FU is metabolized to form fluorodeoxyuridylate (FdUMP) (Harbers $et\ al.$, 1959; Chadwick and Rogers, 1970), the active form of the drug, which occupies the active center of the enzyme that normally converts deoxyuridinemonophosphate to thyminedeoxyribomonophosphate. FdUMP appears to be covalently bound temporarily by following the normal catalytic mechanism by which the process of thymidylate synthesis normally occurs (Hartmann and Heidelberger, 1961); drug binding appears to be enhanced for a long period of time by the presence of the normal coenzyme, tetrahydrofolate (FH_4) (D. Santi, unpublished observations). Normally, the 5 position of uridylate has a hydrogen that is rapidly displaced by the coenzyme methylation process via FH_4. This coenzyme, with the energy provided after the drug binds to the enzyme, cannot readily displace the fluorine, which has an energy of bonding to carbon much higher than that of hydrogen (Pauling, 1960); thus the process of synthesis of thymidylate is temporarily arrested. The turnover time with drug metabolite bound may take half a day, but normally would take a millisecond; for all practical purposes, the enzyme is taken out of commission and is nonfunctional, creating the equivalent of thymineless death in the cell. It also appears that the drug fluorouridine is incorporated into RNA, and this incorporation acts to create abnormal RNA, which may be either an equivalent cytotoxic cause of death of cancer cells or possibly even a major cytotoxic factor in the death of cancer cells.

A second example in this subcategory is the drug MTX, which is readily absorbed, but not as readily discarded by the body. A great portion of the drug binds the plasma proteins (E. S. Henderson $et\ al.$, 1965). For all practical purposes, it is not metabolized in man, although a few minor metabolites may be derived either through gut microbial metabolism or an extremely slow metabolism in man (Zaharko $et\ al.$, 1969). Most of each dose would therefore be expected to be excreted. The vitamin folic acid is rapidly converted metabolically to tetrahydrofolic acid (FH_4) (Burchall, 1971), which acts as the carrier of one-carbon units and is a required cofactor for the synthesis of purines in a variety of methylation reactions, including that of thymidylic acid synthesis (Bertino, 1975; Huennekens and Osborn, 1959; Lorenson $et\ al.$, 1967). The synthesis of purines through folic-dependent reactions is absolutely essential for the biosynthesis of RNA,

DNA, ATP, NAD, CoA, and many of the major genetic and energy-processing molecules in the cell. The drug MTX blocks the conversion of folate into tetrahydrofolate, the carrier of these methyl groups; since this vitamin acts catalytically, a small decrease in its level has an enormous impact in the cell. MTX appears to bind almost irreversibly to the enzyme active center of the enzyme that converts dihydrofolate to tetrahydrofolic acid (Osborne *et al.*, 1958). It is hypothesized that the higher binding is due to the presence of the additional hydrogen bond introduced by the displacement of the hydroxyl group on the normal vitamin with the amino group of the antimetabolite (Huennekens, 1968). This occupation of the enzyme active center is so tight that a single dose of the drug may persist in the tissues for many days, perhaps even weeks (Fountain *et al.*, 1953).

3.3. Blockade of the Enzyme–Substrate Complex by Action on Substrates

A third group of mechanisms is via the prevention of the formation of the proper enzyme–substrate or enzyme–template complex. Two of these processes are alkylation and intercalation. The alkylation process and the intercalation process that we will discuss are based on a loose interpretation of enzyme–substrate complexes, i.e., the inclusion of templates of polynucleotides as cosubstrates.

Most of the effective cancer drugs utilized in the group of covalent alkylators are *bis*(chlorethyl) amines. These drugs include cyclophosphamide (Arnold and Borseaux, 1958), melphalan (Ochoa and Hirschberg, 1967), and mechlorethamine (Kohn *et al.*, 1966). Other alkylators, which are closely related aziridines, include triethylene melamine and triethylenethiophosphoramide (thioTEPA) (Montgomery *et al.*, 1970; Doskocil, 1965). A third group includes the alkylsulfonates or *bis*(methylsulfonates). A new class of agents which has two different functional groups, a nitroso group and an *N*-chloroethyl group, which undergoes a reaction allowing it to be a carbonium ion, are the nitrosoureas, e.g., *bis*(chloroethyl) nitrosourea (BCNU) or cyclohexylchloroethylnitrosourea (CCNU) (Loveless and Hampton, 1969; Ludlum *et al.*, 1976). These drugs act in common to alkylate, to transfer their alkyl groups to biologically important cell constituents, the function of which is then impaired. Their general mechanism of action is summarized as

$$\text{molecule A} + \text{alkylator} \rightarrow \text{molecule A–alkylator}$$

where A can be a cellular amino, carboxyl, sulfhydryl, phosphate, or any base.

Of all the thousands of possible reactions that could occur with alkylators and key cell constituents, the damage seems to be at least in part reversible or repairable, rapidly, if not immediately, by the cell. Some of these reactions seem to be potentially more devastating than others, of which the most important are proposed to be the alkylation of nucleic acid, and particularly the alkylation of purine bases (Brookes and Lawley, 1961). It may be noted that nucleic acid chains can be alkylated at the phosphate backbone and produce strand breakage (Singer,

1975). Complete verification of the intracellular actions of alkylators is still incomplete. The BCNU–CCNU group seems to yield a set of reactions that ultimately transfer an active ethyl carbonium ion to both the 1 nitrogen and 6 amino group of cytidine base in nucleic acids (Ludlum *et al.*, 1976), thus preventing the crucial base-pairing potential of that pyrimidine.

In the case of the chloroethylamines, monochloroethylamines are ineffective as anticancer drugs; therefore, we could conclude that the additional chloroethyl function is crucial. If it is, then the effectiveness of these drugs may require covalent cross-linking. A conclusion that seems to best explain the effectiveness of these drugs is that the alkylated guanine's free chloroethyl again reacts, forming a transient aziridine ring, which then releases from it an active carbonium ion that alkylates an additional DNA chain cross-linking the two DNA chains (Lawley and Brookes, 1965) or ties a chromatin protein to DNA (Puschendorf *et al.*, 1971) (Fig. 3).

Most other mechanisms, e.g., alkylation of enzymes or interlinking DNA guanine and phosphate, may cause transient damage or breakage or miscoding of a single strand of DNA, but can then be repaired by the "cut-and-patch repair" mechanisms that are normally found in cells, a process in which enzymes excise the alkylated bases and fill in the appropriate bases by base-pairing, and finally tie them back into the original DNA chain, executing a complete repair (Setlow and Carrier, 1964; Kohn *et al.*, 1965). But interchain linking, or linking of the alkylated guanine to a chromosome-bound histone or nonhistone protein, produces effects that are not repairable, thus producing extreme devastation to the cell (Fig. 3).

An additional assemblage of natural products and semisynthetic anticancer drugs, most related to antimicrobial antibiotics, act by binding to a nucleic acid template noncovalently. Two such drugs are dactinomycin and doxorubicin. Dactinomycin is an aminophenoxazinone that is substituted by two pentapeptide lactones. It has been suggested that the aminophenoxazine moiety π–π bonds between successive base pairs, especially those with guanine–cytosine purine–pyrimidine bases (Sobell, 1972; Sobell and Jain, 1972; Jain and Sobell, 1972). The affinity is enhanced, in this model, by the H-bonding and other forces securing the pentapeptides to other minor groove components in the polynucleotides.

Doxorubicin consists of a substituted naphthacenequinone with a novel amino sugar affixed. The naphthacenequinone moiety also appears to π–π bond between successive base pairs, especially those having adenine–thymine bases. The appended glycosidic amine may additionally bond to the polynucleotide phosphate, enhancing the affinity of drug to receptor site (Apple, 1973; Waring, 1968, 1970).

3.4. Action on Nonenzymic Protein Receptors

At least two examples of nonenzymic protein receptors for anticancer drugs have been identified: steroid-specific transposition-effector proteins and tubulin protein, such as that found in the cell division spindles. In the former case, the steroid

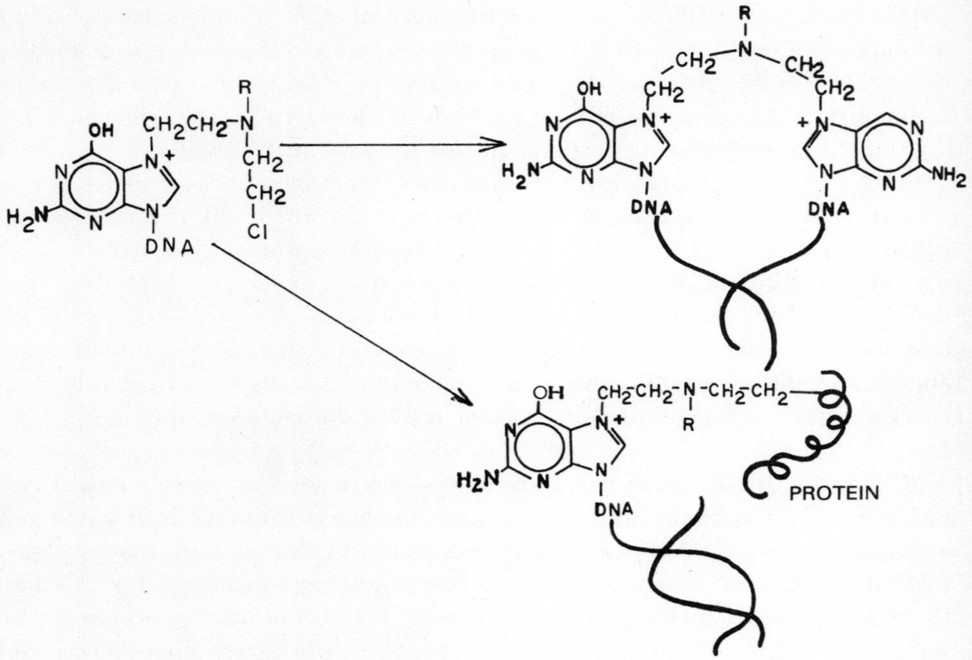

FIGURE 3. Alkylation pathways that could cause irreversible damage.

receptor has two subunits. Following the formation of a steroid–receptor complex and transposition of the complex to the chromosomes, a nonhistone chromosomal protein that normally regulates gene activation combines with one subunit of the steroid–receptor complex. The released steroid receptor subunit can then bind to the DNA, creating an RNA polymerase initiator site (Gorski *et al.*, 1968; Jensen *et al.*, 1971). In the example of corticosteroids acting on a lymphoid cancer cell, this sequence leads to a metabolic imbalance within the cell, leading rapidly to lympholysis. In the example of estrogen steroids acting on breast cancer, cancer cells with measurable receptor protein respond most frequently to estrogen (Karsten *et al.*, 1975).

Colchicine derivatives, vincristine and vinblastine, and the ansamycin maytansine interact with tubulin protein and arrest its normal functions (Owellen *et al.*, 1972, 1976; Wilson, 1975). One of these functions is to pull the chromosomes apart during the telophase stage of the mitotic cycle; when this function is impaired, cell division becomes arrested during the late M phase.

3.5. Reclassification of the Mechanisms for Drug Design

In each of the four activity mechanisms just described, we can clearly define a receptor site (enzyme active center, enzyme allosteric modulation center, substrate/template, or nonenzymic protein) that is an ultimate key to the anticancer effect of the clinically used drug. This reclassification in our thinking about how anticancer drugs work is basic to an improved approach to designing better drugs. It provides an opportunity to really design new, effective drugs, instead of simply happening upon them or blindly appending active moieties via the rules of facile organic chemical synthesis.

611

NEW
ANTICANCER
DRUG
DESIGN:
PAST AND
FUTURE
STRATEGIES

4. Discovery of New Drugs: Screening

4.1. Mouse Tumors: Evaluation

The primary mechanism for discovering new anticancer drugs for human chemotherapy is that of screening through one or several animal cancer models, particularly transplantable mouse cancers. This screening not only provides a basis for comparing different drugs before clinical trial, but allows a miniature mimic in time and scope on which a basic judgment that a drug warrants clinical trial can be made. Yet the limitations of murine cancer models are sufficient to require that those we now have be considered only an important step in the progress toward the better ones that can eventually be developed.

We have relied heavily on the L1210 lymphoid leukemia as a primary screen *in vivo*: drugs given intraperitoneally, usually on a daily schedule, are compared on an arbitrary empirical standard—that the number of days drug-treated animals survive will be over 50% longer than controls given saline or no drug (T/C·100 ≥ 150 or % ILS ≥ 50) (Venditti, 1975). Of course, the drug may show a schedule dependency, and its activity will be missed on the wrong administration schedule. Or the drug may be most active against cancer-cell populations with a low growth fraction; the murine cancers like L1210 have a very high growth fraction. Or the drug may have a high partition coefficient and not be effective on a murine leukemia, while it will be active in a large, solid cancer.

To expand the scope and effectiveness of animal screens, the current trend is not only to select reproducibly transplantable cancers that show a pattern of drug response that parallels the known pattern of human cancer drug responsiveness, but also to include in the preclinical studies selected samples of drug-sensitive and drug-resistant human cancers that can be grown as solid tumors in T-cell-deficient or immunosuppressed mice as a means of making a closer study of human cancers under a variety of conditions and manipulations not otherwise possible (Giovanella, 1976).

Since the L1210 and P388 mouse leukemias are so frequently used for anticancer drug screening, we should review their applicability.

Based on S. K. Carter's tabulation of activity of anticancer drugs against human *solid* cancers, 12 drugs were considered substantially active (S + +); 9 drugs were clearly effective but less so (S +); 12 were marginally active or inactive against most cancers, even though active in one type (S±); and many were inactive in more than one solid cancer type (S −). Of the 21 drugs classed as S + + or S +, 19 passed the minimum activity criteria (>25% ILS, L1210; >50% ILS, P388) for both animal cancer screens (Tables 1 and 2) (Venditti, 1973). Two drugs, clinically active but

TABLE 1
Correlation of Activity in L1210 Screen and Activity in Human Solid Cancers

L1210 % ILS	Human solid CA activity		Total picked from S++ or S+ active drugs in man	
	S++	S+		
200	4	1	5/6	83%
100–199	2	0	2/5	40%
50–99	5	2	7/16	44%
25–49	0	4	4/5	80%
<25	1	2	3/13	23%
≥50% ILS:	11/12 92%	3/9 33%		
≥25% ILS:	11/12 92%	7/9 80%		

not widely accepted, failed this double screen (Fig. 4) (Venditti, 1973). Of the 21, 18 met even more stringent criteria (>50% ILS, L1210; >75% ILS, P388). The degree to which the drugs were active was also predictive: all 6 of 6 drugs giving an ILS of 200% or more in P388 and 5 of 6 giving an ILS of 200% or more in L1210, for a combined total of 11 of 12, or 92%, were in the S+ or S++ category when studied in human cancer patients. If a drug produced a 50–99% ILS in L1210 or P388, then 7 of 16 or 3 of 8, respectively (10 of 24, or 41%, combined), were classified as S+ or S++ in man (Tables 1 and 2) (Venditti, 1973, 1975).

TABLE 2
Correlation of Activity in P388 Screen and Activity in Human Solid Cancers

P388 % ILS	Human solid CA activity		Total picked from S++ and S+ active drugs in man	
	S++	S+		
≥200	5	1	6/6	100%
100–199	4	4	8/14	57%
50–99	1	2	3/8	37%
25–49	1	0	1/6	17%
<25	1	2	3/10	30%
≥100% ILS:	9/12 75%	5/9 56%		
≥50% ILS:	10/12 83%	7/9 78%		
≥25% ILS:	11/12 92%	7/9 78%		

4.2. 50 New Drugs

613

NEW
ANTICANCER
DRUG
DESIGN:
PAST AND
FUTURE
STRATEGIES

The current drug research programs in the United States have led to about 50 new drugs that are moving toward clinical evaluation against cancer. Most of these drugs have come from animal screens here or abroad. Of these drugs, 6 are amino acids (Table 3), 3 are vitamin analogues (Table 4), 4 are pyrimidines (Table 5), 6 are purinelike (Table 6), 13 are probable or possible alkylating agents (Table 7), and the rest are natural products or semisynthetic analogues (Table 8) (Carter, 1975).

What is notable about so many new drugs so active as to be candidate human drugs is that for at least three-fourths of these drugs, there are no publications (as is evident from a recent literature search) that explain either the rationale of their creation or the strategy of their discovery, or their *in vivo* activity, mechanism of action, or even verification of their structures. It is clear that many of these drugs are not the results of rationally based research synthesis programs, but are the products of empirical screening.

Probably half a million chemicals have been studied worldwide as potential anticancer drugs. Activity failures as well as related successes can provide substantial information on new drug design, but we need more analyses of this type to be published from these studies to develop verified major new principles of more successful drug design. Because of the complexity of this analysis, it will take a long time to fully analyze this immense amount of data.

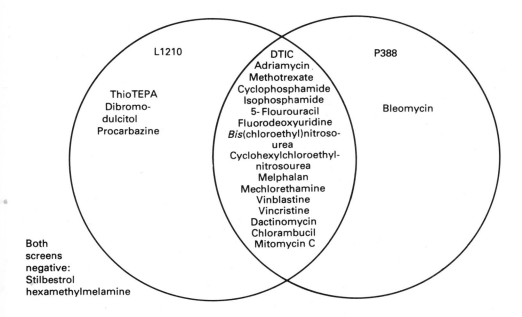

FIGURE 4. Diagram showing how the L1210/P388 screens predicted drugs with clinical effectiveness on solid human cancers (S+ + or S+).

TABLE 3
Amino Acid Analogues

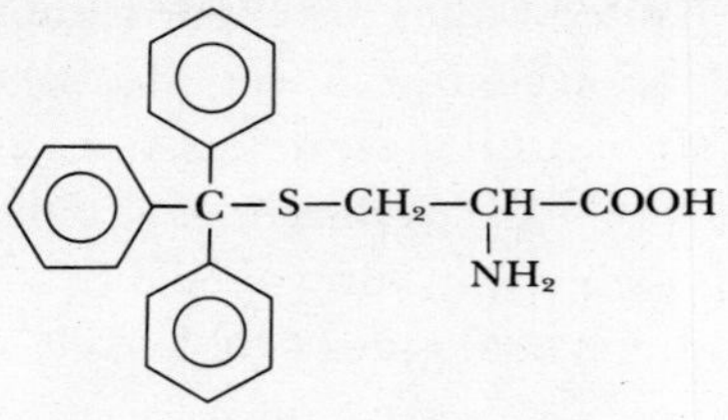

NSC 83265

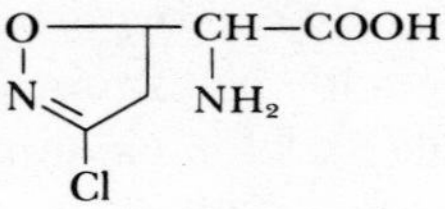

NSC 163501

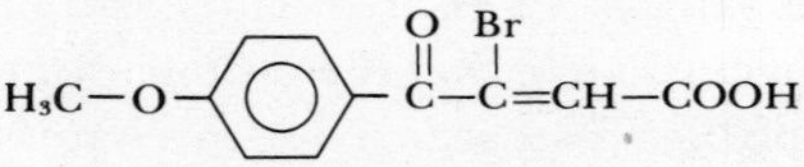

NSC 104801

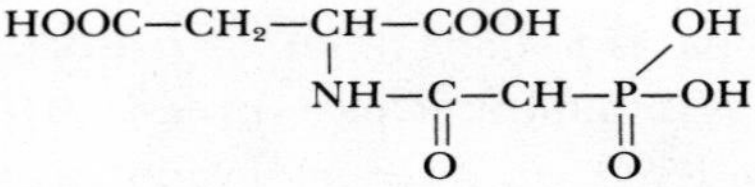

NSC 224131

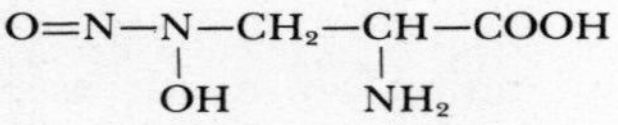

NSC 143647, 153353

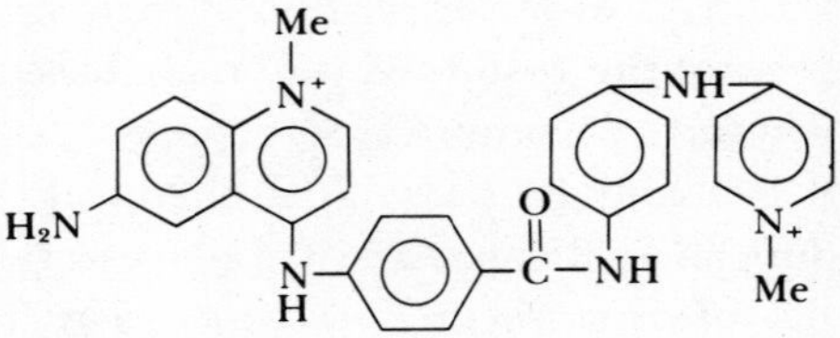

NSC 176319

TABLE 4
Vitamin Analogues

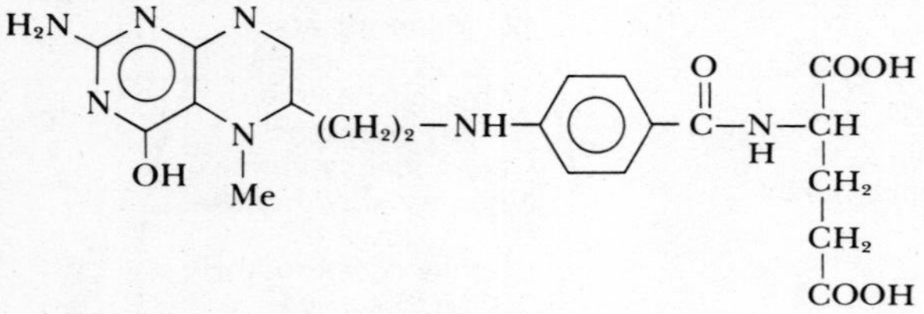

NSC 139490

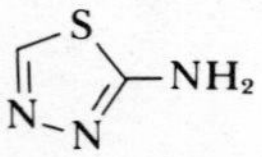

NSC 4728

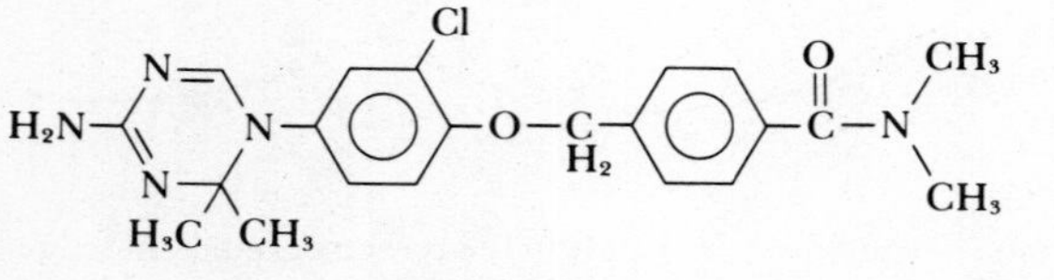

NSC 139105

615

NEW
ANTICANCER
DRUG
DESIGN:
PAST AND
FUTURE
STRATEGIES

TABLE 5
Pyrimidines

NSC 148958

NSC 102816

NSC 126849

NSC 145668

TABLE 6
Purine Structural Analogues

NSC 71851

NSC 143095

NSC 172755

NSC 154020

NSC 118994

NSC 137679

TABLE 7
Possible Alkylating Agents

NSC 73754

NSC 16778

NSC 178248

NSC 16778

NSC 135758

NSC 17211

NSC 169780

NSC 19296

NSC 104800

NSC 249992

NSC 132313

NSC 95466

NSC 24756

TABLE 8
Natural Products and Semisynthetic Analogues

617

NEW
ANTICANCER
DRUG
DESIGN:
PAST AND
FUTURE
STRATEGIES

NSC 126771

NSC 141537

NSC 5159

NSC 141633

NSC 154890

NSC 153858

NSC 163063

NSC 165563

NSC 143057, 238146

NSC 71795

NSC 244393

MARTIN
A. APPLE

4.3. Only a Few New Ideas

Clearly, this is an impressive list of potentially useful new anticancer drugs for man. The number of new ideas related to their discovery is far less impressive. Among those in Table 3, one compound, 224131, was designed as a transition-state inhibitor of a known enzyme target. In Table 4, 139105 was designed by quantitive structure–activity empiricism. In Tables 5 and 6, the structures are mostly simply extensions of previously partly successful ideas. Most of the structures in Table 7 represent new carriers for old alkylating groups, an aspect that can be varied almost infinitely. The last group, Table 8, come mostly from random screening; the activity is usually known before the structure is proved.

Thus, in terms of fresh ideas, the impressiveness of this list leaves much to be desired. It represents the mining of gold after the major nuggets are taken and the quality of ore is rapidly going downhill. These may represent many new leads, or ideas, but it will take time to clarify and verify these possibilities. We cannot now predict how many of these will be clinically acceptable anticancer drugs—certainly half could survive with our current acceptance criteria. What is more important for progress is not that we agree that they work as well (or poorly?) as current drugs, but that they work much better. Since the probability is small that any will be far superior to cyclophosphamide, for example, their current value is mainly to increase the potential for curative combination chemotherapy, or, possibly, selectively affect some generally untreatable cancers (e.g., pancreatic or lung carcinomas). We are fast approaching a point at which the list of usable anticancer drugs will be so long that physicians will need a special residency to learn to select and use them.

4.4. Success Frequency of Screening

While it represents enormous progress from 25 years ago when usable anticancer drugs were unavailable, it provides another kind of judgment when 50 different drugs are used to treat cancer; it says that none is so effective as to be completely satisfactory. The criteria that would allow us to accept 50 drugs as effective will need reexamination.

The screening and serendipity (S&S) approach has led to a number of unarguably successful drug developments for anticancer or antibiotic chemotherapy. The average success rate of this approach has been 0.0001 (*Annual Report of the DCT–NCI*, 1974). This low rate, however, is even as high as it is because it is enriched by having been the result of a survey of a large portion of all the known organic compounds for the first time. Soon the rediscovery problem will arise in this field, as it has in all prior large-scale screening programs. Soon we may enter the era of progressively diminishing return on the screening effort. One summary of the screening effort for new antibiotics showed about a 0.20 success rate in discovering active compounds in 10,000 tries; yet the number of new antibiotics after correcting for duplicates had already dropped the actual success rate to

0.001, and when we require effectiveness in man, however limited, as a criterion, a success rate of 0.0001 begins to look high (Woodruff and McDaniel, 1958). If we now add the criterion of very high effectiveness (e.g., much more effectiveness than currently used chemotherapy in more cancers), we are subject to an empirical observation that as the effectiveness criterion increases linearly, the number of new drugs achieving that criterion decreases exponentially (Hahn, 1975; *U.S. Army Research Program on Malaria Annual Report*, 1973). Drugs substantially better than those we now use clinically would be expected to be uncovered by screening randomly with a success rate below 0.00001, even on an optimistic scale of probability. If even that rate is subject to both exponentially decreasing ability to increase effectiveness and the law of progressively diminishing return, we can only conclude that now is the time to plan to phase out the S&S approaches before they exhaust all our available resources, and plan a more rational successor approach.

5. Physicochemical Correlates of Drug Action: QSAR

5.1. Drug Bonding

The spatial and electronic aspects of different drug structures have long been known to be related to their activities, but not often in obvious or consistent ways. With the mechanism of action unknown and the target receptor undefined, the analysis of the role of structural features of agents and consequent activity remains unclear. However, several proposals for classifying the relationship of structural features to activity of drugs have been developed.

A variety of bonding mechanisms by which drugs interact with receptors and cell membranes include covalent (rarely), ionic, and H bonds (Pauling, 1960). Additionally, a weak electrostatic repulsive (Born) force, a weak but important attractive dipole–dipole (Keesom) force, and an attractive dipole-induced dipole (Debye) force (Settle *et al.*, 1971), as well as an attractive momentary fluctuating dipole (London) force (Heitler and London, 1927; Israelachvili, 1974), play important roles at close range. Since these weak interactions are additive, and a molecule may form many such interactions, the total binding energy may exceed that of many H bonds or even several ionic bonds (Settle *et al.*, 1971). Not only may the addition or deletion of small groups on a drug directly affect the bonding to those groups, but also the steric or spatial relationships are often crucial (e.g., geometric isomerism and enantiomeric selectivity); further, both steric and inductive effects of each moiety in a drug may produce profound effects on the (oft-neglected) weak interactions everywhere around the molecule.

5.2. Quantitative Structure–Activity Relationships

One of the most successful approaches to quantitating the effects of drug structural features on activity has been the Meyer–Overton–Hammet–Taft–Hansch recognition that the degree of drug response is a function of measurable physicochemical parameters that vary in congeners (Overton, 1901; Meyer and Hemmi, 1935; Taft, 1956; Hammet, 1970). The formal statement

$$\text{drug response} = f(\text{hydrophobic}) + f(\text{electronic}) + f(\text{steric}) + f(\text{bonding}) + \text{constant}$$

is as effective a summary of how we measure structure–activity relationships as any now available (Leo *et al.*, 1971; Hansch, 1973). It says we can find features to measure that interact additively; that the most important of these features is the hydrophobic nature of the structure in question, as measured by the nonpolar/polar liquid partition coefficient; that we can assign hydrophobicity to substituents *per se*; that we can measure the way each substituent moiety of the drug affects the electron density of adjacent regions in the structure; that we can quantitate the steric intramolecular effects of substituents on nearby reaction centers and the van der Waals radius of those effects; and that specific bonding of new substituents is quantifiable. The degree of ionization of a series of congeners is not specifically taken into account when it varies extensively, but ionization will, of course, produce measurable shifts in each of the parameters measured.

Adding specificity to this general approach is the Bruice–Free–Wilson derivation of additive substituent constants (Free and Wilson, 1964; Bruice *et al.*, 1956). This derivation does not include only the hydrophobic, electronic, and steric properties in each constant. The limitation of these constants is their poor portability between systems; they do allow an ordering of activating effects of substituents and an empirical basis for predicting many useful structural modifications.

Neither approach tells us anything about the drug's mechanism of action. They tell us instead that empirically derived steric, electronic, and hydrophobic factors of already active drugs can predict increases and decreases in the drug's activity according to definable rules as the structure is modified. They allow the possibility of increasing the success in selecting among options for the "fine-tuning" of molecular-structure modifications among active drug groups. For example, if one were to be able to put any of 40 substituents on the *ortho*, *meta*, or *para* positions of a phenyl ring, one would have $((40)^3)^3$ permutations, or 2.52×10^{14} options. By studying the effects of t-butyl ($-$Sigma, $+$Pi), or CF_3 ($+$Sigma, $+$Pi), SO_2NH_2 ($+$Sigma, $-$Pi), or NH_2 ($-$Sigma, $-$Pi), substituents, one can sometimes determine that three-fourths of the options would not be useful to synthesize, but only those following one of the four sets of Sigma–Pi combinations would be likely to yield more active drugs (Fig. 5) (Hansch and Fujita, 1964; Cammarata and Martin, 1970; Purcell *et al.*, 1973). This approach will fail, of course, when the structural modification precludes effective receptor binding, and the steric, electronic, and other effects then behave unpredictably.

5.3. Bioisosterism

An old empirical approach to chemotherapeutic agents is based on isosteric substitution. Within the structures of an existing normal metabolite or lead drug, a

621

NEW
ANTICANCER
DRUG
DESIGN:
PAST AND
FUTURE
STRATEGIES

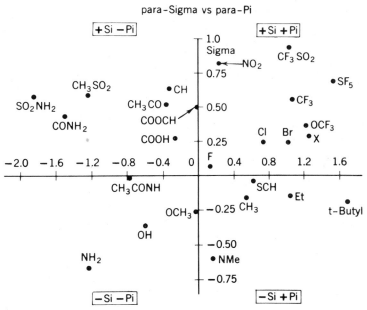

FIGURE 5. Relationship between para-Sigma and para-Pi values. From Purcell *et al.* (1973).

number of atoms can be substituted, creating new compounds with atomic spheres of influence nearly identical to the original compounds (Korolkovas, 1970; Schatz, 1960). If these new compounds are structural analogues of normal metabolites, they sometimes serve as useful chemotherapeutics (Table 9) (Bulkacz *et al.*, 1968).

6. Receptor Targeting and Delivery Approach

6.1. The Crossroads: Screening and Serendipity vs. Receptors

In order to most effectively design new drugs for any purpose, ideally we need to understand clearly both the process or biological activity to be modified and the sequence of events by which drugs elicit their effects. In the absence of either understanding, drug design is successful more by serendipity than by rational design. The historical route to drug discovery has more often followed the route of aspirin and penicillin than rational design. In these cases, the drugs were discovered accidentally (von Gerhardt, 1853; Fleming, 1929), and became widely used decades before the biochemical mechanisms through which each produces a drug effect became elucidated. This does not condemn the S&S route as a way to discover new drugs or improve existing ones; the method is responsible for most of the drugs we now use therapeutically. It is to say that this historical method has provided much useful data that allow us to approach the question of drug design now with more efficiency and rationality than ever before.

TABLE 9
Bioisosteres

Anticancer

Antiviral

Anticancer

Anticancer

Antimicrobial

Antipyretic

Antihistaminic

We previously noted that all known anticancer drugs had target receptors that were nonenzyme proteins, enzyme regulatory sites, enzyme active centers, or enzyme substrates/nucleic acids. We can now often select our target enzyme reaction or receptor site first, design drugs around a receptor affinity first, and modify the drug to improve transmembrane permeability and modify metabolism without negating the desired effect, since we know from the start which portions of the drug molecule can be modified to improve delivery to the target without blocking receptor binding. We are at the crossroads, at a crucial turning point in the history of drug discovery in which we can, and should, consider switching the balance of our approach from the S&S method of the past to the receptor targeting and delivery (RT&D) approach of the future.

6.2. Receptor Targeting and Delivery Strategy

623

NEW
ANTICANCER
DRUG
DESIGN:
PAST AND
FUTURE
STRATEGIES

6.2.1. Background

The model used for this strategy is shown in Fig. 6.

6.2.2. Drug

The drug is assumed to be an organic chemical with a known primary structure and three-dimensional shape that has a variety of measurable properties such as rate of metabolism by human liver P_{450} enzyme complex, pK_as, octanol–water partition coefficient, solubility in bile or urine of various pHs, and albumin binding K_d.

6.2.3. Absorption

Depending on the route of administration, the administered chemical (drug or prodrug) will have to get into the blood by crossing buccal membranes, surviving at stomach acidity, remaining active at intestinal pH and with pancreatic hydrolases, or crossing the membranes involved in intramuscular or subcutaneous administration. Drugs may traverse membranes by active transport against concentration gradients using ATP energy (Kaback, 1972), by facilitated stereospecific diffusion (Storelli *et al.*, 1972), or by diffusion with concentration gradients (Gordon and Kern, 1968). Absorption from the stomach shows a preferential permeability by gastric epithelium to the nonionized form of the drug (Schanker *et al.*, 1957). Evidence is available that molecular size, partition coefficient between lipoid and aqueous milieu, and nonionized forms (at alkaline pH) are important factors in transport across intestinal membranes into the blood (Hogben *et al.*, 1959). Drugs with structures that resemble normal metabolites may be actively transported across intestinal membranes. Orally administered chelators may nonspecifically enhance transport from the intestine to the blood while in the gut (Schanker and Johnson, 1961).

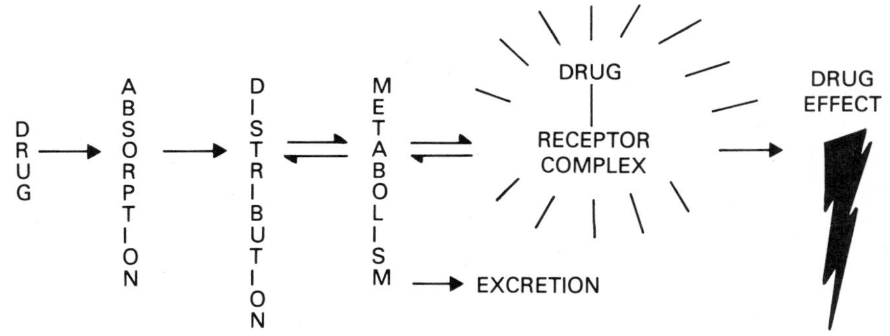

FIGURE 6. Model of receptor targeting and delivery strategy for discovering new anticancer drugs (see the text).

6.2.4. Distribution

Immediate distribution problems, once the drug has entered the blood, involve the degree of plasma protein binding, particularly albumin binding (Keen, 1971). Extensive binding will decrease the free (active) concentration of drug and slow the kinetics of distribution and excretion and the rate of metabolism (B. Martin, 1965). Drug diffusion of the nonionized form into adipose tissue depends on the mass and blood perfusion of body fat and the lipid solubility of the drug. Partitioning into fat changes drug effects by slowing the kinetics of distribution to other sites and slowing excretion. Drugs may enter bone, but the amounts are usually small (Milch *et al.*, 1957). Drugs may distribute into the tissue or muscle mass because the capillary endothelial junctions may have pores over 100Å in size, but distribution into the brain is very limited by tight junctions between endothelial cells (Rall and Zubrod, 1962; Cserr *et al.*, 1970).

6.2.5. Metabolism

An administered drug may be metabolized, i.e., enzymically transformed, so that the active (receptor-binding) form(s) may be created from inactive prodrugs (the administered form), or, second, the administered drug itself may be the active form; in either case, the drug may be (but is not necessarily) metabolized into inactive forms.

All metabolism is of six types, catalyzed by:

1. Oxidoreductases

$$A_{oxidized} + B_{reduced} \rightleftharpoons A_{reduced} + B_{oxidized}$$

2. Hydrolases

$$A—B + H_2O \rightleftharpoons A—OH + B—H$$

3. Ligases

$$NTP + A + B \rightleftharpoons A—B + NDP + Pi$$

4. Transferases

$$A—X + B \rightleftharpoons A + B—X$$

5. Lyases

$$\overset{A—B}{\underset{x\quad y}{\uparrow\quad\uparrow}} \rightleftharpoons A=B + xy$$

6. Isomerases

$$L—cis\text{-}A \rightleftharpoons L—trans\text{-}A \text{ or } D—cis\text{-}A$$

Examples of transferases are glutathione-*S*-transferases, *N*-methyl and *O*-methyl transferases, acetyl transferases, glucuronyl transferases, and sulfo transferases. Examples of hydrolases are the myriad of esterases. Examples of oxidoreductases are amine oxidases, aldehyde oxidases, aldehyde–ketone reductases, aryl hydroxylases, and nitroreductases. Frequently, the drug follows the sequence of oxidoreductase or hydrolase metabolism first, and then a transferase conjugation.

625

NEW
ANTICANCER
DRUG
DESIGN:
PAST AND
FUTURE
STRATEGIES

6.2.6. Drug–Receptor Complex

For most drugs, the proximate active form can exert its effect only on combining with some cell receptor constituent, usually a macromolecular constituent (Cuatrecasas, 1972; Latorre *et al.*, 1970; Bosmann, 1972; Rang, 1971). This is thus the single most important aspect of drug action.

Drug–receptor complex formation can be studied by spectroscopic or dialysis or other physical methods. One may use UV-visible absorption spectroscopy (Klotz, 1946), fluorescence spectroscopy (Chignell, 1970), optical rotatory dispersion and circular dichroism (Chignell, 1969), nuclear magnetic resonance (Fischer and Jardetsky, 1965), electron spin resonance (Sandberg and Piette, 1968), light-scattering (DeRobertis *et al.*, 1969), X-ray diffraction (Sobell and Jain, 1972), and stopped-flow and relaxation spectrometry (King *et al.*, 1969) as spectroscopic variations for such study. One new method using a laser-produced evanescent wave energy total reflection induced fluorescence spectroscopy with Brownian motion emission modulation analysis is so sensitive it can study drug–receptor interactions in solution with atomole quantities (Apple *et al.*, 1976). Applicable dialysis methods include equilibrium dialysis (Klotz *et al.*, 1946), rapid kinetic dialysis, and partition dialysis (Meyer and Guttman, 1970); additional methods, depending on the properties of the receptor and drug ligand, could include ultrafiltration, ultracentrifugation (Richards and Schachman, 1957), polarography (Saroff and Mark, 1953), solubility or precipitation (Ehrenpreiss, 1965), heatburst calorimetry (O'Reilly *et al.*, 1969), electromotive force (Carr, 1973), and enzyme activity.

A number of theories of how a drug–receptor interaction produces a drug effect have developed out of the Langmuir isotherm (Langmuir, 1918) saturation mechanism (Colquhoun, 1973). One theory that can unify and explain many of the anomalies that have led to a history of unverified hypothesizing is the induced-fit notion: as the drug binds, it induces a conformational change in its receptor that leads to the drug effect; the varying degrees of effect with low drug concentrations are due either to a few receptors out of a large receptor population undergoing a full conformational shift or to a large number of receptors undergoing a partial average shift due to the low average frequency of drug–receptor collision. A drug may replace a molecule 10 or 100 times its size, as opiates act to mimic endogenous polypeptide binding to endogenous peptide receptors (Simantov and Snyder, 1976; Loh *et al.*, 1976a,b; Bradbury *et al.*, 1976); this suggests that a few closely juxtaposed loci of different parts of macromolecules may converge on the key receptor area and act as agonists or antagonists of receptor function. Agonists, then, are molecules that induce the "right" conformational change, and antagonists are those that preclude the proper change, by any mechanism, at the receptor "active center" or outside it.

Three of the most important aspects of our receptor consideration here are that (1) receptors are the *sine qua non* of most drug effects, (2) receptors can be isolated, and (3) the degree to which a candidate drug or drug metabolite binds to a receptor can be readily measured *in vitro*. These three independent observations are the foundation for the greatest forthcoming advances in drug design technology.

6.2.7. Excretion

Excretion of a bloodborne drug may be via the lungs, kidneys, or bile. Excretion of many drugs in milk or other forms of sweat is well documented (Knowles, 1965).

Structural size, special structural features, and polarity are major influences on biliary excretion extent and rate. It has been postulated that a critical balance of polar to nonpolar groups leads to extensive biliary excretion (Smith, 1971); molecules that are either very polar or very nonpolar are not easily excreted in bile. An active secretory process may be involved in biliary excretion, but this has not been fully studied. Reabsorption of drugs or metabolites from bile has been documented.

Renal excretion of a drug or its metabolites may involve glomerular filtration or passive or active tubular secretion. An enormous portion of blood perfuses the kidneys every minute (Table 10). Polar drugs, or metabolism to polar products, favor renal excretion of filtered compounds (Weiner, 1967). The pH of urine being formed is a major factor in renal excretion rates of anionic or cationic drugs or their metabolites (Weiner and Mudge, 1964; Milne *et al.*, 1958).

The major variables that affect drug effectiveness are summarized in Fig. 7. What is important for new drug design is to divide all the factors discussed above into two categories, the first being "receptor binding," the second, "all other factors." When drugs are designed to do the first effectively, the remaining manipulations to accommodate to problems raised by other factors are relatively easily performed. Manipulating all the other factors, however, will be effective only to the degree to which the proximate active drug acts on its ultimate receptor. Current research not adequately accounting for this concept may be less productive than research that takes it into account.

TABLE 10

Relationship of Renal Perfusion to Body Mass (Approximate)

Organ	Mass (g)	Blood flow (ml/min)	ml/min/g
Kidney	250–300	1,000–1,500	5
Liver	3,700–4,000	1,500	0.30
Muscle	30,000–35,000	1,200–1,500	0.04
Fat	10,000–15,000	200–300	0.02

627

NEW
ANTICANCER
DRUG
DESIGN:
PAST AND
FUTURE
STRATEGIES

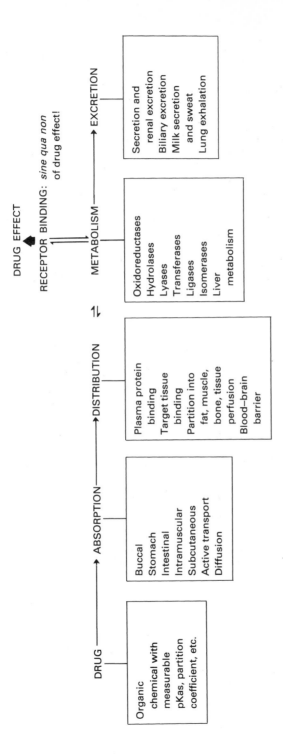

FIGURE 7. Summary of major variables in drug effectiveness.

MARTIN
A. APPLE

7.1. Unknowns and Variables

Current problems in the clinical use of anticancer drugs include: little information on pharmacokinetic and other factors associated with achieving effective concentrations of each drug at receptor sites, narrow therapeutic indices, drug instability, ill-defined metabolism, undefined variability in tumor growth fraction, inadequately studied drug-scheduling optima, almost no systematic and adequate information on how best to combine anticancer drugs, and a lack of predictive tests that select drug-responsive tumors.

An orally administered drug is subject to many variables in achieving solution in a form and at a site available for absorption; most of these variables remain unstudied in man for most anticancer drugs. The distribution, pharmacokinetics, and excretion rates of most anticancer drugs in man are minimally studied and rarely applied to improving administration schedules. The metabolism and properties of excretion of the metabolites of most drugs used for cancer treatment are just now being determined, but little application of this information has been made. Using data on metabolism, it is often possible to design drug congeners that achieve a receptor-binding form but are not further metabolized, so the *in vivo* $t_{1/2}$ of the drug would then become mostly excretion-limited, and the $t_{1/2}$ can be manipulated readily by altering the ionizability and partition coefficient with appropriate chemical structural manipulation. Ariens (1974) has pointed out that in general, nonmetabolizable drugs may often have reduced carcinogenic and mutagenic risks, drug-interaction risks, a prolongation of $t_{1/2}$, fewer animal-to-patient species differences and patient-to-patient variability differences, and reduction in risks of allergenic actions. Any of these considerations would be important, but together they constitute a powerful argument for nonmetabolizability being given consideration in anticancer drug design.

Determining the sensitivity of a tumor to different drugs *in vitro* cannot predict with certainty the effectiveness *in vivo*, the reason being that many other factors, e.g., metabolism and distribution into body fat, will alter the amount of drug getting to the sensitive cells or key receptors. The *in vitro* screening might effectively eliminate insensitive tumors and spare patients' time wasted with drugs that probably will fail.

Drugs for cancer therapy, as a natural consequence of their cytotoxic action and low therapeutic index, produce serious, even life-threatening adverse effects (Salmon and Apple, 1976; Schein *et al.*, 1970). It is improper to call these effects "side effects" of these drugs—they are usually produced by the drugs' normal mechanisms of action being exerted on the noncancer cells with a high renewal rate. Some target tissues of adverse effects are summarized in Table 11. The future progress of anticancer drug chemotherapy may depend on improving the selective toxicity of new drugs.

629

NEW
ANTICANCER
DRUG
DESIGN:
PAST AND
FUTURE
STRATEGIES

TABLE 11

Toxic target organ	Drug producing the overwhelming toxicity
Heart	Doxorubicin, daunorubicin, thalicarpine
Lung	Bleomycin, busulfan
CNS, peripheral nerves	Asparaginase, cycloleucine, azaridine, thalicarpine, vincristine
Kidney	Streptozotocin, cis-Cl$_2$-diamineplatinum
Liver	Mercaptopurine, amethopterin
Intestine	Camptothecin, amethopterin
Bladder	Cyclophosphamide, camptothecin
Testes, ovary	Cyclophosphamide
Bone marrow	Nitrosoureas, most anticancer drugs

7.2. Preclinical Toxicology

It may be noted that toxicity patterns of anticancer drugs are similar, almost predictable, within groups of metabolite structural analogues, steroids, or alkylating agents (Salmon and Apple, 1976). The toxicity patterns become diverse and novel in the group of natural products, alkaloids, and antibiotics (Salmon and Apple, 1976).

Dogs and monkeys are best able to predict the most common adverse effects of new anticancer drugs that occur in man—GI and hematologic toxicities. The true positive rate was about 85% using either dogs or monkeys as predictors of human hematologic toxicities, and the false positive rate was 12–13% (Schein *et al.*, 1970). Among the individual toxicities, dogs predicted true positives with a higher success for thrombocytopenia and anemia, while dogs and monkeys predicted equally for leukopenias.

GI toxicities appear to be best predicted by dogs; their true positive rate is 3 times higher than that of monkeys for diarrhea or vomiting. Overall, dogs show a 92% true positive rate and 8% false positives (Schein *et al.*, 1970). Dogs also predict as adequately as monkeys for neurotoxicities, liver toxicity, renal toxicity, and cardiovascular toxicity. Dogs are probably the animals of first choice for preclinical toxicology of new anticancer drugs; monkeys are a useful adjunct.

7.3. Selective Toxicities

The ability to selectively kill cancer cells occurs to varying degrees with current anticancer drugs. We need more data to derive a clearer understanding of the bases for these selectivities and clarify all the principles of selective toxicity from which new anticancer drug design can be improved.

We have evidence that selective chemotherapeutic toxicity occurs via specific response to drugs based on biochemical differences between two kinds of cells. The use of sulfonamides as chemotherapeutics, taking advantage of the requirement of the target cell for *p*-aminobenzoate to synthesize folate and the absence of this biochemical process in the nontarget tissues, is a classic example. Such clear-cut differences between normal and cancer cells have not so far been evident. Even when differences are apparent (such as reverse transcription), they are not readily exploitable, although clearly promising approaches are being attempted in which new drugs have been shown for the first time to specifically block the *in vivo* development of oncorna-virus-induced cancers (Apple, 1973, 1975*b*). The factor of degrees of differences especially in nucleic acid synthesis rather than absolute all-or-none differences, as a function of degree of malignancy, represents a major success of the state of our current cancer-cell-vs.-normal-cell biochemical difference documentation and limited exploitation.

Selective chemotherapeutic toxicity can occur when the target cell has a unique structure not found in the nontarget cells (Albert, 1975). The effects of penicillin and cycloserine on target cell D-alanine peptide incorporation into cell walls, structures not present in the nontarget cells, are significant examples of this aspect of selective toxicity. Antibody-tagged drugs attempting to exploit the discovery of tumor-specific transplantation antigens, often similar to virus-induced membrane antigens, offer an avenue of further study.

Differences in cell uptake of drugs represent another basis of selective toxicity; e.g., the usefulness or effectiveness of tetracycline, MTX, and radioiodine can be attributed to these differences (Albert, 1975). An example of how uptake and effectiveness are related is shown in Fig. 8 (Kessel *et al.*, 1965, 1968). In this

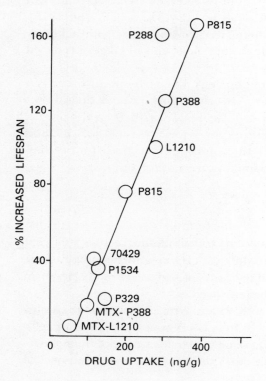

FIGURE 8. Relationship between drug uptake and effectiveness *in vivo* with a variety of murine cancers.

example, we see that the longevity of mice with different cancer types varied over at least a 10-fold range; the uptake of MTX in each tumor type has been measured, and varied at least 6-fold. As the uptake rate increases, the effectiveness against the cancer *in vivo* also increases. Two lines selected for MTX resistance (L1210 and P388) show a 3–4 fold decrease in drug uptake.

631

NEW
ANTICANCER
DRUG
DESIGN:
PAST AND
FUTURE
STRATEGIES

Perhaps the least explored but potentially more vital clinical consideration is that metastases are the major antecedent to the fatal outcome of clinical cancer. How do we prevent or arrest metastases? We have only two confirmed properties that offer major strategic merit: metastases (1) have a maximal growth fraction and (2) induce neoangiogenesis via a novel inductive substance. The first suggests the optimal use of cycle-specific drugs (Schabel, 1975b; Nicolini, 1976). The second suggests that we have a target substance that binds to an endothelial receptor (Folkman, 1974), the identification of which provides a suitable receptor for drug design of potent antagonists.

7.4. Evaluation of Current Anticancer Drugs

Anticancer drugs work best when the tumor mass is least, in most instances; drugs curative in small cancers may do little to extend survival in very advanced cancers. New drugs are ethically studied in voluntarily consenting, evaluable patients whose cancer has progresed beyond current therapy, and thus many evaluations may show a more dismal result than possible for a tumor type under optimal drug use conditions. Drug therapy has, through historical precedent, become the modality of third choice after the more developed modalities of surgery and radiation therapy.

Drug therapy has added immensely to the success trends in cancer treatment. We can now number the cancers in which chemotherapy has tipped the balance to produce some real cures: acute lymphocytic leukemia, Hodgkin's disease, testicular carcinoma, rhabdomysarcoma, Ewing's sarcoma, Wilms's sarcoma, Burkitt's lymphoma, retinoblastoma, choriocarcinoma, skin cancer, histocytic lymphoma, breast carcinoma, and cervical carcinoma. In some instances, the majority of patients with these cancers can be cured only because of drug treatment, e.g., choriocarcinoma, Wilms's sarcoma, and Burkitt's lymphoma.

The real clinical effectiveness of most anticancer drugs has not been adequately compared. No summary can be quantitatively precise; the data are inadequate and not readily compared. Further, the startling variability, such as the same drug being used to treat the same cancer showing a more than 5-fold difference between success rates in small series of patients in the case of 5-FU in intestinal cancer (Moertel and Reitmeier, 1969), suggests that several independent clinical trials will be needed to establish the true effectiveness of single agents for each cancer type and comparable patients. With these caveats, we can summarize the relative effectiveness of current chemotherapy (Table 12). The stage of advancement, a most crucial factor in evaluating drug effectiveness, is not controlled or optimal in these studies, which were mostly done in advanced patients. For

TABLE 12

Percentage of Patients with Cancer of Each Site Showing Significant Objective Responses to Each Drug Used Alone

Drug	Soft tissue sarcomas	Breast carcinoma	Cervix	Colon	Head and neck	Lung (all)	Melanoma	Ovary	Testicle	Stomach	Prostate	Brain (all)	Lymphomas	Acute lymphocytic leukemias	Bladder
Cyclophosphamide	52	34	20	21	36	20	16	a	a	a	15	a	60	40	20
5-Fluorouracil	a	26	23	21	15	b	b	32	27	23	29	b	26	b	35
Adriamycin	25	35	32	b	20	17	b	38	20	26	22	a	78	37	a
Methotrexate	25	34	21	20	47	22	a	25	40	a	a	54	30	40	44
Dactinomycin	25	a	a	15	a	b	35	a	52	a	a	a	50	a	a
Mitomycin C	33	37	22	16	22	23	a	a	a	30	a	a	47	a	25
Melphalan	a	23	a	23	a	b	15	47	57	a	a	a	32	b	a
Vincristine	47	20	29	a	a	14	12	a	a	a	b	57	56	55	a
Bleomycin	a	a	a	a	15	12	b	15	42	a	a	71	50	a	a
Mechlorethamine	36	35	a	12	b	31	a	31	a	16	39	a	63	a	a
Hexamethylmelamine	b	20	28	12	a	20	a	a	a	a	39	a	a	a	30
BCNU	24	21	a	13	16	11	18	a	a	18	15	47	50	a	a
6-Mercaptopurine	a	a	a	a	a	a	a	a	a	a	a	a	37	65	a

[a] Not evaluated adequately.
[b] Less than 10% of patients show objective benefit.

example, Burkitt's lymphoma is usually cured by cyclophosphamide in Stage I or II, but not in Stage IV; thus, Table 12 gives probably the minimum frequency of objective remissions. The data are from the NCI–DCT (Wasserman *et al.*, 1975), and are not comprehensive.

We can see several immediate suggestions from this summary: Many cancer types have not been adequately evaluated with many drugs. The majority of cancers do not respond with remissions. Some cancers, such as lymphomas, are particularly drug-sensitive; others, such as melanoma or lung or colon cancers, are usually quite drug-resistant. For the first time, we can obtain some reasonable idea of the relative effectiveness of many useful drugs in several cancer types.

From this summary, there emerges what might be tentatively called a list of 13 "best" drugs—drugs giving a wide anticancer spectrum or the highest rate of direct effectiveness. The drugs on this list include drugs with many toxic drawbacks (e.g., mitomycin C) or currently limited tumor spectrum (6-MP). The list finds BCNU more effective than its more lipophilic congeners in the overall objective performance. This list includes only three metabolite structure analogues, two acting at active centers of enzymes. Among drugs acting to react directly with DNA, we have 9 of our 13 drugs, 6 of them alkylating agents (Salmon and Apple, 1976). Some drugs have not been evaluated on many cancers. The reason may be, in part, that early uncontrolled trials did not suggest promise; mainly, however, it appears that the studies have just not been conducted.

7.5. Cycle-Phase Specificity and Drug Scheduling

633

NEW
ANTICANCER
DRUG
DESIGN:
PAST AND
FUTURE
STRATEGIES

Another useful principle of clinical drug use is that anticancer drugs seem to act to kill cells (1) only when the cells are in a particular stage of cell division (e.g., Ara-C, hydroxyurea); or (2) only in a particular stage of the cell division cycle, but with a self-limitation due to mechanism of effect (e.g., MTX, 6-MP, 5-FU); or (3) on all cells, in all phases of the mitotic cycle (e.g., cyclophosphamide, doxorubicin, dactinomycin) (Skipper *et al.*, 1970). The importance of knowing this principle is that a basic tenet of clinical drug use, that maximal drug effect is achieved by achieving a maximal product of $C \times t$ (drug Concentration *in vivo* $\times$ time), would be expected only from drugs of the nonspecific type (3) above. In the other cases, the effect of increasing C beyond that needed to kill cancer cells in the susceptible phase would not be to increase effectiveness, since cells in nonsusceptible phases would be unaffected. Thus, the schedule of drug use for drugs effective only in particular stages ("cycle-phase-specific" drugs) would be best if one maintained the drug at a minimally cytocidal concentration long enough for all cells in a tumor to enter the sensitive phase. For many cells in a tumor, this would be one total cycle time. For those cells not in a division cycle in the same tumor, the time and dose would be irrelevant. In theory, all cycle-nonspecific [type (3) above] drugs would be superior to any cycle-specific drug in treating advanced solid cancers (i.e., big enough to see), since the type (3) cycle-nonspecific drug can kill cells cycling or noncycling (i.e., dividing or resting), but a type (1) or type (2) drug can kill only the cycling fraction. In contrast, when tumors are smaller and have mostly cycling cells, such as postsurgical invisible metastases, they might be a good target for cycle-specific drugs (Schabel, 1975*b*).

Examples of data testing the concept of schedule optima are shown in Table 13. The cases represented are extremes, but illustrate the polarity of schedule optima possible (Skipper *et al.*, 1970; Venditti, 1971).

Alkylating drugs and intercalating antibiotics are usually type (3) cycle-nonspecific; drugs acting on enzyme active centers or enzyme regulatory sites are usually type (1) or type (2) cycle-phase-specific drugs.

Perhaps a more useful measure is the ratio of stem cell kill when cells are rapidly proliferating vs. "resting." This ratio is 1.5–2.5 for most alkylating agents, but higher for metabolite structure analogues (e.g., 5-FU = 4.0) (van Putten *et al.*, 1972).

7.6. Gompertzian Growth and Growth Fractions

The population of cancer cells grows almost continuously. The population increases exponentially with time, which provides the illusion of a terminal explosive increase in growth rate. Although there is a substantial increase in cancer cell number, the *rate* of growth is actually continually *decreasing* all through the history of the cancer (van Putten *et al.*, 1972; Laster *et al.*, 1969). Figure 9 illustrates the growth of a cancer that shows an exponential increase in tumor cell

TABLE 13
Cycle Specificity and Dosage Schedule Optima: L1210[a]

Drug[b]	Phase specificity	% ILS	
		Single max. dose	q3h × 8
Cytosine arabinoside	S-phase specific	59	400+
Cyclophosphamide	Nonspecific	400	20

[a] Data from L1210 murine leukemia.

[b] Ara-C given every 3 hr produced some apparent cures; given at a single maximum dose, its effectiveness is minimal, because it drops below an effective level before all cancer cells have entered a sensitive phase. Cyclophosphamide, in contrast, does not have this limitation, and achieves a maximal C × t and selectivity given once.

number with time while growing at a continuously decreasing rate (called *Gompertzian kinetics*) (Salmon and Apple, 1974). At some point, the body has accommodated its maximum burden of cancer cells, and one of the events leading to death will probably occur; this lethal number of cells is over 10^{12}, or 1 kg of cancer (Salmon and Apple, 1976) in many cases.

The rate of growth of tumor is fast when burden is low, slow when body burden is high. The growth fraction, the percentage of the tumor cell population actively in mitosis, is high when the tumor is small and low when the tumor cell population of the body is large.

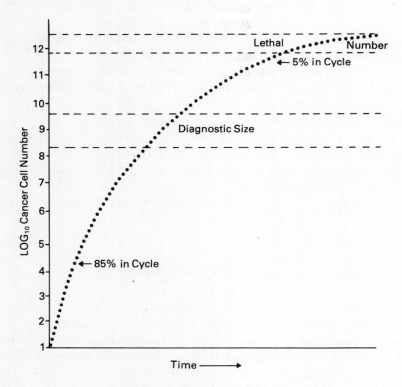

FIGURE 9. Cancer growth *in vivo*.

7.7. Optimizing Single-Drug Use

635

NEW
ANTICANCER
DRUG
DESIGN:
PAST AND
FUTURE
STRATEGIES

The clinical course of cancer is thus the last 2–3 logs of growth, only 5–10 mass doublings, at a rapidly decreasing rate of growth and rapidly diminishing growth fraction of tumor. The immense problems of treatment of this advanced cancer become evident when cycle-phase-specific drugs are employed as first-choice agents, as in advanced colon cancer with 5-FU as a first-choice treatment (Salmon and Apple, 1976; Moore *et al.*, 1968). The success rate is low and, as would be predicted, not curative. Ovarian cancer, which is highly responsive to many alkylating drugs, is also not cured by cycle-phase-specific drugs, but they are given on a one-drug, frequent, low-dose schedule, just the opposite of a predicted more effective schedule. Model experiments in animals indicate that each dose of an anticancer drug kills a specific *fraction*, not a specific number, of surviving cancer cells (i.e., a single dose will cut 10^8 cells to 10^6 or 10^4 to 10^2, although these are quite different numbers of cells killed by the dose) (Skipper *et al.*, 1964).

Each drug also has a toxic effect on normal cells, from which they may eventually recover. The drug therapist must choose (1) the optimal drug(s), (2) the optimal dosage level, (3) the optimal schedule of doses, and (4) the total number of doses. If the chosen drug(s), dosages, schedule, and duration with concomitant tolerable toxicity produce a steady decrease in the number of viable cancer cells, the cancer may be curable. If not, the duration of time the tumor is delayed in reaching a lethal number represents the increased life span of patients, which may be several years.

Given these virtually unapplied developing principles of cycle-phase specificity, Gompertzian growth, growth fraction, fractional cell kill, and inadequate data on the tumor transport, sensitivity, pharmacokinetics, and metabolism of most clinically valuable agents, it is far too early to conclude that the clinical data in Table 12 are final; instead, they will show substantial improvement when judicious use is made of new knowledge about present drugs. These findings will also serve to provide principles on which new drug design can be based to lead to much more effective drugs.

8. Drug Combinations

8.1. Millions of Permutations

The idea of using drug combinations for cancer treatment is a derivation of the prior ideas of antimicrobial combined chemotherapy. In cancer, the idea of sequential blockade of metabolic pathways *in vivo* was proposed as the first basis for combining drugs (Potter, 1951). Early clinical multidrug trials started with lung and testicular cancer at the very beginning of cancer chemotherapy 20 years ago.

The current interest in drug combinations for cancer is an outgrowth both of the history of acute lymphocytic leukemia treatment (Table 14) and of the failure

TABLE 14

Progress in Prognosis Over 20 Years in Acute Lymphocytic Leukemia

Years	Group or investigator	Type of therapy [a]	Median survival
1937–1953	Tivey	Supportive	3.5
1946–1947	Burchenal	Supportive	3.5
1944–1960	Boggs	Supportive pred., MTX, 6-MP	7.0
1956–1957	Hendersen	Pred., MTX, 6-MP	5.0
1961	Boggs	Pred., MTX, 6-MP	12.0
1954–1962	Cutler	Pred., 6-MP, MTX	12.0
1958–1962	ALGB	Pred., MTX, 6-MP, cytoxan	12.0
1959–1963	Burchenal	Pred., MTX, 6-MP, cytoxan	13.0
1955–1963	Zuelzer	Pred., MTX, 6-MP	16.0
1963–1964	NCl	VAMP	24.0
1963–1965	ALGB	Combination of pred., 6-MP, VCR, MTX, cytoxan	24.0
1965–1966	NCI	POMP	33.0
1966–1968	ALGB	Combination pred., VCR, MTX, 6-MP, daunomycin	36.0
1968–1975	St. Jude's	Combination VCR, pred., 6-MP, MTX, cytoxan	46.0

[a] Treatment of acute lymphocytic leukemia has followed the two-decade history of supportive care only (3.5-month survival); discovery, introduction, and improved use of three- and four-drug sequential, one at a time, drug treatments (12–16 month survival); and four- and five-drug combination or concomitant treatment (2–5 year survival); and multidrug plus CNS multimodality therapy (in progress, curative).

to develop rationally designed cancer-selective drugs. Both these influences have led to a variety of often unsystematic trial combinations in patients and to a systematic study in mice using some of the principles we have been discussing. Patient experimentation has led to three-, four-, five-, and even up to eight-drug combination therapy.

We have, depending on the criteria we accept, between 25 and 50 drugs active in cancer chemotherapy. There are 2.54×10^8 permutations of 50 drugs used 5 at a time that could be evaluated. The only strategy possible for evaluating drug combinations is to derive summary principles, an epitome of empirical observations on smaller two- and three- drug groupings. Much groundwork will have to be done in animals, and the chosen animal models will have to include those highly comparable to (or derived from) human solid cancers. Selecting the 15 or 20 most promising drugs for study 2 at a time offers hope of being feasible, since only 380 human trials would be needed to study all potential permutations of 20 drugs used 2 at a time. A comparison of 380 parallel animal studies would provide evidence of the similarities and differences and allow choice of animal models for the next successive step, 20 best drugs used 3 at a time, all the permutations of which can be evaluated in 6840 trials. If ordering proves unimportant or animal data allow prediction of optimal order, we could study the 20 best drugs in all possible best combinations in 1140 trials, at least half of which could be eliminated as unpromising from consistent failure in the two- and three-drug animal trials. We would then, for the first time, have a basis beyond hunch and intuition for pursuing drug combination (concomitant administration) treatment in human cancer.

8.2. Multidrug Rationale

637

NEW
ANTICANCER
DRUG
DESIGN:
PAST AND
FUTURE
STRATEGIES

The current bases for clinical drug combination protocols include the following:

1. Use drugs with widely different mechanisms of action. This basis is not supported by all the evidence. Empirical studies documenting that two alkylating agents can act synergistically (Mayo *et al.*, 1972; Carter, 1972) suggest that this hypothesis might be profitably reexamined.

2. Use drugs with diverse toxicity patterns. This usage has some basis in fact, in that by so doing, one can utilize a full cancerocidal dose and worry less about a lethal pileup of toxicity on one normal target organ. Use of two marrow-toxic drugs at full dosage has been found effective (Frei *et al.*, 1961), however, despite this *a priori* intuition.

3. Use only drugs that themselves are active independently on the target cancer. As a beginning, this is reasonable, but as we learn more, we begin to see uses of second drugs devoid of anticancer effects, such as tetrahydrouridine (Neil *et al.*, 1970), allopurinol (Elion *et al.*, 1963), or folinic acid (Djerassi *et al.*, 1968; Capizzi *et al.*, 1970; Bertino *et al.*, 1971), and must question even this assertion.

Among the pioneer successful drug combinations is the vincristine–MTX–6-MP–prednisone based treatment of childhood acute lymphocytic leukemia. This regimen started the trend toward drug-combination treatment because it had an immediate impact on one of the least treatable cancers (Freireich *et al.*, 1964). A logical argument against its use was that since up to that time we had increased leukemic patient survival by 5-fold by sequential use and failure with each drug alone, and all drug treatments failed in a few months, we might use up all our available drug weapons at once, only to see the disease exacerbate in a few weeks or months, and have no drugs left to continue the treatment. Arrayed against this argument were an *a priori* argument that the antileukemic effects of several drugs at once might be additive, without additive toxicity, and a historical combination-chemotherapy argument that mutation to drug resistance should be independent for each drug, decreasing the chances of a resistant population exponentially with each new drug. The only answer was a test, and the success of the test was evident within two years.

8.3. Multidrug Success

Subsequently, Hodgkin's disease and breast cancer have been treated successfully with drug combinations (DeVita, 1973; Rossi *et al.*, 1976; Greenspan, 1966, Cooper, 1969), and they are now the basis of most new treatment design. The emerging cure of Hodgkin's disease with mechlorethamine–vincristine–procarbazine–prednisone has provided the telling argument leading to combinations of drugs, used earlier and earlier in treatment, becoming the expectation for most present investigation. Important pharmacokinetic considerations for drug-combination optimization are beginning to emerge (Broder and Carbone, 1976; Skipper *et al.*, 1970).

8.4. Unanswered Questions About Multidrug Treatment

We still have many unanswered questions about multidrug therapy. We need systematic evaluations that give clear-cut, decisive answers to these many questions if we are to have any real hope of optimal use of our available anticancer drugs in multidrug regimens. Perhaps answers to some of the following questions will tip the balance to possible cure by optimizing multidrug treatments.

One can approach questions such as which drug first and why? Do we best combine cycle-specific or -nonspecific drugs? Is sequential blockade superior to altogether different mechanisms? What factors contravene the need for different toxicity patterns? Do principles for combining enzyme-active-center-active drugs differ from those of combining drugs acting on DNA? What produces antagonistic drug combinations? How frequent is the production of synergistic toxicity? How many tumor types should be studied in man in initial trials? How many mouse tumors are needed to predict for human drug combinations? What types of drugs are best given simultaneously? Do drugs of one group enhance/block metabolism of another? How do two drugs affect each other's excretion? Can one drug help to selectively protect normal cells from the toxicity of the other? What combinations best prevent the development of resistant clones of tumor *in vivo*? Do drugs that inhibit DNA repair act to potentiate carcinogenicity of other drugs? Is sequential blockade superior/inferior to concurrent or complementary biochemical blockade in creating maximal selectivity? Do we use each drug on its optimal schedule as a single drug?

8.5. Dangerous Drug Combinations

Multiple-drug regimens are now becoming more widely used for cancer drug therapy because of superior results and a wider variety of available drugs. Multiple-drug therapies, however, create a new set of problems: some drugs interact to negate each other's effectiveness; some drugs interact to create new toxicities, or to enhance the toxicity of either agent being used together.

It is also just now being realized that the interactions of nonchemotherapeutics with the newly developed cancer chemotherapeutics can create specific new hazards for the patient; it is thus necessary to be aware if a patient is receiving any cancer chemotherapeutic agent even if he is not being treated for cancer, e.g., the widespread use of MTX for psoriasis.

We may group the mechanisms of adverse drug interactions of noncancer chemotherapeutics with anticancer drugs into those that act by displacement of cancer drug from plasma proteins, those that act metabolically to enhance the cancer drug, those instances in which the cancer drug alters the action of the other drug, and those instances in which the other drug antagonizes the clinically sought activity of the cancer drug (Table 15) (Apple, 1975a).

Due to the inadequacy of study involved in determining the significance of these *in vivo* interactions, one can only prescribe caution in using these drugs together.

639

NEW
ANTICANCER
DRUG
DESIGN:
PAST AND
FUTURE
STRATEGIES

TABLE 15
Potentially Dangerous Interactions in Anticancer Drug Therapy[a]

Interacting drug		Anticancer drug	Adverse effect
Group 1. Displacement interactions in which interacting drug increases anticancer drug toxicity by displacement from plasma proteins			
Aspirin or any salicylate-containing mixture	+	Methotrexate	Pancytopenia
	+	Mercaptopurine	Pancytopenia
	+	Corticosteroids	Leukopenia, gastric ulceration
Barbiturates	+	Methotrexate	Bone marrow depression
Diphenylhydantoin	+	Methotrexate	Bone marrow depression
Phenylbutazone and antiinflammatory pyrazolones	+	Corticosteroids	Leukopenia
Sulfonamides	+	Methotrexate	Pancytopenia, bone marrow depression, bloody diarrhea, aplasia, hepatitis
	+	Mercaptopurine	Bone marrow depression
Tranquilizers	+	Methotrexate	Bone marrow depression
Triamterene	+	Methotrexate	Bone marrow depression
Group 1A. Anticancer drug alters effect of another drug			
Insulin	+	Cyclophosphamide, methotrexate, and probably others	Hypoglycemia
Group 2. Metabolic interactions in which interacting drug increases anticancer drug toxicity by blocking metabolic detoxification or increasing metabolic activation			
Allopurinol	+	Mercaptopurine	Bone marrow aplasia, hepatitis
Barbiturates	+	Cyclophosphamide	Bone marrow depression; also: either can block activation of the other depending on timing
Chlordan, halogenated insecticides	+	Cyclophosphamide	Bone marrow depression
Group 3. Interference in which interacting drug increases anticancer drug effectiveness by blocking activation or increasing metabolic detoxification			
Prednisolone	+	Cyclophosphamide	Decreased cyclophosphamide activation
Chloramphenicol	+	Cyclophosphamide	Decreased cyclophosphamide activation or additive bone marrow toxicity
Antihistamines	+	Corticosteroids	Increased steroid catabolism
Barbiturates	+	Corticosteroids	Increased steroid catabolism
Glutethimide	+	Corticosteroids	Increased steroid catabolism
Group 4. Activity interactions in which anticancer drug alters normal effect of other drugs			
Alcohol	+	Methotrexate	Hepatotoxicity, respiratory failure
	+	Procarbazine	Synergistic potentiation of CNS depression
Tetanus toxoid, other vaccines	+	Cyclophosphamide, methotrexate, corticosteroids	Immunosuppression, failure to develop immunity

(continued)

TABLE 15 (*continued*)

Interacting drug		Anticancer drug	Adverse effect
Penicillin	+	Actinomycin D	Bacteriostasis, failure of penicillin-sensitive bacteria to respond
Barbiturates	+	Actinomycin D	Failure of barbiturate induction of enzymes
	+	Corticosteroids	Increased barbiturate sedation
Anticoagulants	+	Alkylating drugs, antimetabolites	Decreased clotting by induction of thrombocytopenia and inhibition of vitamin K synthesis
Oxytocin	+	Cyclophosphamide	Increased oxytocic effect
Cholinergics (pilocarpine, physostigmine)	+	Cortisteroids	Decreased cholinergic effect
Digitalis	+	Corticosteroids	Increased hypokalemia
Diuretics (furosemide, thiazides)	+	Corticosteroids	Increased hypokalemia
CNS depressants (sedatives, tranquilizers, hypnotics, barbiturates, hypotensives, some antihistamines)	+	Procarbazine	Severe CNS depression, coma, respiratory paralysis
Tricyclic antidepressants	+	Procarbazine	Seizures, hyperpyrexia
Sympathomimetics	+	Procarbazine	Acute hypertensive crisis

a From Apple (1975*a*).

In some instances, the drug combinations can be lethal, and these combinations are probably contraindicated even if the adverse interaction is rare.

Examples of mechanism types include the common displacement of MTX or 6-MP from plasma proteins by salicylates or sulfonamides, enhancing the toxicity of the anticancer drug. Obviously, the degree of effect depends on the dosage and timing of administration of the two drug combinations.

A second type of interaction is illustrated by that proposed for allopurinal–6-MP (Fig. 10). The administered 6-MP is metabolized in two general directions: toward active methylmercaptopurine ribotide and toward inactive thiourate (Caldwell, 1969). The latter path is blocked by the allopurinol frequently given as a preventive for the hyperuricemia that follows chemotherapy, creating excess toxicity of 6-MP. This problem appears to be tentatively solved by cutting the 6-MP dose 4-fold when allopurinol is given concomitantly (Salmon and Apple, 1976; Apple, 1975*a*; Zimmerman *et al.*, 1974).

Some anticancer drugs produce metabolites that affect other drug activity. Procarbazine is metabolized into a MAO inhibitor. Sometimes CNS depressants or

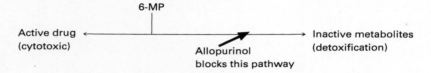

FIGURE 10. Proposed interaction for allopurinol–6-MP.

sympathomimetics will produce bizarre crises if given with procarbazine, this effect being attributed to the drug combination (Apple, 1975a; E. W. Martin, 1971).

Penicillin and the anticancer drug dactinomycin are both able to stop growth of gram-positive bacteria, but dactinomycin is only bacteriostatic, stopping the cell-wall synthesis mechanism by which penicillins act and possibly precluding the penicillin arrest of a susceptible infection (Apple, 1975a; E. W. Martin, 1971).

The existence of these interactions requires that the full drug history, past and present, be known when any anticancer drug is to be given to a patient.

9. Past, Present, and Future

9.1. Tested and Untested Assumptions

The basic premises on which cancer chemotherapy is based are that:

1. A single cancer cell is sufficient to create a lethal tumor.
2. Cancer grows continuously.
3. All cancers can invade or metastasize.
4. Drugs must kill every cancer cell or fail.
5. Anticancer drugs must show selective killing toxicity.
6. In the absence of evidence, hunches will serve to design drug-use protocols.

The basic premises of anticancer drug discovery (over the last half century) are that:

7. Somewhere in nature or among all the world's existing organic chemicals, there exists a magic bullet that will cure cancer.
8. Screening through a chosen animal cancer will uncover that magic bullet.
9. We must screen every existing chemical, including all those new ones created/isolated for other purposes every day.
10. There are no *a priori* bases for intuitive or empirical selection or priority ranking among unscreened chemicals.
11. The active, non-magic-bullet, drugs can be made better by altering their physicochemical properties without first fully determining why they were initially active.

If these premises, the epitome of most current-day anticancer drug science, appear to be phrased to sound like grim satire, the phrasing is intentional.

Where we go from here depends on how many of these premises we accept, what new ones we might add instead. We might easily accept premises (1), (2), and (3), but question all the others; e.g., even if (11) has been demonstrated, it might be far inferior to other strategies. As we progress through the 20th century, we will learn which of these premises was a cornerstone and which were instead castles in the air.

Additional premises to test include:

12. Selective toxicity of anticancer drugs is based on selective concentration in cancer cells.

13. Cycle-phase-specific drugs can be used effectively only for treatment of micrometastases or tumors with a growth fraction of more than 75%.

14. Selective cancer toxicity can be achieved by designing drugs to be activated by carbohydrate catabolic enzymes or amino acid and nucleoside anabolic enzymes.

15. Selective cancer toxicity can be achieved by drug-induced enhanced cancer cell antigenicity.

16. Every drug used clinically in cancer should be given only at its optimal schedule.

17. Human cancers follow Gompertzian kinetics.

18. Negative information is useful for drug design.

19. The more the information available about a drug, the more optimally it will be used.

20. Drug combinations that cure cancer can be developed from rational principles.

21. Learning exhaustively why current anticancer drugs work will allow us to use them as effective leads to improving all existing drugs.

22. Drugs designed first around receptor-binding ultimately will work more effectively and involve less design/synthesis effort than other design bases.

23. Selective curative anticancer effects of new drugs depend on prior intensive biological studies to define the bases on which the drugs can be designed.

24. Both the growth fraction and the optimal drugs of choice shift with each major change in cancer size.

25. A cure for cancer, a "magic bullet," will have to be designed rationally (a corollary, given the inability of random screening thus far to find the magic bullet, is: Any experiment that has failed 250,000 consecutive times should be viewed with suspicion).

9.2. Drug Design Strategy: Cloudy Crystal Ball

Future anticancer drug-design strategy could well start in the domain of biochemical, not physicochemical, measurements. Receptor targets might be chosen with care. Such receptors might include enzymes that are key to the marginal or significant biochemical differences between cancer cells and normally growing counterparts, antigenic identity markers, or noncancer sites, e.g., endothelial cell angiogenesis factor receptor. The receptor function might become exhaustively known, its properties (isolated and *in situ*) carefully defined.

Drugs binding to the receptor might be created *de novo* or as antagonists to known binding agents (e.g., enzyme substrates), following predictive models of receptor functioning and blockade. The receptor-binding antagonists might be studied to determine binding affinity, kinetics of release, contact points between drug candidate antagonists and receptor key to affinity, and so on. The success and failure of the *in vitro* receptor-effective agent as a drug *in vivo* might be exhaustively documented: how and how well the drug is absorbed, plasma protein bound, metabolized, excreted, handled by cancer cells of differing redox potential, and affected by other drugs in combination. From these data, a prescription might be written that suggests structural manipulations at non-receptor-binding sites that would increase absorption, decrease plasma protein binding, block destructive metabolism (or enhance desired metabolism), slow the excretion, be selectively transported into cancer cells, be selectively activated in cancer cells, and synergize the activity of a drug in combination. These prescriptions could be tested by appropriate synthesis of structural congeners. From the feedback of these data, further "fine tuning" of structural features could be prescribed and tested.

These prescriptions should be designed to test all feasible and possible options against each other simultaneously, rather than pursuing each idea one at a time; crucial tests distinguishing multiple viable alternatives could be the rule of experimentation.

The approach that might be taken is illustrated in Fig. 11. Such an approach, the rational science of cancer chemotherapeutic drug discovery, naturally takes

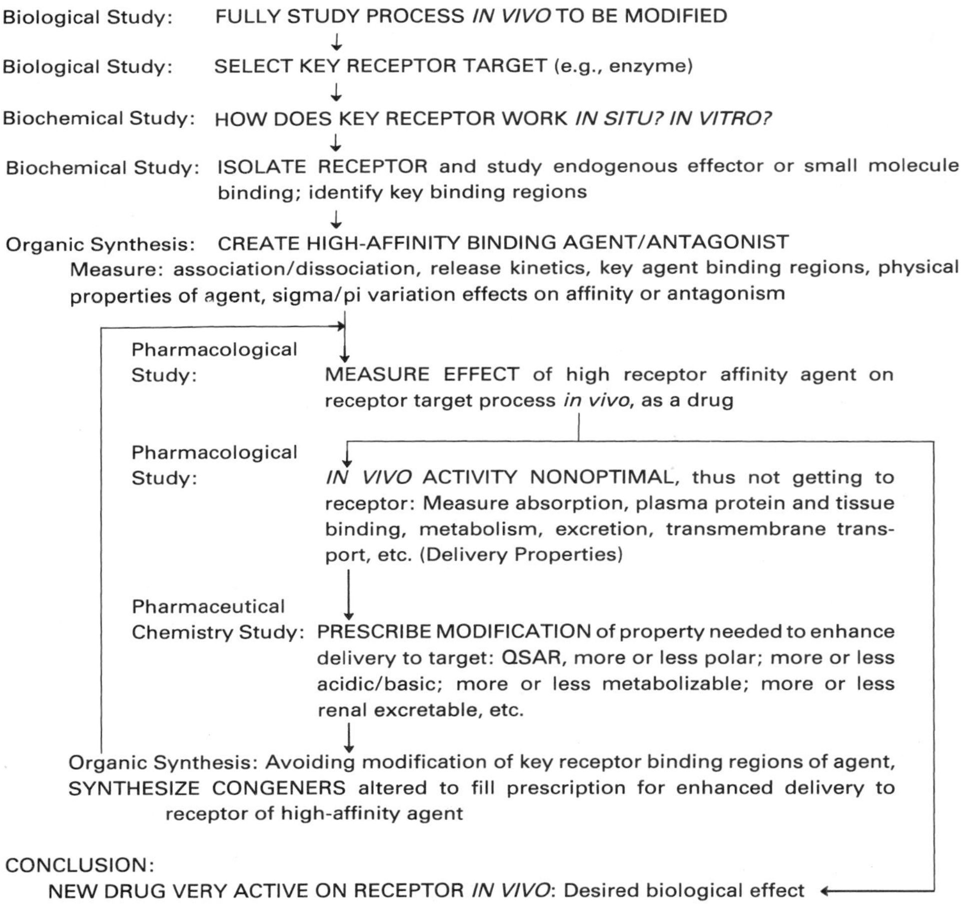

643

NEW
ANTICANCER
DRUG
DESIGN:
PAST AND
FUTURE
STRATEGIES

Biological Study: FULLY STUDY PROCESS *IN VIVO* TO BE MODIFIED
↓
Biological Study: SELECT KEY RECEPTOR TARGET (e.g., enzyme)
↓
Biochemical Study: HOW DOES KEY RECEPTOR WORK *IN SITU? IN VITRO?*
↓
Biochemical Study: ISOLATE RECEPTOR and study endogenous effector or small molecule binding; identify key binding regions
↓
Organic Synthesis: CREATE HIGH-AFFINITY BINDING AGENT/ANTAGONIST
      Measure: association/dissociation, release kinetics, key agent binding regions, physical properties of agent, sigma/pi variation effects on affinity or antagonism

Pharmacological
Study: MEASURE EFFECT of high receptor affinity agent on receptor target process *in vivo*, as a drug

Pharmacological
Study: *IN VIVO* ACTIVITY NONOPTIMAL, thus not getting to receptor: Measure absorption, plasma protein and tissue binding, metabolism, excretion, transmembrane transport, etc. (Delivery Properties)

Pharmaceutical
Chemistry Study: PRESCRIBE MODIFICATION of property needed to enhance delivery to target: QSAR, more or less polar; more or less acidic/basic; more or less metabolizable; more or less renal excretable, etc.

Organic Synthesis: Avoiding modification of key receptor binding regions of agent, SYNTHESIZE CONGENERS altered to fill prescription for enhanced delivery to receptor of high-affinity agent

CONCLUSION:
    NEW DRUG VERY ACTIVE ON RECEPTOR *IN VIVO*: Desired biological effect ←

FIGURE 11. Receptor targeting and delivery strategy (the rational integration of biological, biochemical, pharmacological, pharmaceutical chemical, and organic chemical studies).

some years to develop fully, but predicts that the future fruits of knowledge are more likely to exceed the fruits of ignorance. Further expanding random screening technology is less perspicacious than developing rational design methods. We are in the drug era of the one-at-a-time handmade product; if we take the time now to create new tools of knowledge, even if no new drugs develop out of these tools immediately, we will launch the equivalent impact of the industrial revolution in the field of drug discovery for cancer.

As we stop cursing the darkness to light one candle, and by its light we order "Let the revolution begin," the titles of three books by Thomas Paine, in the following sequence, come to mind as a suitable conclusion to this volume: *The American Crisis, Common Sense, The Age of Reason.*

ACKNOWLEDGMENTS

This research was supported in part by USPHS grant CA 14894-03. The author thanks reviewers Dr. F. Becker and Dr. S. K. Carter, and Winifred Heintz for secretarial assistance.

10. References

ALBERT, A., 1975, Selective toxicity, in: *Pharmacological Basis of Cancer Chemotherapy*, pp. 152–164, Williams and Wilkins, Baltimore.

ALLAN, P., SCHNEBLI, H., AND BENNETT, L., 1966, Conversion of 6-mercaptopurine to 6-methylmercaptopurine ribotide in human epidermoid carcinoma #2 cells in culture, *Biochim. Biophys. Acta* 114: 647–650.

AMES, B., AND GARRY, B., 1959, Coordinate repression of the synthesis of four histidine biosynthetic enzymes by histidine, *Proc. Natl. Acad. Sci.* 45:1453–1460.

ANDERSON, D., 1971, Some characteristics of familial breast cancer, *Cancer* 28:1500.

ANDERVONT, H. B., AND BRYAN, W. F. 1944, Properties of the mouse mammary-tumor agent, *J. Natl. Cancer Inst.* 5:143.

ANNUAL REPORT OF THE DCT–NCI, 1974, U.S. Government Printing Office.

APPLE, M. A., 1973, Review of reverse transcription and its inhibitors, *Annu. Rep. Med. Chem.* 8:251–262.

APPLE, M. 1975a, Avoiding drug interactions in anticancer drug therapy, *Drug Ther.* 5:203–215.

APPLE, M. A. 1975b, Active intervention to prevent cancer with prophylactic drugs *in vivo, J. Clin. Pharmacol.* 15:29–36.

APPLE, M. A., AND GREENBERG, D., 1972, Enzymes as anticancer drugs: Antileukemic effect and substrate inhibition properties of an enzyme catalyzing nucleophilic displacements at N^6 of purines, *Proc. West. Pharmacol. Soc.* 15:143–153.

APPLE, M., FORMICA, J., AND JOHNSON, R. K., 1975, *In vivo* cure of P-388 leukemia and prevention of oncorna virus induced sarcomas by new azetomicins, *Pharmacology* 17:297.

APPLE, M. A., HERCHER, M., HIRSCHFELD, T., AND KEEFE, T., 1976, Microdetection and differentiation of free and intraviral nucleic acids using laser fluorescence microscopy and fluorochrome staining, in: *Immune RNA and Neoplasia* (M. Fink, ed.), pp. 303–316, Academic Press, New York.

ARIENS, E. J., 1974, Design of bioactive compounds, in: *Topics in Current Chemistry*, Vol. LII, pp. 1ff, Springer-Verlag, New York.

ARNOLD, H., AND BORSEAUX, F., 1958, Synthese and Abban zytostatisch wirksamer cyclischer N-phosphamidester des *Bis*(Beta-chloroäthyl)-amins, *Angew. Chem.* 70:539–544.

645

NEW
ANTICANCER
DRUG
DESIGN:
PAST AND
FUTURE
STRATEGIES

ATKINSON, M., MORTON, R., AND MURRAY, A., 1964, Inhibition of adenlyosuccinate synthetase and adenylosuccinate lyase from Ehrlich ascites tumor cells by 6-thioinosine-5'-phosphate, *Biochem. J.* **92**:398–404.

BENNETT, L. L., JR., BROCKMAN, R., SCHNEBLI, H., CHUMLEY, S., DIXON, G. J., SCHABEL, F., DULMADGE, E., SKIPPER, H., MONTGOMERY, J., AND THOMAS, H., 1965, Activity and mechanism of action of 6 methylthiopurine ribonucleoside in cancer cells resistant to 6-mercaptopurine, *Nature London* **205**:1276–1279.

BERTINO, J., 1975, Folate antagonists, in: *Antineoplastic and Immunosuppressive Agents*, Vol. II (A. Sartorelli and D. Johns, eds.), pp. 468–483, Springer-Verlag, New York.

BERTINO, J. R., LEVITT, M., MCCULLOUGH, J., AND CHABNER, B., 1971, New approaches to chemotherapy with folate antagonists: Use of leucovorin rescue and enzymic folate depletion, *Ann. N. Y. Acad. Sci.* **186**:486.

BITTNER, J., AND LITTLE, C. 1937, The transmission of breast and lung cancer in mice, *J. Hered.* **28**:117.

BLOEDORN, F. G., CONLEY, R., CUCCIA, C., AND MERCADO, R., 1961, Combined therapy, irradiation and surgery in the treatment of bronchogenic carcinoma, *Amer. J. Roentgenol.* **85**:875.

BLUMENTHAL, R., CHANGEAUX, J.-P., AND LEFEVER, R., 1970, *C. R. Acad. Sci. (Paris) Ser. D*: **270**:389.

BOSMANN, H. B., 1972, Acetylcholine receptor, *J. Biol. Chem.* **247**:130–145.

BRADBURY, A. F., SMYTH, D., SNELL, C., BIRDSAELL, N., AND HULME, E., 1976, C-fragment of lipotropin has a high affinity for brain opiate receptors, *Nature (London)* **260**:793.

BRODER, L. E., AND CARBONE, P., 1976, Pharmacokinetic considerations in the design of optimal chemotherapeutic regimens for the treatment of breast carcinoma: A conceptual approach, *Med. Pediatr. Oncol.* **2**:11–27.

BROOKES, P., AND LAWLEY, P., 1961, The reaction of mono-and difunctional alkylating agents with nucleic acids, *Biochem. J.* **80**:495–503.

BRUICE, T. C., KHARASCH, N., AND WINZLER, R. J., 1956, *Arch. Biochem. Biophys.* **62**:305.

BULKACZ, F., APPLE, M., CRAIG, J., AND NAIK, A., 1968, Thiophene analogs of sulfanilamide: Bacterial growth inhibitors, *J. Pharm. Sci.* **57**:1017–1021.

BURCHALL, J., 1971, Comparative biochemistry of dihydrofolate reductase, *Ann. N. Y. Acad. Sci.* **186**:143–152.

BUSCH, H., AND STARBUCK, W., 1964, Biochemistry of cancer, *Annu. Rev. Biochem.* **33**:519.

CALDWELL, I., 1969, Ion exchange chromatography of tissue nucleotides, *J. Chromatogr.* **44**:331–341.

CAMMARATA, A., AND MARTIN, A., 1970, Physical properties and biological activities, in: *Medicinal Chemistry* (A. Burger, ed.), pp. 118–163, Wiley-Interscience, New York.

CAPIZZI, R., DECONTI, R., MARSH, J., AND BERTINO, J., 1970, Methotrexate therapy of head and neck cancer: Improvement in therapeutic index by the use of leucovorin "rescue," *Cancer Res.* **30**:1782.

CARR, C. W., 1973, Studies of the binding of small ions in protein solutions with the use of membrane electrodes, *Arch. Biochem. Biophys.* **40**:286–294.

CARTER, S. K. 1972, Rationale of combination chemotherapy, *Eur. J. Cancer* **9**:183.

CARTER, S. K., AND SLAVIK, M., 1974, Chemotherapy of cancer, *Annu. Rev. Pharmacol.* **14**:157.

CARTER, S. K., SLAVIK, M., *et al.* 1975, Minutes of the Phase-I study working groups, Nov. 1975, DCT, NCI.

CASKEY, C., ASHTON, D., AND WYNGAARDEN, J., 1964, The enzymology of feedback inhibition of glutamine phosphoribosylpyrophosphateamidotransferase by purine ribonucleotides, *J. Biol. Chem.* **239**:2570–2579.

CHADWICK, M., AND ROGERS, W., 1970, The distribution of 5-fluoro-2'deoxyuridine-5'monophosphate in mice after 5-fluorouracil administration. *Proc. Amer. Assoc. Cancer Res.* **11**:15.

CHANGEAUX, J. P., GERHART, J., AND SCHACHMAN, H. K., 1968, Allosteric interactions in aspartate transcarbamylase. I. Binding of specific ligands to the native enzyme and its isolated subunits, *Biochemistry*, **7**:531–538.

CHIGNELL, C., 1969, Optical studies of drug–protein complexes, *Mol. Pharmacol.* **5**:244–252, 455–462.

CHIGNELL, C., 1970, Spectroscopic techniques for studying the interactions of drugs with biological systems, *Adv. Drug. Res.* **5**:55–94.

CLINE, M. J., AND HASKELL, C. M., 1975, *Cancer Chemotherapy*, Saunders, Philadelphia, pp. 1–324.

COHEN, J. L., KRANDT, M., SHNIDER, B., MATIAS, P., NORTON, J., AND BAXTER, D., 1971, Radiation plus 5-fluorouracil: Clinical demonstration of an additive effect in bronchogenic carcinoma, *Cancer Chemother. Rep.* **55**:253.

COLQUHOUN, D., 1973, Relation between classical and cooperative models for drug action, in: *Drug Receptors, A Symposium*, pp. 149–182, University Park Press, Baltimore.

COOPER, R. 1969, Combination chemotherapy of hormone resistant breast cancer, *Proc. Amer. Assoc. Cancer Res.* **10**:15.

CRAIG, P. 1971, Interdependence between physical parameters and selection of substituent groups for correlation studies, *J. Med. Chem.* **14**:680–683.

CSERR, H., FENSTERMACHER, J., AND RALL, D., 1970, Permeability of the choroid plexus and blood-brain barrier to urea, in: *Proceedings of the International Colloquium on Urea and Kidney*, Sarasota, pp. 127–137, Excerpta Medica Foundation, Amsterdam.

CUATRECASAS, P., 1972, Affinity chromatography and purification of the insulin receptor of the inner cell membranes, *Proc. Natl. Acad. Sci. U.S.A.* **69**:1277.

DEBYE, P., 1929, *Polar Molecules*, Chemical Catalog Co., New York.

DEROBERTIS, E., GONZALES, J., AND TELLER, D., 1969, The interaction between atropine sulfate and a proteolipid from cerebral cortex studied by light scattering, *FEBS Lett.* **4**:4–8.

DEVITA, V., 1973, Combined drug treatment of Hodgkin's disease: Remission induction, duration and survival; an appraisal, *Natl. Cancer Inst. Monogr.*, No. 36, pp. 373–379.

DEWEY, W. C., AND HUMPHREY, R. M., 1965, Increase in radiosensitivity of ionizing radiation related to replacement of thymidine in mammalian cells with 5-bromodeoxyuridine, *Radiat. Res.* **26**:538–547.

DJERASSI, I., ROYER, G., TREAT, C., AND CARIM, H., 1968, Management of childhood lymphosarcoma and reticulum cell sarcoma with high dose intermittent methotrexate and citrovorum factor, *Proc. Amer. Assoc. Cancer Res.* **9**:18.

DOSKOCIL, J., 1965, Reaction of deoxyribonucleic acid with triethylenemelamine, *Collect. Czech. Chem. Commun.* **30**:2434.

DRUCKREY, H., PREUSSMA, R., IVANKONIE, S., AND SCHMAHL, S., 1967, Organotropic carcinogenic effects of 65 different *N*-nitroso compounds in BD rats, *Z. Krebsforsch.* **69**:103.

EDWARDS, C. L., AND HAYS, R., 1970, Scanning malignant neoplasms with gallium-67, *J. Amer. Med. Assoc.* **212**:1182–1191.

EHRENPREISS, S., 1965, An approach to the molecular basis of nerve activity, *J. Cell. Comp. Physiol.* **66**:159–164.

ELFORD, H., FREESE, M., PASSAMANI, E., AND MORRIS, H. P., 1970, Ribonucleotide reductase and cell proliferation: Variations in ribonucleotide reductase activity with tumor growth rate in a series of rat hepatomas, *J. Biol. Chem.* **245**:228.

ELION, G. B., CALLAHAN, S., AND NATHAN, H., 1963, Potentiation by inhibition of drug degradation: 6-Substituted purines and xanthine oxidase, *Biochem. Pharmacol.* **12**:85–93.

ERIKSON, R. L., AND SZYBALSKI, W., 1963, Molecular radiobiology of human cell lines. III. Radiation sensitizing properties of 5-iododeoxyuridine, *Cancer Res.* **23**:122–131.

FEFER, A., 1974, Tumor immunotherapy, in: *Antineoplastic and Immunosuppressive Agents*, Vol. I (A. Sartorelli and D. Johns, eds.), pp. 527–554, Springer-Verlag, New York.

FEIGELSON, P., 1968, Studies on allosteric regulation of tryptophan oxygenase: Structure and function, *Adv. Enzyme Regul.* **7**:119.

FISCHER, J., AND JARDETSKY, D., 1965, Nuclear magnetic relaxation study of intermolecular complexes. The mechanism of penicillin binding to serum albumin, *J. Amer. Chem. Soc.* **87**:3237–3244.

FLAKS, J. G., ERWIN, M. J., AND BUCHANAN, J. M., 1957, Biosynthesis of the purines. XVIII. 5-Amino-1-ribosyl-4-imidazolecarboxamide 5′-phosphate transformylase and inosinicase. *J. Biol. Chem.* **229**:603–613.

FLEMING, A., 1929, On the bacterial action of cultures of penicillin with special references to their use in the isolation of *B. influenzae*, *Br. J. Exp. Pathol.* **10**:266.

FLETCHER, G., 1970, Irradiation of peripheral lymphatics in conjunction with radical mastectomy, in: *Breast Cancer, Early and Late, Proceedings of the 13th Clinical Conference on Cancer*, pp. 161–169, Year Book Publishers, Houston.

FOLKMAN, M. J., 1974, Tumor angiogenesis factor, *Cancer Res.* **24**:2109–2113.

FOLKMAN, M. J., AND COTNAN, R., 1976, Relation of endothelial proliferation to tumor growth, *Int. Rev. Exp. Pathol.* **16**:207–248.

FOUNTAIN, J., HUTCHISON, D., WARING, G., AND BURCHENAL, J., 1953, Persistence of amethopterin in normal mouse tissues, *Proc. Soc. Exp. Biol. Med.* **83**:369.

FREE, S., AND WILSON, J., 1964, A mathematical contribution to structure–activity studies, *J. Med. Chem.* **7**:395–399.

647

NEW
ANTICANCER
DRUG
DESIGN:
PAST AND
FUTURE
STRATEGIES

FREI, E., FREIREICH, E. J., GEHAN, E., PINKEL, D., HOLLAND, J., SELAWRY, O., HAURANI, F., SPURR, C., HAYES, D., JAMES, G., ROTHBERG, H., SODEE, D., RUNDLES, R., SCHROEDER, L., HOOGSTRATEN, B., WOLMAN. I.. TRAGGIS. D.. COOPER, T., GENDEL, B., EBAUGH, F., AND TAYLOR, R., 1961, Studies of sequential and combination antimetabolite therapy in acute leukemia: 6-Mercaptopurine and methotrexate, *Blood* 18:431.

FREIREICH, E., KARON, M., AND FREI, E., 1964, Quadruple combination therapy (VAMP) for acute lymphocytic leukemia of childhood, *Proc. Amer. Assoc. Cancer Res.* 5:20.

FURTH, J. J., AND COHEN, S., 1968, Inhibition of mammalian DNA polymerase by the 5'-triphosphate of 1-beta-D-arabinofuranosylcytosine and the 9-beta-arabinofuranosyladenine, *Cancer Res.* 28:2061–2067.

GELHORN, A., 1958, The cocarcinogenic activity of cigarette tobacco tar, *Cancer Res.* 18:510.

GERHART, J. C., AND PARDEE, A. G., 1964, Aspartate transcarbamylase, an enzyme designed for feedback inhibition, *Fed. Proc. Fed. Amer. Soc. Exp. Biol.* 23:727–735.

GERHART, J. C., AND SCHACHMAN, H. K., 1965, Distinct subunits for the regulation and catalytic activity of aspartate transcarbamylase, *Biochemistry* 4:1054–1062.

GIOVANELLA, B. C., 1976, Heterotransplantation of human breast carcinomas in "nude" thymus deficient mice, *Proc. Amer. Assoc. Cancer Res.* 17:124.

GOLDIN, A., VENDITTI, J., MANTEL, N., KLINE, I., AND GANG, M. 1968, Evaluation of combination chemotherapy with three drugs, *Cancer Res.* 28:950–960.

GOLDIN, A., VENDITTI, J., AND MANTEL, N. 1974, Combination chemotherapy: Basic considerations, in: *Antineoplastic and Immunosuppressive Agents* (A. Sartorelli and D. Johns, eds.), pp. 411–448, Springer-Verlag, New York.

GORSKI, J., TOBT, D., SHYMALA, G., SMITH, D., AND NOTIDES, A., 1968, Hormone receptors: Studies on the interaction of estrogen with the uterus, *Recent Prog. Horm. Res.* 24:45–80.

GORDON, S. G., AND KERN, F., 1968, The absorption of bile salt and fatty acid by hamster small intestine, *Biochim. Biophys. Acta.* 152:372–379.

GREENSPAN, E. M., 1966, Combination cytotoxic chemotherapy in advanced disseminated breast carcinoma, *J. Mt. Sinai Hosp.* 33:1.

GREENWALD, E. S. 1972, Cancer chemotherapy, *N. Y. State J. Med.* 72: 2541–2556, 2641–2654, 2757–2768.

HAENSZEL, W., LOVELAND, D., AND SIRKIN, M., 1962, Lung cancer mortality as related to residence and smoking histories: White males, *J. Natl. Cancer Inst.* 28:947–1001.

HAHN, F., 1975, Strategy and tactics of the chemotherapeutic drug development, *Naturwissenschaften* 62:449–458.

HALSTED, W. S., 1907, The results of radical operations for the cure of cancer of the breast, *Ann. Surg.* 46:80.

HAMMET, L. P., 1970, *Physical Organic Chemistry*, pp. 1–420, McGraw-Hill, New York.

HAMMOND, E. C., AND HORN, D., 1958, Smoking and death rates: Report on forty-four months follow-up of 187,783 men—II. Death rates by cause, *J. Amer. Med. Assoc.* 166:1294–1308.

HANSCH, C., 1973, Quantitative approaches to pharmacological structure–activity relationships, in: *Structure–Activity Relationships* (C. J. Cavallito, ed.), pp.75–165, Pergamon Press, New York.

HANSCH, C., AND FUJITA, I., 1964, Rho–sigma–pi analysis: A method for correlation of biological activity and chemical structure, *J. Amer. Chem. Soc.* 86:1616–1626.

HARBERS, E., CHAUDHURI, N., AND HEIDELBERGER, C., 1959, Studies on fluorinated pyrimidines VIII. Further biochemical and metabolic investigations, *J. Biol. Chem.* 234:1255–1261.

HARTMAN, S. C., 1970, Purines and pyrimidines, in: *Metabolic Pathways*, Vol. IV (D. M. Greenberg, ed.), 3rd edition, pp. 1–70, Academic Press, New York.

HARTMAN, S. C., AND BUCHANAN, J. M., 1959, Biosynthesis of the purines. XXVI. The identification of the formyl donors of the transformylation reactions, *J. Biol. Chem.* 234:1812–1817.

HARTMANN, K., AND HEIDELBERGER, C., 1961, Studies on fluorinated pyrimidines. VIII. Inhibition of thymidylate synthetase, *J. Biol. Chem.* 236:3006–3013.

HEITLER, W., AND LONDON, F., 1927, Wechselwirkung neutraler Atome und Homöötolare Bindung nach der quanten Mechanik, *Z. Phys.* 44:455–472.

HENDERSON, E., AND SAMAHA, R., 1969, Evidence that drugs in multiple combinations have materially advanced the treatment of human malignancies, *Cancer Res.* 29:2272–2280.

HENDERSON, E. S., ADAMSON, R., AND OLIVERIO, V., 1965, The metabolic fate of tritiated methotrexate: Absorption and excretion in man, *Cancer Res.* 25:1018.

HENDERSON, J., AND KHOO, M., 1965, On the mechanism of feedback inhibition of purine biosynthesis *de novo* in Ehrlich ascites tumor cells *in vitro*, *J. Biol. Chem.* 240:3104–3109.

HOLLAND, J., AND FREI, E., 1974, *Cancer Medicine*, Lea and Febiger, Philadelphia.

HOGBEN, C., TOCCO, D., BRODIE, B. B., AND SCHANKER, C., 1959, On the mechanism of intestinal absorption of drugs, *J. Pharmacol. Exp. Ther.* **125**:275–282.

HUENNEKENS, F. M., 1968, Folate and B_{12} coenzymes, in: *Biological Oxidations* (T. P. Singer, ed.), pp. 439–513, John Wiley and Sons, New York.

HUENNEKENS, F. M., AND OSBORN, M. J., 1959, Folic acid coenzymes and one-carbon metabolism, *Adv. Enzymol.* **21**:369.

ISRAELACHVILI, J. N., 1974, Van der Waals forces in biological systems, *Q. Rev. Biophys.* **6**:341–387.

IUPAC, 1972, *Enzyme Nomenclature: Recommendations of the International Union of Biochemistry on the Nomenclature and Classification in Enzymes*, Elsevier, Amsterdam.

JAIN, S., AND SOBELL, H., 1972, Refinement and further details of the actinomycin–deoxyguanosine crystalline complex, *J. Mol. Biol.* **68**:1–20.

JENSEN, E., NUMATA, M., BRECHER, P., AND DESOMBRE, E., 1971, Hormone–receptor interaction as a guide to biochemical mechanism, in: *Biochemistry of Hormone Action* (R. Smellie, ed.), pp. 133–159, Academic Press, New York.

KABACK, H. R., 1972, Transport across isolated bacterial cytoplasmic membranes, *Biochem. Biophys. Acta* **265**:367–416.

KARSTEN, C. B., ENGELSMAN, E., AND PERSIJN, J., 1975, Clinical value of estrogen receptors in advanced breast cancer, in: *Estrogen Receptors in Human Cancer* (W. McGuire, P. Carbone, and E. Vollmer, eds.), pp. 93–105, Raven Press, New York.

KEEN, P., 1971, Effect of binding to plasma proteins on the distribution, activity and elimination of drugs, in: *Concepts in Biochemical Pharmacology* (B. Brodie and J. Gillette, eds.), pp. 212–233, Springer-Verlag, New York.

KELLOFF, G., HUEBNER, R., CHANG, N., LEE, Y., AND GILDEN, R., 1970, Envelope antigen relationships among three hamster-specific sarcoma viruses and a hamster-specific virus, *J. Gen. Virol.* **9**:19.

KESSEL, D., HALL, T. C., ROBERTS, B. D., AND WODINSKY, I., 1965, Uptake as a determinant of methotrexate response in mouse leukemias, *Science* **150**:752.

KESSEL, D., HALL, T. C., AND ROBERTS, D., 1968, Modes of uptake of methotrexate by normal and leukemic human leukocytes *in vitro* and their relation to drug response, *Cancer Res.* **28**:564.

KING, R., TAYLOR, P., AND BURGEN, A. S. F., 1970, Kinetics of complex formation between carbonic anhydrase and aromatic sulfonamides, *Biochem.* **9**:2638–2645.

KIT, S., 1970, Nucleotides and nucleic acids, in: *Metabolic Pathways* (D. M. Greenberg, ed.), pp. 69–275, Academic Press, New York.

KLIGERMAN, M. M., 1974, Principles of radiation therapy, in: *Cancer Medicine* (J. Holland and E. Frei, eds.), pp. 541–565, Lea and Febiger, Philadelphia.

KLOTZ, I., WALKER, F., AND PIVAN, R., 1946, The binding of organic ions by proteins, *J. Amer. Chem. Soc.* **68**:1486–1490.

KNOWLES, J. A., 1965, Excretion of drugs in milk: A review, *J. Pediatr.* **66**:1068–1082.

KNOX, W. E., 1966, The regulation of tryptophan pyrrolase activity by tryptophan, *Adv. Enzyme Regul.* **4**:287.

KOHN, K., STEIGBIGEL, N., AND SPEARS, C., 1965, Cross-linking and repair of DNA in sensitive and resistant strains of *E. coli* treated with nitrogen mustard, *Proc. Natl. Acad. Sci. U.S.A.* **53**:1154–1161.

KOHN, K., SPEARS, C., AND DOTY, P., 1966, Interstrand crosslinking of DNA by nitrogen mustard, *J. Mol. Biol.* **19**:266–288.

KOROLKOVAS, A., 1970, *Essentials of Molecular Pharmacology*, pp. 54–63, Wiley-Interscience, New York.

LANGMUIR, I., 1918, Evaporation of small spheres, *Phys. Rev.* **12**:368–370.

LASTER, W. R., MAYO, J., SIMPSON-HERRON, L., GRISWOLD, D., LLOYD, H., SCHABEL, F., AND SKIPPER, H., 1969, Success and failure in the treatment of solid tumors II: Kinetic parameters and "cell cure" of moderately advanced CA 755, *Cancer Chemother. Rep. Part 1* **53(3)**:169–188.

LATORRE, J., LUNT, G., AND DEROBERTIS, E., 1970, Isolation of a cholinergic proteolipid receptor from electric tissue, *Proc. Natl. Acad. Sci. U.S.A.* **65**:716.

LAWLEY, P., AND BROOKES, P., 1965, Molecular mechanism of cytotoxic action of difunctional alkylating agents and of resistance to this action, *Nature (London)* **206**:480–483.

LEHMAN, I., 1974, DNA joining enzymes, in: *The Enzymes* (P. Boyer, ed.), Vol. X, pp. 237–259, Academic Press, New York.

LEO, A., HANSCH, C., AND ELKINS, D., 1971, Partition coefficients and their uses, *Chem. Rev.* **71**:525–616.

LEPAGE, G. A., 1960, Incorporation of 6-thioguanine into nucleic acids, *Cancer Res.* **20**:403–408.

649

NEW
ANTICANCER
DRUG
DESIGN:
PAST AND
FUTURE
STRATEGIES

LePage, G. A., 1963, Basic biochemical effects and mechanism of action of 6-thioguanine, *Cancer Res.* **23:**1202–1206.

LePage, G. A., and Jones, M., 1961, Purine thiols as feedback inhibitors of purine synthesis in ascites tumor cells, *Cancer Res.* **21:**642–649.

Lo, C.-H., Farina, F., Morris, H. P., and Weinhouse, S., 1968, Glycolytic regulation in rat liver and hepatomas, *Adv. Enzyme Regul.* **6:**453.

Loh, H., Tseng, L., Holaday, J., and Wei, E., 1976a, Endogenous peptides and opiate actions, in: *Proceedings of the International Symposium on Factors Affecting Actions of Narcotics* (M. Adler, ed.), in press.

Loh, H. H., Tseng, L., Wei, E., and Li, C. H., 1976b, Beta endorphin is a potent analgesic agent, *Proc. Natl. Acad. Sci. U.S.A.* **73:**2895–2898.

Lorenson, M. L., Maley, G. F., and Maley, F., 1967, The purification and properties of thymidylate synthestase from chick embryo extracts, *J. Biol. Chem.* **242:**3332–3345.

Loveless, A., and Hampton, C., 1969, Inactivation and mutation of coliphage T_2 by *N*-methyl- and *N*-ethyl-*N*-nitrosourea, *Mutat. Res.* **7:**1–12.

Ludlum, D., Wang, J., Murphy, M., and Tong, W., 1976, Reaction of 1,3-*bis*(2-chloroethyl)-1-nitrosourea and 1,3-*bis*(2-fluoroethyl)-1-nitrosourea with cytidylic and polycytidylic acids, *Proc. Amer. Assoc. Cancer Res.* **17:**194.

Lukens, L., and Buchanan, J., 1959, Biosynthesis of the purines. XXIV. The enzymatic synthesis of 5-amino-1-ribosyl-4-imidazolecarboxylic acid 5′-phosphate from 5-amino-1-ribosylimidazole 5′-phosphate and carbon dioxide, *J. Biol. Chem.* **234:**1799-1806.

Lukens, L., and Herrington, K., 1957, Enzymic formation of 6-mercaptopurine ribotide, *Biochim. Biophys. Acta* **24:**432–433.

MacMahon, B., Lin, T., Lowe, C., Mirra, A., Raunihar, B., Salber, E., Valaoras, V., and Yuasa, S., 1970, Age at first birth and breast cancer risk, *Bull. W.H.O.* **43:**209.

Martin, B., 1965, Potential effect of the plasma proteins on drug distribution, *Nature (London)* **207:**274.

Martin, E. W., 1971, *Hazards of Medication,* pp. 378–895, J. B. Lippincott, Philadelphia.

Mathé, G., Pomillart, P., and Lapeyraque, F., 1969, Active immunotherapy of L-1210 leukemia applied after the graft of tumor cells, *Br. J. Cancer* **23:**814–824.

Mathé, G., Amiel, J., Schwartzenberg, L., Catton, A., Schneider, ,M., deVassal, F., and Schrumpberger, J. R., 1970, Strategy of the treatment of acute lymphoblastic leukemia: Chemotherapy and immunotherapy, *Recent Results Cancer Res.* **30:**109.

Masironi, R., and Popovic, V., 1967, Differential hypothermia–normothermia as a new tool to enhance the activity of anti-cancer drugs. Radioisotope study, *Acta Isot.* **7:**289–298.

Massey, V., 1953, Studies on fumarase. II. Effects of inorganic anions on fumarase activity, *Biochem. J.* **53:**67–71.

Mayo, J. G., Laster, W. R., Andrews, C., and Schabel, F., 1972, Success and failure in the treatment of solid tumors: "Cure" of metastatic Lewis lung carcinoma with methyl-CCNU and surgery–chemotherapy, *Cancer Chemother. Rep.* **56:**183.

McCollister, R., Gilbert, R., Ashton, D., and Wyngaarden, J., 1964, Pseudo feedback inhibition of purine synthesis by 6-mercaptopurine ribonucleotide and other purine analogs, *J. Biol. Chem.* **239:**1560–1563.

Meyer, K. H., and Hemmi, H., 1935, *Biochem. Z.* **277:**39.

Meyer, M. C., and Guttman, D. E., 1970, Dynamic dialysis as a method for studying protein binding: Evaluation of the method with a number of binding systems, *J. Pharm. Sci.* **59:** 39–48.

Milch, R., Rall, D. P., and Tobie, J., 1957, Bone localization of tetracyclines, *J. Nat. Cancer Inst.* **19:** 87–93.

Miller, J. A., 1970, Carcinogenesis by chemicals: An overview, *Cancer Res.* **30:**559.

Miller, R. W., Lukens, L. N., and Buchanan, J. M., 1959, Biosynthesis of the purines. XXV. The enzymatic cleavage of *N*-(-5-amino-1-ribosyl-4-imidazolylcarbonyl)-L-aspartic acid 5′-phosphate, *J. Biol. Chem.* **234:**1806–1812.

Milne, M., Scribner, B., and Crawford, M., 1958, Non-ionic diffusion and the excretion of weak acids and bases, *Amer. J. Med.* **24:**709–729.

Moertel, C., and Reitmeir, R., 1969, *Advanced Gastrointestinal Cancer: Clinical Management and Chemotherapy,* Harper and Row, New York.

Monod, J., 1960, Formation, induction, répression dans la biosynthèse d'un enzyme, Dynamik des Eiweisses (colloquium), *Ges. Physiol. Chem.* **10:**120–145.

MONOD, J., AND COHN, M., 1952, La biosynthèse induite des enzymes (adaptation enzymatique), *Adv. Enzymol.* **13**:67–119.

MONOD, J., WYMAN, J., AND CHANGEAUX, J., 1965, On the nature of allosteric transitions: A plausible model, *J. Mol. Biol.* **12**:85.

MONTGOMERY, J. A., JOHNSTON, T., AND SHEAHY, Y., 1970, Drugs for neoplastic diseases, in: *Medicinal Chemistry* (A. Burger, ed.), pp. 680–783, John Wiley and Sons, New York.

MOORE, G., BROSS, I., AUSMAN, R., NADLER, S., JONES, R., SLACK, N., AND RIMM, A., 1968, Effects of 5-fluorouracil (NSC 19893) in 389 patients with cancer, *Cancer Chemother. Rep.* **52**:641.

MORRIS, H. P., 1965, Studies in the development, biochemistry and biology of experimental hepatomas, *Adv. Cancer Res.* **9**:228.

NATHANSON, L., HALL, T., SCHILLING, A., AND MILLER, S., 1969, Concurrent combination chemotherapy of human solid tumors: Experience with a three–drug regimen and review of the literature, *Cancer Res.* **29**:419–425.

NEBERT, D. W., AND GELBOIN, H. V., 1968, Substrate-inducible microsomal aryl hydrocarbon hydroxylase in mammalian cell cultures, *J. Biol. Chem.* **243**:6242–6261.

NEIL, G. L., MOXLEY, T., AND MANAK, R., 1970, Enhancement by tetrahydrouridine of 1-α-D-arabinofuranosylcytosine oral activity in L-1210 leukemic mice, *Cancer Res.* **30**:2166-2172.

NICOLINI, C., 1976, The principles and methods of cell synchronization in cancer chemotherapy, *Biochim Biophys. Acta* **458**:243–282.

OCHOA, M., AND HIRSCHBERG, E., 1967, Alkylating agents, in: *Experimental Chemotherapy* (R. Schnitzer and F. Hawkins, eds.), Vol. 5, pp. 1–132, Academic Press, New York.

OPLER, S. R., 1967, Observations on a new virus associated with guinea pig leukemia, *J. Natl. Cancer Inst.* **38**:797.

O'REILLY, R., OHMS, J., AND MOTLEY, C., 1969, Studies on coumarin anticoagulant drugs, *J. Biol. Chem* **244**:1303–1305.

OSBORNE, M., FREEMAN, M., AND HUENNEKENS, F., 1958, Inhibition of dihydrofolic reductase by aminopterin and amethopterin, *Proc. Soc. Exp. Biol. Med.* **97**:429.

OVERTON, E., 1901, *Studien über die Narkose*, p. 45ff, Fischer, Jena.

OWELLEN, R., OWENS, A., AND DONIGIAN, D., 1972, The binding of vincristine, vinblastine and colchicine to tubulin, *Biochem. Biophys. Res. Commun.* **47**:685–691.

OWELLEN, R., HARTKE, C., DICKERSON, R., AND HAINS, F., 1976, Inhibition of tubulin-microtubule polymerization by drugs of the vinca alkaloid class, *Cancer Res.* **36**:1499–1502.

PAULING, L., 1960, *The Nature of the Chemical Bond*, pp. 449–504, Cornell University Press, Ithaca, New York.

PITOT, H. C., 1966, Some biochemical aspects of malignancy, *Annu. Rev. Biochem.* **35-I**:335.

POTTER, V. R., 1951, Sequential blocking of metabolic pathways *in vivo*, *Proc. Soc. Exp. Biol. Med.* **76**:41–46.

POTTER, V., 1969, Recent trends in cancer biochemistry: The importance of studies on fetal tissue, *Can. Cancer Conf.* **8**:9.

POTTER, V., WALKER, P., AND GOODMAN, J., 1972, Survey of current studies on oncogeny as blocked ontogeny, *Gann Monogr.* **13**:121.

PURCELL, W. P., BASS, G. E., AND CLAYTON, J. M., 1973, *Strategy of drug design: A guide to biological activity*, pp. 49 and 50, John Wiley and Sons, New York.

PUSCHENDORF, B., WOLF, H., GRUNICKE, H., 1971, Effect of the alkylating agent tris-ethyleneiminobenzoquinone on the template activity of chromatin and DNA in RNA and DNA polymerase systems, *Biochem. Pharmacol.* **20**:3039–3050.

RALL, D. P., AND ZUBROD, C. G., 1962, Mechanisms of drug absorption and excretion: Passage of drugs in and out of the central nervous system, *Annu. Rev. Pharmacol.* **2**:109.

RANG, H. P., 1971, Drug receptors and their function, *Nature* **231**:91–96.

RAPP, F., AND DUFF, R., 1972, Transformation of hamster cells after infection by inactivated Herpes simplex virus-type 2, in: *Oncogenesis and Herpes Viruses* (P. Biggs *et al.*, eds.), pp. 447–450, IARC, Lyon.

RICHARDS, E. G., AND SCHACHMAN, H., 1957, A differential ultracentritugal technique for measuring small changes in sedimentation coefficients, *J. Amer. Chem. Soc.* **79**:5324–5325.

RICKARD, C. G., POST, J., NORONHA, F., AND BARR, L. M., 1969, A transmissible virus-induced lymphocytic leukemia in the cat, *J. Natl. Cancer Inst.* **42**:937.

ROSSI, A., VALAGUSSA, P., BONADONNA, G., AND VERONESI, U., 1976, Adjuvant treatment with prolonged CMF (CTX-MTX-FU) in operable breast cancer with positive nodes, *Proc. Amer. Cancer Res.* **17**:73.

651

NEW
ANTICANCER
DRUG
DESIGN:
PAST AND
FUTURE
STRATEGIES

ROUS, P., 1911, A sarcoma of the fowl transmissible by an agent separable from the tumor cells, *J. Exp. Med.* **13**:397–411.

ROWE, W. P., HARTLEY, J., LANDER, M., AND TEICH, N., 1971, Noninfectious AKR mouse embryo cell lines in which each cell has the capacity to be activated to produce infectious murine leukemia virus, *Virology* **46**:866.

SALMON, S., AND APPLE, M. A., 1976, Cancer chemotherapy, *Rev. Med. Pharmacol.* **5**:470–503.

SANDBERG, H., AND PIETTE, L., 1968, EPR studies of psychotropic drug interactions at cell membranes, *J. Amer. Chem. Soc.* **75**:1420–1426.

SARIN, P., AND GALLO, R., 1974, RNA directed DNA polymerase in: *MTP International Review of Science: Biochemistry of Nucleic Acids* (K. Burton, ed.), pp. 219–254, University Park Press, Baltimore.

SAROFF, H., AND MARK, H., 1953, Polarographic analysis of the serum albumin–mercury and zinc complexes, *J. Amer. Chem. Soc.* **75**:1420–1426.

SARTORELLI, A. C., AND JOHNS, D. G. (eds.), 1974, *Antineoplastic and Immunosuppressive Agents*, Vol. I, pp. 1–762, Springer-Verlag, New York.

SARTORELLI, A. C., AND JOHNS, D. G. (eds.), 1975, *Antineoplastic and Immunosupressive Agents*, Vol. II, pp. 1–1067, Springer-Verlag, New York.

SCHABEL, F., 1975a, Synergism and antagonism among antitumor agents, in: *Pharmacological Basis of Cancer Chemotherapy*, pp. 596–621, Williams and Wilkins, Baltimore.

SCHABEL, F. M., 1975b, Concepts for the treatment of micrometastases, *Cancer* **35**:15–29.

SCHANKER, L., AND JOHNSON, L., 1961, Increased intestinal absorption of foreign organic compounds in the presence of ethylenediaminetetraacetic acid, *Biochem. Pharmacol.* **8**:420–422.

SCHANKER, L., SHORE, P., BRODIE, B., AND HOGBEN, C., 1957, Absorption of drugs from the stomach: I. The rat, *J. Pharmacol. Exp. Ther.* **120**:528.

SCHATZ, V. B., 1960, Isosterism and bioisosterism as guides to structural variations, in: *Medicinal Chemistry* (A. Burger, ed.), pp. 72–88, Wiley-Interscience, New York.

SCHEIN, P., DAVIS, R., CARTER, S., NEWMAN, J., SCHEIN, D., AND RALL, D., 1970, The evaluation of anticancer drugs in dogs and monkeys for the prediction of qualitative toxicities in man, *Clin. Pharmacol. Ther.* **11**:3.

SCOLNICK, E. M., AND PARKS, W. P., 1973, Isolation and characterization of a primate sarcoma virus: Mechanism of rescue, *Int. J. Cancer* **12**:138.

SETLOW, R., AND CARRIER, W., 1964, The disappearance of thymine dimers from DNA: An error-correcting mechanism, *Proc. Natl. Acad. Sci. U.S.A.* **51**:226–231.

SETTLE, W., HEGEMAN, S., AND FEATHERSTONE, R. M., 1971, Nature of drug–protein interaction, in: *Concepts in Biochemical Pharmacology* (B. Brodie and J. Gillette, eds.), pp. 174–186, Springer-Verlag, New York.

SIMANTOV, R., AND SNYDER, S. H., 1976, A morphine-like peptide "enkephalin" in mammalian brain: Isolation, structure, elucidation, and interactions with opiate receptor, *Proc. Natl. Acad. Sci.* **73**:2515–2519.

SINGER, B., 1975, Reactions of oncogenic alkylating agents with nucleic acids, *Proc. Amer. Assoc. Cancer Res.* **16**:81.

SKIPPER, H., SCHABEL, F., AND WILCOX, W., 1964, Experimental evaluation of potential anticancer agents: On the criteria and kinetics associated with "curability" of experimental leukemia, *Cancer Chemother. Rep.* **35**:1–111.

SKIPPER, H., SCHABEL, F., MELLET, L., MONTGOMERY, J., WILCOFF, L., LLOYD, H., AND BROCKMAN, R., 1970, Implications of the biochemical, cytokinetic, pharmacologic and toxicologic relationships in the design of optimal therapeutic schedules, *Cancer Chemother. Rep.* **54**:431–450.

SMITH, R. L., 1971, Excretion of drugs in bile, in: *Concepts in Biochemical Pharmacology* (B. Brodie and J. Gillette, eds.), Vol. XXVIII/1, p. 367, Springer-Verlag, New York.

SOBELL, H., 1972, The stereochemistry of actinomycin binding to DNA, *Prog. Nucleic Acid Res.* **13**:153.

SOBELL, H., AND JAIN, S., 1972, Stereochemistry of actinomycin binding to DNA: Detailed molecular model of actinomycin–DNA complex and its implications, *J. Mol. Biol.* **68**:21–34.

STORELLI, C., VOGELI, H., AND SEMENZA, G., 1972, Reconstitution of a sucrase-mediated sugar transport system in lipid membranes, *FEBS Lett.* **24**:287–293.

STRAULI, P., 1970, The barrier function of lymph nodes; a review of experimental studies and their implications for cancer surgery, in: *Surgical Oncology* (F. Saegesser and J. Pethavel, eds.), pp. 161–176, Huber, Berne.

TAFT, R. W., 1956, Separation of polar, steric and resonance effects in reactivity, in: *Steric Effects in Organic Chemistry* (M. Newman, ed.), pp. 556–675, John Wiley and Sons, New York.

TEMIN, H. M., AND BALTIMORE, D., 1972, RNA-directed DNA synthesis and RNA tumor viruses, *Adv. Virus Res.* **17:**129–186.

TEMIN, H., AND MIZUTANI, S., 1974, RNA tumor virus DNA polymerases, in: *The Enzymes* (P. Boyer, ed.), pp. 211–236, Academic Press, New York.

UMBARGER, H., 1969, Regulation of amino acid metabolism, *Annu. Rev. Biochem.* **38:**323–371.

UPTON, A. C., 1968, Radiation carcinogenesis, in: *Methods in Cancer Research* (H. Busch, ed.), Vol. IV, pp. 53–82, Academic Press, New York.

U.S. ARMY RESEARCH PROGRAM ON MALARIA ANNUAL REPORT, 1973.

VALERIOTE, F., BRUCE, W., AND MEEKER, B., 1968, A synergistic action of cyclophosphamide and 1,3-bis(2-chloroethyl)-1-nitrosourea on a transplanted murine lymphoma, *J. Natl. Cancer Inst.* **41:**935–944.

VAN PUTTEN, L., LELIEVELD, P., AND KRAM-IDSENGA, L., 1972, Cell-cycle specific and therapeutic effectiveness of cytostatic agents, *Cancer Chemother. Rep.* **56-I**(6):691–700.

VENDITTI, J., 1971, Treatment schedule dependence of experimentally active antileukemic drugs, *Cancer Chemother. Rep. Part 3* **2**(1):35–59.

VENDITTI, J., 1973, Minutes of the Phase-I study working group, Oct. 11, 1973, DCT, NCI.

VENDITTI, J., 1975, Relevance of transplantable animal tumor systems to the selection of new agents for clinical trial, in: *Pharmacological Basis of Cancer Chemotherapy*, pp. 243–270, Williams and Wilkins, Baltimore.

VERONESI, U., 1973, Principles of cancer surgery, in: *Cancer Medicine* (J. Holland and E. Frei, eds.), pp. 521–534, Lea and Febiger, Philadelphia.

VON GERHARDT, C., 1853, Untersuchungen über die wasserfreien organischen Säuren, *Liebigs Ann.* **87:**149.

VON LEYDEN, E., AND BLUMENTHAL, F., 1902, Attempts to immunize humans by inoculation of their own tumor, *Dtsch. Med. Wochenschr.* **28:**637–638.

WARBURG, O., 1956, On respiratory impairment in cancer, *Science* **124:**269.

WARING, M. J., 1968, Drugs which affect the structure and function of DNA, *Nature (London)* **219:**1320.

WARING, M. J., 1970, Variations of the supercoils in closed circular DNA by binding of antibiotics and drugs: Evidence for molecular models involving intercalation, *J. Mol. Biol.* **54:**247.

WASSERMAN, T., COMIS, R., GOLDSMITH, M., HANDELSMAN, H., PENTA, J., SLAVIK, M., SOPER, W., AND CARTER, S., 1975, Tabular analysis of the clinical solid tumors, *Cancer Chemother. Rep. Part 3* **6:**399–419.

WEBER, G., 1966a, The molecular correlation concept: Studies on the metabolic patterns of hepatomas, *Gann Monogr.* **1:**151.

WEBER, G., 1966b, The molecular correlation concept: An experimental and conceptual method in cancer research, in: *Methods in Cancer Research* (H. Busch, ed.), Vol. III, pp. 524–581, Academic Press, New York.

WEBER, G., AND CANTERO, A., 1957, Glucose-6-phosphate utilization in hepatoma, regenerating and newborn rat liver and the liver of fed and fasted rats, *Cancer Res.* **17:**995.

WEBER, G., AND LEA, M., 1966, The molecular correlation concept of neoplasia, *Adv. Enzyme Regul.* **4:**115.

WEINER, I. M., 1967, Mechanisms of drug absorption and excretion, *Annu. Rev. Pharmacol.* **7:**39–56.

WEINER, I., AND MUDGE, G., 1964, Renal tubular mechanisms for excretion of organic acids and bases, *Amer. J. Med.* **36:**743–762.

WEINHOUSE, S., 1960, Enzyme activities and tumor progression, in: *Amino Acids, Proteins and Cancer Biochemistry* (J. Edsall, ed.), pp. 109–119, Academic Press, New York.

WILSON, L., 1975, Microtubules as drug receptors: Pharmacological properties of microtubule protein, *Ann. N. Y. Acad. Sci.* **253:**213–231.

WOLFE, L. G., SMITH, R. K., THIELEN, G., RUBIN, H., KAWAKAMI, T., AND BUSTAD, L., 1971, Induction of tumors in marmoset monkeys by simian sarcoma virus type 1 (Lagothrix), *J. Natl. Cancer Inst.* **47:**115.

WOODRUFF, H., AND MCDANIEL, L., 1958, The antibiotic approach, in: *The Strategy of Chemotherapy*, p. 29, Cambridge University Press, Cambridge.

WYNDER, E. L., 1959, Identification of women at high risk for breast cancer, *Cancer* **24:**1235.

ZAHARKO, D., BRUCKNER, H., AND OLIVERIO, V., 1969, Antibiotics after methotroxate metabolism and excretion, *Science* **166:**887–888.

ZIMMERMAN, T. P., CHUR, L., BUGGE, C. NELSON, D., LYON, G., AND ELION, G., 1974, Identification of 6-methylmercaptopurine ribonucleoside-5'-diphosphate and 5'-triphosphate as metabolites of 6-mercaptopurine in man, *Cancer Res.* **34:**221–224.

Index

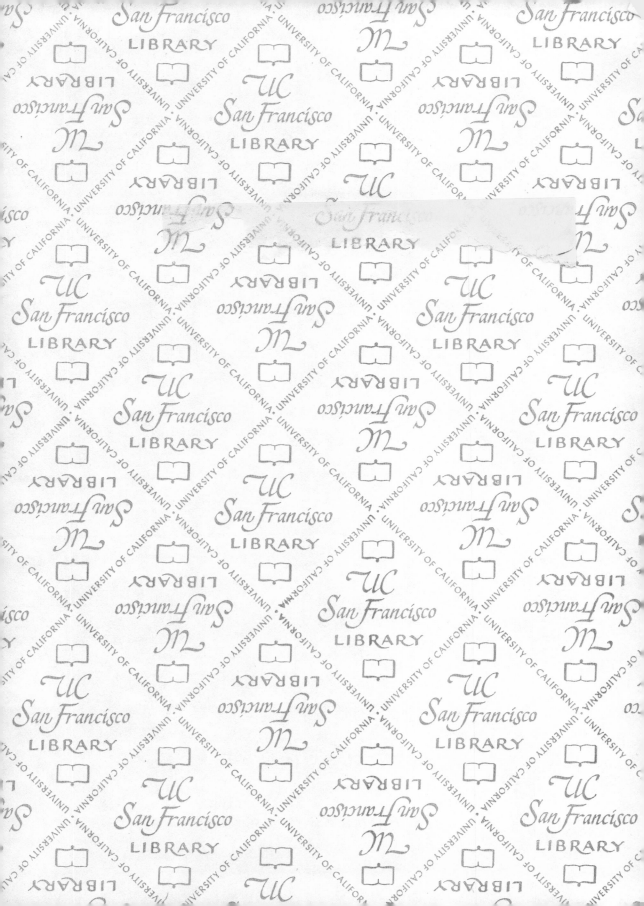